Frontiers in
Hypertension Research

Frontiers in Hypertension Research

Edited by

John H. Laragh
Hilda Altshul Master Professor of Medicine
Director, Cardiovascular Center
Chief, Division of Cardiology
The New York Hospital—Cornell Medical Center
New York, New York

Fritz R. Bühler
Associate Professor of Medicine
Department of Medicine and
  Department of Research
Director of Hypertension Unit
Consultant in Cardiology
University Hospital
Basel, Switzerland

Donald W. Seldin
William Buchanan Professor of Medicine
Chairman of Internal Medicine
University of Texas Health Science Center at Dallas
Chief of the Medical Service
Parkland Memorial Hospital
Dallas, Texas

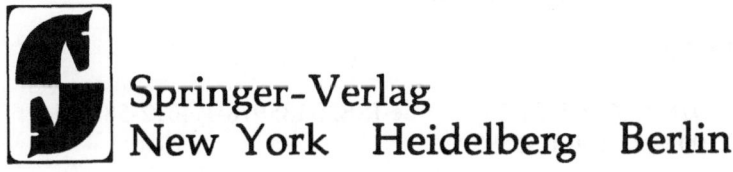
Springer-Verlag
New York   Heidelberg   Berlin

John H. Laragh, M.D.
Director, Cardiovascular Center
New York Hospital
525 East 68th Street
New York, New York 10021 U.S.A.

Fritz Bühler, M.D.
Associate Professor of Medicine
Department of Medicine and
   Department of Research
University Hospital
4031 Basel, Switzerland

Donald W. Seldin, M.D., M.A.C.P.
Chairman of Internal Medicine
University of Texas Health Science Center
   at Dallas
Dallas, Texas, U.S.A.

Proceedings of an International Symposium held May 19–21, 1980 in New York
and sponsored by: USV Laboratories
Division Revlon Health Care Group

Sponsoring Editor: Larry W. Carter
Production: Berta Steiner
Design: Berta Steiner

With 242 Illustrations

Library of Congress Cataloging in Publication Data
Main entry under title:
Frontiers in hypertension research.

   Includes index.
   1. Hypertension—Congresses. I. Laragh, John H.
II. Bühler, Fritz R.   III. Seldin, Donald W.   IV. USV
Pharmaceutical Corp.   Revlon Health Care Group.
[DNLM: 1. Hypertension—Congresses. WG 340 F935   1980]
RC685.H8F76   616.1′32   81–5619
                          AACR2

Printed in the United States of America

9 8 7 6 5 4 3 2 1

ISBN-13: 978-1-4612-5901-5   e-ISBN-13: 978-1-4612-5899-5
DOI: 10.1007/978-1-4612-5899-5

Dedication
Sir George Pickering—A Tribute

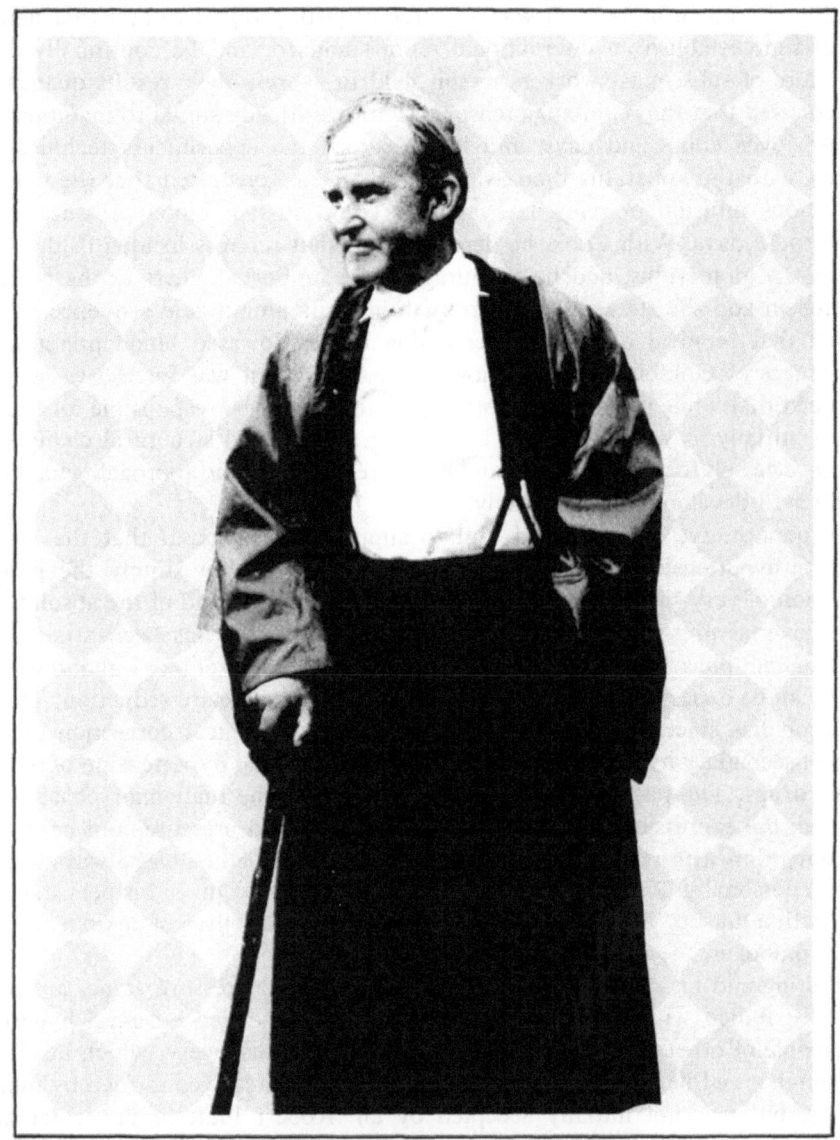

When Sir George Pickering died in Oxford on September 3, 1980, cardiovascular medicine lost one of its most creative and influential personalities of the last fifty years. The present volume records his still penetrating contributions to what was, regrettably, the last major meeting he was to attend.

George Pickering's career was greatly stimulated by his association with Sir Thomas Lewis at University College Hospital, London, in the late 1920s and early 1930s. It was then that he developed fully the method of applying quantitatively basic physiologic principles to clinical medicine, an approach which was to pervade his subsequent work. Withal, he retained a warm and sympathetic bedside manner and was always conscious of the psychologic impact of doctors ("the doctor must never frighten his patient").

The pertinacity with which he strove for precise quantification of clinical and experimental results underlay all his major contributions to medicine. His interests were wide, including peptic ulceration, headache, and temperature regulation, but his greatest achievements were in the field of hypertension.

In the 1930s, following Goldblatt's experiment, he was one of those responsible with Prinzmetal for the rediscovery of renin, which had first been described by Tigerstedt and Bergman in 1898. It was a source of lasting regret to him that he did not at that time establish an international renin standard, and he continually deplored the failure of subsequent workers in this field to express their results quantitatively. He perceived that the renin-angiotensin system was ideally suited to maintain arterial pressure over hours and days, and he pioneered the experiments–technically very difficult with the apparatus then available–which demonstrated that the continuous intravenous infusion of renin into animals could sustain blood pressure elevation for up to 18 days. With Cook, he demonstrated that renin is located in the vascular pole of the glomerulus, and he encouraged and supported Peart in the isolation of angiotensin and the subsequent determination of its amino acid sequence. Pickering showed that removal of the sole remaining kidney lowered blood pressure in the early stages of Goldblatt hypertension in the rabbit, but was ineffective later. Thus he argued that while the renin-angiotensin system might be responsible for the hypertension initially, it was unlikely to be so later. He favored structural changes in the resistance vessels for this latter role and thus foreshadowed the approach which Folkow was later to develop so penetratingly.

The quantitative approach led him to support the proposal that the malignant phase of hypertension is not a separate disease entity, but simply the pathologic expression of very severe blood pressure elevation–a compound of the absolute height of the arterial pressure and the rapidity with which this has been attained. Thus the malignant phase can supervene in hypertension of varied etiology and, most importantly, can be expected to resolve with adequate blood pressure reduction. This latter prediction has since been demonstrated both by the surgical correction of various forms of secondary hypertension and by the use in essential hypertension of antihypertensive drugs. The papilledema and retinal edema of the malignant phase were, he reasoned, the expressions of increased cerebrospinal fluid pressure, and he supported this contention with relevant pressure measurements, which he was always concerned to make personally. Pickering's lumbar puncture technique, given his persistence combined with a marked hereditary tremor, was invariably a source of anxious fascination for the onlooker.

Pickering and his colleagues demonstrated that blood pressure values are continuously distributed within populations and thus that so-called essential hypertension is incapable of other than an arbitrary definition. This discovery, which he described as "though a veil had been lifted," has since been repeatedly confirmed by numerous workers, but was not initially accepted by all. Robert Platt in particular entered the lists, and there followed the famous Pickering-Platt debates of the 1950s. Platt thought that the distribution of blood pressures in the general population was not unimodal. He believed that a single gene, with incomplete dominance, was responsible for the development of high blood pressure with increasing age in some persons. Pickering demonstrated convincingly that the distribution was in fact unimodal, that the tendency to develop high blood pressure was almost certainly inherited in a polygenic fashion and, most importantly, that it was impossible to draw a dividing line between a "normotensive" and a "hypertensive" subset. He summarized his case in "The Nature of Essential Hypertension" in 1961, a book which is a model of cogent, lucid scientific writing.

Pickering went on to emphasize the continuous, quantitative relationship between blood pressure and the incidence of vascular complications—close for stroke, where arterial pressure and age are the predominant pathogenic influences; less close for ischemic heart disease, where blood pressure is but one of several important risk factors. It is often now forgotten how central these concepts are to preventive antihypertensive therapy today.

This work progressed naturally into another fruitful scientific field as he pioneered, together with younger colleagues in Oxford, devices for the continuous measurement of arterial pressure. These revealed the very large fluctuations of pressure which occur during normal daily activities. He was so delighted with the findings that he chose as a cover design for the second edition of his book *High Blood Pressure* a record of arterial pressure during coitus.

As his contributions to the present volume show, he remained to the end unconvinced that moderate dietary salt restriction is effective in reducing arterial pressure. In this view he was greatly influenced by the detailed Medical Research Council Study of 1950, which showed that while severely hypertensive patients in hospital did respond to very strict salt restriction (down to 10–20 mEq/day), a regime that could be tolerated only briefly, blood pressure rose again when salt intake was allowed to rise only to the range 35–50 mEq/day. We remain uncertain whether Pickering's views on this topic will eventually be vindicated; what is sure is that his criticisms will inspire further accurate and definitive studies of the problem.

George Pickering's clarity of thought was evident in both his speech and his writing, which were invariably models of lucidity and style. He deplored clumsiness of expression as betraying confusion of reason. In sharp contrast, his manner of dress seemed of little concern to him. He combined great personal charm with an often ribald and occasionally caustic sense of humor. While never, to my knowledge, unwittingly offensive, he suffered fools not at all. He thrived on controversy and revelled in debate in which he could take, as well as give, hard blows. He was always concerned to distinguish scientific argument from personal animosity; nevertheless, his critique of a paper was often accompanied by a finely wrought vignette of the author's personality, a practice which invariably illuminated insight into the work under consideration.

For me, and I am sure for many others, a day in George Pickering's company always sharpened the wits and warmed the heart. My last memory of him, just a few weeks before his death, is happy and appropriate. We dined together in a Paris restaurant, with George charming my small daughter, recounting slightly bawdy tales, relishing the food and wine, complaining of a deficiency of garlic, and calling loudly for the salt cellar. We shall not, sadly, see his like again.

J.I.S. Robertson

Contents

Session 3
Sodium Metabolism: The Sodium-Potassium Membrane Pump and Volume Overload Hypertension
Chairman: F.R. Bühler

Session 12
Hypertension Mechanisms in Experimental Animals and Their Relevance to Humans
Chairman: F.O. Simpson

Session 13
Hypertension, Vasopressors, and the Susceptibility to Vascular Injury
Chairman: E. Muirhead

Session 16
Converting Enzyme Blockade as a Therapeutic Modality
Chairman: J.H. Laragh

Session 17
Physiologic Effects and Diagnostic Relevance of Acute Converting Enzyme Blockade
Chairman: D.W. Seldin

Session 18
New Approaches to Renin System Blockade
Chairman: R.L. Soffer

Epilogue: After Dinner Science and Friendship

Prologue

The creation of this symposium to discuss, analyze, and then publish the frontiers in hypertension research occurred partly by accident and partly by intent. It could be viewed as another example of chance and prepared minds.

I had in mind to have a modest one-day meeting on hypertension at my home base, The New York Hospital/Cornell Medical Center in New York City. I wanted, in particular, to invite Don Seldin to participate. He had graciously invited me and a number of my research group to Dallas two years ago to exchange views with his faculty on the high blood pressure problem. I was especially anxious to do it again because in my long association with Don I have enjoyed and cherished his passion for knowledge in general and his special interest in renal physiology and hypertensive phenomena. He is the ideal sounding board and critic. He brings to a conference table the broader perspective of a professor of medicine not particularly committed or involved in hypertension research but at the same time extremely interested in its products and their relevance. As is indicated by some of his comments in this volume his ability to interpret data and synthesize their meaning provides another helpful dimension. Don was particularly intrigued, as I was, with Roger Palmer's experiments in the turkey model showing that the form of the pulse wave and the force of cardiac contraction are more important than the absolute pressure level for producing vascular damage.

While I was thinking about arranging my next meeting with Seldin, I met with Fritz Bühler at a symposium in Berne, Switzerland. He expressed interest in having an international symposium where some of the recent clinical trials in hypertension might be discussed along with other selected issues, with the idea of producing a book containing not only the formal presentations but also transcripts of the discussions, and this as quickly as possible so that none of the freshness of the issues would be lost. Don Seldin was also at the meeting in Berne and the three of us agreed that we would like to be involved in such a venture. Fritz Bühler's expertise in the areas of beta receptor blocking drug action, sympathetic nervous system theory and in the conduct and analysis of clinical trials was especially valuable for arranging a number of the scientific sessions. His own pioneering research linking neurogenic activity to the activity of the renin system also served as a springboard in several of the scientific sessions.

It was apparent to all of us that the International Symposium on Hypertension to be held in New Orleans in the Spring of 1980 created an opportunity for us to bring together a large group of distinguished scientists, who might not otherwise be available. Accordingly, we began to construct an agenda and a slate.

Not surprisingly, the size and scope of the project grew overnight. We recognized the possibilities for a working meeting involving the world's most distinguished investigators in the many disciplines of basic or clinical science that compose the field of hypertension research. The opportunity was mouth-watering. We set about to identify at least one scientist from every major laboratory in the world and involve him in this scientific exchange. The responses to our invitations were uniformly enthusiastic, with over 120 scientists participating, most arriving with manuscripts and data in hand.

We foresaw great possibilities for such a meeting. We would bring together under one roof the full range of scientific disciplines involved in hypertension research, ranging from epidemiologists to clinical investigators, to animal physiologists, pharmacologists, cell biologists and biochemists. It would be an opportunity for interdisciplinary cross-fertilization on critical issues. For example, we proposed to look anew at the growing epidemiologic evidence on the value, or lack of value, and the risks of various types of drug therapy. We also wanted to re-examine the value or lack of value of manipulating dietary salt and consider the key issue of whether such interventions were useful or harmful to various subsets of patients.

Within this epidemiologic reference framework the meeting was designed to consider fundamental cellular mechanisms of sodium transport and of vascular tone and their mediation by local chemical transmitters or circulating hormones. The orchestration of these phenomena by control systems involving the nervous system and the renin system and possibly other control systems would also be considered.

In dealing with pathogenesis we decided to re-examine the obviously subtle and still elusive role of the sympathetic nervous system and also to reconsider the role of the renin-angiotensin-aldosterone system as a primary, sustaining, or reactive factor in the spectrum that composes essential hypertension. In particular the question would be examined of the meaning and the role of renin and of volume factors in the pathogenesis of hypertension where renin values are low or normal. We would consider, in the light of new evidence, the possible role of intravascular renin production.

We also would probe the question of the pathogenesis of hypertensive vascular and organ damage and the possibly important role of renin and other vasoconstrictions. The role of blood pressure and blood flow, the role of renin, the role of neither one, but rather of some complex interaction between cardiac output, pulse wave form and resistance vessel activity determined by renin or other vasoconstrictors would be discussed. And finally we would consider the action and relevance and the promise of therapeutic modalities including of course the latest anti-renin drug types as exemplified by the prototype teprotide and captopril.

Operationally, the plan was to have three working days with the discussions to be transcribed and published in entirety. The meeting would be divided into 18 frontier "topics," each of which would be introduced by a position paper of 20 minutes or less followed by a series of short papers of 10 minutes or less on particular aspects of the problem, and then by the discussion period. Our goal was to openly discuss even the most tender areas of dispute while maintaining decorum and friendship in an atmosphere where maximum disagreement could be encouraged with the common goal of sharpening the issues and answers.

The symposium was an incredible success. The staying power of the participants was beyond belief. The discussions were comprehensive and constructive, at times bristling with disagreement. There was some acerbity but the mood was mostly one of friendship and respect built on a commonality of interest, as you will find upon reading these discussions.

The 18 topics covered represent the final choice of what the three editors consider to be the important frontiers in hypertension research. Within this volume they are presented in entirety as they occurred. Unfortunately, however, everything could not be covered. For example, I have a personal regret that time did not allow us to have a session on the factors involved in aldosterone secretion. Moreover, there was no time for discussing the biobehavioral approaches to hypertension. These we can save for another time. Inevitably, too, there were a few scientists who unavoidably could not attend. In these instances, we tried to ensure that their work and viewpoints were recognized.

This symposium never could have become a reality without the marvelous and unqualified support of USV Laboratories Division of the Revlon Health Care Group. No detail was overlooked for making the symposium a success and for maintaining the highest standards of science without any intrusion from commercial interests.

The three full days' sessions were held at the Metropolitan Club. Attendance was by invitation and the press was specifically excluded. Indeed, our sponsors at USV Laboratories insisted that we have total freedom to criticize or discuss their own or any other drug company product, and that the meeting be a forum for absolutely free expression of current thinking on the part of working scientists the world over who are concerned with the high blood pressure problem. All this, I think, is reflected in this present volume.

I did not have to mention more than once the plans for our symposium to Chuck Smith and Herb McDade at Revlon Health Care Group before they evinced great enthusiasm for it. Indeed they jumped at the opportunity to support it. Their enthusiasm was even amplified after they discussed it with John Roelker, the President and Group Executive of Revlon Health Care Group, and with Michel Bergerac, Chairman and Chief Executive of Revlon, Inc. These people not only made the symposium possible, they created a setting where distinguished scientists participated actively with a large pool of their peers for three days and enjoyed their companionship as well in the off-hours and at meals with almost no extraneous distractions. This volume serves as a lasting testimony of what was achieved. Hopefully it will be helpful for research scientists and other people interested in the high blood pressure problem.

The organization of the meeting and all of the attendant details which made it not only scientifically successful but a distinct pleasure for all of the participating scientists were accomplished by my longtime associate, Joan Banes, with the help of Howard Mason, Director of Product Management, USV Laboratories. Mrs. Banes also was responsible for the faithful transcription of all of the discussions and for organizing the entire text into book form. It was a Herculean task well done.

Finally, the scientists of our field were greatly saddened by the death of Sir George Pickering, shortly after he participated in his usual lively manner in the Frontiers meeting. We have lost a leader whose contributions speak for themselves. Fortunately, a piece of his personal integrity and force is captured in this volume in his paper and in his telling comments throughout the regular sessions and during the special evening section transcribed at the end of this book. George was my friend and I will miss him. We are pleased to dedicate this volume to him. I am especially grateful to Bob Robertson for the discerning resume of George's career.

John Laragh

Participants

M. Akhmeteli, M.D.
Chief, Division of Preventive Cardiology
National Cardiology Research Center
Academy of Medical Sciences
Moscow 101387, USSR

Michael H. Alderman, M.D.
Professor of Public Health and
Associate Professor of Medicine
Cornell University Medical College
New York, N.Y. 10021 U.S.A.

John C. Alexander, M.D.
Director of Clinical Research
E.R. Squibb and Sons, Inc.
Princeton, New Jersey 08540 U.S.A.

A. Amery, M.D.
Department of Internal Medicine
University Hospital Sint-Rafäel
Kapucijnenvoer 35
3000 Leuven, Belgium

Richard P. Ames, M.D.
Associate Clinical Professor of Medicine
Columbia University College of Physicians and
    Surgeons
New York, N.Y. 10032 U.S.A.

M.J. Antonaccio, Ph.D.
The Squibb Institute for Medical Research
E.R. Squibb and Sons, Inc.
Princeton, New Jersey 08540 U.S.A.

Steven A. Atlas, M.D.
Assistant Professor Medicine
Cardiovascular Center
Cornell University Medical College
New York, N.Y. 10021 U.S.A.

Carlos R. Ayers, M.D., F.A.C.P., F.A.C.C.
Professor of Medicine
University of Virginia
Head, Hypertension Unit,
University of Virginia Medical Center
Charlottesville, Virginia 22908 U.S.A.

Nigel S. Baber, B.Sc., M.D., M.R.C.P.
Medical Adviser
ICI Pharmaceuticals
Macclesfield, Chesire, SK 10 4TG England

G. Bianchi, M.D.
Istituto di Clinica Medica 1
Università di Milano
20122. Milano, Italy

Willem H. Birkenhäger, M.D.
Professor of Medicine
Erasmus University
Head, Department of Medicine
Zuiderziekenhuis
Rotterdam, 3075 EA The Netherlands

Mordecai P. Blaustein, M.D.
Professor and Chairman
Department of Physiology
University of Maryland School of Medicine
Baltimore, Maryland 24201 U.S.A.

Graham W. Boyd, M.D.
Department of Medicine
Royal Hobart Hospital
Hobart, Tasmania
7000 Australia

Hans R. Brunner, M.D.
Chairman, Department of Nephrology
Centre Hospitalier Universitaire
Vaudois, Lausanne, 1011 Switzerland

Fritz R. Bühler, M.D.
Associate Professor of Medicine
Department of Medicine and Department of Re-
    search
Director of Hypertension Unit
Consultant in Cardiology
University Hospital
4031 Basel, Switzerland

F. Merlin Bumpus, Ph.D.
Research Division
Cleveland, Clinic
9500 Euclid Avenue
Cleveland, Ohio 44106 U.S.A.

Robert M. Carey, M.D., F.A.C.P.
Professor of Internal Medicine
Head, Division of Endocrinology and Metabolism
University of Virginia School of Medicine
Charlottesville, Virginia 22908 U.S.A.

David B. Case, M.D.
Associate Professor Medicine
Director, Clinical Research Center
Cornell University Medical College
New York, N.Y. 10021 U.S.A.

Kevin Catt, M.D., Ph.D.
Endocrinology and Reproduction Research
  Branch
National Institute of Child Health and Human
  Development
National Institutes of Health
Bethesda, Maryland 20205 U.S.A.

Jay Cohn, M.D.
Professor of Medicine
Head, Cardiovascular Division
University of Minnesota
Minneapolis, Minnesota 55455 U.S.A.

A.W. Cowley, Jr., Ph.D.
Professor and Chairman
Department of Physiology
Medical College of Wisconsin
Milwaukee, Wisconsin 53226 U.S.A.

David W. Cushman, Ph.D.
Squibb Institute for Medical Research
Princeton, New Jersey 08540 U.S.A.

Jacques deChamplain, M.D., Ph.D.
Professor, Department of Physiology
Université de Montréal
J.C. Edwards Professor in Cardiovascular Re-
  search, Department of Physiology
Consultant, Nephrology Section and Clinical Re-
  search
Department of Medicine
Hôpital Sacré-Coeur
Montréal, Quebec, C.P. 6208 Canada

Vincent DeQuattro, M.D., F.A.C.P.
Professor of Medicine
Chief, Hypertension Service
Department of Medicine
Los Angeles County–University of Southern Cali-
  fornia Medical Center
Los Angeles, California 90033 U.S.A.

Gerald F. DiBona, M.D., F.A.C.P.
Professor and Vice-Chairman
Department of Internal Medicine
University of Iowa College of Medicine
Chief, Medical Service,
Veterans Administration Medical Center,
Iowa City, Iowa 52240 U.S.A.

Armin G. Distler, M.D.
Associate Professor of Medicine
Department of Internal Medicine
University of Mainz
6500 Mainz, Germany

A.E. Doyle, M.D., F.R.C.P.
Chairman of Department of Medicine
Professor of Medicine
University of Melbourne,
Austin Hospital
Heidelberg, Victoria 3084 Australia

Victor Dzau, M.D.
Assistant Professor of Medicine
Harvard University Medical School
Director, Hypertension Unit
Brigham and Women's Hospital
Boston, Massachusetts 02115 U.S.A.

Haskel E. Eliahou, B.A., M.D.
Associate Professor of Nephrology
Sackler School of Medicine
Tel-Aviv University Medical School
Head, Department of Nephrology
Chaim Sheba Medical Center
Tel-Hashomer, Israel

Ervin G. Erdös, M.D.
Department of Pharmacology
University of Texas
Southwestern Medical School
5323 Harry Hines Boulevard
Dallas, Texas 75235 U.S.A.

Carlos M. Ferrario, M.D.
Associate Head, Department of Hypertension
Cleveland Clinic Research Division
9500 Euclid Avenue
Cleveland, Ohio 44106 U.S.A.

B. Folkow, M.D., Ph.D.
Professor in Physiology
Department of Physiology
University of Göteborg
Göteborg, 40038 Sweden

Edward D. Freis, M.D.
Professor of Medicine
Georgetown University
Senior Medical Investigator
Veterans Administration Medical Center
Washington, D.C. 20422 U.S.A.

J.C. Frölich, M.D.
Head, Department of Clinical Pharmacology
Dr. Margarete Fischer-Bosch Institut für Klinische Pharmakologie
Stuttgart, 7.000 Germany

Curt D. Furberg, M.D.
Chief, Clinical Trials Branch
National Heart, Lung and Blood Institute
Bethesda, Maryland 20205 U.S.A.

Detlev Ganten, M.D., Ph.D.
Professor of Pharmacology and Experimental Medicine
University of Heidelberg, and
Scientific Director
German Institute for Hypertension Research
Heidelberg, 6900 F.R.G.

Haralambos Gavras, M.D.
Professor of Medicine
Boston University School of Medicine
Boston, Massachusetts 02115 U.S.A.

Andreas Gruentzig, M.D.
Department of Medicine (Cardiology)
Emory University Hospital
Atlanta, Georgia 30322 U.S.A.

Arthur C. Guyton, M.D., D.Sc.
Professor and Chairman
Department of Physiology
University of Mississippi Medical Center
Jackson, Mississippi 39216 U.S.A.

Edgar Haber, M.D.
Professor of Medicine
Harvard Medical School
Chief, Cardiac Unit
Massachusetts General Hospital
Boston, Massachusetts 02115 U.S.A.

Francis J. Haddy, M.D., Ph.D.
Professor and Chairman
Department of Physiology
Uniformed Services University
Bethesda, Maryland 20014 U.S.A.

Guenther W. Hausler, M.D.
Associate Professor of Pharmacology
Pharmaceutical Research Department
F. Hoffmann–La Roche and Co., Ltd.
CH 4002 Basel, Switzerland

A. Helgeland, M.D.
Director, Health Service of Norwegian Telecommunication
Oslo, 1 Norway

Norman K. Hollenberg, B.Sc. (Med.), M.D., Ph.D., F.R.C.P. (C)
Professor and Director of Physiologic Research
Department of Radiology
Harvard Medical School
Senior Associate in Medicine
Cardiorenal Division
Peter Bent Brigham Division
Brigham and Women's Hospital
Boston, Massachusetts 02115 U.S.A.

U. Lennart Hulthén, M.D., Ph.D.
Department of Endocrinology
University of Lund
Malmö General Hospital
Malmö, S-21401 Sweden

Tadashi Inagami, Ph.D.
Professor of Biochemistry
Director, Hypertension Center
Department of Biochemistry
Vanderbilt University School of Medicine
Nashville, Tennessee 37232 U.S.A.

W. Januszewicz, M.D.
Professor of Medicine
Department of Angiology
Academy of Medicine
Nowogrodzka 59
Warsaw 02–006, Poland

William B. Kannel, M.D., M.P.H., F.A.C.P., F.A.C.C.
Professor of Medicine
Head, Section of Preventive Medicine and Epidemiology
Boston University School of Medicine
Visiting Physician, University Hospital
Boston University Medical Center
Boston, Massachusetts 02115 U.S.A.

Irwin J. Kopin, M.D.
Chief, Laboratory of Clinical Science
National Institute of Mental Health
Bethesda, Maryland 20205 U.S.A.

Ulla C. Kopp, Ph.D.
Department of Pharmacology
University of Göteborg
Göteborg, Sweden

Paul I. Korner, M.D., F.R.A.C.P., F.A.A.
Director Baker Medical Research Institute
Professor of Medicine
Monash University
Director of Clinical Research Unit
Alfred Hospital
Melbourne, 3181 Australia

Lawrence R. Krakoff, M.D., F.A.C.P.,
    F.A.C.C.
Chief, Hypertension Division
Professor of Medicine
Mount Sinai School of Medicine CUNY
New York, N.Y. 10021 U.S.A.

John H. Laragh, M.D.
Hilda Altshul Master Professor of Medicine
Director, Cardiovascular Center
Chief, Division of Cardiology
Cornell University Medical College
New York, N.Y. 10021 U.S.A.

Robert J. Lefkowitz, M.D.
Professor of Medicine
Duke University Medical Center
Durham, North Carolina 27710 U.S.A.

A.F. Lever, M.B.
Consultant Physician
MRC Blood Pressure Unit and Department of
    Medicine
Western Infirmary
Glasgow, G11 6NT Scotland

W.A. Littler, M.D., F.R.C.P.
Department of Cardiovascular Medicine
University of Birmingham
East Birmingham Hospital
Birmingham, England

Alexander G. Logan, M.D., F.R.C.P. (C)
Associate Professor of Medicine
University of Toronto
Director, Tri-Hospital Hypertension Service
Mount Sinai Hospital
Toronto, Ontario, M5 G1X5 Canada

Friedrich C. Luft, M.D.
Associate Professor of Nephrology
Indiana University Medical Center
Indianapolis, Indiana 46202 U.S.A.

Eugenie Ruth Lumbers, M.D.
Associate Professor, School of Physiology and
    Pharmacology
University of New South Wales
Sydney, Australia 2033

Graham Alexander MacGregor, M.A., M.R.C.P.
Senior Lecturer
Department of Medicine
Charing Cross Hospital Medical School
Honorary Consultant Physician
Blood Pressure Unit
Charing Cross Hospital
London, W5 8RF England

Robert E. McCaa, Ph.D.
Professor of Physiology and Biophysics
University of Mississippi School of Medicine
Jackson, Mississippi 39216 U.S.A.

Herbert McDade
President, International Operations
Revlon Health Care Group
1 Scarsdale Road
Tuckahoe, New York 10707 U.S.A.

Denis G. McDevitt, D.Sc., M.D., F.R.C.P.
Professor of Clinical Pharmacology
The Queen's University of Belfast
Consultant Physician
Belfast City Hospital and Royal Victoria Hospital
Belfast, BT9 7BL Ireland

John C. McGiff, M.D.
Professor and Chairman
Department of Pharmacology
Professor of Medicine
New York Medical College
Valhalla, New York 10595 U.S.A.

Prof. Agrégé Joel Ménard
Service d'Hypertension Artérielle
Hôpital Saint-Joseph
7, Rue Pierre-Larousse
75674 Paris, Cedex 14, France

Philippe Meyer, M.D.
I.N.S.E.R.M. U 7
Department of Physiology and Pharmacology
Hospital Necker
Paris, 75015 France

Alberto Morganti, M.D.
Assistant Professor
Department of Internal Medicine
University of Milan
Milan, 20122 Italy

E.E. Muirhead, M.D.
Chairman and Professor
Department of Pathology
Professor of Medicine
University of Tennessee Center for the Health Sciences
Memphis, Tennessee 38103 U.S.A.

John B. Myers, M.B.B.Ch. (Rand), F.C.P. (SA), B.Sc.
N.H. and M.R.C. Medical Postgraduate Research Scholar
Department of Medicine
Royal Newcastle Hospital and Faculty of Medicine
University of Newcastle
Newcastle, NSW, Australia

Alberto Nasjletti, M.D.
Professor of Pharmacology
University of Tennessee Center for the Health Sciences
Memphis, Tennessee 38103 U.S.A.

Andreas P. Niarchos, M.D., F.A.C.C.
Associate Professor of Medicine
Cardiovascular Center
Cornell University Medical College
New York, N.Y. 10021 U.S.A.

Roger F. Palmer, M.D.
Department of Pharmacology
University of Miami School of Medicine
P.O. Box 520875
Biscayne Annex
Miami, Florida 33152 U.S.A.

Sir George Pickering, F.R.S., M.D., F.R.C.P.
Regius Professor of Medicine Emeritus
University of Oxford
Oxford, England

Thomas G. Pickering, M.D., D.Phil.
Associate Professor of Medicine
Cardiovascular Center
Cornell University Medical College
New York, N.Y. 10021 U.S.A.

Yu. V. Postnov, M.D.
Central Scientific Research Laboratory
USSR Ministry of Health
Moscow 101387 U.S.S.R.

Ian A. Reid, Ph.D.
Associate Professor of Physiology
University of California, San Francisco
San Francisco, California 94143 U.S.A.

John L. Reid, M.D., F.R.C.P.
Regius Professor of Materia Medica
University of Glasgow
Glasgow, G11 6NT Scotland

Donald J. Reis, M.D.
Professor of Neurology
Director, Laboratory of Neurobiology
Cornell University Medical College
New York, N.Y. 10021 U.S.A.

Richard D. Remington, Ph.D.
Dean and Professor of Public Health
University of Michigan School of Public Health
Ann Arbor, Michigan 48109 U.S.A.

John Roelker
President and Group Executive
Revlon Health Care Group
1 Scarsdale Road
Tuckahoe, New York 10707 U.S.A.

Stephen M. Schwartz, M.D., Ph.D.
Associate Professor
Department of Pathology
School of Medicine
University of Washington
Seattle, Washington 98195 U.S.A.

Jean E. Sealey, D.Sc.
Associate Professor of Physiology in Medicine
Cardiovascular Center
Cornell University Medical College
New York, N.Y. 10021 U.S.A.

Donald W. Seldin, M.D., M.A.C.P.
William Buchanan Professor of Medicine
Chairman of Internal Medicine
University of Texas Health Science Center at Dallas
Chief of the Medical Service
Parkland Memorial Hospital
Dallas, Texas 75216 U.S.A.

David G. Shand, Ph.D., M.B.
Department of Pharmacology
Duke University Medical Center
3813 Duke Medical Center
Durham, North Carolina 27710 U.S.A.

I.K. Shkvatasabaya, M.D.
National Cardiology Research Center
Academy of Medical Sciences
Moscow 101387, U.S.S.R.

F.O. Simpson
Clinical Service
Wellcome Medical Research Institute
University of Otago Medical School
P.O. Box 913
Dunedin, New Zealand

Leonard T. Skeggs, Ph.D.
Professor of Biochemistry
Case Western Reserve University and Medical Investigator
Veterans Administration Hospital
Cleveland, Ohio 44106 U.S.A.

Charles G. Smith, Ph.D.
Vice President, Research and Development
Revlon Health Care Group
1 Scarsdale Road
Tuckahoe, New York 10707 U.S.A.

Richard L. Soffer, M.D.
Professor of Biochemistry and Medicine
Cornell University Medical College
1300 York Avenue
New York, N.Y. 10021 U.S.A.

Reuel A. Stallones, M.D.
Professor of Epidemiology
School of Public Health
University of Texas
Houston, Texas 77025 U.S.A.

David H.P. Streeten, M.B., D.Phil, F.R.C.P., F.A.C.P.
Professor of Medicine and Chief, Section of Endocrinology
Department of Medicine
SUNY Upstate Medical Center
Syracuse, New York 13210 U.S.A.

Robert C. Tarazi, M.D.
Vice Chairman, Research Division
Head, Clinical Science Department
Research Division
Cleveland Clinic Foundation
Cleveland, Ohio 44106 U.S.A.

Stanley H. Taylor, B.Sc., M.B.Ch.B., F.R.C.P.
Senior Lecturer in Cardiology
Department of Cardiovascular Studies
University of Leeds
Physician-in-Charge
Cardiac Care Unit
The General Infirmary at Leeds
Leeds, LS1 3EX England

Herbert Thurston, M.D.
Department of Medicine
The General Hospital
Leicester LE 5 4 PW, England

Louis J. Tobian, Jr.
Professor of Medicine
University of Minnesota Hospital and School of Medicine
Minneapolis, Minnesota 55455 U.S.A.

D. Tosteson, M.D.
Dean
Harvard Medical School
Boston, Massachusetts 02115 U.S.A.

Sidney Udenfriend, Ph.D.
Roche Institute of Molecular Biology
Nutley, New Jersey 07110 U.S.A.

Michael A. Weber, M.D., F.A.C.P.
Associate Professor of Medicine
University of California, Irvine
College of Medicine
Irvine, California 90801 U.S.A.
Chief, Section of Clinical Pharmacology and Hypertension
Veterans Administration Medical Center
Long Beach, California U.S.A.

Christopher S. Wilcox, M.A., B.M., B.Ch., Ph.D., M.R.C.P.
Senior Wellcome Clinical Research Fellow
Honorary Senior Lecturer in Medicine
The Medical Unit
St. Mary's Hospital Medical School
London, W2 1NY England

Kenjiro Yamamoto, M.D.
Professor of Pharmacology
Osaka City University Medical School
Osaka, Japan

Yukio Yamori, M.D., Ph.D.
Chairman, Professor of Pathology
Shimane Medical University
Research Director
Japan Stroke Prevention Center
Izumo, 693 Japan

David B. Young, Ph.D.
Professor, Department of Physiology and Biology
University of Mississippi School of Medicine
Jackson, Mississippi 39216 U.S.A.

Alberto Zanchetti, M.D.
Professor of Medicine
Director, Institute of Medical Pathology
Associate Director, Cardiovascular Research Institute
University of Milan
School of Medicine
Milan, 20122 Italy

Contributors

Bengt Åblad, M.D.
Adjunct Professor of Pharmacology
University of Göteborg
Göteborg, Sweden

William Adam, M.B.B.S, PhD., F.R.A.C.P.
Renal Physician
Repatriation Hospital, Heidelberg
Victoria, Australia

Greti Aguilera, M.D.
Endocrinology and Reproduction Research
  Branch
National Institute of Child Health and Human
  Development
National Institutes of Health
Bethesda, Maryland 20205 U.S.A.

F. Alhenc-Gélas, M.D.
I.N.S.E.R.M. U 36
Paris, France

Franz W. Amann, M.D.
Senior Resident, Department of Medicine
University Hospital
Basel, Switzerland

Gunnar H. Anderson, Jr., M.D.
Associate Professor of Medicine
SUNY Upstate Medical Center
Syracuse, N.Y. 13210 U.S.A.

M. Assad, Ph.D.
The Squibb Institute for Medical Research
E.R. Squibb and Sons, Inc.
Princeton, New Jersey 08540 U.S.A.

M. Aurell, M.D.
Associate Professor of Nephrology
Medical Department I
Sahlgren's Hospital
Göteborg, Sweden

Kenneth M. Baker, M.D.
University of Virginia
Charlottesville, Virginia 22908 U.S.A.

A.C. Barger, M.D.
Robert Henry Pfeiffer Professor of Physiology
Harvard Medical School
Boston, Massachusetts 02115 U.S.A.

D.G. Beevers, M.D.
Consultant Physician
Dudley Road Hospital
Birmingham, England

C. Beretta-Piccoli, M.D.
Visiting Research Fellow
MRC Blood Pressure Unit and Department of
  Medicine
Western Infirmary
Glasgow, Scotland

Osmund Bertel, M.D.
Senior Resident
Department of Medicine
University Hospital
Basel, Switzerland

Robert F. Bing, M.B.Ch.B., M.R.C.P.
Lecturer in Medicine
Leicester University, U.K.
Senior Registrar
Leicester Royal Infirmary
Leicester, U.K.

R. Bloch, M.D.
Indiana University Medical Center
Indianapolis, Indiana U.S.A.

Peter Bolli, M.D.
Consultant in Hypertension
Department of Medicine
University Hospital
4031 Basel, Switzerland

Margereta Bramnert, M.D., Ph.D.
Professor of Internal Medicine and Endocrinology
University of Lund
Malmö General Hospital
Malmö, Sweden

Emmanuel L. Bravo, M.D.
Staff, Research Division
Cleveland Clinic
Cleveland, Ohio 44106 U.S.A.

Bennie Brooks
Research Associate
University of Tennessee Center for the Health Sci-
  ences
Baptist Memorial Hospital
Memphis, Tennessee 38103 U.S.A.

K. Bridget Brosnihan, Ph.D.
Associate Staff
Cleveland Clinic Foundation
Research Division
Cleveland, Ohio 44106 U.S.A.

J.J. Brown, M.B.
Consultant Physician
MRC Blood Pressure Unit and Department of
    Medicine
Western Infirmary
Glasgow, Scotland

Peggy S. Brown
Senior Electron Microscopy Technician
University of Tennessee Center for the Health Sci-
    ences
Baptist Memorial Hospital
Memphis, Tennessee 38103 U.S.A.

D.B. Brunner, D.V.M.
Division of Nephrology and Hypertension
Centre Hospitalier Universitaire
Lausanne, Switzerland

Alessandro Capponi, Ph.D.
Endocrinology and Reproduction Research
    Branch
National Institute of Child Health and Human
    Development
National Institutes of Health
Bethesda, Maryland 20205 U.S.A.

George Cardinale, Ph.D.
Roche Institute of Molecular Biology
Nutley, New Jersey 07110 U.S.A.

M.R. Celio, M.D.
Assistant
Department of Anatomy
University of Zürich
Zürich CH8 006 Switzerland

Alice Chatzilias
Technician
University of Toronto
Mt. Sinai Hospital
Toronto, Ontario, Canada

D.L. Clemens, B.S.
Vanderbilt University School of Medicine
Nashville, Tennessee 37232 U.S.A.

David L. Clough, Ph.D.
Assistant Professor of Physiology
Uniformed Services University
Bethesda, Maryland 20014 U.S.A.

Uwe Cordes, M.D.
Associate Professor of Medicine
Division of Endocrinology
Department of Internal Medicine
University of Mainz
6500 Mainz, Germany

P. Corvol, M.D.
I.N.S.E.R.M. U 36
Paris, France

A.M.M. Cumming, S.R.N.
Research Nursing Officer
MRC Blood Pressure Unit and Department of
    Medicine
Western Infirmary
Glasgow, Scotland

D.L. Davies, M.D.
Senior Lecturer
MRC Blood Pressure Unit and Department of
    Medicine
Western Infirmary
Glasgow, Scotland

P. Degoulet, M.D.
I.N.S.E.R.M. U 36
Paris, France

Hugh E. deWardener, M.D., F.R.C.P.
Professor, Department of Medicine
Charing Cross Hospital Medical School
Consultant Physician
Charing Cross Hospital
London W6 8RF England

C.D. DeVaux, Ph.D.
I.N.S.E.R.M. U 36
Paris, France

John G. Dymling, M.D., Ph.D.
Associate Professor of Internal Medicine and En-
    docrinology
Department of Endocrinology
University of Lund
Malmö General Hospital
Malmö, Sweden

Giora Z. Feuerstein, M.Sc.
Visiting Associate, Laboratory of Clinical Science
National Institute of Mental Health
Bethesda, Maryland 20205 U.S.A.

S. Foote
I.N.S.E.R.M. U 36
Paris, France

Andras Foti, Ph.D.
Research Biochemist, Department of Medicine
Los Angeles County—University of Southern California Medical Center
Los Angeles, California 90025 U.S.A.

Fetnat M. Fouad, M.D.
Research Division, Cleveland Clinic
Cleveland, Ohio 44106 U.S.A.

J. Franciosa, M.D.
Scientist
Chief of Cardiology
Veterans Administration Hospital
Philadelphia, Pennsylvania 19123 U.S.A.

R. Fraser, Ph.D.
MRC Blood Pressure Unit and Department of Medicine
Western Infirmary
Glasgow, Scotland

F.X. Galen, Ph.D.
I.N.S.E.R.M. U 36
Paris, France

R.P. Garay, M.D., M.Sc.
Department of Physiology and Pharmacology
Hospital Necker
Paris, France

Irene Gavras, M.D.
Assistant Professor of Medicine
Boston University School of Medicine
Boston, Massachusetts 02115 U.S.A.

D. Goldfarb, M.D.
Chaim Sheba Medical Center
Tel-Hashomer, Israel

David S. Goldstein, M.D., Ph.D.
Clinical Associate, Hypertension-Endocrine Branch
National Heart, Lung, and Blood Institute
National Institutes of Health
Bethesda, Maryland 20205 U.S.A.

John E. Hall, Ph.D.
Associate Professor, Department of Physiology
University of Mississippi Medical Center
Jackson, Mississippi 39216 U.S.A.

M. Hallbäck-Nordlander, M.D.
Assistant Professor, Department of Physiology
University of Göteborg
Göteborg, Sweden

Carlene A. Hamilton, Ph.D.
Research Assistant
Department of Materia Medica
University of Glasgow
Glasgow, Scotland

D.P. Henry, M.D.
Indiana University Medical Center
Lilly Laboratories for Clinical Research
Indianapolis, Indiana 46202 U.S.A.

Peter Hill, Ph.D.
Head, Lipid Metabolism
American Health Foundation
Valhalla, New York 10595 U.S.A.

Shigehisa Hirose, Ph.D.
University of Tsukuba
Tsukuba, Japan

I. Hjermann, M.D.
Assistant Director
Oslo Study
Ullevaal Hospital
Oslo, Norway

Bernt Hökfelt, M.D.
Department of Endocrinology
University of Lund
Malmö General Hospital
Malmö, Sweden

I. Holme
Director, Institute of Medical Statistics
Ullevaal Hospital
Oslo, Norway

Ryoichi Horie, M.D., Ph.D.
Department of Neurosurgery
Shimane Medical University
Associate Director, Clinical Research
Japan Stroke Prevention Center
Izumo, Japan 693

Diana E. Hurlbut, B.S.
Department of Pharmacology
University of California
Irvine, California 90801 U.S.A.

Bryan Christopher Hurst, M.Biol.
Imperial Chemical Industries Ltd.
Mereside, Alderley Park
Macclesfield, Chesire, England

A. Iaina, M.D.
Senior Nephrologist
Chaim Sheba Medical Center
Tel-Hashomer, Israel

Takehiro Igawa, M.Sc.
Department of Pathology
Shimane Medical University
Izumo, Japan

Fumihiko Ikemoto, Ph.D.
Assistant Professor of Pharmacology
Osaka City University Medical School
Osaka, Japan

M.J. Ismay, M.B.B.S.
School of Physiology and Pharmacology
University of New South Wales
Sydney, Australia 2033

T.E. Jackson, M.D.
Department of Physiology
University of Mississippi Medical Center
Jackson, Mississippi 39216 U.S.A.

Marilyn James-Krake, Ph.D.
Research Associate
Washington University School of Medicine
St. Louis, Missouri 63110 U.S.A.

Minoru Kawamura, M.D.
Department of Pharmacology
Osaka City University Medical School
Osaka, Japan

Masahiro Kihara, M.D.
Instructor of Epidemiological Pathology
Shimane Medical University
Research Associate
Japan Stroke Prevention Center
Izumo, Japan

Wolfgang Kiowski, M.D.
Department of Medicine
University Hospital
4031 Basel, Switzerland

W. Kitajima, M.D.
Department of Clinical Pharmacology
Dr. Margarete Fischer-Bosch-Institut für Klini-
   sche Pharmakologie
Stuttgart, Germany

Rainer Kolloch, M.D.
Fellow of American Heart Association
Los Angeles Affiliate
American Heart Association
Los Angeles, California 90025 U.S.A.

U. Kuhlmann, M.D.
Department of Medicine
Emory University
Atlanta, Georgia 30332 U.S.A.

Regine Landmann, M.D.
University Hospital
4031 Basel, Switzerland

Stanley Lang, Ph.D.
Associate Professor of Physiology
Washington University School of Medicine
St. Louis, Missouri 63110 U.S.A.

D. Lau, B.S.
Vanderbilt University School of Medicine
Nashville, Tennessee 37232 U.S.A.

W.B. Lee
School of Physiology and Pharmacology
University of New South Wales
Sydney, Australia 2033

Gastone Leonetti, M.D.
Associate Professor of Medicine
University of Milan
School of Medicine
Milan, Italy

P. Leren, M.D.
Director, Medical Outpatient Clinical
Ullevaal Hospital
Oslo, Norway

Daniel Levine, M.D.
Assistant Professor of Neurology
Director of Electromyography Department
Los Angeles County—University of Southern California Medical Center
Los Angeles, California 90025 U.S.A.

T. Barry Levine, M.D.
Department of Medicine
University of Minnesota
Minneapolis, Minnesota 55455 U.S.A.

J.A. Lewis, M.A., Dip.Stat, F.I.S.
Statistics Section Manager
ICI Pharmaceutical Division
Macclesfield, Cheshire, England

T.E. Lohmeier, Ph.D.
Associate Professor
Department of Physiology
University of Mississippi Medical Center
Jackson, Mississippi 39216 U.S.A.

Jorge A. Lopez-Ovejero, M.D.
Cardiovascular Center
Cornell University Medical College
New York, N.Y. 10021 U.S.A.

S. Lundin
Research Assistant
Department of Physiology
University of Göteborg
Göteborg, Sweden

P.G. Lūnd-Larsen, M.D.
Assistant Director
National Mass Radiography Service
Oslo, Norway

Borwin Lüth, M.D.
Research Associate
Department of Internal Medicine
University of Mainz
6500 Mainz, Germany

D.I. McCloskey, M.B., B.S., D.Sc., D.Phil., F.R.A.C.P.
Associate Professor
School of Physiology and Pharmacology
University of New South Wales
Sydney, Australia 2033

Kafait U. Malik, Ph.D.
Professor of Pharmacology
University of Tennessee Center for the Health Sciences
Memphis, Tennessee 38103 U.S.A.

Joseph S. Mallov, M.D.
Research Fellow in Endocrinology,
Department of Medicine
SUNY Upstate Medical Center
Syracuse, New York
Assistant Attending Physician
Allegheny General Hospital
Pittsburgh, Pennsylvania U.S.A.

Guiseppe Mancia, M.D.
Associate Professor of Medicine
University of Milan School of Medicine
Milan, Italy

Johannes Mann, F.E., M.D.
Department of Pharmacology
University of Heidelberg
Heidelberg, F.R.G.

R.D. Manning, Jr., Ph.D.
Associate Professor
Department of Physiology
University of Mississippi Medical Center
Jackson, Mississippi 39216 U.S.A.

Nirmala Markandu, S.R.N.
Research Technician, Blood Pressure Unit
Department of Medicine
Charing Cross Hospital Medical School
Fulham, London, England

P.A. Mason, Ph.D.
MRC Blood Pressure Unit and Department of Medicine
Western Infirmary
Glasgow, Scotland

Milton Mendlowitz, M.D.
Lowe and Price Professor of Medicine Emeritus
Mount Sinai School of Medicine
New York, N.Y. 10021 U.S.A.

Trefor O. Morgan, M.D., B.S. B.Sc. (Med.) F.R.A.C.P.
Repatriation Hospital
Heidelberg, Victoria, Australia

J.J. Morton, Ph.D.
Scientist
MRC Blood Pressure Unit and Department of
    Medicine
Western Infirmary
Glasgow, Scotland

Yasuo Nara, Ph.D.
Instructor of Biochemical Pathology
Shimane Medical University
Chief, Biochemical Section
Japan Stroke Prevention Center
Izumo, Japan

Ing-Marie Nilsson
University of Göteborg
Göteborg, Sweden

Miguel A. Ondetti, Ph.D.
Squibb Institute for Medical Research
Princeton, New Jersey 08540 U.S.A.

Akira Ooshima, M.D., Ph.D.
Associate Professor of Pathology
Shimane Medical University
Associate Director, Basic Research
Japan Stroke Prevention Center
Izumo, Japan

P.L. Padfield, M.B.
Senior Registrar
MRC Blood Pressure Unit and Department of
    Medicine
Western Infirmary
Glasgow, Scotland

Motilal B. Pamnani, M.D., Ph.D.
Associate Professor of Physiology and Medicine
Uniformed Services University
Bethesda, Maryland 20205 U.S.A.

Judith M. Paulin, B.Sc.
University of Otago
Wellcome Medical Research Institute
Department of Medicine
Medical School
Dunedin, New Zealand

Thomas Philipp, M.D.
Associate Professor of Medicine
Department of Internal Medicine
University of Mainz
6500 Mainz, Germany

James A. Pitcock, M.D.
Clinical Associate Professor, Pathology
University of Tennessee Center for the Health Sci-
    ences
Baptist Memorial Hospital
Memphis, Tennessee 38103 U.S.A.

P.F. Plouin, M.D.
I.N.S.E.R.M. U 36
Paris, France

E.K. Potter, B.Sc.
School of Physiology and Pharmacology
University of New South Wales
Sydney, Australia 2033

Ralph E. Purdy, Ph.D.
Assistant Professor of Medicine
Department of Pharmacology
University of California
Irvine, California 90801 U.S.A.

L.I. Rankin, M.D.
Indiana University Medical Center
Indianapolis, Indiana 46202 U.S.A.

I. Reimann, M.D., Ph.D.
Department of Clinical Pharmacology
Dr. Margarete Fischer-Bosch-Institut für Klin-
    ische Pharmakologie
Stuttgart, Germany

S.E. Ricksten
Research Assistant
Department of Physiology
University of Göteborg
Göteborg, Sweden

D. Robertson, M.D.
Department of Medicine
Vanderbilt University
Nashville, Tennessee 37232 U.S.A.

J.I.S. Robertson, M.B.
Consultant Physician
MRC Blood Pressure Unit and Department of
    Medicine
Western Infirmary
Glasgow, Scotland

B. Rosenkranz, M.D.
Department of Clinical Pharmacology
Dr. Margarete Fischer-Bosch-Institut für Klinische Pharmakologie
Stuttgart, Germany

Joseph E. Roulston, M.A., M.R.S.C.
Senior Biochemist, Department of Medicine
Charing Cross Hospital Medical School
London, England

Bernard Rubin, Ph.D.
Squibb Institute for Medical Research
Princeton, New Jersey 08540 U.S.A.

Sarah Schoentgen, M.Sc.
Research Associate
Department of Medicine
Los Angeles County—University of Southern California Medical Center
Los Angeles, California 90025 U.S.A.

L.G. Siwek, M.D.
Clinical Associate
National Institutes of Health
Bethesda, Maryland 20205 U.S.A.

May Sjölander
University of Göteborg
Göteborg, Sweden

Robert R. Smeby, Ph.D.
Staff, Research Division
Cleveland Clinic Foundation
Cleveland, Ohio 44106 U.S.A.

M.J. Smith, Jr., Ph.D.
Assistant Professor
Department of Physiology
University of Mississippi Medical Center
Jackson, Mississippi U.S.A.

Kenneth Sniderman, M.D.
Assistant Professor of Radiology
Cornell University Medical College
New York, N.Y. 10221 U.S.A.

Thomas A. Sos
Professor of Radiology
Director, Division of Cardiovascular Radiology
Cornell University Medical College
New York, N.Y. 10021 U.S.A.

F. Soubrier, M.D.
I.N.S.E.R.M. U 36
Paris, France

Georg Speck
Department of Pharmacology
University of Heidelberg
Heidelberg, F.R.G.

Sydney Spector, Ph.D.
Roche Institute of Molecular Biology
Nutley, New Jersey 07110 U.S.A.

Eric G. Spokas, Ph.D.
Instructor
Department of Pharmacology
New York Medical College
Valhalla, New York 10595 U.S.A.

Jay Springer, M.D.
Department of Medicine
SUNY Upstate Medical Center
Assistant Attending Physician in Medicine
State University Hospital
Syracuse, New York 13210 U.S.A.

T.J. Stallard, A.I.M.L.T.
Department of Cardiovascular Medicine
University of Birmingham
East Birmingham Hospital
Birmingham, England

Donna M. Standaert, B.S.
Research Technician III
Department of Pathology
School of Medicine
University of Washington
Seattle, Washington 98195 U.S.A.

Andrea Stella, M.D.
Assistant Professor of Medicine
University of Milan
School of Medicine
Milan, Italy

D.D. Stevens
School of Physiology and Pharmacology
University of New South Wales
Sydney, Australia 2033

Martha G. Stoddard, M.D.
University of Virginia
Charlottesville, Virginia 22908 U.S.A.

Patricia Sullivan, RN
Cardiovascular Center
Cornell University Medical College
New York, N.Y. 10021 U.S.A.

Patrick A. Sullivan, M.B., M.R.C.P.
Visiting Scientist, Department of Medicine
Los Angeles County—University of Southern California Medical Center
Los Angeles, California
Consultant Physician
County Hospital
Mallow Co.
Cork, Ireland

Frederick S. Suderlin, M.D.
Research Fellow in Endocrinology
Department of Medicine
SUNY Upstate Medical Center
Syracuse, New York
Staff Physician
Geisinger Medical Center
Danville, Pennsylvania U.S.A.

John D. Swales, F.R.C.P.
Professor of Medicine
University of Leicester
Honorable Consultant Physician
Leicester Royal Infirmary
Leicester, England

Kazuo Takaori, M.D.
Department of Pharmacology
Osaka City University Medical School
Osaka, Japan

Yukio Takii, Ph.D.
Vanderbilt University School of Medicine
Nashville, Tennessee 37232 U.S.A.

M. Thibonnier, M.D.
I.N.S.E.R.M. U 36
Paris, France

P. Thorén, M.D., Ph.D.
Assistant Professor
Department of Physiology
University of Göteborg
Göteborg, Sweden

G.A. Turini, M.D.
Division of Nephrology and Hypertension
Centre Hospitalier Universitaire
Lausanne, Switzerland

Thomas Unger, M.D.
Department of Pharmacology
University of Heidelberg
Heidelberg, F.R.G.

Peter van Brummelen, M.D.
Senior Resident
Afdeling Nierziekten
Academisch Ziekenhuis Leiden
Leiden, The Netherlands

E.D. Vaughan, Jr., M.D.
James J. Colt Professor of Urology
Cornell University Medical College
Chairman, Division of Urology
The New York Hospital
New York, N.Y. 10021 U.S.A.

Gilda Versales, M.D.
Hypertension Research Fellow
Department of Medicine
Los Angeles County—University of Southern California Medical Center
Los Angeles, California 90025 U.S.A.

Nicolas D. Vlachakis, M.D.
Associate Professor of Medicine
Section of Clinical Pharmacology
University of Southern California School of Medicine
Los Angeles, California 90025 U.S.A.

B. Waeber, M.D.
Division of Nephrology and Hypertension
Centre Hospitalier Universitaire
Lausanne, Switzerland

R.D.S. Watson, B.Sc., M.B., M.R.C.P.
Department of Cardiovascular Medicine
University of Birmingham
East Birmingham Hospital
Birmingham, England

J.P. Wauters, M.D.
Division of Nephrology and Hypertension
Centre Hospitalier Universitaire
Lausanne, Switzerland

Myron H. Weinberger, M.D.
Professor of Medicine
Indiana University Medical Center
Director, Specialized Center of Research in Hypertension
Indianapolis, Indiana 46202 U.S.A.

A.E. Weymen, M.D.
Indiana University Medical Center
Indianapolis, Indiana 46202 U.S.A.

Thomas A. Wilson, M.D.
Division of Endocrinology and Metabolism
University of Virginia School of Medicine
Charlottesville, Virginia 22908 U.S.A.

Hideyoshi Yokosawa, Ph.D.
University of Hokkaido
Hokkaido, Japan

J. Young
Technician
MRC Blood Pressure Unit and Department of Medicine
Western Infirmary
Glasgow, Scotland

Hartmut Zschiedrich, M.D.
Research Associate
Department of Internal Medicine
University of Mainz
Mainz, Germany

Frontiers in Hypertension Research: Past, Present and Future

Introduction

John H. Laragh

THE PHENOMENON

A lot has happened since 1895 when Riva-Rocci developed the first practical means for routine blood pressure measurements in the clinical setting. The next inevitable step was the collation of survey type of information. Not surprisingly, it was found that blood pressures were distributed in a normal bell-shaped curve. It was therefore possible to define, for different ages, albeit arbitrarily, a level above which persons were characterized as hypertensive. The standards selected separated out an alarming 10–20% of the adult population. When known causes for the arbitrarily defined high blood pressure were excluded (e.g., kidney and adrenal diseases), the very large residuum was termed "essential" or idiopathic hypertension. It was widely assumed that this biophysical deviation was a single disease. However, it was recognized very early that the function or survival of most people having untreated high blood pressure was not affected appreciably, if at all. Hence, the appropriately popular eponym "benign essential hypertension." Indeed this benign characteristic of the disorder was emphasized in writings of Homer Smith, Perera, Goldring, and Chasis.

Early on, however, it also became appreciated that, on a statistical basis, having a relatively higher blood pressure even within the normal range is on average clearly associated with a shortened survival. This is demonstrable at every decile of life. Such actuarial data have become the basis for life insurance company evaluations and are a yardstick for defining the increased risk of people having an elevated blood pressure. Actually, the figures suggest that this risk is small and not randomly distributed. Some small fraction of the population are actually at greater risk of premature cardiovascular complications and an earlier demise, and this vulnerable subgroup reduces the average chance for survival for the group as a whole. However, the major fraction of those with hypertension are not at greater risk of premature death, and for these people the term "benign" remains appropriate.

Notwithstanding this heterogeneity in risk and survival, it has become common practice for clinicians, research scientists and epidemiologists alike to consider essential hypertension as a single uniform entity, perhaps genetically conditioned. This concept has had a predominant influence on the research and attitudes of twentieth century research on hypertension. In looking back upon this attitude, it seems to me a bit strange that a physical sign such as hypertension would be accepted as likely having only a single basis. Certainly an elevated body temperature would never upfront be considered to reflect a single cause.

THE VINDICATION AND THE PROBLEMS OF EMPIRIC THERAPY

An important research contribution of the past 20 years has been the establishment of the fact that whenever the blood pressure of hypertensive people is effectively reduced, the susceptibility to some of its major cardiovascular complications, stroke, kidney failure and heart failure, can be reduced and useful life significantly prolonged. Most such studies employed not only diuretics but sympatholytic and vasodilator drugs as needed to subdue the blood pressure. This body of research indicates that lowering the blood pressure, by whatever means, appears to be the common denominator for the derived benefit.

More recently, research has begun to sort out the relative value of different types of therapies.

Studies, some of which will be reviewed in this volume, seem to indicate that when diuretic agents are used it is difficult to demonstrate any protection from myocardial infarction, (indeed vulnerability may increase) whereas when beta-adrenergic blocking drugs are the sole antihypertensive agent, considerable protection has been shown. Obviously, for the future, the type of agent used and the means by which the blood pressure is lowered may become increasingly relevant as we learn more about hypertensive mechanisms.

The practical spinoff has been the drafting of universal health care recipes by national health managers. It has even been suggested that not to treat hypertension is irresponsible. Moreover, physicians are told that it is not worth upfront searching for any causes of the hypertension. The main message today is to treat, enthusiastically and vigorously, and for a lifetime.

It is likely that such enthusiasm goes beyond the bounds of available information and, as will be discussed, actually fails to recognize the lack of risk of many hypertensive people as well as the possible lack of commensurate safety of antihypertensive drugs employed for the time periods envisioned, especially in mild disease. As discussed herein, even the safest classes of drugs, diuretics and beta-blockers, have their inherent risks. These are crucial issues which need more thought and which are faced in this volume. It is not likely that we have reached the point where physicians can be advised to trade in their power of reason for a single recipe.

ETIOLOGIC FACTORS

Notwithstanding the persistence of this holistic attitude, research over the years has turned up some hard facts about possible causes. Four pathogenic factors are widely recognized: Broadly speaking, these are the kidneys, dietary sodium, the adrenal cortex, and the nervous system.

THE KIDNEYS

The key role of the kidneys was first pointed out by the studies of Bright in 1826. This relationship was reinforced by a number of investigations, in particular the discovery of renin by Tigerstedt and Bergman in 1898. Their beautifully designed experiments revealed a humoral substance in the kidneys with a powerful capacity to raise blood pressure. However, renin lost its credibility when other established workers failed to confirm the experiment. Renin also failed to survive despite the renewed demonstration of an important role for the kidneys with the studies of Volhard and Fahr in 1914, showing an association between renal necrotizing arteriolitis and malignant hypertension. Indeed, interest in renin and in the kidneys lay fallow until 1934 when Goldblatt produced hypertension by renal artery constriction in the dog. Following these classic studies, interest in renin revived and the original observations were at last confirmed. It did not take long then for Page and Braun-Menendez and their colleagues to independently demonstrate that renin was not a pressor itself but was an enzyme which released a pressor peptide from a plasma substrate. The peptide was then identified as the octapeptide angiotensin II, synthesized, and its formidable pressor properties well characterized.

Despite these important developments interest in renin lagged once again as investigators failed to demonstrate any relationship between the blood pressure and the renin level in clinical or experimental hypertension. The failure of these studies only became explicable when it was shown that renin secretion is the key part of a control system for regulating sodium balance and blood pressure and in which renin levels fluctuate widely according to the dietary sodium intake. Recognition of this relationship has allowed a rational separation of essential hypertension, for purposes of analysis, into low, medium and high renin subgroups. Some of the fruits of this approach are considered in this volume.

Also discussed is a second important reason that the relevance of renin has been so long delayed: methodology. It has only been in the past five years that prorenin has been recognized. The presence in plasma of this substance in amounts 10 times or more greater than active renin is of great current theoretical interest. Moreover, the nonawareness of prorenin in the past 20 years of research has rendered certain widely applied renin methods grossly incorrect, sometimes producing a 10-fold or more variable error in renin values that has confused general understanding.

DIETARY SODIUM AND BLOOD PRESSURE

The influence of sodium intake on blood pressure was recognized in the early 1900s when it became apparent that a low sodium diet could improve edematous states such as congestive heart failure and also lower the blood pressure. This observation reached full definition in the 1940s by Kempner and associates in demonstrating the beneficial effects of a low salt rice diet for treating hypertensive patients. It became apparent that the value of rice was wholly related to its sodium content. A rice diet, or any other stringent low sodium diet, greatly improves or completely corrects the hypertension of about ⅓ or so of all patients with essential hypertension. However, what is often forgotten is that little or no benefit accrues to the remaining majority of patients.

Parallel studies of animal models has demonstrated the amplifying effect of a high sodium diet on blood pressure and vice versa. Strains of rats were developed which are especially sensitive to the pressor effects of a high sodium diet. In a way, the pressor action of a very high sodium diet and the depressor influence of a very low sodium diet pointed again to an important role for the kidneys, since the kidneys are the only route for elimination of sodium. Accordingly, too, the greater occurrence of hypertension in chronic renal diseases can be largely assigned to a failure to excrete normal amounts of sodium.

While sodium is a basic determinant of blood pressure and flow since it is the major determinant of extracellular fluid volume and viscosity, the relevance of changes in dietary intake to blood pressure within the usual ranges selected remains to be clarified. Epidemiologic studies are not definitive. Thus, in societies with little access to salt there seems to be little hypertension. Conversely, societies with higher salt intakes have more hypertension. However, the meaning of such observations is clouded because whenever individuals within a single society are examined, there is no relationship between the level of salt intake and the height of the blood pressure. It appears that extremes of sodium intake not easily achieved in humans are necessary to show any depressor or pressor effect. These issues are discussed in spirited fashion in these proceedings.

ALDOSTERONE

Companion to the key role of the kidneys as both an endocrine organ for renin secretion and an excretory organ for sodium elimination is an important role of the sodium-retaining hormone of the adrenal cortex. This was defined by early research of Selye and his colleagues which established that administration of an adrenal sodium-retaining hormone, DOC, consistently produces hypertension in rats provided there is adequate sodium in the diet. The important role of adrenal aldosterone secretion in supporting human hypertension is now well recognized as are the beneficial effects of blockade, especially in low-renin patients who exhibit inappropriate or absolute excesses of aldosterone secretion. Further definition of the more subtle participation of aldosterone and of the factors that control aldosterone secretion in hypertensive subjects are promising areas for further research.

THE NERVOUS SYSTEM

Besides the endocrine and excretory functions of the kidney and the influence of dietary sodium and of aldosterone secretion, there has been long-standing agreement about the important role of the nervous system in blood pressure control. This involvement is well demonstrated by the value of sedatives, tranquilizers, anesthetic agents and ganglioplegic drugs for lowering blood pressure. Moreover its participation in acute blood pressure phenomena has been elegantly defined by the research of Heymans and his associates which exposed and characterized the carotid and aortic baroceptors and their linkage with a central mediated reflex arc which modulates blood pressure and heart rate. However, notwithstanding a possibly critical role of the nervous system in longer term blood pressure regulation, research to date has failed to identify or characterize any definable unique role of abnormal neural function in chronic human hypertension. There are suggestive data from both animal and human studies, some of which will be discussed herein. We need more data about central or autonomic nervous activity that might act either directly or by affecting other pressor systems. Any participation of the nervous system in long term blood pressure control is obviously subtle, since numerous studies of overt changes in catecholamine hormones in the blood or in the urine have thus far been largely unconvincing. These issues too are reexamined in some depth in this volume.

PERCEPTIONS AND WORKING HYPOTHESES ON THE NATURE OF ESSENTIAL HYPERTENSION

As the data base from experimental, clinical and epidemiological sources grew, it was natural for working scientists to attempt to synthesize their perception of the phenomenon. Practically all of these syntheses have been built on the upfront belief that high blood pressure is a single more or less uniform disorder perhaps genetically conditioned. Thus, the epidemiologic studies of Pickering and his colleagues led him to conclude that hypertension was merely a quantitative deviation, comprising the upper end of a Gaussian distribution curve. In his construction, hypertension was a continuum of the normal blood pressure distribution and the dividing line between it and normotension was purely arbitrary. He perceived it as an inherited phenomenon of polygenic origin. Platt, on the basis of his research, took an opposing position and considered hypertension to be a separate, qualitatively different disorder than normotension because he was able to demonstrate a separate secondary peak in the distribution curve. Looking back on this today, it may not be useful to debate whether hypertension is qualitatively as opposed to quantitatively different from normotension since in fact most diseases (e.g., hyperthyroidism, Cushing's syndrome) are in fact quantitative deviations from the norm. Whatever the case, the analyses of Pickering in describing a continuum between normotension and hypertension are extremely valuable because they define a large grey zone of borderline hypertension. This should be borne in mind whenever new studies are reported in which absolute differences in a biochemical or physical measurement are claimed to clearly separate hypertensive from normotensive people.

Page continues to support the notion that hypertension is a *mosaic* in which, at any given point in time, at least eight different ill-defined factors may or may not dynamically contribute to the maintenance of the hypertension. This theory makes the unprecedented proposal that hypertension in an individual person does not have a single cause, but rather involves multiple defects which intermittently contribute. Although a cascade of reactions to a primary fault is a well-recognized pathologic phenomenon this is not what the mosaic expresses. Whatever its intent, the mosaic theory well reflects the frustration and consternation of investigators in their attempts to unravel the problem. However, its framework lacks sufficient specificity for it to provide a basis for planning new experiments.

An attractive hypothesis about hypertension that certainly deserves further exploration implicates the central and autonomic nervous system and in one approach examines the question of whether chronic hypertension might not be an abnormal conditioned response to environmental or other stimuli as in the classic model of Pavlov. The idea is attractive since blood pressure phenomena in acute settings can be closely linked to emotional and autonomic stimuli, and because we would all like to believe in the central coordination of pressure and flow. At the same time, as of this writing, there are very few definitive experiments with convincing data to support the possibility of a defect in central control.

Research in animal models, pioneered by Folkow, by Ledingham and by Guyton and their respective colleagues points up the possibly key role of the behavior of the arteriolar resistance vessels in chronic hypertension and suggests the possibility that an adaptive or autoregulatory response of these vessels, causing structural changes, perhaps in reaction to overperfusion, perhaps from renal sodium-retention and perhaps autonomically mediated, may be a critical mechanism. These ideas are probed and contested in this volume.

Research of our own group suggests that so-called essential hypertension is a group of disorders that comprise a spectrum of abnormal *vasoconstriction-volume* interactions reflected by renin system behavior. This analytical model is based on data to define the renin-angiotensin-aldosterone system as a cohesive control system for the long term regulation of blood pressure and sodium balance. Accordingly, the patterns revealed by the renin system in individual hypertensive patients define the relative participation of renin or of volume. The patterns show that an absolute or inappropriate excess of renin activity participates through its pressor action in the maintenance of most essential hypertension. Conversely, in some thirty percent with low-renin values a volume factor is often demonstrable. Clinically, this analytical framework enables experiments to be designed for the future identification of other vasoconstrictor substances such as vasopressin or norepinephrine, which might be critically involved in some forms and which can also be expected to produce predictable reactive patterns in renin system behavior. This analytical scaffold differs fundamentally from previous approaches because it presumes that the hypertensive population is heterogeneous both biochemically and pathophysiologically. At the same time it exposes new questions for future research. We need to know for example, why renin secretion so often participates, why it fails to turn itself off and what is the nature of the neurogenic control of it. We also need to understand the reason for the inappropriate volume factor.

Whichever of these or other perceptions prove useful for defining and understanding hypertension, it seems likely that it is no longer profitable to analyze hypertensive phenomena with the presumption that they largely reflect a single disorder. The heterogeneity of human hypertension is strongly apparent, not only from the wide interindividual variation in its natural history and prognosis, but also from the fact that different patients differ widely in their responsiveness or lack of responsiveness to different types of antihypertensive drugs. To an increasing degree, these evidences of heterogeneity can in turn be correlated with differences in pathophysiology and with underlying differences in biochemical patterns as revealed, for example, by studies of the renin-angiotensin-aldosterone control system.

All of this evidence for heterogeneity of essential hypertension is further supported by the numerous impressive exceptions observed in the past in studies of groups of hypertensive patients in which positive correlations have been observed. Thus, while it is certainly true that the low sodium diet greatly benefits a minor fraction of patients with high blood pressure, it is often forgotten that sodium depletion is totally ineffective in other larger fractions. Similarly, it is true that the higher the blood pressure in general the greater is the likelihood of developing stroke, heart attack, or malignant hypertension. However, it must be kept in mind that most of these events can occur with milder or even no hypertension. Conversely, some people with marked hypertension have no vascular complications or impairment of function. Such outstanding exceptions test accepted doctrines (exceptione probot regulum), and, rather than dismiss them, these exceptions should provide real opportunities for future research.

The experience in animal models of hypertension mirrors the human experience in demonstrating that there are many different ways to initiate and sustain chronic hypertension, only some of which are related to dietary salt intake. Unfortunately none of these animal models resembles the spectrum of human essential hypertension. This may be one reason why most of the widely used drugs, including diuretics, beta-blockers, methyl dopa and clonidine, were not identified or predicted to be antihypertensive from animal research. I have always thought that this is partly related to the upright posture. Human hypertension surely has a strong postural component. Whatever the reasons, the lack of a good animal model makes the human experience the final arbiter in the research process. Alexander Pope's "the proper study of mankind is man" certainly is applicable here.

Since it seems that essential hypertension is probably not one disorder, the challenge for the future is to take this group apart and analyze it farther for crucial biochemical and pathophysiologic differences. Perhaps someday, hopefully in the not-too-distant future, we will no longer treat a blood pressure elevation per se. We may be more concerned with whether this elevation is compromising tissue flow or not. Perhaps, as suggested in this volume abnormalities in flow or in the form of the pressure tracing, will be more important mandates for therapy than any deviation in the blood pressure itself.

In the symposium and this record of it, we have tried to re-examine old ideas and introduce new ones. We take a fresh look at the epidemiologic evidence. The role of chemical mediators acting locally or systemically, and the concepts of neural-endocrine linkages and of control system analysis are given special attention. Altogether, the explosion in our knowledge base, especially in the past 20 years or so, suggests that we are moving closer to final solutions for blood pressure phenomena. *Litera scripta manet.*

Session 1
The Variation in Risk Among Hypertensive Patients: Is Broad Scale Therapy to Help Only a Few Justifiable? What Pressure Levels Should Be Treated?

Chairman: J. H. Laragh

Position Paper: The Variation in Risk Among Hypertensive Patients: Is Broad Scale Therapy to Help Only a Few Justifiable? What Pressure Levels Should Be Treated?

M. H. Alderman

Since 75% of all hypertensive persons have mild or moderate elevation of blood pressure, and since available data provide, at best, inconsistent guidance for therapy, it is not surprising that intense interest continues to raise the questions: who should be treated, at what time, and by what means. Often the issue is joined by the straightforward question, "At what level of blood pressure should treatment be instituted?" Unfortunately, however, available knowledge about the nature of high blood pressure suggests that the question is as yet unanswerable (1). The results of epidemiologic and intervention studies reveal a clinical heterogeneity so complex as to defy discrimination of those to be, and those not to be, treated by any device as simple as a single and highly variable physical measure (2).

THE FRAMINGHAM STUDY

Tables constructed from the longitudinal experience of middle-aged adults in Framingham permit estimation of the probability of having a cardiovascular disease event within the following 15 years (3).

Figure 1 depicts graphically the risk of developing cardiovascular disease in 15 years for 35-year-old men and women under different clinical conditions. The "low-risk" 35-year-old man does not smoke, has a cholesterol of 235 mg%, no EKG abnormality or evidence of glucose intolerance. He stands a 15% risk of developing cardiovascular "disease" if his systolic blood pressure is 195 mmHg. A 35-year-old man, however, with the same blood pressure of 195 mmHg, but at "high risk" (cigarette smoker, a cholesterol of 310 mg%, LVH on EKG and glucose intolerance), has an 86% chance of experiencing a cardiovascular disease event over the ensuing 15 years. Thus, two men at the same age and level of pressure can have a sixfold difference in their expectation of disease.

In contrast, a 35-year-old woman with the "low"-risk configuration of associated clinical and behavioral characteristics has only a 6% risk of disease events in 15 years if her blood pressure is 195 mmHg. This is equivalent to the hazard faced by a man with the "low"-risk characteristics, but a systolic blood pressure of 135 mmHg. Thus, this man and woman sharing the same age and risk have blood pressures separated by 60 mmHg. Furthermore, this low-risk woman with a systolic blood pressure of 195 has only one-sixth the risk faced by a "high"-risk man with a systolic blood pressure of 135 mmHg.

These examples demonstrate the enormous variety in natural history of hypertension that is not predicted by blood pressure level. In fact, it is clear that the range of risk within a single blood pressure stratum is enormous, while people with vastly different blood pressures can have exactly the same risk of disease and others with lower pressures can have risks greater than those faced by persons with higher pressures.

These projections suggest that although the height of arterial pressure may distinguish groups in which the aggregate burden of subsequent cardiovascular disease occurrence is different, it also tends to lump together individuals with vastly different life expectations. Moreover, since disease risk is not evenly distributed within blood pressure strata, it seems reasonable to expect that the benefit of any blood pressure reduction might not be uniformly received by all the persons at a given level of blood pressure.

In an attempt to provide a quantitative dimension to this intragroup variability, my colleagues and I have calculated the extent of disease preven-

The Risk of CVD During 15 Years After Age 35 by SBP and Risk Status

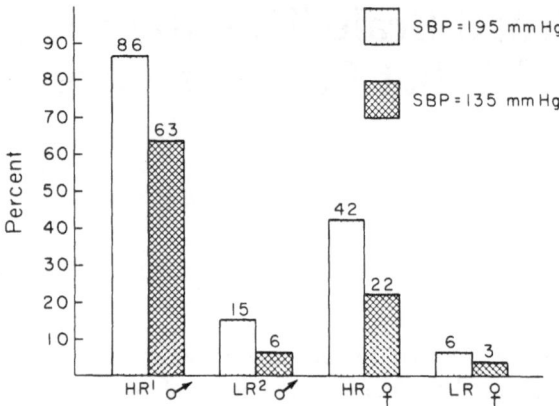

Fig. 1. Risk of developing cardiovascular disease (CVD) in 15 years for men and women aged 35 years by SBP level and risk status. High risk: LVH, cigarette smoker, cholesterol = 310 mg% and glucose intolerance. Low risk: no LVH, nonsmoker, cholesterol = 235 mg% and no glucose intolerance. [Gordon et al. (2)]

tion that might be realized by blood pressure reduction under various clinical and blood pressure circumstances. These calculations depend on the validity of three fundamental assumptions: First, blood pressure declines of the magnitude defined can be achieved and maintained for 15 years. Second, the means employed to manipulate the pressure would not, in themselves, produce harm. Finally, those whose blood pressure was so artificially altered would thereafter enjoy the life experience of one whose blood pressure was naturally at that lower level.

Figure 2 depicts the ratio of nonbenefit to benefited if treatment were begun at age 35 and continued for 15-, 25-, or 30-year periods. In the top, left-hand panel, it can be seen that almost 50, 35-year-old women, with the low-risk configuration, must have their pressure dropped from 165 to 135 mmHg for 15 years without any benefit for every such woman who would benefit from the same treatment. Of course, the odds ratio can change dramatically when other blood pressures and clinical circumstances are considered. In the lower left-hand panel, it can be seen that only three high-risk men need fruitlessly undergo a blood pressure reduction 195–135 for 15 years for each such patient to benefit.

In sum, this arithmetic indicates that, regardless

of the sex, blood pressure level, clinical status, extent of reduction, or length of follow-up, the majority of hypertensive persons can expect to be treated without hope of benefit. Moreover, at the milder levels of pressure and during shorter periods of follow-up, ongoing treatment is likely to benefit only a very small fraction of the persons exposed. These data, based on the best possible interpretation of observed natural history, permit some reasonable predictions about the likely optimal results of intervention trials. The trials themselves suggest that the modest expectations presaged by the Framingham experience have indeed been borne out by empirical investigation.

INTERVENTION TRIALS

VA STUDIES

Completed more than a decade ago, the VA studies were designed to determine the ability of active

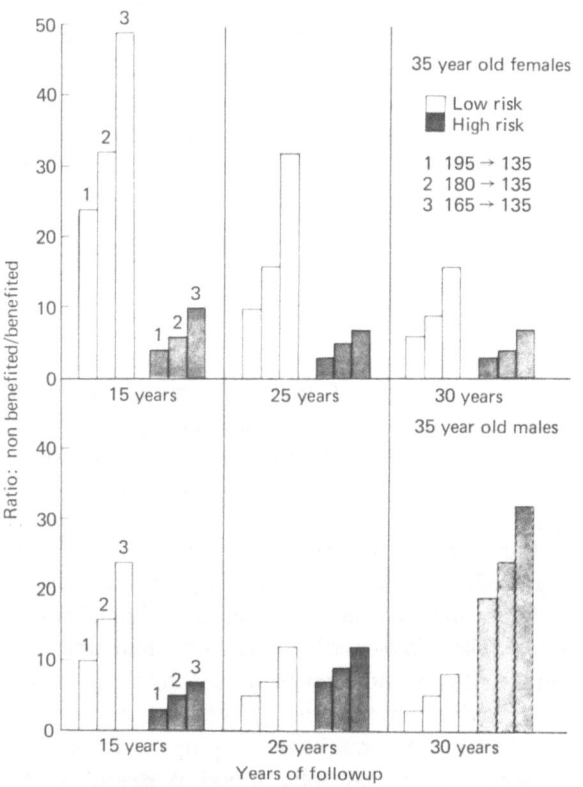

Fig. 2. Relative benefit of various degrees of blood pressure reduction for three periods of follow-up and at two levels of associated risk for 35-year-old males and females. [Gordon et al. (2)]

hypotensive agents to reduce cardiovascular disease morbidity and mortality (4, 5). The power of these studies derives from the precision of their design and elegance of completion. Participants, selected according to rigid criteria, were randomly allocated to either placebo or active treatment. Thereafter, save for their pharmacologic category, all patients received the same follow-up care.

Under the circumstances of this study, particularly the heavy selection basis to "high-risk" patients, it was possible to demonstrate quickly the value of treatment for patients with diastolic pressures in excess of 114 mmHg. At the mild and moderate levels below that range, results were less dramatic and, indeed, in the mild range (90–104 mmHg); no statistically significant benefit of treatment was found. Since the vast bulk of so-called hypertensives resides in that mild blood pressure stratum, it is worth reviewing the more detailed examination of the data provided by E. D. Freis and associates (6).

These data (Fig. 3) depict the variety of natural history that exists within a single blood pressure stratum. For example, male veterans in the placebo group with entry diastolic pressures between 90 and 104 mmHg, who had no evidence of cardiac abnormality at entry, had a risk less than one-half that of a person with the same blood pressure who had evidence of cardiovascular risk abnormality at entry. Other categories of demography and clinical status produced similarly wide variations in actual disease incidence.

It is, therefore, not surprising that, when the benefit of treatment is examined, concomitant variation between subgroups appears. Figure 4, for example, illustrates how patients without cardiovascular abnormalities at entry had little risk of disease and no apparent benefit of therapy. Moreover, in Fig. 5, it can be seen that while older patients in the 90–104-mmHg stratum were at great risk and experienced substantial benefit from treatment, younger persons with the same pressure had little risk and slight benefit through treatment.

These examples of the diversity of both the risk of disease and the benefit to be derived from active therapy are consistent with what might have been expected from the experience in Framingham. Mild high blood pressure does not define a homogeneous cohort. Instead, this group is heterogeneous not only in terms of its demographic, clinical, and behavioral characteristics, but more importantly in the variation of benefit to be realized from treatment. The VA study confirms the expectation that cardiovascular disease events, as well as their reduction through chemotherapy, do not follow a chance pattern, but tend to cluster accord-

VA Study
Incidence of CVD in Untreated Patients

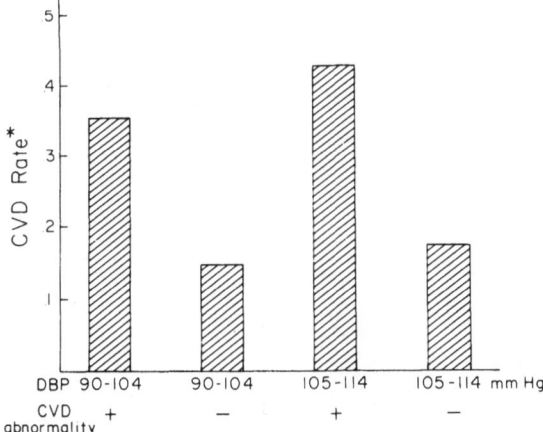

VA Study
CVD Incidence and Benefit of Therapy in Mild Hypertension (90–104 mmHg) by CVD Status

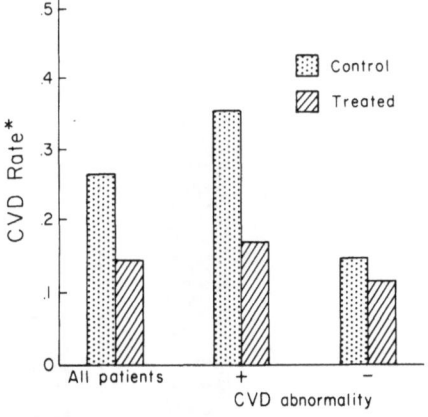

Fig. 3. Incidence of CVD in untreated patients. *Estimated by multiple regression technique. [Veterans Administration Cooperative Study Group on Hypertensive Agents (5)]

Fig. 4. CVD incidence and benefit of therapy in mild hypertension (90–104 mmHg) by CVD status. *Estimated by multiple regression technique. [Veterans Administration Cooperative Study Group on Hypertensive Agents (6)]

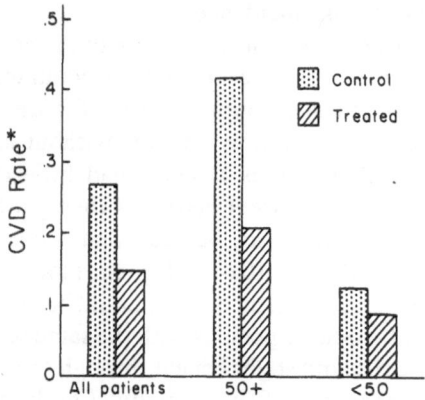

VA Study
CVD Incidence and Benefit of Therapy in Mild Hypertension (90–104 mmHg) by Age

Fig. 5. CVD incidence and benefit of therapy in mild hypertension (90–104 mmHg) by age. *Estimated by multiple regression technique. [Veterans Administration Cooperative Study Group on Hypertensive Agents (6)]

HYPERTENSION DETECTION AND FOLLOW-UP PROGRAM

In the face of this tantalizing, but inconclusive, information, support was mobilized in the early 1970s to undertake studies that might fill the gaps in knowledge.

The Hypertension Detection and Follow-up Program (HDFP) was designed to test the value of antihypertensive therapy for mild hypertensives drawn from the general community (7). Unfortunately, the meaning of its observed outcomes is somewhat clouded by the absence of a control group defined in the conventional sense. Instead of a placebo group, HDFP randomly allocated participants into special or regular care treatment cohorts. The special care (SC) group received vigorous care without cost under conditions designed to maximize compliance to a predetermined, albeit somewhat outmoded, chemotherapeutic regimen. The regular care (RC) group, by contrast, was referred to community physicians to receive treatment in the conventional fashion. Under these circumstances, it is difficult to determine whether any differences in outcomes were due to the hypotensive therapy or the nonspecific benefits of general medical care. As it turned out, deaths ascribed to noncardiovascular events fell by an amount that was approximately 60% of the extent of the decline

ing to the presence or absence of factors other than arterial pressure level. Thus, while demonstrating that blood pressure reduction can reduce morbidity and mortality, the VA study also demonstrated that the level of blood pressure, certainly in the mild and moderate range, is of modest prognostic value and of even less value in determining whom to treat.

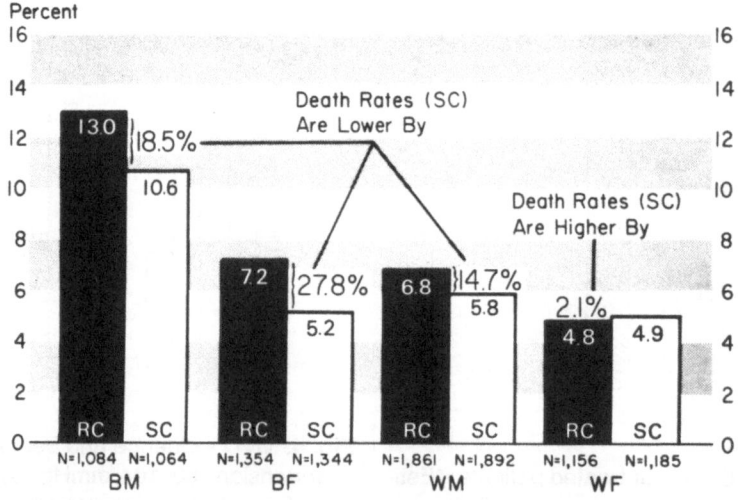

Mortality—All Causes by Sex and Race
5-Year Mortality Rates (%) (HDFP)

Fig. 6. Mortality: All causes by sex and race. BM, black male; WM, white male; BF, black female; WF, white female. [Hypertension Detection and Follow-up Program Cooperative Group (7)]

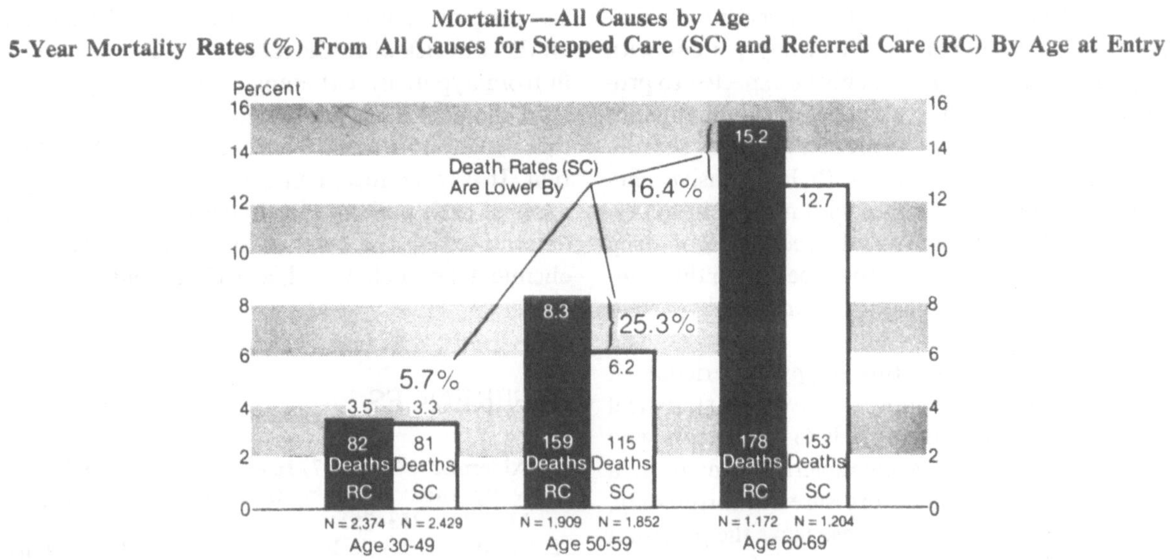

Mortality—All Causes by Age
5-Year Mortality Rates (%) From All Causes for Stepped Care (SC) and Referred Care (RC) By Age at Entry

Fig. 7. Mortality: All causes by age. [Hypertension Detection and Follow-up Program Cooperative Group (7)]

in cardiovascular-related deaths. Thus, it is hard to discount the importance of the nonspecific impact of SC.

Assuming that the decline in mortality was entirely due to the impact of the demonstrated fall in blood pressure, it is still clear that these results do not resolve the issues surrounding treatment of mild hypertension. First, although the difference in all cause mortality in the mild strata was 16%, attack rates were low, and the actual difference in survival over 5 years was approximately 1.5% between the two groups, with more than 92% of all participants surviving. In fact, this difference, was 13 per 1,000 persons over 5 years, or 0.26% per year.

Moreover, when the experience of this mild group was subjected to slightly more detailed scrutiny, the anticipated heterogeneity of the group emerged (Fig. 6) (3). For example, when mortality differences according to sex and race were examined, blacks showed high attack rates and substantial benefit, while white women suffered few deaths and did not seem to benefit from a lowered blood pressure. Furthermore, when the results were depicted according to age, again, as expected, older persons seemed more likely to die and had substantially fewer deaths if they participated in SC (Fig. 7). But those persons under 50 had slight mortality, and this was not reduced by achieving a lower pressure in stepped care.

CONCLUSIONS

What comfort can be drawn from these landmark intervention trials? Both the VA and HDFP studies confirm the hope that reduction of arterial pressure can produce benefit. This is true even at very mild elevations. Unfortunately, at all levels, but more so at increasingly lower levels, the prognostic heterogeneity of persons with the same level of pressure is so great that benefits from wholesale treatment, which are small to begin with, are unevenly distributed. Thus, particularly at mild levels, a uniform treatment plan based on blood pressure level dooms the vast majority of those treated to long-term intervention without hope of benefit. Although treatment is good for some, better means are needed to identify those persons. In the absence of needed precise clinical markers, there is an understandable, but, nevertheless, inappropriate tendency to rely on the single clinical device of blood pressure level to define the need for treatment.

The present inability to attain clinical certainty can perhaps be better perceived in contrast to the situation regarding malignant hypertension. Patients with malignant hypertension could be readily identified by precise diagnostic criteria (8). Moreover, they pursue a uniform course that proceeds rapidly downhill, and when untreated, almost invariably ends fatally. In view of this clinical and prognostic homogeneity, interventions that produced a particular result in any patient with this condition could reasonably be expected to produce a similar result in all patients with malignant hypertension (9). Thus, more than two decades ago, favorable experience with hypotensive chemotherapy in some persons with malignant hypertension led to the universal acceptance of drug therapy which has proved so successful in the management of all patients with malignant hypertension (10).

Extrapolating from this happy experience, it would be tempting to apply the favorable statistical results of current clinical trials to all patients who had the same defining characteristic—namely, a particular level of blood pressure. Unfortunately, the defining marker in this case lacks the precision of the whole syndrome of malignant hypertension. At the mild level, blood pressure is about as specific as temperature in predicting patient outcome or signaling the proper therapy.

Instead of using this deceptively simple unidimensional tool to solve a complex clinical problem, physicians would be better advised to employ all the epidemiologic, clinical, biochemical, and behavioral data at their command to arrive at a management plan for each patient. Neglect, benign or otherwise, has always been, and is today, an unsound medical policy. But in this symptomless, but complex, array of dissimilar clinical situations now conveniently described by the simple rubric of essential hypertension, judicious restraint may sometimes be more advantageous than wholesale and precipitous application of a standardized chemotherapeutic recipe.

SUMMARY

The proper management of mild and moderate hypertension remains a matter of considerable professional disagreement. Major clinical and population research has been largely designed to define a level of blood pressure at which treatment should be initiated. In this paper, studies of the natural history of hypertension and the findings of intervention trials have been reviewed to determine whether the blood pressure level alone is adequate to identify, diagnose, and predict the future course of hypertensive patients.

Observational data suggest that patients defined by mild elevation of blood pressure are a heterogeneous group who do not share a common progno-

sis. Moreover, intervention trials reveal that not all those at risk of cardiovascular disease will benefit from hypotensive therapy. Thus, blood pressure level alone defines neither the group at risk nor those likely to benefit from blood pressure reduction. It is, therefore, concluded that the management of each patient with hypertension should be determined on the basis of available clinical, biochemical, and behavioral, as well as epidemiologic data.

REFERENCES

1. Alderman MH (1977) High blood pressure: Do we really know whom to treat and how? N Engl J Med 296: 753–755
2. Gordon T, Sorlie P, Kannel WB (1971) Framingham study: An epidemiological investigation of cardiovascular disease In: Kannel WB, Gordon T (eds.) Section 27, U.S. Dept. of Health, Education and Welfare. National Institutes of Health, Bethesda, Md
3. Hypertension Detection and Follow-up Program Cooperative Group (1979) Five-year findings of the Hypertension Detection and Follow-up Program: II. Mortality by race-sex and age. JAMA 242: 2572–2576
4. Veterans Administration Cooperative Study Group on Antihypertensive Agents (1967) Effects of treatment on morbidity in hypertension: I. Results in patients with diastolic blood pressure averaging 115 through 129 mmHg. JAMA 202: 1028–1034
5. Veterans Administration Cooperative Study Group on Hypertensive Agents (1970) Effects of treatment on morbidity in hypertension: II. Results in patients with diastolic blood pressure averaging 90 through 114 mmHg. JAMA 213: 1143–1152
6. Veterans Administration Cooperative Study Group on Antihypertensive Agents (1972) Effects of treatment on morbidity in hypertension: III. Influence of age, diastolic pressure, and prior cardiovascular disease; further analysis of side effects. Circulation 45: 991–1004
7. Hypertension Detection and Follow-up Program Cooperative Group (1979) Five-year findings of the Hypertension Detection and Follow-up Program: I. Reduction in mortality of persons with high blood pressure, including mild hypertension. JAMA 242: 2562–2571
8. Kincaid-Smith P, McMichael J, Murphy EA (1958) The clinical course and pathology of hypertension with papilledema (malignant hypertension). J Med 105: 117–153
9. Harington M, Kincaid-Smith P, McMichael J (1959) Results of treatment in malignant hypertension: A seven year experience in 94 cases. Br Med J 2: 969–980
10. Lee TH, Alderman MH (1978) Malignant hypertension: Declining mortality rate in New York City, 1958 to 1974. NY State J Med 78: 1389–1391

Interpretation of the Hypertension Detection and Follow-up Program

Richard D. Remington

Five months ago, the Hypertension Detection and Follow-up Program (HDFP) reported findings for its primary design end point, all cause mortality (1, 2). This community-based randomized trial screened 158,906 individuals aged 30–69 in 14 communities nationwide. Attempts were made to enroll all individuals with blood pressure elevations maintained through two screenings, at home and in the clinic, and high participation rates were achieved. Because very few individuals were to be excluded, it was ethically unfeasible to use placebos, thereby blocking treatment for persons with very high blood pressures. Participants were randomly assigned to stepped care or referred care groups, and the randomization was effective in equating the groups. Referred care participants received a full base-line examination and were then sent to their usual source of care in the community, while participating in annual follow-up examinations under study auspices.

Stepped care participants received a systematic program of increasing dosages and numbers of drugs, beginning with the long-acting diuretic, chlorthalidone. Each member of this group was assigned a goal blood pressure, based on the diastolic level at entry. For those with entry levels 100 or greater, 90 mmHg was the goal. For levels in the 90s, there was a 10-mm reduction defined goal. Thus, some participants were treated to a goal as low as 80 mm.

Toxicity was minimal. No stepped care deaths were attributed to adverse drug reactions, and few hospitalizations occurred for such reasons. Because of the availability of alternative medications specified by the protocol, toxicity rarely prevented the attainment of goal blood pressure.

The reduction in all cause mortality was sizable. Overall, 17% fewer deaths occurred during the 5-year follow-up period in the stepped care as compared to referred care group. Among those with blood pressure 90–104 mmHg, a 20% reduction occurred. Both these differences were statistically significant at the 1% level. Mortality reductions also occurred in the groups with higher entry blood pressures, but the study design ensured groups of modest size at these levels, and, therefore, significance tests in such groups were avoided to preclude misinterpretation of statistical comparisons of inadequate sensitivity to important differences.

Substantial mortality reductions were found for black participants of both sexes, for white males, and for individuals over 40 years of age. Cardiovascular and cerebrovascular mortality were greatly reduced. Younger participants and white females showed little decrease in death rates. However, in both these subgroups, overall mortality was very low, and for white women in the referred care group, treatment and control of blood pressure elevation were more widespread than for the other race–sex subgroups. These findings cannot, therefore, be taken to mean that blood pressure treatment is unwarranted in the young or in white women.

Overall, the HDFP findings support vigorous management by pharmacologic means of individuals with even modest elevations of diastolic blood pressure. In fact, stepped care participants with entry level 90–94 had a mortality reduction of 22% compared to referred care. It has subsequently been reported that reductions also occurred in groups with or without evidence of end-organ damage at base line and in those on or off antihypertensive medication at entry.

In the light of these results, we should reconsider terms such as "mild hypertension" or "benign essential hypertension." If such substantial reductions of mortality are available using inexpensive, safe medication in individuals with diastolic levels barely over 90, are the terms "mild" or "benign" justified?

Surely, there is something distasteful about consigning the younger individual with blood pressure elevations in the 90-mm range to a lifelong drug regimen, even though such a life might well be longer on than off treatment. We must develop improved techniques for preventing blood pressure elevation in the first place. Second, we must look for nonpharmacologic modalities for reducing the lower levels of blood pressure elevation.

A word of caution, however, is in order. Western medicine and public health are probably not sufficiently vigorous in their approach to pharmacologic control of blood pressures in the 90-mm range. Effective and acceptable nonpharmacologic control is either unavailable or at best untested. At present, only pharmacologic intervention has been shown capable of consistently producing sustained blood pressure reductions to within the normal range. Furthermore, radical dietary or lifestyle interventions present problems of patient compliance at least as great, and probably greater, as those attending regular usage of antihypertensive medication. One of the earliest findings of the HDFP (3) was the two- to threefold increase in percentage of hypertensives in US communities detected, treated, and controlled since the early 1970s. However, it is important to recognize that we are still reducing to within normal limits the blood pressures of fewer than one-half the hypertensives in this country. The large majority of those hypertensives have blood pressures in the range formerly called mild hypertension. Furthermore, as shown in another HDFP report (4), the majority of all excess deaths attributable to blood pressure elevation occurs in individuals with these lower pressures.

The message seems clear. Efforts to elucidate mechanisms responsible for elevated blood pressure must continue as must efforts directed toward developing effective and acceptable methods for primary prevention and nonpharmacologic control of high blood pressure. However, these efforts must not be allowed to impede our progress toward delivering the increased longevity and higher quality of life available through mass pharmacologic control of elevated blood pressure, including modestly elevated blood pressure.

SUMMARY

In December 1979, the HDFP reported results for its primary end point, all cause mortality. This nationwide, community-based trial screened 158,906 individuals aged 30–69 in 14 localities. Hypertensives were randomly assigned to referred care by their regular physicians or to stepped care, a systematic program of medication designed to reduce the blood pressure to a predetermined goal.

Results established a 17% reduction in all cause mortality in stepped compared to referred care, with minimal toxicity. Individuals with base-line diastolic blood pressure 90–104 mmHg showed an even larger mortality reduction of 20%. These reductions were substantial for black participants of both sexes, for white males, and for participants above age 40. White women and younger participants showed little decrease below already low mortality rates.

These results justify a vigorous approach to pharmacologic control of hypertensive patients, even those with diastolic blood pressure in the 90-mm range. At present, fewer than one-half the hypertensives in US communities are detected, treated, and controlled. While research efforts to prevent high blood pressure and to control blood pressure elevation by nonpharmacologic means must continue, current treatment practices should be altered to include vigorous pharmacologic management of all hypertensives, designed to bring the blood pressure to within the normal range. This specifically applies to those patients formerly labeled "mild" hypertensives.

REFERENCES

1. Hypertension Detection and Follow-up Program Cooperative Group (1979) Five-year findings of the Hypertension Detection and Follow-up Program: I. Reduction in mortality of persons with high blood pressure, including mild hypertension. JAMA 242: 2562–2571
2. Hypertension Detection and Follow-up Program Cooperative Group (1979) Five-year findings of the Hypertension Detection and Follow-up Program: II. Mortality by race-sex and age. JAMA 242: 2572–2577
3. Hypertension Detection and Follow-up Program Cooperative Group (1977) Blood pressure studies in 14 communities: A two-stage screen for hypertension. JAMA 237: 2385–2391
4. Hypertension Detection and Follow-up Program Cooperative Group (1977) The Hypertension Detection and Follow-up Program: A progress report. Circ Res 40(Suppl 1): 106–109

Implications of Framingham Study Data for Treatment of Hypertension: Impact of Other Risk Factors

William B. Kannel

The recent findings of the Hypertension Detection and Follow-up Program (HDFP) extend the evidence that early detection and control of hypertension can substantially reduce cardiovascular morbidity and mortality and prolong life (1). In particular, it has now been demonstrated that treatment of even mild degrees of hypertension (i.e., 90–104 mmHg diastolic pressure) can reduce cardiovascular sequelae. Furthermore, it has been shown that more rigorous goals pay dividends in a greater reduction in mortality. This finding is quite consistent with epidemiologic data from Framingham, which have indicated a continuum of risk with a 30% increment for each 10-mmHg increase in pressure throughout the blood pressure range and including "normotensive" values (Fig. 1). This has indicated that the lower the pressure, the lower the risk, even within the borderline or normal range.

Mild degrees of hypertension have been shown to double the risk of a cardiovascular event (Table 1). This is true at all ages and in both sexes. It is also true whether the pressure elevation is systolic or diastolic in nature and whether labile or fixed. For any given average pressure, risk of cardiovascular events is unaffected by the degree of variability of the pressure (Table 2).

The focus of *diastolic* pressure in the trials of antihypertensive therapy is unfortunate. Diastolic hypertension has been widely and justifiably accepted as a cause of cardiovascular mortality (1–5). However, it has also been accepted that the cardiovascular sequelae of hypertension derive chiefly from the diastolic pressure component. Prospective data suggest that, if anything, systolic pressure is actually the more powerful contributor to cardiovascular disease (Fig. 2). Even *isolated* systolic hypertension has been shown to be associated with an increased risk (Table 3), particularly in the elderly where it is highly prevalent.

Thus, even mild degrees of hypertension, whether labile or fixed, systolic or diastolic, can be dangerous in the elderly as well as the young and in either sex. It is now shown that vigorous treatment to reduce pressures to well within the normal range is most beneficial (Fig. 3). Also, some 10% of the adult population has diastolic pressures exceeding 90 mmHg on repeat screening of which 70% is in the 90–104-mmHg range. Because of the higher prevalence of this milder hypertension, almost 60% of the excess mortality attributable to hypertension comes from this pressure range (Fig. 4). Hence, this mild hypertension constitutes a major public health problem. However, even though the HDFP showed few dangerous side effects in controlling mild hypertension, one won-

Actual and Smoothed Probability of CVD According to Systolic Blood Pressure Level: Men and Women 45–64 Framingham Study

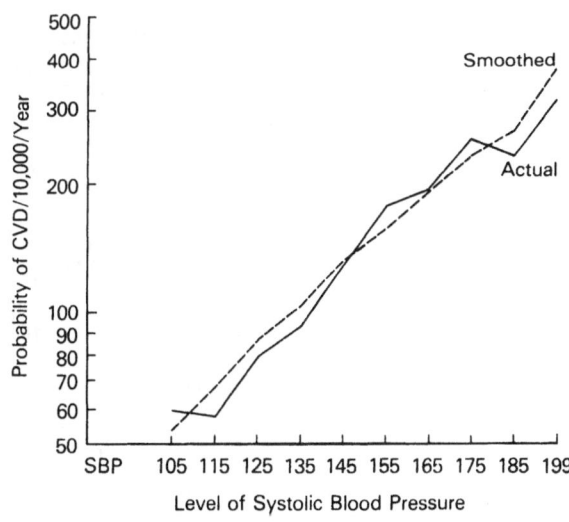

Fig. 1. Actual and smoothed probability of CVD according to systolic blood pressure level: Men and women 45–64. Framingham study.

Table 1. Risk of cardiovascular disease according to hypertensive status and age.

Hypertensive status	Average annual incidence per 1,000					
	Men			Women		
	45–54	55–64	65–74	45–54	55–64	65–74
Normal	8.6	15.6	17.1	2.7	6.1	8.6
Borderline	14.5	30.4	32.7	6.1	14.4	22.5
Hypertension	23.6	43.9	51.0	9.7	23.7	35.6

Framingham study: 20-year follow-up. Men and women 45–74.

Table 2. Regression of incidence of cardiovascular disease on systolic pressure level, degree of lability, and age.

Category	Standardized regression coefficients	
	Men	Women
Age	0.303*	0.458*
Systolic BP level	0.357*	0.420*
Systolic BP lability	0.027	0.080

Framingham study: 20-year follow-up. Men and women 45–74.
* $p = <0.001$.

ders about the impact on the quality of life in terms of cost, inconvenience, nasal stuffiness, dry mouth, lethargy, sleep disturbance, and impotence.

A preventive approach to such a highly prevalent condition as mild hypertension would require public health measures to reduce its incidence in the general population through hygienic means such as sodium restriction, weight control, avoidance of alcohol, and more exercise. When it comes to drugs, it is imperative to focus treatment of mild hypertension on a high-risk subgroup because there is no way to adequately monitor such treatment for the huge numbers of persons involved, if all are to be placed on treatment.

Substantial epidemiologic evidence indicates that the increased risk of the mild hypertensives is concentrated in those with associated cardiovascular risk factors (Fig. 5). Thus, the risk varies widely at any blood pressure level according to HDL and LDL lipid values (Fig. 6). It also varies in relation to cigarette habit, glucose tolerance, and whether or not there is target organ involvement (Fig. 5).

Data from the MRFIT, USPHS multicenter trial and VA–NHLBI studies of hypertension sug-

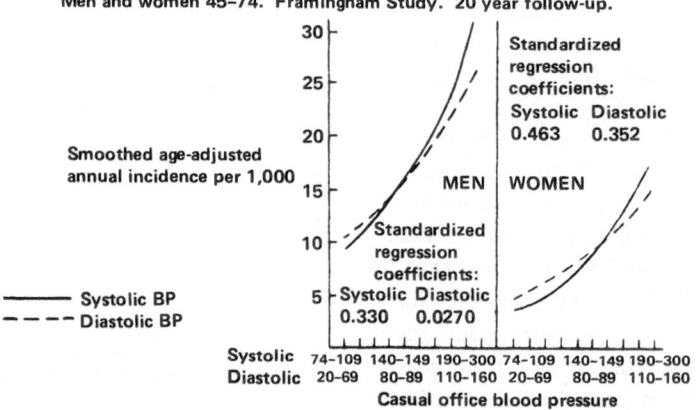

INCIDENCE OF CORONARY HEART DISEASE ACCORDING TO SYSTOLIC VS DIASTOLIC BP
Men and women 45–74. Framingham Study. 20 year follow-up.

Fig. 2. Incidence of CHD according to systolic versus diastolic blood pressure. Framingham study: 20-year follow-up. Men and women 47–74. (Reproduced with permission from Ann NY Acad Sci 304: 135, March 30, 1978.)

Table 3. Two-year morbidity and mortality associated with isolated systolic hypertension.

Category	Men		Women	
	Rate per 1,000	Factor of incr. risk	Rate per 1,000	Factor of incr. risk
Death (all causes)	56	2.0	29	2.0
Cardiovascular mortality	30	1.8	24	4.7
Cardiovascular morbidity	114	3.6	50	3.8

Framingham study: 20-year follow-up. Men and women 55–74. Excludes persons having diastolic BP ⩾ 95 mmHg at any time over 20 years. Risk ratio = ratio of rates in isolated systolic HBP and normotensives.

gest that among mild hypertensive subjects 20% will have cardiomegaly and EKG changes, with 4% renal involvement. Approximately one-third will have elevated cholesterol values and will smoke cigarettes.

It would seem reasonable to focus attention on the mild hypertensive with a poor cardiovascular risk profile. Even here, hygienic measures should be tried first and drug treatment instituted only in those who fail to achieve a reduction in overall risk by hygienic means. It is important to recognize that the risk of a cigarette-smoking hypertensive can be reduced by 50% just by getting him to quit (Table 4).

Pharmacotherapy can be reserved for the mild hypertensives who cannot, or will not, reduce their

risk through hygienic measures. In the subject with a poor cardiovascular risk profile, the risk

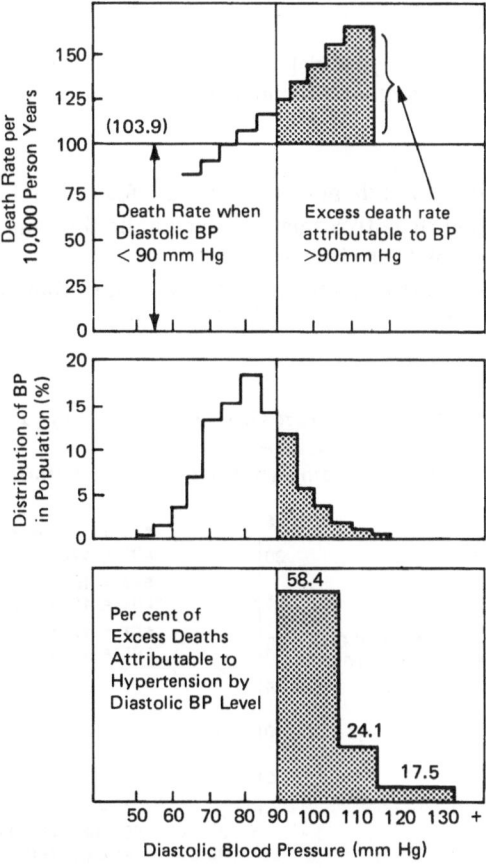

Percentage of deaths attributable to hypertension by diastolic blood pressure level

Fig. 4. Percent deaths attributable to hypertension by diastolic blood pressure. (Reproduced with permission from Ann NY Acad Sci 304: 254–266, 1979.)

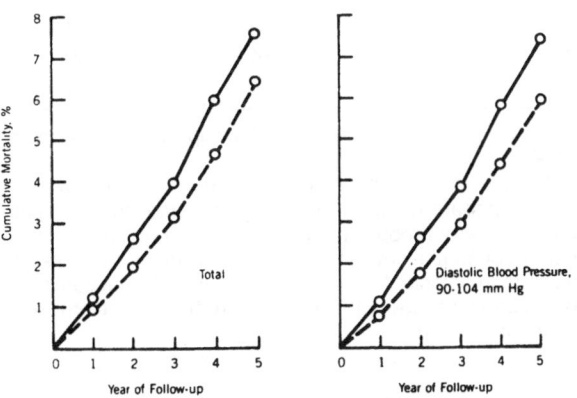

Fig. 3. Hypertension Detection and Follow-up Program: Life-table cumulative mortality, total versus stratum 1 (diastolic pressure 90–104 mmHg). *Dashed line,* stepped care; *solid line,* referred care.

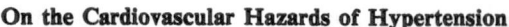

On the Cardiovascular Hazards of Hypertension

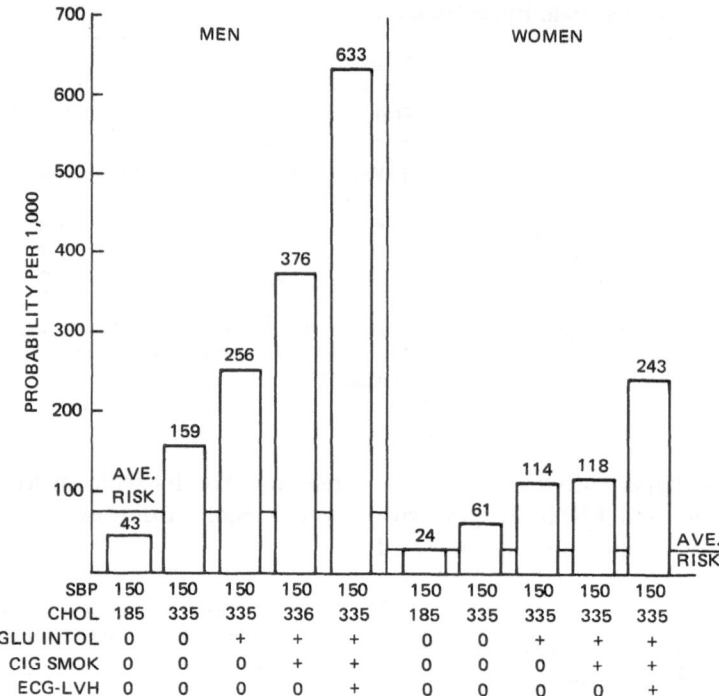

Fig. 5. Eight-year risk of cardiovascular disease at 150 mmHg. Systolic pressure according to level of other risk factors. Framingham study: 18-year follow-up. Men and women aged 45.

is high enough and subjects are few enough to warrant drug treatment, replacing the shotgun approach with a clean rifle shot.

The HDFP reports have now indicated that even coronary heart disease (CHD) incidence can be

Risk of Coronary Heart Disease According to Levels of HDL-Cholesterol
Men aged 55. Framingham Study. 24-year follow-up.

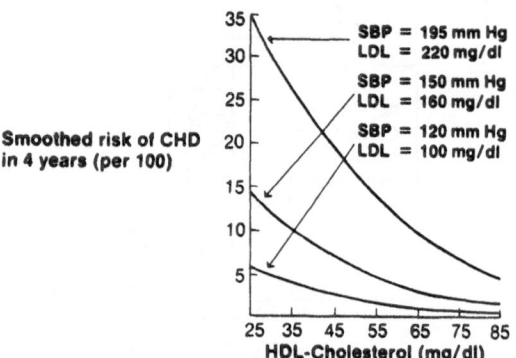

Fig. 6. Risk of coronary heart disease according to levels of HDL cholesterol. (Reproduced with permission from Ann Intern Med 90: 88, 1979.)

Table 4. Percent decreased risk of coronary attacks in hypertensives on quitting smoking.

No. cigarettes per day (pkg)	Estimated decrease in coronary attacks in 2 years on quitting smoking (%)	
	Men	Women
½	19	24
1	34	40
2	57	64

Framingham study: 20-year follow-up. Men and women 35–64.

Method of estimation: (P1 − P2)/P1 × 100 where: P1 = probability of an event while smoking specified amount; P2 = probability of an event for non-smoker with same concommitant variables. P1 and P2 are calculated using the coefficients of a six-variable logistic function: high blood pressure, age, EKG–LVH, cigarettes, cholesterol, glucose intolerance.

reduced along with mortality, that treatment of mild as well as severe hypertension is efficacious. All this has been shown comparing specially treated hypertensives not with a placebo group, but with those treated with usual care by a private physician. The results, then, represent an *underestimate* of the potential benefits of treatment. It is interesting that the study did not show any substantial benefit for patients under 50 with mild hypertension. However, white women showed a lesser impact as well, and they are the best compliers to treatment. Hence, the regular treatment group probably was receiving maximum benefit and consequently differed little from the special intervention group in adherence to treatment.

The fact that overall mortality as well as cardiovascular mortality was improved is reassuring but also consistent with improved overall medical care. The differences between the special care and those who received the usual care in this HDFP trial indicate the value of a careful follow-up, surveillance, and control of hypertensive patients. Evidently, a treatment goal should be set and vigorously pursued. The HDFP study showed major benefits in blacks, indicating an opportunity for greater improvements in that segment of the population. The study also demonstrates the importance of effective use of drugs, frequent regular visits, and intensive follow-up. It is interesting that in the group receiving regular care, there was a progressive improvement in mortality as the trial proceeded. This suggests that mortality improved as physicians improved their management of hypertension, and as their patients came to expect closer control.

We are now at a point where there is a need for a trial to determine if milder degrees of hypertension can be controlled with hygienic measures such as weight control, sodium restriction, avoidance of alcohol, and exercise. It would also be helpful to know if mild hypertensives, once controlled, can be eased off drugs with such hygienic measures. Furthermore, we need more information on the efficacy of treating isolated systolic hypertension, particularly in the elderly.

It is now clear that a little hypertension can be lethal and that vigorous normalization of the pressure prolongs life and reduces the cardiovascular sequelae of hypertension including CHD. There is little excuse for not treating hypertension, including mild hypertension. However, although all hypertensives should be treated, most will require only hygienic measures such as weight reduction, salt restriction, avoidance of cigarettes, and a diet low in saturated fat and cholesterol. For those with a persistent poor cardiovascular risk profile

whose pressures remain high, vigorous drug treatment would seem clearly in order.

SUMMARY

It is now established that treatment of even mild degrees of hypertension can reduce cardiovascular sequelae and that more rigorous goals pay dividends in reduced mortality. This finding is quite consistent with epidemiologic data, which indicate that the lower the pressure, the lower the risk, even within the borderline range. Mild hypertension is associated with a double risk of cardiovascular disease and almost 60% of the excess mortality attributable to hypertension comes from this category; hence, it constitutes a major public health problem.

Epidemiologic evidence indicates that the increased risk of mild hypertension is concentrated in those with associated cardiovascular risk factors and attention should be focused on these. While all mild hypertensives should be treated, most will require only hygienic measures such as weight reduction, sodium restriction, avoidance of cigarettes, less saturated fat and cholesterol in their diet, and more exercise. Only for those whose cardiovascular risk profile remains poor, and whose elevated pressures persist, vigorous drug treatment would appear justified.

REFERENCES

1. Hypertension Detection and Follow-up Program Cooperative Group (1979) Five-year findings of the Hypertension Detection and Follow-up Program: I. Reduction in mortality of persons with high blood pressure, including mild hypertension. JAMA 242: 2562–2571
2. Kannel WB, Dawber TR (1974) Hypertension as an ingredient of a cardiovascular risk profile. Br J Hosp Med 2: 508–524
3. Apostilides A, Blaufox MD, Borhani NO, Cutter G, Daugherty S, Lewin AJ, Polk BF (1979) Mild Hypertensives in the Hypertension Detection and Follow-up Program. Ann NY Acad Sci 304: 254–266
4. Veterans Administration Cooperative Study Group on Antihypertensive Agents (1967) Effects of treatment on morbidity in hypertension: I. Results in patients with diastolic blood pressures averaging 115–129 mmHg. JAMA 202: 1028–1034
5. Koch-Weser J (1973) The therapeutic challenge of systolic hypertension. N Engl J Med 289: 481

Factors Affecting Morbidity and Mortality and the Risk Factor Concept

Reuel A. Stallones

Commonly, the efficacy of therapy is evaluated as the proportion of those persons who were improved from among those who were treated. This, by itself, is not an adequate measure of overall effectiveness of therapy, for it says nothing about whether those persons who might be expected to benefit from treatment are actually treated. The impact of treatment on a community is, therefore, a function of its efficacy, narrowly defined, and of its availability and acceptance. Treatment of high blood pressure has advanced greatly in recent years, and, to some of us, the most notable aspect of the advance has been the extension into the general population of programs to detect and treat persons with asymptomatic hypertension. However, if we were able to extend the best available therapeutic management to all members of entire communities, we would still fall far short of an optimal strategy. The importance of continued effort to understand and modify the environmental causes of hypertension is not diminished by the success of treatment.

Epidemiologic research has explored a number of facets of causation of elevated blood pressure (1, 2), but no unambiguous approaches to prevention have been discovered. However, some very important observations have been uncovered in this research effort:

1) N. A. Scotch (3) reported that Zulu who migrated to an urban center, Durban, had higher blood pressures than those who grew up in the city, and that both of these groups had higher average values than Zulu who remained on the reservation. Although this finding has not been widely replicated, and, indeed, not always found when sought (4, 5), neither does it sit completely in isolation. For example, Tokelauan children living in New Zealand had higher blood pressures than their counterparts living on the home atoll in the South Pacific, and the differences could not be explained fully by variations in weight or urinary sodium excretion (6).

2) A number of populations have been found in which older adults do not have higher average blood pressures than younger adults (7). These groups are, by and large, small, exotic, and isolated from Western industrial civilization. However, the failure to show a rise in mean blood pressure with increasing age is not an attribute of all small, exotic, and isolated communities, and we have not identified factors that will predict the phenomenon.

3) Since 1949, in the United States, rates of mortality attributed to hypertension and diseases strongly associated with hypertension have been decreasing steeply for both sexes and all races. The decline is log linear with a change in slope in 1968, which is more probably due to a modification of the system for classifying cause of death than to any change in the biology of the disease or its medical management. A reduction in mortality from hypertension is not certainly a reflection of a reduction in the frequency of hypertension, but no better explanation is apparent.

Taken together, the observations present the apparent contradiction that groups of people entering an urban, industrial culture may sometimes, but not always, show an increase in blood pressure that may become increasingly severe with advancing age, while the population of one of the most highly urban countries in the world probably has experienced a major reduction in blood pressure. None of these findings is explicable given our present knowledge of the epidemiology of hypertension, but they indicate clearly that whatever the genetic contribution to hypertension may be, the condition is controlled by environmental factors, and is, therefore, potentially preventable.

The search for environmental determinants of hypertension could follow many paths, and one of the most promising is the study of blood pressure in children. We do not know whether a relative elevation of blood pressure in childhood is a foretoken of adult hypertension. To pursue this question in studies of individuals is important, but even with efficient study designs, the research must extend over several years. Community-based cross-sectional investigations, although plagued by problems of cohort effects and differential survivorship, can provide answers to some equally important questions quickly and inexpensively. In all populations observed, blood pressure rises rapidly during the period of active growth, with a sharp reduction in the slope of the curve between 15 and 20 years of age. Therefore, to characterize a community, or a subset of a community, we need measures of the slope and the variance of blood pressure in juveniles, the slope and the variance of blood pressure in adults, and the magnitude of the blood pressure at the interception of the juvenile and adult curves. A specific hypothesis to test is that, in a community, the age-related change in average blood pressure of groups of children is predictive of the average blood pressure of adults, or of the rate of increase associated with aging in the adult population. If the hypothesis is correct, children might be especially valuable study subjects, for they may reflect the effects of environmental differences and environmental changes more sensitively than adults, with less confusion introduced by multiple confounding variables.

SUMMARY

Strong evidence exists that blood pressure is strongly affected by environmental factors, but our knowledge of these influences is rudimentary. Prevention of hypertension and its complications is so much more advantageous than long-term treatment that research to define the environmental influences and to discover how they may be modified should be pursued vigorously.

REFERENCES

1. Stamler J (1978) Epidemiology and treatment of hypertension. In: Carlson RJ, Cunningham R (eds) Future directions in health care: A new public policy. Ballinger, Cambridge, Mass
2. Smith WM (1977) Epidemiology of hypertension. Med Clin North Am 61: 467–486
3. Scotch NA (1963) Sociocultural factors in the epidemiology of Zulu hypertension. Am J Public Health 53: 1204–1213
4. Reed D, Labarthe D, Stallones R (1970) Health effects of westernization and migration among Chamorros. Am J Epidemiol 92: 94–112
5. Labarthe D, Reed D, Brody J, Stallones R (1973) Health effects of modernization in Palau. Am J Epidemiol 98: 161–174
6. Beaglehole R, Eyles E, Salmond C, Prior I (1978) Blood pressure in Tokelauan children in two contrasting environments. Am J Epidemiol 108: 283–288
7. Epstein F, Eckoff R (1967) The epidemiology of high blood pressure—geographic distribution and etiological factors. In: Stamler J, Stamler R, Pullman T (eds) The epidemiology of hypertension. Grune & Stratton, New York

Australian Therapeutic Trial in Mild Hypertension

A. E. Doyle

The Australian National Blood Pressure Study was a controlled therapeutic trial of antihypertensive drug treatment in 3,427 men and women aged 30–69 years. The subjects were recruited from the general population by community screening. Persons whose average diastolic blood pressure (DBP), measured twice on each of two occasions, was within the defined mild range, and who had no exclusion factors (Table 1), were eligible to enter the study. The defined mild range of hypertension was an average DBP of 95–109 mmHg with a systolic blood pressure (SBP) of less than 200 mmHg. Eligible subjects who agreed to enter the study were randomly allocated with stratification of age and sex to take either pharmacologically active tablets or matching placebo tablets.

All subjects in the study were treated at special clinics for an average period of 4 years. They attended the clinics at two weekly intervals during stabilization and then at four monthly intervals,

or more frequently, if at any visit DBP was 110 mmHg or more or SBP was 200 mmHg or more. If at three such successive visits within a 6-week period the blood pressure remained above these thresholds, definitive antihypertensive treatment was given. This was not a trial end point and these subjects, 198 in the placebo group and 4 in the active group, were kept in the study in their original treatment classification. Any trial end points (Table 2) that occurred were counted against the trial regimen to which they had been randomized originally.

At each four monthly visit, blood pressure was measured, tablet doses were adjusted if necessary, and evidence for trial end points and treatment side effects was sought. A full clinical biochemical and electrocardiogram examination was made annually. Trial end points were reviewed by a special committee unaware of the subject's treatment

Table 1. Exclusion factors.

First screening visit
  On treatment for hypertension in past 3 months

Second screening visit
  Angina pectoris by Rose questionnaire
  History of myocardial infarction in past 3 months
  History of stroke
  Pregnancy
  Taking estrogen and progesterone in combination
  Asthma, diabetes, gout

Clinic visit
  Primary cause of hypertension
  Evidence of cerebrovascular disease, transient cerebral ischemic attacks, acute coronary insufficiency, plasma creatinine > 2 mg/dl
  Other serious complications of hypertension
  EKG evidence of myocardial ischemia
  Any potentially fatal disease
  Taking tricyclic antidepressants

Table 2. Trial end points.

Fatal
  Death from any cause (cause of death specified)
    a) Cardiovascular*
    b) Other

Nonfatal
  Thrombotic or hemorrhagic cerebrovascular disease
  Transient cerebral ischemic attacks with observed neurologic signs
  Myocardial infarction by WHO category I or II
  Other ischemic heart disease by Rose questionnaire or defined EKG criteria
  Congestive cardiac failure
  Dissecting aneurysm of the aorta
  Retinal hemorrhages, exudates, or papilledema
  Hypertensive encephalopathy
  Onset of renal failure with plasma creatinine elevated above 2 mg/dl

* Cardiovascular deaths are limited to those caused by the conditions listed under nonfatal trial end points (TEP).

group and blood pressure. An EKG committee, similarly blind, reported on all tracings. The occurrence of any trial end point terminated the subjects participation in the study.

RESULTS

PREMATURE WITHDRAWALS

The status of the trial population at the end of the study is shown in Table 3. Approximately one-third prematurely stopped the regimen to which they had been randomized. There were no significant differences between the entry characteristics of the subjects in the active and placebo groups in those who stopped prematurely, and the rates of subsequent trial end points were not significantly different between the two groups. Of the 88 subjects lost to follow-up, 42 were in the active and 46 were in the placebo group. None had been registered as a death in Australia. The fact that in subjects who prematurely stopped their regimen the match between the active and placebo groups in regard to entry characteristics, trial end-point rates, types of end points, and reasons for stopping makes it unlikely that factors associated with premature stopping biased the results.

TRIAL END POINTS

The cumulative occurrence of total trial end points and of all deaths for subjects continuing on their regimen is shown in Fig. 1. Differences between

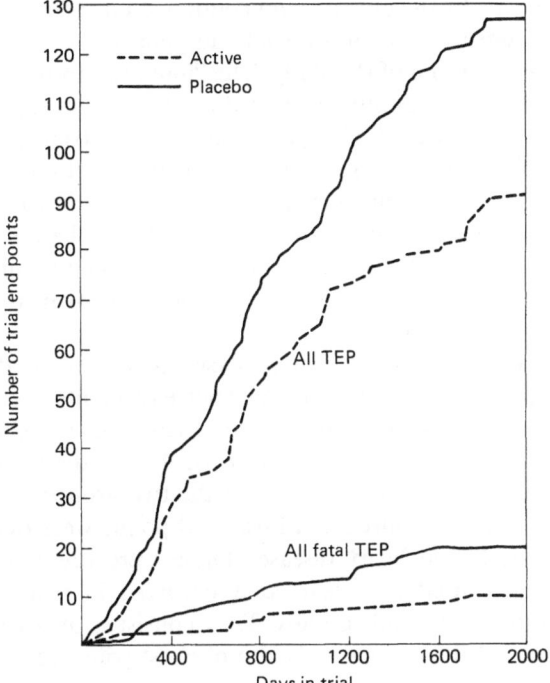

Cumulative Incidence of Trial End Points

Fig. 1. Cumulative incidence of trial end points.

the groups emerged early, and when analyzed by life-table analysis (1), were significant for all trial end points ($p < 0.01$) and for all deaths ($P < 0.05$).

Two types of analysis of end points were made. The "on-treatment" analysis takes into account the experience, prior to stopping, of the 1,209 who

Table 3. Incidence of trial end points.

Category	Intention to treat				On treatment			
	Active N = 1,721		Placebo N = 1,706		Active N = 1,721		Placebo N = 1,706	
	No.	Rate	No.	Rate	No.	Rate	No.	Rate
Fatal TEP								
Cardiovascular	8	1.1	18	2.6*	4	0.8	13	2.5*
Noncardiovascular	17	2.4	17	2.5	5	0.9	6	1.2
Total fatal	25	3.5	35	5.1	9	1.7	19	3.7**
Nonfatal TEP	113	16.2	133	19.4	82	15.5	108	20.8*
All TEP	138	19.7	168	24.5**	91	17.2	127	24.5***

Rates per 1,000 person-years' exposure to risk.
* $p < 0.025$; ** $p < 0.05$; *** $p < 0.01$.

prematurely stopped their regimen and also that of the 2,218 subjects who continued on their trial regimen either until a trial end point occurred or until the end of the study. The "intention-to-treat" analysis takes into account the person-years exposure to risk of all 3,427 subjects and trial end points that occurred either before or after stopping in the 3,339 subjects whose status was known at the end of the trial. In the two analyses, the rates of both cardiovascular deaths and trial end points were significantly lower in the active than in the placebo group.

In the on-treatment analysis, the rates of all deaths and of all nonfatal trial end points were significantly lower in the active than in the placebo group (Table 3). Noncardiovascular deaths were similarly distributed between the two groups.

Over two-thirds of all trial end points were due to ischemic heart disease. These were predominantly nonfatal events that occurred in similar numbers in both groups. They consisted of myocardial infarctions, episodes of chest pain accom-

panied by EKG changes, and angina pectoris as assessed by a positive response to the Rose questionnaire.

In contrast, the incidence of all types of cerebrovascular events was significantly lower in the active than in the placebo group, both for fatal and nonfatal strokes (Table 4). There were fewer trial end points in the active than in the placebo groups in men and women considered separately and in those over and under 50 years of age at entry.

BLOOD PRESSURE LEVELS

For each subject, the average of all diastolic pressures recorded after commencing tablets has been estimated. In both active and placebo groups, the average DBP while on tablets was lower than the screening DBP, and the higher the screening pressure, the greater the fall. For each screening DBP class, the fall was greater in the active than in the placebo group (Table 5).

The relationship between average DBPs during

Table 4. Numbers of trial end points by diagnostic categories.

Category	A Intention to treat		B On treatment		In premature withdrawals after stopping (A–B)	
	Active	Placebo	Active	Placebo	Active	Placebo
Ischemic heart disease						
Fatal	5	11	2	8	3	3
Nonfatal						
Myocardial infarction	28	22	18	17	10	5
Others	65	76	50	63	15	13
Total	98	109	70	88	28	21
Cerebrovascular events						
Fatal	3	6	2	4	1	2
Nonfatal						
Hemorrhage or thrombosis	10	16	7	13	3	3
Transient cerebral ischemic attacks	4	9	3	8	1	1
Total	17	31	12	25	5	6
Other fatal						
Aortic aneurysm	0	1	0	1	0	0
Noncardiovascular						
Neoplasm	9	8	1	2	8	6
Other	8	9	4	4	4	5
Other nonfatal						
Retinopathy	2	5	1	4	1	1
Congestive cardiac failure	3	3	2	1	1	2
Renal failure	1	2	1	2	0	0
Total	138	168	91	127	47	41

Table 5. Blood pressure levels throughout the trial.

Screening diastolic pressure (mmHg)	No. of subjects[a]		Mean of screening DBP (mmHg)		Mean of average DBP (mmHg) while on trial regimen		Mean of fall in DBP (mmHg)[b]	
	Active	Placebo	Active	Placebo	Active	Placebo	Active	Placebo
95–99	756	763	96.9	97.0	87.2	92.1	9.7	5.0
100–104	558	563	101.9	101.9	88.8	94.5	13.1	7.4
105–109	320	291	106.7	106.7	90.2	97.5	16.5	9.2
Total	1,633	1,617	100.5	100.4	88.3	93.9	12.2	6.6

[a] Does not include the 176 subjects who did not have any blood pressure readings after entry.
[b] Difference between screening DBP and average DBP.

the therapeutic regimen and trial end points occurring at each class of blood pressure is shown in Table 6. In the active group, 64% of subjects had average diastolic pressures during the study of less than 90 mmHg and 4.7% had average DBP above 100 mmHg. In the placebo group, 25% had average DBP below 90 mmHg and 20% above 100 mmHg. In both groups, the numbers of trial end points were lowest in the classes with lower average DBP. Although there was a significant difference in the incidence of trial end points between the active and placebo group for the total groups $\chi^2 = 6.6$ $p < 0.01$, the incidence of trial end points in the two groups subdivided for average DBP was significantly different only for the groups with average DBP above 100 mmHg $\chi^2 = 6.4$ $p < 0.05$.

DISCUSSION

The data from this study have shown a significant reduction in cardiovascular mortality and morbidity in patients with mild hypertension free from preexisting cardiovascular disease treated with antihypertensive drugs.

The overall cardiovascular mortality in both the actively treated and placebo-treated groups was considerably lower than in either of the groups of the Hypertension Detection and Follow-up Program (HDFP) stratum 1 (2). The subjects in the two groups were similar in entry characteristics except that patients with previous stroke, myocardial infarction, EKG changes, and diabetes and receiving antihypertensive drugs were excluded from the Australian study but included in the HDFP. It seems very likely that the presence of preexisting complications of hypertension was the cause of the much greater mortality from cardiovascular disease in the HDFP. If this is so, it further emphasizes the need for treatment of hypertension to commence before vascular disease has become clinically evident.

The differences in the numbers of trial end points between the active and placebo groups were mainly due to a reduced incidence of stroke in the treated group. Although deaths from myocardial infarction were lower in the actively treated group, there was no difference in the incidence of nonfatal episodes of ischemic heart disease between the two groups.

The data on the relationship between DBPs during the trial and the incidence of trial end points strongly suggest that the lower incidence of trial

Table 6. Relationship between diastolic blood pressures during treatment and trial end points.

Average DBP	Active				Placebo			
	No.	%	TEP	%	No.	%	TEP	%
≤ 89	1,044	64	53	5.0	407	25	23	5.2
90– 94	370	23	23	6.1	482	30	26	5.7
95– 99	143	9	12	8.4	412	25	32	7.4
≥100	77	4	3	4.0	316	20	46	12.1
	1,634		91		1,617		127	

end points in the treated group is closely related to the lower levels of blood pressure achieved. Average blood pressures below 90 mmHg were achieved in 64% of the treated group, but in 25% of the placebo group. In this group of patients, the incidence of trial end points was similar irrespective of the treatment regimen.

In both groups, the incidence of trial end points increased as average diastolic pressures increased. The evidence suggests that diastolic pressures remain persistently above 95 mmHg in about half the placebo-treated group, and that it is this group which experiences the highest incidence of cardiovascular complications. It is likely that the incidence of trial end points was also reduced in the placebo group because patients whose DBPs exceeded 110 mmHg were given active treatment. There were 198 subjects (12.2%) in the placebo group in this category.

The data suggest that patients identified as having mild hypertension without overt cardiovascular disease, whose blood pressures remain persistently above 95 mmHg, are those most likely to benefit from antihypertensive drug treatment and that treatment of such patients may be mainly expected to reduce the incidence of cerebrovascular complications.

SUMMARY

The Australian National Blood Pressure Study was a controlled therapeutic trial of the effects of antihypertensive drug treatment in 3,427 persons aged 60–69 years.

There was a significant reduction in both cardiovascular morbidity and mortality in the treated group, mainly due to a reduction in the incidence of stroke. There was no difference in the incidence of nonfatal episodes of ischemic heart disease between the groups.

In both the active and the placebo groups, the incidence of trial end points increased with increasing average diastolic pressures during the study.

In the placebo group, diastolic pressures remained persistently above 95 mmHg in about half the subjects, and these persons experienced the highest incidence of cardiovascular complications.

ACKNOWLEDGMENTS

The study was initiated and administered by the National Heart Foundation of Australia and jointly sponsored by the National Health and Medical Research Council of Australia, the Life Insurance Medical Research Fund of Australia and New Zealand, the Victorian Government, the Clive and Vera Ramaciotti Foundations, and the Raine Medical Research Foundation of Western Australia.

Management Committee: R. Reader (Chairman), G. E. Bauer, A. E. Doyle, K. W. Edmondson, S. Hunyor, T. H. Hurley, P. I. Korner, P. W. Leighton, R. R. H. Lovell, M. G. McCall, J. M. McPhie, M. J. Rand, H. M. Whyte. Study Centre Directors: J. A. Abernethy, Jenny Baker, Margaret Bullen, Rupert Edwards, Gwen Francis, Margaret Lamb, Mary Stewart. Statisticians: G. Santow, C. Fazekas. Consultant in design: R. Prineas. Computer programmers: W. Clapton, H. Knight. Ethics Committee: K. Brewer, M. Crawford, P. W. Leighton, P. J. Nestel. Trial End Point Review Committee: R. J. Craig, J. McPhie, J. Waddy. EKG Committee: G. E. Bauer, P. Caspari, S. Hunyor.

REFERENCES

1. Cox RD (1972) Regression models and life tables. J R Stat Soc (Series B) 34: 187–220
2. Hypertension Detection and Follow-up Program Cooperative Group (1979) Five-year findings of the hypertension detection and follow-up program: I. Reduction in mortality of persons with high blood pressure, including mild hypertension. JAMA 242: 2562–2571

Treatment of Borderline and Mild Hypertension: The Oslo Study

A. Helgeland, I. Hjermann, I. Holme, P. G. Lund-Larsen, and P. Leren

A 5-year controlled trial to evaluate drug treatment of borderline and mild hypertension was started in 1972 (1). The background for this study was based on the results of the treatment of mild hypertension in the Veterans Administration (VA) study (2); which showed that for a blood pressure range of 90–104 mmHg a) a small gain in cardiovascular incidence b) no gain in coronary heart disease.

In contrast to the VA study, the participants in the present study were symptom-free, middle-aged men without known cardiovascular disease. The study groups included a total of 785 men, aged 40–49, with SBP 150–179 and DBP < 110, 406 who were randomized to a drug treatment and a control group, of 379 men. The trial was open and no placebo was given to the controls.

Drug treatment started with hydrochlorothiazide (HCTH) 50 mg daily. Alpha methyldopa (250–750 mg b.i.d.) was added when blood pressure remained above 140/90 mmHg. When side effects occurred, alpha methyldopa was replaced by propranolol (40–160 mg b.i.d.). No systematic intervention was performed on other risk factors.

During the trial, the following drug-induced effects on lipid and uric acid metabolism were observed:

1) Men on thiazide alone experienced no significant triglyceride increase and only a moderate increase in uric acid. However, those with pronounced increase in uric acid also presented a triglyceride increase (3).

2) Men on combination treatment had a stronger increase in triglycerides and uric acid. The combination thiazide–propranolol showed the highest increase in triglycerides and uric acid (4). The men on thiazide–methyldopa reacted as those treated with thiazide alone in regard to effect on triglycerides and uric acid.

A substantial part of the increase in triglycerides and uric acid was confined to men gaining weight during treatment. However, in comparing all those with corresponding weight increase, the thiazide–propranolol-treated men showed a much stronger increase in triglycerides and uric acid than those with the same weight increase on thiazide plus methyldopa, thiazide alone, or in the control group (3, 4).

3) Men on thiazide–propranolol combination experienced a reduced HDL cholesterol level compared with men on other treatment (5). These results are consistent with the reported inverse correlation between HDL cholesterol and triglycerides (6).

4) The study shows that propranolol seems to be responsible for the greatest part of the described lipid changes when using the propranolol–thiazide combination. This contention is confirmed in a recently published study showing a distinct increase of triglycerides and a decrease in HDL cholesterol in men treated with propranolol alone (7).

No serious drug-induced side effects were observed. At 4-years, a questionnaire was mailed to the participants from an independent institution to evaluate possible drug-related complaints against complaints in the untreated controls (8). The treated men more often had drowsiness, fatigue, impotence, and gout. However, regarding gastrointestinal complaints and skin, nose, and throat symptoms, there was no difference between the two groups. Diabetes occurred in one patient treated with the thiazide–propranolol combination.

An "ethical roof" of SBP 180 mmHg and/or DBP 110 mmHg was established for offering treatment in the control group. Sixty-five controls experienced such a blood pressure increase, and thus had drug treatment during the trial.

A difference in SBP of about 17 mmHg and in DBP of about 10 mmHg between the treatment and control group was maintained throughout the study.

At the end of the trial all participants had been observed for at least 5 years; the mean observation time was 66 months.

There was a reduction in blood pressure-related cardiovascular complications in the treatment group: cerebrovascular events (0 versus 7 in the control group); dissecting aneurysms (0 versus 2); congestive heart failure (0 versus 1); and EKG changes with marked left ventricular hypertrophy (0 versus 7). No preventive effect on coronary heart disease events was observed (20 versus 13). There was no effect on major cardiovascular events comparing groups as established by randomization. Regarding total cardiovascular events, there was a small difference in favor of the drug group (6.2% versus 9.0%; $p > 0.10$). In subgroups with DBP above 100 mmHg, there was a small reduction in total cardiovascular events in favor of the drug group (7.6% versus 16.4%; $p = >0.06$).

There was no difference in mortality between treated and controls. With the relatively small study groups and the short observation period, it was not reasonable to expect a mortality difference; therefore, valid conclusions regarding the influence on mortality of antihypertensive treatment of borderline and mild hypertension should not be drawn.

SUMMARY

Results are presented from a 5-year controlled drug treatment trial of borderline and mild hypertension in symptom-free, middle-aged men without target organ damage. Between 1972 and 1973, 785 men (aged 40–49) were randomized to a drug treatment and a control group, 406 and 379 men, respectively. Drug treatment consisted of HCTH 50 mg daily. If adequate blood pressure reduction was not achieved, alpha-methyldopa was added. If side effects occurred, alpha-methyldopa was replaced by propranolol. The mean observation time was $5\frac{1}{2}$ years.

There was no effect on total mortality and major cardiovascular events. However, subdividing groups, treated men with DBP above 100 mmHg had a reduction in total cardiovascular events. Regarding blood pressure-related events (cerebrovas-

cular disease, congestive heart failure, dissecting aortic aneurysms), there was good protection. There was no effect on coronary heart disease.

REFERENCES

1. Helgeland A (1980) Treatment of mild hypertension: A 5-year controlled drug trial. The Oslo study. Am J Med 69: 725–732
2. Veterans Administration Cooperative Study Group on Antihypertensive Agents (1970) Effects of treatment on morbidity in hypertension: II. Results in patients with diastolic blood pressure averaging 90 through 114 mmHg. JAMA 213: 1143
3. Helgeland A, Hjermann I, Holme I, et al (1978) Serum triglycerides and serum uric acid in untreated and thiazide treated patients with mild hypertension: The Oslo study. Am J Med 64: 34
4. Helgeland A, Hjermann I, Leren P, et al (1978) Possible metabolic side effects of beta adrenergic blocking drugs. Br Med J 1: 828
5. Helgeland A, Hjermann I, Leren P, et al (1978) High density lipoprotein cholesterol and antihypertensive drugs: The Oslo study. Br Med J 2: 403
6. Miller GJ, Miller NE (1975) Plasma-high-density-lipoprotein concentration and development of ischaemic heart disease. Lancet 1: 16
7. Leren P, Foss PD, Helgeland A, et al (1980) Effect of propranolol and prazosin on blood lipids: The Oslo study. Lancet 2: 4–6
8. Baksaas I, Helgeland A (1980) Patient reactions to information and motivation factors in longterm treatment with antihypertensive drugs. Acta Med Scand 207: 407

DISCUSSION

Dr. Laragh (New York) (Chairman): The impression that I get from hearing of the clinical trials, Dr. Remington, yours as well as the Australian and Oslo experiences, is that in mild hypertension if there is any benefit, you are in a situation where only 1% or 2% are helped, or as Dr. Doyle says, 1.5 out of a 100 in the HDFP. This means to me that 98 or 99 people out of 100 are being treated for no purpose in order to benefit the 1% or 2%. Of course too, this putative "benefit" requires the use of drugs that are ostensibly wholly safe and have no problems intrinsic of their own. Maybe I would ask Drs. Remington, Doyle, and Helgeland to comment about this issue. We also have Professor Akhmeteli from the Soviet Union here for a comment.

Dr. Remington (Ann Arbor, Mich.): Dr. Laragh, that's an interesting question. One or two things put some balance into that figure. First, there is a substantial percentage reduction in all-cause mortality and I think these results are consistent across the trials. Second, Dr. Stallones made a comment shortly after your question, John. Prevention in Western societies has been a very well accepted kind of concept. We haven't hesitated to advocate mass immunization against poliomyelitis in an instance in which the overall mortality, and even the overall rate of morbidity, from paralytic poliomyelitis was low and in a case in which there was even some toxicity associated with the immunization program itself. If we continue to study these current findings, namely, that treatment with a simple diuretic will normalize the blood pressure of the vast majority of mild hypertensives at very low cost (less than 5 cents a day) in this country, and with negligible or manageable side reactions, then the withholding of that mortality benefit would seem to many of us to be unjustifiable.

Dr. Laragh: I see the reasoning and again I think what it requires is that the drug therapy have no intrusive effects of its own. I mean absolutely zero because 99 people out of 100 are being treated who aren't at any risk.

Dr. Doyle (Melbourne, Australia): I think that raises an important point. The beauty about these trials is that you can, depending on your personality, make of them exactly what you want to. If you are therapeutically conservative, you can say it obviously isn't worth it. If you're a rabid enthusiast, you can say it obviously is. I think there is one other point relating to the point you made that if some drug does in fact have an adverse effect on mortality, it might very well be that you are substituting one kind of death for another and you would be burying it completely. We would never know that. The data from our study and from others would not really allow one to say whether you were saving some by reducing their blood pressure and killing others by giving them a drug.

Dr. Young (Jackson, Miss.): I think it is important to point out in these 5-year trials you have not proved a benefit, but neither have you proved there is a lack of benefit of treatment. I would also like to point out that because I'm 35 years old, I'm not interested in 5-year survival. I am interested in survival of a much longer period of time. Since hypertension is a disease which probably causes damage over many years, I think these

5-year studies may be too brief to come to any definitive conclusion.

Dr. Laragh: Does anybody want to respond to this comment?

Dr. Doyle: Well, I think you really have to try and answer one question at a time basically. The first question that we chose to ask is: "Is there any evidence that if you have just mild hypertension and nothing else, will drug treatment make a difference?" I think the answer is clearly yes, but not much. The question you are asking is if you take 1,000, 35-year-old men who are anxious about their future, and treat half of them, will one-half be immortal? I think that is going to take a long time, and we really need to get some young people to design the study.

Dr. Udenfriend (Nutley, New Jersey): The trouble is that you have all been talking about patients where the design of the experiments is difficult. In experimental animals, one can show pretty clearly that the vascular effects are a function of pressure multiplied by time. These are the variables. In rats, one might have to try to equate the time with that in humans. This has not been done carefully. It might be that in humans, the time and the pressures necessary are higher than in rats. The previous discussant made a fine point there. Is 2, 3, or 5 years an adequate time for follow-up? And second, one of the speakers showed some data that bothered me because the selection of the patients may not have been adequate. In one group of controls, just putting them on placebo lowered their pressures remarkably. Was that an in-house study? I could imagine that would happen as an in-patient, but why should placebo lower the effect of out-patients in the slightest? What kind of placebos were used?

Dr. Remington: It's worse than that Dr. Udenfriend, much worse. The most miraculous cure for high blood pressure yet found is to take a second blood pressure. About a third of hypertensives are normalized.

Dr. Udenfriend: I feel that that is not good experimentation. Marked placebo responders should be dropped from the study. In other words, the proper patients weren't taken for the study.

Dr. Kannel (Boston, Mass.): I just wanted to point out that at our last cardiovascular epidemiology meeting somebody reanalyzed the coronary drug project data, and the question arose as to whether the benefits to antilipemic therapy were occurring in the subgroups of good adherers to the therapy. They made the mistake of looking at the good adherers to the placebo, and found a beneficial response in the good adherers to the antilipemic therapy, but they found an equally good response to adherence to placebo. This suggests that if you participate in a trial, what you should do is contrive to be in the placebo group and adhere to the treatment because that will improve your mortality. So there is obviously something going on in these trials that has to do with general medical care.

Dr. Alderman (New York): Getting back to the point about the variability of the natural history of the disease and the potential influences other than treatment that play a role, there is evidence from a variety of studies, in Czechoslovakia, for example, where 100 persons with diastolic blood pressures consistently in excess of 100 between the ages of 20 and 30 were remeasured 20 years later; a third of those patients had normalized blood pressure without any treatment during the intervening period. None of those persons had died of cardiovascular disease and only a small fraction of them had any evidence of increase of their blood pressure. So there is a lot we don't know about the predictability of any blood pressure taken at any point of time and in view of the small incremental benefit as opposed to the proportional reduction, I think the notion of a single standardized approach to therapy might be hard to sustain on the basis of the data that we have now.

Dr. Boyd (Hobart, Tasmania): I wonder whether one of the missing factors here is the rate of rise of blood pressure. Whether through structural or functional arteriolar changes, patients whose blood pressure rose early for example might develop an increased rate of pressure rise and then finish up years later with much more hypertension and, therefore, a much higher risk of large vessel disease than those whose early blood pressure observations remained stable. Could I, therefore, ask Dr. Kannel whether in follow-up patients whose blood pressure rises more develop more large vessel disease?

Dr. Kannel: I'm not sure I can give a clear answer to that. All we can say is that the risk associated with hypertension is related to the pressure. It appears to be a time–dose product of the level of pressure (i.e., the time exposed to a particular level). It's difficult to know whether the risk is related to rate of rise in pressure as against the level of pressure attained. This is being analyzed currently at NHLBI, but is a very complex statisti-cal issue requiring rather high-level mathematical and statistical manipulations. We do have a couple of people trying to work on this question of whether the rate of rise predicts the ultimate level attained independent of the starting level of pressure. It's an extremely complex issue to which I can't give you a straightforward answer.

Dr. Eliahou (Tel Hashomer, Israel): It's a little surprising that weight reduction has not been considered as a separate therapeutic entity in all these large studies. Just to put things into perspective, may I say in a long-term follow-up study of over 100 patients, it is enough to reduce half of the overweight, to get two-thirds of the patients in the normotensive range. (Eliahou HE. Unpublished data)

Dr. Helgeland (Oslo, Norway): The intention of our study was to investigate the effect of the drugs, not the effect of a combined intervention on hypertension, diet, weight reduction, and smoking. You have to have very large studies if you want to evaluate the different factors in multifactorial intervention trials.

Dr. Lever (Glasgow, Scotland): I am involved in the Medical Research Council trial of hypertensive drugs. The trial has two control groups. One gets supervision and the other gets supervision and a placebo tablet. The fall in blood pressure in the two groups is exactly the same. So returning to the question of the mechanism of the placebo effects, which is usually attributed to the placebo tablet, I suggest it is not the tablet, but some other aspect of the supervision. Perhaps the patient is getting more familiar with the doctor.

Dr. Akhmeteli (Moscow, U.S.S.R.): I would like to give a short account of our experience in the Soviet Union. We are having a large trial study in an organized population. Specifically, we are studying male factory workers, aged 40–54 years. We have not yet finished the study. However, we are in the third year. We have a group in which intervention is carried out and a comparable group in the other factories where we are screening the population but not taking special treatment actions. However, the group is under the medical care of the factory medical staff. Conclusions at this stage are the following: First, these studies are visible, and more and more cities are joining the corporate study. The second point is that we are able within a short period of time, at least in the years that we are following, to influence the level of blood pressure, and we are bringing the blood pressure down in the group under treatment.

During the same time, we don't see any reasonable decrease in the blood pressure level in the control group in the factories where no special treatment programs are carried out and only screening is being performed. Finally, we fully agree with the opinion expressed here that it is absolutely impossible to take care of all the mild hypertensives on drug treatment, as the level of hypertension in the adults is very high in my country too and certainly it is unbelievable how we could manage to handle millions of people on the drug treatment. Therefore, our attention is also on the attempt to differentiate those would be more prone to develop complications compared with those who may be surviving without our special drug treatment. However, we understand how difficult and challenging the task is in front of us. On these lines, we will continue our studies because the final aim is to adopt these schemes to the basic care facilities in the community.

Dr. Folkow (Göteborg, Sweden): I know one should be careful to draw parallels between man and rats, but the rats really have some virtues. Their life-span is short, they are genetically homogeneous, they have to take their drugs, and one can have them in a controlled environment. Dr. L. Weiss in our lab compared the SHR, which were under hypotensive treatment from the age of weaning up to the age of 8 months, with entirely untreated SHR. No treatment was given after 8 months of age, but arterial pressure remained lower in these rats than in their untreated brothers and sisters though modestly higher than the normotensive controls. At the age of nearly 2 years, 75% of those not treated had died, but only 25% during the early period of treatment [Weiss L (1974) Acta Physiol Scand 91: 393–408]. If I were a rat, I would have preferred to be among those who survived because of this early period of hypotensive treatment. Considering man's long lifespan, 5 years of observation is probably too short for judging the long-term consequences.

Dr. Doyle: Could I just comment on what would happen if Dr. Folkow was a rat. I think the first point is that he wouldn't get myocardial infarction, and I'm sure you know that nobody denies that in human hypertension you can reduce the pressure-related events. The real problem is that they are swamped by the others, such as ischemic heart disease, which are not so closely related to pressure.

Dr. Korner (Prahran, Australia): I just wonder whether one could look at the various trials in another kind of way. In all the groups receiving treatment, there were, in fact, quite a lot of cardiovascular events in both the fatal and nonfatal categories. I wonder whether what we are really seeing in these various trials of mild hypertension represents the limit of what can be achieved by the kind of nonspecific therapy that we are currently using. If we look at the data this way, they represent a challenge for finding out more about the causes of the various subsets in our heterogeneous population of hypertensive patients.

Dr. Laragh: Would any of the panelists like to respond to that?

Dr. Remington: I think that is certainly a reasonable challenge for the future. That work has to go on, as I tried to indicate in my discussion and we need to know more. But we will never have complete knowledge. And let me play one more numbers game with everyone. We estimate from the HDFP, considering both the percentage and the absolute reduction in mortality, that if hypertensives in this country on a mass basis were to receive stepped care, the annual reduction in numbers of deaths in this country in the age range of 30–69 would be at least 65,000. For comparison, that's roughly the total number of deaths at these ages from the fourth leading cause of death in the United States, accidents.

Dr. Helgeland: When we look at the multifactorial risk profile presented by the Framingham study, it is a crucial point, I think, that we reduce the blood pressure but also change the lipid profile of some of the participants against the lipoprotein type IV with some of our most used drugs.

Dr. Laragh: Dr. Alderman would you like to make a closing comment?

Dr. Alderman (New York): A number of important points have been raised in this spirited discussion. I certainly agree with the statement that prevention is an accepted medical function in this country. However, I am not certain that a single bolus of prevention, such as vaccination, with well-defined side effects and limitations is, in fact, comparable to long-term antihypertensive therapy. Although it is often claimed that a single diuretic tablet controls blood pressure for most mild hypertensives, the available data indicate, in fact, that the majority of even patients with mild hypertension ultimately require two or more drugs to achieve blood pressure control. The long-term hazards of these potent agents (diuretics included) are, of course, unknown, but the immediate inconvenience and unpleasantness are certainly appreciable. [Morgan TO, Adams WR, Hodgson M, et al (1980) Med J Aust 2: 27–31]

Dr. Remington has extrapolated from the HDFP Study to suggest that indiscriminate application of the stepped care approach to all those with mild hypertension would produce a substantial reduction in cardiovascular mortality. While statistically accurate, this kind of mathematics ignores the limitations of the basic study. Of only 5 years duration, it might have been too short to permit the emergence of severe toxicity associated with the subtle metabolic derangements caused by antihypertensive chemotherapy. Secondly, by its design, HDFP did not distinguish between the effects of drugs and the superior overall medical care available to stepped care patients. In fact, about 60% of the reduction in cardiovascular mortality occurred in the non-cardiovascular category.

Beyond this, however, the critical issue is that any unimodal chemopharmacologic approach to the management of patients with hypertension implies that a level of pressure defines a homogeneous cohort. Reality is quite the contrary, however, and, as astute observers have recognized for half a century or more, persons with high blood pressure are a remarkably heterogeneous and hardy lot. Specifically, patients with the same blood pressure level can have vastly different courses and outcomes. At the mild level, as HDFP has confirmed, the vast majority are at no apparent risk. Moreover, even this small risk is not evenly distributed but can be shown to cluster according to certain demographic clinical and biochemical characteristics.

The stepped care approach imposes a uniformity upon clinical practice that is unjustified by the facts. Blood pressure alone simply does not provide a sufficiently precise guide to either the initiation or the type of therapy required. As a practical guide, Dr. Boyd's suggestion that a rising pressure may be a tip-off to timing the need to start treatment may be quite useful.

Session 2
Dietary Sodium and Human Hypertension

Chairman: A. E. Doyle

Position Paper: Dietary Sodium and Human Hypertension

Sir George Pickering

Albutt (1) defined his hyperpiesis, which we now term essential hypertension, as "a malady in which at or towards middle life blood pressure rises excessively"—a definition that has never been improved. The cause of this excessive rise is the outstanding problem concerning the malady. Two main possibilities exist: The cause may be genetic or environmental. Of these, the environmental hypothesis is much more attractive because it suggests possibilities for prevention and treatment. Up to now, no environmental factor of significance other than overnutrition has been identified in Western societies. Persons whose blood pressure tends to rise fastest in middle age also tend to put on weight (2). Conversely, weight reduction in the obese usually leads to a fall of arterial pressure (3).

The different patterns of rise of arterial pressure with age are illustrated in Fig. 1, which shows the frequency distribution curves for females arranged by age in decades in our population samples (4). In each decade, the distribution is continuous; there is no sudden break. With each decade, the curves spread out and move to the right. Arterial pressure seems to rise with age, but it rises more in some subjects than in others. In 1973, Harlan et al. (2) showed that "tracking" of arterial pressure tends to occur in a population; those subjects who rank in the top tenth in one examination tend to remain in that position subsequently. Zinner et al. (5) demonstrated that this tracking is likely to show familial aggregation and is thus probably inherited.

Two other points need emphasizing. First, there is no natural dividing line between normal blood pressure and hypertension. As I have stressed elsewhere—and as the World Health Organization has just recognized—any dividing line is an artifact. Inspection of the curves shows that almost any

Reprinted from Cardiovascular Reviews and Reports 1: 13–17, 1980.

ratio between affected and unaffected can be obtained by choosing an appropriate dividing line and an appropriate age. This is the mistake that led Weitz (6) and Platt (7) into believing that hypertension is inherited through a Mendelian dominant gene. Dahl, as we shall see, overlooked this

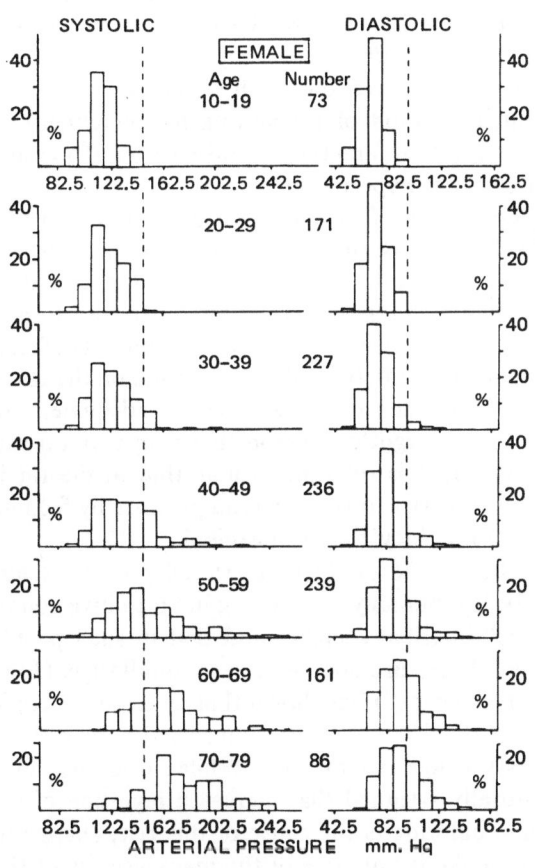

Fig. 1. Frequency distribution curves of systolic and diastolic pressure in females of the population sample investigated by Hamilton et al. (4).

fundamental pitfall when he sought evidence for salt intake as the cause of hypertension.

By far the most popular environmental factor that has been invoked is excessive intake of sodium chloride. A theoretical reason for this is that it conforms to Guyton's popular theory of autoregulation (8). According to the argument, excessive intake of salt increases extracellular fluid volume, plasma volume, and cardiac output. This leads to an increase in arterial pressure, which in turn leads to adaptive changes in peripheral blood vessels, some effected through the baroreceptor reflexes. This vasoconstriction results in an increased peripheral resistance that eventually maintains the arterial pressure as the cardiac output returns to normal. Each of these steps is small. The whole is viewed as a cascade effect. The most important step concerns the kidney. The rise in intravascular pressure leads to an increased glomerular filtration rate and ultimately to a pressure diuresis that goes on until the excess salt and its accompanying water have been excreted. This process is fundamental to all physiology and results in *"la fixité du milieu intérieur,"* which Claude Bernard saw as *"la condition de la vie libre."*

Excessive ingestion of salt would be a most convenient method of accounting for increments in plasma volume and thus for raised arterial pressure in essential hypertension.

Four lines of evidence are cited in support of this hypothesis: the study of primitive peoples, the study of salt intake in Western societies, the effect of gross salt restriction on arterial pressure, and the effect of ingestion of excessive amounts of salt. I shall deliberately omit the literature on the effect of salt on rats for the simple but adequate, and too often forgotten, reason that man is not a rat. However, it is relevant to note that in the rat it is much easier to raise arterial pressure by feeding salt if a kidney has been excised.

There is no doubt that arterial pressure tends to be low in many races living in "primitive conditions" in tribal societies and that in such people arterial pressure does not rise in middle age. However, Shaper (9) has shown that when such people adopt the lifestyle of Western societies their blood pressure does rise with age. While enthusiasts have naturally assumed that increased ingestion of sodium chloride is the cause of this rise, change in salt intake is only one of the many aspects of the differences of the two lifestyles. Having visited some of these peoples, I would certainly not consider salt intake as the prime reason for the difference. In my opinion, the great contrast is between the certainty of behavior in a society ruled by ritual and taboo and the uncertainty in Western societies, in which life is a series of individual choices and decisions. Primitive peoples living in tribal societies differ in so many particulars that to select salt intake as the culprit is to me just bad science. Prior (10), Beaglehole (11), and their colleagues are looking more closely into the most important factor leading to the rise in arterial pressure as migrants from the Pacific Islands become incorporated into the civilized society of New Zealand.

Dahl and Love (12) sought evidence that increased salt intake was associated with hypertension. They submitted a questionnaire to the staff of the Brookhaven Laboratory to ascertain whether they added salt to their food before tasting (high-salt intake), sometimes added salt (average intake), or never added salt (low intake). The arterial pressures were measured by Love during annual medical examinations. The average arterial pressures were as follows: in the low-intake group, 116.6/68.5; in the average-intake group, 115.1/70.2; and in the high-intake group, 114.9/70.4. I regard this as clear evidence that salt did not affect arterial pressure. Dahl and Love, however, thought otherwise. Accepting 140/90 or greater as an indication of hypertension, they found the percentages of hypertensives to be 0, 8, and 13 in the three dietary groups. They, therefore, argued that a sodium intake in excess of a certain level seemed to be necessary for the development of hypertension.

Dahl and Love (13) went on to explore his hypothesis on a wide geographic scale. He produced a celebrated diagram (Fig. 2) showing a linear relationship between the average daily salt intake and the percentage of hypertensives in a population. Two points, the Eskimo and northern Japan, are dead on the line. The others, the Marshall Islands, North America, and southern Japan, are very close. Unfortunately, Dahl published none of the data; he neither defined what he meant by hypertension nor gave the age range of the population he studied. As seen in Fig. 1, the frequency distribution curves in a population sample are such that any ratio may be obtained for the presence or absence of hypertension in a population by selecting a suitable dividing line and suitable age range. I regard his diagram as a work of the imagination but of no value as evidence. Dahl's work was re-

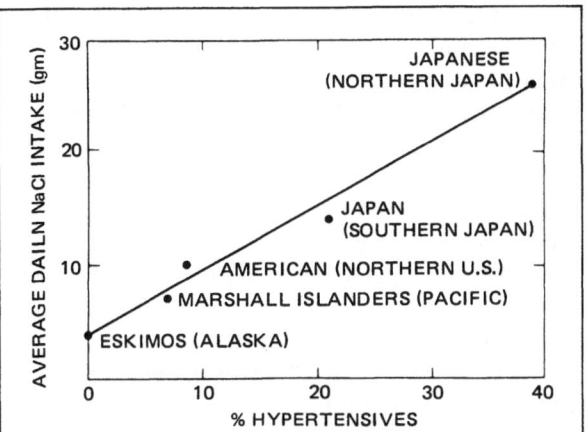

Fig. 2. Dahl's diagram showing the alleged relationship between salt intake and hypertension among different peoples. [Dahl and Love (13)]

peated by Miall (14) in his study with Oldham et al. (15) of their population sample in South Wales. Table 1 summarizes their results.

Miall restricted his measurements to postmenopausal women. Because sodium is not retained in the human body, the 24-h excretion is the same as the 24-h intake. In fact, high- and low-salt eaters selected in Dahl's dietary history show no differences in sodium excretion. His questionnaire is clearly erroneous as an index of salt ingestion. Moreover, salt excretion is almost the same in persons with arterial pressures above 200 mmHg and those under 150 mmHg, the highest sodium figures in each case being found with the lowest arterial pressures. The Framingham group got similar and completely convincing results (16). Table 2 shows that arterial pressure is uninfluenced by the 24-h

Table 2. Twenty-four hour urine sodium excretion compared to blood pressure, Framingham heart study.

Category	Na excretion (converted to g NaCl)			
	<8	8–10.4	10.5–12.9	>13
No. of persons	41	55	45	44
Age	44	44	44	45
Bp	131/85	139/89	13787	139/88
Persons with HBP	8(20%)	13(24%)	12(27%)	16(36%)

Source: Courtesy of Dawber et al. (16).

sodium excretion, and Table 3 shows that the dietary history is valueless as a guide to sodium intake. Individuals with the highest pressures in a population excrete no more salt in 24 h than those with the lowest pressures. This has also been shown by Thomas et al. (7) in a study of workers at the Atomic Energy Research Establishment in Harwell, England, in Milton, New Zealand, by Simpson and his colleagues (18), and in a study by Bind et al. (19). These observations are so consistent that we conclude with some certainty that in Western societies excessive salt intake is not the cause of essential hypertension.

Two other questions need answering. Will restriction of salt intake lower arterial pressure, and will excessive salt intake raise it? The answer to each question is yes, but the changes have to be extreme. Early French workers such as Widal (20) and Ambard and Beaujard (21) found that in nephritis it was possible to change weight and arterial pressure by withholding or feeding salt. They attributed the effect to chloride. Allen and Sherrill

Table 1. Dietary salt history, blood pressure, and urine sodium excretion, postmenopausal women in South Wales.

Dietary history of salt	SBP >200 mmHG		SBP >150 mmHg	
	No.	Na excretion/ 24 h (mEq)	No.	Na excretion/ 24 h (mEq)
Low	26	123.1	61	130.7
High	23	122.1	43	146.3

Source: Miall (14).

Table 3. Twenty-four hour urine sodium excretion compared to sodium intake by diet history, Framingham heart study.

Diet	Na excretion		
	Low	Medium	High
Low	2	1	1
Medium	3	16	4
High	3	6	3
Total	8	23	8

Low <3 g Na/day; high >6 g Na/day.
Source: Courtesy of Dawber et al. (16).

(22) got similar effects and also attributed them to chloride restriction. Volhard (23), who found the same, was a great advocate of a salt-free diet, which his patients hated. When I visited his clinic in 1931, the expression "lying like a saltless" was used to describe the difference between what the "saltless" told Volhard about the salt they were eating and what their neighbors actually saw them eat. When I returned home, and particularly after Kempner's experience (24), I tried to repeat the observations on salt, edema, and blood pressure. I found it quite easy to demonstrate that withholding salt in edematous patients reduced their weight, but I only found one patient in whom I could prove that reducing salt would lower arterial pressure. I did learn, however, that my patients, too, hated the diet, and I was not tough enough to force it on them.

The first really successful salt-restrictive regimen was Kempner's rice and fruit diet (24). As originally conceived, the diet had other properties, but it transpired that a sodium content of about 5 mEq/day, and certainly of less than 10 mEq/day, was its essential property. Kempner showed that this diet, which contained a daily intake of 200 mg chloride and 150 mg sodium, would reduce arterial pressure, heart size, and retinopathy in patients with severe hypertension, including those in the malignant phase. The urinary sodium fell 4–0.01 g/liter. The serum sodium was 142.8 mEq/liter before treatment and 141.7 mEq/liter afterward. Kempner's results, though disputed by some researchers, were confirmed by others, for example, the Medical Research Council (MRC) and Watkin et al. (25). Watkin and his colleagues confirmed Kempner's findings in a careful study of 50 patients on the Columbia service of the Goldwater Hospital in New York; however, they found that there was a prompt return of arterial pressure with as little as 1 g sodium chloride/day. They wrote: "The critical tolerance level of sodium intake with respect to blood pressure is extremely low in patients in the advanced stage of hypertension. In fact it is so low that it has not been convincingly demonstrated that effective dietary sodium levels can be achieved by other than the rice–fruit diet or equivalent extremely restricted regime. Such dietary restrictions impose such hardships on the patient that only a minority can sustain a sufficient low-sodium intake to obtain persistently salutary effects. With resumption of a normal diet, blood pressures rapidly return to

pretreatment levels. Many patients complain bitterly about anorexia. Lassitude and weakness were often pronounced."

The reason that Kempner succeeded with his diet when others failed is simple. He collected 24-h urine specimens in each patient. Before he went to the ward to see his patients, he found out how much sodium they were excreting. Woe betide those who had erred! They did not dare to repeat it. The very careful work done at that time, particularly by Watkin and his co-workers, and by the MRC, established beyond a reasonable doubt that a daily diet containing less than 10 mEq sodium would reduce arterial pressure but that larger amounts of sodium in the diet would restore it. Recently, claims have been made that a lesser restriction of sodium is effective (26, 27). These papers have been criticized by Simpson (28), justifiably in my opinion. I consider the older work to stand.

The idea that salt restriction might lower arterial pressure has received support from the undoubted ability of thiazide diuretics to reduce arterial pressure. The outstanding effect of these drugs is to increase the excretion of salt. At first, their action is accompanied by a fall in plasma volume and extracellular fluid volume, but these return to normal while the effect on the blood pressure continues. Bing et al. (19) found that in 36 patients with hypertension, the sodium excretion was the same as in normal controls and "no effect was observed in two years' treatment with bendrofluazide." However, the plasma renin rose progressively over the 2 years of therapy. In seven patients, the sodium excretion at the end of 2 years was more than 45 mEq/24 h greater than before treatment. The blood pressure fall in these patients was no less than in those in whom the change of sodium excretion was smaller.

Kirkendall and his associates (29) gave diets containing 10, 210, and 410 mEq sodium to eight normal volunteers for periods of 4 weeks. The salt excretion paralleled the intake. There was no significant change in arterial pressure in either supine or upright positions, though total exchangeable sodium and inulin space showed the expected changes. On the other hand, the same group (30) found that change from the low- (10 mEq) to the high- (410 mEq) sodium diet did produce a change of about 10 mmHg in borderline hypertension. Kawasaki et al. (31) changed the daily salt intake 9–249 mEq in 19 patients with idiopathic hypertension. Nine were salt sensitive, changing their pressures on an average 17.6 mmHg, while ten were insensitive, changing their pressures on an average 4.1 mmHg. Luft et al. (32) administered 10, 100, 300, 600, 800, 1,200, and 1,600 mEq sodium/day. The highest level had to be given intravenously. The arterial pressure showed no significant or constant changes up to 800 mEq but rose with the highest doses—intakes that civilized man probably never achieves naturally.

Taking all these studies together, it seems justifiable to conclude that humans, like Dahl's rats, vary in their sensitivity to salt. Most people, including those with mild or severe hypertension, show a fall of pressure when salt is restricted to 10 mEq (0.58 g)/day. However, this intake is distasteful, produces loss of appetite and weakness, and, therefore, is naturally not selected by those living in Western societies.

It is possible that a very few people respond with a small fall of pressure to salt restriction of the order of 1 g/day. Above this level, however, there is no evidence of any effect of salt intake on arterial pressure until intakes reach levels that are far above those consumed under natural conditions. Within the range ingested by most Westerners, there is no evidence that the amount of salt influences arterial pressure.

What all this work emphasizes is the remarkable ability of the normal human body to regulate the sodium content of its plasma despite enormous changes in sodium intake. Indeed, there is perhaps no better example of Claude Bernard's concept of *la fixité du milieu intérieur* than the plasma sodium. In maintaining the constancy of the plasma sodium, the kidneys play a prominent part. Changing the arterial pressure through changes in dietary sodium is much easier in subjects whose renal function is impaired. In the extreme example of the patient without kidneys who is kept alive on repeated hemodialysis, the arterial pressure may be raised or lowered by adjusting the gain or loss of sodium to the body.

Harm arising from excessive salt intake is, in my opinion, extremely rare. Minor degrees of salt deficiency—enough to cause asthenia and apathy—are common in hot weather, after severe exercise, and after diarrhea. Severe salt deficiency is a very dangerous condition, particularly in diabetic ketosis and after surgery, which the saline infusions of modern therapy are designed to prevent.

The data summarized here allow the conclusion that manipulating the dietary salt intake within the range of 2–10 g/day or recommending that Americans reduce their salt intake 10–6 g is utterly meaningless. Admonitions to avoid a saltshaker seem rather silly, and taking salt out of canned foods could be dangerous, considering its preservative value.

This review illustrates that it is only at the very extremes of intake that salt has any impact, and these are not likely to concern the average citizen of Western society.

SUMMARY

Four lines of evidence, all poorly substantiated, have been traditionally cited in support of the theory that excessive salt intake is related to essential hypertension in man. First, epidemiologic studies of primitive peoples have revealed many societies where both salt intake and blood pressure are lower than in westernized societies, but because there are so many other differences between such societies, it is hard to prove that the relationship between salt and pressure is causal. Furthermore, most epidemiologic surveys of westernized societies have shown no correlations between salt intake and blood pressure. Second, the effects of gross salt restriction on blood pressure have been variable and generally disappointing, even using extreme diets such as the Kempner rice diet. Individuals vary greatly in their response to salt intake. Third, animal experiments are of doubtful relevance to man. Fourth, experiments where salt intake has been increased have shown that blood pressure rises only at levels of salt intake that are much higher than occur normally.

It is concluded that minor manipulations of salt intake have no place in the prevention of hypertension.

REFERENCES

1. Allbutt TC (1915) Diseases of the arteries, including angina pectoris. Macmillan, London
2. Harlan WR, Oberman A, Mitchell RE, et al (1973) A thirty year study of blood pressure in a white male cohort. In: Onesti G, Kim KE, Moyer JH

(eds) Hypertension: Mechanisms and management. Grune & Stratton, New York

3. Reisin E, Abel R, Modan M, et al (1978) The effect of weight loss without salt restriction on the reduction of blood pressure in overweight hypertensive patients. N Engl J Med 298: 1

4. Hamilton M, Pickering GW, Roberts JAF, et al (1954) The aetiology of essential hypertension: I. The arterial pressure in the general population. Clin Sci Mol Med 13: 11

5. Zinner SH, Levy PS, Kass EH (1971) Familial aggregation of blood pressure in childhood. N Engl J Med 284: 402

6. Weitz W (1923) Zur Ätiologie der genuinen oder vaskulären Hypertension. Z Klin Med 96: 151

7. Platt R (1963) Heredity and hypertension. Lancet 1: 899

8. Guyton AC (1977) Personal views on mechanisms of hypertension. In: Genest J, Koiw G, Kuchel O (eds) Hypertension. McGraw-Hill, New York

9. Shaper AG (1967) Blood pressure studies in East Africa. In: Stamler J, Stamler R, Pullman TN (eds) Epidemiology of hypertension. Grune & Stratton, New York

10. Prior AM, Evans JG, Harvey HP, et al (1968) Sodium intake and blood pressure in two Polynesian populations. N Engl J Med 279: 515

11. Beaglehole R, Salmond CE, Hooper A, et al (1977) Blood pressure and social interaction in Tokelauan migrants in New Zealand. J Chronic Dis 30: 803

12. Dahl LK, Love RM (1954) Evidence for relationship between sodium (chloride) intake and human hypertension. Arch Intern Med 94: 525

13. Dahl LK, Love RM (1961) Possible risk of chronic excess salt consumption in the pathogenesis of essential hypertension. Am J Cardiol 8: 571

14. Miall WE (1959) Follow-up study of arterial pressure in the population of a Welsh mining valley. Br Med J 2: 1204

15. Oldham PD, Pickering GW, Roberts JAF, et al (1960) The nature of essential hypertension. Lancet 1: 1085

16. Dawber TR, Kannel WB, Kagan A, et al (1967) Environmental factors in hypertension. In: Stamler J, Stamler R, Pullman TN (eds) Epidemiology of hypertension. Grune & Stratton, New York

17. Thomas GW, Ledingham JGG, Beilin LJ, et al (1978) Reduced renin in hypertension. Kidney Int 13: 513

18. Simpson FO, Waal-Manning HJ, Bolli P, et al (1978) Relationship of blood pressure to sodium excretion in a population survey. Clin Sci Mol Med 55: 373

19. Bing RF, Thurston H, Swales JD (1979) Salt intake and diuretic treatment of hypertension. Lancet 2: 121

20. Widal F (1903) Role du chlorure de sodium dans la pathogénie de certains oedèmes britiques. La Semaine Medicale 23: 199

21. Ambard L, Beaujard E (1904) Causes de l'hypertension arterielle. Archives Generales Medicine 1: 520

22. Allen FM, Sherrill JW (1922) The treatment of arterial hypertension. J Metabol Res 2: 429

23. Volhard F (1931) Nieren und Ableitende Harnwege. In: von Bergmann G, St Staehelin R (eds) Handbuch der Inneren Medizin, Vol 6. Springer, Berlin, p. 1

24. Kempner W (1948) Treatment of hypertensive vascular disease with rice diet. Am J Med 4: 545

25. Watkin DM, Froeb HF, Hatch FT, et al (1959) Effects of diet in essential hypertension. Am J Med 26: 428

26. Parijs J, Joosens JV, van der Linden L, et al (1973) Moderate sodium restriction and diuretics in the treatment of hypertension. Am Heart J 85: 22

27. Morgan T, Adam W, Gillies A, et al (1978) Hypertension treated by salt restriction. Lancet 1: 227

28. Simpson FO (1979) Salt and hypertension: A sceptical review of the evidence. In: Proceedings of the 6th meeting of the international society of hypertension, Göteborg, Sweden Clinical Science 57: (Suppl 5) 4635, Medical Research Society and the Biochemical Society, London

29. Kirkendall WM, Conner WE, Abboud F, et al (1976) The effect of dietary sodium chloride on blood pressure, body fluids, electrolytes, renal function and serum lipids of normotensive man. J Lab Clin Med 87: 418

30. Mark AL, Lawton WJ, Aboud FM, et al (1975) Effects of high and low sodium intake on arterial pressure and forearm vascular resistance in borderline hypertension. Circ Res 36(Suppl 1): 194

31. Kawasaki T, Delea CS, Bartter FC, et al (1978) The effect of high sodium and low sodium intakes on blood pressures and other related variables in human subjects with idiopathic hypertension. Am J Med 64: 193

32. Murray RH, Luft FC, Bloch R, Weyman AE (1978) Blood pressure responses to extremes of sodium intake in normal man. Proc Soc Exp Biol Med 159: 432

Sodium Deprivation as an Approach to Hypertension

Edward D. Freis

ROLE OF SODIUM IN HYPERTENSION

There are certain key pieces of information that seem to be crucial in understanding the role of sodium in hypertension. These key points also seem to be frequently misinterpreted. A summary of these points will be the subject of my discussion.

The first key point is that there seems to be an influence of sodium on blood pressure *only* below a sodium intake of approximately 75 mEq/day. This point is supported by data from studies of patients on sodium-restricted diets and epidemiologic studies of unacculturated peoples. There appears to be no correlation, however, between sodium intake and blood pressure above the approximate level of 75 mEq/day (1, 2). For example, in studies on free-living populations in the United States (3) and in Great Britain (4), the dietary intake of sodium was almost always above 100 mEq/day and there was no correlation between sodium excretion and level of blood pressure. Whether the diet contains 150 or 500 mEq does not seem to make any important difference, although there is a little evidence to suggest that at extremely high intakes of sodium there might be an additional hypertensive effect (5). The important point is, however, that there is an influence of sodium ingestion on blood pressure, but it is primarily operative below 75 mEq/day. The demonstration of no correlation between sodium intake and blood pressure with diets containing more than 75 mEq sodium/day does not in any way negate a relationship between salt and hypertension. There is a definite relationship between sodium and hypertension but it is present only at low levels of sodium intake. The absence of a relationship at higher levels should not be taken as evidence that sodium plays no role in hypertension.

The second important point is that the antihypertensive effects of sodium depletion are associated with a reduction in plasma and extracellular fluid volume (1, 6). In this respect, diets very low in sodium have similar effects on volume as do the diuretics (7). It is a striking fact that the rice and fruit diet and the thiazide diuretics both reduce plasma and extracellular fluid volume by approximately 10%–15%. Present evidence suggests that the antihypertensive effects of the diuretics depend on reduction in plasma and extracellular volumes. If the antihypertensive effects of low-sodium diets are also dependent on reduction of these volumes, which seems likely, then it is obvious that sodium must be severely restricted in order to achieve a reduction of plasma and extracellular volume. This probably explains why it is necessary to restrict sodium rather severely in order to obtain an antihypertensive effect.

A third important consideration with respect to sodium in hypertension is the variability of pressor responsiveness to sodium in the general population. This consideration was first noted by Dahl who selectively bred strains of rats who were either salt sensitive or salt responsive (8). More recently, Bartter's group has shown a similar spectrum of sodium responsiveness in hypertensive patients, the blood pressure of some patients being quite reactive to the addition of sodium to a low-sodium diet, whereas the blood pressure of other patients was resistant to such dietary manipulation (9). Thus, sodium may or may not be more important in the blood pressure control of certain individuals as compared to others depending on whether they are constitutionally sodium sensitive or sodium resistant.

The fourth point is that although the salt which occurs naturally in foods is sufficient for our survival without any need for extra sodium, the fact remains that most animals, including man, crave salt in their diet. Because of this salt appetite, it is difficult to enforce a low-sodium diet, and, when it is attempted, compliance generally is very poor. Therefore, low-sodium diet therapy does not represent a practical approach toward the long-term control of hypertension. Some investigators have claimed success with the use of diets moderately low in sodium, such as those below 140 mEq/day when combined with low doses of diuretics. This has been done to avoid thiazide-induced hypokalemia. I do not feel that the advantages are great enough to warrant imposing a restrictive diet that may or may not be followed. One suspects that the low-sodium diet is more often prescribed than it is observed.

A fifth point is that the patient populations studied with low-sodium diets were different 30 years ago than they are today. The early studies were carried out in hospitalized patients with severe hypertension who were given the rice and fruit diet. Early workers such as Watkin et al. (1) and Murphy (6) proved that the antihypertensive effectiveness of the diet was due to its low-sodium content. Watkin found that raising the sodium content of the diet from approximately 8–30 mEg/day nullified the antihypertensive effect of the diet.

Today, on the other hand, we hear that Hunt and Margie (2) have controlled hypertension with diets containing as much as 60–70 mEq sodium/day. Parijs from Belgium has also reported that simply reducing the salt content of the diet 10–5 g resulted in a lowering of blood pressure, although admittedly the degrees of lowering were not very great (10). A similar small reduction of blood pressure during moderate sodium restriction was observed by Morgan et al. (11). Why is it that diets used in recent times by Hunt and others were effective, whereas 30 years ago these and even more restricted diets were ineffective?

An obvious difference is in the type of patients studied in 1950 and recently. As indicated above, the 1950 studies included patients with very severe and life-threatening hypertension. In modern studies, patients have mostly mild or, at most, moderate hypertension. According to Hunt, mild hypertensives respond more readily to diets containing 60–75 mEq sodium than do patients with moderate hypertension (2). Hunt did not treat any patients with severe hypertension such as were studied by Watkin et al. (1) and Murphy (9) 30 years ago. These former studies, therefore, are not particularly relevant to today's investigations. Since the severity of the hypertension is an important determinant of the antihypertensive response to sodium restriction, it is quite possible that lesser degrees of sodium restriction might be effective in lowering the blood pressure of mild hypertensives than were required in severe hypertensives.

The amount of sodium restriction required to lower blood pressure in mild hypertension has not yet been elucidated, although the available evidence suggests that the intake should not exceed 75 mEq/day.

There is a need at the present time for controlled trials on the effects of moderate sodium restriction in patients with mild hypertension. The available trials do not contain an appropriate control group. This is important because of the downward drift of blood pressure that occurs over time without any specific treatment, especially in patients with mild hypertension. Hunt did observe his patients for a month before starting the diet, which should help eliminate some who spontaneously revert to normal blood pressure.

If the five points noted above are kept in mind, they should help to clarify some of the confusion and conflicting claims that exist today with respect to the role of sodium in hypertension.

SUMMARY

This critique stresses five key points with respect to the role of sodium in hypertension. The points are as follows: 1) The correlation between dietary sodium and blood pressure is not a continuum. The relationship only holds below an intake of 75 mEq sodium/day; 2) the reason for the above statement may be due to the fact that the antihypertensive effect of sodium restriction seems to be caused at least in part by a reduction in plasma and extracellular fluid volumes; 3) patients differ markedly in sodium responsiveness; some are sodium sensitive, whereas others are sodium resistant; 4) low-sodium diets do not offer a practical approach to treatment because most patients will not follow a restricted diet for more than a few weeks; and 5) it is not justified to extrapolate the results of older studies of severe dietary restriction in patients with severe hypertension to current studies of moderate sodium restriction in patients with mild hypertension.

REFERENCES

1. Watkin DM, Fraeb HR, Gutman AB (1950) Effects of diet in essential hypertension: II. Results with

unmodified Kempner rice diet in fifty hospitalized patients. Am J Med 9: 441

2. Hunt JC, Margie JD (1980) Influence of diet in hypertension. In: Hypertension update: Mechanisms, epidemiology, evaluation and management. From the Ed. Bd. of Dialogues in Hypertension. HLS Press, Bloomfield, NJ, p 197

3. Dawber TR, Kannel WB, Kagan A, et al (1967) Environmental factors in hypertension. In: Stamler J, Stamler R, Pullman, TN (eds) Epidemiology of hypertension. Grune & Stratton, New York, p 255

4. Miall WE (1959) Follow-up study of arterial pressure in the population of a Welsh mining valley. Br Med J 2: 1204

5. Sasaki N (1964) The relationship of salt intake to hypertension in the Japanese. Geriatrics 19: 735

6. Murphy RJF (1950) The effect of "rice diet" on plasma volume and extracellular fluid space in hypertensive subjects. J Clin Invest 29: 912

7. Wilson IM, Freis ED (1959) Relationship between plasma and extracellular fluid volume depletion and the antihypertensive effects of chlorothiazide. Circulation 20: 1028

8. Dahl L, Heine M, Tassinari L (1962) Effect of chronic excess salt ingestion: Evidence that genetic factors play an important role in susceptibility to experimental hypertension. J Exp Med 115: 1172

9. Kawasaki T, Delea CS, Bartter FC, Smith H (1978) The effect of high-sodium and low-sodium intakes on blood pressure and other variables in human subjects with ideopathic hypertension. Am J Med 64: 193

10. Parijs J, Joosens JV, VanderLinden L, Verstreken G, Amery AKPC (1973) Moderate Sodium restriction and diuretics in the treatment of hypertension. Am Heart J 85: 22

11. Morgan T, Gillies A, Morgan G, Adam W, Wilson M, Carney S (1978) Hypertension treated by salt restriction. Lancet 1: 227

Sodium and Other Dietary Factors in Experimental and Human Hypertension: The Japanese Experience

Yukio Yamori, Yasuo Nara, Masahiro Kihara, Ryoichi Horie, and Akira Ooshima

Stroke is the most preponderant cause of death in Japan, while myocardial infarction is the first cause of death in Western countries. Epidemiologic studies have indicated that stroke incidence in Japan, which is closely related to hypertension itself, is rather inversely correlated with serum cholesterol levels that are generally far lower than those of the populations in Western countries; the mean of the various populations in Japan is mostly below 200 mg/dl. Since the stroke incidence is higher in rural inhabitants in Japan who are taking less cholesterol and protein, but excess salt (the mean daily intake is mostly over 12 g, not infrequently over 20 g), salt excess seems to be more closely related to high stroke incidence.

On the other hand, of the unique animal models, that is, stroke-prone spontaneously hypertensive rats (SHRSP) (1, 2), that develop cerebrovascular lesions, nearly 100% were established in Japan in 1974. Since then it has become possible to analyze "experimentally" not only the pathogenesis but also the risk factors of stroke, the prediction and prevention in SHRSP (3). We have confirmed in these models that the adverse effect of salt excess is influenced by genetic predisposition as well as by other nutritional factors such as protein and lipid intakes. We further analyzed the relationship of blood pressure or stroke incidence with dietary intakes of salt or protein by a 24-h urinalysis in the rural population in Japan in order to extrapolate the experimental findings in animal models to humans.

EXPERIMENTAL STUDIES IN ANIMAL MODELS (SHR, SHRSP)

IMPORTANCE OF GENE—ENVIRONMENT INTERACTION

Salt sensitivity was different among SHR substrains, and SHRSP showed greater increases in blood pressure than most of the stroke-resistant substrains of SHR or normotensive Wistar–Kyoto rats (WKY) (Fig. 1) (4). Moreover, the effect of excess salt intake on stroke incidence was greater in SHR substrains with higher spontaneous incidence of stroke (4). These experimental findings indicate that salt sensitivity and stroke proneness may be closely related to salt metabolism (3, 4). In fact, slight impairment of renal salt handling was noted in SHRSP in the pre- or early hypertensive stage (5). Therefore, the adverse effect of salt may be marked in the individual rats or probably in humans with such a disposition, and the early detection of this disposition seems to be important in the prevention of hypertension or stroke.

INTERACTION OF VARIOUS NUTRITIONAL FACTORS

Analyses on the effect of salt loading on SHRSP fed various protein diets clearly showed that adverse effects of salt was augmented by a low-protein diet (6–8). It has been proven that high-protein diet feeding prevents the development of severe hypertension and decreases stroke incidence (7, 8). The mechanism of prevention of stroke by high-protein diet feeding has been studied further: Fish protein, especially sulfoaminoacids and tyrosine, decreases blood pressure centrally and attenuates the development of severe hypertension. It also accelerates renal sodium excretion and, therefore, counteracts the adverse effect of excess salt intake. Soybean protein, although it does not affect blood pressure, improves the physical characteristics of arterial walls in SHRSP fed on enough protein from a young age (3).

In SHRSP fed a high-fat cholesterol (HFC) diet, the incidence of arterionecrotic-thrombogenic stroke was decreased (9, 10). The reduction of stroke incidence in these SHRSP was ascribed to the attenuation of severe hypertension, the mechanism of which might be due to the reduction of

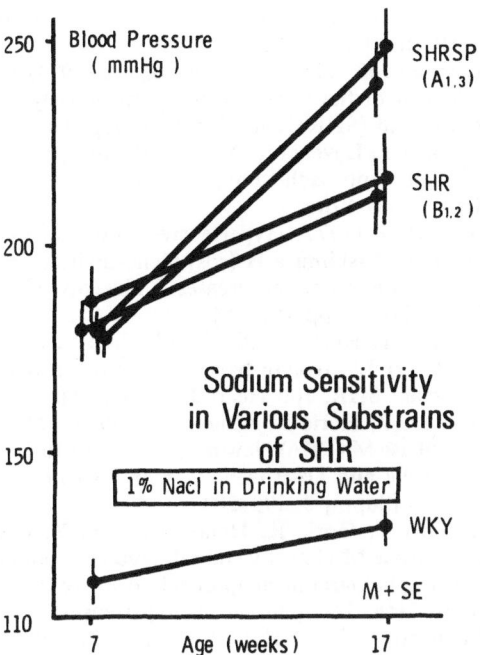

Fig. 1. Na sensitivity in various substains of SHR.

EPIDEMIOLOGIC STUDIES IN RURAL INHABITANTS

RELATION OF DIETARY SODIUM TO HYPERTENSION OR STROKE

First, in search of a better scientific evaluation of dietary Na and protein intake, Na, inorganic sulfate from sulfoaminoacids, and urea nitrogen from aminoacids were checked in a 24-h urine deposit obtained from volunteers fed on both high- or low-salt and high- or low-protein diets. Since the urinary Na/creatinine ratio and sulfate/creatinine ratio were proven to be closely related to dietary salt and protein intakes, these urinalyses were applied for the nutritional survey of two farming and fishing villages, where the stroke incidences were so markedly different—high in the farming and low in the fishing village (3).

A 24-h urine deposit was collected from 111 males and females aged 40–50. Their diastolic blood pressures were significantly higher in the farming than in the fishing village. Urinalyses showed that urinary sulfate derived from animal protein was significantly lower in the farming village, although urinary sodium and urea nitrogen were not different in the two villages. This observation confirmed our experimental data in animal models, which indicated that greater animal protein intake attenuates hypertension and reduces stroke incidence.

Furthermore, multiple regression analyses proved that systolic blood pressures were significantly correlated not only with age, sex, and obesity, but also with urinary Na/K or sulfate/urea

vascular reactivity to pressor substances in SHRSP fed on a HFC diet (11). These experimental data are consistent with epidemiologic findings that the incidence of stroke due to arterionecrosis (not atherosclerosis) is high in Japan where hypertension is not always accompanied by hypercholesterolemia, whereas myocardial infarction is more preponderant than stroke in Western countries where marked hypercholesterolemia is very common.

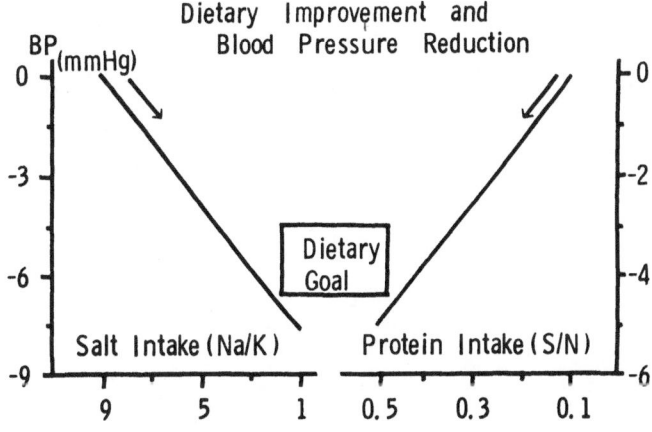

Fig. 2. Correlation between blood pressure and Na/K ratio or inorganic S/N ratio.

nitrogen (S/N) ratios. These are the first epidemiologic data in the world indicating that Na and animal protein intake are, positively or inversely, correlated with blood pressure in "one community" (Fig. 2).

DIETARY GOALS FOR THE JAPANESE

The regression analyses, thus obtained, suggest that urinary Na/K ratios should be reduced, while urinary S/N ratios should be increased for nutritionally reducing blood pressure. Thus, less salt and more protein intake are the goal for our dietary improvement in Japan.

SUMMARY

Since animal models for cardiovascular diseases were established, risk factors can be analyzed not only epidemiologically, but also experimentally. The evidence that was confirmed both experimentally and epidemiologically indicates that excess salt intake, excess lipid intake, and relative protein deficiency are definitely risk factors, which should be improved for the prevention of cardiovascular diseases.

REFERENCES

1. Yamori Y, Nagaoka A, Okamoto K (1974) Importance of genetic factors in hypertensive cerebrovascular lesions: An evidence obtained by successive selective breeding of stroke-prone and resistant SHR. Jpn Circ J 38: 1095–1110
2. Okamoto K, Yamori Y, Nagaoka A (1974) Establishment of the stroke-prone spontaneously hypertensive rat (SHR). Circ Res 34, (Suppl 1): 143–153
3. Yamori Y, Lovenberg W, Freis E (eds) (1979) Prophylactic approach to hypertensive diseases. Raven Press, New York
4. Yamori Y (1977) Hypertensive strains of rat. In: Inoue E, Nishimura H (eds) Gene-environment interaction in common diseases. University of Tokyo Press, Tokyo, pp 151–154
5. Yamori Y, Horie R, Ohtaka M, Nara Y, Ooshima A (1979) Electrolyte balance in stroke-prone and -resistant SHR. Jpn Heart J 20(Suppl 1): 65–67
6. Yamori Y, Horie R, Akiguchi I, Ohtaka M, Nara Y, Fukase M (1976) New models of SHR for studies on stroke and atherogenesis. Clin Exp Pharmacol Physiol [Suppl] 3: 199–203
7. Yamori Y, Horie R, Handa H, Nara Y, Ohtaka M, Fukase M (1977) Cerebral circulation and electroencephalographical approach to stroke in stroke-prone SHR. In: Spontaneous hypertension. DHEW Publication No. (NIH) 77-1179, pp 279–286
8. Yamori Y, Horie R, Akiguchi I, Nara Y, Ohtaka M, Fukase M (1977) Pathogenetic mechanism of stroke in stroke-prone SHR. In: de Jong W (ed) Progress in brain research, Vol 47: Hypertension and brain mechanisms. Elsevier, Amsterdam, pp 219–234
9. Yamori Y, Horie R, Nara Y, Ikeda K (1977) Prophylactic trials for stroke in stroke-prone SHR: I. Effects of fat, protein and amino acids. Jpn Heart J 18: 551–553
10. Yamori Y, Horie R, Ohtaka M, Nara Y, Fukase M (1976) Effect of hypercholesterolemic diet on the incidence of cerebrovascular and myocardial lesions in spontaneously hypertensive rats. Clin Exp Pharmacol Physiol [Suppl] 3: 205–208
11. Yamori Y, Horie R (1977) Vascular reactivity in pathological states. In: Shibata S, Canier O (eds) Factors influencing vascular reactivity. Igaku-Shoin, Tokyo

Metabolic Risks of Diuretic Therapy

Richard P. Ames and Peter Hill

Hypertension, like hypercholesterolemia, is a major risk factor for coronary heart disease (CHD). A characteristic such as hypertension attains risk factor status for CHD if its presence correlates with a high incidence of subsequent myocardial infarction. Although statistical correlation does not prove causation, the association suggests potentially fruitful avenues for research and possible prevention of the condition. Thus, one benefit of the treatment of hypertension was expected to be a reduction of CHD. Two sizable and lengthy placebo-controlled trials failed to demonstrate the expected reduction in CHD (1, 2). A trial of huge proportions was required to document the decrease in CHD and thereby substantiate the causal relationship between the two conditions (3). Does the difficulty in decreasing CHD mean that hypertension plays only a minor contributory role in the pathogenesis of CHD? Where can we now look for additional reductions in CHD? In an ongoing inquiry into these questions, we previously reported that diuretic drugs, when used in the treatment of hypertension, cause an increase in serum lipid concentrations (4). Two short-term studies have confirmed our observations (5, 6), but one large trial reported no change in serum lipids after 3 years of treatment with hydrochlorothiazide (7). To evaluate the durability of the effect of diuretics on serum lipids, we report herein our observations for intervals of treatment up to 18 months in duration, the longest periods for which we have treated sizable numbers of patients continuously with single agents. In addition, as part of a search for mechanisms of the effect, we report measurements of fasting serum insulin concentrations before and during treatment.

PATIENTS

The patients included in this report have, with few exceptions, uncomplicated primary hypertension. Individuals with clinically evident concomitant disease were excluded. These patients were referred to us by a multiphasic screening center and by other patients. Some patients responded to newspaper advertisements, and many have been included in previous publications (4, 8). This report brings our experience with several diuretics up to date. All patients who had fasting blood sampled before or after as well as during diuretic treatment were included in this analysis. The details of the patients in the diuretic groups are listed in Table 1. Many of the patients have received several diuretics in serial fashion and thereby enter into more than one of the treatment groups. Most of this treatment was conducted in an open, that is, nonrandomized, nonblinded, manner.

METHODS

Our methods for measurement of total serum cholesterol and triglyceride were described previously (8). Glucose was determined by autoanalyzer methods (9). High-density lipoprotein (HDL) cholesterol was estimated by the same method as total cholesterol after precipitation of serum with heparin and manganese (10). HDL cholesterol was measured in 10 patients treated with chlorthalidone, 26 treated with hydrochlorothiazide, and 12 treated with furosemide. Serum insulin was determined by radioimmunoassay using commercial kits (11).

All clinical and laboratory measurements taken before, or at least 3 weeks after, discontinuation of antihypertensive therapy were averaged and used as the control value for each individual. Measurements obtained during successive 6-month intervals of continuous single-agent diuretic therapy were compared to the control values. If multiple, measurements for each patient were averaged during each 6-month interval.

Table 1. Details of patients during diuretic treatment.

Category	Chlorthal.	H-thiazide.	Spirono.	Furosemide
Number	41	54	27	14
Male–female	21–20	29–25	16–11	10– 4
Black–white	17–24	15–39	7–20	7– 7
Age (years)*	49 ± 10	51 ± 13	56 ± 10	51 ± 12
Relative weight (% above ideal)*	16 ± 18	15 ± 15	12 ± 15	19 ± 35
Systolic blood pressure (mmHg)*	163 ± 20	162 ± 21	165 ± 25	157 ± 28
Diastolic blood pressure (mmHg)*	103 ± 11	100 ± 13	97 ± 13	104 ± 11
Total cholesterol (mg/dl)*	221 ± 37	225 ± 38	224 ± 44	233 ± 44
Fasting triglyceride (mg/dl)*	109 ± 51	142 ± 102	116 ± 58	128 ± 64
HDL cholesterol (mg/dl)*	47 ± 12	48 ± 16	ND	66 ± 16

ND, not determined.
* Mean ± SD.

In the statistical analysis, treatment values were compared to control values using paired data t-tests. When fewer than 20 persons comprised a group, means that were statistically different at the 5% level of confidence were checked by non-parametric tests (i.e., the Wilcoxon signed rank test) before accepting statistical significance. The association between changes in variables during treatment was analyzed by linear regression using the method of least squares or Pearson's product moment correlation (12).

RESULTS

Figures 1 and 2 summarize the effects of chlorthalidone, hydrochlorothiazide, and spironolactone on total cholesterol and triglyceride. Chlorthalidone caused an increase in cholesterol and triglyceride of approximately 15 and 35 mg/dl, respectively, during continuous treatment up to 12 months in duration. Hydrochlorothiazide caused an increase in cholesterol of 10 and 47 mg/dl in the first and third 6-month intervals, respectively, of continuous treatment. In the 12–18 month interval, triglyceride was also increased. HDL cholesterol did not change during treatment with chlorthalidone or hydrochlorothiazide. Spironolactone did not cause an increase in total cholesterol. Rather, it increased triglyceride by 28 mg/dl during the 6–12 month interval of treatment. We have studied furosemide only recently. During treatment ranging up to 6 months in duration, it produced no change in total cholesterol or triglyceride (Table 2). In contrast to chlorthalidone and hydrochlo-

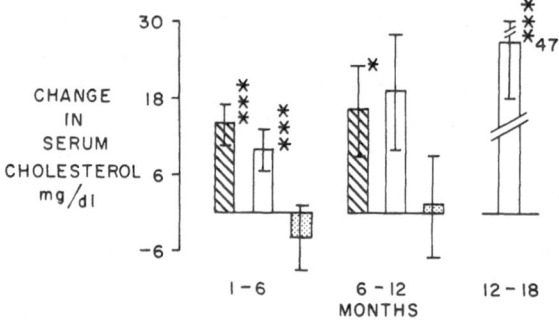

Fig. 1. The bars represent the average change in total serum cholesterol from the base-line value for measurements obtained during successive 6-month intervals following the start of individual diuretic drugs. For chlorthalidone ▨, 40 persons were studied in the first treatment interval and 9 in the second. For hydrochlorothiazide ▢, 53 persons were studied in the first, 23 in the second, and 9 in the third treatment interval. For spironolactone ▨, 26 individuals were studied in the first and 12 in the second treatment period. ⁑, $p < 0.001$; * $p < 0.05$ versus baseline values.

rothiazide, furosemide caused a decrease in HDL cholesterol. HDL cholesterol was not measured during treatment with spironolactone.

The total cholesterol to HDL cholesterol (TC/HDL) ratio, a strong predictor of CHD (13), was not increased by any individual diuretic. Combining the diuretics, the TC/HDL ratio increased significantly (4.76–5.06, $p < 0.05$).

We measured fasting insulin before and during treatment with chlorthalidone and hydrochlorothiazide. Insulin increased with both diuretics (Fig. 3). During the 12–18-month interval of treatment

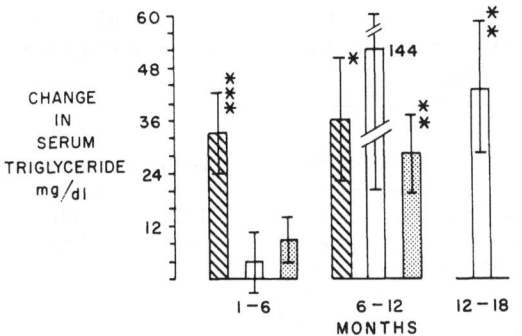

Fig. 2. Changes in serum triglyceride from control values, studied in the same patients as in Fig. 1, are displayed in similar fashion as cholesterol in Fig. 1. Triglyceride increased significantly in at least one treatment interval for each drug. The dose of diuretic did not vary appreciably among treatment periods. (see Table 3). ▨, Chlorthalidone; ◻, hydrochlorothiazide; ▦, spironolactone. $\overset{*}{\underset{*}{*}}$ $p < 0.001$; $\overset{*}{*}$ $p < 0.025$; * $p < 0.05$ versus base-line values.

Table 2. Serum lipids before and during treatment of hypertension with furosemide ($N = 13$).

Serum lipid	Control (mg/dl)	Treatment (mg/dl)
Total cholesterol	233	236
Triglyceride	128	166
HDL cholesterol	67	60*

* $p > 0.05$ versus control value.

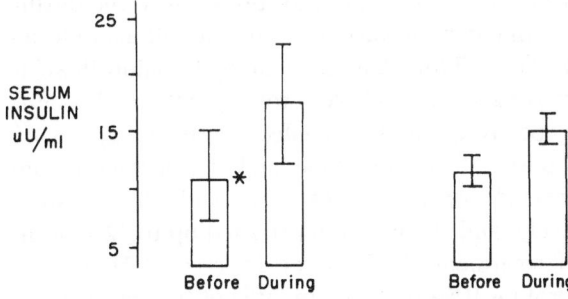

Fig. 3. The bars represent the serum concentration of fasting insulin before and during the first 6-month interval of treatment with chlorthalidone ($N = 13$, $p < 0.05$) and hydrochlorothiazide ($N = 41$, $p < 0.01$). * Mean ± SEM.

with hydrochlorothiazide, insulin was also significantly increased (control 10, treatment 23 μU/ml, $p < 0.05$) in the 8 patients having paired measurements. Fasting blood sugar was not changed during these intervals except for the first 6 months of treatment with hydrochlorothiazide (control 103, treatment 107 mg/dl, $p < 0.01$).

DISCUSSION

This study extends our previous observations on serum lipid changes during diuretic treatment of hypertension by showing that the increases continue in our population for up to 18 months of therapy. In addition, HDL cholesterol measurements are now available. Chlorthalidone and hydrochlorothiazide caused no change, in agreement with a previous report (14). However, furosemide caused a decrease in HDL cholesterol. Thus, all the diuretics that we have reported to date have caused a change in the serum concentration of one or more lipids. Peculiarly, each diuretic has caused a different pattern of change. The clinical importance as well as the mechanisms of these responses remains for further study.

Searching for mechanisms of the lipid disturbance, we examined serum insulin concentrations because insulin may stimulate hepatic triglyceride synthesis (15). Fasting insulin increased during diuretic treatment. Despite the higher insulin concentrations, fasting blood sugar was either unchanged or higher. This finding suggests that insulin resistance regularly develops during diuretic treatment. Alternatively, inactive insulin may be secreted during diuretic therapy. We found no correlation between changes in insulin and changes in serum lipids during treatment. Of interest, insulin may represent yet another risk factor for CHD (16).

A possible clue to the mechanism of the increase in triglyceride may be found in the linear relationship that existed between it and the decrease in systolic blood pressure in patients treated with chlorthalidone (Fig. 4). This relationship did not obtain with the other diuretic drugs, but in contrast to chlorthalidone, neither hydrochlorothiazide nor furosemide increased serum triglyceride. If the increase in triglyceride is hemodynamically triggered, as suggested by the correlation, perhaps the absence of an effect of hydrochlorothiazide

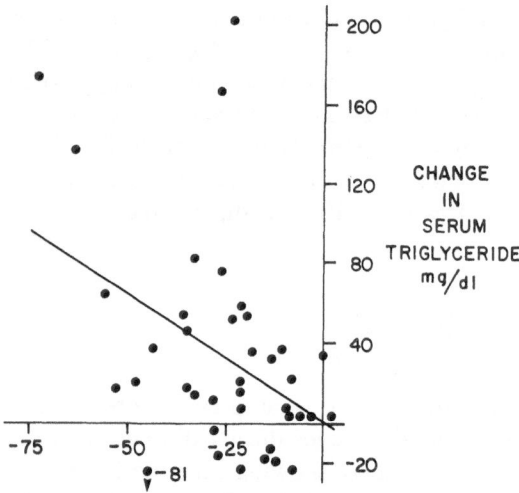

CHANGE IN SYSTOLIC BLOOD PRESSURE mm Hg

Fig. 4. Inverse correlation of the change in triglyceride as a function of the change in systolic blood pressure during the first 6-month period of treatment with chlorthalidone. $r = -0.39$, $N = .39$, $p < 0.02$, $y = 0.43-1.3X$.

and furosemide on triglyceride is explained by the smaller decrease in blood pressure that they induced (Table 3); that is, a large drop in systolic blood pressure may be required before triglyceride rises.

Although the average increase in total cholesterol during diuretic therapy was not large, a subgroup of diuretic-treated patients have more notable elevations. One such subgroup, identified previously, comprises patients less than 50 years of age (17). In this subgroup, the increase in cholesterol averaged 28 mg/dl, and the increase offset the benefit to coronary risk status conferred by the lowering of systolic blood pressure according

Table 3. Changes in blood pressure and drug dose during the first 6 months of treatment.

Drug	ΔSBP (mmHg)	ΔDBP (mmHg)	Dose (mg/day)
Chlorthalidone (C)	−26*	−13***	62
Hydrochlorothiazide (HC)	−16**	−8**	54
Spironolactone (S)	−18**	−7**	58
Furosemide (F)	0	+4	72

SBP, systolic blood pressure; DBP, diastolic blood pressure.
* $p < 0.005$ versus HC and F; ** $p < 0.01$ versus F; *** $p < 0.05$ versus other drugs.

Table 4. Probability of myocardial infarction based on risk factors before and during diuretic therapy.

Risk factors	Before	During	If chol. unchanged
SBP (mmHg)	157	140	140
Chol. (mg/dl)	208	236	208
Probability (%)			
Male age 35	0.9	1.0	0.7
Male age 65	10.1	8.6	8.4

Chol., serum cholesterol.
Source: Gordon and Kannel (18).

to the risk tables (Table 4) (18). In older patients, an increase in cholesterol of this magnitude would not greatly influence the probability of subsequent myocardial infarction (13, 18). This may explain, in part, why the benefit in mortality accrued only to patients over 50 years of age in the Hypertension Detection and Follow-up Program, a study in which diuretics represented first-line drug therapy. Younger patients had no decrease in mortality rate (19). Alternative therapeutic regimens may be required to improve mortality statistics in younger patients with hypertension.

SUMMARY

Because treatment of hypertension based on diuretic drugs does not greatly improve mortality from ischemic heart disease, we studied fasting serum total cholesterol, triglyceride, HDL cholesterol, and insulin concentrations before and during treatment with various common sulfonamide diuretics. Chlorthalidone and hydrochlorothiazide increased total cholesterol by 6% and 4.5%, respectively, and the effect persisted up to 18 months. Chlorthalidone and spironolactone increased triglyceride by 30% and 28%, respectively, and the increase persisted up to 12 months of treatment. Furosemide lowered HDL cholesterol by 10% during 6 months of treatment. Insulin levels increased during treatment with chlorthalidone and hydrochlorothiazide by 57% and 23%, respectively. There was no correlation between changes in lipids and insulin. The increase in triglyceride correlated with the change in systolic blood pressure during treatment with chlorthalidone ($r = -0.39$, $p < 0.02$). The data suggest that attention to lipid metabolism and other metabolic derangements may be needed to bring about further gains against CHD during the treatment of hypertension.

REFERENCES

1. Veterans Administration Cooperative Study Group on Antihypertensive Agents (1970) Effects of treatment on morbidity in hypertension: II. Results in patients with diastolic blood pressure averaging 90 through 114 mmHg. JAMA 213: 1143–1152
2. Smith WM (1977) Treatment of mild hypertension: Results of a ten-year intervention trial. Circ Res 40(Suppl 1): 98–105
3. Hypertension Detection and Follow-up Program Cooperative Group (1979) Five-year findings of the Hypertension Detection and Follow-up Program: I. Reduction in mortality of persons with high blood pressure, including mild hypertension. JAMA 242: 2562–2571
4. Ames RP, Hill P (1976) Increase in serum lipids during the treatment of hypertension with chlorthalidone. Lancet 1: 721–723
5. Gluck Z, Baumgartner G, Weidmann P, Peheim E, Bachmann C, Mordasini R, Flammer J, Keusch G (1978) Increased ratio between serum B- and A-lipoproteins during diuretic therapy: An adverse effect? Clin Sci Mol Med 55: 325S–328S
6. Bauer JH, Brooks CS, Burch RN (1979) Study of ticrynafen and hydrochlorothiazide alone and with propranolol in hypertensive man. Postgrad Med Communications 73–86
7. Helgeland A, Hjermann I, Holme I, Leren P (1978) Serum triglycerides and serum uric acid in untreated and thiazide-treated patients with mild hypertension. Am J Med 64: 34–38
8. Ames RP, Hill P (1976) Elevation of serum lipid levels during diuretic therapy of hypertension. Am J Med 61: 748–757
9. Hunter WH (1967) Automated simultaneous determination of blood glucose and urea. J Med Lab Technol 24: 293–300
10. Friedewald WT, Levy RI, Frederickson DS (1972) Estimation of the concentration of low density lipoprotein cholesterol without the use of preparative ultracentrifugation. Clin Chem 18: 499–502
11. Yalow RS, Berson SA (1960) The immunoassay of endogenous plasma insulin in man. J Clin Invest 39: 1157–1175
12. Colton T (1974) Statistics in medicine. Little, Brown, Boston, Mass, p 219
13. Kannel WB, Castelli WP, Gordon T (1979) Cholesterol in the prediction of atherosclerotic disease. Ann Intern Med 90: 85–91
14. Perry HM Jr, Goldman AI, Schnaper HW, Fitz AE, Frohlich ED, Steele B, Richman HG, Tosch T, Lavin MA (1979) Effects of chlorthalidone and reserpine in the treatment of mild hypertension: Induced changes with emphasis on blood pressure and chemistry. In: Gross F, Strasser T (eds) Mild hypertension: Natural history and management. Pitman Medical, Bath, pp 206–220
15. Olefsky JM, Farquhar JW, Reaven GM (1974) Reappraisal of the role of insulin in hypertriglyceridemia. Am J Med 57: 551–560
16. Pyorala K, Nikkila EA, Taskinen MR, Siltanen P, Punsar S (1979) Plasma insulin as coronary heart disease risk factor (abstr). Am J Cardiol 43: 436
17. Ames RP, Hill P (1978) Raised serum lipid concentrations during diuretic treatment of hypertension: A study of predictive indexes. Clin Sci Mol Med 55(Suppl 4): 311S–314S
18. Gordon T, Kannel WB (1973) Coronary risk handbook. American Heart Association, New York
19. Hypertension Detection and Follow-up Program Cooperative Group (1979) Five-year findings of the Hypertension Detection and Follow-up Program: II. Mortality by race-sex and age. JAMA 242: 2572–2577

Sodium and Blood Pressure: A New Zealand Study

F. O. Simpson and Judith Paulin

It is an attractive thought that hypertension could be prevented by reducing the intake of salt. The saving in human suffering from vascular disease and in money spent on antihypertensive drugs would be enormous. However, most people like a good deal of salt in their food and it seemed to us that before leaning heavily on people to persuade them to reduce salt intake, we had an obligation to obtain evidence that salt eating really is harmful.

Accordingly, when the opportunity presented itself, we did a survey in the small town of Milton, 50 km south of Dunedin. (1, 2) Among other things we measured BP (three measurements over 5 min; subject seated; electronic version of London School of Hygiene blind manometer), height and weight, and 24-h excretion of Na, K, and Cr. We also collected data on the taking of oral contraceptives and antihypertensive medication, but it makes little difference to the analyses whether these subjects are included are not.

BP rose with age, as in all Western communities, particularly the systolic and particularly in the women. The mean intake of Na was 173 mEq/24 h for men and 140 mEq/24 hr for women. These values were very similar to those found for patients referred to the Dunedin Hypertension Clinic. Multiple regression analysis showed that both systolic and diastolic pressures were related to age, body mass index (Quetelet's), and pulse rate but not to Na output, Na/K ratio, or Na/Cr ratio. The use of Na/height ratio made very little difference, though it is probably a more logical parameter to use as kidney size is likely to be related to height; a tall person should have more reserve capacity to handle a Na load than a short person. Na excretion is quite strongly related to body weight and to body mass index, probably reflecting the amount of food eaten.

The original report of these findings (3) and the subsequent discussion (4) seemed to add some fuel to the controversy over salt and hypertension. Certainly it is a subject that needs discussing. If it is true that most hypertension could be abolished by reducing average Na intake to less than 70 mEq/day, then we should be doing much more about it. If it is not true, then we should stop worrying about it.

The problem is to sort out hard fact from cherished theory. Originally it was said that people who used the salt shaker heavily were more hypertensive than those who did not (5). This could not be confirmed (6), and certainly inquiry about salt added at the table is a highly unreliable guide to 24-h output of Na. Dahl (7) then said that the estimation of salt-shaker use was only helpful if it reflected the total amount of salt eaten daily. The clear implication was, and still is, that within a population those people who eat large amounts of salt are more liable to become hypertensive than those who eat less. But, as we all know, this has not really proved to be the case. One study in Australia reported that male hypertensives referred to a clinic had higher 24-h Na excretion than normotensive or mildly hypertensive people (male and female) in a population survey (8). But as previously reviewed (4), a number of other studies have failed to demonstrate any correlation between Na intake (assessed as 24-h Na output) and blood pressure within a population, or to demonstrate any difference between hypertensives and normotensives in a given population. Indeed, one study showed that sodium output was actually *lower* in 50-year-old men with hypertension than in normotensive men of the same age (9).

The question arises of course as to whether 24-h collections of urine for Na are inherently so inaccurate that they are unreliable as measures of Na intake. We asked a subgroup of subjects (those with the 12 highest and the 12 lowest Na excretions, and 43 others selected on criteria irrelevant to BP or Na) in the Milton survey to collect another 24-h urine 2 months later. In a simple correlation analysis comparing the first and second values for Na excretion in these subjects, there was a highly significant correlation, r value being 0.72 (Fig. 1); the slope of the line is less than 45°, in keeping with some regression toward the mean, as is not unexpected considering that the highest and lowest excretors of Na had been selected. Whether this result is taken as indicating good or poor repeatability probably depends on one's point of view. Twenty-four hour urine collections have their problems, but we have really no better guide to Na intake. In our 1978 survey, we did not do 24-h collections of urine, but we obtained samples of the second voiding of urine in the morning by the women (no breakfast having been eaten). Na/K ratio in these spot urines (but not Na/Cr ratio) turned out to be slightly, though significantly, related to systolic BP. However, the variance of these ratios was very high (Table 1) and the values ranged 0.5–74.0 for Na/Cr and 0.09–10.39 for Na/K. It seems probable that something other than Na intake was affecting the findings (e.g., the effect of change of posture on renal function).

Another possible reason for failure to find a link between salt and hypertension within a population is that only some people are genetically susceptible to salt-induced hypertension (10); the work showing, for instance, abnormalities in erythrocyte

Table 1. Na/Cr and Na/K ratios in the second morning voiding of urine by women in the 1978 Milton survey.

Age	N	Na/Cr (mEq)*	Na/K (mEq)*
16–19	48	10.2 ± 6.16	2.2 ± 1.69
20–29	132	12.0 ± 10.11	1.6 ± 0.98
30–39	114	10.9 ± 6.95	1.6 ± 1.05
40–49	89	11.6 ± 6.45	1.8 ± 1.08
50–59	93	13.5 ± 12.17	1.9 ± 1.49
60–69	86	14.0 ± 10.59	2.1 ± 1.46
70 +	46	15.3 ± 10.37	2.6 ± 1.81
Total	608	12.4 ± 9.49	1.9 ± 1.33

* Mean ± SD.

membrane binding of Ca^{2+} in hypertensives (11) and of abnormalities in erythrocyte membrane Na^{+}/K^{+} fluxes in families with hypertension is certainly exciting (12), but the facts are as yet by no means clear. In addition, hypertension is relatively so common after the age of 50 that it is difficult to accept that genetic factors would obscure the picture entirely.

It has been suggested that Na excretion may be reduced in hypertensive subjects because of a defect in the hypertensive kidney. But it cannot be as simple as that, because the subjects in epidemiologic studies must be presumed to be in Na equilibrium.

A further possibility is that subjects who know they are hypertensive deliberately eat less salt be-

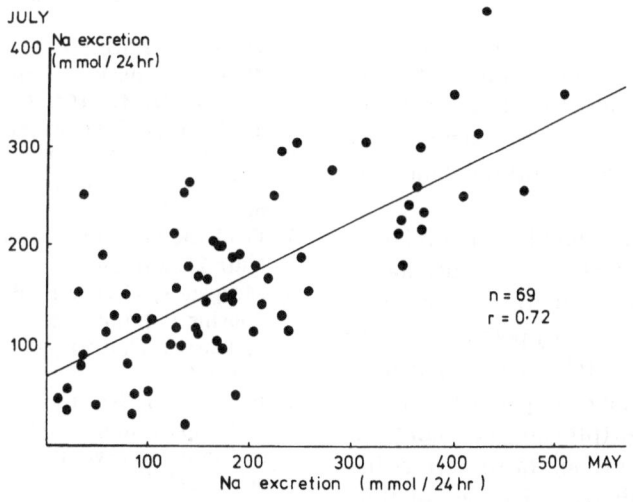

Fig. 1. Relationship between a single 24-hour sodium excretion value in May 1975 and a second one in July 1975.

cause they have heard it is bad for them, and this may happen in some cases. However, the subjects studied by Berglund et al. (9) did not know that they were hypertensive, and the same was the case in many subjects in our study in 1975.

Finally, there is the possibility that when people become hypertensive, they instinctively take less salt (13). This could, for instance, be due to a damping down of the renin angiotensin system; angiotensin is reported to increase salt appetite in animals (14). Such a trend, toward less salt appetite as BP rises, would certainly prove a link between Na and hypertension within a very difficult population, and it has to be accepted as a possible explanation of the hitherto negative findings.

Thus, if there is a link between salt intake and hypertension in man, we probably have to postulate that: a) there are genetic differences in susceptibility (which do not seem unreasonable); and b) when a person becomes hypertensive, salt appetite is reduced slightly compared with other people in the same community. There is nothing wrong with the latter as a working hypothesis, or (less kindly put) as a final fall-back position for the salt theory of hypertension, but it is certainly not proved.

SUMMARY

A community study on 1,200 adults in Milton, a small town near Dunedin, showed a highly significant relationship of blood pressure (BP) to age and body mass (Quetelet's) index, but not to 24-h sodium output. The use of sodium/potassium (Na/K), sodium/creatinine (Na/Cr), or height Na/ratio did not alter the picture significantly. Mean daily Na output was 173 mEq for men and 140 mEq for women.

Possible causes for the failure to find a relationship between Na excretion and BP include: inaccuracies in the data or unrepresentativeness of single-day collections of urine (certainly possible); genetic differences in susceptibility (also possible); deliberate reduction in salt intake by persons knowing that they are hypertensive (probably not significant in this population at the time); instinctive reduction in salt intake as BP rises. The last of these causes would certainly make it impossible to find a relationship between salt intake and BP within a population. It is also possible that salt intake, at least at the level found in this population, is not an important factor in causing hypertension. Further data are required.

ACKNOWLEDGMENTS

The Milton surveys were supported by the National Heart Foundation of New Zealand and the Medical Research Council of New Zealand. The surveys were a collaborative effort by many colleagues. The author is grateful to Dr Ailsa Goulding, Department of Medicine, for the 1978 urinary Na, K, and Cr values.

REFERENCES

1. Simpson FO, Nye ER, Bolli P, Waal-Manning Hendrika J, Goulding AW, Phelan EL, de Hamel FA, Stewart RDH, Spears GFS, Leek GM, Stewart AC (1978) The Milton survey: I. General methods, height, weight and 24-hour excretion of sodium, potassium, calcium, magnesium and creatinine. NZ Med J 87: 379–382
2. Simpson FO, Waal-Manning HJ, Bolli P, Spears GFS (1978) The Milton survey: II. Blood pressure and heart rate. NZ Med J 88: 1–4
3. Simpson FO, Waal-Manning HJ, Bolli P, Phelan EL, Spears GFS (1978) Relationship of blood pressure to sodium excretion in a population survey. Clin Sci Mol Med 55: 373S–375S
4. Simpson FO (1979) Salt and hypertension: A sceptical review of the evidence. Clin Sci Mol Med 57: 463S–469S
5. Dahl LK, Love RA (1957) Etiological role of sodium chloride intake in essential hypertension in humans. JAMA 164: 397–399
6. Tobian L (1974) Current status of salt in hypertension. In: Paul O (ed) Epidemiology and control of hypertension. Symposium Specialists, Miami, Fla, pp 131–146
7. Dahl LK (1972) Salt and hypertension. Am J Clin Nutr 25: 231–244
8. Morgan T, Carney S, Wilson M (1975) Interrelationship in humans between sodium intake and hypertension. Clin Exp Pharmacol Physiol [Suppl] 2: 127–129
9. Berglund G, Wikstrand J, Wallentin I, Wilhelmsen L (1976) Sodium excretion and sympathetic activity in relation to severity of hypertensive disease. Lancet 1: 324–328
10. Tobian L (1979) Interrelationships of sodium and hypertension. In: Onesti G, Klimt CR (eds) Hypertension: Determinants, complications, and interven-

tion. Fifth Hahnemann International Symposium on Hypertension. Grune & Stratton, New York

11. Gulak PV, Boriskina GM, Postnov YV (1979) Ca^{2+}-binding to erythrocyte membrane of hypertensive men and rats: Effects of acetylcholine and eserine. Experientia 35: 1471–1472

12. Garay RP, Dagher G, Pernollet MG, Devynck MA, Meyer P (1980) Inherited defect in a Na^+, K^+ co-transport system in erythrocytes from essential hypertensive patients. Nature 284: 281–283

13. Morgen T (1979) In round table 2: Salt intake and hypertension. Clin Sci Mol Med 57: 479S

14. Fitzsimons JT (1978) Angiotensin, thirst, and sodium appetite: Retrospect and prospect. Fed Proc 37: 2669–2675

Blood Pressure in Sodium Fed Humans

Myron H. Weinberger, Friedrich C. Luft, Richard Bloch, David P. Henry, Arthur E. Weyman, and Laura I. Rankin

Evidence for a relationship between sodium intake and arterial blood pressure in humans is largely circumstantial (1). Epidemiologic studies demonstrating a spectrum of association between magnitude of sodium intake and blood pressure (2, 3) may have been limited by potential genetic factors. We performed a series of experiments to determine: a) whether acute sodium loading can raise blood pressure in normotensive men; b) to examine the threshold as well as possible racial differences of blood pressure response to sodium; and c) to define the mechanisms by which blood pressure changes were induced and compensated for, and to explore the potential significance of such observations to hypertension.

MATERIALS AND METHODS

In the first of 2 experiments, 14 normotensive men (aged 18–40 years) without a family history of hypertension were studied. Seven of the subjects were white and seven black. The experimental protocols were approved by the Indiana University Human Use Committee and each subject voluntarily participated in the study and provided informed consent after detailed explanation of the procedures to be performed. The subjects received a constant diet containing 10 mEq sodium, 80 mEq potassium, 65 g protein, 50 g fat, 270 g carbohydrate, 400 mg calcium, and 1,000 mg phosphorus daily. Dietary sodium intake was maintained at 10 mEq for 7 days; then, supplemental sodium chloride was added to provide 300 mEq/day for 3 days (all 14 subjects), 600 mEq/day for 3 days (6 subjects), 800 mEq/day for 3 days (8 subjects), 1,200 mEq/day for 3 days (6 subjects), and 1,500

mEq/day for 3 days (8 subjects). To achieve the sodium intake of 1,200 and 1,500 mEq/day, 800 mEq/day were given orally, and supplemental sodium was given intravenously in the form of normal (0.9%) saline at night. Fluid intake (distilled water) was allowed *ad libitum*.

The subjects were weighed every morning before breakfast after voiding. Blood pressure was measured by the indirect auscultatory technique three times daily after 5 min of supine rest. Mean arterial pressure was calculated by adding one-third the pulse pressure to the diastolic pressure. Twenty-four hour urine collections were obtained daily in acetic acid for determination of sodium, potassium, creatinine, and norepinephrine. At 7:00 AM of the final day at each level of sodium intake, blood samples were obtained following 2 h of ambulation for hematocrit, creatinine, sodium, potassium, plasma renin activity, aldosterone, and norepinephrine. Stroke index and cardiac index were measured noninvasively by echocardiography on the final day at each level of sodium intake (4). In six of the subjects, a second study was performed, identical to the first except that urinary potassium losses that occurred at higher levels of sodium intake were prevented by administration of oral potassium daily. The amount was calculated from the previous day's urinary losses.

Sodium and potassium concentrations in plasma and urine were measured by a flame photometer (Instrumentation Laboratories, Boston, Mass.). Creatinine was measured by an automated technique (Technicon, Chauncey, New York). Plasma renin activity and plasma aldosterone were measured by radioimmunoassay (5) and plasma and urinary norepinephrine concentrations by a radioenzymatic technique (6). The data were analyzed statistically by two-way repeated measures analysis of variance.

RESULTS

On the final day of each level of sodium intake, urinary sodium excretion approached balance. Potassium was retained during the low-sodium period of both studies. In the first study, urinary potassium losses were seen at sodium intakes of 600 mEq/day and higher; in the second study, such losses were replaced daily to avoid potassium depletion and to evaluate the effect of potassium on the blood pressure response to sodium loading. Cumulative sodium balance in study 1 was not significantly different between blacks and whites [1,163 ± 172 (SEM) mEq and 1,084 ± 268 mEq, respectively]. No significant racial differences in sodium balance were seen in study 2 (blacks 1,375 ± 518; white 1,001 ± 534). However, whites lost significantly more ($p < 0.01$) potassium (356 ± 58 mEq) than did blacks (45 ± 60 mEq) during the first experiment. In the second study, potassium losses were prevented by dietary potassium supplementation. Changes in body weight were similar between races in both studies. No consistent changes in plasma sodium or potassium were observed during either study.

Changes in mean arterial blood pressure for the entire group in both studies are shown in Table 1. A significant interaction ($p < 0.05$) between sodium intake and blood pressure was observed in both studies. Furthermore, changes in blood pressure from the lowest to highest sodium intake levels were correlated with cumulative sodium balance ($r = 0.52$, $p < 0.03$). When potassium depletion was prevented in the second study, mean arterial pressure was significantly lower ($p < 0.05$) at the 800- and 1,500-mEq levels when compared to the initial study. Differences in theshold and magnitude of blood pressure responses to sodium

intake were observed between black and white subjects in both studies. The whites developed a significant ($p < 0.05$) increase in systolic and diastolic pressure at the 1,200-mEq/day level of study 1 when compared to the 10-mEq/day intake, whereas the blacks developed significant increases ($p < 0.05$) at the 800-mEq/day intake. In the second study, significant changes in blood pressure were seen only in blacks who had higher ($p < 0.05$) systolic pressures at the end of the 1,500-mEq/day period.

DISCUSSION

The observations from the present study clearly show that arterial blood pressure can be raised acutely in normotensive man by increasing sodium intake to very high levels. In conjunction with previous reports (7–10), this study indicates that massive increases in sodium intake are necessary to consistently elevate the blood pressure of normotensive subjects. In the present study, we were able to identify significant differences in the blood pressure response to dietary sodium loading of black and white subjects. Coupled with the known increased prevalence of hypertension among black Americans, these observations suggest that a genetic predisposition to salt sensitivity of blood pressure may also exist in man. A previous report from our laboratory (11) indicated that blacks excreted an intravenous salt load less well than whites and that their plasma–renin activity was more suppressed by the salt load compared to whites. Since in the present and previous studies (12) blacks and whites had similar creatinine and PAH clearances, and since their levels of renin and aldosterone were not different, some other fac-

Table 1. Blood pressure responses to sodium loading.

Sodium intake (mEq/24 h)	No potassium replacement		Potassium replacement	
	Systolic	Diastolic	Systolic	Diastolic
	(mmHg)		(mmHg)	
10	111 ± 2	69 ± 3	114 ± 2	67 ± 5
300	116 ± 2	71 ± 3	115 ± 3	65 ± 5
800	121 ± 3	76 ± 3	122 ± 4	69 ± 5
1,500	131 ± 4	85 ± 3	124 ± 4	72 ± 5

Significant increases ($p < 0.05$) in stroke index and in cardiac index were seen in both studies. Pulse rate decreased significantly ($p < 0.05$) in both experiments.

tor must be responsible for the observed differences.

In the present study, whites and blacks developed similar degrees of sodium retention following sodium loading. In contrast, blacks differed from whites in their excretory pattern of potassium. During the 10-mEq/day period, both groups were in net-positive potassium balance; however, the blacks accumulated more potassium than did whites. With the onset of sodium loading in study 1, all subjects excreted increasing amounts of potassium; however, the whites did so to a greater degree. The kaliuretic response following sodium loading in both groups of subjects may be attributed to increased sodium delivery to the distal nephron (13). It is also possible that some of the kaliuresis may have followed physical displacement of potassium from intracellular stores by sodium (9). By the end of study 1, whites had lost significantly more potassium than blacks. These differences cannot be explained by differences in natriuresis, plasma renin activity, or plasma aldosterone concentration. Racial differences in potassium excretion have been previously observed by Langford and Watson (14) who found that although blacks and whites excreted similar amounts of sodium, blacks excreted less potassium. Their observations suggest that blacks ingest less potassium than whites. In addition, we reported that following an acute intravenous saline infusion, or after furosemide, blacks consistently excreted less potassium than whites (11). These differences and those observed in the first experiment of the present study are probably not related to a lower total body potassium content in blacks. Meneely et al. (15) and Cohn and colleagues (16) found that black men and women had higher total body potassium content than whites. Thus, it would appear that blacks have potassium regulatory mechanisms different from those of whites.

In the first series of experiments, it was apparent that increases in blood pressure with sodium loading were accompanied by appreciable urinary losses of potassium, particularly in white subjects. Six subjects agreed to be restudied under conditions in which losses of potassium were prevented. These six subjects failed to increase their blood pressure with sodium loading to the same degree when potassium loss was prevented. The mechanism responsible for this blunting of the blood pressure-raising effect of sodium in the second study is not clear.

In summary, these observations demonstrate that sodium excess can raise blood pressure in normotensive men. Differences in sensitivity and magnitude of the blood pressure response can be seen between black and white men. The prevention of potassium loss consequent to massive sodium loading attenuates the rise in blood pressure. The renin aldosterone system and the sympathetic nervous system are markedly suppressed by massive sodium loading and do not appear to participate in the increase in blood pressure. Finally, the increase in arterial pressure seen with sodium loading appears to correlate with an increase in cardiac index. Further examination of factors that may reduce the ability of the kidney to excrete sodium would appear to be relevant to clarify more fully the role of sodium in the pathogenesis of hypertension.

SUMMARY

Fourteen normotensive men (seven black, seven white) were studied following equilibration during dietary sodium intake of 10, 300, 600, 800, 1,200, and 1,500 mEq sodium/day. Significant ($p < 0.05$) increases in mean arterial blood pressure were seen after sodium intake of 800 mEq/day. Blood pressure increased at lower levels of sodium intake (800 mEq/day) and to a greater magnitude (21 mmHg) in blacks than in whites (1,200 mEq/day; 13 mmHg). Sodium loading was associated with marked suppression of plasma renin activity, aldosterone, and norepinephrine and increases in cardiac index. At higher levels of sodium intake, urinary potassium loss was seen. A subsequent experiment replacing urinary potassium losses as they occurred in six subjects demonstrated attenuation of the blood pressure increases seen in response to dietary sodium loading. These studies demonstrate a potential role for sodium and potassium in blood pressure regulation in normotensive man, and suggest that heterogeneity of response may be involved in the development of hypertension in individuals predisposed to avid sodium conservation.

REFERENCES

1. Freis ED (1975) Salt, volume and the prevention of hypertension. Circulation 53: 589–595

2. Tobian L (1978) Salt and hypertension. Ann NY Acad Sci 304: 178–197
3. Michell AR (1978) Salt appetite, salt intake and hypertension. Perspect Biol Med 21: 335–347
4. Feigenbaum H, Popp RL, Wolfe SB, Troy BL, Pombo JF, Haine CL, Dodge HT (1972) Ultrasound measurements of the left ventricle. Arch Intern Med 129: 461–467
5. Weinberger MH, Kem DC, Gomez-Sanchez C, Kramer NJ, Martin BT, Nugent CA (1975) The effect of dexamethasone on the control of plasma aldosterone concentration in normal recumbent man. J Lab Clin Med 85: 957–967
6. Henry DP, Starman BT, Johnson DG, Williams RH (1975) A sensitive radioenzymatic assay for norepinephrine in tissue and plasma. Life Sci 16: 375–384
7. McDonough J, Wilhelm CM (1954) The effect of excess salt intake on human blood pressure. Am J Dig Dis 21: 180–181
8. McQuarrie I, Thompson WH, Anderson JA (1936) Effects of excessive ingestion of sodium and potassium salt in carbohydrate metabolism and blood pressure in diabetic children. J Nutr 11: 77–101
9. Kirkendall WM, Conner WE, Abboud F, Rastogi SP, Anderson TA, Fry M (1976) The effect of dietary sodium chloride on blood pressure, body fluids, electrolytes, renal function, and serum lipids of normotensive man. J Lab Clin Med 87: 418–434
10. Dahl LK (1972) Salt and hypertension. Am J Clin Nutr 25: 231–244
11. Luft FC, Grim CE, Higgins JT, Weinberger MH (1977) Differences in response to sodium administration in normotensive white and black subjects. J Lab Clin Med 90: 555–562
12. Luft FC, Rankin LI, Bloch R, Weyman AE, Willis LR, Murray RH, Grim CE, Weinberger MH (1979) Cardiovascular and humoral responses to extremes of sodium intake in normal black and white men. Circulation 60: 697–706
13. Diezi J, Michoud P, Aceves J (1973) Micropuncture study of electrolyte transport across capillary collecting duct of the rat. Am J Physiol 224: 623–634
14. Langford HG, Watson RC (1973) Electrolytes, environment and blood pressure. Clin Sci Mol Med 45: 1115–1135
15. Meneely GR, Heyssel RM, Ball COT (1963) Analysis of factors affecting body composition determined from potassium content of 915 normal subjects. Ann NY Acad Sci 110: 271–281
16. Cohn SH, Abesamis C, Zani I, Aloia JF, Yasumura S, Ellis KJ (1977) Body elemental composition: Comparison between black and white adults. Clin J Physiol 232: E419–E422

Adverse Effects of Diuretic Therapy

T. Morgan, J. Myers, and W. Adam

INTRODUCTION

This study reports our experience with the use of thiazide diuretics compared with other drugs in the treatment of mild hypertension and reports an increased number of myocardial infarcts in the thiazide-treated group. The patients in the study were all men born between 1900 and 1925 and entered into the study between 1972 and 1978. After several blood pressure readings, patients were divided into three groups according to the diastolic blood pressure. The only exclusion to entry into the study was the presence of a neoplasm, severe psychiatric disturbance, physical incapacity, or the presence of a disease likely to cause death within 2 years. Vascular diseases or previous vascular accidents were not an exclusion. A total of 373 patients entered the study and were subdivided as in Table 1 and then, within each group, were randomly assigned to different therapeutic regimens. The effect of these regimens on blood pressure has been reported previously (1), and is briefly summarized in Table 1. The status of all subjects at 1 November 1978 was known at the time of this analysis. The data have been analyzed, taking note of the age of the patient and the time of entry, and compared between the different groups and with the "normal" Australian population. These results have recently been reported (2).

RESULTS

The mortality of the different groups is expressed in Table 2 as per 100,000 patient days; in Table 3, the mortality is compared with that predicted for a group of similar age and entry point.

In these tables, it can be observed that one group is markedly different from the others. The group with mild hypertension treated with thiazide diuretics has an increased overall mortality compared with all other groups. This increased mortal-

Table 1. Allocation of patients to different groups.

Group	Therapy	N	Diastolic blood pressure (mmHg)	Initial blood pressure (mmHg)	Last blood pressure (mmHg)
I.	None	104	<95	144/88	151/93
II.	None	42	≥95, <110	155/102	156/101
	Diet	35		155/102	145/95
	Thiazide	55		164/104	146/94
	β-Blocker	40		164/105	144/94
III.	Thiazide	51	>110	178/118	146/94
	β-Blocker	46		173/117	144/93

Diet = advice regarding salt restriction.

Table 2. Mortality rate of each group per 100,000 days in the study.

Group	Mortality rate
I. No therapy	7.91
II. No therapy	9.25
Diet	8.00
Thiazide	19.23*
β-Blocker	7.66
III. Thiazide	6.03
β-Blocker	9.97

* $p < 0.01$.

Table 4. Total number of infarcts or sudden death in each group.

Group	No. of patients	Fatal	Nonfatal	Total
I. No therapy	104	3	5	8
II. No therapy	42	2	3	5
Diet	35	2	3	5
Thiazide	55	10	1	11
β-Blocker	40	4	3	7
III. Thiazide	51	2	3	5
β-Blocker	46	2	3	5

ity was due to an increased number of deaths from myocardial infarction or sudden death (Table 3). The patients with diastolic blood pressure $\geqslant 110$ mmHg treated with a thiazide diuretic did not show this effect. In Table 4, the number of nonfatal myocardial infarcts in each group is indicated. The data for this table are not as rigorous as in the mortality estimation and are an underestimation.

Patients given thiazide diuretics were not routinely given potassium supplements. Serum potassium was measured at 6-month intervals. The mean serum potassium of all patients who died of myocardial infarction or sudden death was 4.4 mEq/liter at their visit prior to death. Thus, hypokalemia did not appear to be a factor in the cause of death.

No significant difference was seen between the initial plasma renin activity of patients who died of a myocardial infarct and age-matched controls.

DISCUSSION

Elderly patients, many with vascular disease, who had a diastolic blood pressure between 95 and 110 mmHg had an increased mortality when treated with a thiazide diuretic. This increased mortality was due to myocardial infarction or sudden death. It appeared to be an increased number of fatal infarcts rather than a marked increase in the number of myocardial infarcts. The same observation was not seen in patients with more severe hypertension, and for a long time this suggested to us that this may be an artefact. The finding may be fortuitous, but it is possible that it is a correct finding. If confirmed in studies presently underway, it would have important therapeutic implications. It could be an explanation of the failure of most studies to show a reduction in myocardial

Table 3. Number of deaths in each group compared with expected number of deaths normalized for 100 patients in each group.

Group	Total deaths Predicted	Total deaths Actual	Myocardial infarcts Predicted	Myocardial infarcts Actual
I. No therapy	12.8	10.6	7.1	2.9
II. No therapy	10.7	11.9	6.2	4.8
Diet	10.0	11.4	6.6	5.7
Thiazide	12.3	23.6*	6.9	18.1*
β-Blocker	11.0	10.0	6.8	10.0
III. Thiazide	10.3	7.8	6.3	3.9
β-Blocker	7.3	10.8	4.6	4.3

* $p < 0.01$.

infarction after therapy for hypertension though other vascular complications are markedly reduced.

SUMMARY

This study reports on the experience with the use of thiazide diuretics in the treatment of mild hypertension as compared with other regimens of treatment in three groups of hypertensive men all born between 1900 and 1925. In the group with mild hypertension (DBP >95 to >110) those treated with thiazide diuretics had an increased overall mortality compared with all other treatment or control groups.

ACKNOWLEDGMENTS

This study was supported by the Australian Department of Veterans' Affairs.

REFERENCES

1. Morgan T, Gillies A, Morgan G, Adam W, Wilson M, and Carney S (1978) Hypertension treated by salt restriction. Lancet 1: 227
2. Morgan T, Adam WR, Hodgson M, Gibberd RW (in press) Failure of therapy to improve prognosis in elderly males with hypertension. Med J Aust

DISCUSSION

Dr. Doyle (Melbourne, Australia) (Chairman): It seems to be fairly clearly established that if one looks at hypertensives as one group and normotensives as another group, it is very difficult to discern any systematic changes in salt excretion or salt intake between these groups of patients. On the other hand, as several speakers have mentioned, there is the possibility of undefined genetic differences or differences in sensitivity between one group and the other. In addition, we have the fascinating differences in thiazides as opposed to salt depletion. Do thiazides have other effects? They appear to have effects on lipids, and they

appear, in the last paper (T. Morgan and J. Myers) at least, to be dangerous. I think we might try and take this discussion in two segments if you are agreeable to that. First, to discuss factors relating to salt intake in hypertension and, second, to perhaps look more closely at the thiazide diuretics.

Dr. Tobian (Minneapolis, Minn.): I feel a flash of understanding on hearing these talks and I would like to try it on the audience here.

I have always wondered why hypertensives did not eat less salt. According to the concept that their kidneys have difficulty getting rid of salt, there should be a tendency to increase body sodium which ought to reduce salt appetite. If that hypothesis is correct, you would expect that they should eat less salt. However, they do not. In a few studies it was shown they ate less, but in large studies like Dr. Simpson just showed us indicated they ate about the same amount of salt. Another part of his data may offer the reason why hypertensives do not eat less salt. Hypertensives are fatter. Fatter people eat more sodium in general. One effect would thus offset the other, and it should come out just about even that hypertensives eat about the same amount of salt as normotensives. Of course, this doesn't disprove at all the concept that salt has something to do with hypertension. It is just not only the amount of salt in the diet that does it, but the capacity of the kidney for the rapid excretion of the salt.

Dr. Simpson (Dunedin, New Zealand): I think what Dr. Tobian says is very reasonable. The only problem is that it is putting the whole burden, as it were, on the matter of whether there are genetic differences in salt handling in our population and again whether these differences form a graded characteristic or are a present or absent type of characteristic. It does seem a little difficult to fit the data into either of these two models, unless you simultaneously postulate that hypertensives tend to eat less salt as they become more hypertensive.

Dr. Bianchi (Milan, Italy): Perhaps an important factor should be discussed when evaluating the effect of sodium intake on blood pressure, and that is the influence of age. There are three observations in this regard. It was shown by Louis Dahl many years ago, that it is possible to produce a stable hypertension by just feeding one sensitive rat with a high-salt diet for 1 week when it is young, and the hypertension could last for all its life without any need for higher salt intake. This is the first observation. The second observation is the common experience for those trying to produce experimental hypertension in rats by treating them with salt and DOCA. You in fact have to treat the rats when they are very young because it is impossible to produce hypertension if you treat adult rats. A third observation comes from my clinical experience, and I am wondering if it is the experience of others here in the audience; that is, if you look at patients ingesting an excess of licorice or other mineralocorticoid, resulting in hypertension, the blood pressure is much higher in young people than in older people. If you keep these three observations in mind, perhaps we could explain the discrepancy that has been shown this morning; that is, it is possible to find a correlation between the salt intake in blood pressure when you look at different populations. Let us say when you correlate the blood pressure and the salt intake of a given population, it is impossible to find a correlation when you study individual patients of the same population. Now, if you admit that you need a high salt intake from an early age to obtain an effect on blood pressure, you might explain this discrepancy; in fact it is likely that the subjects of a given population eat the high or low amount of salt since an early age when the effect of blood pressure may occur. On the contrary, the different salt intakes occurring in adult hypertensive patients of a given population may be the result of habits acquired at a later age.

Dr. Yamori (Izumo, Japan): When we induced experimental hypertension in younger animals, the effect was greater, and I think it depends on the ability of the vasculature to induce adaptive structural changes. That is, the protein synthesis of arterial walls is greater in younger rats, so that the adverse effect of the salt is greater when it is taken excessively by young rats or people.

Dr. Udenfriend (Nutley, New Jersey): We have produced animals that have a maintained hypertension after DOCA and salt are withdrawn. So has Dr. William Hollander (Boston University). If you treat such animals successfully for several months with an antihypertensive drug and then remove the drug, these previously hypertensive animals remain normotensive for life; therefore, it is an effect on the vessel walls of the hypertension. This can be reversed permanently by giving an antihypertensive drug effectively for a sufficiently long period of time.

Dr. Bianchi: I think that you still have to explain why you find a correlation between salt intake and blood pressure among different populations while you do not find a correlation in individual patients of a given population.

Dr. Simpson: Dr. Bianchi's theory is almost unprovable because it would require longitudinal studies from childhood. One of the problems with it for the sodium activists, in your theory, as I understand it, is that it would really make no difference in adult life whether the sodium intake was reduced. That is, the damage would have been done in childhood so sodium intake in adult life would not matter any more.

Dr. Bianchi: This is what the three groups of experiments I mentioned earlier suggest to me.

Dr. Birkenhager (Rotterdam, The Netherlands): I was very much intrigued by Dr. Luft's paper. We have been shifting salt intake in mild hypertensives within a much narrower range (50–150 mEq), and from that experience we calculated that a net difference in salt balance amounting to 1 g was equivalent to 1 mmHg mean arterial pressure. Dr. Luft, I wonder whether you could figure out whether that fits with your data over a much wider range of sodium intake? I might add another question in that you presumably have seen a recent paper by Dr. S. Julius and his group about a biphasic relationship between salt intake and norepinephrine response [Nicholls MG, Kiowski W, Zweifler AY, et al (1980) Hypertension 2: 29]? Plasma norepinephrine was high with a very low sodium intake of approximately 10 mEq, then going down at a level of 100 mEq salt and then going up again at a level of 300 mEq. Now that is rather conflicting with your data. I wonder whether you have also varied the sequence of your dietary intakes as Dr. Julius and his co-workers did.

Dr. Luft (Indianapolis, Ind.): Yes I'm aware of Dr. Julius' paper and I'm really not able to explain the discrepancy. I think one of the major criticisms of our study is that we didn't randomize the dietary sequence. We didn't do that because of technical constraints; that is, the length of the study would have been considerably prolonged. A 1 g sodium accumulation caused approximately 0.6-mmHg increase in mean blood pressure.

Dr. J. Reid (Glasgow, Scotland): I would like to go back to the sodium dose–response relationship that Dr. Simpson introduced and the study from Indiana extends. It is important to interpret some of the experimental data in the stroke-prone and nonstroke prone SHR in terms of salt intake. I would like to ask Dr. Yamori about the salt intake in his rats given 1% salt in drinking water. My rapid calculation is that they would be taking approximately 3–5 g/kg NaCl a day. That would be equivalent in man to an intake of several hundred grams of sodium a day. Therefore, the rats fed 1% and Dahl rats fed 4% and 8% sodium chloride diets are on enormous sodium intakes which might not be comparable or relevant to human behavior.

Dr. Yamori: Yes, I think compared to humans, the intake of salt is high in rats. But, experimentally we can see the effect of salt within a short period under such conditions. As an experimental system, I think it is good.

Dr. J. Reid: Well, I'm not strictly happy. I would like to see the salt-intake range in animals examined to see whether more moderate and comparable salt intakes do have this dramatic effect on morbidity and mortality. I suspect they wouldn't and I suspect this effect is only seen, as in the studies reported from Indiana, at the very high intakes.

Dr. Yamori: If we give smaller doses of salt to rats, it takes a longer time to see the clear effect. However, the life-span is so short in rats that we have to administer a relatively higher dose of salt.

Dr. Tobian: In feeding Dahl rats, the 4% NaCl diet corresponds to a 20-g daily salt intake for 150-lb men. The 8%-NaCl diet would, of course, be twice as great.

Dr. MacGregor (London, England): If Sir Pickering accepts that a high-sodium intake is important in raising blood pressure, whereas a low-sodium intake is not, I would like to ask where is the cutoff point in this normally distributed variable that makes him claim that sodium intake is unimportant in our normal diet?

Sir George Pickering (Oxford, England): I think that Dr. Luft's data made it fairly clear to me that in most human subjects there is a range of sodium intake between approximately 10 and 250 mEq/day within which an increase or a decrease in sodium intake has very little or no effect on blood pressure. Below that range, a decrease reduces blood pressure, but it is very difficult to push it below that range because people feel so beastly on it. We know a lot about the symptoms of salt deficiency. McCance and his pupils showed that you lose your appetite and taste, and you become extremely weak. I would like to ask Dr.

Luft what were the symptoms of too much salt, because this is something that has been studied by very few people; and getting up to these enormous intakes, which you can only do apparently by supplementary intravenous injections, introduces a new range into human behavior about which I would like to learn more.

I would also like to make two other points. First, of course, is that rats and man differ and, second, that there are genetic differences. We know a great deal about their existence. What we don't know much about is in this respect whether the differences represent a continuous distribution or a discontinuous distribution, and I'm not going to guess.

Dr. Doyle: Dr. Luft, what does salt poisoning feel like?

Dr. Luft: Very briefly, I don't think that our study really addresses the question about whether hypertensive individuals respond to sodium restriction. We had really remarkably few symptoms indeed on either end of the spectrum. In order to inject all that sodium, we had to drink a great deal of free water to avoid diarrhea. We had no respiratory symptoms. The major problem, quite frankly, was nocturia and related sleeplessness. Actually, we had no other specific discomfort.

Dr. Freis (Washington, D. C.): I would like to ask Dr. Luft if he began to see an elevation of blood pressure at the time the diet reached a level in which there was an expansion of extracellular volume, and whether there was a correlation between extracellular volume expansion or weight gain and blood pressure rise as he increased the sodium intake.

Dr. Luft: We unfortunately weren't able to measure extracellular volume directly, but as reflected by weight gain the answer is yes.

Dr. Zanchetti (Milan, Italy): I think this issue of salt and hypertension has two different aspects. One is a heuristic one concerning the etiology or the pathogenesis of hypertension. A lot of support in favor of salt as an etiologic factor has come from Dahl's salt-sensitive rats as mentioned earlier. In this context, it may be worth mentioning that some experiments done by Dr. Friedman in Dahl's laboratory showed that these animals are prone to hypertension, not only to sodium-caused hypertension. Indeed, rats of the sodium-sensitive strain could also have developed hypertension when they were maintained on moderate salt but exposed to stressful operant-conditioning procedures. Thus, this strain of rats seems to be really prone to hypertension, whichever the insult that the environment provides to these animals. The second aspect of the issue is a therapeutic one, management of hypertension. The idea of controlling hypertension by a change in the diet and without giving drugs may seem a very appealing one, but I would like to advance a word of caution in this context, because certainly our life habits are deeply inherited, not in our genes but in our culture, and changing our life habits is going to be more difficult, probably less successful, and certainly implying greater psychological violence than giving a pill.

Dr. DeQuattro (Los Angeles, Cal.): I would like to carry Dr. Zanchetti's remarks on Dahl rats back toward man again. Bartter reported that there are some salt-sensitive borderline hypertensive patients who become more hypertensive on a 250-mg Na^+ diet. He thus found a salt-sensitive subgroup. Further, Julius and his colleagues [Nicholls MG, Kiowski W, Zweifler AY, et al (1980) Hypertension 2: 29] found that catecholamines may increase in some hypertensives as you go up the scale on sodium diet. There may be a biphasic catecholamine response in some hypertensives who have a response in the sympathetic nervous system to salt; thus, their blood pressures are salt sensitive because of their sympathetic nervous system response. We have all seen certain patients who reduce their blood pressure moderately and sometimes markedly by just reducing sodium. It is going to take much more convincing data for me to believe that salt doesn't make some impact on blood pressure, especially in some patients.

Dr. Birkenhager: I would like to support Dr. DeQuattro. Much as I loathe to disagree with Sir George, I simply have to reiterate some of our findings; otherwise his ideas will keep afloat I'm afraid. I don't think you need to reduce salt intake to the very low levels of the order of 10 mEq/day in order to lower pressure. When we varied sodium intake between 50 and 150 mEq during a careful metabolic ward study, we found significant changes in arterial blood pressure. By the way, in this study, we got rid of the "curiosity reflex." So the changes in blood pressure we observed were really due to modest variations in salt intake and sodium balance.

Dr. Laragh: I am sure we all agree that sodium ions act hydraulically as the major determinant of all blood pressure phenomena simply because the amount of sodium in the body is the major determinant of the extracellular fluid and blood volumes. However, it is also clear from what we have heard thus far that the body is organized so that it is only at the very extremes of high or low intakes that blood pressure can be appreciably changed. Thus, homeostasis is organized so that we comfortably ingest and excrete what are large excesses of sodium over what seem to be needed. For most of us, this is not only not harmful, but is perhaps beneficial because it assures a high level of flow to the microcirculation and tissues, and it can protect us from a variety of threats such as severe exercise, diarrheas, fever, heat stroke, or diabetic coma.

There is no convincing evidence, as Sir George has stated, that manipulating dietary sodium intake within the habitual ranges (e.g., 2–10 g daily) makes any difference. Moreover, we should not forget as Dr. Yamori's studies bear out, that the protein intake rather than the high sodium intake may be the critical factor in the Japanese or in his experimental animals. Actually, the Japanese now live significantly longer than do Americans, despite their twice-as-high sodium intake.

It is quite true as Kempner described and Dr. DeQuattro suggested that there are certain patients (perhaps 30% of essential hypertension) in whom stringent sodium deprivation or diuretic therapy is dramatically beneficial. We, and others, believe these comprise the low-renin patient subgroup. This means to me that all so-called essential hypertension is not all alike so that sodium deprivation is only appropriate for those who respond and in whom, to me, an underlying volume excess is suggested. However, just because sodium deprivation is so dramatic in a minor subgroup, it does not follow that everybody with high blood pressure should be subjected to this treatment. To be sure, if the depletion is drastic enough, it will lower pressure to some degree in all of us. For this, the tradeoff is dehydration and shock. To me, this is boring a hole in the floor to fix a leak in the ceiling. The real goal of antihypertensive therapy is of course to reduce pressure while maintaining or improving flow. This means using primary agents directed at correcting the increased peripheral resistance.

Dr. Myers (New South Wales, Australia): I also wish to not be too contrary to Sir George, but I would like to ask him whether some of his patients treated on drugs don't also feel the same symptoms he described with salt reduction. The second point is that the modern concept that salt reduction is not salt reduction in the concept of which perhaps we have been talking (i.e., severe salt restriction); but it is the replacement of a high-salt-containing diet with a more balanced diet containing less sodium and more potassium and a change from the high-salt diet to a more vegetarian diet that would give better health, and certainly if I changed from one to the other makes me feel better. But also in patients it is effective in lowering the blood pressure.

Sir George Pickering: May I say that my experience with a low-salt diet is a very limited one. It took place many years ago when we had no other effective treatment for hypertension and it was a matter of life or death. I, therefore, persisted in trying to get my patients to eat as little sodium as Kempner employed with his rice diet. I found it extremely hard work because my patients hated it and thus I failed. And I learned then what a terrible experience being on a low-salt diet is. You have to buy special food, you have to carry it with you, you can't go out to dinner, and you can't have people to dine in your house. It seems to me that there ought to be one principal objective in treatment, namely, the objective of the declaration of independence, life, liberty, and the pursuit of happiness. A salt-free diet may give you life. I'm not sure about that, but it certainly deprives you of liberty and the pursuit of happiness.

Session 3
Sodium Metabolism: The Sodium-Potassium Membrane Pump and Volume Overload Hypertension

Chairman: F. R. Bühler

Position Paper: Sodium Metabolism: The Sodium-Potassium Membrane Pump and Volume Overload Hypertension

Francis J. Haddy, Motilal B. Pamnani, and David L. Clough

The mechanism of salt-dependent, volume-overloaded hypertension is particularly troublesome (1–3). Renin levels are low, and the responses to converting enzyme inhibitors and angiotensin antagonists are minimal. Catecholamine levels are not helpful; in fact, plasma catecholamine levels decrease as a function of salt intake in normal subjects. Long-term autoregulation subsequent to increased cardiac output and overperfusion of tissues has been considered, but increase in total peripheral resistance and blood pressure have been observed in the absence of increased cardiac output.

Recent studies in our laboratory suggest reduced sodium–potassium (Na–K) pump activity in the cardiovascular muscle of animals with investigator-induced low-renin hypertension. This finding is of interest because induced suppression of the Na–K pump in the cardiovascular muscle of normal animals, with the cardiac glycosides, for example, reproduces some of the changes seen in experimental low-renin hypertension. These changes include vasoconstriction, increased vascular sensitivity to vasoactive agents, increased cardiac contractility, and raised blood pressure (particularly if diuresis cannot occur). Thus, it is possible that the pump suppression and hypertension are causally related.

In this short review, we will first describe the Na–K pump, and then present the evidence for pump suppression in animals with experimental low-renin hypertension. We will next describe the hemodynamic effects of induced pump suppression in normal animals, and then speculate on the mechanism of the pump suppression seen in animals with low-renin hypertension. Finally, we will summarize the few studies on Na–K pump activity in hypertensive man.

Na–K PUMP

It is now widely believed that the high concentration of potassium and the low concentration of sodium in intracellular fluid relative to extracellular fluid results to a large extent from the activity of a pump in the cell membrane. This pump actively transports potassium ions into, and sodium ions out of, the cell, and the pump is stimulated by the addition of potassium ions to the extracellular fluid and of sodium ions to the intracellular fluid. The pump is inhibited by lowering the extracellular potassium concentration or the intracellular sodium concentration. It is also inhibited by cold or by adding cardiac glycosides, such as ouabain, to the extracellular fluid.

When the cells are broken and the membranes isolated, an enzyme can be demonstrated that splits adenosine triphosphate. This enzyme is activated by sodium and potassium and, hence, is called Na^+,K^+–ATPase. Like the Na–K pump in the intact cell, the Na^+,K^+–ATPase is inhibited by low concentrations of potassium or sodium and by exposure to cold or ouabain. It is, therefore, thought that this enzyme occupies a central position in the operation of the pump. By splitting intracellular adenosine triphosphate, it provides the energy for potassium and sodium transport.

In many cells, the pump is electrogenic (i.e., it affects the membrane potential). Increasing the speed of pumping hyperpolarizes the membrane, whereas decreasing the speed of pumping depolarizes the membrane. These effects are thought to result from the transfer of charge across the cell membrane due to unequal pumping rates for sodium and potassium (more sodium ions are normally transported out than potassium ions in per pump cycle). Thus, reduction of the pump speed by lowering the external potassium concentration or by administration of ouabain results in an accumulation of net positive charge on the inside and, hence, depolarization. The concentrations of sodium and potassium in the cell need not change measurably for this effect; all that is needed is charge separation. The vascular smooth muscle cell is among those cells with an electrogenic pump.

EVIDENCE FOR PUMP SUPPRESSION

We have tested pump activity in the cardiovascular muscle of animals with experimental hypertension by two methods, rubidium uptake and Na^+,K^+–ATPase activity. Rubidium is an ion that can substitute for potassium in active transport by the pump across cell membranes. It is used in the study of pump activity because its radioactive form has a longer half-life and a lower energy emission than the radioactive form of potassium. The ouabain-sensitive rudidium uptake is that uptake related to active transport, because ouabain inhibits the Na–K pump which is responsible for active transport. This technique had been used successfully to estimate pump activity in heart and brain. Pamnani adapted the myocardial rubidium uptake

technique to blood vessels, and then we applied the technique to mesenteric arteries and veins of dogs with one-kidney, one-wrapped hypertension. In this study (4), mesenteric arteries and veins were taken from the animals and immediately placed in a cold, potassium-free Krebs-Henseleit to stop the Na–K pump. They were then transferred to a warm solution containing nonradioactive rubidium to start up the pump. The solution also contained radioactive rubidium and its uptake was measured 16 min later. Uptake by ouabain-treated vessels was subtracted from this value to give ouabain-sensitive uptake, which reflects the activity of the Na–K pump. Ouabain-sensitive uptake by both arteries and veins from hypertensive animals was less than that by vessels from normotensive animals (Fig. 1). The ouabain-insensitive uptake (uptake by ouabain-treated vessels), which probably reflects distribution in extracellular space and passive penetration into the cell, was much less than the ouabain-sensitive uptake and not different in the two groups of animals. Thus, the defect was only in the ouabain-sensitive Na–K pump. Since this defect was also present in veins, it did not appear to be secondary to increased pressure.

We next examined Na^+,K^+–ATPase activity in a similar model of low-renin hypertension. Like Na–K pump activity in intact cells, total ATPase

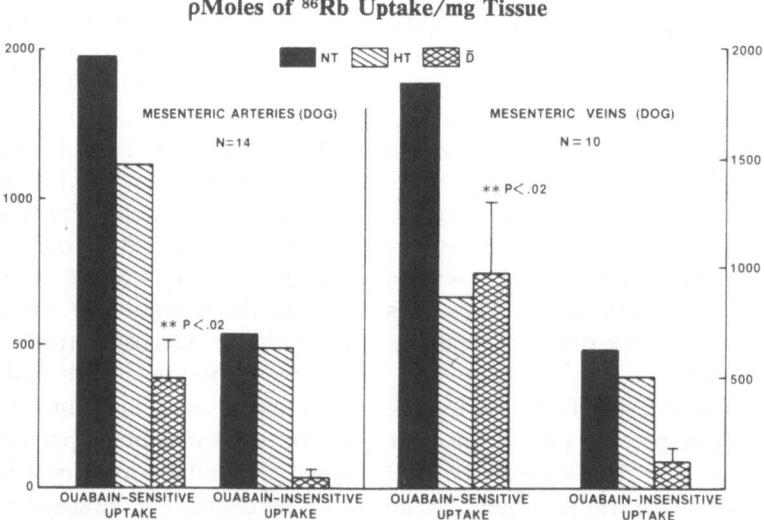

Fig. 1. Rubidium uptake (pmol/mg tissue) by mesenteric arteries and veins of dogs with one-kidney, one-wrapped hypertension. *Left-hand panel*, arteries; *right*, veins. Each panel shows the ouabain-sensitive and ouabain-insensitive rubidium uptake from sham-operated normotensive animals (■), hypertensive animals (▨), and the difference (▩). The ouabain-sensitive uptake reflects Na–K pump activity. [Adapted from Overbeck et al. (4)]

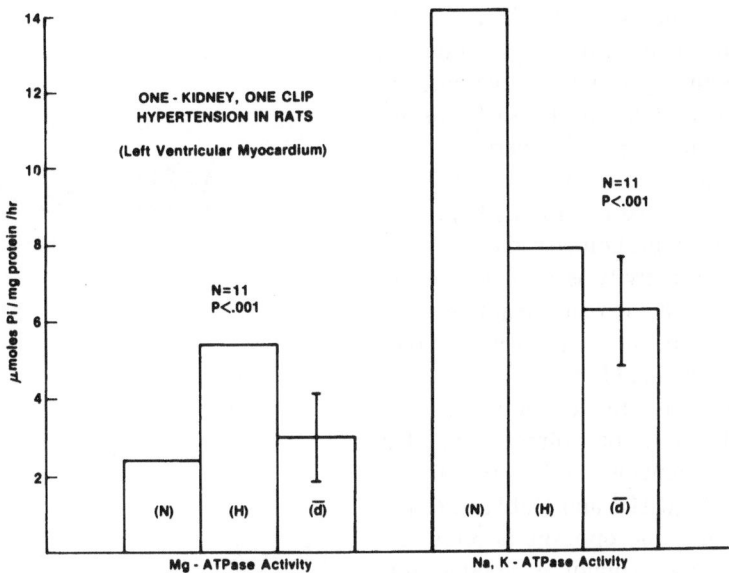

Fig. 2. Na⁺,K⁺-ATPase activity in left-ventricular microsomes of rats with one-kidney, one-clip hypertension. N, normotensive control animals; H, hypertensive animals; d, difference. [Adapted from Clough et al. (5)]

activity of isolated sarcolemma is inhibited by ouabain and removal of potassium. Any residual activity is due to Mg^{2+}–ATPase. Na^+,K^+–ATPase activity is then the difference between total ATPase and Mg^{2+}–ATPase activities. While there are practical difficulties in the measurement of Na^+,K^+–ATPase activity in blood vessels, this is not the case for myocardium. Therefore, Clough et al. measured Na^+,K^+–ATPase activity in microsomes isolated from the left (5, 6) and right (6)

ventricles of rats with one-kidney, one-clip hypertension and found it suppressed in both the high- and low-pressure chambers. The findings in the high-pressure chamber are presented in Fig. 2.

We have subsequently examined ouabain-sensitive rubidium uptake and Na^+,K^+–ATPase activity in a variety of models of experimental hypertension, some investigator-induced and some genetic in origin. The findings are summarized in Table 1 (7–12). It is apparent that ouabain-sensi-

Table 1. $Na^+–K^+$ pump activity in blood vessels and heart of animals with various types of experimental hypertension.

Type	Blood vessel[a] ouabain-sensitive rubidium uptake	Ref.	Ventricular Na^+,K^+-ATPase activity	Ref.
One-kidney, one-wrapped (dog)	↓	4		
One-kidney, one-clip (rat)	↓	b	↓	5, 6
One-kidney, DOCA, salt (rat)	↓	7	↓	8
Reduced renal mass (rat)	↓	9	↓	b
Acute renoprival (rat)			↓	10
One-kidney, dexamethasone (rat)	↑	7	↑	b
SHR (rat)				
vs. WKY	↑	11	↔	b
vs. Wistar	↔	11	↔	b
Dahl S (rat)				
vs. Dahl R (low-salt)	↑	12	↑	b
vs. Dahl R (high-salt)	↑	12	↔	b

[a] Mesenteric arteries and veins in the dog, tail artery in the rat.
[b] D. Clough, M. B. Pamnani, and F. J. Haddy (unpublished observation).

tive rubidium uptake and Na$^+$,K$^+$–ATPase activity are reduced only in the investigator-induced, nongenetic, low-renin, presumably volume-expanded, forms of hypertension. These forms include one-kidney, one-wrapped hypertension in the dog and a) one-kidney, one-clip, b) one-kidney, DOCA, salt, and c) reduced renal mass hypertension in the rat. Earlier preliminary data suggest that Na$^+$,K$^+$–ATPase activity is also reduced in the heart of the rat with acute renoprival hypertension. On the other hand, ouabain-sensitive rubidium uptake and Na$^+$,K$^+$–ATPase activity are not reduced in one form of investigator-induced hypertension not considered to be volume expanded (dexamethasone hypertension) and in two forms of genetic hypertension (SHR and Dahl salt sensitive). In fact, here just the opposite is often the case (ouabain-insensitive rubidium uptake, not shown in Table 1, is also increased, suggesting that the increased pump activity might be secondary to increased intracellular sodium concentration subsequent to increased permeability). Thus, it appears that pump activity is reduced only in the nongenetic, low-renin, presumably volume-expanded, forms of experimental hypertension. Pump activity seems to decrease following maneuvers that interfere with water and salt excretion by the kidney, either mechanical (renal mass reduction, renal artery constriction) or functional (administration of DOCA).

Jones and Hart (13) had previously reported increased ^{42}K efflux from ^{42}K-loaded arteries [and, more recently, from ^{42}K-loaded veins (14)] isolated from rats with one-kidney, DOCA, salt hypertension but suggested that this results from increased permeability of the cell membrane to potassium.

HEMODYNAMIC EFFECTS OF INDUCED PUMP SUPPRESSION

Suppression of the Na–K pump in cardiovascular muscle has long been known to increase cardiac contractility and produce vasoconstriction. It has more recently been shown that pump suppression also increases the responses of blood vessels to vasoactive agents and substantially increases blood pressure if diuresis cannot occur. The mechanism of these changes is not entirely clear, but the changes are not unlike those seen in certain forms of volume-expanded hypertension.

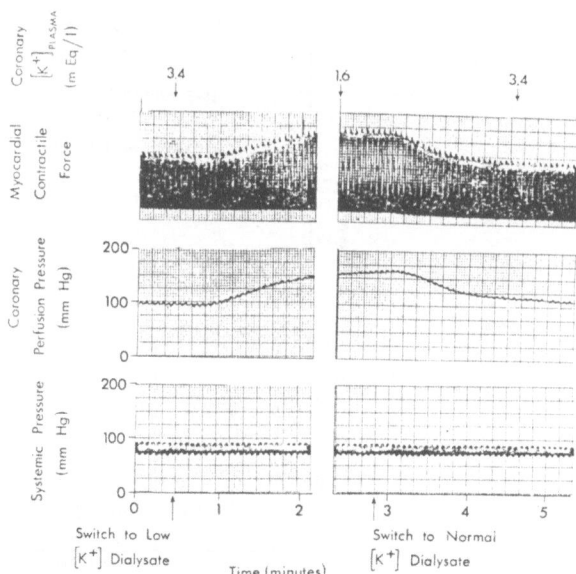

Fig. 3. Typical effects of local hypokalemia on left-ventricular contractile force, left-common coronary artery perfusion pressure, and systemic arterial pressure in the dog heart. Left-common coronary artery was perfused at constant flow with arterial blood, and this blood was rendered hypokalemic with a hemodialyzer interposed in the perfusion line. [Brace et al. (15)]

Two ways to induce pump suppression in normal animals is to lower the extracellular potassium concentration and administer cardiac glycosides. Figure 3 shows the effect of acute hypokalemia on left-ventricular contractile force and left-common coronary artery perfusion pressure at constant flow in the dog heart (15). Both increase promptly on inducing hypokalemia and promptly return to normal on returning potassium concentration to normal. Except for time course, the changes produced by intracoronary administration of ouabain are similar (15). Local hypokalemia and ouabain administration also increase resistance in quiescent forelimb, gracilis muscle and kidney (16–20). In gracilis muscle, the increase in resistance has been shown to progress with the degree of hypokalemia (18, 19) (Fig. 4). The cardiac glycosides and decreased extracellular potassium concentration also contract isolated vascular smooth muscle (see references in 3, 21).

They also increase the responses of blood vessels to vasoconstrictor stimuli. Arteries and veins isolated in a bath initially respond to electrical stimulation and a variety of vasoactive agents more

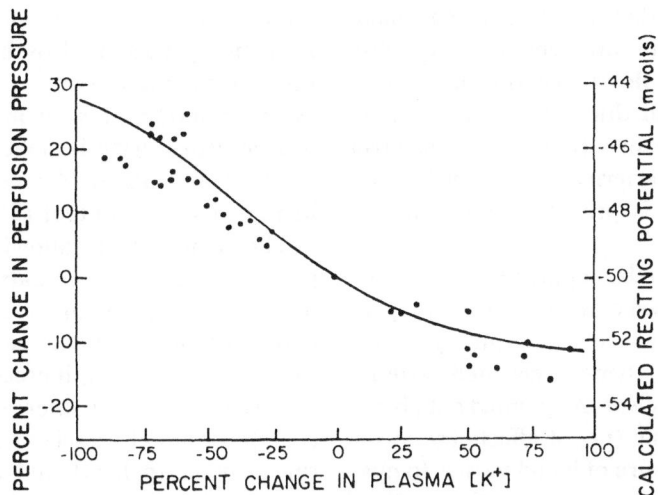

Fig. 4. Effects of local hypokalemia and hyperkalemia on perfusion pressure at constant flow in gracilis muscle of dog. *Dots,* initial change (after approximately 1–5 min) in perfusion pressure in 31 animals on locally altering the arterial plasma potassium concentration about the normal 4 mEq/liter with a hemodialyzer interposed in the perfusion line; *solid line,* calculated membrane potential of the vascular smooth cell. [Brace (19)]

vigorously when exposed to ouabain or low potassium (22, 23) (Fig. 5). Later on, responses are suppressed. An enhanced resistance response to norepinephrine also occurs in the dog forelimb early during a local infusion of ouabain (24). Later on, however, the response is depressed and this is also the case during local hypokalemia (18). It may be that increased responses to vasoactive

agents occur only with mild pump suppression and before the transmembrane ion gradients run down.

Suppression of the Na–K pump will also raise blood pressure, particularly if fluid loss is not allowed to occur. Intravenous infusion of ouabain, for example, into the normal anesthetized dog produces only a slight rise in blood pressure under

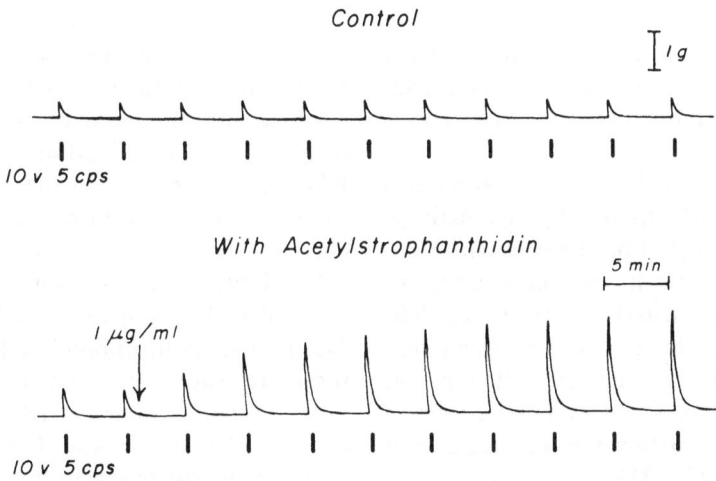

Fig. 5. Potentiation of adrenergic venomotor responses in dog saphenous vein by acetylstrophanthidin. Response of two strips from same saphenous vein to electrical stimulus. *Top,* contractile response of control strip remained unaltered; *bottom,* progressive increase in contractile response of other strip after addition of acetylstrophanthidin (1 µg/ml) to bath. [Brender et al. (23)]

usual conditions, but when water balance is maintained (by infusing fluid intravenously at the precise rate of the urine flow), the rise in pressure is quite impressive and due entirely to a rise in total peripheral resistance (25). This maneuver mimics the abnormal arterial pressure–urine volume relationship that is present in most models of hypertension (26).

The mechanism whereby suppression of the Na–K pump causes increased cardiac contractility, vasoconstriction, increased vessel sensitivity to vasoactive agents, and, hence, elevated arterial pressure is not entirely clear. As pointed out above, the pump is electrogenic (i.e., it affects the membrane potential). Exposure of blood vessels to ouabain or low potassium increases the sodium content, decreases the potassium content, and depolarizes the membrane (19, 21, 27–31), and the changes in membrane potential correlate with the changes in tension or resistance (19, 27–29) (Fig. 4). Thus, one possibility is that the vasoconstriction results from a voltage-dependent increase in the permeability of the cell membrane to calcium (15, 17, 19, 21, 27–29, 31). According to this scheme, the cell is more sensitive to vasoactive agents because the membrane potential is closer to the threshold potential. It is, however, difficult to explain the positive inotropic effect in heart via this scheme, and for this reason and others some investigators favor an explanation that utilizes the Na–calcium (Na–Ca) exchange mechanism (32). In this scheme, the pump suppression raises intracellular sodium concentration, resulting in a lowered transmembrane sodium gradient and, hence, decreased energy for calcium extrusion from the cell. The decreased efflux raises intracellular calcium concentration and, hence, contractility.

Ouabain and low-potassium concentration also reduce norepinephrine uptake by sympathetic nerve endings (33), suggesting the possibility that increased contractility results from higher concentration of norepinephrine in the neuroeffector cleft. This, however, cannot be a complete explanation because ouabain and potassium are still active on blood vessels in the presence of norepinephrine depletion or blockade and in vessels that are devoid of adrenergic nerves (21, 31).

While acute in vitro pump suppression increases cell water in some tissues, this does not seem to be the case for blood vessels (34). Addition of ouabain to, or withdrawal of, potassium from medium-bathing isolated blood vessels causes sodium gain and potassium loss but does not influence the water content. On the other hand, prolonged in vivo pump suppression may in fact cause arteries to gain water. Arteries taken from dogs who have received digoxin for 4 weeks appear to have an increased water content (35).

The changes seen following induced pump suppression in normal animals, described above, are not unlike those seen in experimental low-renin hypertension (2, 3). Increased cardiac contractility, vasoconstriction, increased vascular responses to vasoactive agents, increased sodium and water content of blood vessels, depletion of norepinephrine content in heart and blood vessels, and increased blood pressure all occur in this type of hypertension. Increased cardiac contractility has been observed early in the course of one-kidney, one-clip hypertension. Decreased norepinephrine content of heart and blood vessels has been observed in a variety of types of experimental low-renin hypertension.

MECHANISM OF PUMP SUPPRESSION

As pointed out above, suppression of the Na–K pump in experimental hypertension does not seem to be secondary to elevated pressure because it also occurs in right ventricle and veins where the pressure has not been shown to be elevated. It seems to be present only in the nongenetic, low-renin, presumably volume-expanded, forms of experimental hypertension. Acute volume expansion *per se* mimics the pump changes seen in these animals; that is, saline loading reduces rubidium uptake by arteries of normal rats to roughly the same extent as seen in rats with one-kidney, one-clip and one-kidney, DOCA, salt hypertension (36). Similar changes occur when volume is expanded with an isotonic solution of mannitol (M. B. Pamnani, unpublished observation). Furthermore, supernates of boiled plasma from the saline-expanded animals reduce rubidium uptake when applied to arteries from another rat (36). The same is true of plasma from volume-expanded dogs; that is, rubidium uptake by rat tail arteries is decreased when exposed to supernates of boiled plasma from volume-expanded dogs. Finally, serum from dogs with one-kidney, one-wrapped hypertension increases the sodium content of rabbit aortic media explants (37).

All of these findings suggest that the pump suppression observed in animals with experimental low-renin hypertension results from an unknown heat-stable humoral agent evoked by the volume expansion *per se*.

What is the nature of this agent? In our previous reviews (1–3), we tended to favor the natriuretic factor because its plasma level rises with volume and because it suppresses sodium pump activity in the renal tubule. Blaustein (38) also considers the natriuretic factor to be a good possibility. The factor is heat stable and appears to be a low-molecular weight, acidic peptide formed from a precursor molecule (39). It probably comes from brain (40) and may be released in response to distention of the pulmonary vascular bed (41).

Old and recent literature, in fact, suggests the presence of an unknown, slowly acting pressor and sensitizing agent in the blood of animals with low-renin hypertension (for references, see 3). In 1940, Solandt cross circulated blood between two dogs, one with one-kidney, one-clip or one-kidney, one-wrapped hypertension and the other smaller and acutely nephrectomized, and found that pressure rose in the small acutely nephrectomized animal. The pressor response was delayed in onset, taking about 1 h to appear. In 1953, Gordon et al. circulated blood for 30–60 min between two rabbits, one with one-kidney, one-clip hypertension and the other salt loaded but normotensive, and found that pressure rose in the normotensive salt-loaded assay rabbit. The response was delayed in onset and prolonged. The maximum rise in pressure was not reached until 2–3 h after completion of the 30–60-min cross circulation. Gordon, however, was unable to reproduce those results at a later date (personal communication).

In 1965, Hinke noted that plasma from rats with uninephrectomy-DOCA-salt hypertension increased the vasoconstrictor response of an isolated perfused rat tail artery to norepinephrine. Something in the plasma made the norepinephrine more active. In 1969, Dahl et al. placed their salt-resistant rat in parabiosis with their salt-sensitive rat and found that the resistant rat also developed hypertension when both animals were fed salt or when one-kidney, one-clip hypertension was produced in the sensitive strain. Something crossed from one animal to the other. They speculated that a common pathogenic mechanism exists in both salt and renal hypertension and suggested that many of the apparent anomalies of the angiotensin–aldosterone system in hypertension could be explained if a sodium-excreting hormone were postulated that had the capacity of also inducing hypertension when produced by a hypertension-prone subject.

In 1972, Mizukoshi and Michelakis reported that plasma from hypertensive subjects, particularly those with low-renin essential hypertension, slowly raised the blood pressure and increased the pressor responses to angiotensin and norepinephrine in an assay rat. In 1975, they showed that the same was the case for plasma from dogs with one-kidney, one-clip hypertension and that the active plasma factor appears to be a polypeptide or a small protein. Injection of 15 μl hypertensive plasma into the pentolinium-treated, nephrectomized rat produced a slow, prolonged increase in pressure and also increased the pressor response to angiotensin. More recently, they extended their studies to rats with one-kidney, one-clip hypertension and to dogs with one-kidney, one-wrapped hypertension and showed that plasma from the rats also contains a factor with slow pressor and sensitizing activity. Plasma from the dogs increased the vasoconstrictor response to norepinephrine in small mesenteric arteries isolated from rats. Fractionation of the plasma showed that the active substance has a molecular weight of approximately 1,000. While it is not easy to understand how the activity in 15 μl plasma, when injected intravenously in a whole rat, could produce a rise in blood pressure and increased pressor sensitivity, the findings have been confirmed by another group of investigators using plasma from other models of low-renin hypertension.

Meneely's group used the Michelakis technique to show that serum from the common laboratory rat with dietary salt hypertension also contains a factor that enhances the pressor activity of norepinephrine. The activity of the agent is slow in onset and continues for at least 3 h. It is heat stable and active after repeated freezing and thawing. More recently, they showed that 20 μl serum from SHR fed a diet containing 1.0%–1.25% sodium chloride potentiates the pressor effect of norepinephrine when injected into the bioassay animals.

Bloom et al. reported a similar effect of plasma from patients with normal-renin essential hypertension; that is, plasma perfused through an isolated femoral artery from a rabbit increased the vasoconstrictor repsonse to norepinephrine. Kurz et al. found a similar effect of blood from rabbits with 3-day-old one-kidney, one-clip hypertension; that is, infusion of 43 ml blood from these animals into bioassay rabbits made the bioassay animals more sensitive to the pressor action of intravenously injected norepinephrine (blood from control animals did not).

Finally, Tobian et al. recently reported that perfusion of kidneys from normal rats with blood from Dahl salt-sensitive rats results in 16% higher renal vascular resistance than perfusion with blood from Dahl salt-resistant rats.

Thus, it appears that we must seriously consider the possible role of an unknown slowly acting humoral pressor, vasoconstrictor, and sensitizing agent in the genesis of low-renin hypertension. The possible relationship between this agent, the humoral suppressor of the pump observed on acute volume expansion, and natriuretic hormone deserves study.

Na–K PUMP ACTIVITY IN HYPERTENSIVE MAN

There have been no studies of pump activity in the cardiovascular tissues of hypertensive man, but increased sodium content in arterial wall (42) and studies of white and red blood cells suggest that a pump defect may exist in some hypertensive subjects (see 2 for complete references). Of particular interest is the observation by Edmondson et al. (43) that the rate constant for total sodium efflux from isolated leukocytes procured from patients with uncomplicated essential hypertension is suppressed. This defect lies in the ouabain-sensitive portion of sodium efflux, remains despite numerous washings, and is accompanied by significant increases in the intracellular sodium and water contents. Elevated intracellular sodium concentration in leukocytes from patients with essential hypertension has also been reported by Araoye et al. (44) and Tartagni et al. (45). Garay and Meyer (46) recently found reduced sodium efflux from washed sodium-loaded red cells obtained from patients with severe essential hypertension. Plasma renin activity was not reported in these four studies.

Borghetti et al. (47) found an increased ratio of exchangeable sodium to exchangeable potassium and low-plasma renin activity in 20% of patients with essential hypertension. Exaggerated natriuresis has been observed in hypertensive man by many investigators. A recent systematic appraisal of this response in the various forms of human hypertension shows that increased fractional sodium excretion is peculiar to low-renin essential hypertension and primary aldosteronism and is not related to mean arterial pressure alone (48). It is not increased in normal-renin and high-renin essential hypertension. Thus increased fractional excretion of sodium occurs in the same types of hypertension, that is, the volume-expanded varieties in which Michelakis found the highest plasma concentration of the low-molecular weight, slowly acting pressor substance (see above). It is noteworthy that the natriuretic activity of material isolated from the urine of human hypertensive subjects, who respond to a salt-loading procedure with exaggerated natriuresis, is significantly higher than that from normotensive subjects responding to the same procedure (49). An attempt should be made to determine whether these several observations are related.

SUMMARY

Ouabain-sensitive rubidium uptake and Na^+, K^+–ATPase activity have been used to assess Na–K pump activity in cardiovascular muscle of animals with various types of experimental hypertension. The findings suggest that pump activity is suppressed in the nongenetic, low-renin, presumably volume-expanded forms. This finding is of interest because induced pump suppression in cardiovascular muscle of normal animals, with ouabain, for example, results in vasoconstriction, increased responsiveness of blood vessels to vasoconstrictor agents, and increased myocardial contractility, changes not unlike those in experimental low-renin hypertension. Other findings suggest that the pump suppression observed in animals with experimental low-renin hypertension results from an unknown, heat-stable, humoral agent evoked by the volume expansion *per se*. The old and recent literature suggest the presence of an unknown, heat-stable, low-molecular weight, slowly acting pressor and sensitizing agent in the blood of animals with low-renin hypertension. Volume expansion is known to release natriuretic hormone, a low-molecular weight, heat-stable, acidic peptide, which suppresses Na–K pump activity in the renal tubule. These three observations may be related. Na–K pump activity has not been studied in the cardiovascular muscle of hypertensive man, but studies in white and red blood cells suggest that this will be a fertile area for future study.

REFERENCES

1. Haddy FJ, Overbeck JW (1976) The role of humoral factors in volume expanded hypertension. Life Sci 19: 935–948
2. Haddy F, Pamnani M, Clough D (1978) The sodium-potassium pump in volume expanded hypertension. Clin Exp Hypertension 1: 295–336
3. Haddy FJ, Pamnani MB, Clough DL (1979) Humoral factors and the sodium-potassium pump in volume expanded hypertension. Life Sci 24: 2105–2118
4. Overbeck HW, Pamnani MB, Akera T, Brody TM, Haddy FJ (1976) Depressed function of a ouabain-sensitive sodium-potassium pump in blood vessels from renal hypertensive dogs. Circ Res 38(Suppl II): 48–52
5. Clough DL, Pamnani MB, Overbeck HW, Haddy FJ (1977) Decreased myocardial Na,K–ATPase in rats with one-kidney Goldblatt hypertension. Fed Proc 36: 491
6. Clough DL, Pamnani MB, Overbeck HW, Haddy FJ (1977) Decreased Na,K–ATPase in right ventricular myocardium of rats with one-kidney Goldblatt hypertension. Physiologist 20: 18
7. Pamnani MB, Clough DL, Haddy FJ (1978) Altered activity of sodium-potassium pump in arteries of rats with steroid hypertension. Clin Sci Mol Med 55: 41S–43S
8. Clough DL, Pamnani MB, Haddy FJ (1978) Decreased Na,K–ATPase activity in left ventricular myocardium of rats with one-kidney DOCA-saline hypertension. Clin Res 26: 361
9. Huot S, Pamnani M, Clough D, Haddy F (1980) Depressed Na$^+$–K$^+$ pump activity in tail arteries of reduced renal mass hypertensive rats. Fed Proc 39: 1188
10. Nivatpumin T, Scheuer J, Bhan AK, Penpargkul S (1973) Effects of acute uremia on myocardial function in rats. Clin Res 21: 952
11. Pamnani MB, Clough DL, Haddy FJ (1979) Na$^+$–K$^+$ pump activity in tail arteries of spontaneously hypertensive rats. Jpn Heart J 20(Suppl I): 228–230
12. Pamnani M, Clough D, Huot S, Haddy F (1980) Vascular Na$^+$–K$^+$ pump in Dahl S and R rats. Fed Proc 39: 812
13. Jones AW, Hart HG (1975) Altered ion transport in aortic smooth muscle during deoxycorticosterone acetate hypertension in the rat. Circ Res 37: 333–341
14. Tsay SL, Jones AW (1978) Effect of pressure vs DOCA on ^{42}K efflux in vascular smooth muscle from the rat. Fed Proc 37: 902
15. Brace RA, Anderson DK, Chen WT, Scott JB, Haddy FJ (1974) Local effects of hypokalemia on coronary resistance and myocardial contractile force. Am J Physiol 227: 590–597
16. Haddy FJ, Scott JB, Florio MA, Daugherty RM Jr, Huizenga JN (1963) Local vascular effects of hypokalemia, alkalosis, hypercalcemia, and hypomagnesemia. Am J Physiol 204: 202–212
17. Chen WT, Brace RA, Scott JB, Anderson DK, Haddy FJ (1972) The mechanism of the vasodilator action of potassium. Proc Soc Exp Biol Med 140: 820–824
18. Anderson DK, Roth SA, Brace RA, Radowski D, Haddy FJ, Scott JB (1972) Effect of hypokalemia and hypomagnesemia produced by hemodialysis on vascular resistance in canine skeletal muscle. Circ Res 31: 165–173
19. Brace RA (1974) Time course and mechanisms of the acute effects of hypokalemia and hyperkalemia on vascular resistance. Proc Soc Exp Biol Med 145: 1389–1394
20. Nyhof R, Dabney J, Haddy FJ (1978) Effect of ouabain on skin and skeletal muscular vascular beds in the dog forelimb. Proc Soc Exp Biol Med 158: 161–165
21. Haddy FJ (1975) Potassium and blood vessels. Life Sci 16: 1489–1498
22. Leonard E (1957) Alteration of contractile response of artery strips by a potassium-free solution, cardiac glycosides and changes in stimulation frequency. Am J Physiol 189:185–190
23. Brender D, Vanhoutte PM, Shepherd JT (1969) Potentiation of adrenergic venomotor responses in dogs by cardiac glycosides. Circ Res 25: 597–606
24. O'Neill J, Inciarte D, Swindall B, Haddy F (1980) Effect of ouabain on norepinephrine vasoconstriction in the dog forelimb. Fed Proc 39: 582
25. Haddy FJ, Scott JB (1973) Mechanism of the acute pressor action of hypokalemia, hypomagnesemia, and hypo-osmolality. Am Heart J 85: 655–661
26. Guyton AC, Coleman TG, Cowley AW Jr, Manning RD Jr, Norman RA Jr, Ferguson JD (1974) A systems analysis approach to understanding long-range arterial blood pressure control and hypertension. Circ Res 35: 159–176
27. Hendrickx H, Casteels R (1974) Electrogenic sodium pump in arterial smooth muscle cells. Pfluegers Arch 346: 299–306
28. Anderson DK (1976) Cell potential and sodium-potassium pump in vascular smooth muscle. Fed Proc 35: 1294–1297
29. Siegel G, Roedel H, Nolte J, Hofer HW, Bertsche O (1976) In: Bülbring E, Shuba MF (eds) Physiology of smooth muscle. Raven Press, New York, pp 19–39

30. Hermsmeyer K (1976) Electrogenesis of increased norepinephrine sensitivity of arterial vascular muscle in hypertension. Circ Res 38: 362–367

31. Haddy FJ (1978) The mechanism of potassium vasodilatation. In: Vanhoutte PM, Leusen I (eds) Mechanisms of vasodilatation. Karger, Basel, pp 200–205

32. Reuter H, Blaustein MP, Haeusler G (1973) Na-Ca exchange and tension development in arterial smooth muscle. Philos Trans R Soc Lond [Biol] 265: 87–94

33. Sharma VK, Banerjee SP (1977) Inhibition of [^{3}H]norepinephrine uptake in peripheral organs of some mammalian species by ouabain. Eur J Pharmacol 41: 417–429

34. Macknight ADC, Leaf A (1977) Regulation of cellular volume. Physiol Rev 57: 510–573

35. Overbeck HW, Pamnani MB, Ku DD (1977) Suppression of the ouabain-sensitive sodium-potassium pump in arterial smooth muscle. Proc Intl Union Physiol Sci 13: 573

36. Pamnani MB, Clough DL, Steffen RP, Haddy FJ (1978) Depressed Na^+–K^+ pump activity in tail arteries from acutely volume expanded rats. Physiologist 21: 88

37. Simon G (1979) Angiopathic serum factor in perinephritic hypertensive dogs. Hypertension 1: 197–201

38. Blaustein M (1977) Sodium ions, calcium ions, blood pressure regulation, and hypertension: A reassessment and a hypothesis. Am J Physiol 232: C165–C173

39. Gruber KA, Buckalew VM Jr (1978) Further characterization and evidence for a precursor in the formation of plasma antinatriferic factor. Proc Soc Exp Biol Med 159: 463–467

40. Bealer S, Haywood JR, Johnson AK, Gruber, KA, Buckalew VM, Brody MJ (1979) Impaired natriuresis and secretion of natriuretic hormone in rats with lesions of the anteroventral 3rd ventricle. Fed Proc 38: 1232

41. Epstein M (1976) Cardiovascular and renal effects of head-out water immersion in man. Circ Res 39: 619–628

42. Tobian L (1960) Interrelationship of electrolytes, juxtaglomerular cells and hypertension. Physiol Rev 40: 280–312

43. Edmundson RPS, Thomas RD, Hilton PJ, Patrick J, Jones NF (1975) Abnormal leukocyte composition and sodium transport in essential hypertension. Lancet 1: 1003–1009

44. Araoye MA, Khatri IM, Yao LL, Freis ED (1978) Leukocyte intracellular cations in hypertension: Effect of antihypertensive drugs. Am Heart J 96: 731–738

45. Tartagni F, Ambrosioni E, Montebugnoli L, Magnani B (1978) A new method for intralymphocytic sodium concentration. In: Proceedings of the fifth meeting of the international society on hypertension. Clin Sci Mol Med 55: 268

46. Garay RP, Meyer P (1979) A new test showing abnormal net Na^+ and K^+ fluxes in erythrocytes of essential hypertensive patients. Lancet 1: 349–353

47. Borghetti A, Bruschi G, Mutti A, Biggi A, Coruzzi P, Novarini A (1978) Abnormalities of body electrolytes and aldosterone secretion in essential hypertension. In: Proceedings of the fifth meeting of the international society on hypertension, Clin Sci Mol Med 55: 37

48. Luft, FC, Grim CE, Willis LR, Higgins JT, Weinberger MH (1977) Natriuretic response to saline infusion in normotensive and hypertensive man. Circulation 55: 779–784

49. Viskoper JR, Czaczkes JW, Schwartz N, Ullmann TD (1971) Natriuretic activity of a substance isolated from human urine during the excretion of a salt load. Comparison of hypertensive and normotensive subjects. Nephron 8: 540–548

Erythrocyte Sodium Extrusion in Primary Hypertension

Ricardo P. Garay and Philippe Meyer

A new method capable of determining net Na^+ and K^+ fluxes across red blood cell membranes has been described in our laboratory. This method has enabled us to demonstrate, in Na^+-loaded/K^+-depleted erythrocytes, the existence of major abnormalities characteristic of essential (primary) hypertension (1, 2).

PRIMARY HUMAN HYPERTENSION

In January 1980, 88 essential hypertensives had been investigated in our laboratory, and it appears that: a) primary hypertension is constantly associated with a decreased erythrocyte net Na^+/K^+ flux ratio as compared to our control population, which consisted of 33 normotensives strictly devoid of familial hypertension ($\ominus$ normotensives); b) in contrast, the erythrocyte test was found to be normal in 23 cases of true secondary hypertension, thus conferring to the erythrocyte cation flux measurement, an important value in the laboratory distinction between primary and secondary hypertension.

FAMILIAL PATTERN

A positive erythrocyte test was also present in the offspring of essential hypertensives. Twenty-six out of 46 children born of 1 hypertensive parent, and 8 out of 12 children born of 2 hypertensive parents, had the erythrocyte abnormality.

The corresponding percentages of 56% and 75% are suggestive of a dominant and monogenic inheritability. The presence of a positive erythrocyte test at each generation of the 14 hypertensive families investigated in detail is also compatible with this mode of transmission (3).

No close association was found between the erythrocyte defect and either any haplotype of the major histocompatibility complex HLA or any major erythrocyte blood group.

These various findings, together with the observation that no erythrocyte flux abnormality was encountered in subjects belonging to normotensive families (as well as with the presence of similar erythrocyte defects in genetically hypertensive rats mentioned later in this chapter), demonstrate a close association between hypertension and the net Na^+ and K^+ erythrocyte alteration. One may, therefore, propose that the $\oplus$ normotensives (i.e., the normotensives with a reduced Na^+/K^+ net flux ratio born of hypertensive parents) are subjects that are hypertension-prone.

The detection of positive erythrocyte tests in the offspring of hypertensive parents may, accordingly, constitute the basis of a selective primary prevention: The presence of the erythrocyte defect could indicate appropriate medical measures, such as alimentary Na^+ restriction and strict medical care during estrogen contraception and pregnancy in $\oplus$ females.

MOLECULAR ANALYSIS

It is now accepted that Na^+ transport across the erythrocyte membrane is ensured by passive permeability (Na^+ leak) and by three specific mechanisms: Na^+,K^+–ATPase, Na^+,K^+–co-transport, and Na^+,Na^+–countertransport. The Na^+, K^+–ATPase and Na^+,K^+–co-transport are inhibited by ouabain and furosemide, respectively, thus permitting the measurement of the respective participation of the two mechanisms in the process of intracellular Na$^+$ extrusion.

A marked reduction in the Na$^+$,K$^+$–co-transport was demonstrated in all essential hypertensives and in the $\oplus$normotensive subjects born of hypertensive parents. The Na$^+$ and K$^+$ leaks were found to be identical to those of controls ($\ominus$normotensives), whereas the Na$^+$,K$^+$–ATPase activity was increased in most of the benign hypertensives and the $\oplus$ normotensives. Binding experiments performed with ^{3}H-ouabain did not show that this ATPase activation stemmed from an increased number of pump unities (4).

These abnormalities are interpreted as follows: a) the deficit of the Na$^+$,K$^+$–co-transport is one of the membrane mechanisms transmitted genetically in primary hypertension; b) the Na$^+$,K$^+$–ATPase activation could be a secondary event preventing the tendency of intracellular Na$^+$ accumulation brought about by the deficit of the Na$^+$,K$^+$–co-transport; c) permanent intracellular Na$^+$ accumulation may, therefore, occur at a late stage. Other membrane abnormalities have been described in erythrocytes of hypertensive patients and of some of their relatives, such as an increased activity of the Na–Na exchange (5) and a reduction in calcium binding (6). It is not possible at this stage to define the relationship existing between these abnormalities and the deficit in the Na$^+$,K$^+$–co-transport described in our laboratory.

GENETIC HYPERTENSION OF THE RAT

A reduced active Na$^+$ extrusion has been also described in varieties of genetically hypertensive rats (7), supporting a further link between the erythrocyte membrane defect and primary hypertension. In the Okamoto SHR, the reduction in net Na$^+$ efflux is present at 4 weeks of age before the apparition of a marked hypertension, demonstrating that the erythrocyte alteration cannot be the simple consequence of the blood pressure increase. Reduction of the net Na$^+$ extrusion also occurs in the salt-sensitive H substrain of the Sabra Wistar colony of the Jewish University of Jerusalem as compared to the control N salt-resistant substrain.

In two other varieties of genetically hypertensive rats (Milan and Lyon strains) in which hypertension is less severe, the Na$^+$ net extrusion appears

identical to that of controls, but the net K$^+$ influx is markedly increased, possibly in relation to an enhanced Na$^+$,K$^+$–ATPase.

THEORETICAL IMPLICATIONS

According to the above clinical and experimental investigations, the membrane defect alters the intracellular Na$^+$ homeostasis and leads to a transitory or permanent increase in intracellular Na$^+$ concentration.

In excitable cells, such as catecholaminergic neurons and vascular smooth muscle cells, the activity of the transmembrane Na$^+$–Ca$^+$ exchange system characteristic of these cells is such that any increase in intracellular Na$^+$ content leads subsequently to a rise in intracellular Ca^{2+} concentration (8). Such an increase in intracellular calcium may explain the development of hypertension since it triggers the various mechanisms capable of increasing blood pressure permanently. Several observations indicate that the cell membrane is altered in various tissues both in essential human hypertension and in the genetic hypertension of the rat. In human primary hypertension, membrane defects in white blood cells (9) and in platelets (10) are associated with erythrocyte membrane abnormalities. In genetically hypertensive rats, abnormal membrane properties have been described in smooth muscle cells (11), erythrocytes (12), adipocytes (13) and hepatocytes (M. A. Devynck, M. G. Pernollet, P. Meyer, unpublished observations). Further investigation is needed to understand these abnormalities at a molecular level and to define the common biochemical feature.

However, it now seems possible to emphasize the pathogenic importance of membrane alterations in excitable cells and to propose that they may represent the genetically determined mechanism of primary hypertension.

SUMMARY

In 1978–1979, we reported that erythrocytes of essential hypertensives were not functionally normal: after K$^+$ depletion and Na$^+$ enrichment, net Na$^+$ extrusion and net K$^+$ influx were reduced and increased, respectively, indicating a reduction of net Na^+/K^+ flux ratio. These abnormalities appear to be secondary to a deficiency in the Na^+,K^+–co-transport. It was soon observed that the erythrocyte abnormality ($\oplus$ test) was specific of primary hypertension and occurred in some young offspring of essential hypertensives.

We described the frequency of $\oplus$ tests in children born of hypertensive parents: 52% when one parent was normotensive; 74% when two parents were hypertensive. Males and females were equally affected. Thus, the pattern of the genetic transmission appears to follow a Mendelian, dominant and autosomic mode.

We found it necessary to demonstrate irrevocably that the erythrocyte abnormality is genetically linked with primary hypertension, excluding at the same time any fortuitous familial agglutination, as the above results suggest that the erythrocyte test can be a tool permitting a true primary and selective prevention.

Several substrains of genetically hypertensive rats were, therefore, investigated. A reduction of net Na^+ efflux, similar to that observed in essential hypertensives, was indeed observed in two varieties of genetically hypertensive rats (the Okamoto and the hypertension-prone Sabra substrains) compared with their respective genetic controls. The erythrocyte abnormality was present in young rats before the development of significant elevation in blood pressure, demonstrating again that the erythrocyte alteration is not a consequence of hypertension.

It is still uncertain whether the functional perturbations of rat erythrocytes should be attributed to a deficit in the Na^+,K^+–co-transport, as recognized in man. However, several biochemical abnormalities are already described in rat erythrocytes consisting of increased calcium passive influx probably ensured by a reduction of the Ca^{2+} binding sites at the internal side of the membrane and decreased ATP-dependent Ca^{2+} extrusion. Thus, the intracellular concentrations of Na^+ and Ca^{2+} will have a tendency to rise.

The membrane defect leading to an intracellular enrichment in Na^+ thus appears of major significance. In erythrocytes, this defect represents a biochemical marker of essential hypertension. In excitable cells, it may represent the innate factor of hypertension which permits the expression of environmental factors, such as Na^+ excess.

REFERENCES

1. Garay RP, Meyer P (1979) A new test showing abnormal net Na^+ and K^+ fluxes in erythrocytes of essential hypertensive patients. Lancet 1: 349–353
2. Garay RP, Elghozi JL, Dagher G, Meyer P (1980) Laboratory distinction between essential and secondary hypertension by measurement of erythrocyte cation fluxes. New Engl J Med 302: 769
3. Meyer P, Bellet M, Dagher G, Garay RP (1981) A genetic study of abnormal cation transport in essential hypertension (in press)
4. Garay RP, Dagher G, Pernollet MG, Devynck MA, Meyer P (1980) Inherited defect in a Na^+,K^+–co-transport system in erythrocytes from essential hypertensive patients. Nature 284: 281
5. Canessa M, Adragna N, Solomon H, Connolly T, Tosteson D (1980) Increased sodium-lithium countertransport in red cells of patients with essential hypertension. New Engl J Med 302: 772
6. Postnov YV, Orlov SN, Shevchenko AS, Adler AM (1977) Altered sodium permeability, calcium binding and Na,K–ATPase activity in red blood cell membranes in essential hypertension. Pfluegers Arch 371: 263
7. De Mendonca M, Grichois ML, Garay RP, Sassard J, Ben-Ishay D, Meyer, P (in press) Abnormal net Na^+ and K^+ fluxes in erythrocytes of three varieties of genetically hypertensive rats. Proc Natl Acad Sci USA
8. Blaustein MP (1977) Sodium ions, calcium ions, blood pressure regulation and hypertension: A reassessment and a hypothesis. Am J Physiol 232(2): C165
9. Edmondson RPS, Thomas RD, Hilton PJ, Jones NH (1975) Abnormal leukocyte composition and Na transport in essential hypertension. Lancet 1: 1003
10. Mattiasson I, Mattiasson B, Hood B (1979) The efflux rate of norepinephrine from platelets and its relation to blood pressure. Life Sci 2: 2265
11. Kwan CY, Belbeck L, Daniel EE (1980) Abnormal biochemistry of vascular smooth muscle plasma membrane isolated from hypertensive rats. Mol Pharmacol 17: 137
12. Postnov YV, Orlov S, Pokudin NI (1979) Decrease of calcium binding in the red blood cell membranes in spontaneously hypertensive rats and in essential hypertension. Pfluegers Arch 379: 191
13. Postnov YV, Orlov SN (1979) Features of intracellular calcium distribution in the adipose tissue of spontaneously hypertensive rats (SHR). Experientia 35: 1480

Sodium Countertransport and Co-Transport in Human Red Cell Membranes

D. C. Tosteson

At least three kinds of coupled Na transport are known to occur in human red cell membranes. One is outward movement of Na coupled with inward movement of K and the hydrolysis of ATP through the Na–K pump (for recent reviews see refs. 1 and 2). Two other types of coupled Na transport do not derive energy from the hydrolysis of ATP, but rather from the gradient in electrochemical potential of another participating ion. If the other participating ion must be located on the opposite, or *trans*, side of the membrane, the process is called exchange or countertransport. If it is on the same, or *cis*, side of the membrane, it is called co-transport. This short paper describes observations of an Na–Na exchange system that can perform Na–Li countertransport (3) and a Na–K co-transport system (4) in human red cells from normal subjects and from persons suffering from hypertension.

Na–Li countertransport involves a 1:1 exchange of Na for Li ions (5). It occurs on a system that promotes exchange of Na for Na and will accept Li but no other cation so far tested (6). The concentration of external Li necessary to produce half-maximal Li influx through this transport pathway is 1.5 mM, whereas the corresponding value for external Na is 25 mM. These measures of the affinities of the system for Na and Li do not differ appreciably in red cells from different individuals, but the maximum rates of transport do show substantial interindividual differences. In some persons with mania, the maximum rate of Na–Li countertransport is very low (7). These interindividual differences are, at least in part, under genetic control (8).

We have recently reported measurements of the maximum rate of Na–Li countertransport in the red cells of patients suffering from hypertension as compared with normal human subjects (9). Red cells were loaded to contain approximately 12 mEq Li/liter cells by incubating them for 3 h at 37°C in a medium containing 140 mM LiCl. During the loading, the red cell Na concentration fell to approximately 5 mEq/liter cells. There was no significant difference between hypertensive and normal subjects in the mean intercellular Li, Na, and K concentrations before and after loading. The efflux of Li from the loaded cells was measured both into a medium containing no Na (MgCl₂-sucrose substitution) and into one containing 150 mM NaCl. The difference between these two values (i.e., the external Na-stimulated Li efflux) was taken to be a measure of the maximum rate of Na–Li countertransport. In a group of 36 hypertensive patients, the mean (±SEM) value for the maximum rate of Na–Li countertransport was 0.55 ± 0.02 as compared with 0.24 ± 0.02 for a group of 26 normotensive subjects. Na–Li countertransport was also increased in red cells from first-degree relatives of patients with essential hypertension, but not in red cells from patients with secondary hypertension. These results raised the possibility that the genes coding for the Na–Li countertransport system might also be involved in predisposition to hypertension. We are currently exploring this possibility.

Evidence suggesting the presence of a Na–K co-transport system in human red cells has been accumulating for many years. Hoffman and Kregenow (10) first reported net-outward uphill Na transport from human red cells in the presence of ouabain. Sachs (11) confirmed their observations and noted that the process was inhibited by external K and by furosemide. Wiley and Cooper (4) noted stimulation of both furosemide-sensitive K influx by external Na and furosemide-sensitive Na influx by external K and suggested the presence of Na–K co-transport. Garay et al. (12) have reported ouabain-insensitive, net-uphill Na transport from human red cells loaded by the *p*-chloromercuribenzoate (PCMBS) method (13) to contain approximately 80 mEq Na/liter cells. We have recently shown that ouabain-insensitive, furosemide-sensitive net-inward or outward uphill movement of Na or K can be driven by an appropriate gradient of the co-ion (14).

Garay and Meyer (15) have also shown that the ouabain-resistant furosemide-sensitive, external K-sensitive outward movement of Na is reduced in Na-loaded red cells from patients with essential hypertension. They suggest that this lesion in red cell Na transport is the result of deficient Na–K co-transport in the red cell membranes of patients with essential hypertension. At present, they assay the Na–K co-transport system by measuring furosemide-inhibited K and Na loss from cells loaded by the PCMBS method to contain 20–30 mEq/liter cells of both Na and K (choline replacement). Because they have also observed deficient co-transport in members of the families of hypertensives, they have speculated about the relationship between the genes that code for co-transport and genetic predisposition to essential hypertension.

These observations of increased Na–Li countertransport and decreased Na–K co-transport in the red cells of patients with essential hypertension raise several interesting questions. First, are these two different transport systems or two different aspects of the same system? At present, there is no definite evidence for a link between the two pathways. Indeed, the fact that the countertransport is inhibited by phloretin, while the co-transport is reduced by furosemide argues against, but does not rule out, such a link (16). Do these two transport processes use different transport proteins or does one or both involve either of the two integral proteins of the human red cell membrane that are known to perform ion transport—the Na–K ATPase that promotes ouabain-sensitive active transport of Na and K and band 3 that promotes exchange of Cl and HCO_3? Again, there are no data that rule these possibilities in or out. Are the abnormalities in these cation transport pathways observed in hypertension an accommodation to the increased blood pressure or are they expressions of a membrane disorder that is part of the pathogenesis of the disorder?

Several investigations have speculated about the latter possibility (15, 17, 18). At least two general lines of conjecture have been put forward. In one line, an increased intracellular Na concentration

in vascular smooth muscle leads to reduced extrusion of Ca with a consequent increase in tension developed by the actomyosin filaments [e.g., (17)]. Another plausible line is that the Na–Ca exchange system functions not as an outwardly directed Ca pump, but rather as an inwardly directed Ca leak in vascular smooth muscle cells. This would occur if other processes maintained the intracellular Ca concentration at a value less than that specified by the equilibrium position of the Na–Ca exchange system. If such conditions obtain, an increase in the maximum rate of Na–Ca exchange, comparable to that observed in the maximum rate of Na–Li exchange in the red cells of patients with essential hypertension, would increase the inward movement of Ca and, thus, intracellular Ca concentration and vascular smooth muscle tone. To distinguish between these and other possibilities will require further research.

SUMMARY

Na–Li countertransport in human red cells takes place on a Na–Na exchange system that is insensitive to ouabain but inhibited by phloretin. The system promotes one for one Na–Na, or Na–Li exchange, but does not accept K or any other cation thus far tested. The system has a 20-fold greater affinity for Li than Na and shows saturation kinetics. The maximum transport rate varies considerably between individuals and is, at least partially, under genetic control. We report measurements of the maximum rate of Li–Na countertransport in red cells taken from 26 normal control subjects and from 36 patients suffering from essential hypertension. The assay was made by loading the cells to contain approximately 10 mM Li and measuring the Li efflux into a medium with and without Na. The external Na-stimulated Li efflux was taken as a measure of the maximum rate of Li–Na countertransport. The mean maximum rate was more than twice as great in the hypertensive than in the normal control subjects. The difference between the two groups was also clear after one week of severe restriction of Na in the diet.

REFERENCES

1. Caviares JD (1977) The sodium pump in human red cells. In: Ellory JC, Lew VL (eds) Membrane

transport in red cells. Academic Press, London, pp 1–37

2. Sarkadi B, Tosteson DC (1979) Active cation transport in human red cells. In: Tosteson DC (ed) Membrane transport in biology, Vol II. Springer, Heidelberg, pp 117–160

3. Haas M, Schooler J, Tosteson DC (1975) Coupling of lithium to sodium transport in human red cells. Nature 258: 424–427

4. Wiley JS, Cooper RA (1974) A furosemide-sensitive cotransport of sodium plus potassium in the human red cell. J Clin Invest 53: 745–755

5. Sarkadi B, Alifimoff JK, Gunn RB, Tosteson DC (1978) Kinetics and stoichiometry of Na-dependent Li transport in human red blood cells. J Gen Physiol 72: 249–265

6. Pandey GN, Sarkadi B, Haas M, Gunn RB, Davis JM, Tosteson DC (1978) Lithium transport pathways in human red blood cells J Gen Physiol 72: 233–247

7. Pandey GN, Ostrow DG, Haas M, Dorus E, Casper RC, Davis JM, Tosteson DC (1977) Abnormal lithium and sodium transport in erythrocytes of a manic patient and some members of his family. Proc Natl Acad Sci USA 74: 3607–3611

8. Pandey GN, Dorus E, Davis JM, Tosteson DC (1979) Lithium transport in human red blood cells: Genetic and clinical aspects. Arch Gen Psychiatry 36: 902–908

9. Canessa M, Adragna N, Solomon HS, Connolly TM, Tosteson DC (1980) Increased Na–Li counter-transport in red cells of patients with essential hypertension. New Engl J Med 302: 772–776

10. Hoffman JF, Kregenow F (1966) The characterization of new energy-dependent cation transport processes in red blood cells. Ann NY Acad Sci 137: 566

11. Sachs JR (1971) Ouabain-insensitive Na movements in the human red blood cell. J Gen Physiol 57: 259–282

12. Garay RP, Dagher G, Pernollet MG, Devynck MA, Meyer P (1980) Inherited defect in a (Na + K) co-transport system in erythrocytes from essential hypertensive patients. Nature 284: 281–282

13. Garrahan PJ, Rega AF (1967) Cation loading of red blood cells J Physiol (Lond) 193: 459

14. Bize I, Canessa M, Tosteson DC Na–K co-transport in human red cells (in preparation)

15. Garay RP, Meyer P (1979) A new test showing abnormal net Na and K fluxes in erythrocytes of essential hypertensive patients. Lancet 1: 349–353

16. Canessa M, Bize I, Adragna N, Garay R, Tosteson DC (1980) Countertransport and cotransport of Na, Li and K in human red cells. Fed Proc 39: 1842

17. Blaustein MP (1977) Na, Ca, blood pressure regulation and hypertension: A re-assessment and a hypothesis. Am J Physiol 232: C165–C173

18. Postnov YU, Orlov SN, Shevchenko A, Adler AM (1977) Altered Na permeability, Ca binding and Na-K ATPase activity in the red blood cell membrane in essential hypertension. Pfluegers Arch 371: 263–269

Cellular Basis of Sodium-Induced Hypertension

Mordecai P. Blaustein, Stanley Lang, and Marilyn James-Kracke

It is, surely, unnecessary for me to discuss in this forum the alarming prevalence of hypertensive cardiovascular disease in the acculturated societies of the world. It is also unnecessary for me to reemphasize the importance of determining the pathophysiology of the disease (or diseases) so that we can, hopefully, institute appropriate preventive measures.

The contributions of genetic factors and of high-salt diet and abnormal salt metabolism are certainly well documented. In this context, the two preceding chapters (Garay and Mayer; and Tosteson) may provide important new insights into these factors; their hypotheses, therefore, deserve the most careful scrutiny.

However, despite the uncertainty about these hypotheses, there are several well-documented observations that red and white blood cell sodium concentrations and sodium-to-potassium ratios (Na/K) are elevated in many patients with essential hypertension (1, 2). These observations have raised the possibility that abnormal Na concentrations and Na/K ratios may also be present in most other tissues in these patients. Such abnormalities are difficult to detect in some tissues because separation of intra- and extracellular electrolytes is fraught with error and uncertainty. Nevertheless, it is reasonable to assume, as a working hypothesis, that such abnormalities are present, and to make a concerted effort to detect these abnormalities.

As pointed out elsewhere (3–5), a simple and rational explanation of the cellular mechanisms underlying the increased peripheral resistance of essential hypertension follows directly from this assumption. The key appears to lie in the interrelationship between Na and Ca ions in the regulation of the intracellular free Ca^{2+} concentration ($[Ca^{2+}]_i$) and maintained tension (tone) in vascular smooth muscle (3). These ideas rest on the well-documented evidence that a rise in $[Ca^{2+}]_i$ is the factor that triggers an increase in vascular smooth muscle tension (6).

Three hypotheses have been put forth to account for a relationship between cellular Na metabolism and tone in vascular smooth muscle:

1) An increase in $[Na^+]_i$ (the intracellular Na^+ concentration) in the presynaptic terminals of the sympathetic neurons that innervate vascular smooth muscle promotes enhanced Ca-dependent norepinephrine release (7) via a Na–Ca exchange mechanism (8). The norepinephrine, acting on α-receptors, would be expected to increase $[Ca^{2+}]_i$ by increasing Ca influx and by releasing Ca from intracellular stores in the smooth muscle fibers (9).

2) Partial inhibition of Na–K exchange pumps, which are electrogenic in vascular smooth muscle (10), may slightly depolarize the muscle fibers. This should increase $[Ca^{2+}]_i$ by promoting Ca entry through voltage-sensitive Ca channels (11).

3) When $[Na^+]_i$ is elevated in vascular smooth muscle cells, either because of increased (leak) entry or decreased extrusion (via Na–K exchange pumps), $[Ca^{2+}]_i$ will also be elevated. This occurs because there is a smaller Na electrochemical gradient to drive net Ca extrusion via Na–Ca exchange (12).

In all of these hypotheses, the final common path involves a rise in smooth muscle $[Ca^{2+}]_i$. As noted above, this will, in turn, be expected to enhance vascular smooth muscle tone directly. Our immediate objective is to evaluate the possible contributions of these three proposed mechanisms.

There is evidence that inhibition of Na extrusion from sympathetic neurons leads to the enhancement of catecholamine release (7). This is apparently the result of net Ca gain by the nerve terminals, via an Na–Ca exchange mechanism. The rise in $[Ca^{2+}]_i$ in the terminals would be expected to accelerate transmitter release. This suggests that mechanism #1 may contribute to the increase in tone when Na metabolism is altered. However, a number of workers have observed a relationship between Na metabolism and vascular tone even when α-adrenergic receptors are blocked, or when catecholamine stores are depleted (13). Clearly, then, other factors must also be involved.

Haddy and Overbeck (11) have suggested that depolarization, due directly to inhibition of electrogenic Na–K pumps, may be the primary factor relating Na metabolism to vascular tone. However, several considerations indicate that this depolarization cannot play a role under realistic in vivo conditions primarily because *in the steady state, the pumped efflux of Na must equal the rate of Na entry.* Therefore, unless the entry rate is reduced, the (net) Na–K pump current must return to its original steady-state value during a prolonged period of partial pump inhibition. In other words, inhibition of some of the pumps (e.g., by a natriuretic hormone) should *transiently* reduce the outward Na–K pump current. But, $[Na^+]_i$ will then rise until the pump current returns to about its initial level, and Na efflux again equals influx. Accordingly, the Na–K pump current *will not be reduced* significantly when the pumps are slightly inhibited for a prolonged period of time. Under these circumstances, $[Na^+]_i$ will rise slightly, and $[K^+]_i$ will fall, to new steady-state levels. The fall in the $[K^+]_o/[K^+]_i$ ratio (and, therefore, the potassium equilibrium potential E_K) may, however, produce a small depolarization. One possibility is that this depolarization could open voltage-sensitive Ca channels and permit Ca to enter the muscle fibers and enhance contraction. But some observations indicate that small depolarizations from the normal resting potential do not markedly increase Ca entry (Figs. 1 and 2).

Figure 1 shows the effect of the extracellular K concentration on the perfusion pressure in the isolated hindquarters of a rat perfused with Krebs-Henseleit solution at a constant flow rate (see ref. 13 for details). Note that when $[K^+]_o$ was reduced from 5.9 mM to (nominally) "0," the perfusion pressure (and peripheral resistance) increased; this is an indication that vascular tone increased. On the other hand, when $[K^+]_o$ was increased from 5.9 to 11.8 mM, the perfusion pressure fell (and peripheral resistance decreased); clearly, vascular tone decreased under these circumstances. However, as shown in Fig. 2, increasing $[K^+]_o$ from 5.9 to 11.8 mM may be expected to depolarize vascular smooth muscle fibers by a few millivolts. Obviously, this small depolarization is insufficient to open voltage-sensitive Ca channels, presumably because their threshold is somewhat higher. When $[K^+]_o$ is increased to 15–20 mM, a marked increase in perfusion pressure is observed, presumably because the attendant depolarization is then sufficient to open the Ca channels. But clearly, for small depolarizations, the depolarization and contraction can be dissociated.

How, then, can we explain the paradoxical vascular smooth muscle relaxation when $[K^+]_o$ is increased from 5.9 to 11.8 mM? And how can we explain the contraction that is observed when $[K^+]_o$ is reduced below 5.9 mM, or when the Na–K pumps are inhibited slightly? The most parsimonious explanation centers on the fact that $[Na^+]_i$ should fall when $[K^+]_o$ is increased and the Na–K pumps are stimulated. Conversely, $[Na^+]_i$ should rise when the pumps are inhibited (e.g., by cardiotonic steroids or a reduction in $[K^+]_o$).

There is considerable evidence that Ca efflux from vascular smooth muscle involves a Na–Ca exchange mechanism that derives its energy, at

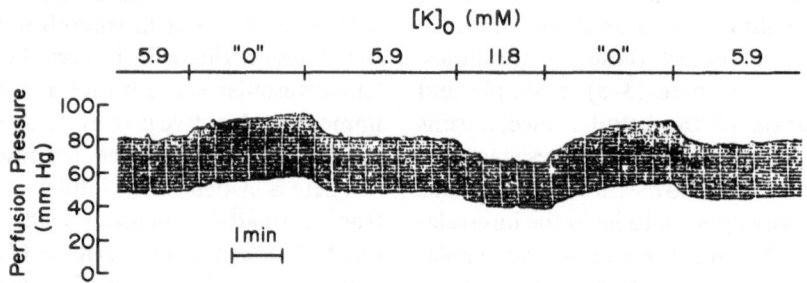

Fig. 1. Effects of increased and reduced $[K]_o$ on arterial perfusion pressure in the isolated hindquarter of a reserpine-treated rat during constant flow perfusion. Red cell-free fluids were used for this experiment.

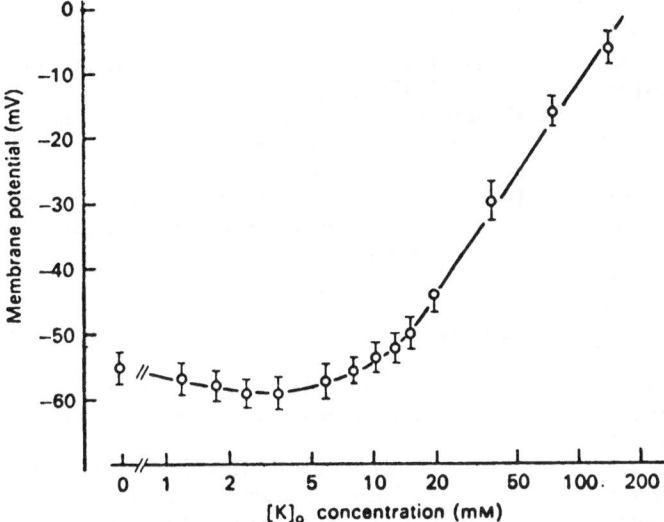

Fig. 2. Effect of the external K concentration ([K]$_o$) on the membrane potential of smooth muscle cells in the main pulmonary artery of the rabbit. The membrane potentials were measured with intracellular microelectrodes [Modified from Casteels et al. (14)]

least in part, from the Na electrochemical gradient across the plasma membrane (3, 12). This implies that [Ca^{2+}]$_i$ is exquisitely sensitive to changes in [Na$^+$]$_i$, and that the parallel rise and fall in [Na$^+$]$_i$ and [Ca^{2+}]$_i$ are governed by a power law relationship (3). Moreover, if [Ca^{2+}]$_i$ is maintained above the contraction threshold, the changes in [Ca^{2+}]$_i$ (resulting from changes in [Na$^+$]$_i$) will be immediately translated into changes in vascular tone (3).

The foregoing considerations lead to the conclusion that any factors that enhance (leak) Na entry, or inhibit Na extrusion in vascular smooth muscle, will increase [Ca^{2+}]$_i$ and vascular tone primarily by altering [Na$^+$]$_i$ and effecting a change in the [Ca^{2+}]$_o$/[Ca^{2+}]$_i$ gradient via the Na–Ca exchange mechanism. This mechanism may be a critical link in the interrelationship between sodium ions and the increased peripheral vascular resistance of arterial hypertension.

SUMMARY

Elucidation of the mechanisms underlying the well-documented relationship between salt and hypertension should greatly enhance our understanding of the pathophysiology of this disease. A key factor in this relationship may be the Na–Ca exchange mechanism that helps to regulate the intracellular Ca concentration ([Ca^{2+}]$_i$) in vascular smooth muscle. We expect that, either because of increased leak entry or decreased extrusion (as suggested by others), intracellular Na levels may be slightly elevated in many hypertensive patients.

As a result, [Ca^{2+}]$_i$ will also be elevated because the Ca electrochemical gradient across the plasma membrane is tightly coupled to the Na gradient via Na–Ca exchange. Since Ca^{2+} is the immediate trigger for contraction, the increased [Ca^{2+}]$_i$ would be expected to increase smooth muscle tone (and peripheral vascular resistance). This hypothesis provides a straightforward explanation for the relationship between salt metabolism and the increased peripheral vascular resistance that is the primary manifestation of hypertension.

ACKNOWLEDGMENTS

We thank Drs. B. K. Krueger and W. J. Lederer for helpful comments. The original research mentioned in this article was supported by grants from the AHA, MDA, NINCDS and NSF.

REFERENCES

1. Losse H, Wehmeyer H, Wessels F (1960) Der Wasser and Electrolytgehalt von Erythocyten bei arterieller Hypertonie. Klin Wochenshr 38: 393–395
2. Edmondson RPS, Thomas RD, Hilton PJ, Patrick J, Jones NF (1975) Abnormal leucocyte composition and sodium transport in essential hypertension. Lancet 1: 1003–1005
3. Blaustein MP (1977) Sodium ions, calcium ions, blood pressure regulation and hypertension: A reassessment and a hypothesis. Am J Physiol 232: C165–C173

4. Blaustein MP (1980) How does sodium cause hypertension? A hypothesis. In: Zumkley H, Losse H (eds) Proceedings of first international symposium on intracellular electrolytes and arterial hypertension. Georg Thieme Verlag, Stuttgart

5. Blaustein MP, Lang S, James-Kracke M (1980) Sodium ions, calcium transport, and the control of vascular tone. In: Zumkley H, Losse H (eds) Proceedings of first international symposium on intracellular electrolytes and arterial hypertension. Georg Thieme Verlag, Stuttgart

6. Filo RS, Bohr FF, Ruegg JC (1965) Glycerinated skeletal and smooth muscle: Calcium and magnesium dependence. Science 147: 1581–1583

7. Bonaccorsi A, Hermsmeyer K, Smith CB, Bohr DF (1977) Norepinephrine release in isolated arteries induced by K-free solution. Am J Physiol 232: H140–H145

8. Blaustein MP (1974) The interrelationship between sodium and calcium fluxes across cell membranes. Rev Physiol Biochem Pharmacol 70: 33–82

9. Deth R, van Breemen C (1974) Relative contributions of Ca^{2+} influx and cellular Ca^{2+} release during drug-induced activation of the rabbit aorta. Pfluegers Arch 48: 13–22

10. Hendrickx H, Casteels R (1974) Electrogenic sodium pump in arterial smooth muscle cells. Pfluegers Arch 346: 299–306

11. Haddy, FJ, Overbeck HW (1976) The role of humoral agents in volume expanded hypertension. Life Sci 19: 935–948

12. Reuter H, Blaustein MP, Haeusler G (1973) Na–Ca exchange and tension development in arterial smooth muscle. Philos Trans R Soc Lond [Biol] 265: 87–94

13. Lang S, Blaustein MP (in press) The role of the sodium pump in the control of vascular tone. Circ Res

14. Casteels R, Kitamura K, Kuriyama H, Suzuki H (1972) Excitation-contraction coupling in the smooth muscle cells of the rabbit main pulmonary artery. J Physiol (Lond) 271: 63–79

Alteration of Cell Membrane Control over Intracellular Calcium in Essential Hypertension and in Spontaneously Hypertensive Rats

Yu. V. Postnov

In recent years, a series of facts have shown that cell membranes may be considered a basic determinant that can activate blood pressure control systems. These facts concern both essential hypertension in humans and spontaneous hypertension in rats. In both types of pathology, there is now evidence that a cell membrane defect is not restricted to the arterial wall, but is a part of a more widespread pattern. The first indication of this appeared in the study concerning passive permeability of the erythrocyte membrane for sodium and potassium ions. It was found, particularly by our group, that passive permeability of the erythrocyte membrane for these cations increased considerably in both types of hypertension (1, 2). These data agreed with the findings of Losse et al. (3) who earlier found an increase of sodium content in red blood cells (RBC) in essential hypertensive patients.

Further studies showed that the increased passive permeability of the RBC membrane to monovalent cations is associated with a change in the distribution of calcium ions in the membrane. It was found that calcium binding by the inner part of the erythrocyte membrane is lowered both in spontaneously hypertensive rats (SHR) and in essential hypertension (by 48% and 28%, respectively) (4).

It seems that altered Ca^{2+} binding of the inner part of the RBC membrane is directly related to its passive premeability for monovalent cations. We found, for instance, that a considerable increase of permeability for sodium and potassium ions can be induced by calcium depletion of the inner part of the RBC membrane. Diminishing the amount of membrane-bound calcium by EDTA results in considerable increase of sodium and potassium permeability of the membrane (2). After these results were obtained for erythrocytes, it was natural to assume that these are just fragments of a more widespread cell membrane alteration.

Abnormalities of the monovalent cation transport and membrane calcium handling were later demonstrated in vascular smooth muscle in spontaneous hypertension by Jones (5) in the United States and by Aoki et al. (6) in Japan. However, these data were related to the hypertrophied contractile cells with a highly developed contractile apparatus activated in hypertension. The changes may be due either to cell hypertrophy or to a secondary effect of the troponin–myosin complex activation (in other words, a secondary effect of hypertension).

Some time ago, we obtained data that demonstrated the abnormalities of membrane calcium handling in "noncontractile" cells of SHR, namely, in cells of adipose tissue that are known to be very diffusely spread in the body (7).

The in vitro study of kinetics of $^{45}Ca^{2+}$ efflux from adipose tissue reveals the presence of three pools of exchangeable calcium. The two most slowly exchangeable pools relate to intracellular calcium (mitochondria, endoplasmic reticulum, and the inner part of the plasma membrane). A rapidly exchangeable pool A relates to extracellular calcium. It was found that calcium content in the intracellular pools of adipose tissue in SHR are increased substantially. Adrenalectomy increased this difference (7). It seems that in this connection, the hypertrophy of the adrenal cortex in this type of hypertension may represent a means of compensating for a cell membrane defect (maybe via sodium transport correction).

A similar study was carried out in patients with essential hypertension subjected to surgical intervention for chronic cholecystitis. Calcium distribution in adipose tissue of the omentum major was investigated. The results also gave clear evidence of enlarged intracellular calcium pools in hypertensive patients as compared to the normotensive group (Fig. 1). The similarity of the results obtained in hypertensive animals and in humans with essential hypertension is striking (8).

It was found that SHR have a lowered CA-binding ability of the plasma membrane of adipocytes and a considerably decreased Ca-accumulating ability of the endoplasmic reticulum. Remarkably, however, calcium accumulation by mitochondria proved to be enhanced (9). Because the calcium pool in mitochondria is much larger than all other pools, one may think that an increased content of intracellular calcium in adipocytes in both types of hypertension is due mainly to mitochondria caused by a permanent excess of free calcium due to the insufficiency of Ca accumulation by the endoplasmic reticulum and plasma membrane. Thus, it is the measure of compensation (or correction) of this defect.

The data on erythrocytes and adipocytes support the view that changes in smooth muscles and myocardiocytes (6, 10) are particular manifestations of typical widespread membrane pathology. The pathogenetic role of this membrane defect is not limited to being a constant cause of the activation of the actomyosin complex in the contractile cells of the cardiovascular system. More importantly, the general membrane defect may be a con-

stant source of the activation of the peripheral part of the sympathetic nervous system. Some recent findings support this suggestion. It is known that an increase in calcium concentration suppresses the activity of membrane adenylate cyclase. It was found by our group that this enzyme is inhibited (or suppressed) in adipocytes of hypertensive rats. It was shown that isoproterenol stimulation of membrane adenylate cyclase in adipocyte ghosts results in a decreased formation of cyclic AMP in hypertensive rats as compared to normotensive controls (11). Therefore, a more powerful sympathetic impulse may be needed for normal lipolysis (generally for normal energetic supply of the specific tissues). We feel that here may be the cause of the hitherto unexplained hyperactivity of the postganglionic part of the sympathetic nervous system in these types of hypertension.

But one may ask if membrane alterations are a consequence of enhanced sympathetic activity. In our most recent study, we show that if peripheral immunosympathectomy is performed on newborn SHR, then hypertension does not develop, but calcium distribution in adipocytes remains altered (Fig. 2) (12). These data support the view that membrane function alteration concerning membrane calcium handling is not a consequence of increased sympathetic activity.

The Size of Extracellular (A) and Intracellular (B and C) Calcium Pools in Adipose Tissue in Hypertensive and Normotensive Patients

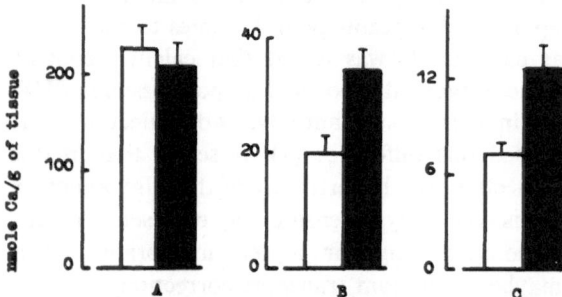

Fig. 1. The size of extracellular (A) and intracellular (B and C) calcium pools in adipose tissue in hypertensive and normotensive patients. □, Normotensive patients ($N = 13$); ■, hypertensive patients ($N = 13$); ⊤, mean ± SD.

The Size of Intracellular Calcium Pools (S_B and S_C) in Adipose Tissue of Intact (1) and NGF-Antiserum Treated (2) rats

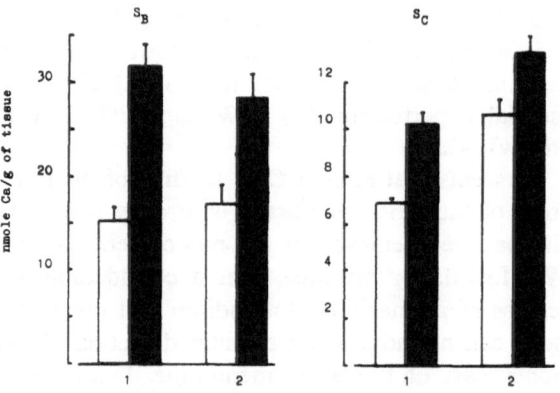

Fig. 2. The size of intracellular calcium pools (S_B and S_C) in adipose tissue of intact (1) and nerve growth factor antiserum-treated (2) rats. □, normotensive Kyoto-Wistar Rats; ■, SHR; ⊤, mean ± SE.

SUMMARY

We are arriving at the conclusion that in SHR as well as in human essential hypertension, there is a cell membrane defect that does not seem to be an isolated phenomenon limited to the cardiovascular contracting cells, but also takes place in RBC and in adipocytes.

The general feature of this membrane defect (at the present stage of our knowledge) is an alteration of Ca binding and Ca-accumulating ability of cell membranes and mitochondria resulting in the deficiency of membrane control over intracellular calcium.

The pathogenetic significance of this defect is probably not limited to the constant activation of the actomyosin complex in the cells of the cardiovascular system. Altered intracellular calcium distribution in a large and sensitive target for the sympathetic system (adipose tissue) may affect the functional state of its peripheral part and provide hyperactivity of postganglionic sympathetic neurons.

REFERENCES

1. Postnov YuV, Orlov SN, Shevchenko AS (1975) Alteration of the erythrocyte membrane permeability in rats with spontaneous genetic hypertension (in Russian). Cardiology (Moscow) 15(10): 88–92
2. Postnov YuV, Orlov SN, Shevchenko AS, Adler AM (1977) Altered sodium permeability, calcium binding and Na–K-ATPase activity in red blood cell membrane in essential hypertension. Pfluegers Arch 371: 263–269
3. Losse H, Wehmeyer H, Zumkley H (1966) The behaviour of the intracellular electrolytes in arterial hypertension. In: Electrolytes and cardiovascular diseases. Karger, Basel/New York, pp 174–197
4. Postnov YuV, Orlov SN, Pokudin NI (1979) Decrease of calcium binding by the red blood cell membrane in spontaneously hypertensive rats and in essential hypertension. Pfluegers Arch 379: 191–195
5. Jones AW (1973) Altered ion transport in vascular smooth muscle from spontaneously hypertensive rats: Influence of aldosterone, norepinephrine and angiotensin. Circ Res 34, 35(Suppl I): 62–69
6. Aoki K, Ikedo N, Yamashita K, Tazumi K, Sato I, Hotta K (1974) Cardiovascular contraction in spontaneously hypertensive rats: Ca^{2+} interaction of myofibrils and subcellular membrane of heart and arterial smooth muscle. Jpn Circ J 38: 1115–1119
7. Postnov YuV, Orlov SN (1979) Features of intracellular calcium distribution in the adipose tissue of spontaneously hypertensive rats (SHR). Experientia 35: 1480–1481
8. Postnov YuV, Orlov SN, Pokudin, NI (1980) Alteration of intracellular calcium distribution in the adipose tissue in essential hypertension (in Russian). Cardiology (Moscow) 20(8): 65–67
9. Postnov YuV, Orlov SN (1980) Evidence of altered calcium accumulation and calcium binding by the membranes of adipocytes in spontaneously hypertensive rats. Pfluegers Arch 385: 85–89
10. Wei W-J, Janis RA, Daniel EE (1976) Studies of subcellular fraction from mesenteric arteries of spontaneously hypertensive rats: Alteration in both calcium uptake and enzyme activities. Blood Vessels 13: 293–308
11. Postnov YuV, Reznikova MB (1980) Phosphodiesterase and adenylate cyclase activity in adipocytes of spontaneously hypertensive rats. In: Seventh Scientific Meeting of the International Society of Hypertension, New Orleans, May 11–14, p 104
12. Postnov YuV, Orlov SN, Pokudin NI (in press) Peripheral immunosympathectomy in spontaneously hypertensive rats: Altered intracellular calcium distribution in adipose tissue in the absence of hypertension (in Russian). Cardiology (Moscow) 20(9)

A Circulating Sodium Transport Inhibitor in Essential Hypertension

G. A. MacGregor and H. E. de Wardener

Dahl et al. (1) first proposed in 1969 that an explanation of results of experiments they had performed in parabiotic rats could be that a "saluretic substance" was present which also had the capacity to raise the blood pressure. This hypothesis was extended by Haddy and Overbeck (2) in 1976 who suggested that the rise in blood pressure which occurs with volume expansion might be due to an increase in a circulating sodium transport inhibitor which, while increasing sodium excretion, would cause a rise in blood pressure. There was at this time, however, no explanation of how such an inhibitor could cause a rise in blood pressure. One year later, Blaustein (3) suggested a possible mechanism whereby a sodium transport inhibitor could, through an effect on intracellular sodium and thereby intracellular calcium, cause an increase in the tone of the smooth muscle in the arteriolar wall and the eventual development of hypertension. De Wardener and MacGregor (4) have recently proposed that Dahl's hypothesis can be further extended to explain the development of essential hypertension. This paper outlines this extended hypothesis and presents some of the supporting evidence.

OUTLINE OF DAHL'S HYPOTHESIS AS APPLIED TO ESSENTIAL HYPERTENSION

Dahl's hypothesis (4) proposes that development of essential hypertension in man is due to an inherited defect in the ability of the kidney to eliminate sodium (Fig. 1). As sodium intake increases to levels above 50 mEq/day, there is a tendency for an increase in extracellular volume. This gives rise to an increased secretion of a circulating sodium transport inhibitor that acts on the kidney to in-

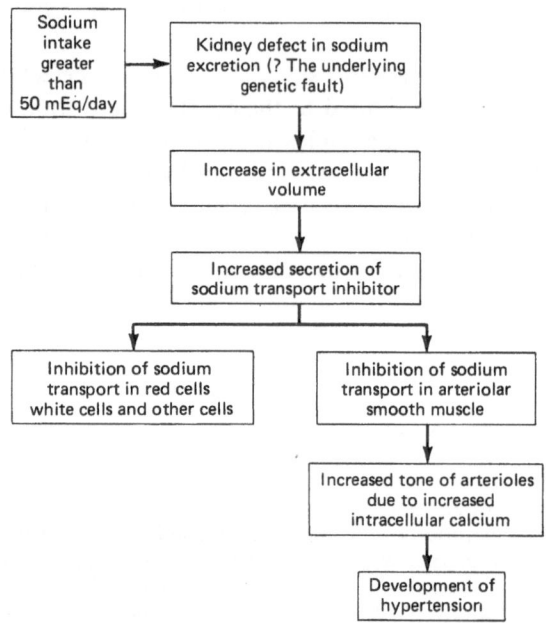

Fig. 1. Dahl's hypothesis applied to essential hypertension.

crease the secretion of sodium and thereby attempts to correct the tendency for an increase in extracellular volume. There is, therefore, in these patients a continuous state of correction of a tendency for volume expansion. This sodium transport inhibitor also inhibits sodium transport in the arteriolar smooth muscle. Inhibition of sodium transport gives rise to an increase in intracellular sodium which, by the mechanism Blaustein (3) has outlined, causes a rise in intracellular calcium and an increase in tone of the smooth muscle cell, leading eventually to the development of hypertension. The rate of development and the height of the blood pressure will, therefore, according to the hypothesis, depend on the sodium intake and the severity of the inherited defect in eliminating sodium from the kidney.

EVIDENCE FOR SODIUM INTAKE

While there is controversy about the importance of sodium intake in the development of essential hypertension, the prevalence of essential hypertension is directly related to sodium intake (5) and urinary sodium excretion (6–11). Studies in three communities have shown that high blood pressure is unknown when sodium intake is below 50 mEq/day (6–8). One objection to the accumulating evidence that sodium intake is important in the development of hypertension has been that within a community there is no relationship between the prevalence of hypertension and sodium intake (11–13). But this relationship could only occur if all individuals in the community were equally liable to develop high blood pressure and there was a very wide range of sodium intake.

A GENETIC DEFECT IN THE KIDNEY

The hereditary nature of essential hypertension in man is well known (14). There is in man no direct evidence that the genetic fault lies in the kidney. But the kidney cross-transplantation experiments performed in the Dahl salt-sensitive and salt-resistant rats (15–17) and the Milan spontaneously hypertensive and normotensive rats (18–20) clearly indicate that the blood pressure goes with the kidney. And the association between sodium intake and the prevalence of hypertension in the stock colony rat (21, 22), the Dahl salt-sensitive hypertensive rat (23, 24), and the retention of sodium that occurs in the Milan spontaneously hypertensive rat during the development of hypertension (25–27) suggests that the underlying abnormality in the rat kidney is the difficulty in eliminating sodium.

EVIDENCE FOR A CONTINUOUS STATE OF CORRECTION OF A TENDENCY FOR VOLUME EXPANSION

If there is a difficulty in excreting sodium in essential hypertension, then there will be a tendency for an increase in extracellular volume that the hypothesis proposes is being continuously corrected by the presence of an increased concentration of circulating sodium transport inhibitor, which, by inhibiting sodium reabsorption in the tubule, will increase sodium excretion. This would explain why in essential hypertension extracellular fluid volume measurements are within normal limits (28). Evidence in man with essential hypertension that there is a continuous state of correction of volume expansion is circumstantial, but is supported by the finding that all patients with essential hypertension have an accelerated natriuresis when challenged with sodium (29, 30), which is unrelated to changes in colloid osmotic or hydrostatic pressures in the kidney (31) and is greatest in patients with the lowest plasma renin activity (32). An exaggerated natriuresis occurs in normal subjects who are salt loaded, or who have been given mineralocorticoids (33), and in patients with primary aldosteronism (34), situations where there is a state of continuous correction of a tendency for volume expansion.

The finding that approximately 30%–50% of patients with essential hypertension have a low-plasma renin activity (35) is also suggestive of a corrected state of volume expansion.

INHIBITION OF SODIUM TRANSPORT IN THE ARTERIOLES

There is no direct evidence in man that sodium transport is inhibited in the smooth muscle of the arterioles of patients with essential hypertension, apart from the original finding of Tobian and Binion (36) of an increase in the sodium content of renal arteries in patients with hypertension. The mechanism whereby an increase in the concentration of a circulating sodium transport inhibitor might cause an increase in the tone of smooth muscle arteriole has been reviewed by Blaustein (3). Theoretical calculations by Blaustein of the sensitivity of this system show that a very small rise in intracellular sodium would give a rise in intracellular calcium concentration, which, in turn, would increase the resting tone of vascular smooth muscle by approximately 50% (3).

EVIDENCE FOR INHIBITION OF SODIUM TRANSPORT IN RED AND WHITE CELLS

Abnormalities in sodium transport in red cells in man with essential hypertension were first reported in 1960 (37) and have been confirmed by many others (38–42). More recently, abnormalities in sodium transport in both leukocytes and lymphocytes have been reported (43–46). The methodology of measuring sodium transport in red and white cells has been as varied as the findings and interpretations. Most of the reported abnormalities could be explained by a reduction in net sodium transport. This could be compatible with an increased concentration of a sodium transport inhibitor. Recent work using ^{22}Na has confirmed that in essential hypertension there is an impairment of sodium efflux in both white and red cells in patients with essential hypertension (47, 48). It was also confirmed that in the white cells, this impairment of total sodium efflux rate constant is due to a reduction in the ouabain-sensitive component (47) as originally described by Edmondson et al. (43). If the hypothesis is correct, it should be possible to demonstrate that there is an increase in the concentration of a sodium transport inhibitor in the plasma of hypertensive patients when compared to that of normotensive subjects. Cross-incubation experiments where the red and white cells of normotensive subjects have been incubated in the plasma of hypertensive patients show that the normal white cells acquire the same abnormalities of sodium transport as the cells of the hypertensive patients (47). They also show that this sodium transport inhibitor in the plasma of hypertensives affected the ouabain-sensitive component of the total sodium efflux rate constant, suggesting that the sodium transport inhibitor present in the plasma of hypertensive patients is an ouabain-like substance (47). Similar experiments in red cells failed to show any effect of hypertensive plasma on normotensive red cells, which may be due to a difference in the conditions for the experiments with red cells as compared to those for white cells (48). It might also be expected, according to the hypothesis, that the abnormality in sodium transport in the white cells would be greatest in those whose kidneys have the greatest tendency for sodium retention, therefore, the greatest tendency for extracellular fluid volume expansion, and, thus,

the highest level of circulating sodium transport inhibitor. Such patients will have a less reactive renin–angiotensin system to sodium restriction. The impairment of leukocyte sodium transport, therefore, should be greatest in hypertensive patients with a subnormal response of the renin–angiotensin system to sodium restriction. This conclusion has recently been demonstrated to be correct (49).

ALTERNATIVE HYPOTHESES

Neither the autoregulatory hypothesis of Ledingham (50), the neurogenic hypothesis of Dickinson (51), nor the structural hypothesis of Folkow (52) incorporate an explanation of the widespread alterations that are now being described in cell membrane transport in essential hypertension. The only alternative hypothesis to Dahl's hypothesis that does include an explanation of these membrane abnormalities is that they are due to an inherited defect in the cell membrane which is present in all cells (53). This alternative hypothesis does not explain:

1) why sodium intake is related to the prevalence of high blood pressure;
2) that plasma in hypertensive man can alter the vascular reactivity of the rat into which it is injected (54);
3) why the defect in sodium transport in red cells and leukocytes is not present in patients treated with diuretics (38, 44); and
4) that the plasma from patients with essential hypertension reduces the total sodium efflux rate constant in white cells of normotensive subjects to the same level as those found in essential hypertension (47).

Nevertheless, the different defects in cell membrane transport now being described in essential hypertension indicate that these two hypotheses may not necessarily be exclusive.

SUMMARY

There is increasing evidence, in patients with essential hypertension, of an abnormality of sodium transport that may be responsible for the development of high blood pressure. A hypothesis suggesting that the abnormalities in sodium transport are due to a circulating sodium transport inhibitor is proposed, and some of the evidence supporting the hypothesis is discussed.

REFERENCES

1. Dahl LK, Knudsen KD, Iwai J (1969) Humoral transmission of hypertension: Evidence from parabiosis. Circ Res 24, 25(Suppl I): 21–33
2. Haddy FJ, Overbeck HW (1976) The role of humoral agents in volume expanded hypertension. Life Sci 19: 935–948
3. Blaustein MP (1977) Sodium ions, calcium ions, blood pressure regulation, and hypertension: A reassessment and a hypothesis. Am J Physiol 232(3): C165–C173
4. de Wardener HE, MacGregor GA (1980) Hypothesis: Further observations on Dahl's hypothesis that a saluretic substance may be responsible for a sustained rise in arterial pressure. Its possible role in essential hypertension. Kidney Int (in press)
5. Gleibermann L (1973) Blood pressure and dietary salt in human populations. Ecol Food Nutr 2: 143
6. Dahl LK (1961) Possible role of chronic excess salt consumption in the pathogenesis of essential hypertension. Am J Cardiol 8: 571–575
7. Sinnett PF, Whyte HM (1973) Epidemiological studies in a total highland population, Tukisenta, New Guinea: Cardiovascular disease and relevant clinical, electrocardiographic, radiological and biochemical findings. J Chronic Dis 26: 265–290
8. Oliver WJ, Cohen EL, Neel JV (1975) Blood pressure, sodium intake, and sodium related hormones in the Yanomamo Indians: A "no-salt" culture. Circulation 52: 146–151
9. Fukuda T (1954) Investigation on hypertension in farm villages in Akita prefecture: Chiba, Igakki, Zasshi (J Chiba Med Soc) 29: 490–502
10. Takamatsu M (1955) Figure of body fluid of farmers in the northeastern districts viewed from angle of water and salt metabolism. J Sci Lab (Rodo Kagaku) 31: 349–370
11. Sasaki N (1964) The relationship of salt intake to hypertension in the Japanese. Geriatrics 19: 735–744
12. Miall WE (1959) Follow-up study of arterial pressure in the population of a Welsh mining valley. Br Med J 2: 1204–1210
13. Simpson FO, Waal-Manning HJ, Bolli P, Phelan EL, Spears GFS (1978) Relationship of blood pressure to sodium excretion in a population survey. Clin Sci Mol Med 55: 373S–375S
14. Pickering G (ed) (1968) High blood pressure, Vol 12, 2nd ed. Churchill London, pp 236–290
15. Tobian L, Coffee K, McCrea P, Dahl LK (1966) A comparison of the antihypertensive potency of kidneys from one strain of rats susceptible to salt hypertension and kidneys from another strain resistant to it. J Clin Invest 45: 1080
16. Dahl LK, Heine M, Thompson K (1972) Genetic influence of renal homografts on the blood pressure of rats from different strains. Proc Soc Exp Biol Med 140: 852–856
17. Dahl LK, Heine M, Thompson K (1974) Genetic influence of the kidneys on blood pressure: Evidence from chronic renal homografts in rats with opposite predispositions to hypertension. Circ Res 34: 94–101
18. Bianchi G, Fox U, Di Francesco GF, Bardi U, Radice M (1973) The hypertensive role of the kidney in spontaneously hypertensive rats. Clin Sci Mol Med 45: 135–139
19. Bianchi G, Fox U, Di Francesco GF, Giovanetti AM, Pagetti D (1974) Blood pressure changes produced by kidney cross-transplantation between spontaneously hypertensive rats and normotensive rats. Clin Sci Mol Med 47: 435–448
20. Fox U, Bianchi G (1976) The primary role of the kidney in causing the blood pressure difference between the Milan hypertensive strain (MHS) and normotensive rats. Clin Exp Pharmacol Physiol [Suppl] 3: 71–74
21. Meneely GR, Tucker RG, Darby WJ, Auerbach SH (1953) Chronic sodium chloride toxicity: Hypertension, renal and vascular lesions. Ann Intern Med 39: 991–998
22. Smirk FH, Hall WH (1958) Inherited hypertension in rats. Nature 182: 727–728
23. Dahl LK, Heine M, Tassinar L (1962) Effects of chronic excess salt ingestion: Evidence that genetic factors play an important role in susceptibility to experimental hypertension. J Exp Med 115: 1173–1190
24. Dahl LK, Schackow E (1964) Effects of chronic excess salt ingestion: Experimental hypertension in the rat. Can Med Assoc J 90: 155–160
25. Bianchi G, Fox U, Imbasciati E (1974) The development of a new strain of spontaneously hypertensive rats. Life Sci 14: 339–347
26. Bianchi G, Baer PG, Fox U, Duzzi L, Pagetti D, Giovannetti AM (1975) Changes in renin, water balance, and sodium balance during development of high blood pressure in genetically hypertensive rats. Circ Res 36, 37(Suppl I): 153–161
27. Bianchi G, Baer PG, Fox U, Guidi E (1977) The role of the kidney in the rat with genetic hypertension. Postgrad Med J 53(Suppl II): 123–135
28. Schalekamp MA, Beevers DG, Kolsters G, Lebel M, Fraser R, Birkenhager WH (1974) Body-fluid volume in low-renin hypertension. Lancet 2: 310–311
29. Baldwin DS, Biggs AW, Goldring W, Hulet WH, Chasis H (1958) Exaggerated natriuresis in essential hypertension. Am J Med 24: 893–902
30. Lowenstein J, Beranbaum ER, Chasis H, Baldwin DS (1970) Intrarenal pressure and exaggerated na-

triuresis in essential hypertension. Clin Sci 38: 359–374

31. Willassen Y, Ofstad J (1978) Renal sodium excretion and peritubular capillary starling forces (PCSF) in essential hypertension. In: Sixth international congress of nephrology. Karger, Basel

32. Krakoff LR, Goodwin FJ, Baer L, Torres M, Laragh JH (1970) The role of renin in the exaggerated natriuresis of hypertension. Circulation 42: 335–345

33. Rovner DR, Conn JW, Knopf RF, Cohen EL, Hsueh M.T.-Y. (1965) Nature of renal escape from the sodium-retaining effect of aldosterone in primary aldosteronism and in normal subjects. J Clin Endocrinol Metab 25: 53–64

34. Biglieri EG, McIllroy MB (1966) Abnormalities of renal function and circulatory reflexes in primary aldosteronism. Circulation 33: 78–86

35. Dunn MJ, Tannen RL (1974) Low renin hypertension. Kidney Int 5: 317–325

36. Tobian L Jr, Binion JT (1952) Tissue cations and water in arterial hypertension. Circulation 5: 754–758

37. Losse H, Wehmeyer H, Wessels F (1960) The water and electrolyte content of erythrocytes in arterial hypertension. Klin Wochenschr 38: 393–395

38. von Gessler U (1962) Intra- und extrazelluläre Elektrolytveränderungen bei essentieller Hypertonie vor und nach Behandlung. Z Kreislaufforsch 51: 177–183

39. Wessels VF, Junge-Hüsling G, Losse H (1967) Untersuchungen zur Natriumpermeabilität der Erythro zyten bei Hypertonikern und Normotonikern mit familiärer Hochdruckbelastung. Z Kreislaufforsch 56: 374–380

40. Postnov YV, Orlov SN, Shevchenko A, Adler AM (1977) Altered sodium permeability, calcium binding and Na–K–ATPase activity in the red blood cell membrane in essential hypertension. Pfluegers Arch 371: 263–269

41. Garay RP, Meyer P (1979) A new test showing abnormal net Na^+ and K^+ fluxes in erythrocytes of essential hypertensive patients. Lancet 1: 349–353

42. Henningsen NC, Mattsson S, Nosslin B, Nelson D, Ohlsson O (1979) Abnormal whole-body and cellular (erythrocytes) turnover of $^{22}Na^+$ in normotensive relatives of probands with established essential hypertension. Clin Sci 57: 321S–324S

43. Edmondson RPS, Thomas RD, Hilton PJ, Patrick J, Jones NF (1975) Abnormal leucocyte composition and sodium transport in essential hypertension. Lancet 1: 1003–1005

44. Thomas RD, Edmondson RPS, Hilton PJ, Jones NF (1975) Abnormal sodium transport in leucocytes from patients with essential hypertension and the effect of treatment. Clin Sci Mol Med 48: 169S–170S

45. Ambrosioni E, Tartagni F, Montebugnoli L, Magnani B (1979) Intralymphocytic sodium in hypertensive patients: A significant correlation. Clin Sci 57: 325S–327S

46. Araoye MA, Khatri IM, Yao LLY, Freis ED (1978)

Intracellular sodium in hypertensive patients. Clin Res 26: 53

47. Poston L, Sewell RB, Williams R, Richardson P, de Wardener HE (1980) The effect of (1) a low molecular weight natriuretic substance and (2) serum from hypertensive patients on the sodium transport of leucocytes from normal subjects. In: Zumkley H, Losse H (eds) Intracellular electrolytes and arterial hypertension. Georg Thieme Verlag, Stuttgart, pp 93–95

48. Clarkson EM, MacGregor GA, de Wardener HE (1980) Observations using red cells on the natriferic properties of plasma from normotensive and hypertensive individuals, and of the low molecular weight natriuretic substance obtained from human urine. In: Zumkley H, Losse H (eds) Intracellular electrolytes and arterial hypertension. Georg Thieme Verlag, Stuttgart, pp 95–97

49. Edmonson RPS, MacGregor GA (1980) Leucocyte cation transport: Its relationship to the renin angiotensin system in essential hypertension. In: Zumkley H, Losse H (eds) Intracellular electrolytes and arterial hypertension. Georg Thieme Verlag, Stuttgart, pp 187–193

50. Ledingham JM (1971) Blood pressure regulation in renal failure. J R Coll Physicians Lond 5(2): 103–134

51. Dickinson CJ (1965) Neurogenic hypertension. Blackwell, Oxford

52. Folkow B (1978) Cardiovascular structural adaptation: Its role in the initiation and maintenance of primary hypertension. Clin Sci Mol Med 55: 3S–22S

53. Garay RP, De Mendonca M, Elghozi JL, Devynck MA, Dagher G, Pernollet MG, Gricnois ML, Ben-Ishay D, Meyer P (1979) Clinical and pathological relevance of erythrocyte cation fluxes measurement in hypertension. Clin Sci 57: 329S–331S

54. Michelakis AM, Mizukoshi H, Huang C, Murakami K, Inagami T (1975) Further studies on the existence of a sensitizing factor to pressor agents in hypertension. J Clin Endocrinol Metab 41: 90–96

DISCUSSION

Dr. Bühler (Basel, Switzerland) (Chairman): One question is whether these different sodium transport defects represent a genetic marker or are a causative factor of hypertension. Alternatively, too, these different pump derangements may be a consequence of the hypertensive disease process. To start the discussion, I should like to ask Drs. Meyer and Tosteson whether they feel that they could link up their own findings with a pathogenetic defect in circulating cells of hypertensive patients or with a change in intracellular calcium concentration as suggested by Dr. Blaustein's work.

Dr. P. Meyer (Paris, France): Well, if the membrane defect that we demonstrated in blood cells expresses a diffuse membrane abnormality, then in excitable cells with a high surface volume ratio (neurons, smooth muscle cells), the reduction—even small—in sodium extrusion would increase, according to the NA–Ca exchange, the intracellular calcium concentration. This phenomenon could result in the molecular events leading to vasoconstriction and hypertension.

Dr. Tosteson (Boston, Mass.): As Dr. Blaustein made clear in his discussion, if the Na–Ca exchange is in proportion to the ratio of intra- to extracellular sodium concentration, then anything that changes the intracellular sodium concentration will modify the calcium distribution. A question that our own data on the exchange system raises is whether changes in the maximum rate of the exchange system could also have comparable effects. I would like to illustrate a way it could. There will be an equilibrium position for the Na–Ca system that will depend on the stoichiometry of the Na–Ca exchange system which seems to be such that three sodium ions exchange for one calcium ion. If this is the correct transport reaction, then equilibrium will be reached when the ratio of intra- to extracellular calcium concentration equals the cube of the sodium concentration ratio, that is:

$$\frac{[Ca]_i}{[Ca]_o} = \left\{\frac{[Na]_i}{[Na]_o}\right\}^3$$

This system can function either as a pump or as a leak for calcium. If the calcium ratio is greater than the value given by this relationship, then the system will function as a calcium pump and will extrude calcium until this relationship is obeyed. Conversely, if the calcium concentration is less than the equilibrium value, then the Na–Ca exchange system will function as a leak for calcium. In vascular smooth muscle, it is not clear whether the Na–Ca exchange system functions mainly as a calcium pump or as a calcium leak. If the latter conditions obtain, an increase in the maximum exchange capacity of the system would increase intracellular calcium concentrations and, thus, the tension developed by the actomyosin fibers. In this case, the increase in smooth muscle calcium content would not be secondary to a change in the intracellular sodium concentration, as proposed by Blaustein, but rather due to an increased num-

ber and/or turnover of Na–Ca exchange sites. It is plausible, but clearly speculative, to propose that the increased maximum Na–Li exchange that we have reported in red cells reflects increased maximum Na–Ca exchange in vascular smooth muscle leading directly to increased calcium movement into the cells without a prior increase in cellular sodium.

Dr. J. Myers (New South Wales, Australia): I wish to make it clear that when physiologic measurements of sodium efflux rate constant or of the Na–K ATPase pump mechanism are made, dietary sodium intake must be taken into account.

We found [Fitzgibbon W, Morgan T, Myers J (in press) International Society of Hypertension, New Orleans, Clin Sci Suppl] that there was an inverse correlation between sodium intake and red cell total sodium efflux rate constant in hypertensive patients. No such correlation occurred in normotensive controls. The importance of this finding is that it demonstrates for the first time in man that dietary sodium may affect the regulation of cellular sodium transport.

An implication of this inverse effect could be that regulation of the sodium pump mechanism is more variable in patients with hypertension, either due to a lack of a controlling factor in hypertensive persons or to the presence of a controlling factor in normotensives. This may be a plasma factor such as natriuretic hormone as proposed by Haddy and Overbeck [Haddy FJ, Overbeck HW (1976) Life Sci 19: 935–948]. Time unfortunately does not permit discussion of our more recent findings. However, based on the present data, the following mechanism could be proposed for hypertension. A high-salt intake affects the sodium pump, which may present cellular mechanisms at a higher level. This could result in an increased reactivity in cardiac muscle and vascular smooth muscle, particularly in renal vascular smooth muscle, and, by potentiating the effects of salt and the interaction between salt and catecholamines on sodium metabolism at the cellular level, lead to the development of hypertension in genetically predisposed persons.

Dr. Reis (New York): The evidence for potential defects of the cell membrane in hypertension is attractive: It suggests a unified field theory, namely, that there is a single membrane defect. Moreover, if there is a gene coding for hypertension, this abnormal membrane may be what it is coding for. A better question, however, is: If indeed there is a widespread membrane defect in hypertension that affects every cell, why don't patients with hypertension have many more things wrong with their bodies than they do? Why is the principal abnormality of hypertension strictly an abnormality of arterial pressure?

Dr. Blaustein (Baltimore, Md.): Dr. Reis has raised a good point. One possibility is that the defect is simply manifested in smooth muscle cells, whereas, in most other kinds of cells, the defect is well compensated for. In the case of the smooth muscle cells, the compensation may be much more difficult; furthermore, as I indicated in my talk, the tension effects are exquisitely sensitive to the calcium concentration and, therefore, to *any* change in the intracellular sodium concentration because of Na–Ca exchange. In essence, we would expect a direct translation between the sodium transport and the maintenance of tone in the smooth muscle cell. It may well turn out that there are other small defects, as a result of the raised intracellular sodium levels, in other cells as well, but these just haven't been very obvious. And, finally, there is the possibility that we are looking at a spectrum of changes with no specific cutoff; thus, individuals may manifest the transport defect(s) to a variable extent.

Dr. Laragh (New York): I would like to ask any or all of the members of the group one or two questions that have bothered me. Apparently, we have heard described and related to hypertension at least three different sodium transport defects or mechanisms. That is, the one described by Dr. Meyer and his group is different than that described by Dr. Tosteson. Granted, there are correlations between them, but they are not duplicable. Then there is the mechanism proposed by Drs. Haddy and MacGregor, still another one which involves abnormal Na^+,K^+–ATPase activity. So there are, I gather, at least three different pump mechanisms implicated. The second problem that I would like to have the group pull together is the fact that Drs. MacGregor and Haddy find their lesion only in a particular volume expansion subtype of hypertension, whereas the lesions described by Drs. Meyer and Tosteson and their co-workers seem to occur across the board in common hypertension. Finally, the comment of Dr. Myers, if I heard him correctly, suggests that sodium in the diet changes the activity so that to point the direction in this frontier area it would help us all to understand whether we're studying the same thing

or something different and what the fundamental differences may be. Also, I wonder how specific these in vitro abnormalities may be since Dr. Tosteson's group, I believe, has already described similar abnormalities in normotensive manic-depressed patients [Pandey et al. (1977) Proc Natl Acad Sci USA].

Dr. Meyer: Thank you for these questions. 1) The relationship between the various pump activities is indeed still uncertain despite the fact that the Na,K-cotransport deficit and the increased Na, Li-countertransport appear to vary in parallel; 2) The depression of the Na,K–ATPase activity in essential hypertension is still debated. We found a normal Na,K–ATPase in most of the patients and an increased Na pump in some benign hypertensives [Garay RP et al (1980) Nature 284: 283]; 3) The deficit in Na,K-cotransport which appears as a hallmark of essential hypertension is not affected by environmental factors. It is also found in primary hypertension of the rat as we have shown [De Mendonca M et al (1980) Proc Natl Acad Sci USA 77: 4283]; 4) Dr. Tosteson did not find the same abnormality in manic and hypertensive patients, but just the opposite, decreased Na,Li-countertransport in the former and increased in the latter.

Dr. Haddy (Bethesda, Md.): There are several ways in which intracellular sodium and, hence, calcium concentrations can rise and lead to vasoconstriction. For example, they can rise because of suppression of the Na–K pump, as we propose for the low-renin models of hypertension, or they can rise because of increased permeability of the cell membrane to sodium, as appears to be the case in the genetic models. Intracellular calcium concentration might also rise because of suppression of Ca^{2+}–ATPase, as emphasized by Daniel and others. As has been pointed out before, there are a number of paths to vasoconstriction and, hence, hypertension.

Dr. Tosteson: I too want to respond to Dr. Laragh's plea for clarity about the different kinds of sodium transport abnormalities in hypertension that have been reported. In the case of two kinds of red cell sodium transport that have been studied in Paris and in our own lab, the relationship between them is unknown and now under investigation. We haven't yet identified the transport protein on which they go. In regard to the question of different subgroups, we do not find Na–Li countertransport elevated in secondary hypertension due to renal disease. I would like to make one comment to Dr. Reis who asked if there is a generalized membrane defect: Why don't we see more wrong? I think that you could ask that same question about any complex syndrome where there are polygenic contributing factors. Clearly, the genetic abnormalities are not great. If they were great, they would not be compatible with survival as long as these subjects live. It doesn't seem to me that anything that has been observed is inconsistent with the idea that there are several genes each producing modest abnormalities that working together lead to the syndrome.

Dr. Bühler: Dr. Tosteson, I wonder whether you measured the same transport defect as Dr. Meyer's group. If so, did you find in your observations a similarly sharp separation between normotensive and hypertensive subjects? Shouldn't there be a large borderline zone? Clinically there is a large pool of such people in whom it is hard to be sure that they truly have hypertension.

Dr. Tosteson: Yes, I think that if you look carefully at their data, there is an overlap between the higher hypertensives and the lower normotensives in the maximum rate of Na–K co-transport. Our preliminary data fall into that region of overlap.

Dr. Folkow (Göteborg, Sweden): One of the most striking differences between early essential hypertension of man or SHR and their respective normotensive controls is a modest increased responsiveness of limbic–hypothalamic–bulbar centers to alerting or stressful stimuli, a deviation which clearly is localized to these central nervous structures as it expresses itself as an accentuated sympathetic discharge, etc. Dr. Postnov, do you think that such a quantitative deviation, present in both SHR and the perhaps most common variant of early human primary hypertension, could also ultimately be dependent on a membrane deviation in the responsible central autonomic neurons, of a nature largely similar to that noted in the different types of blood cells?

Dr. Postnov (Moscow, U.S.S.R.): It could be, one may suggest that changes of the peripheral sympathetic neurons caused by membrane abnormalities may modify the functional state of the lymbic hypothalamic centers.

Dr. MacGregor (London, England): In further answer to Dr. Laragh's question, I think it is important to demonstrate a raised intracellular sodium concentration and also to measure sodium transport under physiologic conditions. Unless this is done one cannot be certain that the abnormalities in sodium transport being described are involved in the development of hypertension.

Session 4
Regulation of Blood Pressure by Prostaglandin-Kinin Interactions

Chairman: R.L. Soffer

Position Paper: Regulation of Blood Pressure by Prostaglandin-Kinin Interactions

John C. McGiff and Eric G. Spokas

Functional coupling of the kallikrein–kinin system with prostaglandins amplifies the vasodilator and diuretic actions of kinins and may be essential to some of the effects of these peptide hormones on blood vessels and renal function (1). Together, prostaglandins and kinins constitute a major blood pressure-regulating system which opposes the effects of circulating hormones, such as angiotensins, ADH, epinephrine, and mineralocorticoids, and of excitation of the adrenergic nervous system (2). Important interactions of prostaglandins and kinins that can lower blood pressure occur within the kidney and blood vessels where they contribute to the regulation of extracellular fluid volume and vascular reactivity. A principal objective of this position paper is to examine the interrelationships of vasoactive polypeptides and arachidonic acid metabolites in terms of the regulation of blood pressure. The central nervous system has been neglected out of ignorance; some of the most important vasodepressor mechanisms involving kinins and prostaglandins presumably occur within the brain, an area of great potential for future studies.

To understand how the interactions of prostaglandins and kinins relate to blood pressure regulation, it is necessary to consider the effects of vasoactive polypeptides on prostaglandin synthesis and metabolism, as well as to define the anatomic compartments where these interactions take place. Interactions of angiotensins and ADH with prostaglandins will also be considered because of their importance to blood volume and vascular tone, major determinants of the levels of blood pressure.

Kinins as well as angiotensins and ADH can release prostaglandins from tissues. Release denotes increased prostaglandin synthesis which results in immediate entry of the newly synthesized prostaglandin into the extracellular compartment (3). This effect of peptide hormones on prostaglandin synthesis depends on their capacity to activate tissue acylhydrolases, such as phospholipase A_2, which liberate arachidonic acid from phospholipids. The transformation of arachidonic acid by the prostaglandin synthesizing complex is initiated by the cyclooxygenase which generates prostaglandin cyclic endoperoxides (4). The latter, PGG_2 and PGH_2, are transformed to stable and labile endproducts which vary with tissues, diseases, and experimental conditions. Two of the labile products of the cyclic endoperoxide intermediates are thromboxane A_2 (TxA_2), a vasoconstrictor, and a vasodilator agent, prostacyclin (PGI_2). TxA_2 is generated by the platelet when aggregating (5) or by the kidney when injured (6). PGI_2 is synthesized by normal vascular tissues (7). Decreased production of PGI_2, described in blood vessels obtained from rabbits with experimental atherosclerosis, was suggested to predispose to vascular disease (8).

In addition to their capacity to induce prostaglandin synthesis, kinins and angiotensins may also affect the activity of a prostaglandin metabolizing enzyme which determines the ratio of two of the more stable species, PGE_2 and $PGF_{2\alpha}$. Thus, vasoactive polypeptides have the ability to increase the activity of PGE–9–ketoreductase, an enzyme which catalyzes reduction of the 9–keto position of PGE_2, forming $PGF_{2\alpha}$ (9). Whether $PGF_{2\alpha}$ or PGE_2 is a major product of enhanced prostaglandin synthesis is of vital consequence to blood pressure control. PGE_2 is vasodilator and diuretic and decreases adrenergic nervous activity (3), whereas $PGF_{2\alpha}$ constricts blood vessels and augments adrenergic nervous activity (10). Thus, an effect of vasoacitve peptides that favors the production of $PGF_{2\alpha}$, rather than PGE_2, can lead to elevation of blood pressure. Further, the action of vasoactive polypeptides on PGE–9–ketoreductase may be secondary to stimulation of guanylyl cyclase. A vascular mechanism involving cyclic GMP in the action of kinins has been suggested by Wong et al. (11) who have shown that cyclic GMP mimics the effects of bradykinin on PGE–9–ketoreductase activity of mesenteric blood vessels. Increased tissue levels of cyclic GMP have been associated with constriction of blood vessels (12) and hypertension (13).

Release of prostaglandins by kinins and angiotensins, therefore, can result in changes in the direction, intensity, and range of the effects of the peptide hormones (Fig. 1) as prostaglandins may, subject to experimental conditions, inhibit, augment, and even mediate the actions of the polypeptide. The modulator function of prostaglandins is the principal basis for their antihypertensive effects, inhibition of pressor hormones and augmentation of depressor hormones. The ability of prostaglandins of the E series to antagonize the vasoconstrictor action of pressor hormones is independent of the vasodilator action of the prostaglandin (14). Indeed, PGE_2 can inhibit the vasoconstrictor response to adrenergic nerve stimulation in the rabbit kidney at a concentration 200-fold less than that which dilates this vascular bed (15). When interpreting these findings, it is important to recall that prostaglandins probably act primarily as agents mediating mechanisms of defense; that is, they are released by a variety of stimuli which alter the basal or resting state of the animal (16).

As the enzymes that regulate the breakdown of the prostaglandin endoperoxides are distributed differentially within the tissues, segregation of their major products such as TxA_2, PGI_2, PGE_2, and PGD_2 to an anatomic compartment occurs. For example, within the lung, the predominant prostaglandin differs for the respiratory tree (PGE_2) and pulmonary vasculature (PGI_2) (17, 18). The anatomic compartmentalization of the major end-products of endoperoxides has particular significance for renal function. Thus, the primary formation of PGI_2 by the vascular compartment (19) of the kidney is crucially related to the regulation of renal blood flow and to interactions with the renin–angiotensin system (20), just as the production of PGE_2 by the cells lining or near the urinary compartment is related to the control of salt and water excretion and to interactions with the kallikrein–kinin system (20) (Fig. 2). The formation of PGE_2 within the medulla (21) is significant in view of the importance of this prostaglandin to inhibition of ADH (22) and to regulation of medullary blood flow (23), effects of PGE_2 that facilitate water excretion.

It is quite likely that disease states and unphysiologic conditions will influence the activity of those enzymes which regulate the breakdown of prostaglandin endoperoxides, favoring the generation of products not ordinarily associated with a tissue. Thus, TxA_2 is generated by the kidney only after

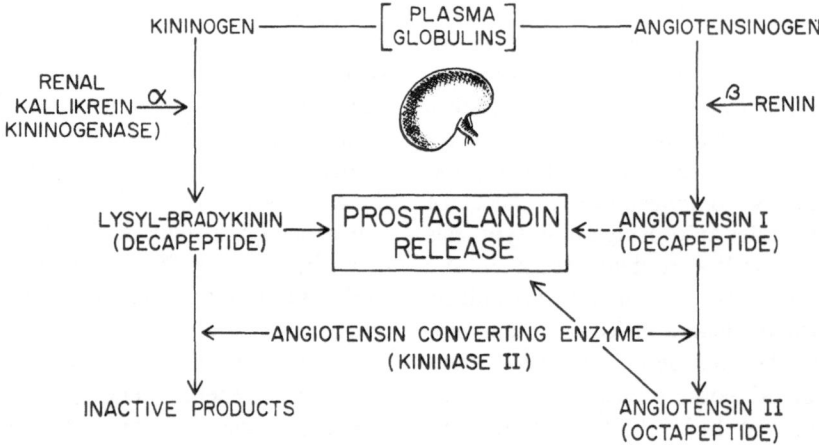

Fig. 1. The symbols α and β above the arrows proceeding from kallikrein and renin, respectively, refer to adrenergic mechanisms that participate in the regulation of kallikrein (α) and renin (β) release. The major products of each system are capable of releasing prostaglandins. Angiotensin-converting enzyme, which increases the activity of the renin–angiotensin system by conversion of angiotensin I to the more active form, angiotensin II, correspondingly reduces the activity of the kallikrein–kinin system by degrading kinins to inactive products.

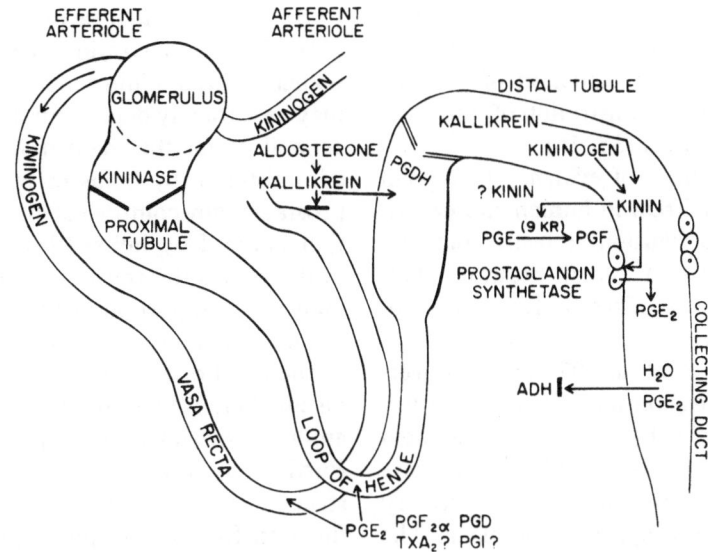

Fig. 2. Kinin–prostaglandin interactions in the nephron. The generation of kinins in the distal part of the nephron and in the collecting ducts can result in the release of PGE₂ which inhibits the effect of ADH and thereby facilitates the excretion of solute-free water. PGDH, prostaglandin 15-hydroxydehydrogenase; 9 KR, PGE-9-ketoreductase.

renal injury (6). It is also important to recognize the differential capacity of tissues, even vascular tissues, to produce PGI_2. Synthesis of PGI_2 by the ductus arteriosus accounts for more than 90% of the products of arachidonic acid metabolism in this tissue (24). In contrast, the umbilical artery and vein show a greater capacity to synthesize PGE_2 and $PGF_{2\alpha}$ than PGI_2 (25). Major-resistance blood vessels, such as the mesenteric and renal arteries, including their primary, secondary, and tertiary branches, generate relatively large amounts of PGE_2 and $PGF_{2\alpha}$, a capacity comparable to the synthesis of PGI_2 by these blood vessels (19, 26). PGE_2, unlike PGI_2, may act as a modulator whereby the responses of the vasculature and transporting epithelia to hormones and nervous activity are modified according to the local requirements of tissues. For example, PGE_2 and $PGF_{2\alpha}$ probably participate in those intrinsic mechanisms regulating the microcirculation, particularly adjustment of local blood flow to changing metabolic requirements of a tissue, as well as to local autoregulatory mechanisms that stabilize blood flow to a tissue (27).

In this regard, the interactions of prostaglandins and kinins have effects primarily at the tissue or local level. The functional effects of their interactions are registered within the organ or tissue of origin. Thus, altered vascular reactivity and changes in salt and water excretion occur as a result of prostaglandin–kinin interactions within the vascular wall and the renal distal tubule, respectively. However, PGI_2, unlike PGE_2 and $PGF_{2\alpha}$, escapes degradation on passage across the pulmonary circulation (28) and, therefore, may act as a circulating hormone if released into the blood stream in sufficient quantities. Because of the rapid degradation of PGI_2 within the vasculature (29), circulating levels may not have biologic significance either in terms of preventing platelet aggregation or decreasing vascular tone (30). Nonetheless, the possibility exists that PGI_2 is released intermittently either from the lungs (31) by chemoreceptor stimulation or from organs such as the kidney in response to activation of the renin–angiotensin system (32).

In 1973, we advanced the working hypothesis that a deficiency in one or more components of the kallikrein–kinin–prostaglandin system, which normally mediates an antihypertensive function, could contribute to the development of hypertension (2). This could arise from a primary deficiency in the kallikrein–kinin system which results in a secondary deficiency in prostaglandin production, if the coupling of kinins with prostaglandins is as close as some studies suggest (33, 34). Hypertension could also arise from a primary reduction in the capacity of the body to synthesize prostaglandins, as evidenced by induction of elevated blood pressure during administration of inhibitors of prostaglandin synthesis (35, 36).

There are several lines of evidence that point to a deficiency of kallikrein in human and experimental forms of hypertension as being contributory to the elevation of blood pressure. This association was first recognized by Elliot and Nuzum (37) more than 40 years ago and was confirmed by Margolius et al. in 1972 (38). Subjects with essential hypertension not only excreted less kallikrein than normal subjects, but demonstrated decreased responsiveness to stimuli that increase kallikrein excretion (39). The lowest excretory rates were found in the hypertensive black. The normotensive black excreted less kallikrein when compared to normal white subjects matched for age and sex (40). These differences were not related to variations in salt or water intake, as urinary sodium and potassium excretion and urine volume were not different among the groups. Further, urinary kallikrein excretion correlated with renal blood flow in all groups except normotensive blacks on a low-sodium diet (41). However, when cognizance was taken of the renin–angiotensin system acting as a determinant of renal blood flow, the ratio—urinary kallikrein/plasma renin activity (PRA)—was correlated with renal blood flow for all subjects. Because of the importance of renal mechanisms to the initiation and maintenance of the hypertensive state, it is important to review the relationships between the kallikrein–kinin and prostaglandin systems within the kidney. The renal vasodilator–diuretic effects of kinins are among their most prominent biologic properties (42). Prostaglandins may contribute to, or even mediate, some of the effects of kinins on renal function.

Bradykinin is a potent stimulus to prostaglandin generation, an effect first demonstrated in the kidney (42). Release of prostaglandins from the kidney, evoked by infusion of bradykinin into the renal artery, is associated with renal vasodilatation and increased excretion of salt and water. The contributions of prostaglandins to the renal vascular actions of kinins are uncertain. In the canine isolated blood-perfused kidney, a significant, albeit small, component of the renal vasodilator action of bradykinin was related to a prostaglandin mechanism (1). However, the vasodilator response to bradykinin for the kidney in situ was considered to be independent of a prostaglandin mechanism (43). The demonstration of a prostaglandin component in bradykinin-induced renal vasodilatation may be critically dependent on electrolyte balance, as well as on the manner in which the kinin is administered, by bolus or by infusion. Thus, the prostaglandin component in the renal vasodilatation induced by infused bradykinin may become evident only after the first 2 min, becoming increasingly more important as the infusion is continued.

The contribution of the released prostaglandin to the renal excretory effects of bradykinin is also disputed (1, 44) because of differences in responses among experimental preparations and species. Further, there are inherent limitations in reconstructing the local effects of a hormone on organ function from the response produced by infusion of the exogenous hormone into the arterial supply of that organ. For example, the influence of increased activity of the renal kallikrein–kinin system on excretion of salt and water may be restricted to the distal nephron as kallikrein normally enters the tubular fluid in the distal convolution (45) (Fig. 2). Thus, studies based on infusion of exogenous bradykinin into the renal artery cannot mimic the effects of activation of the renal kallikrein–kinin system. It is possible, however, to activate the renal kallikrein–kinin system and then determine the effects of increased levels of endogenous kinin or renal function. Inhibition of angiotension-converting enzyme that is identical to kininase II (46)—the principal kinin-degradative enzyme—elevated the activity of the renal kallikrein–kinin system, indicated by a surge of kinins into the urine and venous effluent, and caused concomitantly a several-fold increase in salt and water excretion (47). Administration of mineralocorticoids also increases the activity of the renal kallikrein–kinin system, and effect reversed by the kallikrein inhibitor, aprotinin (Trasylol) (34). Either deoxycorticosterone acetate (DOCA) or aldosterone, given over a period of 10 days, produced an initial transient antinatriuresis; a diuresis appeared on the second day of steroid administration and persisted for the remainder of treatment, associated with a threefold increase in excretion of kallikrein and PGE$_2$. Injection of aprotinin during mineralocorticoid treatment caused a rapid decline in urinary kallikrein activity and secondary decreases in excretion of PGE$_2$, sodium, and water. While the reduction of PGE$_2$ excretion and urinary kallikrein activity could be sustained by a maintenance dose of aprotinin, sodium and water excretion returned to the levels observed before administration of the kallikrein inhibitor. This study indicates a close coupling intrarenally between the kallikrein–kinin and prostaglandin systems. Changes in urinary kallikrein activity preceded major changes in excretion of PGE_2, an index of the activity of the renal prostaglandin system. It also suggests the importance of kinins and PGE_2 to the excretion of free water, at least on an intermediate term basis, since the antidiuresis lasted only several days despite continued depression of kallikrein and PGE_2 excretion. Enhanced excretion of free water in response to bradykinin has been suggested to operate through a prostaglandin-dependent mechanism, because this effect could be abolished by indomethacin in the canine blood-perfused isolated kidney (1). A study conducted in the conscious rabbit provided additional evidence that the renal kallikrein–kinin system may play an important role in the excretion of free water (48). Increased sodium intake in the face of unchanged fluid intake did not affect kallikrein excretion in the rabbit, whereas, when sodium intake was held constant, variations in fluid intake were positively correlated with kallikrein excretion. An important conclusion from these studies is that in the basal state, the activity of the prostaglandin system within the kidney is regulated primarily by the kallikrein–kinin system. However, when the animal is stressed, the renin-angiotensin system may supercede the kallikrein-kinin system in regulating the activity of the renal prostaglandin system (16).

The interrelationship of the prostaglandin and the renin–angiotensin systems is complex and involves the regulation of renin release as well as modulation of the actions of angiotensins. A relationship between these systems was first described in 1970 (49). Infusion of angiotensin II into the renal artery increased the concentrations of prostaglandins in renal venous blood, associated with blunting of the renal vasoconstrictor and antidiuretic actions of angiotensin II. PGE_2 was tentatively identified as the prostaglandin which modulated the renal actions of angiotensin (50). When angiotensin II did not release prostaglandins from the kidney, the renal effects of angiotensin II were not attenuated. Further, inhibition of the release of prostaglandins by treatment with indomethacin also caused sustained vasoconstriction and antidiuresis during infusion of angiotensin II (51). Based

on these studies, it was concluded that release of PGE_2 by angiotensin modulated the effects of the peptide hormone on renal function.

The focus of prostaglandin interactions with the renin–angiotensin system shifted in 1974 when the participation of prostaglandins in the regulation of renin release was demonstrated (52). Administration of arachidonic acid was shown to increase renin release, an effect prevented by indomethacin. Most investigators now accept the participation of a prostaglandin-dependent component in renin release operating in concert with tubular, neural, and mechanical factors (53). This mechanism has been held by some to be the final common pathway for the multiple signals capable of releasing renin (54). Resolution of the issue awaits further studies as does identification of the prostaglandin which subserves the renin-releasing mechanism. As PGI_2 is the principal product of arachidonic acid metabolism in all of the arterial elements thus far examined in the kidney, including interlobular arteries with attached afferent arterioles (19), it has been suggested to be the arachidonic acid metabolite which functions in the renin-releasing mechanism (55). However, PGI_2, an unstable compound, has been shown to be oxidized in the liver to a more stable product, most likely 6–keto–PGE_1 (56) (Fig. 3). Oxidation of PGI_2 via 9-hydroxyprostaglandin dehydrogenase may also occur in the kidney (57). Activity of this enzyme was highest in the cortex and lowest in the papilla, corresponding to the zonal distribution of renin. The capacity of 6-keto-PGE_1 to release renin from renal cortical slices was found to be equal to, or greater than that of, PGI_2 (58). This finding raised the possibility that effects previously attributed to PGI_2 may have resulted from its enzymic transformation to 6-keto-PGE_1, a conversion that may explain the long duration of action of PGI_2 (59).

Prostaglandin interactions with the renin–angiotensin system have been proposed to serve a primary defensive role which protects organ function in the face of increased activity of the renin-angiotensin system. In the dog subjected to the stresses of anesthesia and laparotomy, PGE_2 levels in renal venous blood were greatly increased and positively correlated with plasma renin levels (16). The contribution of prostaglandins to the support of the renal circulation, when the renin–angiotensin system was stimulated in the acutely stressed animal, was demonstrated by inhibition of prostaglandin synthesis (60). Administration of indome-

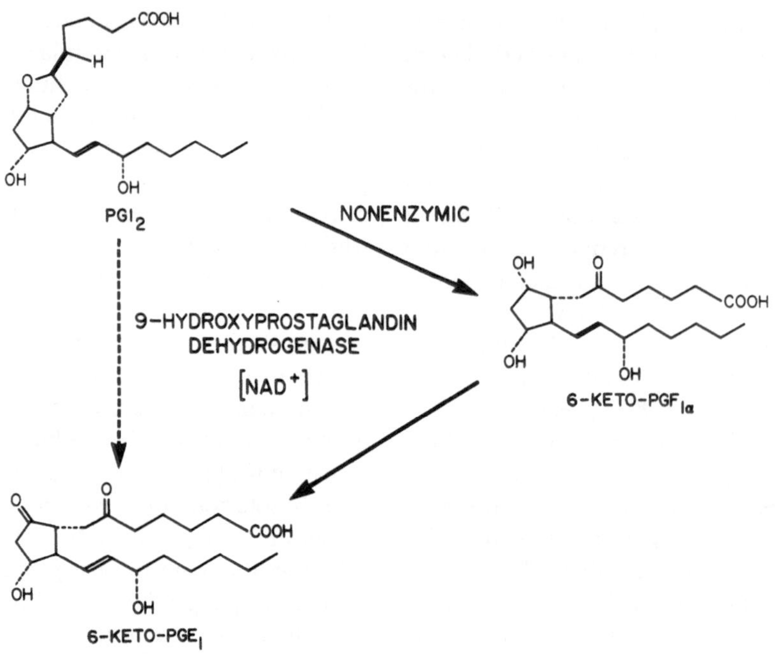

Fig. 3. Chemical structures of PGI_2, 6-keto $PGF_{1\alpha}$, and 6-keto PGE_1. Spontaneous hydrolysis of PGI_2 forms 6-keto $PGF_{1\alpha}$, which differs from 6-keto PGE_1 in the substituent at C-9. The enzyme 9-hydroxyprostaglandin dehydrogenase catalyzes the oxidation of 6-keto $PGF_{1\alpha}$. Alternatively, 6-keto PGE_1 may be formed from PGI_2 through an unknown intermediary pathway.

thacin under these conditions caused a precipitous reduction in renal blood flow which correlated with a decline in efflux of PGE_2 into the renal vein. In contrast, in the resting dog, not subjected to trauma, administration of indomethacin did not affect renal blood (16).

A prostaglandin-dependent mechanism also determines the intrarenal distribution of blood flow, herein providing another example of their generally accepted role as local hormones (61). In the canine isolated kidney perfused with blood, the levels of PGE_2 in the perfusate correlated with increased blood flow to the inner cortex. Administration of indomethacin caused a disproportionate reduction of blood flow to the inner cortex and a redistribution of renal blood flow from the inner to the outer cortex.

We conclude that activation of the renin–angiotensin system need not result in the elevation of blood pressure unless those prostaglandin-dependent mechanisms which contribute to the regulation of the circulation are compromised. The capacity of the kidney and vascular tissues to synthesize prostaglandins is important to the maintenance of normal blood pressure, particularly when considered together with the kallikrein–kinin system. The contribution of prostaglandins to the control of blood pressure is suggested by the demonstration that nonsteroidal antiinflammatory drugs can cause hypertension in animals (35) and in man (36) and increase further the elevated blood pressure in hypertensive man (62).

SUMMARY

Prostaglandins contribute to the control of extracellular fluid volume, vascular tone, and the renal circulation. Kinins can initiate the prostaglandin cascade through liberation of arachidonic acid by stimulating acylhydrolases and can also influence the activity of prostaglandin metabolizing enzymes. The final products of the cascade—TxA_2, PGI_2, PGD_2, and PGE_2—arise from enzymic transformation of the cyclic endoperoxide intermediates in a tissue-specific manner; that is, the enzymes are compartmentalized with activities directed by physiologic and pathologic conditions. Interactions of the prostaglandin and kallikrein–

kinin systems in blood vessels and in the tubular and vascular compartments of the kidney, which may be affected by the background activity of the renin–angiotensin–aldosterone system, are determinants of vascular reactivity, renal blood flow, and salt and water excretion. The range and intensity of the biologic activities of kinins and angiotensins are governed by prostaglandins, effects directly related to the regulation of blood pressure.

ACKNOWLEDGMENTS

This work was supported by USPHS grant HL–25394–02 and an American Heart Associate Research Grant, Westchester/Putnam Chapter. E. G. Spokas is a recipient of a National Kidney Foundation Fellowship.

We thank Dr. John Quilley and Mrs. Caroline Quilley for their criticism of the manuscript. We thank Donna Centi and Sallie McGiff for preparation of the manuscript.

REFERENCES

1. McGiff JC, Itskovitz HD, Terragno NA (1975) The actions of bradykinin and eledoisin in the canine isolated kidney: Relationships to prostaglandins. Clin Sci Mol Med 49: 125–131
2. McGiff JC, Nasjletti A (1973) Renal prostaglandins and the regulation of blood pressure. In: Kahn RH, Lands WEM (eds) Prostaglandins and cyclic AMP biological actions and clinical applications. Academic Press, New York/London, pp 119–151
3. McGiff JC, Itskovitz HD (1973) Prostaglandins and the kidney. Circ Res 33: 479–488
4. Hamberg M, Samuelsson B (1974) Prostaglandin endoperoxides: Novel transformations of arachidonic acid in human platelets. Proc Natl Acad Sci USA 71: 3400–3404
5. Hamberg M, Svensson J, Samuelsson B (1975) Thromboxanes: A new group of biologically active compounds derived from prostaglandin endoperoxides. Proc Natl Acad Sci USA 72: 2994–2998
6. Morrison AR, Nishikawa K, Needleman P (1977) Unmasking of thromboxane A_2 synthesis by ureteral obstruction in the rabbit kidney. Nature 267: 259–260
7. Moncada S, Gryglewski RJ, Bunting S, Vane JR (1976) An enzyme isolated from arteries transforms prostaglandin endoperoxides to an unstable substance that inhibits platelet aggregation. Nature 263: 663–665
8. Dembinska-Kiec A, Gryglewska T, Zmuda A, Gry-glewski RJ (1977) The generation of prostacyclin by arteries and by the coronary vascular bed is reduced in experimental atherosclerosis in rabbits. Prostaglandins 14: 1025–1034
9. Wong PY-K, Terragno DA, Terragno NA, McGiff JC (1977) Dual effects of bradykinin on prostaglandin metabolism: Relationship to the dissimilar vascular actions of kinins. Prostaglandins 13: 1113–1125
10. Ducharme DW, Weeks JR, Montgomery RG (1968) Studies on the mechanism of the hypertensive effect of prostaglandin $F_{2\alpha}$. J Pharmacol Exp Ther 160: 1–10
11. Wong PY-K, McGiff JC, Terragno NA (1977) Polypeptides: Vascular actions as modified by prostaglandins. In: Berti F, Samuelsson B, Velo GP (eds) Prostaglandins and thromboxanes. Plenum, New York, pp 251–264
12. Dunham EW, Haddox MK, Goldberg ND (1974) Alteration of vein cyclic 3',5' nucleotide concentrations during changes in contractility. Proc Natl Acad Sci USA 71: 815–819
13. Amer MS, Gomoll AW, Perhach JL Jr, Ferguson HC, McKinney GR (1974) Aberrations of cyclic nucleotide metabolism in the hearts and vessels of hypertensive rats. Proc Natl Acad Sci USA 71: 4930–4934
14. Weiner R, Kaley G (1969) Influence of prostaglandin E_1 on the terminal vascular bed. Am J Physiol 217: 563–566
15. Malik KU, McGiff JC (1975) Modulation by prostaglandins of adrenergic transmission in the isolated perfused rabbit and rat kidney. Circ Res 36: 599–609
16. Terragno NA, Terragno DA, McGiff JC (1977) Contribution of prostaglandins to the renal circulation in conscious, anesthetized and laparotomized dogs. Circ Res 40: 590–595
17. Gryglewski RJ, Dembinska-Kiec A, Grodzinska L (1977) Generation of prostaglandin and thromboxane-like substances by large airways and lung parenchyma. In: Berti F, Samuelsson B, Velo GP (eds) Prostaglandins and thromboxanes. Plenum, New York
18. Leffler CW, Hessler JR, Terragno NA (1980) Ventilation-induced release of prostaglandinlike material from fetal lungs. Am J Physiol 238: 282–286
19. Terragno NA, Terragno A, Early JA, Roberts MA, McGiff JC (1978) Endogenous prostaglandin synthesis inhibitor in the renal cortex: Effects on production of prostacyclin by renal blood vessels. Clin Sci Mol Med 55: 199S–202S
20. McGiff JC, Wong PY-K (1979) Compartmentalization of prostaglandins and prostacyclin within the kidney: Implications for renal function. Fed Proc 38: 89–93
21. Muirhead EE, Germain G, Leach BE, Pitcock JA, Stephenson P, Brooks B, Brosius WL, Daniels EG, Hinman JW (1972) Production of renomedullary prostaglandins by renomedullary interstitial cells grown in tissue culture. Circ Res 30, 31(suppl II): 161–172

22. Grantham JJ, Orloff J (1968) Effect of prostaglandin E_1 on the permeability response of the isolated collecting tubule to vasopressin, adenosine 3',5'-monophosphate and theophylline. J Clin Invest 47: 1154–1161

23. Itskovitz HD, McGiff JC (1974) Hormonal regulation of the renal circulation. Circ Res 34, 35(Suppl I): 65–73

24. Terragno NA, Terragno A, McGiff JC, Rodriguez DJ (1977) Synthesis of prostaglandins by the ductus arteriosus of the bovine fetus. Prostaglandins 14: 721–727

25. Terragno, NA, Terragno A (1979) Prostaglandin metabolism in the fetal and maternal vasculature. Fed Proc 38: 75–77

26. Terragno, NA, McGiff JC, Smigel M, Terragno A (1978) Patterns of prostaglandin production in the bovine fetal and maternal vasculature. Prostaglandins 16: 847–855

27. Messina EJ, Kaley G (1980) Microcirculatory responses to prostacyclin and PGE_2 in the rat cremaster muscle. In: Samuelsson B, Ramwell PW, Paoletti R (eds) Advances in prostaglandin and thromboxane research, Vol 7. Raven Press, New York, pp 719–722

28. Moncada S, Korbut R, Bunting S, Vane JR (1978) Prostacyclin is a circulating hormone. Nature 273: 767–768

29. Wong PY-K, Sun FF, McGiff JC (1978) Metabolism of prostacyclin in blood vessels. J Biol Chem 253: 5555–5557

30. Steer ML, MacIntyre DE, Levine L, Salzman EW (1980) Is prostacyclin a physiologically important circulating anti-platelet agent? Nature 283: 194–195

31. Gryglewski R, Korbut R, Ocetkiewicz A (1978) Generation of prostacyclin by lungs *in vivo* and its release into the arterial circulation. Nature 273: 765–767

32. Shebuski RJ, Aiken JW (1980) Angiotensin II-induced renal prostacyclin release suppresses platelet aggregation in the anesthetized dog. In: Samuelsson B, Ramwell PW, Paoletti R (eds) Advances in prostaglandin and thromboxane research, Vol 7. Raven Press, New York, pp 1149–1152

33. Colina-Chourio J, McGiff JC, Miller MP, Nasjletti A (1976) Possible influence of intrarenal generation of kinins on prostaglandin release from the rabbit perfused kidney. Br J Pharmacol 58: 165–172

34. Nasjletti A, McGiff JC, Colina-Chourio J (1978) Interrelations of the renal kallikrein-kinin system and renal prostaglandins in the conscious rat. Circ Res 43: 799–807

35. Colina-Chourio J, McGiff JC, Nasjletti A (1979) Effect of indomethacin on blood pressure in the normotensive unanesthetized rabbit: Possible relation to prostaglandin synthesis inhibition. Clin Sci 57: 359–365

36. Wennmalm Å (1978) Influence of indomethacin on the systemic and pulmonary vascular resistance in man. Clin Sci Mol Med 54: 141–145

37. Elliot AH, Nuzum FR (1934) Urinary excretion of a depressor substance (kallikrein of Frey and Kraut) in arterial hypertension. Endocrinology 18: 462–474

38. Margolius HR, Geller RG, de Jong W, Pisano JJ, Sjoerdsma A (1972) Urinary kallikrein excretion in hypertension. Circ Res 30, 31(Suppl I): 125–131

39. Margolius HS, Horwitz D, Pisano JJ, Keiser HR (1976) Relationships among urinary kallikrein, mineralocorticoids and human hypertensive disease. Fed Proc 35: 203–206

40. Zinner SH, Margolius HS, Rosner B, Keiser HR, Kass EH (1976) Familial aggregation of urinary kallikrein concentration in childhood: Relation to blood pressure, race and urinary electrolytes. Am J Epidemiol 104: 124–132

41. Levy SB, Lilley JJ, Frigon RP, Stone RA (1977) Urinary kallikrein and plasma renin activity as determinants of renal blood flow. J Clin Invest 60: 129–138

42. McGiff JC, Terragno NA, Malik KU, Lonigro AJ (1972) Release of a prostaglandin E-like substance from canine kidney by bradykinin. Circ Res 31: 36–43

43. Lonigro AJ, Hegemann MH, Stephenson AH, Fry CL (1978) Inhibition of prostaglandin synthesis by indomethacin augments the renal vasodilator response to bradykinin in the anesthetized dog. Circ Res 43: 447–455

44. Blasingham MC, Nasjletti A (1979) Contribution of renal prostaglandins to the natriuretic action of bradykinin in the dog. Am J Physiol 237(3): F182–F187

45. Carretero OA, Scicli AG (1976) Renal kallikrein: Its localization and possible role in renal function. Fed Proc 35: 194–198

46. Erdös EG (1976) The kinins; a status report. Biochem Pharmacol 25: 1563–1569

47. Nasjletti A, Colina-Chourio J, McGiff JC (1975) Disappearance of bradykinin in the renal circulation of dogs. Circ Res 37: 59–65

48. Mills IH, Ward PE (1975) The relationship between kallikrein and water excretion and the conditional relationship between kallikrein and sodium excretion. J Physiol (Lond) 246: 695–707

49. McGiff JC, Crowshaw K, Terragno NA, Lonigro AJ (1970) Release of a prostaglandin-like substance into renal venous blood in response to angiotensin II. Circ Res 26, 27(Suppl I): 121–129

50. McGiff JC, Malik KU, Terragno NA (1976) Prostaglandins as determinants of vascular reactivity. Fed Proc 35: 2382–2387

51. Aiken JW, Vane JR (1974) Intrarenal prostaglandin release attenuates the renal vasoconstrictor activity of angiotensin. J Pharmacol Exp Ther 184: 678–687

52. Larsson C, Weber P, Änggard E (1974) Arachidonic acid increases and indomethacin decreases plasma renin activity in the rabbit. Eur J Pharmacol 28: 391–394

53. Data JL, Gerber JG, Crum WJ, Frölich JC, Hollifield JW, Nies AS (1978) The prostaglandin system: A role in canine baroreceptor control of renin release. Circ Res 42: 454–458

54. Weber PC, Scherer B, Lang HH, Held H, Schnermann J (1978) Renal prostaglandins and renin release relationship to regulation of electrolyte excretion and blood pressure. In: Proceedings of the seventh international congress of nephrology, Montreal, June 18–23. Karger, Basel, pp 99–106

55. Whorton AR, Misono K, Hollifield J, Frolich JC, Inagami T, Oates JA (1977) Prostaglandins and renin release: Stimulation of renin release from rabbit renal cortical slices by PGI$_2$. Prostaglandins 14: 1095–1104

56. Wong PY-K, Malik KU, Desiderio DM, McGiff JC, Sun FF (1980) Hepatic metabolism of prostacyclin (PGI$_2$) in the rabbit: Formation of a potent novel inhibitor of platelet aggregation. Biochem Biophys Res Commun 93: 486–494

57. Pace-Asciak C (1975) Prostaglandin 9-hydroxydehydrogenase activity in the adult rat kidney: Identification, assay, pathway and some enzyme properties. J Biol Chem 250: 2789–2794

58. Spokas EG, Ferreri NR, Wong PY-K, McGiff JC (1980) Effect of 6-keto prostaglandin E$_1$ (6-keto-PGE$_1$) on renin release from rabbit renal cortical slices (abstr). Circulation 62:

59. Szczeklik A, Gryglewski RJ, Nizankowska E, Nizankowski R, Musial J (1978) Pulmonary and antiplatelet effects of intravenous and inhaled prostacyclin in man. Prostaglandins 16: 651–660

60. Lonigro AJ, Itskovitz HD, Crowshaw K, McGiff JC (1973) Dependency of renal blood flow on prostaglandin synthesis in the dog. Circ Res 32: 712–717

61. Itskovitz HD, Terragno NA, McGiff JC (1974) Effect of a renal prostaglandin on distribution of blood flow in the isolated canine kidney. Circ Res 34: 770–776

62. Ylitalo, P, Pitkäjärvi T, Metsä-Ketelä T, Vapaatalo H (1978) The effect of inhibition of prostaglandin synthesis on plasma renin activity and blood pressure in essential hypertension. Prostaglandins Med 1: 479–488

Prostaglandins in Human Hypertension: Relationships to Renin, Sodium, and Antihypertensive Drug Action

J. C. Frölich, D. Robertson, W. Kitajima, B. Rosenkranz, and I. Reimann

Ever since pharmacologic experiments have shown the blood pressure-lowering effect of prostaglandins (PGs), attempts have been made to elucidate a role of endogenous PGs in regulation of blood pressure (for review, see ref. 1) and mediation of antihypertensive drug effects. Of the initial candidates, PGA_2 and PGE_2, the former has largely vanished from serious consideration, as its levels in vivo are undetectably low by specific methodology (2, 3) and levels of renal medulla have been shown to result from in vitro dehydration of PGE_2 (4).

Assessment of PGE_2 levels of renal medulla in vitro has shown that spontaneously hypertensive rats (SHR) are different from normal rats (5), but the relevance of this finding is unknown. In vivo studies in the rat have shown that in contrast to other species, PGE is a renal vasoconstrictor (6); in the New Zealand hypertensive rat, raised renal PGE_2 levels caused by a reduction in its metabolism have been suggested to cause hypertension (6). In all other species tested, PGE_2 will lower blood pressure and reduce renal vascular resistance.

The following discussion presents new data on PGE_2 synthesis in human hypertension. In addition, the interactions between the prostaglandin system and some drugs useful in the therapy of hypertension will be described.

PGE_2 SYNTHESIS IN HUMAN HYPERTENSION

PGE_2 synthesis in man can be assessed by measuring PGE_2 levels in urine (7) or by measuring the major urinary metabolite of PGE_2, PGE–M (8, 9). Measurement of urinary PGE_2 represents renal PGE_2 synthesis in females. In males, measurement

of urinary PGE_2 can lead to erroneous results due to contamination with seminal fluid, the richest known source of PGE_2 in man. PGE_2 has been shown to be decreased in hypertensive subjects (10). However, because of the problems associated with measurement of urinary PGE_2 by radioimmunoassay with levels from 2- to 28-fold higher measured by RIA than by gas chromatography–mass spectrometry (GC–MS) (11), we have decided to measure PGE–M by GC–MS (12) in male hypertensive and control volunteers.

Seventeen volunteers were studied, five normal controls, seven patients with low-renin, and five patients with high-renin essential hypertension. All subjects were Caucasian and male except for one female with low-renin essential hypertension. (For definition of high- and low-renin status and essential hypertension, see ref. 13.) The participants of the study were brought into balance on a 150–mEq Na^+ diet and subsequently on a 10-mEq Na^+ diet. Dietary balance was assessed by measuring 24-h urinary sodium excretion.

We found that patients with low-renin essential hypertension excrete significantly less PGE–M than patients with high-renin essential hypertension (Fig. 1). For all subjects studied, there was a modest increase in PGE–M when they were placed on a 10-mEq Na^+ diet (Fig. 2). This increase was too small to be statistically significant for each group alone and there was no correlation between the percent change of plasma renin activity (PRA) and PGE–M.

Our data show that in addition to the biochemical parameters known to be different in patients stratified according to their renin status, PGE synthesis also follows this pattern. This finding emphasizes the significance of stratification of hypertensive patients according to renin status which has been shown to be important in diagnosis and therapy of hypertension (14). Investigation of the PG system in hypertensive patients must

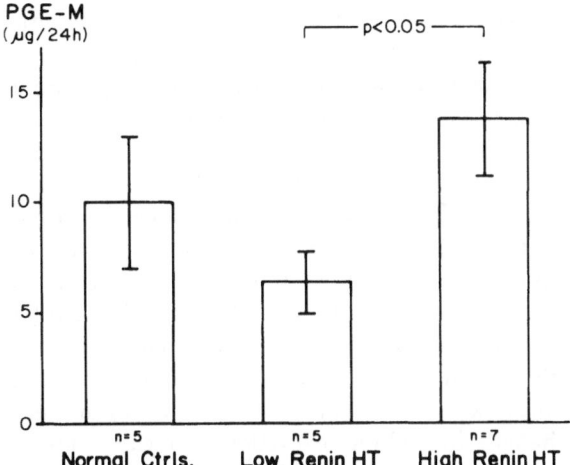

Fig 1. Excretion of PGE–M in normal controls and patients with low-, high-, and normal-renin essential hypertension.

take into account not only age and sex differences but also the renin classification.

The reasons for the difference in PGE_2 biosynthesis between the two groups of hypertensive patients are not obvious. PGE–M is only in part derived from renally synthesized PGE_2, because we have found patients with Bartter's syndrome to excrete threefold more PGE_2 in their urine in the face of normal PGE–M levels (11). Angiotensin II has been shown to enhance renal PGE_2 biosynthesis (15), which is reflected in increased urinary PGE_2 (16); however, no data are available on its effects on PGE–M in vivo. There is uncertainty as to the importance of this PG in regulation of vascular resistance. Although the abnormally

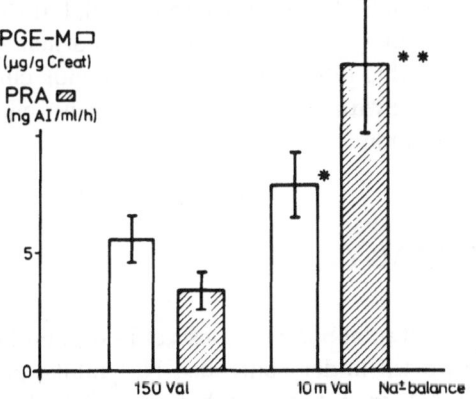

Fig. 2. Effect of reduced Na intake on PGE–M and PRA in patients ($N = 13$) with essential hypertension. Mean ± SE, *$p < 0.05$; **$p < 0.01$.

reduced pressor response to angiotensin II in patients with Bartter's syndrome could be normalized by indomethacin, and these patients were found to excrete excessive amounts of PGE_2 with their urine (17), this does not necessarily indicate a role of PGE_2 in causing the angiotensin II resistance. Nevertheless, it is noteworthy that the human organism synthesizes approximately ten times more PGE_2 than prostecyclin (PGI_2) based on measurement of the respective urinary metabolites (18). It is of course also possible that both PGE_2 and PGI_2 are contributing to the regulation of vascular resistance. However, although angiotensin II can increase renal PGE_2 synthesis, and this increased PG synthesis significantly reduces renal vascular resistance (19), renal PGI_2 synthesis may not be affected by angiotensin in the anesthetized dog determined by measuring 6–keto–$PGF_{1\alpha}$ in urine (W. Kitajima, unpublished observation). Thus, we would like to propose that the renal vasodilatory PGs, PGE_2 and PGI_2, are regulated differently and independently in the kidney. This may apply to other tissues as well.

RELATIONSHIP BETWEEN RENAL RENIN RELEASE AND PG SYNTHESIS

Infusion experiments utilizing PGs had resulted in conflicting data on renal renin release (for review, see ref. 20). Infusion of arachidonic acid, the precursor of the bis-enoic PGs, however, consistently leads to an increase in renal venous PRA, which could be blocked by PG synthesis inhibitors (21, 22).

We have studied the role of renal PGs in renin release in man. In patients with hypertension and normal volunteers, we found that indomethacin would lower PRA, aldosterone and sodium excretion, as well as block the acute rise of PRA following intravenous administration of furosemide (23). Although the reduction of PRA during chronic indomethacin administration could perhaps have resulted from sodium retention, this appeared to be a less likely explanation for the blockade of furosemide-induced renin release.

In order to clarify the role of sodium in the reduction of PRA by PG inhibition, experiments were carried out in normal volunteers on 10–mEq Na^+ balance. Indomethacin caused suppression of

PG synthesis but had no effect on Na$^+$ balance, PRA, or aldosterone (24).

As sodium depletion is associated with significantly increased catecholamine levels, it was conceivable that they provided the major stimulus for renin release in this situation and that this catecholamine-induced renin release was independent of the PG system. This hypothesis was tested in two ways.

In hypertensive subjects on 10–mEq Na$^+$ balance, beta-receptor-mediated renin release was blocked by propranolol and the effect of indomethacin assessed. Under these conditions, blockade of PG synthesis caused a greater than 70% reduction of supine and upright PRA but had no effect on Na$^+$ excretion (7, 25). This study shows that inhibition of PG synthesis can cause suppression of PRA independently of sodium retention.

In the second experiment carried out in normal volunteers on 10–mEq Na$^+$ balance, indomethacin had no effect on stimulation of PRA by isoproterenol (25), lending further support to the concept that in man, in contrast to some animals (26), renin release mediated by stimulation of the beta-receptor is not dependent on a PG mechanism (7). Studies on the mechanism responsible for PG-dependent renin release carried out in 1977 revealed that the baroreceptor is dependent on a normally functioning renal cyclooxygenase system (27). As PGE$_2$ was the only product of renal cortical cyclooxygenase known at that time to cause renin release, we measured its levels in renal venous blood during baroreceptor-stimulated renin release. Because no increase of PGE$_2$ release was observed (20), we reinvestigated renal cortical PG synthesis and discovered that a prominent product of renal cortical cyclooxygenase is PGI$_2$ (28). We found subsequently that PGI$_2$ stimulates renin release in vitro with a molar effectivity similar to isoproterenol. These findings led to the formulation of a hypothesis that PG-dependent renin release is mediated by PGI$_2$ (7).

pindolol in rabbits (24, 29). This drug interaction is potentially of clinical significance. The extrapolation that the antihypertensive effect of propranolol could be mediated by PGs (24), however, is not supported by a study we carried out in seven hypertensive patients. These patients were placed on a 10–mEq Na$^+$ diet until in balance. Propranolol reduced their blood pressure from an average value of 168/104–146/96 mmHg. Administration of indomethacin reduced PGE–M by 60% but had no effect on blood pressure or sodium balance. We have shown previously that indomethacin can cause sodium retention (23), and even small changes in sodium excretion can cause loss of blood pressure control in hypertensive patients.

Both hydralazine and minoxidil have been shown to cause release of prostaglandin-like material from the dog kidney in vivo and their antihypertensive effect was largely abolished by indomethacin (30). In contrast, in guinea pig, rat, rabbit, and rat, indomethacin had only negligible effects on the blood pressure-lowering effect of hydralazine (30). In man, the acute effect of hydralazine seems little affected by blockade of PG synthesis (I. Reimann and J. C. Frölich, unpublished observation).

The diuretic and natriuretic effects of furosemide can be reduced in man by pretreatment with indomethacin (23). The natriuretic effect of intravenous furosemide was found to be reduce by approximately 25% by indomethacin (23). Interpretation of this finding needs to take into consideration not only the effect of indomethacin on PG biosynthesis, but also its effect on tubular transport systems. Thus, furosemide needs to be excreted into the tubular lumen to reach its receptor. Indomethacin has been shown to reduce the urinary concentration of furosemide to a small, but significant, extent (23). In patients with normal renal function, this interaction seems of minor clinical importance with respect to the therapeutic efficacy of furosemide.

MODIFICATION OF ANTIHYPERTENSIVE DRUG EFFECTS BY INHIBITION OF PG SYNTHESIS

The antihypertensive effect of propranolol can be antagonized by indomethacin in man and that of

SUMMARY

The rate of total body synthesis of PGE$_2$ and PGE$_1$ was assessed under controlled Na$^+$ intake of 150 mEq/24 h in patients with low- and high-renin hypertension. For this, the major urinary metabolite of PGE$_1$ and PGE$_2$ was measured by stable isotope dilution assay utilizing GC–MS. It was found that patients with high-renin essential hypertension excrete significantly more of the metabolite than patients with low-renin essential hypertension. Similarly, reduction of Na$^+$ intake to 10 mEq/24 h tended to increase PGE–M. Thus, classification according to renin status is a prerequisit to studying the PG system in hypertension. Furthermore, in addition to other parameters, PGs are following the renin stratification. PG's role in renin regulation is discussed and the clinical importance of Na$^+$ retention by inhibitors of renal cyclooxygenase demonstrated.

ACKNOWLEDGMENTS

This work was supported by the Robert Bosch Foundation, Stuttgart, Germany, and NIH grant HL-14192.

REFERENCES

1. Frölich JC, Gill JR, McGiff JC, Needleman P, Nies AS (1979) Prostaglandins: Subgroup report of the Hypertension Task Force. DHEW Publication No (NIH) 79–1629, US Government Printing Office, Washington, DC, pp 1–98
2. Frölich JC, Sweetman BJ, Carr K, Hollifield JW, Oates JA (1975) Assessment of the levels of PGA$_2$ in human plasma by gas chromatography-mass spectrometry. Prostaglandins 10: 185
3. Frölich JC (1977) Gas chromatography-mass spectrometry of prostaglandins. In: Ramwell P (ed) The prostaglandins, Vol 3. Plenum, New York, pp 1–39
4. Frölich JC, Sweetman BJ, Carr K, Oates JA (1975) Prostaglandin synthesis in rabbit renal medulla. Life Sci 17: 1105–1112
5. Dunn MJ, Howe D, Harrison M (1976) Renal prostaglandin production in the spontaneously hypertensive rat. J Clin Invest 58: 862–870
6. Armstrong JM, Blackwell, GJ, Flower RJ, McGiff JC, Mullane KM, Vane JR (1976) Genetic hypertension in rats is accompanied by a defect in renal prostaglandin catabolism. Nature 260: 582–586
7. Frölich JC, Whorton AR, Walker L, Smigel M, Oates JA, France, R, Hollifield JW, Data JL, Gerber JG, Nies AS, Williams W, Robertson GL (1978) Renal prostaglandins: Regional differences in synthesis and role in renin release of ADH action. In: Proceedings of the seventh international congress of nephrology, Montreal. Karger, Basel, pp 107–114
8. Hamberg M (1972) Inhibition of prostaglandin synthesis in man. Biochem Biophys Res Commun 49: 720–726
9. Seyberth HW, Sweetman BJ, Frölich JC (1976) Assessment of the quantitative analysis of the major urinary metabolite of prostaglandin E in man. Prostaglandins 11: 381–397
10. Abe K, Yasujima M, Chiba S, Orokawa N, Ito T, Yoshinaga K (1977) Effect of furosemide on urinary excretion of prostaglandin E in normal volunteers and patients with essential hypertension. Prostaglandins 14 (3): 513
11. Gill JR, Frölich JC, Bowden RE, Taylor AA, Keiser HR, Seyberth HW, Oates JA, Bartter FC (1976) Bartter's syndrome: A disorder characterized by high urinary prostaglandins and a dependence of hyperreninemia on prostaglandin synthesis. Am J Med 61: 43–51
12. Frölich JC (1976) Gas chromatography-mass spectrometry of prostaglandins. In: Ramwell P (ed) The prostaglandins, Vol 3. Plenum, New York, pp 1–39
13. Hollifield JW, Sherman K, Vander Zwagg R, Shand DG (1976) Proposed mechanism of propranolol's antihypertensive effect in essential hypertension. N Engl J Med 295: 68–73
14. Laragh JH, Sealey JE (1977) Renin-sodium profiling: Why, how, and when in clinical practice. Cardiovasc Med 2: 1053–1075
15. McGiff JS, Crowshaw K, Terragno NA, Lonigro AJ (1970) Release of a prostaglandin-like substance into renal venous blood in response to angiotensin II. Circ Res 27(Suppl I): 1
16. Frölich JC, Wilson TW, Sweetman BJ, Nies AS, Carr K, Watson JT, Oates JA (1975) Urinary prostaglandins: Identification and origin. J Clin Invest 55: 763–770
17. Bartter FC, Gill JR, Frölich JC, Bowden RE, Hollifield JE, Radfar N, Keiser HR, Oates JA, Taylor AA (1976) Prostaglandins are overproduced by the kidneys and mediate hyperreninemia in Bartter's syndrome. Trans Assoc Am Physicians 89: 77–91
18. Rosenkranz B, Fischer C, Reimann I, Weimer KE, Beck G, Frölich JC (in press) Identification of the major metabolite of prostacyclin and 6–keto–prostaglandin F$_1$ in man. Biochim Biophys Acta
19. Aiden JW, Vane JR (1973) Intrarenal prostaglandin release attenuates the renal vasoconstrictor activity of angiotensin. J Pharmacol Exp Ther 184: 678–687
20. Frölich JC (in press) Prostaglandins: Role in renin regulation and mediation of antihypertensive drug effects.
21. Larsson C, Weber P, Änggård E (1974) Arachidonic acid increases and indomethacin decreases plasma renin activity in the rabbit. Eur J Pharmacol 28: 391
22. Weber P, Holzgreve H, Stephan R, Herbst R (1975) Plasma renin activity and renal sodium and water excretion following infusion of arachidonic acid in rats. Eur J Pharmacol 34: 299
23. Frölich JC, Hollifield JW, Dormois JC, Seyberth

HJ, Michelakis AM, Oates JA (1976) Suppression of plasma renin acitivity by indomethacin in man. Circ Res 39: 447–452

24. Durao V, Prata MM, Concalves LMP (1977) Modification of antihypertensive effect of β-adrenoceptor-blocking agents by inhibition of endogenous prostaglandin synthesis. Lancet 2: 1005–1007

25. Frölich JC, Hollifield JW, Vesper BS, Shand DG, Wilson JP, Seyberth HJ, Frölich WH, Oates JA (1979) Reduction of plasma renin activity by inhibition of the fatty acid cyclooxygenase: Independence of sodium retention. Circ Res 44: 781–787

26. Campbell WB, Graham RM, Jackson EK (1979) Role of renal prostaglandins in sympathetically mediated renin release in the rat. J Clin Invest 64: 448–456

27. Data SS, Crump WS, Hollifield JW, Frölich JC, Nies AS (1978) Prostaglandins: A role in baroreceptor control of renin release. Circ Res 42: 454–458

28. Whorton AR, Smigel M, Oates JA, Frölich JC (1978) Regional differences in prostaglandin formation by the kidney: Prostacyclin is a major prostaglandin of renal cortex. Biochim Biophys Acta 529: 176

29. Durao V, Rico JMGT (1977) Modification by indomethacin of the blood pressure lowering effect of pindolol and propranolol in conscious rabbits. Eur J Pharmacol 43: 377–381

30. Häusler G, Gerold M (1979) Increased levels of prostaglandin-like material in the canine blood during arterial hypotension produced by hydralazine, dihydralazine and minoxidil. Naunyn Schmiedebergs Arch Pharmacol 310: 155–167

Interaction of Kinins and Renal Prostaglandins

Alberto Nasjletti and Kafait U. Malik

A kallikrein that cleaves the peptide lysyl-bradyki-nin from a protein substrate is synthesized by the kidney and is released into urine (1). The nonapep-tide bradykinin increases renal prostaglandin syn-thesis by stimulating the deacylation process that makes available free arachidonic acid for conver-sion to cyclic endoperoxides, the precursors of prostaglandins and thromboxane A_2 (2). This pa-per discusses the evidence and significance of an interaction between the renal kallikrein–kinin and prostaglandin systems.

EFFECT OF ALTERATIONS IN THE ACTIVITY OF THE RENAL KALLIKREIN–KININ SYSTEM ON RENAL PROSTAGLANDINS

Evidence linking the renal kallikrein–kinin and prostaglandin systems comes from studies on the effect of kallikrein inhibition on urinary prosta-glandin excretion. In the rat, daily administration of the kallikrein inhibitor, aprotinin (100,000 U/day) reduced the urinary excretion of PGE_2 by 63% and 67% after 1 and 3 days of treatment; this was associated with decreased kallikrein activ-ity in both urine and renal tissue (3). Similarly, aprotinin reduced urine PGE_2 excretion in rats that had been pretreated with DOCA to increase both renal kallikrein and basal renal PGE_2 produc-tion (3). Aprotinin also reduced the urinary excre-tion rate of PGE_2 in the rat during acute saline loading, which increases the basal excretion of PGE_2, and in the nonvolume-expanded animal (4). Inasmuch as the effect of aprotinin in lowering urine PGE_2 excretion is most likely related to re-duction of intrarenal kinin formation, these obser-vations suggest that a product of renal kallikrein activity promotes production of PGE_2 by the kid-ney.

Consonant with this conclusion are the results of a recent study of the effect of inhibition of pep-tidyl dipeptidase (kininase II or angiotensin I-con-verting enzyme) on urine PGE_2 excretion in the rat pretreated with DOCA (5). Inhibition of this enzyme reduces intrarenal kinin degradation, re-sulting in increased kinin levels within the kidney reflected by augmentation of urinary kinin excre-tion (1). Infusion of the peptidyl dipeptidase inhib-itor teprotide (SQ–20881, 1.2 mg/day, s.c., for 6 days) into rats pretreated with DOCA (5 mg/day for 10 days) increased urine PGE_2 excretion (5). This effect of teprotide may relate to augmentation of renal prostaglandin production consequent to a rise in renal kinin levels. If so, this would suggest that kinins generated within the kidney cause stim-ulation of renal prostaglandin production, which implies coupling of the renal kallikrein–kinin and prostaglandin systems.

The regions within the kidney where the kalli-krein–kinin and prostaglandin systems interact are not established, nor is the route followed by lysyl-bradykinin to sites of prostaglandin synthesis. Since renal kallikrein is a cortical enzyme (1), it is conceivable that its peptide product promotes prostaglandin synthesis in renal cortical structures. Also, it is possible that lysyl-bradykinin produced in the distal nephron travels via the tubule to the renal medulla where the peptide stimulates pro-duction of prostaglandins in cellular elements asso-ciated with the collecting tubules, the medullary interstitium, and blood vessels.

KININ–PROSTAGLANDIN INTERACTION IN RELATION TO RENAL FUNCTION

Renal arterial infusion of bradykinin stimulates renal synthesis of PGE_2 and PGI_2, and this is associated with effects on renal hemodynamics and excretory functions similar to those of arachidonic acid, PGE_2, and PGI_2 (2, 6). That many of the renal actions of kinins are reduced by inhibitors of cyclooxygenase suggests involvement of prostaglandins in the actions of the peptide.

Blasingham and Nasjletti (6) examined the effects on renal function of prostaglandin synthesis stimulation by bradykinin; they assessed the changes in renal hemodynamic and excretory functions induced by intrarenal infusion of bradykinin (10 ng/min/kg) in the sodium-replete dog anesthetized with pentobarbital, before and during inhibition of prostaglandin synthesis by sodium meclofenamate (5 mg/kg). Before meclofenamate, bradykinin increased the urinary output of a "PGE"-like substance associated with elevation of renal blood flow, urine flow, and sodium excretion, but affected neither arterial blood pressure nor glomerular filtration. Administration of meclofenamate did not affect the bradykinin-induced increase in renal blood flow and urine volume, but suppressed the evoked output of PGE and blunted the associated natriuresis. In contrast, in another group of dogs, meclofenamate did not affect the natriuresis effected by an equidilator dose of PGE_2 (5 ng/min/kg) infused intrarenally. Two conclusions may be derived from this study. First, prostaglandins produced by the kidney during bradykinin infusion do not appear, under these experimental conditions, to contribute to either the vasodilatory or the diuretic actions of the kinin. Second, bradykinin stimulates synthesis of a prostaglandin, probably PGE_2, which augments urinary sodium excretion and mediates the natriuretic action of the peptide.

Malik and Nasjletti (7) studied the contribution of prostaglandins to the effects of kinins on the reactivity of the renal vasculature to adrenergic stimuli. In the isolated lapine kidney perfused with Tyrode's solution, bradykinin at 1–100 ng/ml reduced the vasoconstriction produced by norepinephrine or by electrical stimulation of renal sympathetic nerves and greatly enhanced the renal output of a PGE-like material (7). Indomethacin (1 μg/ml) suppressed the basal and the bradykinin-evoked output of prostaglandins and diminished the inhibitory action of the peptide on the renal vasoconstrictor response to both adrenergic stimuli (7). Similar observations have been made in the in situ kidney of the dog (8). These observations suggest that bradykinin reduces the reactivity of the renal vasculature to sympathetic stimuli by a mechanism related to prostaglandin synthesis. It would appear, then, that bradykinin stimulates production by the kidney of one or more prostaglandins that attenuate adrenergically induced renal vasoconstriction.

SUMMARY

The kallikrein–kinin and prostaglandin systems interact within the kidney: a) Kinins generated intrarenally promote synthesis of renal prostaglandins; and b) prostaglandins produced by the kidney during infusion of bradykinin mediate the action of the peptide to increase urinary sodium excretion and to reduce the reactivity of the renal vasculature to adrenergic stimuli. Thus, the renal kallikrein–kinin and prostaglandin systems' interaction may be a feature of mechanisms that promote excretion of sodium and protect the renal circulation from vasoconstrictor influences.

ACKNOWLEDGMENTS

This work was supported by USPHS grants HL–18579 and HL–19134. A. Nasjletti and K. U. Malik are the recipients of the USPHS Career Research Development Award 1 K04 HL–00163 and 5 K04 HL–99142, respectively.

REFERENCES

1. Carretero OA, Scicli AG (1980) The renal kallikrein–kinin system. Am J Physiol 238: F247–F255
2. Nasjletti A, Malik KU (1979) Relationships between the kallikrein–kinin and prostaglandin systems. Life Sci 25: 99–110
3. Nasjletti A, McGiff JC, Colina-Chourio J (1978) Interrelations of the renal kallikrein–kinin system and renal prostaglandins in the conscious rat. Circ Res 43: 799–807
4. Kramer HJ, Moch T, Von Sicherer L, Dusing R (1979) Effects of aprotinin on renal function and urinary prostaglandin excretion in conscious rats after acute saline loading. Clin Sci 56: 547–553
5. Barr JG, Diz D, Kauker ML, Nasjletti A (1980) Effect of SQ-20881 on urinary prostaglandin excretion in the conscious rat (abstr). Fed Proc 39: 827
6. Blasingham MC, Nasjletti A (1979) Contribution

of renal prostaglandins to the natriuretic action of bradykinin in the dog. Am J Physiol 237: F182–F187

7. Malik KU, Nasjletti A (1979) Attenuation by bradykinin of adrenergically induced vasoconstriction in the isolated perfused rabbit kidney: Relationship to prostaglandin synthesis. Br J Pharmacol 67: 269–275

8. Susic H, Nasjletti A, Malik KU (in press) Inhibition of bradykinin of the vascular effects of pressor hormones in the canine kidney: Relationship to prostaglandins. Clin Sci

DISCUSSION

Dr. Soffer (New York): (Chairman): I would like to ask Dr. Frohlich a question about his Fig. 2. Do you suppose there is a separate enzyme that's involved in the generation of each metabolite or can some of them be formed chemically from their precursor?

Dr. Frohlich (Stuttgart, F.R.G.): The chemical formation of any of these metabolites occurs only at the level of the conversion of prostacyclin to 6–keto–PGF$_{1\alpha}$. All of the others are synthesized biochemically. We don't know enough about the specificity of the individual enzymes that are involved partly because we don't know exactly where each of these metabolic steps is taking place. For example, we know that beta-oxidation is very active in the liver and in the kidney, but whether the beta-oxidation that is responsible for the formation of dinor–6–keto–PGH$_{1\alpha}$ is the result of hepatic or kidney metabolism is at the present time unknown.

Dr. McGiff (Valhalla, New York): There is another metabolite of prostacyclin that I would like to address that is important in the vasculature (i.e., 6,15–diketo–PGH$_{1\alpha}$. It may well be that the intravenous administration of prostacyclin prevented its interaction with the metabolizing enzyme 15–hydroxy prostaglandin dehydrogenase, which is found in abundance in the vasculature and results in generation of this metabolite. One must recognize the limitations imposed by clinical studies. However, generation of endogenous prostacyclin is associated with simultaneous release of 6,15–diketo–PGF$_{1\alpha}$.

Gryglewski (personal communication) chal-

lenged the isolated lung with angiotensin II and showed release of large amounts of 6,15–diketo. Any attempts to measure prostacyclin release that fail to take into account major metabolites of PGI$_2$ err to that degree.

Dr. Nasjletti (Memphis, Tenn.): Dr. Frohlich, does the state of sodium balance affect the profile of prostaglandins produced by either the kidney or some other tissues?

Dr. Frohlich: These studies in man are difficult to perform, as simple as they may appear. PGM, as I have indicated, is a metabolite reflecting total body synthesis of PGE$_2$, and we don't yet know to what extent it originates from the kidney. I would like to point out that in the patients with Bartter's syndrome who have grossly elevated urinary PGE$_2$ levels, we did not, with the exception of one patient, see that PGE–M was elevated, and that's the reason why we think this relationship between renin and PGE$_2$ in Bartter's-syndrome patients is probably something that is different from that between PGE–M and the low- and high-renin hypertensives. With respect to the question of profiles of prostaglandins under various conditions in urine, we don't yet have any data or prostacyclin. The reason is that the data, until just a few weeks ago, was lacking a rational approach to this issue. I also think that due to the work we have now done we have eliminated, or at least put a large question mark behind, the usefulness of measuring 6–keto–PGF$_{1\alpha}$ in urine as a measure of renal PGI$_2$ synthesis because we have now shown that it can very well originate from prerenal sites. Therefore, it probably does not carry the specificity as an indicator of renal synthesis that we have previously shown to exist for PGF$_{2\alpha}$ and PGE$_2$ when they are excreted in the urine. I think it will require more effort to determine exactly what the source of the 6–PGF$_{1\alpha}$ is that we are measuring in urine. But with respect to PGE$_2$ and PGF$_{2\alpha}$, there are data that have been published to show that these prostaglandins do change as sodium balance changes. However, it has not been studied in detail just what those factors are. Because aldosterone, the kallikrein–kinin, and angiotensin II levels change as you change sodium balance, a detailed analysis of each factor needs to be performed.

Session 5
The Concept of Whole Body Autoregulation and the Dominant Role of the Kidneys for Long-Term Blood Pressure Regulation

Chairman: A. A. Zanchetti

Position Paper: The Concept of Whole Body Autoregulation and the Dominant Role of the Kidneys for Long-term Blood Pressure Regulation

Arthur C. Guyton, John E. Hall, Thomas E. Lohmeier,
R. Davis Manning, Jr., and Thomas E. Jackson

This paper addresses two different topics: a) the concept of whole body autoregulation; and b) the role of the kidneys for long-term blood pressure regulation. In the minds of most persons in the field of hypertension research, these are interdependent phenomena. However, this is quite untrue. One of the purposes of this paper will be to point out the independence of these two phenomena, to show that each one of them can function independently of the other—though, at times, they do function together.

WHOLE BODY AUTOREGULATION

LOCAL CONTROL OF BLOOD FLOW AND THE AUTOREGULATION PHENOMENON

The mechanism of whole-body autoregulation begins at the level of each individual tissue. It has long been known that each tissue has within itself a complex local blood flow-regulating mechanism. In general, the flow is regulated in accord with a tissue's need for new blood. In the great majority of the tissues, there is an extremely strong relationship between the need of the tissues for oxygen and the rate of blood flow (1); that is, if the tissue utilizes an excess of oxygen, or if the blood is failing to deliver adequate quantities of oxygen, the local blood vessels will dilate and the flow will increase. Obviously, this is an intrinsic negative feedback control system for regulating local blood flow in relation to tissue need for oxygen. However, oxygen delivery is not the only object of the local blood flow control system. Local feedback mechanisms also exist for control of tissue carbon dioxide concentration and tissue pH in almost all tissues of the body, but especially so in the brain. And, in some organs, highly specialized local control systems also exist; for instance, an elaborate control mechanism functions to control renal blood flow in response to changes in the composition of electrolytes in the fluids of the distal tubules.

Regardless of the precise mechanism utilized by each respective tissue for control of its local blood flow, a multitude of different experiments has now demonstrated that local blood flow regulation is universally present in the body tissues. Thus, it is said that blood flow through the tissues is "autoregulated."

SHORT-TERM AND LONG-TERM AUTOREGULATION

Some of the mechanisms for autoregulation of blood flow function within seconds, while others require weeks or even months to become fully developed. For instance, when the amount of oxygen in the arterial blood is severely and suddenly decreased, local tissue blood flow in most areas of the body will increase to a new level within 30 s to 1 min, an effect that obviously helps to prevent acute tissue nutritional deficiency. However, this acute mechanism often is not powerful enough to correct more than a small part of the deficiency. Yet, continued deficiency will lead gradually to increased sizes of the tissue vessels and even to increased numbers of vessels (reviewed in ref. 2). These changes begin to occur within a few days, but they do not become fully developed for as long as several weeks to several months. Nevertheless, by the time the vascularity of the tissue has thus increased, the tissue blood flow deficiency will often then be almost fully corrected. In summary, acute autoregulation often is not very powerful, but it can occur within minutes. On the other hand, long-term autoregulation, which requires weeks or months to occur, can be extremely powerful.

OVERALL AUTOREGULATION IN THE WHOLE BODY

It is a simple step from local tissue blood flow autoregulation in all areas of the body to the phenomenon of whole-body autoregulation. If blood flow in each tissue is autoregulated, then it is axiomatic that blood flow in the whole body also will be autoregulated. Furthermore, since blood flow in the whole body is equal to the cardiac output, cardiac output too is autoregulated.

Figure 1 illustrates two examples of whole-body autoregulation. These experiments were performed in dogs whose heads had been removed to eliminate all nervous reflexes so that the phenomenon of whole-body autoregulation could be studied independently of nervous reflex complications (3). The top three curves of this figure show the effect on cardiac output and oxygen consumption caused by suddenly decreasing the arterial pressure from a mean level of 120–60 mmHg by removing blood from the circulation. The immediate effect was to decrease the cardiac output to one-half normal. And, at the same time, the oxygen consumption decreased by approximately 25% because of inadequate delivery of blood to the tissues. However,

during the ensuing 30–45 min, the cardiac output returned about 80% of the way back to its original level, even though the arterial pressure was kept continually at the low level of 60 mmHg. At the same time that the cardiac output returned almost to normal, the oxygen consumption returned so nearly to normal that we were unable to measure any remaining abnormality. Thus, it is clear from this experiment that the intrinsic ability of the tissues of the whole body to regulate their own blood flow overcame almost completely the effect of decreased arterial pressure to diminish the flow.

The bottom three curves of Fig. 1 illustrate exactly the opposite experiment. The arterial pressure had been held at a pressure of 60 mmHg for 1 h until both cardiac output and oxygen consumption had reached steady levels. Then, by adding blood to the circulation, the arterial pressure was raised to 100 mmHg and maintained at this level for the remainder of the experiment. The immediate effect was approximately 50% increase in cardiac output and 25% increase in oxygen consumption. However, during the ensuing ½ h to 45 min, both of these again returned either to, or very nearly to, the control levels. Thus, after an appropriate period of compensation, one finds

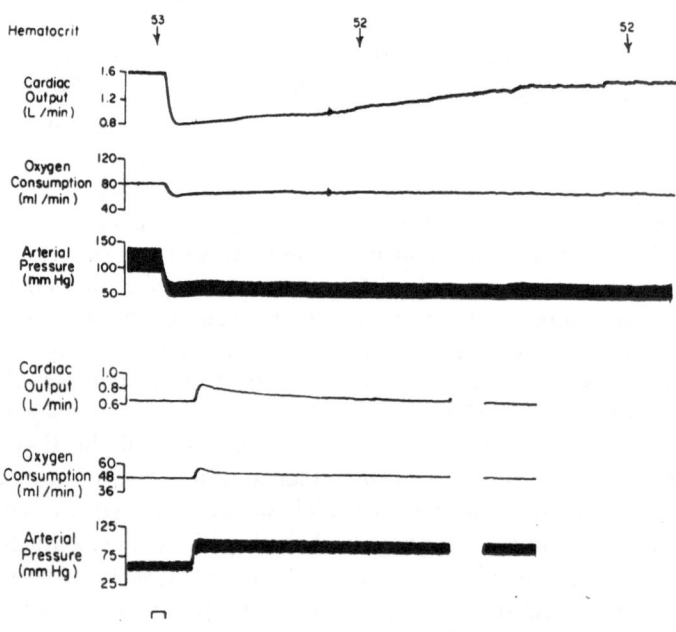

Fig. 1. Two experiments illustrating the phenomenon of whole-body autoregulation. The upper three curves show the effect of decreasing the arterial pressure to one-half normal by removing blood from a headless dog. Note the initial fall in cardiac output but then return almost to normal in 30–45 min. Opposite results are shown in the bottom three curves in which the arterial pressure was increased. [Modified from Granger and Guyton (3)]

relatively little effect of arterial pressure on the whole-body blood flow.

EFFECT OF AUTOREGULATION TO INCREASE THE TOTAL PERIPHERAL RESISTANCE WHEN THE CARDIAC OUTPUT INCREASES

Our discussion of autoregulation thus far hardly explains why this phenomenon has become so important in the minds of some hypertension research workers. However, an important consequence of autoregulation has often been overlooked: If the cardiac output is great enough to supply the tissues with an overabundance of blood flow, then the arterioles in all tissue areas of the body begin to constrict, attempting to reduce their local blood flows back to the appropriate levels. This constriction obviously increases the total peripheral resistance. This phenomenon is shown diagrammatically in Fig. 2. In the middle of this figure is a hypothetical curve in which the control cardiac output is 5 liters/min, but the output is then increased by 10%, up to 5½ liters/ min, and maintained at this elevated level for the remainder of the experiment. The effect on arterial pressure is also illustrated, showing that the 10% increase in cardiac output increases the arterial

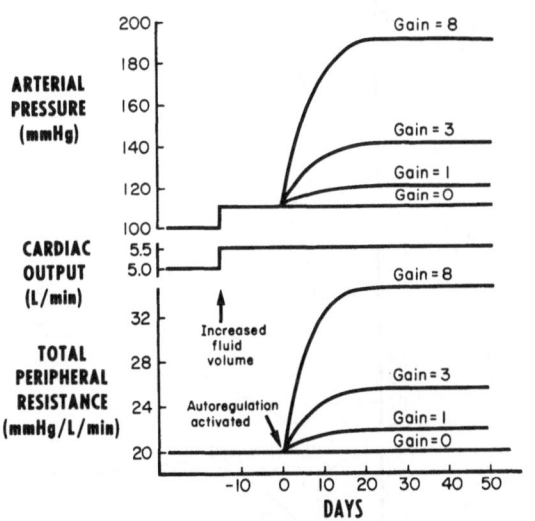

Fig. 2. Analysis of the effect of autoregulation on arterial pressure when the cardiac output is increased by 10%. Note that before autoregulation is activated, the arterial pressure also rises 10%. But when autoregulation is activated, on day 0, total peripheral resistance and arterial pressure both rise markedly, the degree of rise depending on the autoregulatory gain. [Guyton (2)]

pressure from 100 to 110 mmHg, also a 10% increase. This is the effect that would be observed were there no change whatsoever in the total peripheral resistance. However, Fig. 2 also shows the effect that would occur if, approximately 15 days after the initial increase in cardiac output, the phenomenon of autoregulation were then suddenly activated. Since there is an excess cardiac output of 10%, and, therefore, excess blood flow through the local tissue areas also of 10%, activation of the autoregulation mechanism would then cause progressive vasoconstriction in an attempt to decrease the cardiac output back toward normal. However, if the cause of the increased cardiac output persisted so that the output would not return back toward normal, the increase in peripheral resistance would continue to increase up to some limit determined by the intrinsic ability of the local vascular control systems to respond to excess blood flow. If a 10% increase in cardiac output causes a 10% increase in total peripheral resistance, then the autoregulatory gain is said to be 1. If a 10% increase in cardiac output increases the total peripheral resistance 30%, then the gain is 3. And, likewise, a gain of 8 means that there will be eight times as much increase in total peripheral resistance as there is increase in cardiac output. Therefore, beginning at day 0 in the figure, the effect of the 10% excess cardiac output plus the secondary autoregulation on both total peripheral resistance and arterial pressure is illustrated by two separate families of curves, representing different levels of gain. Thus, one can see that an autoregulatory gain of 1 will approximately double the effect of an increase in cardiac output on arterial pressure. Even more important, an autoregulatory gain of 8 will cause almost ten times as much increase in arterial pressure for a given increase in cardiac output as would be true if there were no autoregulatory gain at all.

AUTOREGULATION AS A CAUSE OF HIGH TOTAL PERIPHERAL RESISTANCE IN HYPERTENSION

When methods first became available for widespread measurement of cardiac output, it was immediately recognized that the cardiac output is usually very near to normal in almost all hypertensive patients, while the total peripheral resistance is greatly elevated. This naturally led to the assumption that the cause of hypertension in almost all instances is a primary increase in total peripheral resistance. The next logical step was a search for a vasoconstrictor factor in patients with hypertension. But after many years of search, the primary vasoconstrictor principle is still elusive. Take two separate examples: First, many investigators postulated primary constriction of the arterioles caused by sympathetic signals. However, the vast experience of Smithwick (4) and others with sympathectomy operations failed to show that the total peripheral resistance could be decreased by interrupting the sympathetic outflow to the vast majority of the resistance vessels. Second, the discovery of the renin–angiotensin system led for a while to the belief that the increased total peripheral resistance in many, if not most, hypertensive patients was caused by the effect of angiotensin on the arterioles. However, we now know that more than half of hypertensive patients have normal or low renins rather than high renins (5).

Therefore, in the absence of proof of a direct vasoconstrictor principle in hypertension, and yet knowing that the total peripheral resistance is high in almost all hypertensive patients, many investigators began to wonder whether or not the elevated total peripheral resistance in most instances of hypertension might not result from the autoregulation phenomenon. The first experiments suggesting that this might be true were those of Houck (6) who showed that enhanced extracellular fluid volume in anephric, dialyzed dogs led first to increased cardiac output and arterial pressure, and then several days later to increased total peripheral resistance while the cardiac output returned back toward normal. This was followed by a series of other experiments and clinical observations (7, 8) all of which demonstrated that initial enhancement of body fluid volume is followed by the same sequence as that observed by Houck. And, experiments by Langston (9), Douglas (10), Coleman (11), Cowley (12), and Manning (13) in our laboratory have now shown that at the onset of volume-loading hypertension, the arterial pressure rises before the total peripheral resistance increases and that this is followed a few days later by increased total peripheral resistance and return of the cardiac output back toward normal.

Figure 3 illustrates a composite of the results obtained in these experiments performed in the following way: First, approximately 70% of the kidney mass of a dog was removed (removal of one whole kidney and the two poles of the opposite

kidney). Second, after the dog had become equilibrated to its new renal state, its salt intake was then increased to five to seven times normal. This increase caused considerable retention of salt and water in the extracellular fluids, and the results were those illustrated in Fig. 3. Note especially the initial increases in the fluid volumes, cardiac output, and arterial pressure. Then later the total peripheral resistance rose to a very high level, while the cardiac output and other factors related to excess body fluid volumes returned toward normal. In the final state, the increase in cardiac output was so slight that the increase was almost impossible to measure; indeed, in the clinical setting, one would suspect that it would actually be impossible to prove an elevated cardiac output. On the other hand, the total peripheral resistance was clearly elevated. Therefore, volume-loading hypertension is a high-resistance type of hypertension, not a high-cardiac output type, but the high

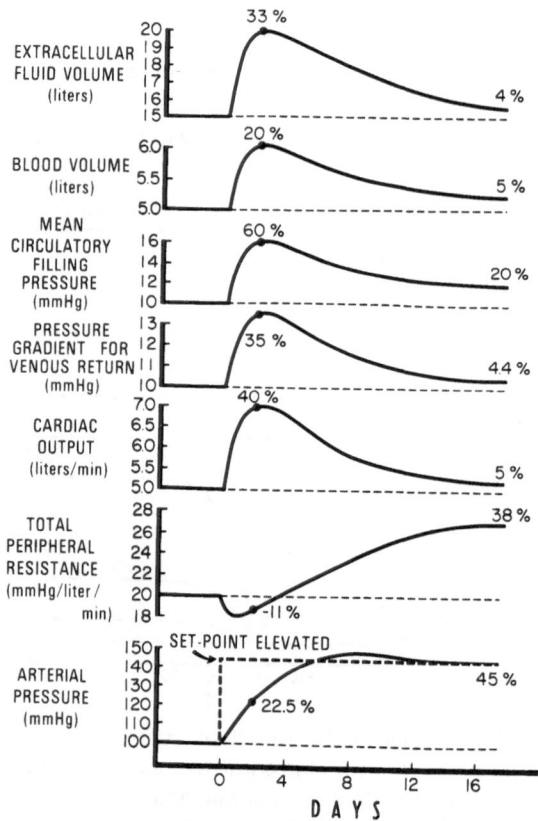

Fig. 3. Sequential changes in hemodynamic variables during the onset of volume-loading hypertension. These are average results from a series of experiments over the past 20 years. [Guyton (2)]

resistance develops *after* the hypertension develops and, therefore, *is not* the initiating cause of the hypertension.

Thus, it seems clear that hypertension caused by volume loading is characterized by high total peripheral resistance. Obviously, this could account for the vast number of hypertension patients who have very high total peripheral resistances but in whom no specific vasoconstrictor factor can be found. All that would be necessary would be an initial excess of cardiac output. This would then be followed by increased total peripheral resistance. And once the increase in total peripheral resistance has occurred, the cardiac output will return essentially to normal. Once this stage of the hypertension has been reached (which probably normally occurs within a few weeks to a few months), measurements of cardiac output would be useless in determining whether the increased total peripheral resistance was primary to the hypertension or secondary to it.

DOMINANT ROLE OF THE KIDNEYS FOR LONG-TERM BLOOD PRESSURE REGULATION

Beginning in the mid-1960s and continuing to the present, we have put forward the notion that the kidneys not only play an important role in arterial pressure control, but indeed that the kidney-volume-pressure feedback control mechanism plays such a dominant role that in the long-run, it completely overrides the nonrenal pressure control systems (2, 14, 15). This overriding capability of the kidney control system has been the subject of much debate. However, three separate kidney transplant experiments in recent years have lent much new credence to this concept. These were transplants in three different rat models of hypertension: in the Dahl rats with salt-sensitive hypertension (16), the Bianchi strain of spontaneously hypertensive rats (17), and the Okamoto strain of spontaneously hypertertensive rats (18). In each of these rat models, transplantation of the kidneys of hypertensive rats into normotensive rats caused hypertension in the transplanted rats. Conversely, transplantation of normal kidneys into the hypertensive rats caused normotension. Thus, the hypertension follows the kidneys.

Our original and continued belief that the kidneys play a dominant role in blood pressure control has been based on both experimental and theoretical analyses of the hemodynamics of arterial pressure control. Therefore, let us review the original logic and some of the experimental data that have led to our conclusion that the kidneys play an overriding, dominant role in long-term regulation of arterial pressure.

THE KIDNEY-VOLUME-PRESSURE FEEDBACK CONTROL SYSTEM

Beginning with the lowest animals that had functioning kidneys, a very fundamental mechanism for pressure control developed: An increase in arterial pressure increases the rate at which the kidneys excrete fluid and electrolytes. This reduces the volume of fluid in the body and, therefore, reduces the pressure back toward normal. Conversely, when the arterial pressure falls too low, fluid is retained in the body, the blood volume increases, and the arterial pressure returns again back toward normal.

Thus, all animals with functioning kidneys have an intrinsic fluid-volume, hemodynamic mechanism for pressure control. In higher animals, still other pressure control mechanisms have been superimposed, so much so that many investigators have suggested that the basic intrinsic kidney-volume-pressure control mechanism might have become totally subjugated to the wills of the more recently added controllers. The remainder of this paper will explore whether or not this is true.

PRESSURE-NATRIURESIS AND PRESSURE-DIURESIS MECHANISM AS THE BASIS OF KIDNEY CONTROL OF PRESSURE

Studies from many different laboratories have demonstrated that urinary output of sodium is highly dependent on the arterial pressure. The solid curve of Fig. 4 illustrates this effect. This is a composite curve of the average results from numerous different laboratories, but mainly from Selkurt et al. (19). It shows that an increase in arterial pressure 100–200 mmHg will increase the kidney output of sodium by approximately sevenfold. Conversely, decreasing the arterial pressure down to approximately 50 mmHg will reduce urinary sodium output essentially to zero. This is called the pressure-natriuresis phenomenon. The solid curve of Fig. 4 could also depict almost quan-

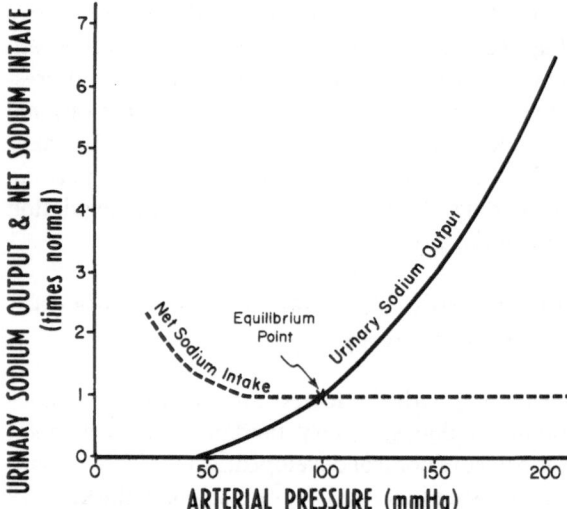

Fig. 4. A pressure-analysis diagram showing the relationship between arterial pressure and urinary sodium output and the "equilibrium point" at which the urinary sodium output curve crosses the intake level. It is only at the pressure level of the equilibrium point that indefinite balance between sodium intake and output can be achieved. [Guyton (2)]

titatively the relationship between arterial pressure and volume output as well, which is the pressure-diuresis phenomenon.

CRITICAL PRESSURE LEVEL AT WHICH BALANCE IS ACHIEVED BETWEEN INTAKE AND OUTPUT OF SODIUM

Clearly, it would be impossible for a person to live indefinitely if his sodium output were forever greater than his sodium intake. Likewise, it would be equally impossible for him to live if his sodium intake were greater than his sodium output. Now, let us assume for the sake of argument that the two curves of Fig. 4 represent the unvarying relationships between arterial pressure and sodium intake on the one hand and sodium output on the other hand. It immediately becomes obvious that there is only one pressure level, the level at which the two curves cross each other, at which the intake and output of sodium can remain exactly equal day in and day out. In this figure, this pressure level is 100 mmHg. The crossing point of the two curves, therefore, is called the "equilibrium point."

PRINCIPLE OF "INFINITE GAIN" FOR PRESSURE CONTROL

Let us continue to assume that the two curves of Fig. 4 are unchangeable, but also hypothesize that the person's arterial pressure for some transient reason increases to 150 mmHg. This increase would cause the sodium output to be three times the sodium intake. Consequently, there would be a net loss of sodium from the body and consequently a progressively decreasing extracellular fluid volume, decreasing blood volume, decreasing cardiac output, and decreasing arterial pressure. Once the arterial pressure should fall to the 100-mmHg level, then the sodium output and intake would once again be equal, and the pressure would stabilize at this point. Conversely, if the arterial pressure should fall to some value below normal, the intake of sodium would predominate until the pressure should rise to the 100-mmHg level, at which time equilibrium between intake and output of sodium would once again obtain.

Therefore, if the two curves of Fig. 4 were indeed invariable, then the arterial pressure would always reapproach the 100-mmHg pressure level, and the kidney-sodium-volume-pressure control mechanism would never stop acting until this pressure level should be achieved. Thus, the pressure always reapproaches the equilibrium point between the two curves, and *it does so with infinite feedback gain* because the system never stops working until the pressure returns always to the same exact pressure level.

Now, let us change the argument somewhat to assume that the two curves of Fig. 4 are not invariable, but that either one of them can change. For instance, assume that the urinary sodium output curve shifts to the right by 50 mmHg; then the equilibrium point would be at 150 mmHg rather than 100 mmHg. Does this invalidate the infinite-gain principle? The answer to this is, no. Instead, the kidney-sodium-volume-pressure control mechanism will now control the arterial pressure to the level of 150 mmHg with infinite gain. Thus, the gain of the feedback control system is still infinite, but the "set-point" has been changed 100–150 mmHg.

TWO LAWS OF PRESSURE CONTROL

Note Figure 5, but at first pay no attention to the multiple curves shown to the right in the figure.

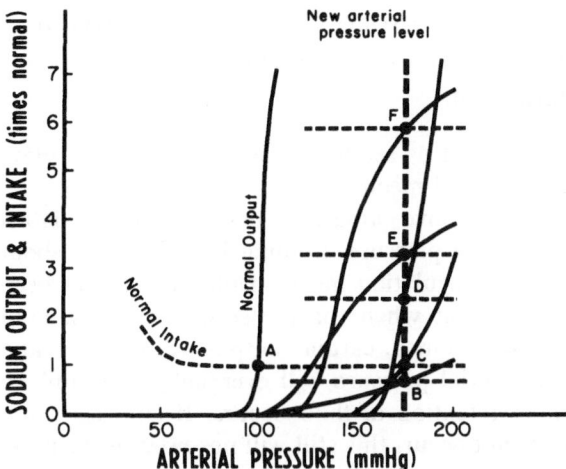

Fig. 5. A pressure-analysis diagram used to explain the two basic laws of arterial pressure control (explained in the text). [Guyton (2)]

To the left are two curves, one labeled "normal intake" and the other labeled "normal output." These two curves again show the relationships between arterial pressure and sodium output and intake. However, the normal output curve is much steeper than the curve shown in Fig. 4. The reason for this is that this new curve represents not only the direct effect of arterial pressure on kidney output of sodium as measured in the isolated kidney, but this direct effect plus several indirect effects of the pressure as well operating through the hormonal systems of the normal functioning body. The equilibrium point at which the two curves cross each other, point A, is still at an arterial pressure level of 100 mmHg. Furthermore, the infinite-gain principle still applies, and the arterial pressure will be controlled with infinite gain at this pressure level of 100 mmHg.

There are two basic laws of pressure control tha can be derived from Figs. 4 and 5 and from the infinite-gain principle of pressure control by the kidney-sodium-volume-pressure system:

LAW NO. 1: It is impossible to develop hypertension unless the equilibrium point is shifted to a high pressure level. Thus, in Fig. 5, let us assume that a person has hypertension with a mean arterial pressure of 175 mmHg. It would be impossible for this person to maintain this hypertensive state unless the equilibrium point for balance between sodium intake and output were also at 175 mmHg.

Points B through F represent five different equilibrium points, showing both low and high intakes of sodium as well as sodium output curves that are either depressed or shifted far to the right. But, in each instance, the equilibrium between intake and output, as represented by points B through F, all lie at the 175-mmHg pressure level.

LAW NO. 2: If the equilibrium point for balance between intake and output of sodium increases to a hypertensive level, then the person will develop hypertension up to the pressure level of the equilibrium point. Figure 5 also substantiates this law. If the renal function crosses the intake level of sodium at any one of the points B through F, then it is clear that the equilibrium point for balance between intake and output of sodium has now been increased to 175 mmHg. The infinite-gain principle for pressure control requires that sodium be retained until the arterial pressure rises to 175 mmHg. Only then, will sodium retention cease. (One might wonder what would have happened if the arterial pressure failed to rise to the 175-mmHg level? The answer to this is that sodium would continue to be retained forever, and the clinical picture would be that of typical progressive decompensated heart failure. But if the heart is strong enough, the excess volume will eventually raise the pressure to the level of the equilibrium point.)

TWO LONG-TERM DETERMINANTS OF ARTERIAL PRESSURE

Now, we can add one more step of logic. Since the equilibrium point for pressure control is determined by the crossing point of the sodium output and intake curves, these two curves are, in fact, the two long-term determinants of the arterial pressure level.

And, we can go still one step further. The salt intake in most persons is determined mainly by habit or by dietary availability of salt, and in general this intake remains almost constant throughout life. If this is true, then the single real determinant of the arterial pressure level is the character of the renal sodium output curve, a curve that is frequently called the "renal function curve." If the renal function curve is depressed, or if it is shifted to higher pressure levels, then hypertension will ensue.

Furthermore, since the renal function curve is

a characteristic of the kidneys, it now becomes clear why we were led to the conclusion early in our hemodynamic investigations of hypertension that the kidneys almost always must be involved in some way if chronic hypertension is to develop.

FACTORS THAT CAN SHIFT THE RENAL FUNCTION CURVE TO HIGHER PRESSURE LEVELS

We do not have to look far for the different changes in renal function that can cause the renal function curve to shift to high pressure levels. These can be divided into two major categories: a) those that tend to reduce glomerular filtration; and b) those that tend to *increase* tubular reabsorption of sodium and water. The factors that tend to reduce glomerular filtration are:

1) Increased renal vascular resistance
2) Sympathetic stimulation of the kidneys
3) Effect of angiotensin on the kidneys to cause vascular constriction
4) Pathologic effects in the kidneys to increase vascular resistance
5) Pathologic effects to decrease the glomerular filtration coefficient
6) Increased plasma colloid osmotic pressure

Factors that increase tubular reabsorption are:

1) Effect of aldosterone to increase sodium reabsorption
2) Effect of angiotensin to increase both water and salt reabsorption
3) Effect of still other undiscovered factors to increase reabsorption.

It will be clear from the above lists that some of these factors that cause the renal function curve to shift to hypertensive levels are either pathologic or functional abnormalities of the kidneys themselves. Others derive from outside the kidneys.

The point of the above analyses and of the exercise in logic that we have presented is mainly to show that, in the end, it is impossible to develop hypertension without involvement of the kidneys either by intrinsic changes in the kidneys themselves or by the effects of extrinsic factors on the kidneys.

ROLE OF AUTOREGULATION IN THE RENAL MECHANISM FOR ARTERIAL PRESSURE CONTROL

Finally, let us see what role autoregulation plays in the renal mechanism for pressure control.

In the above paragraphs describing renal control of arterial pressure, nothing has been said about the autoregulation mechanism. All that has been said is that when the pressure is too low, fluid will be retained, cardiac output will increase, and the arterial pressure will eventually rise until no more retention of fluid occurs. If autoregulation does not occur, this still will not prevent the renal mechanism from causing hypertension. However, in the absence of any change in total peripheral resistance, to raise the arterial pressure 50%, the cardiac output must also rise 50%. On the other hand, if autoregulation occurs and has a gain as high as 5–10 (gains that are very likely on the basis of experiments), then a cardiac output of only 3%–8% could result in very severe hypertension because of the multiplying effect that autoregulation has to increase arterial pressure when cardiac output is enhanced.

But, let us also present still another scenario. If damage occurs to the kidneys, this may cause a tendency to retain salt and water but at the same time cause the kidneys to secrete renin. Then angiotensin is formed and causes increased total peripheral resistance. If enough angiotensin is formed, the arterial pressure might rise acutely—before any salt retention occurs—to a level above the pressure level of the equilibrium point for sodium intake and output balance. But at the same time, the pressure level of the equilibrium point itself is increased a lesser amount. In this case, the excess pressure would actually cause salt and water to be excreted from the circulation, thus leading to reduced extracellular fluid volume, reduced blood volume, and reduced cardiac output. Yet, it is still the equilibrium point for balance between salt intake and output that establishes the level at which the pressure will be controlled. If the reader does not understand this, he should pause and think it through, because the kidney-volume-pressure control mechanism still functions to determine the final arterial pressure level even in such conditions as this—despite the low blood volume and low cardiac output.

Also, the autoregulation phenomenon is still

functional as well. The increased total peripheral resistance, in this instance, is not caused by autoregulation but instead by the direct effect of the vasoconstrictor agent angiotensin. But, the angiotensin is attempting to reduce the blood flow to the tissues below their desires. Therefore, autoregulation now operates in exactly backward direction, this time preventing too much decrease in the tissue blood flow. This might be called *negative autoregulation* because it actually opposes the effect of the vasoconstrictor agent to increase the arterial pressure, which is in contrast to the positive effect that autoregulation has to increase the arterial pressure in the volume-loading type of hypertension. Here again, one needs to think through this mechanism, because the literature is replete with misstatements about the role of autoregulation in hypertension.

SUMMARY

In this paper, we have discussed the basic fundamentals of the autoregulation process itself and the dominant role of the kidneys in long-term arterial pressure regulation. Basically, the phenomenon of autoregulation means the ability of the body's tissues to control their own blood flows in relation to their local needs. When the cardiac output is too high, excess blood flows through the tissues, and the local intrinsic blood flow regulatory mechanisms then cause marked increase in total peripheral resistance in an attempt to return the tissue blood flow back to normal. This obviously exacerbates the hypertension caused by enhanced cardiac output.

The dominant role of the kidneys for long-term control of arterial pressure results from the effect of increased pressure to increase the kidney output of salt and water. Whenever the pressure is too high, if hypertension is to be maintained, it is essential that some abnormality occur to prevent the kidneys from removing salt and water from the body. This can result either from intrinsic abnormalities of kidney function or from extrinsic factors that affect kidney function. But, in any case, the kidney must be involved either directly or indirectly.

It is especially interesting that even in low-volume, low-cardiac output hypertension caused by vasoconstrictor agents such as angiotensin, the kidney-volume mechanism for pressure control still determines the pressure level at which the arterial pressure will stabilize. However, if such a vasoconstrictor agent attempts to raise the pressure to a level higher than the pressure "set-point" level of the kidney-volume-pressure control mechanism, this latter mechanism will actually reduce the blood volume until the pressure falls back to its set-point, thus leading to low-volume, low-cardiac hypertension.

REFERENCES

1. Guyton AC, Ross JM, Carrier O Jr, Walker JR (1964) Evidence for tissue oxygen demand as the major factor causing autoregulation. Circ Res 14(1): 60–69
2. Guyton AC (1980) Arterial pressure and hypertension. Saunders, Philadelphia, Pa
3. Granger HJ, Guyton AC (1969) Autoregulation of the total systemic circulation following destruction of the central nervous system in the dog. Circ Res 25: 379–388
4. Smithwick RH (1951) Hypertensive cardiovascular disease: The effect of thoracolumbar splanchnicectomy upon mortality and survival rates. JAMA 147: 1611–1615
5. Kolsters G, Schalekamp MADH, Birkenhager WH, Lever AF (1975) Renin and renal function in benign essential hypertension: Evidence for a renal abnormality. In: Berglund G, Hansson L, Werko L, Lindgren A, Soner AB (eds) Pathophysiology and management of arterial hypertension, Molndal, Sweden, p 54
6. Houck CR (1954) Effect of hydration and dehydration and hypertension in chronic bilaterally nephrectomized dog. Am J Physiol 176: 183–189
7. Borst JGG, Borst-DeGeus A (1963) Hypertension explained by Starling's theory of circulatory homeostasis. Lancet 1: 677–682
8. Ledingham JM, Cohen RD (1964) Changes in the extracellular fluid volume and cardiac output during the development of experimental renal hypertension. Can Med Assoc J 90: 292–294
9. Langston JB, Guyton AC, Douglas BH, Dorsett PE (1963) Effect of changes in salt intake on arterial pressure and renal function in nephrectomized dogs. Circ Res 12: 508–513
10. Douglas BH, Guyton AC, Langston JB, Bishop VS (1964) Hypertension caused by salt loading: II. Fluid volume and tissue pressure changes. Am J Physiol 207: 669–671
11. Coleman TG, Guyton AC (1969) Hypertension caused by salt loading in the dog: III. Onset transients of cardiac output and other circulatory variables. Circ Res 25: 152–160

12. Cowley AW Jr, Guyton AC (1974) Baroreceptor reflex contribution in angiotensin II induced hypertension. Circulation 50(3): 60

13. Manning RD Jr, Coleman TG, Guyton AC, Norman RA Jr, McCaa RE (1979) Essential role of mean circulatory filling pressure in salt-induced hypertension. Am J Physiol 236: R40–R47

14. Guyton AC, Coleman TG (1967) Long-term regulation of the circulation: Interrelationships with body fluid volumes. In: Reeve EB, Guyton AC (eds) Physical bases of circulatory transport-regulation and exchange. Saunders, Philadelphia, Pa, pp 179–201

15. Guyton AC, Coleman TG, Cowley AW Jr, Manning RD Jr, Norman RA Jr, Ferguson JD (1974) A systems analysis approach to understanding long-range arterial blood pressure control and hypertension. Circ Res 35: 159–176

16. Dahl LK, Heine M (1975) Primary role of renal homografts in setting blood pressure levels in rats. Circ Res 36: 692–696

17. Bianchi G, Fox U, KiFrancesco GF, Giovanetti AM, Pagetti D (1974) Blood pressure changes produced by kidney cross-transplantation between spontaneously hypertensive rats (SHR) and normotensive rats (NR). Clin Sci Mol Med 47: 435–448

18. Kawabe K, Watanabe TX, Shiono K, Sokabe H (1978) Influence on blood pressure of renal isografts between spontaneously hypertensive and normotensive rats, utilizing the F_1 hybrids. Jpn Heart J 19: 886–894

19. Selkurt EE, Hall PW, Spencer MP (1949) Influence of graded arterial pressure decrement on renal clearance of creatinine, σ-amino hippurate and sodium. Am J Physiol 159: 369–378

Regulation of Renal Blood Flow by Chloride

C. S. Wilcox

We observed that infusion of a hypertonic sodium chloride solution into one renal artery of an anesthetized dog elicited progressive renal vasoconstriction in that kidney (1). The infusion raised the plasma sodium chloride concentration (P_{NaCl}) at the kidney by 15–25 mEq/liter, and after 15–30 min, it reduced the renal blood flow (RBF) and glomerular filtration rate (GFR) by some 14% below previous levels. The renal vasoconstriction was related not only to the rise in P_{NaCl}, but also to the degree of metabolic acidosis and hemodilution that accompanied the infusions (1). Changes in NaCl excretion also correlated closely with the rise in P_{NaCl}, the degree of metabolic acidosis, and the degree of hemodilution, suggesting that RBF and tubular NaCl reabsorption might be related (2, 3). Indeed, Gerber et al. (4) observed that inhibition of NaCl reabsorption with furosemide inhibited the renal vasoconstriction produced by an infusion of hypertonic NaCl solution in the dog. Micropuncture experiments in rats by Thurau and Schnermann (5) have demonstrated that increased delivery of chloride to the loop of Henle, with subsequent reabsorption there, can reduce the nephron blood flow and GFR.

Subsequent experiments tested whether the renal vasoconstriction that develops during an infusion of hypertonic saline was related to the increase in plasma osmolality, P_{Na} or P_{Cl} (6). Forty-seven greyhounds were anesthetized and the "experimental" kidney denervated by resection and reanastamosis (7). Fluid was infused into this renal artery at 0.1 ml/min/kg. Initially, the fluid was 0.154-M NaCl solution, but for 30 min, it was changed to a 1.232-M solution of either NaCl, $NaHCO_3$, Na acetate, NH_4Cl, NH_4 acetate, or dextrose. RBF was assessed from the clearance of ^{125}I-Hippuran, corrected for its renal extraction. The plasma composition at the experimental kidney was assessed from samples obtained from the renal vein after correction for urinary losses (7). Results obtained 15–30 min after starting the hypertonic infusions were contrasted with those obtained previously during the infusion of 0.154-M saline and are presented in Table 1.

The results show that the infusions raised the osmolality of the plasma perfusing the experimental kidney by approximately 13% (the precise increase was dependent on the RBF). The infusion of hypertonic dextrose solution increased RBF by 15% ± 13%. Equally hypertonic solutions of Na acetate and $NaHCO_3$ also increased RBF, and the changes in RBF were not significantly ($p \geqslant 0.1$) different from dextrose. This finding suggests that hyperosmolality leads to renal vasodilatation and, further, that the changes in RBF that occur during hypernatremia may be attributed simply to hyperosmolality. On the other hand, the infusions of hypertonic NaCl and NH_4Cl solutions led to highly significant reductions in RBF. This indicates that hyperchloremia, in contrast to hypernatremia, elicits renal vasoconstriction which overrides the vasodilatation characteristic of hypertonic infusions. Finally, RBF was lower during the infusion of NH_4 acetate than Na acetate and also during the infusion of NH_4Cl than NaCl, suggesting that high plasma levels of ammonium ions may provoke renal vasoconstriction. Overall, the changes in RBF produced by the infusions correlated with the changes in P_{Cl} ($r = -0.61$, $N = 47$, $p < 0.001$), but not with the changes in P_{Na} ($r = -0.03$, $N = 47$, NS). The falls in RBF during infusion of NaCl or NH_4Cl were greater at the experimental kidneys than at the kidneys remaining in situ, indicating that the renal vasoconstriction was a response to the local increases in P_{Cl} (greater at the experimental kidney) rather than to the systemic effects of the infusions (manifest at both kidneys). In further experiments, these same six hypertonic solutions were infused into

Table 1. Changes in RBF and plasma composition during intrarenal–arterial infusions.

Infusion	No. of exp.	RBF (%)	P_{osmol} (mosmol/liter)	P_{Na} (mEq/liter)	P_{Cl} (mEq/liter)
Na acetate	6	$+28 \pm 18$ ($p < 0.01$)	$+33 \pm 8$	$+19 \pm 3$	-5 ± 3
Dextrose	9	$+15 \pm 13$ ($p < 0.005$)	$+30 \pm 12$	-6 ± 2	-6 ± 2
$NaHCO_3$	5	$+8 \pm 8$ ($p < 0.05$)	$+39 \pm 13$	$+21 \pm 4$	-4 ± 1
NH_4 acetate	5	$+5 \pm 25$ (NS)	$+38 \pm 8$	-1 ± 1	-7 ± 3
NaCl	16	-15 ± 9 ($p < 0.0005$)	$+42 \pm 14$	$+22 \pm 7$	$+22 \pm 5$
NH_4Cl	6	-44 ± 24 ($p < 0.005$)	$+46 \pm 17$	-1 ± 1	$+28 \pm 7$

Results from 47 experiments in which an intrarenal–arterial infusion of 0.154 M NaCl solution was changed to one of the six 1.232 M solutions listed. The mean ($\pm$ SD) initial value for RBF was 17.6 ± 5.8 ml/min/kg BW/kidney. The mean ($\pm$ SD) percentage changes in the RBF during the infusions are shown (with their levels of statistical significance). The mean ($\pm$ SD) absolute changes in plasma osmolality, plasma sodium, and chloride concentrations at the experimental kidney follow. There are no significant changes in mean arterial blood pressure during the infusion of any of these solutions.

a femoral artery and were found to produce only vasodilatation in the femoral vascular bed. Thus, these experiments suggest the presence of an intrarenal mechanism that elicits vasoconstriction during increases in chloride concentration and that may be specific for the kidney. This renal vasoconstriction was accompanied by a reduction in GFR which might have stabilized the loads of NaCl and fluid delivered to the distal nephron (1).

We have also studied the changes in renal hemodynamics in response to two other stimuli, metabolic acidosis and hemodulution, that lead to increased delivery of NaCl and fluid to the distal nephron.

In micropuncture experiments on rats, we used double-barreled, ion-selective microelectrodes to measure in vivo the membrane potential and intracellular potassium ion activity of proximal tubular cells. Rats made acidotic by gavage with HN_4Cl showed a reduction in both membrane potential and intracellular potassium ion activity (8). Using free-flow micropuncture methods, we found that the acidotic rats had a reduction in proximal tubular sodium and fluid reabsorption and a fall in GFR (C. S. Wilcox, unpublished observations). In experiments on anesthetized dogs, we also observed that a hyperchloremic metabolic acidosis reduced RBF and GFR (1). This renal vasoconstriction during metabolic acidosis might be secondary to the alterations produced in proximal

tubular cell function which resulted in increased delivery of fluid to the loop of Henle. Again, reduction in GFR accompanied the vasoconstriction, tending to stabilize the distal tubular NaCl and fluid load.

In the rat, a reduction in hematocrit produced by exchange transfusion of blood for plasma reduces fluid reabsorption by the proximal tubule (9). We investigated the changes in renal hemodynamics that occur in the dog following similar acute isovolemic changes in hematocrit (10). After hemodilution, there was an abrupt increase in RBF, probably a consequence of the fall in blood viscosity. This was overcome, however, by a renal vasoconstriction that restored RBF and GFR to previous levels over 20–40 min. Again, the adjustments that occurred in renal vascular resistance and GFR should stabilize the NaCl and fluid load presented to the distal nephron.

These experiments have demonstrated that an infusion of hypertonic saline, induction of a metabolic acidosis, or hemodilution all increase the delivery of fluid or NaCl from the proximal nephron and cause renal vasoconstriction and a restriction of the GFR. This response can be elicited specifically by increasing the chloride load. A diagrammatic representation of the proposed sequence of events is presented in Fig. 1. Further work is required to determine the role of this intrarenal process which regulates renal vascular tone in the

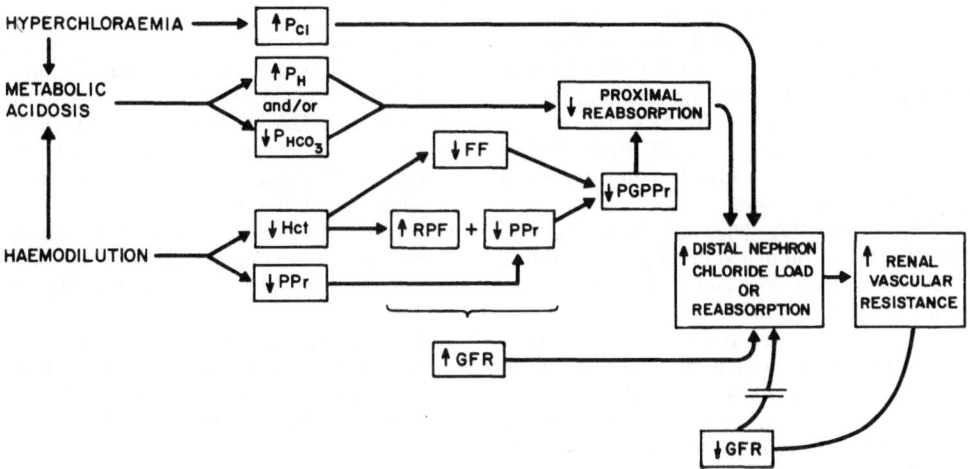

Fig. 1. Diagrammatic representation of the proposed sequence of events whereby the distal nephron chloride load is stabilized during increments in chloride delivery produced by hyperchloremia, metabolic acidosis, or hemodilution. During hyperchloremia, there is an increase in the chloride concentration of the filtrate and thereby the nephron chloride load. During metabolic acidosis, the plasma concentration of hydrogen ion (P_H) is increased but bicarbonate (P_{HCO_3}) is decreased. There is a reduction in proximal tubular fluid reabsorption which augments distal fluid and NaCl delivery. During hemodilution, a fall in hematocrit (Hct) increases the renal plasma flow (RPF), which should increase the GFR and the distal fluid and NaCl delivery. Moreover, proximal fluid reabsorption is reduced, probably a consequence of the fall in filtration fraction (FF) and postglomerular plasma protein concentration (PGPPr), and this should augment further the distal delivery of fluid and NaCl. Likewise, a fall in plasma protein concentration (PPr) should increase GFR and reduce proximal fluid reabsorption, thereby increasing the distal delivery of fluid and NaCl. The increased distal chloride load or rate of reabsorption elicits renal vasoconstriction which reduces the GFR and stabilizes the distal delivery of NaCl and fluid.

regulation of extracellular fluid volume and blood pressure.

SUMMARY

We have investigated the regulation of renal vascular resistance and GFR and their relationship to tubular NaCl reabsorption. The infusion of hypertonic NaCl solutions into one renal artery of anesthetized dogs led to a progressive renal vasoconstriction with a fall in GFR. This response could be mimicked by other chloride-containing solutions, whereas other sodium-containing solutions elicited only vasodilatation (a response characteristic of plasma hyperosmolality). In micropuncture experiments on rats, metabolic acidosis was found to impair proximal tubular fluid reabsorption, to increase the distal fluid and NaCl delivery, and to reduce the GFR. Likewise, in the dog, metabolic acidosis produced renal vasoconstriction and a reduction in GFR. Finally, hemodi-

lution, which also reduces proximal tubular fluid reabsorption, was found in the dog to elicit a slowly developing renal vasoconstriction that abolished any rise in GFR. Thus, hyperchloremia, metabolic acidosis, and hemodilution all increase distal chloride delivery and elicit renal vasoconstriction. It is proposed that these stimuli may elicit intrarenal vasoconstriction which reduces the GFR and stabilizes the distal delivery of NaCl and fluid.

ACKNOWLEDGMENTS

C. S. Wilcox gratefully acknowledges a Senior Wellcome Research Fellowship and a grant from the National Kidney Research Trust.

REFERENCES

1. Nashat FS, Tappin JW, Wilcox CS (1976) The renal blood flow and the glomerular filtration rate of

anaesthetized dogs during acute changes in plasma sodium concentration. J Physiol 256: 731–745

2. Nashat FS, Tappin JW, Wilcox CS (1976) Plasma sodium concentration and sodium excretion in the anaesthetized dog. J Physiol 254: 183–202

3. Gordon D, Nashat FS, Wilcox CS (1979) Analytical techniques applied to the study of sodium excretion in dogs. Kidney Int 15: 446

4. Gerber JG, Branch RA, Nies AS, Hollifield JW, Gerkens JF (1979) Influence of hypertonic saline on canine renal blood flow and renin release. Am J Physiol 237: F441–F446

5. Schnermann J, Osswald H, Hermle M (1976) Activation of tubulo-glomerular feed-back by chloride transport. Pfluegers Arch 362: 229–240

6. Wilcox CS (1979) Separate effects of acute increase in plasma sodium or chloride on renal blood flow rate. Fed Proc 38: 1311

7. Wilcox CS (1978) The effect of increasing plasma magnesium concentration on renin release from the dog's kidney: Interactions with calcium and sodium. J Physiol 284: 203–217

8. Cemerikic DA, Wilcox CS, Giebisch G (1979) Intracellular potential and K^+ activity of rat kidney proximal tubular cells in metabolic and respiratory acidosis. Kidney Int 16: 809

9. Brenner BM, Galla JH (1971) Influence of postglomerular hematocrit and protein concentration on rat nephron fluid transfer Am J Physiol 220: 148–156

10. Nashat FS, Scholefield FR, Tappin JW, Wilcox CS (1969) The effect of changes in haematocrit on the intra-renal distribution of blood flow in the dog's kidney. J Physiol 201: 639–655

Action of Angiotensin II on Renal Blood Flow and Urinary Sodium Excretion

Robert E. McCaa

It is well established that the active component of the renin–angiotensin system, angiotensin II, has at least three major functions: a) It increases intrarenal vascular resistance; b) acts on the renal tubules to conserve sodium; and c) stimulates aldosterone secretion. Recently, we evaluated quantitatively the role of the renin–angiotensin system in the maintenance of renal blood flow, urinary sodium excretion, plasma aldosterone concentration, and arterial blood pressure during sodium deficiency. Our studies were performed in intact conscious dogs maintained on long-term administration of the angiotensin I-converting enzyme inhibitor, captopril (1). In response to long-term captopril administration in sodium-deficient dogs, arterial blood pressure decreased from 103 ± 5 to 67 ± 2 mmHg ($p < 0.001$), plasma aldosterone concentration decreased from 36.4 ± 6.8 to 14.2 ± 3.4 ng/dl ($p < 0.001$), urinary sodium excretion increased from 0.65 ± 0.26 to 4.8 ± 1.2 mEq/day ($p < 0.001$), effective renal plasma flow increased from 136 ± 6 to 154 ± 8 ml/min ($p < 0.01$) and remained elevated during long-term captopril administration, while glomerular filtration rate decreased from 65 ± 9 to 36 ± 7 ml/min ($p < 0.001$) and remained below control levels until arterial blood pressure returned to normal after captopril administration was discontinued. Also, during long-term captopril administration, the concentration of kinins in the blood increased from 0.17 ± 0.02 to 0.41 ± 0.05 ng/ml ($p < 0.001$), urinary kinin excretion increased from 7.2 ± 1.5 to 31.4 ± 3.2 μg/day ($p < 0.01$), and urinary kallikrein activity decreased from 23.6 ± 3.1 to 5.3 ± 1.2 EU/day ($p < 0.001$). This significant increase in circulating and renal concentration of kinins during long-term administration of captopril suggests that the hypotensive and natriuretic actions of the angiotensin I-converting enzyme inhibitor could be due in part to both inhibition of angiotensin II formation and the accumulation of kinins.

To evaluate quantitatively the role of angiotensin II in mediating the hypotensive and natriuretic actions of captopril, we determined the response of arterial blood pressure, urinary sodium excretion, and plasma aldosterone concentration to angiotensin II infusion in sodium-deficient dogs maintained on captopril (Fig. 1). Sodium-deficient dogs were maintained on continuous captopril infusion (400 mg/day) for 7 days (2). After 7 days of captopril infusion, arterial blood pressure decreased from 102 ± 3 to 68 ± 4 mmHg ($p < 0.001$), urinary sodium excretion increased from 0.69 ± 0.24 to 7.8 ± 1.6 mEq/day ($p < 0.001$), and plasma aldosterone concentration decreased from 37.8 ± 6.5 to 16.3 ± 3.6 ng/dl ($p < 0.001$). During the next 7 days, the animals were maintained on captopril infusion at the rate of 400 mg/day and angiotensin II infusion at the rate of 3 ng/kg/min. In response to angiotensin II infusion (3 ng/kg/min), arterial blood pressure increased from 68 ± 4 to 86 ± 3 mmHg ($p < 0.001$), urinary sodium excretion decreased from 7.8 ± 1.6 to 1.7 ± 0.9 mEq/day ($p < 0.001$), and plasma aldosterone concentration increased from 16.3 ± 3.6 to 27.5 ± 5.2 ng/dl ($p < 0.001$) within 24 h after beginning angiotensin II infusion. During the next 48 h of continuous angiotensin II infusion, arterial blood pressure increased to 96 ± 3 mmHg, urinary sodium excretion decreased to 0.53 ± 0.21 mEq/day, and plasma aldosterone concentration increased to 34.3 ± 6.4 ng/dl.

Inhibition of angiotensin II formation with captopril administration in sodium-deficient dogs resulted in a marked decrease in intrarenal vascular resistance, an increase in renal blood flow, an increase in urinary sodium excretion, and a decrease in arterial blood pressure. Angiotensin II infusion at the low rate of 3 ng/kg/min into sodium-defi-

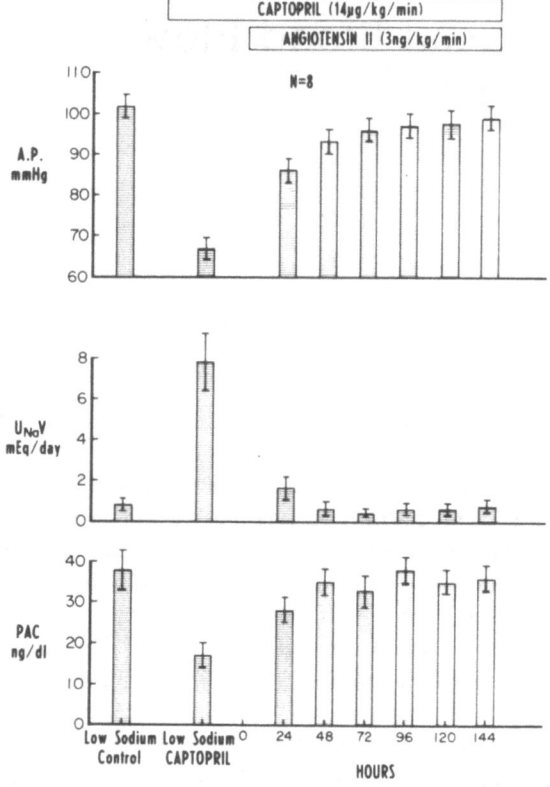

Fig. 1. Response of arterial blood pressure (AP), urinary sodium excretion (U$_{Na}$V), and plasma aldosterone concentration (PAC) to continuous angiotensin infusion (3 ng/kg/min) in sodium-deficient dogs maintained on continuous captopril infusion (14 μg/kg/min). Vertical lines, ± SE; N, number of dogs studied.

cient dogs maintained on captopril administration increased intrarenal vascular resistance, induced sodium retention, stimulated aldosterone secretion, and restored arterial blood pressure to levels that existed in untreated sodium-deficient dogs. However, angiotensin II infusion at rates higher than 5 ng/kg/min increased urinary sodium excre-

tion due to pressure-induced natriuresis. These studies indicate that the hypotensive and natriuretic actions of inhibitors of angiotensin I-converting enzyme (kininase II) are due to the inhibition of angiotensin II formation and not to increased circulating and renal concentration of kinins.

SUMMARY

Inhibition of angiotensin II formation and increased circulating and renal concentration of kinins both produce hypotensive and natriuretic effects in normal, sodium-deficient, and experimental renovascular hypertensive animals. Despite the sustained increase in circulating and renal concentration of kinins in sodium-deficient dogs maintained on captopril, angiotensin II infusion at the rate of 3 ng/kg/min restored arterial blood pressure, urinary sodium excretion, and plasma aldosterone concentration to the levels that existed in untreated sodium-deficient dogs. These data demonstrate that the hypotensive and natriuretic actions of inhibitors of angiotensin I-converting enzyme (kininase II) are due to the decrease in circulating and renal concentration of angiotensin II and not to the accumulation of circulating and renal kinins.

REFERENCES

1. McCaa RE, Hall JE, McCaa CS (1978) The effects of angiotensin I-converting enzyme inhibitors on arterial blood pressure and urinary sodium excretion. Circ Res 43(Suppl I): I–32–I–39
2. McCaa RE (1980) Specificity of converting enzyme inhibition. In: Gross F, Vogel H (eds) Enzymatic release of vasoactive peptides. Raven Press, New York, pp 383–399

Neural Regulation of Renal Function

Gerald F. DiBona

Histochemical, histofluorescence, and ultrastructural studies indicate that the mammalian kidney receives an essentially exclusive adrenergic innervation. Adrenergic neuroeffector junctions have been observed on both glomerular and nonglomerular vascular elements, proximal and distal tubular epithelial cells, and renin-containing juxtaglomerular granular cells (1, 2). These extensive morphologic studies form the basis for consideration of the direct effects of changes in efferent renal sympathetic nerve activity on renal tubular sodium and water reabsorption and renin release independent of alterations in renal hemodynamics. Additionally, the role of the afferent and efferent renal innervation in mediating compensatory adaptive responses of the kidney is of interest as a physiologic renorenal reflex.

Renal clearance, micropuncture, and nerve recording studies in the anesthetized dog and rat have demonstrated that both increases and decreases in efferent renal sympathetic nerve activity, produced either directly or reflexly, cause parallel changes in renal tubular sodium and water reabsorption in the absence of changes in glomerular filtration rate, renal blood flow, or its intrarenal distribution. The neuroadrenergic specificity of this effect is demonstrated by its abolition with the sympathetic blocking agents, phenoxybenzamine or guanethidine, or sectioning of the afferent neural pathways of the reflex responses. The response is not mediated by neurogenically released angiotensin II or prostaglandins since it occurs despite renal blockade to angiotensin II or inhibition of prostaglandin synthesis. The proximal convoluted tubule has been identified as one site of action of this effect. The important physiologic role of this neuroregulatory system is further demonstrated by studies in unanesthetized dogs, which show that reflex manipulations of efferent renal sympathetic nerve activity also produce similar parallel changes in renal tubular sodium and water reabsorption independent of renal hemodynamic alterations (reviewed in refs. 3–9). Thus, several lines of evidence indicate that the efferent renal sympathetic nerves via adrenergic neuroeffector junctions on renal tubular epithelial cells participate in the physiologic regulation of tubular sodium and water reabsorption.

Employing levels of direct electrical stimulation of the efferent renal sympathetic nerves which do not change renal blood flow, glomerular filtration rate, or urinary sodium excretion (10 V, 0.5 ms, 0.5 Hz), a direct neurogenic mechanism for renin release has been demonstrated. This renin release is completely abolished by renal arterial administration of either the nonselective beta-adrenergic receptor blocking agent, propranolol, or the selective beta-1 receptor blocking agents, metroprolol or atenolol (9). In addition, levels of efferent renal sympathetic nerve stimulation that are also subthreshold for renin release (10 V, 1.0 ms, 0.25 Hz) significantly augment the renin release response to either decreased renal perfusion pressure or increased ureteral pressure; this augmentation is also blocked by propranolol or metoprolol (9). Thus, levels of efferent renal sympathetic nerve activity that do not change renal hemodynamics can directly increase renin release independent of any input stimuli to either the renal baroreceptor or macula densa receptor.

Responses occurring in one kidney produced by interventions on the other kidney and that are mediated by neurohumoral mechanisms are called renorenal reflexes. Renal denervation produces an ipsilateral diuresis and natriuresis that is accompanied by a compensatory antidiuresis and antinatriuresis from the contralateral kidney. This contralateral response is mediated by increased efferent renal sympathetic nerve activity since renal nerve recordings demonstrate a 47% increase in efferent activity and the compensatory antidiuresis and antinatriuresis are abolished by renal denervation (9). Ureteral occlusion produces an increase in ipsilateral renal blood flow and a decrease in contralateral renal blood flow. Denervation of either kidney abolishes the contralateral renal vasoconstriction without affecting the ipsilateral renal vasodilatation. Combined renal hemodynamic and nerve recording studies indicate that renal mechanoreceptors, stimulated by increased intrarenal pressure produced by ureteral occlusion, send signals via the ipsilateral afferent renal nerves to supraspinal centers. The efferent limb is via the efferent renal sympathetic nerves to the contralateral kidney (9).

These several investigations indicate that the renal innervation contributes significantly to the overall physiologic regulation of several important aspects of renal function: tubular sodium and water reabsorption, renin release, and renorenal reflex compensatory responses.

SUMMARY

Increases or decreases in efferent renal sympathetic nerve traffic, produced directly or reflexly, cause parallel changes in renal tubular sodium reabsorption independent of changes in renal hemodynamics or humoral factors. This response is mediated by alpha-adrenoceptors located on adrenergic neuroeffector junctions in direct contact with the basement membrane of renal tubular epithelial cells. The proximal convoluted tubule has been identified as a locus of this effect. Levels of efferent renal sympathetic nerve stimulation that do not affect renal hemodynamics or tubular sodium reabsorption (circa 0.5 Hz) increase renin release by direct activation of beta-adrenoceptors located on the juxtaglomerular granular cells. Levels of efferent renal sympathetic nerve activity that do not affect renin release along (circa 0.25 Hz) can augment and potentiate the renin release response to other stimuli to the baroreceptor and macula densa mechanisms. Renorenal reflexes consist of an intrarenal receptor (mechanoreceptor, chemoreceptor) with afferent signals traveling via afferent renal nerves to spinal cord and supraspinal centers and efferent signals traveling via efferent renal sympathetic nerves to both contralateral and ipsilateral kidneys. These renorenal reflexes are able to participate in compensatory and adaptive responses wherein one kidney exhibits an alteration in function in response to an intervention on the opposite kidney.

ACKNOWLEDGMENTS

This work was supported by Public Health Service Grants AM-15843 and Program Project HL-14388, and grants from the Iowa Heart Association and the Veterans Administration.

REFERENCES

1. Barajas L (1978) Innervation of the renal cortex. Fed Proc 37: 1192–1201
2. Barajas L (1979) Anatomy of the juxtaglomerular apparatus. Am J Physiol 237: F333–F343
3. Hillemand B, Leroy J, Joly J-P, Le Grix A (1976) Les retentissements in systeme nerveux sur le rein. Sem Hop Paris 52: 958–963, 1163–1172
4. DiBona GF (1977) Neurogenic regulation of renal tubular sodium reabsorption. Am J Physiol 233: F73–F81
5. DiBona GF (1978) Symposium: Neural control of renal functions. Fed Proc 37: 1192–1221
6. Gottschalk CW (1978) Symposium: Control of kidney function by the nervous system. In: Proceedings of the seventh international congress of nephrology, Montreal. Karger, Basel, WJ 300 IN846P 1978 pp 544–571
7. Linden RJ (1978) Neurocirculatory control of sodium and water excretion. In: Dickinson CJ, Marks J (eds) Developments in cardiovascular medicine. MTP Press, Lancaster, U.K., pp 191–203
8. Gottschalk CW (1979) Renal nerves and sodium excretion. Annu Rev Physiol 41: 229–240
9. DiBona GF (1980) Function of the renal nerves. Rev Physiol Biochem Pharmacol (in press)

Renal Perfusion and Vascular Reactivity in Essential Hypertension

Norman K. Hollenberg

Systems analysis has underscored the role the kidney must play in *sustaining* a blood pressure rise, however initiated (1). I will focus on the possibility that the renal blood supply is implicated in "essential" hypertension, and review preliminary evidence on the nature of the participation. As to whether the renal perfusion is involved in *initiating* the process, the answer remains beyond us.

RENAL PERFUSION IN ESSENTIAL HYPERTENSION

The relationship of partial occlusion of the renal artery to hypertension raised the possibility that essential hypertension is due to reduced renal perfusion (2, 3). Clearance techniques led Smith et al. (4) to conclude: "the evidence in man argues against primacy of renal ischemia in the pathogenesis of essential hypertension," based on eight studies involving hundreds of patients. Not that the method failed to reveal many essential hypertension in whom renal perfusion and function were reduced: Indeed, Smith's study revealed a diodrast clearance that was less than the average normal value in 57 of 60 patients (5). Renal perfusion in most patients, however, was in the normal range. Renal biopsy or necropsy examination also may reveal normal vessels, despite even long-standing hypertension (6–8). Why then has debate continued about renal perfusion in the pathogenesis?

The answer lies in the inherent weakness in the methods of evaluation. Histology suffers from an important sampling problem and will not identify vasoconstriction. Blood flow measurement also has limitations: There is a large normal range even after correction for age and gender (9). Clearance studies require a prolonged steady-state, and assume normal active tubular transport. Both have contributed to variability.

Recent interest in the renal blood supply, moreover, has expanded to include regional intrarenal perfusion rates. New methods based on indicator transit through the kidney after intraarterial injection of either a dye, with venous sampling, or a radioactive tracer, with residue detection by external counting, provide an accurate, convenient method for measuring mean renal blood flow; the character of indicator transit has also provided an index of intrarenal perfusion patterns (10–12).

Because long-standing hypertension impacts on the microvasculature (6–8), we need information on renal blood flow early in the course, which is difficult to document: Symptoms occur late. We performed an analysis on a large group of normal and hypertensive subjects who were under 35 years of age (13). At this age, examinations performed at school, for employment, for the military, for insurance, contraception, and pregnancy made it possible to bracket the onset of hypertension with greater precision than later in life. Moreover, a prolonged duration is unlikely in the young. Restricting the age range also reduced the coefficient of variation for normal renal blood flow, which varies strikingly with age, and in an alinear fashion (9).

Despite a documented duration of hypertension of less than 2 years in over 50% of the 83 patients with essential hypertension and less than 1 year in one-third of them, mean renal blood flow was reduced in the patients from a normal median and mode of 3.5–4.0 ml/g/min to 2.5–3.0 ml/g/min ($p < 0.001$). A Gaussian distribution was evident in the normal subjects, but not in the patients. The mode in two-thirds was reduced by 20% from the expected, identical to the 20% average blood flow reduction in young patients with renovascular hypertension (13).

RENAL VASCULAR TONE IN ESSENTIAL HYPERTENSION

There is in essential hypertension a frequent reduction in cortical perfusion whether the index employed is xenon or krypton washout (10–18) or the character of dye transit across the kidney (19, 20). The reduction in cortical blood flow could reflect either parenchymal atrophy due to organic microvasculature disease or vasoconstriction (20).

How can we assay vascular tone? We have employed three approaches, each of which suggests that active vasoconstriction plays an important, perhaps primary, role in the reduction in renal blood flow in most patients. Our premise was that an organic lesion, reflecting permanent vascular damage, would be associated with a fixed reduction in renal blood flow. Conversely, a functional abnormality might induce a more variable abnormality. Fixed, organic lesions should be unresponsive to vasodilators, whereas a functional abnormality might show an enhanced response. All investigation has led to one conclusion: There is, indeed, increased vascular tone in the renal bed of most patients with essential hypertension.

Differences in renal perfusion in sequential measurements of blood flow in the same kidney made minutes apart clearly cannot be attributed to organic changes. We demonstrated such a difference in essential hypertension (13). In normal subjects, an absolute average difference on repeated renal blood flow measurement was 40 ± 8 ml/g/min. In 18 patients with essential hypertension, there was a more than twofold larger difference (86 ± 15 ml/g/min), which was not present in the kidney contralateral to significant renal artery stenosis: Thus, this abnormality was attributable to the "essential" element rather than to the elevated blood pressure *per se*. Strong confirmation can be found in a study reported earlier (21); reanalysis revealed a threefold larger variability of renal perfusion in patients with essential hypertension.

All analytic method for assessing the instability of xenon transit through the human kidney based on engineering principles of wave-form analysis has revealed a striking increase in the variability of xenon washout through the kidney in essential hypertension. Such an abnormality could be attributable only to short-term, active vasoconstriction. Green dye concentration in the renin vein during intraarterial infusion in essential hypertension showed a similar phenomenon (20).

A dose-related increase in blood flow occurred in response to acetylcholine and dopamine in normal man: The renal response was blunted strikingly when organic microvascular disease might have been expected to contribute to the abnormal renal perfusion, in malignant hypertension, chronic pyelonephritis, and polycystic kidney disease (22). Conversely, the response to both agents was potentiated in 9 of 13 (69%) patients with mild essential hypertension. An equivalent potentiation was induced by increasing renal vascular tone with angiotensin.

The potentiated response to acetylcholine and to dopamine was associated with the reversal of the small vessel abnormalities in the renal arteriogram.

WHAT MEDIATES THE INCREASE IN RENAL VASCULAR TONE IN ESSENTIAL HYPERTENSION?

There are several candidates that mediate the increase in renal vascular tone. Enhanced vascular reactivity to pressor stimuli has been well documented (23, 24). If renal smooth muscle reactivity were enhanced in essential hypertension, even normal amounts of angiotensin and norepinephrine would increase renal vascular tone. Evidence that plasma renin activity and angiotensin formation (25) and sympathetic nervous system activity (26) are increased in some patients with essential hypertension implicates these factors in at least some patients. As yet unidentified vasoconstrictor factors could also be responsible (27).

In view of interest in renal hemodynamics and in vascular reactivity, there have been surprisingly few studies on renal vascular reactivity in essential hypertension. Indeed, the most studied vascular beds, of the extremity, may not participate in parallel (28). Of the studies on renal vascular reactivity, none have utilized the optimal approach, an intraarterial infusion, not surprising in view of the inaccessibility of the renal artery. The renal response to norepinephrine administered intravenously was normal in essential hypertension (29). Moreover, a reduced renal vascular response to angiotensin administered intravenously was associated with a reversal of the renal functional effects of angiotensin (30). Conversely, there is a striking increase in the renal vascular response to nonpharmacologic stimuli, emotion and exercise, in essential hypertension (28, 31).

Access to the renal artery at selective renal arteriography has made it possible to assess the renal vascular response to angiotensin in doses too small to induce a systemic response (32–34). A normal dose-related renal blood flow reduction was modified by maneuvers known to activate the renin-angiotensin system, such as altering sodium intake (32), potassium intake (33), and oral contraceptives (34).

Preliminary studies in essential hypertension have revealed a potentiated response. Such an observation provides a mechanism by which enhanced renal vascular tone may be sustained without an increased concentration of either angiotension or norepinephrine. To the extent that the concentration of either hormones is increased in some patients, the tendency to an increase in renal vascular tone would be potentiated.

Phentolamine, the alpha-adrenergic blocking agent, failed to increase renal blood flow in normal subjects when infused into the renal artery in doses sufficient to block a large dose of norepinephrine (22), but increased renal blood flow in six of nine patients with essential hypertension (22). Again, the selective arteriogram was in excellent accord. As a nonspecific effect, phentolamine induces vasoconstriction; thus, it seems likely that vasodilatation reflects reversal of an adrenergic response (35).

The mixed evidence implicating sympathetic nervous system activity in the pathogenesis of essential hypertension may reflect regional, rather than generalized, autonomic activation. Tests for generalized activation may thus be inadequate. Regionally differentiated activation may lead to a highly selective increase in renal vascular resistance (36). Preliminary observations based on the measurement of norepinephrine in arterial and renal venous plasma suggest that in some patients, increased renal norepinephrine release occurs. Catecholamine release is normal in others, but the increase in tone could reflect a potentiated vascular response to a normal local concentration.

We have also documented an enhanced renal vascular response to a converting enzyme inhibitor, SQ 20881, in essential hypertension (37).

Moreover, SQ 20881 is the first vasodilator reported which increases glomerular filtration rate and sodium excretion as renal blood flow rises (38). Whether this response is due to reversing angiotensin-mediated renal vasoconstriction or reflects other actions of this class of agent, such as reduced bradykinin degradation or activation of prostaglandin synthetase, is not clear. The renal vascular response to the oral-converting enzyme inhibitor, captopril, is similar.

CONCLUSION

Despite promising clues, the contribution of the renal vascular bed to the pathogenesis and maintenance of essential hypertension remains ill defined. We can be encouraged by recent advances, including improved techniques for the measurement of renal blood flow; for cardiovascular catheterization and angiography; in pharmacology that provide a range of agents for interruption of the renin–angiotensin system; and improved assay techniques, especially for catecholamines and angiotensin II in biological fluids. A coordinated application of these methods should make it possible to make the rigorous assessment that this question surely merits.

SUMMARY

Current concepts suggest a pivotal role for the kidney in *sustaining* hypertension from any source or etiology. The possibility that the renal vasculature also participates in the *induction* of essential hypertension has been the subject of continuing interest for decades. Recent evidence suggests that a functional abnormality resulting in increased renal vascular tone is present in approximately two-thirds of patients with uncomplicated essential hypertension. Available evidence will not allow us to identify the possible mediator. At least some evidence is available for sympathetic nervous system activity operating directly on the vascular smooth muscle: inappropriate activation of the renin–angiotensin system with a local vasoconstrictor action of angiotensin on the renal vessels; or enhanced intrinsic reactivity of the renal vessels resulting in an inappropriately large response to normal concentrations of either or both mediator. Other possible candidates include abnormalities of the prostaglandin or kinin systems. A perfectly normal renal arterial tree, free of organic abnormality or an increase in tone due to active vasoconstriction, is distinctly unusual in the untreated patient with essential hypertension—and may never be present once therapy is initiated.

ACKNOWLEDGMENTS

Personal research reported in this essay was supported by grants from the National Institutes of Health (HL-14944, HL-11668, GM-18674, HL-07236, HL-05832) and the National Aeronautics and Space Administration (NSG-9078). Metabolic studies were performed on and supported by the Clinical Research Center (RR-00888).

REFERENCES

1. Guyton AC, Coleman TG, Cowley AW, Scheel KW, Manning RD, Norman RA (1972) Arterial pressure regulation; overriding dominance of the kidneys in long-term regulation and in hypertension. Am J Med 52: 584
2. Goldblatt H (1964) Hypertension due to renal ischemia. Bull NY Acad Med 40: 745
3. Stamey TA (1963) Renovascular hypertension. Williams & Wilkins, Baltimore, Md
4. Smith HW, Goldring W, Chasis H, Ranges HA, Bradley SE (1943) The application of saturation methods to the study of glomerular and tubular function in the human kidney. J Mt Sinai Hosp 10: 59
5. Goldring W, Chasis H, Ranges HA, Smith HW (1941) Effective renal blood flow in subjects with essential hypertension. J Clin Invest 20: 637
6. Bell ET (1951) The pathological anatomy in primary hypertension. In: Hypertension, a symposium. University of Minnesota Press, Minneapolis, Minn
7. Saltz M, Sommers SC, Smithwick RH (1957) Clinicopathologic correlations of renal biopsies from essential hypertensive patients. Circulation 16: 207
8. Tracy RE (1970) Quantitative measures of the severity of hypertensive nephrosclerosis. Am J Epidemiol 91: 25
9. Wesson LG Jr (1969) Renal hemodynamics in physiological states. In: Physiology of the human kidney. Grune & Stratton, New York, p 96
10. Grunfeld JP, Raphael JC, Bankir L (1971) Intrarenal distribution of blood flow. In: Hamburger J, Crosnier J, Maxwell MH (eds) Advances in nephrology. Year Book, Chicago, Ill
11. Hollenberg NK, Mangel R, Fung H (1976) The assessment of intrarenal perfusion with radioxenon: A critical review of analytical factors and their implications in man. Semin Nucl Med 6: 193
12. Hollenberg NK, Adams DF (1976) The renal circulation in hypertensive disease. Am J Med 60: 773
13. Hollenberg NK, Borucki LJ, Adams DF (1978) The renal vasculature in early essential hypertension: Evidence for a pathogenetic role. Medicine 57: 167
14. Case DB, Casarella WJ, Hassar M, Laragh JH, Cannon PJ (1972) Renal circulation and renin secretion in normal and low renin essential hypertension. Circulation 46: 11
15. Dell RB, Sciacca R, Lieberman K, Case DB, Cannon PJ (1973) A weighted least-squares technique for the analysis of kinetic data and its application to the study of renal ^{133}xenon washout in dogs and man. Circ Res 32: 71
16. Blaufox MD, Fromowitz A, Lee HB, Meng CH, Elkin M (1970) Renal blood flow and renin activity in renal venous blood in essential hypertension. Circ Res 27: 913
17. Inasaka T (1969) Studies in the intrarenal distribution of blood flow with ^{133}Xe in diseased human kidney. Jpn Circ J 33: 735
18. Ladefoged J, Pedersen F (1969) Renal blood flow in patients with hypertension. Clin Sci 37: 253
19. Logan AG, Velasquez MT, Cohn JN (1973) Renal cortical blood flow, cortical fraction, and cortical blood volume in hypertensive subjects. Circulation 67: 1306
20. Lowenstein J, Steinmetz PR, Effros RM, Demeester M, Chasis H, Baldwin DS, Gomez DM (1967) The distribution of intrarenal blood flow in normal and hypertensive man. Circulation 35: 250
21. Kioschos JM, Kirkendall WM, Valenca MR, Fritz AE (1967) Unilateral renal hemodynamics and characteristics of dye-dilution curves in patients with essential hypertension and renal disease, Circulation 35: 229
22. Hollenberg NK, Adams DF, Solomon H, Chenitz WR, Burger BM, Abrams HL, Merrill JP (1975) Renal vascular tone in essential and secondary hypertension: Hemodynamic and angiographic responses to vasodilators. Medicine 54: 29
23. Doyle AE, Fraser JRE (1961) Vascular reactivity in hypertension. Circ Res 9: 755
24. Mendlowitz M (1967) Vascular reactivity in essential and renal hypertension in man. Am Heart J 73: 121
25. Laragh JH (1973) Vasoconstriction-volume analysis for understanding and treating hypertension: The use of renin and aldosterone profiles. Am J Med 55: 261
26. Engelman K, Portnoy B, Sjoerdsma A (1970) Plasma catecholamine concentrations in patients with hypertension. Circ Res [Suppl] 27: 1
27. Fasciolo JC, Risler NR (1974) Reduction of the pressor effect of angiotensin and norepinephrine by

a renal peptide in anesthetized rats. Circ Res [Suppl] 34, 35: 1

28. Brod J, Fencl V, Hejl Z, Zirka J, Ulrych M (1962) General and regional haemodynamic pattern underlying essential hypertension. Clin Sci 23: 339

29. Gombos EA, Hulet WH, Bopp P, Goldring W, Baldwin DS, Chasis H (1962) Reactivity of renal and systemic circulations to vasoconstrictor agents in normotensive and hypertensive subjects. J Clin Invest 41: 203

30. Peart WS, Brown JJ (1961) Effect of angiotensin (hypertension or angiotonin) on urine flow and electrolyte excretion in hypertensive patients. Lancet 1: 28

31. Wolf SJ, Pfeiffer P, Ripley HS, Winter UW, Wolff HG (1948) Hypertension as a reaction pattern to stress: Variation in blood pressure and renal blood flow. Ann Intern Med 29: 1056

32. Hollenberg NK, Solomon HS, Adams DF, Abrams HL, Merrill JP (1972) Renal vascular response to angiotensin and norepinephrine in normal man: The effect of salt intake. Circ Res 31: 750

33. Hollenberg NK, Williams GH, Burger BM, Hooshmand I (1975) Potassium's influence on the renal vasculature, the adrenal, and their responsiveness to angiotensin II in normal man. Clin Sci Mol Med 49: 527

34. Hollenberg NK, Williams GH, Burger B, Chenitz, WR, Hooshmand I, Adams DF (1976) Renal blood flow and its response to angiotensin II: An interaction between oral contraceptive agents, sodium intake, and the renin-angiotensin system in healthy young women. Circ Res 38: 35

35. Hilliard CC, Bagwell EE, Daniell HB (1972) Effects of sympathetic and central nervous system alterations on the blood pressure responses to phentolamine. J. Pharmacol Exp Ther 180: 743

36. Folkow B, Johansson B, Lofving B (1961) Aspects of functional differentiation of the sympatho-adrenergic control of the cardiovascular system. Medicina Experimentalis 4: 321

37. Williams GH, Hollenberg NK, (1977) Accentuated vascular and endocrine response to SQ 20881 in hypertension. New Engl J Med 297: 184

38. Hollenberg NK, Swartz SL, Passan DR, Williams GH (1979) Increased glomerular filtration rate following converting enzyme inhibition in essential hypertension. New Engl J Med 301: 9

Does Hypertension Develop Through Long-term Autoregulation?

Paul I. Korner

The common usage of the term autoregulation of blood flow refers to the ability of vascular beds to regulate blood flow in accordance with changing needs. Different authors have placed different emphasis on the role in autoregulation of myogenic tone, chemical stimuli, and local hormones (for review, see refs. 1 and 2). The distinctive feature of such local autoregulation is that it is rapid, with a time-course of minutes rather than hours or days. For example, in "whole-body autoregulation," blood flow adjustments to step changes in blood pressure were completed in 20–60 min (3). In isolated organ systems with more uniform properties of the blood vessels, the autoregulatory adjustments were much faster (i.e., 3–5 min) (2, 4).

It has recently been suggested that a special type of long-term autoregulation is important in the pathogenesis of hypertension (5–9).

The *autoregulation theory of hypertension* postulates that in the early development of hypertension, the rise in blood pressure is entirely mediated through a rise in cardiac output, which occurs most commonly through disturbances in the body's fluid balance ("volume" factors). The rise in blood pressure then triggers a myogenic response in the resistance vessels, producing an "autoregulatory" rise in total peripheral resistance (TPR), which eventually leads to restoration of cardiac output. From experimental studies on volume overloading in humans and dogs with marked renal impairment, it takes 1–2 weeks before the rise in blood pressure is mediated entirely through increased TPR (6, 10, 11).

The autoregulation theory of hypertension thus postulates a mechanism whereby changes in cardiac output become transformed into changes in vascular resistance. In broad terms, since the cardiac output changes are often brought about by alterations in body fluid volume, the autoregulation theory's importance lies in the close interrelationship that it postulates between "volume" and "constrictor" factors.

Initial support for the autoregulation theory of hypertension came from clinical studies showing that in a relatively high proportion of young hypertensive patients, the cardiac output tended to be elevated (12). Some longitudinal studies have been reported which show a tendency for cardiac output to decrease and TPR to increase (13), but these studies lack age-matched controls and it is difficult to be certain what the role of age changes *per se* is from these studies. Therefore, tests of the theory have had to rely on experimental studies. The results of several provide support for the autoregulation theory (7–9, 11, 14–16), but there are others where its postulates have not been fulfilled (5, 7–9, 17–22).

The point at issue is whether a) constrictor and volume factors (i.e., cardiac output) can each produce long-term elevation of blood pressure independently of one another or whether b) volume and constrictor factors are always closely interrelated through the process of *long-term autoregulation*. In this paper, I wish to discuss briefly results obtained in rabbits with cellophane wrap hypertension which suggest that TPR and cardiac output can each exert independent long-term effects on blood pressure. In one experiment, we studied the changes occurring during the *development* of hypertension (18), whereas in the other we altered volume factors during stable *established* hypertension (22).

DEVELOPMENT OF CELLOPHANE WRAP HYPERTENSION

In the first experiment, the time-course of changes in blood pressure, cardiac output (Doppler flowmeter), and TPR was studied before, and for 32 days, after either cellophane wrapping of both kidneys or sham operation (18). In the first postoperative week, cardiac output increased by approximately 10%, but the changes were exactly the same in cellophane-wrapped and sham-operated rabbits (Fig. 1, left). We concluded that the elevation of cardiac output was a nonspecific consequence of operation and was irrelevant in the development of hypertension. A rise in cardiac output did not occur in every rabbit of either cellophane-wrapped or sham-operated groups; whether or not it occurred in a given wrapped animal, made no difference to the subsequent magnitude and time-course of blood pressure and TPR changes (18). In the wrapped animals, the cardiac output declined after the first 7–10 days and reached a value of approximately 75% of control by day 32, compared with 95% of control observed in sham-operated animals (Fig. 1, left). The reason for the fall in cardiac output in wrapped rabbits was not clear, but appeared to be partly due to a tendency to lose weight compared with sham-operated rabbits (18).

Through the entire observation period of 32 days after operation, the arterial pressure and TPR were each significantly higher in the cellophane-wrapped rabbits than in the sham-operated animals. The elevation in blood pressure was due to elevation in TPR from the earliest stage of development of hypertension. The rises in both the blood

pressure and TPR were small at first, but increased progressively with time (Fig. 1, left).

The important feature of the experimental design of this study was the presence of a matched control group. Without this control group, the initial rise in cardiac output and the gradual rise in TPR could have been regarded as providing support for the autoregulation theory. However, the experimental design provided strong support for the conclusion that the elevation of TPR was not causally related to rise in cardiac output (18). One problem in interpreting the results of numerous experimental studies is that in many the need for a matched control group has been considered unnecessary, owing to the serial observations made before and after onset of hypertension. In my view, a control group is always necessary to assess time-related effects in chronic experiments.

ALTERATION OF VOLUME FACTORS

In this experiment, the dietary sodium intake was altered but only after renal wrap hypertension had become established at a stable level of blood pres-

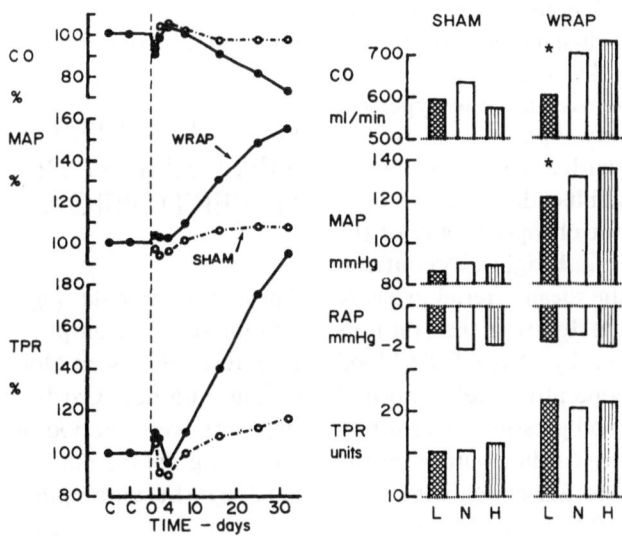

Fig. 1. Left: Average changes (% of control) in cardiac output (CO), mean arterial pressure (MAP), and total peripheral resistance (TPR) on two control days (C) and on days 4, 8, 16, 25, and 32 following renal wrapping (ten rabbits) or sham operation (nine rabbits). [Based on results of Fletcher et al. (18)] **Right:** Average values of hemodynamic variables in ten sham-operated and ten renal-wrapped rabbits. Each animal was studied at the end of 2 weeks on low- (L), normal- (N), and high- (H) dietary sodium. CO, ml/min; MAP, mmHg; RAP, right arterial pressure, mmHg; TPR, units. * $p < 0.05$ from value on normal salt. [Based on results of Korner et al. (22)]

sure (22). Rabbits were maintained on a "normal"-salt diet before, and for 6 weeks after, either renal cellophane wrapping or sham operation. The wrap- and sham-operated rabbits each contained two subgroups: a) five rabbits with bilateral cellophane wrap and five with one kidney wrapped plus the other removed; b) five rabbits with both kidneys exposed at sham operation and five with only one kidney exposed plus the other removed. After 6 weeks, the main part of the experiment began and every animal spent 2 weeks each on low-, normal-, and high-sodium diet which contained 1, 9, and 50 mEq/100 g of food, respectively. The pellets used in the diet were identical in composition except for the sodium concentrations; the animals were allowed tap water plus pellets *ad libitum*. Hemodynamic and metabolic measurements were made at the end of each 2-week period. A Latin square experimental design was used to eliminate bias due to order of diets. In the normotensive sham-operated rabbits, plasma renin concentration (PRC) averaged 7.1, 5.4, and 4.3 ng/ml/h on low-, normal-, and high-sodium diets, whereas in the hypertensive animals, the corresponding values averaged 8.5, 4.5, and 3.0 ng/ml/h with the values on low sodium slightly higher and the values on high sodium slightly lower than in the normotensive group (22). Urinary sodium output per day was slightly greater in sham-operated than in hypertensive rabbits on the normal- and high-salt diets, presumably due to a difference in intakes (22).

In neither the normotensive nor the hypertensive rabbits were there any differences in the responses of the subgroups with different renal mass. In the sham-operated rabbits, the different diets did not produce significant changes in any of the hemodynamic variables (Fig. 1, right). By contrast, in hypertensive rabbits, the mean arterial pressure on low sodium was 12 mmHg lower than on normal and high sodium (i.e., by 25% of the blood pressure rise from the preoperative level on normal salt). The reduction in blood pressure was entirely accounted for by the lower cardiac output on the low-sodium diet which was associated with a reduction in blood volume (22). In the hypertensive rabbits on normal- and high-salt cardiac output and stroke, volumes were higher than in sham-operated animals on the same diet (22). The reduction in cardiac output on the low-sodium diet brought this variable into the range of sham-operated rabbits. The TPR did not alter with changes

in intake of salt either in the hypertensive rabbits or in the sham-operated group (Fig. 1, right).

In this experiment, changes in cardiac output exerted prolonged effects on blood pressure independently of resistance changes. This is in accord with findings on steroid hypertension in the dog where blood pressure elevation was maintained in some animals for many weeks and was entirely due to elevation of cardiac output (17). Prolonged experimental steroid hypertension (21) in sheep is also usually maintained solely through elevation of cardiac output over several weeks (B. A. Scoggins, personal communication).

Our results are contrary to the predictions of the autoregulation theory where, after 2 weeks on each salt diet, one would have expected relatively little difference in cardiac output but that the TPR would be greatest on high sodium and lowest on low sodium. The feature of the experimental design was that volume factors were experimentally varied only after constrictor factors had reached stable levels. In many of the earlier studies, the experimental designs employed would not have permitted a distinction whether volume or constrictor factors were independent or interrelated. Many of the studies were performed during *development* of experimental hypertension, and early cardiac output changes would appear to become transformed into an elevated TPR even if volume and constrictor factors were independent, but altered, at different rates.

CONCLUSIONS AND SUGGESTED MECHANISM OF WRAP HYPERTENSION

These experiments suggest that constrictor and volume (cardiac output) factors can each produce long-term effects on blood pressure independently of one another. Cardiac output can alter blood pressure over a period of at least 2 weeks without triggering the type of hemodynamic pattern envisaged by the autoregulation theory of hypertension. In the experiment on the development of hypertension, volume factors were the same in wrap and sham rabbits so that the experiment highlighted the importance of constrictor factors as the predominant cause of the rise in blood pressure. In the second experiment, resistance had become constant in established hypertension, thus permitting assessment of the role of experimentally altering volume factors. We cannot be certain that our results apply to other models of experimental hypertension or to human hypertension, but it would seem reasonable to assume that they do, at any rate, as a working hypothesis.

It has always been difficult to explain why in the development of cellophane wrap hypertension, the onset of the hypertension (and TPR) should be relatively slow. One attractive feature of the theory of long-term autoregulation has been that it appeared to provide a reasonable explanation for this delay. In cellophane wrap hypertension, hormonal constrictor mechanisms have not been obvious. For example, in the detailed study of Campbell et al. (23), no changes in plasma renin activity and PRC were observed over an observation period of several weeks. We propose an alternative explanation that the renal compression which occurs in cellophane wrap hypertension is a very gradual process. It takes 4–6 weeks before the kidney becomes encased by a firm fibrous capsule that weighs approximately 25%–30% of the renal parenchymal mass (22). In the dog, this fibrous capsule exerts a tissue pressure of approximately 30 mmHg (24), which would create a renal hemodynamic pattern rather analogous to one-kidney Goldblatt hypertension model where the renal artery stenosis gradient is slowly increased (18, 25).

A further factor involved in the rise of the systemic blood pressure is the hypertrophy of the media of the resistance vessels as first suggested by Folkow (26). This hypertrophy becomes an "amplifier" of constrictor stimuli and enhances the narrowing of the vascular lumen produced by a given stimulus. We have found that in rabbits with wrap hypertension, the vascular amplifier in the hindlimb doubles the rise in resistance produced by a given dose of constrictor hormone in a nonspecific manner with similar amplification produced by norepinephrine, angiotensin II, and vasopressin (27, 28). The amplification of the overall vascular amplifier is somewhat smaller, about 1.5 (29). The important point is that the pathophysiologic change of vascular hypertrophy probably occurs in response to an increase in blood pressure, be it due to constrictor or to volume factors. In the development of hypertension, the gradually increasing gain of the vascular amplifier contributes to further elevation of blood pressure and still more medial hypertrophy until a new steady-state is eventually established. In man, this pathophysiologic change can be almost completely reversed by antihypertensive treatment (30). However, once treatment stops, hypertension rapidly returns.

In conclusion, autoregulation is a short-term process important in the moment-to-moment control of blood flow. The experimental evidence discussed suggests that volume and constrictor factors can each exert independent long-term effects on blood pressure and not the closely interrelated effects suggested by the long-term autoregulation theory of hypertension. Rises in blood pressure due to either mechanism will eventually produce pathophysiologic changes in vessel geometry, leading to exaggerated vascular responses to normal stimuli.

SUMMARY

Two experiments are discussed in relation to the autoregulation theory of hypertension. In the first, we studied the time-course of changes in blood pressure, cardiac output, and TPR before, and for 32 days after, bilateral renal cellophane wrapping or sham operation (i.e., during development of hypertension. Through the entire observation period, mean arterial pressure and TPR were each significantly higher in wrapped rabbits than in sham-operated animals, though both groups had initially identical changes in cardiac output. In the second experiment, volume factors were varied 6 weeks after operation in sham-operated and wrapped rabbits; in the latter group, hypertension had become stable at this time. Each animal was on three diets with 2 weeks on each; the diets differed in salt content (approximately 0.5, 7, and 30 mEq/day). Variation in salt intake produced no change in hemodynamic variables in the sham-operated group. In the hypertensive rabbits, arterial pressure and cardiac output were higher on normal and high salt than on low salt. On the low salt, the fall in blood pressure was entirely through reduction in cardiac output and TPR was the same on every diet. Both experiments are inconsistent with the autoregulation theory of hypertension. They show that volume and constrictor factors each exert independent long-term effects on blood pressure and not the closely interrelated effects suggested by the theory.

ACKNOWLEDGMENT

This work was supported by a grant from the Australian National Health and Medical Research Council.

REFERENCES

1. Johnson PC, (1964) Review of previous studies and current theories of autoregulation. Circ Res 14, 15(Suppl I): 2–9
2. Berne RM (1964) Metabolic regulation of blood flow. Circ Res 14, 15(Suppl I): 261–268
3. Granger HT, Guyton AC (1969) Autoregulation of the total systemic circulation following destruction of the central nervous system in the dog. Circ Res 25: 379–388
4. Johnson PC (1968) Autoregulatory responses of cat's mesenteric arterioles measured in vivo. Circ Res 22: 199–212
5. Ledingham JM, Pelling D (1967) Cardiac output and peripheral resistance in experimental renal hypertension. Circ Res 20, 21(Suppl II): 187–198
6. Coleman TG, Cowley AW Jr, Guyton AC (1974) Experimental hypertension and the long-term control of arterial pressure. In: Guyton AC, Jones CE (eds) Cardiovascular physiology (MTP international review of science–physiology, Series I, Vol 1.) University Park Press, Baltimore, pp 259–297
7. Korner PI, Fletcher PJ (1977) Role of the heart in causing and maintaining hypertension. Cardiovasc Med 2: 139–155
8. Gross F, Dietz R (1979) The significance of volume and cardiac output in the pathogenesis of hypertension. Clin Sci 57: 59S–67S
9. Ferrario CM, Page IH, McCubbin JW (1970) Increased cardiac output as a contributing factor in experimental renal hypertension in dogs. Circ Res 27: 799–810
10. Coleman TG, Bower JD, Langford HG, Guyton AC (1970) Regulation of arterial pressure in the anephric state. Circulation 62: 509–514
11. Coleman TG, Guyton AC (1969) Hypertension caused by salt loading in the dog. Circ Res 25: 153–160
12. Widimský J, Fejfarová MH, Fejfar Z (1957) Changes of cardiac output in hypertensive disease. Cardiologia 31: 381–389
13. Eich RH, Cuddy RP, Smulyan H, Lyons RH (1966) Hemodynamics in labile hypertension: A follow-up study. Circulation 34: 299–307
14. Ledingham JM, Cohen RD (1964) Changes in the extracellular fluid volume and cardiac output during the development of experimental hypertension. Can Med Assoc J 90: 292–294
15. Ferrario CM (1974) Contribution of cardiac output and peripheral resistance to experimental hypertension. Am J Physiol 226: 711–717
16. Bianchi G, Tilde Tenconi L, Lucca R (1970) Effect in the conscious dog of constriction of the renal artery to a sole remaining kidney on haemodynamics, sodium balance, body fluid volume, plasma renin concentration and pressor responsiveness to angiotensin. Clin Sci 38: 741–766
17. Bravo EL, Tarazi RC, Dustan HP (1977) Multifactorial analysis of chronic hypertension induced by electrolyte-active steroids in trained unanesthetised dogs. Circ Res 40(Suppl I): 104–145
18. Fletcher PJ, Korner PI, Angus JA, Oliver JR (1976) Changes in cardiac output and total peripheral resistance during development of renal hypertension in the rabbits: Lack of conformity with the autoregulation theory. Circ Res 39: 633–639
19. Korner PI, Anderson WP, Johnston CI, Angus JA, Fletcher PJ (1978) Role of cardiac output in the pathogenesis of hypertension. In: Proceedings of the seventh international congress of nephrology, Montreal. Karger, Basel, pp 517–523
20. Stephens GA, Davis JO, Freeman RH, De Forrest JM, Early DM (1979) Hemodynamic, fluid and electrolyte changes in sodium-depleted one-kidney hypertensive dogs. Circ Res 44: 316–321
21. Scoggins BA, Allen KJF, Coghlan JP, Denton DA, Graham WF, Humphrey TJ, Whitworth JA (1979) Haemodynamics of ACTH-induced hypertension in sheep. Clin Sci 57: 333S–336S
22. Korner PI, Oliver JR, Casley DJ (1980) Effect of dietary salt on hemodynamics of established renal hypertension in the rabbit: Implications for the autoregulation theory of hypertension. Hypertension (in press)
23. Campbell DJ, Skinner SL, Day AJ (1973) Cellophane perinephritis hypertension and its reversal in rabbits: Effect on plasma renin, renin substrate and renal mass. Circ Res 33: 105–112
24. Brace RA, Jackson TE, Ferguson JD, Norman RA Jr, Guyton AC (1974) Pressure generated by scar tissue contractions: Perinephritis hypertension. IRCS (Cardiovascular) 2: 1683
25. Anderson WP, Korner PI, Johnston CI (1979) Acute angiotensin II-mediated restoration of distal renal artery pressure in renal artery stenosis and its relationship to the development of sustained one-kidney hypertension in conscious dogs. Hypertension 1: 292–298
26. Folkow B (1978) Cardiovascular structural adaptations: Its role in the initiation and maintenance of primary hypertension. Clin Sci Mol Med 55: 3S–22S
27. West MJ, Angus, JA, Korner PI (1975) Estimation of non-autonomic and autonomic components of iliac bed vascular resistance in renal hypertensive rabbits. Cardiovasc Res 9: 697–706
28. Angus JA, West MJ, Korner PI (1976) Assessment of autonomic and non-autonomic components of resting hindlimb vascular resistance and reactivity to pressor substances in renal hypertensive rabbits. Clin Sci Mol Med 51: 57S–59S
29. West MJ (1974) Studies in experimental renal hypertension and some aspects of human essential hy-

pertension. PhD thesis, University of Sydney, pp 88–100

30. Jennings GL, Korner PI, Esler MD (1979) Effect of 1 year's therapy in essential hypertension systemic haemodynamics studies before and after "total" autonomic blockade. Clin Sci 57: 11S–13S

DISCUSSION

Dr. Zanchetti (Milan, Italy) (Chairman): From being too often associated with the more vague, and at least less persuasive, concept of long-term autoregulation, I think that the pressure–natriuresis story can be interpreted in two different ways. If we believe that it begins directly in the kidney, then the concept of autoregulation is necessary in order to explain how a primary change within the kidney, subsequent sodium retention, and volume increase are going to cause the hemodynamic pattern of elevated resistance that is typical of hypertension. But, the story in my mind can also be read in a different way. It can start outside of the kidney from some agent, not necessarily in the sympathetic system, but any kind of agent which can act simultaneously on both the pressure–natriuresis curve and on peripheral vascular resistance. In this case, we still have hypertension with increased peripheral resistance and without necessarily implying any volume expansion, which has never been found in essential hypertension. But according to the different balances of peripheral extrarenal and renal vasoconstriction, there will be a greater or smaller reduction in volume, no change in volume, or even an increase in volume; in no case shall we need the concept of autoregulation. This is the story as can be read in pheochromocytoma. Pheochromocytoma could be, in principle, a better model for essential hypertension than renal insufficiency or Conn's syndrome. If we can spend a few minutes' discussion, I think it would be convenient to discuss separately the pressure–natriuresis problem and the autoregulation hypothesis. Is there someone here willing to define the theory of pressure–natriuresis?

Dr. Doyle (Heidelberg, Australia): I feel that we are very privileged in being here at the final interment of this hypothesis. I think that the data Dr. Guyton showed us in relation to the SHR where we have an animal that has high blood pressure and is perfectly capable of controlling his sodium without any hint at all of the relationship between pressure and natriuresis really illustrates exactly how unpivotal the role of the kidney is. What we are really seeing, of course, is these animals are hypertensive while they retain a perfectly normal capacity to excrete sodium irrespective of blood pressure. Now I suspect that in all cases, other than perhaps the situation in which two-thirds of both kidneys have been removed, that that is in fact the normal situation.

Dr. Guyton (Jackson, Miss.): I am surprised that you would say that this is the interment of the hypothesis because, if you had looked at the renal function curves carefully, you would have seen that in the SHR it is only at the higher pressure that the kidneys will excrete sodium—that at the lower pressures they won't excrete, they turn off, and the blood volume then increases. Thus, in fact, they require the higher pressure to excrete sodium normally.

Dr. Boyd (Hobart, Australia): Like Dr. Korner, I am very puzzled by the long time-course of Dr. Guyton's so-called autoregulation, and I agree that we should be very careful about calling it that. An alternative explanation of the gradually increasing resistance after volume loading is that the increased blood pressure which results from the elevated cardiac output could, through Dr. Folkow's related mechanisms, bring about structural changes in the arterioles. Could I, therefore, ask Dr. Folkow whether he has ever seen structural arteriolar changes over such a time-course in hypertension, particularly those due to a volume load.

Dr. Folkow (Göteborg, Sweden): Concerning the exchange between Drs. Doyle and Guyton, I think it is fair to say that both have a point. In adult SHR with established hypertension, the renal excretion curve is in fact displaced in parallel toward a higher pressure level, but in *young* SHR with less hypertension, it is essentially equal to that in normotensive controls. Actually, in the course of SHR hypertension, the renal curve gradually shifts to the right simply because there occurs the same structural increase of the preglomerular resistance as afflicts *all* other systemic precapillary resistance vessels, being an adaptive response to the increased load. This correspondingly raises the *ratio* between the pre- and postglomerular resistances in SHR and, hence, calls for a higher arterial pressure to maintain effective glomerular filtration pressure. This renal resetting is, however, in my view *secondary* and *not* primary in SHR hypertension.

Dr. Simpson (Dunedin, New Zealand): Dr. Guyton: If the line is as vertical as you showed us, does that not mean that the kidney cannot be primarily responsible in that particular model?

Dr. Guyton: The line is almost vertical because of the active feedback control exerted by the renin–angiotensin system. If we increase the pressure rapidly, in the time before this system can be activated, the curve is not vertical at all. It is vertical only when the sodium load is increased day after day and the curve is progressively recorded. The difference between the SHR and the normal rat is that everything about renal function operates at a much higher pressure level.

Dr. Korner (Prahran, Australia): As Dr. Guyton knows, I don't agree with him on the long-term autoregulation theory, but I do agree with him on the part of the role of the kidneys. For example, in our model of cellophane wrap hypertension the reason why our animals were more susceptible to high and normal salt than sham-operated rabbits was because they had a slightly depressed glomerular filtration rate which was about 20% down from their prewrap value. We believe that this is an important "renal" reason in this model for the greater salt susceptibility in contrast to the absolutely normal renal function and absence of hemodynamic changes in sham-operated rabbits on all levels of salt.

Dr. Lumbers (Sydney, Australia): I wonder if I could change the subject and ask Dr. Wilcox what he postulates is the mechanism by which increased chloride delivery to the tubules causes an increase in renal vascular resistance?

Dr. Wilcox (London, England): We are investigating this. We measured the renin concentrations and the rate of renin release into renal blood and lymph. In our preparation, the renin levels start rather low probably because of fluid administered to the animals during the surgical preparation. There is no evidence for a release of renin or angiotensin I into the lymph or the renal venous blood in response to infusions of hypertonic saline.

Dr. Zanchetti: Dr. Wilcox, I would like to ask a question about these interesting data. In your presentation, you used the similar responses you found with sodium chloride and ammonium chloride as supporting your conclusion that it is chloride, rather than sodium, which induces renal vasoconstriction. Then you mentioned in the dis-

cussion that ammonium chloride is probably acting because of the acidosis it induces; so these data are not really going to be a support of the chloride hypothesis. Indeed, there could be two different mechanisms: One could be either sodium or chloride, and the other one could be acidosis.

Dr. Wilcox: When ammonium chloride was infused into the renal artery, there was no change in the blood pH across the kidney. In the micropuncture experiments in rats, however, the ammonium chloride was given by gavage and produced a pronounced acidosis. The effects of hyperchloremia and acidosis are closely related, however, and are being studied further.

Dr. Birkenhager (Rotterdam, The Netherlands): I would like to go back to Dr. Guyton and ask him why he associates the steepness of the blood pressure sodium excretion curve with the renin–angiotensin system and not with the adrenergic system? You have performed many studies in this area. It is quite obvious that the shape of the pressure–natriuresis is influenced by the adrenergic system.

Dr. Guyton: Yes, relative to the steepness of the curve, as I showed in one of my figures, we were able to demonstrate that the renin–angiotensin feedback mechanism is one of the major factors causing this steepness. However, I did make a mistake in emphasizing that this in the *only* mechanism, because the aldosterone feedback mechanism can also steepen the curve, and I am sure that catecholamine feedback can do as well. The thing that has worried me about the catecholamine system is that most of the sensors (such as the baroreceptors) that elicit the catecholamine response reset with a few days; therefore, this would be a short-term type of steepening of the curve rather than long-term. Yet, if anyone can find a sensor that causes reflex stimulation of catecholamines and that does not adapt, then I would be perfectly happy to accept that catecholamines participate in steepening the curve.

Finally, I want to challenge Dr. Korner, because all of his experiments have been multivariate types of experiments. They have been the Goldblatt type of experiment in which everyone has failed to demonstrate the autoregulation concept. Why haven't you performed pure volume-loading hypertension experiments rather than the multivariate type? I issue this challenge because those who do the volume type of hypertension find autoregulation, while we and many other investigators have shown that there are too many variables in the Goldblatt type of hypertension to allow consistent demonstration of autoregulation.

We should also note that the best evidence for long-term autoregulation comes from patients with coarctation of the aorta. We cannot forget the evidence that patients with this condition have high pressure in their upper body and low pressure in the lower body, and, yet, the data that are available thus far show that these patients have normal blood flow in both these areas. This is certainly the best evidence of all for long-term autoregulation.

Dr. Korner: All I would like to say is that I don't think that our experiments are multivariate. In our first study on *development* of hypertension, one could conceivably regard it in that way because both volume and resistance changed. However, we were lucky in that the volume (i.e., cardiac output) changed by the same amount in the control group, so that we had a situation where the cause of the hypertension was an increase in resistance factors, with volume held mostly constant. Accordingly, in the second study we started the experiment when conditions had become constant and we had reached constant resistance. It was only then that we varied volume by dietary salt. I have no doubt as to the facts of Dr. Guyton's volume-loading experiment but I have a lot of doubt about their interpretation. When these two factors (i.e., volume and constriction factors) are changing so quickly, it is impossible to say whether they are independent or interrelated. They could be quite independent and just change at different rates. This needs to be tested experimentally. To answer the question that we addressed, one must look at the problem under relatively stable conditions where each factor can be *experimentally* changed, one at a time. Our dietary salt experiments are, I believe, a sort of moderate volume loading; indeed our animals did show appropriate blood volume changes.

Dr. Guyton: what about coarctation of the aorta? This is a steady-state condition, very much so.

Dr. Korner: I don't know about coarctation of the aorta.

Dr. Zanchetti: Normalization of blood flow to the lower part of the body in coarctation of the aorta is strictly dependent on the development of collateral blood flow through the intercostal and other arteries. When the coarctation is very long and all these collateral vessels cannot develop, you don't find such a good blood flow to the lower part of the body.

Dr. Tosteson (Boston, Mass.): Dr. Guyton, I am confused. You have spoken about the mechanisms producing the steepness of the curves, but what about the mechanisms producing the shift of the curve? Why does the SHR operate at a higher pressure?

Dr. Guyton: We would agree very much with Dr. Folkow's studies which show that this results from structural changes in the vasculature of the SHR kidney.

Dr. Folkow: I have a comment concerning Dr. Guyton's statement that catecholamine mechanisms should not be capable of maintaining a long-term regulation of cardiovascular events. Actually during all my 58 years of life, the adrenergic vasoconstrictor fibers have, by means of their tonic activity, served me (and all other people) quite well without yielding, and I would at this moment drop to the floor by fainting, if this were not the case. I think that you greatly underestimate the power and endurance of the cardiovascular adrenergic nerve system, and parallels should *not* be drawn to norepinephrine infusions which is quite another matter.

Dr. Guyton: I am afraid that I did not make myself clear. I was referring to the blood pressure sensors that activate the catecholamine system, such as the baroreceptors that do adapt, not to the catecholamine receptors.

Dr. Laragh (New York): Dr. DiBona, did I misinterpret that last experiment of yours where you postulated an afferent signal going from one kidney to the other? My second question is, have you done your studies with angiotensin absent, such as after captopril?

Dr. DiBona (Oslo, Norway, and Iowa City, Ia.): First, the experiment does indicate renal afferent signals to the contralateral kidney. We have other data also indicating afferent signals from the kidney both in response to mechanoreceptor stimuli as well as chemoreceptor stimuli. Second, we have not looked at the responses in the presence of angiotensin blockade.

Dr. Zanchetti: As you know, in our laboratory we have a lot of experience with these renal chemoreceptors, and Recondati at the recent New Orleans international hypertension meeting showed that when these chemoreceptors are activated, there is increased discharge in the contralateral renal nerve. Stella Golin and I have recently tested electrical stimulation of the central stump of one renal nerve and studied diuresis and natriuresis of the contralateral kidney, comparing them with those of the ipsilateral kidney, which is obviously denervated. We observed some increased diuresis and natriuresis, but these changes were equal in the two kidneys, and seem to be due mostly to the increase in blood pressure induced by renal nerve stimulation. Thus, this increase seems to be an example of pressure natriuresis. Therefore, the problem of renorenal reflexes is still unsolved and has to be studied further.

Dr. Zanchetti (concluding remarks): This session has debated very important concepts, and I think we need some further discussion. I am glad that Dr. Guyton opened his presentation by saying that this session was centered not around one, but around two concepts not necessarily connected: One is the pressure–natriuresis concept, the other the long-term autoregulation hypothesis. It has always been my impression that the importance and the strength of persuasion of the pressure–natriuresis concept has suffered somewhat by being linked to the long-term autoregulation concept. As we have seen, however, both concepts have proven valuable for interpreting hypertensive phenomena and, more particularly, for designing experiments to answer new questions.

Session 6
Vasoconstriction and Volume Factors in Renovascular Hypertension

Chairman: H. R. Brunner

Position Paper: Vasoconstriction and Volume Factors in Renovascular Hypertension

Haralambos Gavras, Irene Gavras, and Hans R. Brunner

Interest in the pathogenesis of renovascular hypertension has remained strong since Goldblatt's famous experiment in 1934 where by constricting one renal artery, he produced hypertension that was reversed by clamp removal or nephrectomy. The role of a pressor mechanism via the renin–angiotensin system in this type of hypertension has been vigorously supported and refuted with equally convincing arguments over the years. In support of renin's contribution to the development and maintenance of renovascular hypertension are the facts that it can be readily produced experimentally by clamping of one renal artery, thus stimulating oversecretion of renin (1); it is frequently characterized by high levels of plasma renin activity (PRA) (2); it can frequently be cured by removal or revascularization of the affected kidney (3); it can be prevented (4) or reversed (5, 6) by administration of various angiotensin inhibitors after the experimental procedure that produces severe stenosis of the renal artery. Against renin's role are the findings that PRA is sometimes found to be in the normal or even subnormal range (7), and there is no correlation between PRA levels and the degree of hypertension (8); that corrective or ablative surgery is not always successful in curing hypertension (3); that angiotensin blockade does not always produce a fall in blood pressure (5, 9)—in fact, the competitive antagonists of angiotensin II that possess partial agonistic effects may occasionally increase, rather than decrease, the arterial pressure, a reaction characteristic of the low-renin hypertension state attributed to sodium overload (10).

In addition, there are other vasoconstrictor mechanisms that may contribute to renovascular hypertension. Arginine vasopressin (AVP) was found to be five times higher than normal in the plasma of rats with renovascular hypertension. In most of these animals, a specific AVP antiserum produced a transient fall in blood pressure similar to that obtained by angiotensin II antiserum (11).

The central nervous system apparently also plays a role in the induction and maintenance of renovascular hypertension. Damage of the specific angiotensin-sensitive sites of the brain prevents the development of renal hypertension (12), raising the possibility of a centrally mediated vasoconstrictor effect of high levels of circulating angiotensin II. This effect may be partially due to central sympathetic vasomotor discharge in addition to the pressor activity of angiotensin itself (13).

Peripheral sympathetic stimulation has also been demonstrated in acute renovascular hypertension, with circulating catecholamine levels rising in parallel to those of PRA (14). Whether this stimulation of plasma norepinephrine and epinephrine represents an additional causative factor triggered off by renal artery constriction, or whether it is a result secondary to activation of the central sympathetic neurons (13) or the adrenal medulla (15) by the stimulated renin–angiotensin system, is not clear. It is even possible that such activation may in fact partially play a protective role rather than exert an additional detrimental action on certain vascular beds, as will be discussed later.

Finally, evidence has been presented supporting the existence of various ill-defined pressor substances of renal origin with properties distinct from those of renin, such as renopressin (16), corticotensin (17), nephrotensin (18), etc., which may be activated by renal artery constriction.

As with most types of hypertension, sodium plays an important role in the development and maintenance of renovascular hypertension. Metabolic studies have shown that a positive sodium and water balance occurs soon after clipping of a renal artery (19–21), probably as a result of secondary hyperaldosteronism following angiotensin stimulation. Sodium-deficient diet starting immediately after placing a clip on one renal artery prevented the development of hypertension (22), whereas sodium depletion at a later stage of established hypertension did not affect the level, but only changed the mechanism maintaining high blood pressure (9, 23). It has been shown that sodium retention is more pronounced in certain types of renovascular disease than in others (24). And after release of renal artery constriction, there is profuse diuresis with negative sodium and fluid balance and a fall in cardiac output while blood pressure decreases progressively to normal (21, 25). However, the exact mode of action by which sodium accumulation affects the level of arterial pressure is still unclear. Theories include intravascular fluid volume expansion (26), retention of sodium and fluid by mucopolysaccharides within the vascular wall with thickening (water-logging) of certain layers and concomitant narrowing of the lumen (27), heightened reactivity of the vascular smooth muscle to normal or subnormal levels of circulating vasoconstrictor substances (28), and possible stimulation of vasopressor substances by the sodium ion itself (29).

The following is a brief review of the experimental work exploring the various hypertensive mechanisms incriminated in different types of renal artery disease. Three models have been used most frequently for these studies: acute hypertension induced by a previously implanted constricting device (i.e., an inflatable cuff or a clamp fitted with a stainless spring); chronic hypertension induced by application of a silver clip or steel clamp or by plication of one renal artery, with the contralateral kidney either left intact (two-kidney model) or removed (one-kidney model).

ACUTE HYPERTENSION

Immediately after constriction of one renal artery in unanesthetized animals [with one or two kidneys (14, 19–21)], there is always a sharp rise in blood pressure accompanied by an increase in PRA and peripheral vascular resistance. Thus, the predominant role of angiotensin II-related vasoconstriction at this early phase appears to be incontrovertible. Circulating plasma catecholamines were also found to be elevated, with epinephrine being far more stimulated than norepinephrine (14).

Whether this is a primary effect of renal artery constriction or the result of secondary stimulation of central sympathetic neurons (13) or the adrenal medulla (15) by angiotensin II, cannot be determined from the available data. Neither is it known whether catecholamines aggravate the vasoconstriction or, on the contrary, play a protective role, at least in certain organs, by blunting the detrimental effect of angiotensin II. Indeed, in baroreceptor denervated dogs, the development of renovascular hypertension was accelerated (21), although the final level of blood pressure was similar to that obtained in intact dogs. On the other hand, dogs pretreated with alpha- and beta-adrenoceptor blockade exhibited a lesser blood pressure elevation after acute renal artery occlusion than intact animals (14). Interestingly, a redistribution of regional blood flow occurred after occlusion, with angiotensin-sensitive vascular beds (30) (e.g., the renal, adrenal, and cerebral circulation) exhibiting relatively more increase in local vascular resistance than nonsensitive beds (e.g., the musculoskeletal and cutaneous regions). However, the coronary vasculature that is also highly sensitive to the constrictor effect of angiotensin II developed significant increase in diastolic arteriolar resistance only in the alpha- and beta-blocked animals, but not in the intact ones; furthermore, after teprotide injection, the coronary resistance in the adrenergic-blocked animals decreased again, whereas, in intact ones it remained practically unchanged (14). Interestingly, it has also been found that in acute blood pressure elevation leading to hypertensive encephalopathy, simultaneous sympathetic stimulation attenuates the damage to the blood-brain barrier (31). Taken together, these data suggest that adrenergic stimulation accompanying the stimulation of the renin–angiotensin system after acute renal artery stenosis, may not necessarily accentuate the generalized vasoconstriction, but, on the contrary, may protect certain vascular regions depending on their varying sensitivity to the pressor effect of each hormone. In other words, vascular regions such as cerebral and coronary vessels, with heightened pressor response to angiotensin (30) and relative insensitivity to the pressor effect of catecholamines (32), may be afforded partial protection by the parallel increase in sympathetic activity. Since epinephrine, known to have combined alpha- (constrictor) and beta- (dilator) adrenergic activity, was stimulated threefold to final levels approximately twice as high as those of norepinephrine, it is reasonable to speculate that epinephrine may be the protective agent. Musculoskeletal regions, on the contrary, are far more sensitive to the pressor effect of catecholamines and less sensitive to that of angiotensin than the heart, kidney, and brain, so that the additive effect of the two systems would tend to produce more pronounced vasoconstriction.

Cardiac output and heart rate was found in most studies to remain unchanged or decreased immediately after renal artery stenosis (14, 20), though one study reported an increase in cardiac output (19). Since angiotensin II has a direct-positive inotropic effect on the myocardium (tending to augment cardiac output, but the concomitantly elevated peripheral vascular resistance tends to decrease cardiac output), it is conceivable that in most cases, the two opposite actions may balance out; but occasionally one or the other may prevail. Within a few hours, however, there was always an elevation in plasma aldosterone, which, combined with the dipsogenic effect of elevated angiotensin II, led to sodium and fluid retention, with definite increase in blood volume and cardiac output both in one-kidney (20, 21) and two-kidney models (19).

CHRONIC RENOVASCULAR HYPERTENSION

Between the acute and the established phase of renovascular hypertension, a number of hemodynamic and humoral adjustments have been described, including alterations in cardiac output, vascular resistance, PRA and plasma aldosterone levels, metabolic balance of fluid, and electrolytes (19–21). Throughout these changes, blood pressure remains elevated but is sustained by different mechanisms depending on the experimental model (one- or two-kidney) and on the time lapse between the induction of renal artery stenosis and the performance of the studies. Species differences may also play a role, because the speed of evolution through successive stages of renovascular disease may be different in rats, rabbits, sheep, and dogs. Early studies revealed high levels of circulating renin in the two-kidney model, but low levels in the one-kidney model (2). The use of angiotensin II blockade (either with competitive antagonists or with inhibitors of the converting enzyme) pro-

vided proof that two different mechanisms were acting to maintain high blood pressure in the two different models: The two-kidney model responded to angiotensin blockade with a fall in blood pressure, whereas the one-kidney model exhibited no change in blood pressure (5, 6), indicating that the former model had angiotensin-dependent hypertension, but the latter did not. Since significantly more exchangeable sodium has been found in the latter model, it was suggested that the one-kidney renovascular type has a sodium-dependent hypertension (24). Yet, administration of a converting enzyme inhibitor was clearly shown to prevent or reverse the onset of hypertension in the one-kidney type (4), suggesting that in its very early phase this type also might have gone through a stage of angiotensin dependency.

In order to elucidate further the interplay of these two mechanisms and their time sequence, the following experiments were carried out (9, 23). One-kidney renovascular rats at 4 weeks' postsurgery received infusion of saralasin which, as expected, produced no change or slight increase in blood pressure, indicating that angiotensin was not responsible for the maintenance of high blood pressure. If, however, these animals were previously submitted to sodium deprivation at the stage of established hypertension, their blood pressure did not change, but they responded to saralasin infusion with a fall in blood pressure in the manner characteristic of renin-dependent hypertension. If they were subsequently allowed access to 1% saline as drinking water, they avidly drank large amounts; repeat infusion of saralasin 24 h later produced again the response characteristic of nonrenin-dependent hypertension (i.e., increase or lack of change in arterial pressure).

When the two-kidney animals (which at 4 weeks were known to have renin-dependent hypertension), were maintained on regular rat chow for 16 weeks, infusion of saralasin at that stage produced a response similar to that observed earlier in the one-kidney model (i.e., lack of change or slight increase in blood pressure). If they were deprived of sodium before the infusion of saralasin, they too behaved like the one-kidney model; their blood pressure was converted to renin-dependent type by sodium depletion, but would again become nonrenin-dependent as soon as they were repleted with sodium.

These findings reconciled seemingly conflicting earlier observations by indicating that both models apparently followed similar stages of evolution, the main difference being in the duration of each stage. Thus, the sequence of events leading to established renovascular hypertension could be constructed as follows: Severe constriction of one renal artery leads to stimulation of the renin–angiotensin–aldosterone system with hypertension initially being due mostly to the vasopressor effect of angiotensin. This stage is of very short duration in the one-kidney model because secondary hyperaldosteronism causes retention of sodium and fluid—provided that salt is readily available—and hypertension is soon converted to the sodium-dependent type. The two-kidney model with adequate healthy renal parenchyma is capable of excreting the salt and fluid load for a longer period of time; but continuing uncontrolled hypertension causes subtle progressive vascular and parenchymal damage to the kidneys, eventually affecting their excretory capacity and leading to sodium retention. At that stage, renin's contribution in either model can only be uncovered by sodium depletion.

Severity of hypertension depends on the degree of renal artery stenosis and resulting reduction of renal blood flow (33). Excessive elevation of blood pressure may induce acute, malignant-phase hypertension heralded by loss of weight, excessive loss of sodium and water with hemoconcentration, and marked rise in PRA (34). Interestingly, the same findings, except elevation of PRA, characterize malignant hypertension of mineralocorticoid origin, which is induced by a totally different mechanism (35). If at the malignant stage the renovascular animals are offered 0.9% saline instead of drinking water, blood pressure rises further, but, surprisingly, their general condition improves and the process of malignant microvascular lesions is arrested (34).

These data, taken together with the findings from the deoxycorticosterone acetate (DOCA-salt) model of hypertension, suggest that both in renovascular and in mineralocorticoid hypertension, the most important factor determining vascular damage may not be the level of blood pressure but the concomitant humoral changes. These include stimulation of vasoconstrictor hormones such as renin and vasopressin (36) as well as sodium kinetics. It is pertinent to mention here our preliminary experiments in which we found that an acute sodium load induced marked blood pressure elevation attributable not to intravascular fluid volume expansion, but to intense vasoconstriction due to vasopressin (29). Furthermore, there is evidence to suggest the existence of at least one additional pressor substance of renal origin, as mentioned earlier, with properties different from those of renin (16).

RENOVASCULAR HYPERTENSION IN MAN

If extrapolation is permitted from experimental models to human renovascular disease, the analogy between various stages of the experimental form and various known clinical entities could be presented as follows.

The typical renovascular hypertension of recent, abrupt onset in a young individual resembles mostly the acute or early phase two-kidney–one-clip model. It is characterized by high peripheral PRA, secondary hyperaldosteronism as attested by the commonly found spontaneous hypokalemia, and intact renal parenchyma in both sides, with excessive renin secretion from the stenotic kidney and normally suppressed renin release from the nonstenotic kidney. This type documentedly has the highest probability of success with corrective surgery (37)—equivalent to the release of the constricting cuff or clip in the experimental model.

The other extreme is hypertension of long duration in a more advanced age, with a stenotic lesion in one renal artery but with a variable degree of renal parenchymal damage due to chronic nephrosclerosis. At this point, the excretory capacity of the kidneys may have gradually diminished, leading to subtle chronic sodium retention. PRA may have returned to the normal range or become suppressed to subnormal levels. Infusion of the competitive antagonist of angiotensin II, saralasin, at this point produces either no response or a pressor response to various levels, characteristic of the state of sodium overload (10). In addition, structural changes of the arteriolar wall resulting from chronic blood pressure elevation are also contributing further to the maintenance of hypertension, which at this stage is probably not reversible. Indeed, corrective surgery to restore blood flow to the stenotic kidney or ablation of a contracted kidney in long-standing hypertension is far less likely to lead to cure of hypertension in cases where base-line PRA is no longer elevated. This is the rationale for the diagnostic significance of the saralasin test in hypertension (38), which has been advocated as a screening test for the detection of renovascular hypertension potentially amenable to surgical correction. (However, since the lateralization of renin output from the affected side is also a prerequisite to indicating surgical curability of hypertension, and since essential hypertension of the high-renin type is far more common in an unselected population than renal artery disease, the value of the saralasin test is limited accordingly.) Whether at this stage chronic renovascular hypertension is maintained through fluid volume expansion, or whether sodium accumulation activates other vasoconstrictive substances such as vasopressin, has not been determined. Moreover, the possible contribution of ill-defined vasoconstrictors of renal origin such as renopressin (16) or, possibly, lack of renal vasodilators such as certain prostaglandins (39) remains to be explored.

SUMMARY

Different hypertensive mechanisms seem to be operative in the various stages of renal vascular hypertension. Experimentally, acute constriction of one renal artery is accompanied by stimulation of the renin–angiotensin system as well as marked elevation of circulating norepinephrine and epinephrine. Chronic renovascular disease follows after an intermediate phase characterized by hemodynamic and humoral adjustments, including changes in cardiac output, vascular resistance, plasma renin and aldosterone levels, and metabolic balance of fluid and electrolytes. In the chronic established phase, hypertension appears to be sustained by an interplay of renin and sodium: In earlier stages, renin-mediated vasoconstriction predominates, whereas in later stages hypertension becomes sodium dependent and the renin factor can be unmasked only after sodium depletion. The one-kidney and two-kidney types seem to differ mainly in the speed of transition through each of these stages.

ACKNOWLEDGMENTS

This work was supported in part by USPHS grant HL-18318. H. Gavras is an Established Investigator of the American Heart Association.

REFERENCES

1. Goldblatt H, Lynch J, Hanzal RF, et al (1934) Studies on experimental hypertension: I. The production of persistent elevation of systolic blood pressure by means of renal ischemia. J Exp Med 59: 347–380
2. Schaechtelin G, Regoli D, Gross F (1963) Bioassay of circulating renin-like pressor material by isovolemic cross-circulation. Am J Physiol 205: 303–306
3. Kaufman JJ (1979) Renovascular hypertension: The UCLA experience. J Urol 121: 139–144
4. Miller ED, Samuels AI, Haber E, Barger AC (1972) Inhibition of angiotensin conversion in experimental renovascular hypertension. Science 177: 1108–1109
5. Brunner HR, Kirshmann JD, Sealey JE, Laragh JH (1971) Hypertension of renal origin: Evidence for two different mechanisms. Science 174: 1344–1346
6. Krieger EM, Salgando HC, Assan CJ, Green LLJ, Ferreira SH (1971) Potential screening test for detection of overactivity of renin-angiotensin system. Lancet 1: 269–271
7. Marks LS, Maxwell MH (1975) Renal vein renin value and limitations in the prediction of operative results. Urol Clin North Am 2: 311–325
8. Gross F (1971) The renin-angiotensin system and hypertension. Ann Intern Med 75: 777–787
9. Gavras H, Brunner HR, Thurston H, Laragh JH (1975) Reciprocation of renin dependency with sodium volume dependency in renal hypertension. Science 188: 1316–1317
10. Gavras H, Ribeiro AB, Gavras I, Brunner HR (1976) Reciprocal relation between renin dependency and sodium dependency in essential hypertension. New Engl J Med 295: 1278–1283
11. Möhring J, Möhring B, Petri M, Haack D (1978) Plasma vasopressin concentration and effects of vasopressin antiserum on blood pressure in rats with malignant two-kidney Goldblatt hypertension. Circ Res 42: 17–22
12. Buggy J, Fink GD, Johnson AK, Brody MJ (1977) Prevention of the development of renal hypertension by anteroventral third ventricular tissue-lesions. Circ Res 25(Suppl I): 110–117
13. Ferrario CM, Gildenberg PL, McCubbin JW (1972) Cardiovascular effects of angiotensin mediated by the central nervous system. Circ Res 30: 257–262
14. Gavras H, Liang C (1980) Acute renovascular hypertension in conscious dogs: Interaction of the renin-angiotensin system and sympathetic nervous system in systemic hemodynamic and regional blood flow responses. Circ Res 47: 356–365
15. Peach MJ (1971) Adrenal medullary stimulation induced by angiotensin I, angiotensin II and analogues. Circ Res 28, 29(Suppl II): 107–116
16. Skeggs LT, Kahn JR, Levine M, Dorer FE, Lentz KE (1977) Chronic one-kidney hypertension in rabbits: III. Renopressin, a new hypertensive substance. Circ Res 40: 143–149
17. Fasciolo JC, Risler NR, Totel G (1972) Corticotensins: Pressor peptides from the kidney. In: Genest

J, Koiw E (eds) Hypertension 1972. Springer, Berlin, pp 177–182

18. Grollman A, Krishnamurty VSR (1973) Differentiation of nephrotensin from angiotensin I and III. Proc Soc Exp Biol Med 143: 85–88
19. Maxwell MH, Lupu AN, Viskoper RJ, Aravena LA, Waks UA (1977) Mechanism of hypertension during the acute and intermediate phases of the one-clip two-kidney model in the dog. Circ Res 25(Suppl I): 24–28
20. Bianchi G, Tenconi LT, Lucca R (1970) Effect in the conscious dog of constriction of the renal artery to a sole remaining kidney on hemodynamics, sodium balance, body fluid volumes, plasma renin concentration and pressor responsiveness to angiotensin. Clin Sci 38: 741–766
21. Liard J-F, Cowley AW, McCaa RE, McCaa CS, Guyton AC (1974) Renin, aldosterone, body fluid volumes, and the baroreceptor reflex in the development and reversal of Goldblatt hypertension in conscious dogs. Circ Res 34: 549–560
22. Miksche LW, Miksche U, Gross F (1970) Effect of sodium restriction on renal hypertension and on renin activity in the rat. Circ Res 27: 973–984
23. Gavras H, Brunner HR, Vaughan ED, Laragh JH (1973) Antiotensin-sodium interaction in blood pressure maintenance of renal hypertensive and normotensive rats. Science 180: 1369–1372
24. Tobian L, Coffee K, McCrea P (1969) Contrasting exchangeable sodium in rats with different types of Goldblatt hypertension. Am J Physiol 217: 458–460
25. Ledingham JM, Cohen RD (1962) Circulatory changes during the reversal of experimental hypertension. Clin Sci 22: 69–77
26. Laragh JH (1973) Vasoconstriction-volume analysis for understanding and treating hypertension: The use of renin and aldosterone profiles. Am J Med 55: 261–274
27. Zelis R, Mason DT (1970) Compensatory mechanisms in congestive heart failure—The role of the peripheral resistance vessels. N Engl J Med 282: 962
28. Brunner HR, Chang P, Wallach R, Sealey JE, Laragh JH (1972) Angiotensin II vascular receptors: Their avidity in relationship to sodium balance, the autonomic nervous system and hypertension. J Clin Invest 51: 58–67
29. Hatzinikolaou P, Gavras H (1980) Sodium induced elevation of blood pressure in the anephric state (abstr). Clin Res 28: 329A
30. Gavras H, Liang C, Brunner HR (1978) Redistribution of regional blood flow after inhibition of the angiotensin converting enzyme. Circ Res 43(Suppl I): 59–63
31. Heistad DD, Marcus MD (1979) Effect of sympathetic stimulation on permeability of the blood-brain barrier to albumin during acute hypertension in cats. Circ Res 45: 331–338
32. Mark AL, Abboud FM, Schmid PG, Heistad DD, Mayer HE (1972) Differences in direct effects of adrenergic stimuli on coronary, cutaneous and muscular vessels. J Clin Invest 51: 279–287
33. Lupu AN, Maxwell MH, Kaufman JJ (1977) Mechanisms of hypertension during the chronic phase of the one-clip, two-kidney model in the dog. Circ Res 25(Suppl I): 57–61
34. Dauda G, Möhring J, Hofbauer KG, Homsy E, Miksche U, Orth H, Gross F (1973) The vicious circle in acute malignant hypertension of rats. Clin Sci Mol Med 45: 251S–255S
35. Gavras H, Brunner HR, Laragh JH, Vaughan ED, Koss M, Cote LJ, Gavras I (1975) Malignant hypertension resulting from deoxycorticosterone and salt excess: The role of renin and sodium in vascular changes. Circ Res 36: 300–309
36. Möhring H, Möhring B, Petri M, Haak D (1977) Vasopressor role of ADH in the pathogenesis of malignant DOC hypertension. Am J Physiol 232: F260–F269
37. Vaughan ED, Bühler FR, Laragh JH, Sealey JE, Baer L, Bard RH (1973) Renin measurements to indicate hypersecretion and contralateral suppression, estimate renal plasma flow and score for surgical curability. Am J Med 55: 402–414
38. Streeten DHP, Anderson GH (1979) Outpatient experience with saralasin. Kidney Int 15: S-44–S-52
39. Lee JB (1973) Hypertension, natriuresis and the renomedullary prostaglandins: An overview. Prostaglandins 3: 551

Intrarenal Resistance in Experimental Benign and Malignant Hypertension

Victor J. Dzau, Leland G. Siwek, and A. Clifford Barger

In 1934, Goldblatt et al. (1) reported that renal ischemia produced by constriction of the renal artery resulted in the development of benign hypertension. Since then, many investigators have confirmed their basic observations but have noted that hypertension could be produced without significant diminution of renal blood flow (2, 3). On the other hand, malignant hypertension is usually accompanied by severe renal ischemia, acute renal failure, and a high-renin state (4). Although several investigators have examined the changes in renal blood flow in experimental hypertension (3, 5, 6), a more detailed and sequential analysis of renal hemodynamics in benign and malignant hypertension, and, in particular, the transition from the benign to the malignant phase, is warranted. In the present study, we examined the changes in renal arterial pressure, renal blood flow, and intrarenal vascular resistance a) immediately after a single renal artery constriction, b) throughout benign hypertension, and c) during malignant phase of hypertension. We studied the pathogenetic factors responsible for these changes, in particular, the vasoconstrictor–volume relationship.

METHOD

Conscious, trained dogs on normal sodium intake (80 mEq Na/day) were uninephrectomized, and catheters chronically implanted in the renal artery, aorta, and inferior vena cava. In addition, an electromagnetic flow probe and a silastic occluder cuff were placed around the renal artery.

ACUTE RENAL ARTERY CONSTRICTION EXPERIMENTS

Renal artery stenosis was produced by inflation of occluder cuff, producing an aortorenal gradient. Reduction of renal perfusion pressure in a stepwise fashion in 5–20 mmHg increments from control (100 mmHg) to 30 was performed in different experiments ($N = 21$). Each decrement was maintained for 20 min.

BENIGN RENAL HYPERTENSION

Renal perfusion pressure was rapidly reduced in a single stage to a predetermined level (50–80 mmHg) by renal artery constriction according to the method of Tagawa et al. (2) ($N = 6$). Renal artery constriction was maintained for 10–14 days.

EXPERIMENTAL MALIGNANT HYPERTENSION

Mild progressive renal artery constriction was performed in 11 dogs. A 5-mmHg reduction of renal perfusion pressure below preconstriction pressure each day for 10–14 days was achieved by daily incremental cuff inflation according to the protocol described by Dzau et al. (7). At the end of 10–14 days, the constricting cuff was deflated.

Plasma renin activity (PRA) was determined by radioimmunoassay of Haber et al. (8), and plasma volume was measured by the Evans blue dye method. Blockade of the intrarenal renin–angiotensin system was performed by infusion of the nonapeptide-converting enzyme inhibitor (teprotide) or angiotensin II antagonist (Sar[1] Ala[8] angiotensin II) into the renal artery at increasing rates (starting at 0.5 μg/kg/min) until a barely detectable drop in systemic pressure was observed.

Intrarenal vascular resistance was determined by the following equation:

$$R_R = \frac{P_{RA} - P_{RV}}{RBF}$$

where: R_R = intrarenal vascular resistance; P_{RA} = mean renal arterial pressure; P_{RV} = mean renal venous pressure; and R_{BF} = renal blood flow.

RESULTS

INTRARENAL HEMODYNAMIC CHANGES IMMEDIATELY AFTER RENAL ARTERY CONSTRICTION

When renal perfusion pressure was lowered from 100 to 70 mmHg, renal blood flow remained unchanged as autoregulatory renal vasodilatation occurred. Further reduction of perfusion pressure resulted in decline of renal flow in a linear fashion. At 55 mmHg, vasodilatation reached its maximum as intrarenal resistance decreased to 50% ± 8% of control. PRA increased inversely with perfusion pressure from control of 1 ± 0.02 to 7.5 ± 0.8 ng angiotensin I/ml/h at renal perfusion pressure of 30 mmHg. Intrarenal infusion of teprotide or saralasin resulted in further decrease in intrarenal resistance ($p < 0.005$).

BENIGN ONE-KIDNEY–ONE-CLIP RENOVASCULAR HYPERTENSION

Benign hypertension was produced by rapid inflation of constricting cuff reducing renal pressure to 50–80 mmHg. The systemic and renal hemodynamic response were similar for this range of renal pressure. Renal vasodilatation occurred immediately after the renal artery constriction. Thirty minutes to several hours after constriction, renal arterial pressure rose toward control level as intrarenal resistance increased slightly above control. These parameters remained relatively constant throughout chronic hypertension. PRA rose immediately after artery constriction and returned to normal in 2–3 days. Sodium and water retention accompanied by plasma volume expansion occurred within 3 days (Fig. 1). Intrarenal infusions of teprotide or saralasin resulted in fall in intrarenal resistance within the first 3 days but failed to do so during the chronic phase of hypertension (Fig. 2). In benign hypertension, deflation of constricting cuff resulted in immediate diuresis and natriuresis with restoration of blood pressure to normal in 2–3 days.

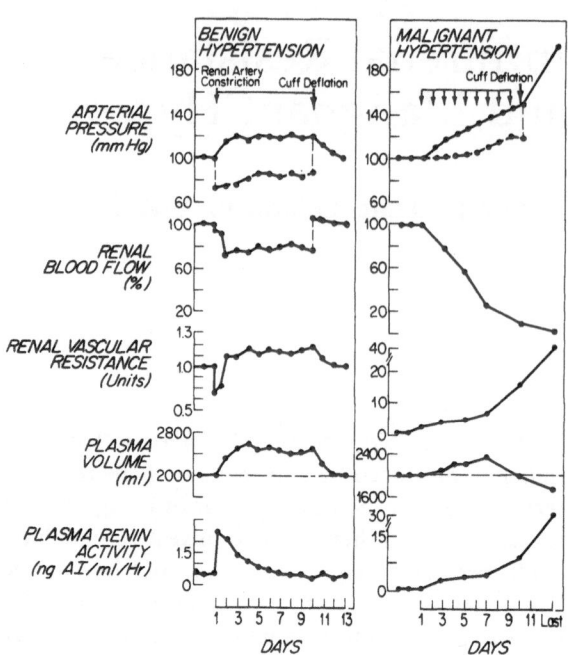

Fig. 1. Sequential changes in systemic and renal hemodynamics, PRA, and plasma volume in experimental benign and malignant hypertension.

MALIGNANT HYPERTENSION

During the first 3–5 experimental days, the response to mild progressive renal artery constriction was similar to that of single-stage constriction (Fig. 1). Moderate increases in systemic blood pressure, PRA, and renal vascular resistance were observed in both models during this period. An initial increase in plasma volume was also seen here by day 5. However, further constriction resulted in marked increase in PRA, blood pressure, intrarenal resistance associated with natriuresis, diuresis, and plasma volume contraction. Clinical signs of malignant hypertension were evident. Despite removal of gradient, natriuresis and diuresis increased, resulting in further volume contraction, a greater than 30-fold rise in PRA as well as a 40-fold increase in renal resistance.

To determine whether the rise in intrarenal resistance was the result of angiotensin II-induced vasoconstriction, teprotide or saralasin was infused intrarenally in four dogs. A small decrease in renal resistance was observed on days 3 and 5, whereas marked reduction occurred on day 7 (Fig. 2) as renal blood flow rose from 25% ± 3% to

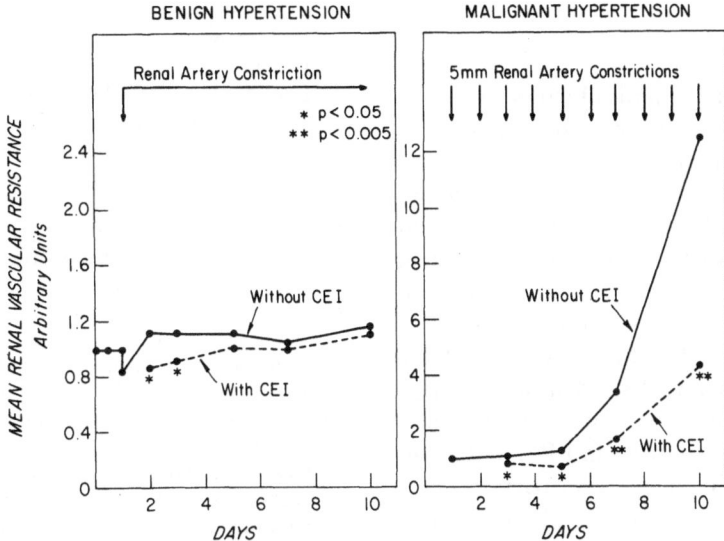

Fig. 2. Effect of intrarenal blockade of renin–angiotensin system on renal vascular resistance in benign and malignant hypertension. ————, without teprotide Converting Enzyme Inhibitor (CEI), — — —, with intrarenal infusion of teprotide.

56% ± 7% of control and day 10 as renal flow increased from 8% ± 0.8 to 25% ± 2% of control. The response was similar with both blockers.

DISCUSSION

The sequential renal hemodynamic changes during experimental benign and malignant renal hypertension are elucidated in this study. Immediately following renal hypotension, renal vasodilatation occurs. However, within hours, intrarenal vascular resistance returns to control and in fact rises above control. This renal vasoconstrictor response appears to be angiotensin II dependent and is reversible with the intrarenal blockade of the renin–angiotensin system. After 3–5 days, intrarenal administration of teprotide or saralasin can no longer reduce renal vascular resistance. Parallel to this, systemic hypertension is no longer renin dependent but is volume dependent as PRA returns to normal and plasma volume increases (2, 9–11). Similar changes in intrarenal resistance have also been observed by Harris and Ayers (5) and Anderson et al. (6). Ayers et al. (12) further demonstrated that sodium depletion at this stage reversed this pro-

cess, making renal vasoconstriction again angiotensin II dependent. These data suggest a renin–angiotensin II volume-interdependent mechanism controlling renal vascular resistance. Since the changes in renal hemodynamics are moderate in benign hypertension, release of cuff resulted in restoration of normal renal function and reversal of hypertension.

During the transition from benign to malignant hypertension, two factors appear to be important: a) increasing angiotensin II-dependent renal vasoconstriction; and b) the development of natriuresis and diuresis resulting in plasma volume contraction. When sufficient reduction in renal function occurs due to decreasing renal blood flow, increasing angiotensin II or rising renal prostaglandins, natriuresis develops. The volume depletion further stimulates renin release. Thus a vicious cycle of volume contraction, renin secretion, and vasoconstriction develops during malignant hypertension (13, 14). When the vicious cycle is established and vascular damage has occurred, renal ischemia and malignant hypertension may be irreversible despite cuff deflation. These observations also emphasize that a small pressure gradient does not necessarily signify a modest degree of stenosis but may be a reflection of high intrarenal resistance.

SUMMARY

Sequential renal hemodynamic changes were studied in the uninephrectomized dog immediately after renal artery constriction, throughout chronic benign hypertension, and during malignant hypertension. Renal vasodilatation occurred immediately after renal artery constriction. However, within hours, intrarenal resistance rose above control. The vasoconstriction was angiotensin II dependent and associated with a rise in systemic PRA but became volume dependent after 3 days. During the transition from benign to malignant hypertension, marked increase in PRA and angiotensin II-dependent renal vasoconstriction developed associated with natriuresis, plasma volume contraction, and a vicious cycle of hyperreninemia and severe vascular damage.

ACKNOWLEDGMENTS

We thank Dr. Edgar Haber for his advice, Squibb Laboratories for a generous supply of teprotide, and Merck, Sharp & Dohme for thrombolysin. Supported in part by NIH grants HL-19467 and HL-02493, and a gift from R. J. Reynolds Industries.

REFERENCES

1. Goldblatt H, Lynch J, Hanzal RF, Summerville WW (1934) Studies of experimental hypertension: I. Production of persistent elevation of systolic blood pressure by means of renal ischemia. J Exp Med 59: 347–479
2. Tagawa H, Gutmann FD, Haber E, Miller ED, Samuels AI, Barger AC (1974) Reversible renovascular hypertension and renal arterial pressure. Proc Soc Exp Biol Med 146: 975–982
3. Ferrario CM, McCubbin JW (1973) Renal blood flow and perfusion pressure before and after development of renal hypertension. Am J Physiol 224: 102–109
4. Laragh JH (1960) The role of aldosterone in man: Evidence of regulation of electrolyte balance and arterial pressure by renal-adrenal system which may be involved in malignant hypertension. JAMA 174: 293
5. Harris RC, Ayers CR (1972) Renal hemodynamics and plasma renin activity after renal artery constriction in conscious dogs. Circ Res 31: 520–530
6. Anderson WP, Koerner PI, Johnston CI (1979) Acute angiotensin II-mediated restoration of distal renal artery pressure in renal artery stenosis and its relationship to the development of sustained one-kidney hypertension in conscious dogs. Hypertension 1: 292–298
7. Dzau VJ, Rosen S, Haber E, Barger AC (1979) Pathogenesis of malignant hypertension induced by mild progressive renal artery stenosis. Am J Cardiol 43: 1066
8. Haber E, Koerner P, Page LB, Kliman E, Purnode A (1969) Application of a radioimmunoassay for angiotensin I to the physiologic measurement of plasma renin activity in normal human subjects. J Clin Endocrinol Metab 29: 1349–1355
9. Brunner HR, Kirshman JD, Sealey JE, Laragh JH (1971) Hypertension of renal origin: Evidence for two different mechanisms. Science 174: 1344–1346
10. Gavras H, Brunner HR, Vaughan ED Jr, Laragh JH (1973) Angiotensin-sodium interaction in blood pressure maintenance of renal hypertensive and normotensive rats. Science 180: 1369–1372
11. Rocchini AP, Barger AC (1979) Renovascular hypertension in sodium-depleted dogs: Role of renin and carotid sinus reflex. Am J Physiol 236: H101–H107
12. Ayers CR, Katholi RE, Vaughan ED, Carey RM (1977) Intrarenal renin angiotensin sodium-interdependent mechanism controlling post clamp renal artery pressure and renin release in the conscious dog with chronic one-kidney Goldblatt hypertension. Circ Res 40: 238–242
13. Dauda G, Mohring J, Hofbauer KG, Momsy E, Miksche U, Orth H, Gross F (1973) The viscious circle in acute malignant hypertension of rats. Clin Sci Molec Med [Suppl] 45: 2515–2555
14. Mohring J, Mohring B, Petri M, Hack D, Hackenthal E (1975) Studies of the pathogenesis of the malignant course of hypertension in rats. Kidney Int 8: S174–S180

Renal Mechanisms in the Pathogenesis of Essential Hypertension

Giuseppe Bianchi

The purpose of this short review on the role of renal mechanisms in the pathogenesis of socalled "essential" hypertension is to focus on some findings that, taken together, begin to delineate the functional pattern of a kidney that is genetically structured to produce (or to contribute to) the development of a type of essential hypertension. To do this, experimental data for rats of different strains [Milan hypertensive strain (MHS), Milan normotensive strain (MNS), Dahl salt-resistant strain (DR), Dahl salt-sensitive strain (DS), spontaneously hypertensive rat strain (Kyoto) (SHR), Wistar-Kyoto strain (WKY)] with spontaneous or hereditary types of hypertension will be discussed together with those for humans with essential hypertension; and the sons of hypertensive parents, assumed to be in the prehypertensive stage, will be compared to sons of normotensive parents. Particular emphasis will be given to the studies carried out during the prehypertensive stage because there are well-known secondary kidney function changes produced by high blood pressure *per se* (1–4). The data may be grouped under the following four categories:

1) *Kidney cross transplantation* between normotensive and hypertensive rats of three strains (MHS, DS, and SHR) showed that the kidney from a hypertensive animal caused a higher blood pressure level in the recipient than transplantation of a corresponding control kidney (5–8). Moreover, in two strains (MHS and DS), this effect was present even when the kidney was removed from the rat in the prehypertensive stage, excluding secondary kidney changes (7, 9). In humans, an analogous study was set up to compare, retrospectively, two groups of recipients of kidney grafts from donors belonging to hypertensive or normotensive families. The two groups of patients were well matched for age, sex, body-surface area, blood pressure, and duration of dialysis before transplan-

tation, original kidney disease, and familial hypertension. During the initial months after transplantation, the two groups had almost the same blood pressure, plasma creatinine, and monthly steroid requirements, but the antihypertensive therapy required was significantly greater in the recipients of kidneys removed from donors with hypertensive families (10).

2) *Renal blood flow:* Because of the well-known pressor effect of renal ischemia, it is important in the prehypertensive stage to assess the renal blood flow of a rat or a human with a kidney that, in some way, is genetically structured to produce a higher blood pressure level. These measurements in MHS and MNS showed that the absolute renal blood flow was almost the same in the two strains, but was significantly ($p < 0.05$) greater when expressed as percentage of cardiac output in MHS (11). This percentage was almost the same in the two strains when hypertension had fully developed and became lower in older MHS (12). Figure 1 shows that sons of hypertensive parents have greater renal blood flow than those of normotensive parents at equal cardiac output (13). Thus, like rats, humans have a larger redistribution of blood flow to the kidney in the prehypertensive stage. A larger renal blood flow in the early stages of human hypertension was also found by others in a subgroup of patients (14). Moreover, it is well-known that the renal blood flow tends to decrease as hypertension and age progress in humans as well as in rats (15).

3) *Renal excretion of a sodium load:* In humans, the excretion of a sodium load is faster in hypertensives than in normotensives (16–19), and it is even faster in low-renin hypertensive parents (19). The renal sodium excretion after an isotonic saline infusion is also faster in MHS and DS rats at the prehypertensive stage than in controls (20, 21), just as in sons of hypertensive parents compared

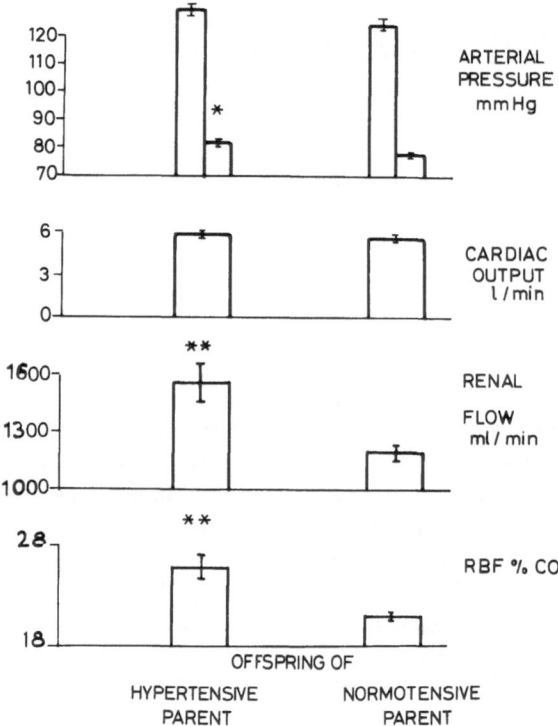

Fig. 1. Systolic and diastolic arterial pressure, cardiac output, and renal blood flow expressed as the absolute value and as the percent value of the cardiac output (RBF % CO) in sons of hypertensive parents and in those of normotensive parents. Mean ± SEM. [See Bianchi et al. (13) for details]

with sons of normotensive parents (22). However, when hypertonic saline is infused into DS rats under the same experimental conditions, a lower sodium excretion is observed than in DR. Moreover, an isolated kidney removed from a DS rat requires a higher perfusion pressure than a DS kidney to excrete the same amount of sodium (23). MHS, studied in a dehydrated condition, showed a greater ability to retain sodium than did MNS (G. Bianchi and L. Duzzi, unpublished observation). Recently, it has been shown that sons of hypertensive parents retain more sodium than those of normotensive parents when studied under certain experimental conditions (24). All these observations indicate that even in the prehypertensive stage, there is abnormal handling of sodium by the kidney. This abnormality is similar to the observation of increased excretion when studied under more physiologic conditions.

4) *Plasma renin:* the plasma renin of MHS is lower than that of MNS in the prehypertensive

stage (25), and it has been shown recently that renin secretion is also lower in MHS at this stage (26). As hypertension develops in the MHS, the differences in plasma renin tend to decrease, but the plasma renin of the MHS remains lower throughout the development of hypertension. In humans, patients with mild, recent onset essential hypertension and low plasma renin tend to have greater renal plasma flow (15), and renal excretion of a sodium load is also faster in low-renin patients than in those with normal plasma renin, again like the MHS (19).

These findings indicate that modification of kidney function can produce a type of essential hypertension in rats and, perhaps, in humans. Whatever the explanation for these findings, they do demonstrate that the functional pattern of a kidney genetically structured to favor the development of an essential type of hypertension may be completely different from what we would expect from the experimental data for renal hypertension. These kidneys have high blood flow, excrete a sodium load faster, and secrete less renin, all findings that are just the opposite of what one would expect from the results obtained in different types of experimental renal hypertension. New insight may be obtained by studying the mechanisms that underly the shift from an increase of renal sodium excretion to a decrease when the type of load is changed. An increase in renal blood flow and a decrease in renin secretion in the MHS were considered in our previous hypothesis to be secondary changes produced by the lower glomerular filtration in the prehypertensive stage (27). However, the changes in renal sodium excretion discussed above are more difficult to reconcile with this hypothesis. It is more likely that they are due to a defect in tubular transport mechanisms; this would fit better with recent findings about sodium and potassium transport through the cell membrane in essential hypertension (28–30).

A full discussion of the possible interrelationships between cell membrane transport and the factors so far discussed is beyond the scope of this short review. However, one may speculate that a genetic modification of the cell membrane transport which results in a tendency toward a higher cytosolic calcium ion activity may be an alternative explanation for the lower renin secretion (31, 32), the faster sodium excretion (33), and the subsequent development of vascular smooth muscle contraction (34, 35). The initial renal vasodilatation might be due to the very low intrarenal generation of renin that, for an initial period of time, may counteract the tendency toward an increase of vascular smooth muscle tone caused by the elevation of cytosolic calcium ion activity.

SUMMARY

Prehypertensive rats or humans prone to develop an essential type of hypertension showed four main differences from appropriately selected controls:

1) After kidney transplantation, the arterial pressure and the requirements for antihypertensive therapy to control blood pressure were higher in the recipients of their kidneys than in those receiving kidneys from controls.

2) The renal flow fraction of the cardiac output was greater than in controls.

3) The renal sodium excretion after an isotonic saline load was faster than in controls.

4) Plasma renin and renal renin secretion were definitely lower in rats. This has also been demonstrated in some subgroups of humans.

Whatever the explanations for these observations, they do suggest that kidney function of prehypertensive rats and humans prone to develop essential hypertension is abnormal and that this abnormality could be responsible, at least in part, for the subsequent increase in blood pressure.

ACKNOWLEDGMENT

This work was supported in part by grant no. 78.01995.04.115.5593 of the CNR of Italy.

REFERENCES

1. Wilson C, Byrom FB (1941) The vicious cycle in chronic Bright's disease: Experimental evidence from the hypertensive rat. J Med 10: 65–93
2. Friedman B, Jarman J, Klemperer P (1941) Sustained hypertension following experimental unilateral renal injuries. Effects of nephrectomy. Am J Med Sci 202: 20–24
3. Ljungqvist A (1969) Intrarenal vascular alterations and the persistence of experimental hypertension. Acta Pathol Microbiol Scand 76: 561–574
4. Koletsky S, Rivera-Velez JM (1970) Factors determining the success or failure of nephrectomy in experimental renal hypertension. J Lab Clin Med 76: 54–65
5. Bianchi G, Fox U, Di Francesco GF, Bardi U, Radice M (1973) The hypertensive role of the kidney in spontaneously hypertensive rats. Clin Sci Mol Med 45: 135S–139S
6. Bianchi G, Fox U, Di Francesco GF, Giovanetti AM, Pagetti D (1974) Blood pressure changes produced by kidney cross-transplantation between spontaneously hypertensive rats and normotensive rats. Clin Sci Mol Med 47: 435–448
7. Dahl LK, Heine M (1975) Primary role of renal homografts in setting chronic blood pressure levels in rats. Circ Res 36: 692–696
8. Kawabe K, Watanabe TX, Shiono K, Sokabe H (1979) Role of the kidney in the pathogenesis of SHR, and other hypertensive rats determined by renal isografts. Jpn Heart J 20(Suppl I): 87–89
9. Fox U, Bianchi G (1976) The primary role of the kidney in causing the blood pressure difference between the Milan hypertensive strain (MHS) and normotensive rats. Clin Exp Pharmacol Physiol [Suppl] 3: 71–74
10. Guidi E, Bianchi G, Dallosta V, Cantaluppi A, Vallino F, Polli E (1980) The influence of familial hypertension of the donor on the blood pressure and antihypertensive therapy of kidney graft recipients (abstr). In: seventh scientific meeting of the International Society of Hypertension, New Orleans, La, May 11–14
11. Bianchi G, Caravaggi AM, Cusi D, Barlassina C, Lupi GP, Duzzi L, Gatti M, Ferrari P, Velis O (1980) Is an abnormal kidney development involved in the pathogenesis of essential hypertension? In: Giovannelli G (ed) Proceedings of the international symposium on juvenile hypertension. Raven Press, New York
12. Caravaggi AM, Minotti E, Ferrari P, Bianchi G (in preparation) Renal blood flow changes with age in MHS and MNS
13. Bianchi G, Gatti M, Ferrari P, Picotti GB, Colombo G, Velis O, Cusi D, Lupi GP, Barlassina C, Bracchi G, Gori D, Mazzei D (1979) A renal abnormality as a possible cause of "essential" hypertension. Lancet, 1: 173–177
14. Hollenberg NK, Borucki LJ, Adams DF (1978) The renal vasculature in early essential hypertension: Evidence for a pathogenetic role. Medicine 57(2): 167–178
15. Hollenberg NK, Adams DF (1976) The renal circulation in hypertensive disease. Am J Med 60: 773–784
16. Cottier PT, Weller JM, Hoobler SW (1958) Effect of an intravenous sodium chloride load on renal hemodynamics and electrolyte excretion in essential hypertension. Circulation 17: 750–760
17. Lowenstein J, Beranbaum ER, Chasis H, Baldwin DS (1970) Intrarenal pressure and exaggerated natriuresis in essential hypertension. Clin Sci 38: 359–374

18. Schalekamp MADH, Krauss XH, Schalekamp-Kuyken MPA, Kolsters G, Birkenhäger WH (1971) Studies on the mechanism of hypernatriuresis in essential hypertension in relation to measurements of plasma renin concentration, body fluid compartments and renal function. Clin Sci 41: 219–231

19. Krakoff LR, Goodwin FJ, Baer L, Torres M, Laragh JH (1970) The role of renin in the exaggerated natriuresis of hypertension. Circulation 52: 335–345

20. Bianchi G, Baer PG, Fox U, Pagetti D (1976) Kidney function and blood pressure in a genetic type of hypertension. In: Proceedings of the sixth congress of nephrology, Florence, 1975. Karger, Basel, pp 274–283

21. Ben-Ishay D, Knudsen KD, Dahl LK (1973) Exaggerated response to isotonic saline loading in genetically hypertension-prone rats. J Lab Clin Med 82(4): 597–604

22. Wiggins RC, Basar I, Slater JDH (1978) Effect of arterial pressure and inheritance on the sodium excretory capacity of normal young men. Clin Sci Mol Med 54: 639–647

23. Tobian L (1979) The kidney, sodium, volume and hypertension. In: Bianchi G, Bazzato G (eds) The kidney in arterial hypertension. Bunge Scientific Publishers, University Park Press, Baltimore

24. Grim CE, Luft FC, Miller JZ, Brown PL, Gannon MA, Weinberger MH (1979) Effects of sodium loading and depletion in normotensive first-degree relatives of essential hypertensives. J Lab Clin Med 94: 764–771

25. Bianchi G, Baer PG, Fox U, Duzzi L, Pagetti D, Giovanetti AM (1975) Changes in renin, water balance, and sodium balance during development of high blood pressure in genetically hypertensive rats. Circ Res 36, 37(Suppl I): I-153–I-161

26. Caravaggi AM, Duzzi L, Bianchi G (in preparation) Renin secretion in Milan hypertensive rats

27. Baer PG, Bianchi G, Duzzi L (1978) Renal micropuncture study of normotensive and Milan hypertensive rats before and after development of hypertension. Kidney Int 13: 452–466

28. Garay RP, Meyer P (1979) A new test showing abnormal net Na$^+$ and K$^+$ fluxes in erythrocytes of essential hypertensive patients. Lancet 1: 349–353

29. Canessa M, Adragna N, Solomon H, Connolly TM, Tosteson DC (in press) Sodium-lithium countertransport is increased in red cells of patients with essential hypertension. New Engl J Med

30. De Mendoça M, Grichois ML, Garay RP, Ben-Ishay D, Sassard J, Bianchi G, Caravaggi AM, Meyer P (submitted) Abnormal net sodium and potassium fluxes in erythrocytes of four varieties of genetically hypertensive rats.

31. Park CS, Malvin RL (1978) Calcium in the control of renin release. Am J Physiol 235: F22–F25

32. Logan AG, Chatzilias A (1980) The role of calcium in the control of renin release from the isolated rat kidney. Can J Physiol Pharmacol 58: 60–66

33. Taylor A, Windhager EE (1979) Possible role of cytosolic calcium and Na–Ca exchange in regulation of transepithelial sodium transport. Am J Physiol 236(6): F505–F512

34. Mordecai BP (1977) Sodium ions, calcium ions, blood pressure regulation, and hypertension: A reassessment and a hypothesis. Am J Physiol 232(3): C165–C173

35. Van Breemen C, Aaronson P, Loutzenhiser R (1979) Sodium-calcium interactions in mammalian smooth muscle. Pharmacol Rev 30(2): 167–208

Renal Venous Renin Secretory Patterns Before and After Percutaneous Transluminal Angioplasty: Verification of Analytic Criteria

E. Darracott Vaughan, Jr., Thomas A. Sos, Kenneth W. Sniderman, Thomas G. Pickering, David B. Case, Jean E. Sealey, and John H. Laragh

In 1964, Dotter and Judkins (1) introduced the concept that atherosclerotic vascular lesions could be remolded by percutaneous transluminal angioplasty (PTA). The technique has gained recent impetus with the development of a double-lumen dilating balloon catheter (2). Renal arterial lesions secondary to either atherosclerosis (3) or fibromuscular disease (4) have been dilated with gratifying reduction in blood pressure and low morbidity.

In 1973, we reported three characteristics of renovascular hypertension that accurately predicted subsequent reversal of hypertension following successful renal arterial revascularization: a) high peripheral plasma renin activity level (PRA) when indexed against sodium excretion; b) absence of renin secretion from the opposite kidney (renal vein renin–inferior vena cava renin = 0); and c) abnormally high ipsilateral renal vein renin concentration relative to the inferior vena cava renin (renal vein renin–inferior vena cava renin divided by the inferior vena cava renin $\geqslant$ 0.50) (5).

Percutaneous transluminal angioplasty provides a unique opportunity to study the effect of restoration of renal blood flow (RBF) on renin secretion and renal vein to inferior vena cava (IVC) renin relationships. Moreover, it has allowed us to verify the concepts that we had previously proposed to identify curable renovascular hypertension.

MATERIALS AND METHODS

Over an 18-month period, 16 hypertensive patients with renal artery stenosis underwent successful PTA at the New York Hospital–Cornell University Medical Center. PTA was carried out by Drs. T.A. Sos or K. W. Sniderman in the division of cardiovascular radiology. The majority of patients have been followed in the Cardiovascular Center.

Cure following PTA is defined as a blood pressure less than 160/95 mmHg without treatment and improvement as a blood pressure less than 160/95 mmHg with minimum medication.

When possible, renal vein renin collections were obtained prior to or at the time of PTA, immediately after PTA, and 3–6 months following PTA. PRA was determined by the radioimmunoassay method of Sealey and Laragh (6).

RESULTS

BLOOD PRESSURE RESPONSE TO SUCCESSFUL PTA

At present, 10 of the 16 patients who had successful PTA maintain a blood pressure <160/95 mmHg without antihypertensive medications (63%), and 4 patients require less medication for blood pressure control (25%) than required before PTA. Two patients have not demonstrated a fall in blood pressure. One patient sustained a polar renal infarct and the second had a lesion of questionable physiologic significance. However, the post-PTA follow-up has been less than 6 months in six cases. Hence, it is premature to give a true success rate at this point.

RENAL VEIN RENIN RESPONSE TO SUCCESSFUL PTA

Prio to PTA, 12 patients demonstrated an ipsilateral renal vein renin concentration at least 50% greater than the IVC renin and the absence of renin secretion from the contralateral kidney. Eleven of the 12 patients had elevated peripheral PRA indexed against sodium excretion. Two of the remaining four patients were selected because of increasing renal failure and two had branch

Table 1. Change in renal vein renin relative to IVC renin concentration immediately following successful PTA.

Patient	Pre-PTA					Immediately post-PTA				
	PRA[a] involved kidney	PRA opposite kidney	IVC renin	$\frac{V-A^b}{A}$ involved	$\frac{V-A}{A}$ opposite	PRA involved kidney	PRA opposite kidney	IVC renin	$\frac{V-A}{A}$ involved	$\frac{V-A}{A}$ opposite
1	65	12	12	4.41	0	10	5.7	5.7	0.75	0
2	31	8.6	10	2.10	0	9.5	6.3	6.3	0.50	0
3	62	42	42	0.48	0	41	29	29	0.41	0
4	37	10	9.9	2.70	0	11	7.2	7.2	0.52	0
5	114	28	20	2.80	0	15	12	12	0.25	0
6	11	2.9	3.1	2.55	0	5.9	4.2	4.2	0.40	0

[a] ng/ml/h.
[b] $\frac{\text{Renal vein}-\text{IVC}}{\text{IVC}}$.

Table 2. Renal vein renin and IVC renin concentration 3–6 months following successful PTA.

	Pre-PTA					3–6 months post-PTA				
Patient	PRA involved kidney	PRA opposite kidney	IVC renin	$\frac{V-A}{A}$ involved	$\frac{V-A}{A}$ opposite	PRA involved kidney	PRA opposite kidney	IVC renin	$\frac{V-A}{A}$ involved	$\frac{V-A}{A}$ involved
1	65	12	12	4.41	0	1.8	1.5	1.3	0.38	0.15
2	31	8.6	10	2.1	0	2.0	2.5	1.8/1.9[a]	0.11	0.32
3	70	25	24/23	1.92	0.09	3.2	3.3	2.5/2.6	0.28	0.27
4	62	42	42	0.48	0	0.53	0.51	0.44/0.43	0.21	0.19
5	37	10	9.9	2.70	0	3.4	4.0	3.3/3.0	0.03	0.33

[a] IVC renin levels drawn with each matching renal vein renin level.

disease (1 failed to have a fall in blood pressure after PTA).

We were able to monitor the acute effect of successful PTA and restoration of RBF on renal vein renin and IVC renin in six patients (Table 1). Prior to PTA, all patients had a renal vein renin concentration higher than the caval level (A) only from the involved side. Hence, there was unilateral renin secretion. Also note that the IVC renin level, an index of renin secretion, was greater than 10 ng/ml/min in five of six patients. Thirty minutes following PTA, there was a marked reduction in renin concentration from the involved kidney. The fall in IVC renin in five of six patients indicates that the fall in renin concentration was due to a fall in absolute renin secretion as well as the expected rise in RBF. Note that the fall in the (V–A)/A relationship was to approximately 0.50, a value previously predicted to occur in the setting of unilateral renin secretion and normal blood flow (5, 7). In addition, contralateral renin suppression persisted; the opposite renal vein renin remained purely a reflectin of the arterial renin input.

Five patients returned for repeat renal vein and IVC sampling 3–6 months following PTA (Table 2). The reduction in circulating (IVC) PRA was dramatic with all values being below 3.5 ng/ml/min. Of equal interest is the observation that there was bilateral contribution of renin secretion in all cases as shown by the bilateral increment of renal vein renin above IVC renin. Hence, contralateral suppression of renin was a characteristic of renovascular hypertension which reversed following successful PTA. Moreover, the increment from each kidney, approximately 25%, is characteristic of the renin secretory pattern found in patients with essential hypertension (7).

DISCUSSION

Renal arterial disease is commonly found in both normotensive and hypertensive patients (8). It is now accepted that the functional significance of the renal arterial lesion must be proven before intervention is recommended. Accordingly, we previously developed criteria to identify potentially curable patients with renal arterial disease based on characteristics of experimental two-kidney-one-clip Goldblatt hypertension in rats (9). Although these criteria have been met with clinical

success (5, 10), we previously were unable to validate the underlying hypotheses because sequential sampling was impossible with surgical intervention.

First, the hallmark of curable renovascular hypertension should be hypersecretion of renin. Since the peripheral PRA is determined by the rate of renin secretion, then a high-peripheral PRA indexed against the 24-h urinary sodium should indicate increased renin secretion. Indeed, the peripheral PRA was elevated in 12 of 16 patients. Although the peripheral PRA indexed against sodium could not be monitored, the IVC renin fell immediately following PTA and was normal <3.5 ng/ml/h in all patients studied 3–6 months following PTA. The peripheral PRA has been shown to fall to normal following successful revascularization (5). In fact, the persistence of a high PRA strongly suggests technical failure (10).

Second, in experimental models there is absence of renal renin in the kidney opposite to the one with renal arterial narrowing. In the clinical setting, this characteristic is demonstrated by the absence of a renal vein renin increment from the opposite kidney—i.e., there is contralateral suppression of renin release. This phenomenon has been established as the second characteristic of renovascular hypertension. The present study supports this concept in two ways. First, contralateral suppression was present in all cases studied acutely and immediately following successful PTA, the contralateral renal vein renin concentration and IVC renin moved in parallel. Second, and more striking, contralateral suppression did not persist following successful PTA. Three to six months following PTA, there was bilateral renin secretion characteristic of that observed in patients with essential hypertension. Taken together, these observations strongly support the concept that contralateral suppression is a valid characteristic of renovascular hypertension.

Finally, based on studies in patients with essential hypertension who show a bilateral renal vein renin increment above IVC renin of approximately 25% from both kidneys, we postulated that a total increment of 50% was necessary to maintain a given peripheral renin level. Moreover, this increment would remain constant regardless of the amount of renin secretion unless there was a reduction in RBF. If the blood flow is reduced, the higher the concentration and the higher the calculated increment. Successful PTA restores blood flow toward normal. Accordingly, immediately following successful PTA, the ipsilateral (V–A)/A fell toward 0.50, indicating continued renin secretion with restoration of blood flow. The fall in IVC renin reflected the decreased renin secretion. However, as predicted, the renal vein renin ratio did not approach unity.

Taken together, successful PTA has given us a unique opportunity to validate further a number of concepts that we have found clinically valuable in identifying patients with renovascular hypertension.

SUMMARY

Sixteen hypertensive patients with renal artery stenosis underwent successful PTA. Fourteen of the 16 had cure or improvement of blood pressure following successful PTA. Immediately following successful PTA, there was usually a dramatic fall in the circulating renin (PRA), indicating a decrease in renin secretion. The ipsilateral renal vein renin concentration fell to a level approximately 50% above the circulating value. There was no renin secretion from the opposite kidney immediately after PTA. Three months later, renin secretion was normal and both kidneys contributed to total renin secretion with values approximately 25% greater than the circulating level. Taken together, these observations document quantitative criteria for the unilateral hypersecretion of renin which characterizes potentially curable renovascular hypertension is corrected following successful PTA, and there is return to a normal bilateral renin secretory pattern.

REFERENCES

1. Dotter CT, Judkins MP (1964) Transluminal treatment of arteriosclerotic obstruction. Circulation 30: 654
2. Gruntzig A, Hopff H (1974) Perkutane rekanalistation chronischer arterieller verslusse mit einem neuen dilatation: Modifikation der Dotter-Technik. Dtsch Med Wochenschr 99: 2502
3. Grutzig A, Kuhlmann U, Vetter W, Lutolf U, Meier B, Siegenthaler W (1978) Treatment of renovascular hypertension with percutaneous transluminal dilation of a renal-artery stenosis. Lancet 1: 801
4. Millan VG, Mast WE, Madias NE (1979) Nonsurgical treatment of severe hypertension due to renal-artery intimal fibroplasia by percutaneous transluminal angioplasty. New Engl J Med 300: 1371
5. Vaughan ED Jr, Buhler FR, Laragh JH, Sealey JE, Baer L, Bard RH (1973) Renovascular hypertension: Renin measurements to indicate hypersecretion and contralateral suppression, estimate renal plasma flow and score for surgical curability. Am J Med 55: 402
6. Sealey JE, Laragh JH (1977) How to do a plasma renin assay. Cardiovasc Med 2: 1079
7. Sealey JE, Buhler FR, Laragh JH, Vaughan ED Jr (1973) The physiology of renin secretion rate and renal plasma flow from peripheral and renal vein renin. Am J Med 55: 391
8. Eyler WR, Clark ME, Garman JE, Rian EL, Menninger KE (1962) Angiography of the renal areas including a comparative study of renal arterial stenosis with and without hypertension. Radiology 78: 897
9. Vaughan ED Jr (1976) Identifying surgically curable renovascular hypertension. Cardiovasc Med 1: 195
10. Vaughan ED Jr, Carey RM, Ayers CR, Peach MJ, Tegtmeyer CJ, Wellons MA Jr (1979) A physiologic definition of blood pressure response to renal revascularization in patients with renovascular hypertension. Kidney Int 15: S-83

DISCUSSION

Dr. Brunner (Lausanne, Switzerland) (Chairman): Dr. Bianchi, in your transplantation studies were the recipient patients matched for blood pressure?

Dr. Bianchi (Milan, Italy): Yes, they were matched. Before the transplantation, the blood pressure of the two groups was almost the same.

Dr. Streeten (Syracuse, New York): I would like to ask about the plasma volume in the chronic state of renal artery stenosis, because there is considerable difference of opinion expressed in the literature. Dr. Dzau showed that plasma volume increased acutely after induction of this lesion and he also showed that plasma volume in malignant hypertensive animals tended to fall as they became sicker toward the end of their course. We have studied plasma volume in human patients with unilateral renal artery stenosis under carefully controlled conditions of sodium intake and when they were in metabolic balance on a 200-mEq sodium daily intake. The patients under these conditions had a high plasma volume. Interestingly enough, these patients with chronic renal artery stenosis, when subsequently placed on a 10-mEq sodium diet daily, lost more sodium than essential hypertensive patients, so that their plasma volume fell to normal. Is it possible that in Dr. Dzau's malignant hypertensive animals, plasma volume falls not so much because of natriuresis, but because they stop eating, and thus have a sharply reduced sodium intake?

Dr. Dzau (Boston, Mass.): That's possible, but the natriuresis actually occurred before the animals had clinical evidence of malignant hypertension; that is, they were eating well at the onset of natriuresis.

Dr. Gavras (Boston, Mass.): Dr. Möhring has done some metabolic balances on the same subject, and he indicated to me that during the actual period of natriuresis and diuresis these animals were still eating when they were entering the phase of malignant hypertension. So in rats, I don't think its a weight loss, but a fluid loss. Thus, the malignant phase is preceded by paroxysms of pressure-natriuresis in both renovascular and DOC-salt hypertensions. [Gavras H, Brunner HR, Laragh JH, et al (1975) Circ Res 36: 300–309] Moreover, Möhring has also shown that saline administration reverses the malignant phase and improves the hypertension. [Dauda G, Möhring J, Hofbauer KG, et al (1973) Clin Sci Mol Med 45: 251S–255S]

Dr. Korner (Prahran, Australia): There are two comments I would like to make about Dr. Dzau's interesting paper. First, the vasodilator phase followed by vasoconstriction is in agreement with data that Dr. W. Anderson and I obtained in the conscious dog. My comment relates to his chronic benign hypertension experiments. What causes the rise in renal and systemic vascular resistance and why does the high-renin phase last for so short a time? A study that we have recently completed addressed the question of the contribution of the renal artery stenosis itself to the overall rise in resistance in a similar model. At about the same degree of hypertension you demonstrated, we found that it contributes approximately half the rise in total peripheral resistance. One has always assumed that this early rise in resistance is entirely angiotensin mediated, but if you actually plot stenosis resistance against either change in angiotensin II or against the rise in blood pressure, you obtain excellent correlations. Our contention is that this third factor, stenosis, is critically important and is the reason why the hypertension becomes renin independent so rapidly. Because of the hydraulic

complexity, the stenosis has to be very tight before hypertension develops. It should be no great surprise to anybody that the stenosis contributes to the resistance. We found it incredible that there are no data on this important point until our recent study.

Dr. Dzau: Dr. Korner, that's a very interesting point. When we first performed the malignant hypertension experiments, we were indeed concerned that we might be producing a highly severe stenosis that occluded renal blood flow. However, when we calculated cuff resistance and the intrarenal resistance, using an analogy of resistance in series, we found that the intrarenal resistance accounted for 20 times the total renal resistance during malignant hypertension. As far as the benign hypertension is concerned, the cuff resistance could account for 50% of total resistance. However, in this present study, I reported only renal vascular resistance, that is the renal artery pressure minus renal venous pressure by renal blood flow and not total resistance. Indeed, the renal vascular resistance is elevated. As far as speculating a mechanism for the rise in resistance in the chronic phase, I believe that this possibly could be a sodium-dependent mechanism similar to that discussed in Session 2 on sodium and hypertension.

Dr. Brunner: I do not quite understand Dr. Korner's point because, if you give captopril or any other renin inhibitor and you put a clamp on the renal artery, you don't get an increase in blood pressure despite the increase in resistance you first described.

Dr. Korner: I certainly don't wish to go into the full details of the hydraulic complexity of stenosis. The point is that when you give captopril, you are not getting the same change in stenosis resistance and the same reduction in renal artery diameter when you don't give captopril. The problem of stenosis and its hydraulics has been very well worked out by others. The factors that are important are aortic pressure, flow, and, above all, the hydraulic resistance of the distal vascular bed which makes the characteristics of stenosis very nonlinear. When you give captopril, you don't get a rise in systemic blood pressure and you keep the distal bed dilated so that when you reduce stenosis resistance to some nominal value of 70 or 80 mmHg, you have a smaller reduction in diameter than if the renin–angiotensin system had not been inhibited. Under these conditions, the renal artery stenosis resistance will be much less, and that's why everyone has thought the angiotensin II was the entire cause of the initial pressure rise. The secret is the complex hydrodynamic properties of the renal artery stenosis.

Dr. Dzau: May I try to answer that question also? We infused renin system-blocking agents intrarenally with minimal spillover of these agents systemically; that is, we progressively stepped up the infusion rates and stopped when we just barely got a detectable drop in systemic pressure. Thus, the pressure proximal to stenosis remained relatively constant, so I really don't think changes in systemic pressure are a major factor in our case.

Dr. Bühler (Basel, Switzerland): Dr. Gavras, you have left us with the notion that in the later development phase of renovascular hypertension, there is primarily a sodium and not a renin–angiotensin vasoconstrictor component. Yet, you have shown us results that saralasin blockade did not change blood pressure. However, a neutral response to saralasin usually indicates the presence of some angiotensin-mediated vasoconstriction; as due to saralasin's partial agonistic effect, one would expect a pressor effect wherever renin is not involved. Second, how do you reconcile these observations with your own earlier results showing that captopril can normalize blood pressure in chronic human renovascular hypertension?

Dr. Gavras: If we repeat those experiments with converting enzyme inhibitor we get the same kind of response. Other people have also repeated those experiments. Dr. J. O. Davis, for instance, recently found similar results in dogs. He has repeated some of his earlier experiments from the early 1970s with the same results, and I believe he also used converting enzyme inhibitors.

Dr. Bühler: You can lower blood pressure in renovascular hypertensive man with captopril, which clearly indicates that there is a renin factor even in the long-term phase.

Dr. Gavras: We also have seen cases with very low-renin levels that won't respond. However, none of the renovascular hypertensives that we studied had low-renin levels. All of them had "normal" to high levels of renin. Again, we get into the same argument. How much captopril works with renin, how much works otherwise? I believe it works primarily through renin.

Dr. Birkenhager (Rotterdam, The Netherlands): I would like to comment on Dr. Bianchi's elegant study in the prehypertensives. When you first reported your results, we were rather skeptical about the increased renal blood flows in part of the prehypertensives, and we set out to refute your findings. We took a slightly different look since there is no guarantee that all siblings are in fact prehypertensive. We, therefore, took a dozen young subjects who had already proven that they could be hypertensive at one moment in life and had returned to the normotensive state at the time of the study. We compared this group to a dozen-matched normotensives who had been normal during a preceding time of observation. Like yourself, we found a significantly increased renal blood flow in our hypertensives as well as some degree of renin suppression. We have no explanation for these phenomena, and I think neither have you, when you related this to cell membranes.

Dr. Bianchi: The explanation we gave was that the lower intrarenal generation of renin could be responsible for the increased blood flow. The sequence was: a lower filtration coefficient, a lower glomerular filtration, a lower delivery of sodium and chloride to the macula densa, a lower secretion of renin, and, then, an intrarenal vasodilatation. The development of hypertension normalizes the delivery to the macula densa. We have shown that this occurs in our rats by the micropuncture technique. We have seen that the lower glomerular filtration coefficient was normalized after the development of the difference in blood pressure. So this was our explanation, but, as I have said already, it is difficult to reconcile the increase in sodium excretion found at this age with this hypothesis even though you can explain the increase in sodium excretion through an increase in blood flow, as it has been shown by L. Early and co-workers. I think that all these observations taken together might be best explained by some changes in intracellular calcium concentration as was discussed in Session 3.

Dr. MacGregor (London, England): Mechanisms that maintain blood pressure in normal subjects may also partly maintain blood pressure in renovascular hypertension, so that just because a drug lowers blood pressure to normal in these patients does not necessarily imply that the drug is working through the mechanism whereby the blood pressure is raised. I wonder whether there were adequate control animals on the normal- and low-sodium diet?

Dr. Gavras: Normal dogs given saralasin or converting enzyme with regular sodium intake had no blood pressure response. In sodium-depleted dogs, blood pressure fell 20–30 mmHg. With rats we get identical results.

Dr. Ames (New York): Dr. Pickering, I can understand how your patients who meet your renin criteria would respond to your balloon procedure. I wonder if there are any patients who don't meet your criteria who might also benefit. As I recall, a few years ago M. Maxwell had some data on patients who didn't meet the renin criteria but who actually responded with a lowering of blood pressure following open operations on the renal artery. Do you have any data on that?

Dr. T. G. Pickering (New York): Seven patients with bilateral disease whom I didn't mention, have had bilateral dilatations and have shown improvement. The Maxwell group report that you mention

I think showed that two patients with a neutral response to saralasin were cured surgically. [Marks LS, Maxwell M, Kaufman JJ (1977) Lancet 1, 615–617] Since we now know that saralasin is an agonist, a neutral response in fact is evidence for renin participation.

Dr. Simpson (Dunedin, New Zealand): I would like to come back to the work of Drs. Bianchi and Birkenhager on young hypertensives. Knowing the correlation between blood pressure and obesity and between blood pressure and heart rate in these young people, could I ask if there was any difference in body weight between children of hypertensive and children of normotensive parents?

Dr. Bianchi: The body weight was the same and the body surface area and the height were the same in the two groups.

Session 7
The Renin-Angiotensin-Aldosterone System for Blood Pressure Regulation and for Subdividing Patients to Reveal and Analyze Different Forms of Hypertension

Chairman: A. Amery

Position Paper: The Renin-Angiotensin-Aldosterone System for Blood Pressure Regulation and for Subdividing Patients to Reveal and Analyze Different Forms of Hypertension

John H. Laragh

A sustaining or causal role for renin in essential hypertension has at least begun to gain credence along with the concept that essential hypertension is not a single clinical entity. Indeed, only recently has renin secretion been implicated in renovascular hypertension; renin measurements were not included even in the broad 1972 evaluation of renovascular hypertension formulated by the National Cooperative Study Group (1).

The change is based on two decades of research documenting the renin-angiotensin-aldosterone axis as a biologic control system simultaneously regulating arterial pressure and sodium balance. The analytic approach emerging from that research, while not precluding roles for other important factors, assumes that the patterns expressed by the renin system always have diagnostic meaning because as a true control system it will either cause, support, or react to any hypertensive state in a predictable way.

DISCOVERY OF THE SYSTEM

Exposure of renin secretion as part of a biologic system goes back to 1960 when it was discovered that patients with malignant hypertension secrete massive excesses of aldosterone (2). This was shown at operation to be associated not with an adrenal tumor, as in primary aldosteronism, but instead with bilateral hyperplasia. Studies in normal volunteers (3) then showed that angiotensin II is a specific and powerful stimulus for aldosterone secretion. Angiotensin II is the product of renin's enzymatic action on a plasma substrate and it is a most potent natural pressor substance.

This research suggested (4) that malignant hypertension is based on a vicious circle beginning with critical renal damage. This causes excessive secretion of renin, which in turn leads to excessive angiotensin and aldosterone in the blood; these changes account for the severe hypertension, hypokalemia, and escalating vasculopathy of this lethal condition (Fig. 1). It was also hypothesized that the newly revealed renin-angiotensin-aldosterone control system was linked to normal blood pressure regulation and might be implicated in the pathogenesis of the spectrum of hypertensive disorders.

HOW THE RENIN SYSTEM OPERATES

It is now evident that renin is normally secreted in response to reduced renal perfusion due either to local reduction in renal blood flow or a lowered systemic arterial blood pressure. Such events as shock, hemorrhage, heart failure, or even sodium depletion can lead to a reduced flow in the distal renal tubule (5).

Having no physiologic action of its own, renin acts enzymatically on a circulating plasma protein to release the inactive decapeptide angiotensin I, which is then rapidly hydrolyzed to the active octapeptide angiotensin II by pulmonary, plasma, or tissue converting enzymes. Angiotensin II's powerful pressor effect quickly raises blood pressure by constricting the arterioles. At the same time it stimulates aldosterone secretion, which in slower fashion causes renal sodium retention with potassium excretion. The resulting water retention and expanding extracellular fluid volume restores flow and further supports the blood pressure.

This combination of angiotensin-vasoconstriction and aldosterone-induced volume expansion restores systemic blood flow and renal perfusion, shutting off the signal that began the cycle. This

The Renal-Adrenal Axis in Malignant Hypertension

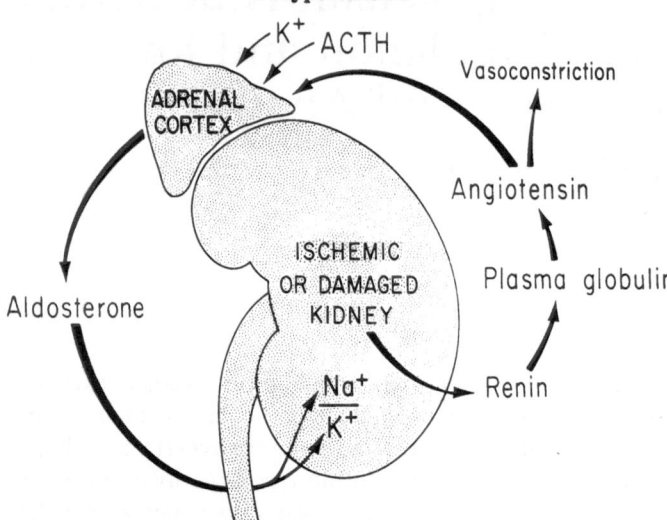

Fig. 1. The renal–adrenal axis, a hormonal cascade involving renin, angiotensin, and aldosterone for regulation of sodium and potassium balance and blood pressure. The interaction is depicted as it was first discovered in the studies of patients with malignant hypertension in whom, because of defective feedback, it is involved in causation. The syndrome is associated with massive oversecretion of aldosterone consequent to an unabated renin release. [Drawn from Laragh (3)]

negative feedback loop involves baroreceptors in the afferent renal arterioles and a sodium-load receptor in the macula densa portion of the renal tubules (6). Beta-adrenergic activity (7) mediates an efferent limb to the renin-containing juxtaglomerular cells of the baroreceptor communication (8).

STUDYING THE RENIN SYSTEM

It became obvious that the level of renin activity should be referenced to the current state of sodium balance, since renin and aldosterone secretion fluctuate widely in response to normal variations in salt intake. We therefore evolved a method in which plasma renin activity values are related to the 24-hr urinary sodium excretion to determine their normalcy (8), or to be more exact, their appropriateness to current physiologic factors. The 24-hr urinary sodium measurement is a reliable indicator of salt intake and balance. This means of analyzing the normalcy of renin activity is called the renin-sodium profile (Fig. 2). Collecting blood samples in ambulatory patients allows us to include postural stimuli and also assures standard conditions. The assay method we recommend is now readily available (9), is relatively simple and reliable, and it is sensitive enough to fully discriminate the subnormal range.

PRACTICAL GUIDELINES: HOW TO MEASURE PLASMA RENIN ACTIVITY

One of the reasons for the long delay in appreciating the role of the renin system in human hypertension has surely been methodological. It is unfortunate but true that three renin assays widely applied over the past 10 years or so (Table 1) contain large sources of error that make many of their results inaccurate or incorrect. The errors built into two of these three methods resulted from an unawareness of the presence in plasma of large amounts of inactive renin (i.e., prorenin) (10), which is converted to active renin by the acid treatment step, thereby misleading the active renin measurement in a variable way, sometimes by a factor of twenty or more.

The third unreliable method, which has been rather widely used, lacks sensitivity and consistency in identifying low-renin patients (Table 1). One fault is the lack of pH control. A rise in pH during incubation can lead to cessation of renin activity. Another fault involves poor angiotensinase inhibition. Also, this method employs BAL as an angiotensinase inhibitor; the compound is now known to inhibit renin activity (11). Fortunately, all these problems are easily solvable (9) (Table 1) so that, in future research, broader and fuller definition of the role of active renin in normal physiology and in diagnosis will be possible.

Plasma Renin and Aldosterone Excretion in Relation to Sodium Balance
Essential Hypertension
219 Patients

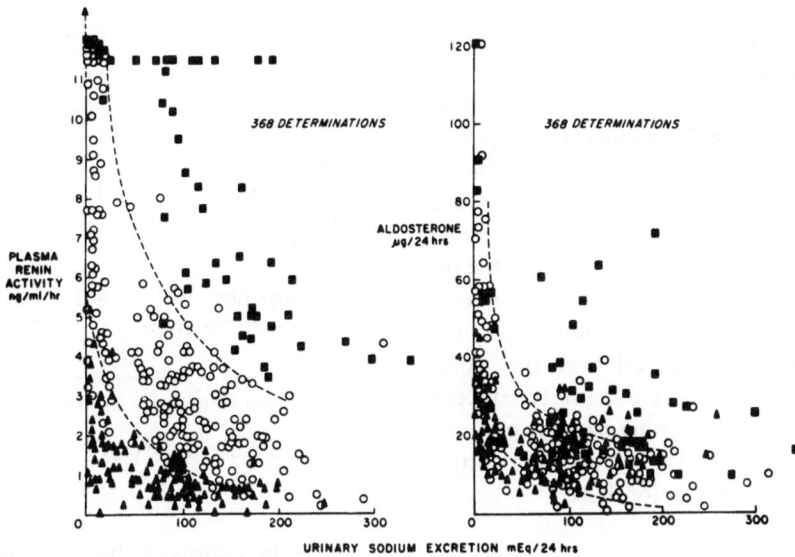

Fig. 2. Relation of the noon ambulatory plasma renin activity and of the corresponding daily urinary aldosterone excretion *(right panel)* to the concurrent daily rate of urinary sodium excretion. The dashed lines define the normal channel derived from the study of normotensive people. A total of 219 patients with untreated essential hypertension were studied, some on several occasions at different levels of sodium intake. ▲, low-renin; ○, normal-renin; ■, high-renin essential hypertension. Three major subgroups are defined by the appropriateness or normalcy of the plasma renin activity to the rate of sodium excretion which is used as an index of dietary intake and of sodium balance. Additional abnormal subgroups are defined when aldosterone *(right panel)* is included in the analysis. [Brunner et al. (14)]

Table 1. Three inaccurate or insensitive renin assays.

Method	Faults	Resulting problem
Skinner (1967)	Acid treatment activates inactive plasma renin.	Results can be 1–20 times too high with inconsistency in this error. Patients with PRA = 0 (i.e., anephric or primary aldosteronism) will appear to have active plasma renin. Renin will not appear to fall with beta-blockade.
Brown et al. (1946)	Same	Same
Haber et al. (1972)	No pH control during incubation—as pH rises renin is destroyed. Incomplete angiotensinase inhibition by BAL + 8-OH-quinoline. BAL also inhibits renin activity.	Generally less accurate, especially so for defining low-renin values.

Solution: The renin assay used should control pH at the optimum for human renin (5.5–6.0) during the incubation and use EDTA plus either DFP or PMSF to inhibit angiotensinases and allow prolonged incubations (18 h) for the low values. (9).

THE RENIN SYSTEM IN UNUSUAL FORMS OF HYPERTENSION

Renin-sodium profiling reveals characteristic abnormalities in the renin system in *malignant hypertension* (8), *primary aldosteronism, renovascular hypertension* (1), and oral *contraceptive hypertension* (12). Moreover, the fundamental diagnostic value of peripheral and renal vein renin studies in surgically curable renovascular hypertension (1), and for the diagnosis of surgically curable primary aldosteronism (8) due to autonomous oversecretion of an adenoma, is appreciated and used in modern medical practice all over the world. However, there has been less unanimity concerning the involvement of the renin system in common essential hypertension and therefore this subject merits more detailed discussion here.

ANGIOTENSIN II AS A VECTOR IN ESSENTIAL HYPERTENSION

Recognizing the existence of the renin-aldosterone system and its important pathogenic role in malignant hypertension and in renovascular hypertension we wondered if lesser, more subtle excesses of renin, leading therefore to milder increases in angiotensin II levels, might be causally involved in mediating the chronic, less fulminant forms of human hypertension such as common essential hypertension.

To study this question, we gave continuous intravenous infusions of either angiotensin or norepinephrine into normal volunteers under balance ward conditions for periods up to 11 days in amounts to produce a mild sustained elevation of blood pressure (13). With norepinephrine (Table 2) it was difficult to sustain an elevated blood pressure even with increasing dosages. The blood pressure tended to fall back to normal as paroxyms of natriuresis were induced. In sharp contrast, blood pressure elevations were maintained with angiotensin, and to our great surprise, with diminishingly small doses as aldosterone-activated sodium retention and weight gain progressed. Thus the aldosterone-sodium limb of the renin control system produces auto-induced sodium retention to reinforce the maintenance of blood pressure and flow (Table 2).

Table 2. Prolonged angiotensin and norepinephrine infusions.

	Angiotensin		Norepinephrine	
	First day	Last day	First day	Last day
Normal subjects				
Dose µg/min*	1.1	0.73	4.9	8.4
Net sodium balance (mEq)	+ 200		− 34	
Cirrhosis				
Dose µg/min*	9.3	16.4	26.2	29.4
Net sodium balance (mEq)	− 327		− 41	

* Duration of infusions = 2–11 days; BP = 155/90 during infusions.
Data from Ames et al. (13).

These data showed that circulating angiotensin II in relatively small amounts can sustain an elevated arterial pressure, whereas circulating norepinephrine, the only other humoral candidate to date, fails to do so. This research was contrary to the popular thinking that angiotensin exhibited tachyphylaxis, so that it could sustain chronic hypertension. The results encouraged us to pursue the role of angiotensin in mediating essential hypertension.

THE RENIN SYSTEM IN EVALUATING ESSENTIAL HYPERTENSION

Let me here summarize other subsequent findings that led to the conviction that renin participates in most forms of essential hypertension and that such participation can be identified, quantified, related to relevant changes in pathophysiology, and treated.

To begin with, the method of study described above—the use of the "renin-sodium profile"—has, when rigorously observed, shown that patients with essential hypertension are biochemically heterogeneous. When referenced to salt balance status, about 30% have low plasma renin activity, about 55% have medium renin, and about 15% high renin levels (14) (Fig. 2).

Companion clinical studies suggest that this biochemical heterogeneity correlates with differences in clinical course and prognosis (14, 15). Despite a degree of hypertension actually greater than that of medium-renin patients, low-renin patients appear to experience fewer heart attacks and strokes and they also have even fewer heart attacks or strokes than do high-renin patients. Moreover, studies the world over have confirmed the observation that low-renin patients are significantly older than patients in the other subgroups. This suggests that the relative absence of renin activity, with its attendant vasoconstriction, confers a measure of protection from cardiovascular damage.

These suggestions become rather compelling in the light of strong clinical and experimental evidence that an increased plasma renin activity, directly or indirectly, predisposes to vascular injury. In high-renin states such as malignant hypertension, renin-secreting tumors (16) and frequently in renovascular hypertension (17, 18) vascular damage is striking. Moreover, injection of renin and sodium in laboratory animals severely damages the cardiovascular system, particularly in the heart, brain, and kidneys (19, 20). Various acute clinical situations associated with high-renin levels are also associated with stroke or heart attack. These include renal trauma or an acute closure of a renal artery graft or a rebound high plasma renin level following a saralasin infusion (21). True, the connection may be circumstantial, but so is that between hypertension and excessive mortality. Indeed, it may help explain why many hypertensive patients ultimately prove not to have been at any greater risk and to a method for identifying them in advance. This relationship is discussed in more detail elsewhere in this volume (see Session 13).

The acceptance of renin's importance in essential hypertension also may have been delayed by the long-standing notion that this condition is a single disease with a common etiology and pathophysiology. It would follow from this monolithic viewpoint that if renin were involved it would be uniformly involved and could be consistently related to the blood pressure. This turns out not to be so; renin levels vary widely in patients with essential hypertension and when the data for the whole group are lumped together no correlation can be shown between renin levels and blood pressure levels. However, if one assumes different subgroups of patients, direct correlations between renin and blood pressure emerge for the medium

and high renin subgroups. These relationships are lost when the low-renin subgroup of patients are included in the analysis.

Adding to the confusion too is the finding that so many patients with essential hypertension exhibit plasma renin activity levels that are ostensibly "normal" when compared with those of normal volunteers. Actually the presence of a "normal" blood level of a substance does not mean that it is therefore inert or inoperative. This confusion is considerably clarified when one asks if "business as usual" in a control system facing excesses in the parameter it is supposed to control, does indeed represent normal activity. When the blood pressure is raised in normal people or animal models by non-renin factors, renin levels will fall as the renin system correctly turns itself off. Accordingly, in a state of hypertension, if the renin system is not involved it should turn itself off completely. In this context, renin actually only seems to behave properly in the low-renin subgroup of patients.

PHARMACOLOGIC PROOF OF RENIN INVOLVEMENT IN ESSENTIAL HYPERTENSION

Having demonstrated the usefulness of renin-sodium profiling for revealing biochemical and associated epidemiological heterogeneity among patients with essential hypertension, the stage was set to perform more definitive physiologic studies to expose and quantify the renin involvement in so-called essential hypertension. To accomplish this goal we identified and applied three different types of pharmacologic probes all of which act to block renin system activity.

BETA-ADRENORECEPTOR BLOCKADE OF RENIN SECRETION

In 1972 Bühler and associates (7) provided the first evidence that plasma renin helps maintain the elevated pressure of many patients with essential hypertension. They found that the degree to which propranolol, the beta-adrenergic blocking agent, lowered blood pressure was directly related to the height of the pretreatment plasma renin level and also to the degree to which the drug reduced the renin level. In fact, propranolol monotherapy was either partially or completely effective in more than half of an unselected group of untreated patients, those with high or normal renin profiles. The selective effectiveness of beat receptor blockers in lowering pressure in high- and medium-renin patients and also the converse—their ineffectiveness in low-renin patients—has been generally verified (22). Moreover the reports that some beta-blockers fail to lower renin secretion have either been retracted or refuted (22a) and it is now generally recognized that all beta-blockers suppress renin secretion.

SARALASIN

The participation of renin activity in essential hypertension revealed by beta blockade was confirmed and extended by the administration of other agents with specific ability to blockade the renin system at different points. Saralasin is an octapeptide analog of angiotensin that competes for angiotensin receptor sites, thereby blocking its pressor action (23). However, like many competitive antagonists, saralasin itself turned out to have a mild pressor effect of its own (24). Therefore, the blood pressure response to saralasin administration can lead to a gross underestimation of true renin participation (24, 25). Because of this, we and others who used saralasin as a guide identified a renin factor in only about 15% of patients, i.e., those with the high renin levels (Fig. 3). This is to be contrasted with an estimated renin factor in some 50% of patients with essential hypertension as implied from the depressor responses to propranolol (7).

CONVERTING ENZYME INHIBITION: TEPROTIDE AND CAPTOPRIL

The next inhibitor to be tested was a converting enzyme inhibitor, which blocks the formation of angiotensin II from the decapeptide, but which has no pressor action of its own. We first evaluated the nonapeptide inhibitor, teprotide or SQ 20881. This compound has to be given parenterally and

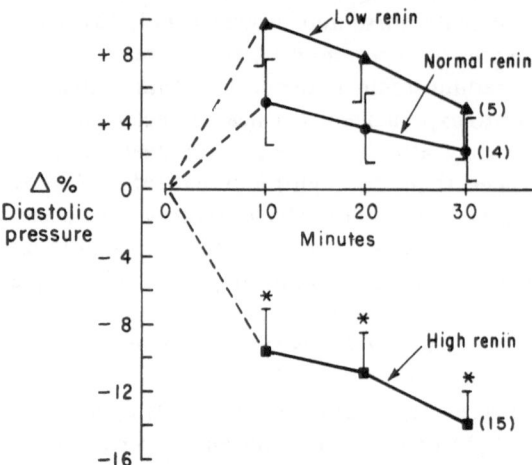

Effect of Saralasin on Diastolic Pressure

Fig. 3. Percent changes in DBP in low- (5 patients), normal- (14 patients), and high- (15 patients) renin subclasses after 10, 20, and 30 min saralasin infusion while on a normal dietary sodium intake. When analyzed by group, normal- and low-renin patients exhibited pressor responses, whereas high-renin patients had depressor responses. *$p < 0.005$. [Redrawn from Case et al. (23)]

acts almost immediately. Our experience with this agent began in 1973 and it comprises 89 patients (25–27). The depressor responses induced by this nonapeptide exposed and defined the participation of the renin system even more clearly than did propranolol, for it indicated that an active renin factor is involved in sustaining or causing the high blood pressure of up to 70% of patients with essential hypertension (Fig. 4). This included the high-renin and most of the medium-renin patients. Again, no significant depressor responses were observed in the low-renin subgroup. Actually all the high-renin and 91% of the medium-renin group exhibited significant responses and in about half of the responders the hypertension was fully corrected.

The more recent introduction of an orally active form of the converting enzyme inhibitor (28, 29), captopril, has now most dramatically confirmed the relationships developed from using the intravenous agent and has shown too that they are valid over the long term. Both captopril's relative freedom from unwanted physiologic side effects and its ability to lower pressure while actually improving flow suggests a higher order of specificity than heretofore possible (See also Sessions 16, 17).

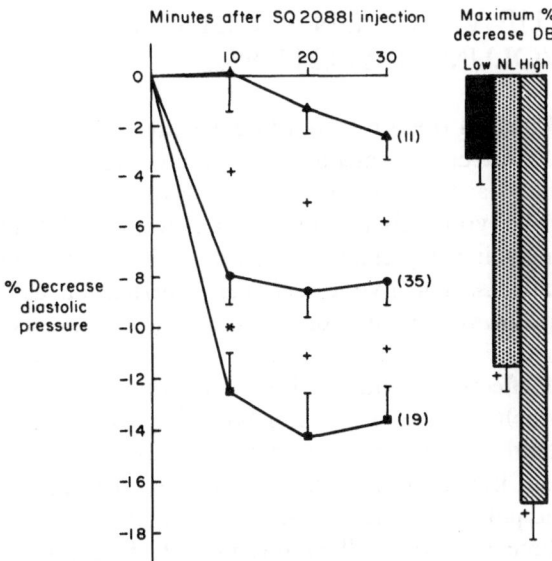

Fig. 4. Depressor responses to converting enzyme blockade in 65-seated hypertensive patients. *Left panel:* represents the time-course of the diastolic pressure changes, comparing the value of the low-renin (▲), normal-renin (●), and high-renin (■) patients. *Right panel:* compares the maximal percent decreases in diastolic blood pressure (DBP) of the three subgroups. The data show a striking antihypertensive effect in high-renin patients, a lesser but still impressive action in most normal-renin patients, and no significant antihypertensive action in low-renin patients. $*p < 0.05$; $+p < 0.01$. [Case et al. (26)]

All our experiences with pharmacologic blockade of the renin system using four different probes are mutually reinforcing. We know from our large experience with both the nonapeptide and then with long-term captopril therapy that the reductions in blood pressure are closely related to induced decrements in angiotensin II formation. Accordingly, it is extremely likely that the decrements in renin secretion produced by propranolol (7) are also critically involved in its antihypertensive action.

From a practical standpoint it is relevant that with all three types of anti-renin agents, the degree of depressor activity can be predicted by a properly performed renin-sodium profile. Accordingly, the cumulative experience shows that the plasma renin level is a true indicator of the active pressor contribution caused by renin-angiotensin vasoconstriction.

Significantly, the converses are also true. All

of these different types of anti-renin agents are either totally ineffective, or only slightly effective, in those 30% of people with essential hypertension whose renin values are low. Moreover, as one would expect, these anti-renin system agents are also ineffective in lowering pressure in primary aldosteronism, and in anephric humans, two other situations characterized by low to absent renin levels. These low-renin patients respond instead to sodium depletion induced by diet, diuretics or dialysis, thus demonstrating that their high blood pressure is predominantly volume-dependent.

DISSECTION OF VASOCONSTRICTION AND VOLUME FACTORS

The reciprocity between vasoconstriction and volume that was dramatically demonstrated in this series of studies appears to have broad applications. Thus, for example, when renin-vasoconstriction is opposed with a vasodilator drug such as hydralazine, minoxidil or nitroprusside, the renin system reacts and induces salt and water retention via amplified aldosterone secretion. In the same way, diuretics, uniquely effective in low-renin patients, can be ineffective in high-renin patients or even pressor, presumably by triggering a reactive renin overshoot in response to volume depletion. This see-saw relationship explains why diuretic-resistant patients respond to the addition of an anti-renin drug and why some medium- or high-renin patients need a diuretic to cope with reactive sodium retention (24). However, the majority of patients will respond to a single agent, providing it is the correct one for their physiologic lesion. A worldwide literature has accumulated to verify the selectivity of beta-receptor blockers and of diuretics when given to different subgroups of patients as defined by renin testing (22).

This reactive reciprocity helps explain why many patients do not respond to traditional trial and error therapy: the agent prescribed may be inappropriate to deal with the factors behind their hypertension. They have not been sufficiently analyzed for the relative contribution of vasoconstriction and volume to their condition. Thus diuretics are usually ineffective in high-renin vasoconstriction-dependent hypertension, and so is renin blockade ineffective in low-renin volume-dependent hypertension (25, 28).

VASOCONSTRICTION AND VOLUME FACTORS IN RENAL HYPERTENSION

On another front, renin system blockade in animal and human forms of renovascular hypertension has defined exactly the same interplay between vasoconstriction and volume factors. When one-kidney is clipped with the opposite kidney untouched, the hypertension model is renin dependent (30). This form resembles surgically-curable human renovascular hypertension, since nephrectomy or vascular repair is curative. The animal with one kidney-clipped and the opposite kidney removed exhibits a low renin level and its hypertension is instead volume dependent (31). The human counterparts, patients with chronic bilateral kidney disease and reduced renal mass, is similar because they exhibit medium or low renin levels and often respond to sodium depletion alone. In others anti-renin therapy may have to be added to cope with reactive increases in renin secretion. Accordingly, the peripheral renin profile becomes a primary screening test for surgically curable forms of renovascular hypertension (1) in which there is unilateral hypersecretion of renin. Practically, this allows the physician to defer the necessity for the more invasive tests of pyelography and arteriography until the need is definitively established by renal-vein renin studies.

THE VASOCONSTRICTION-VOLUME HYPOTHESIS

When all these research findings are put together a construction emerges that we have come to call the Vasoconstriction-Volume Hypothesis (32). This hypothesis provides a framework useful for analyzing, explaining, and treating all hypertensive patients. The hypothesis sees hypertension as a spectrum ranging from a predominant excess of arterial vasoconstriction to a predominant excess of effective volume, with intermediate forms in which relative excesses of both may overlap and jointly contribute to high blood pressure. Malignant hypertension and primary aldosteronism are the polar extremes of the spectrum and the other clinical entities fall at intermediate points (Fig. 5). Renin profiling can generally suggest which type of hypertension prevails within this spectrum. Just as important, those exceptions to the rule who do not respond to anti-renin or anti-volume therapy are set apart by this analysis for further study.

According to the vasoconstriction-volume hypothesis all hypertension is in fact sustained by an increased total peripheral resistance. However the analysis proposes that gross differences in the degree of vasoconstriction help explain observed differences in pathophysiology. Thus low-renin patients have an overfilling or sodium-volume dependent form of hypertension (i.e. corrected by diuretics) and so, for a similar degree of high blood pressure, exhibit better flow than do high-renin patients, who have more vasoconstriction and poorer tissue flow sometimes to the point of overt tissue ischemia.

The Vasoconstriction-Volume Spectrum in Hypertension

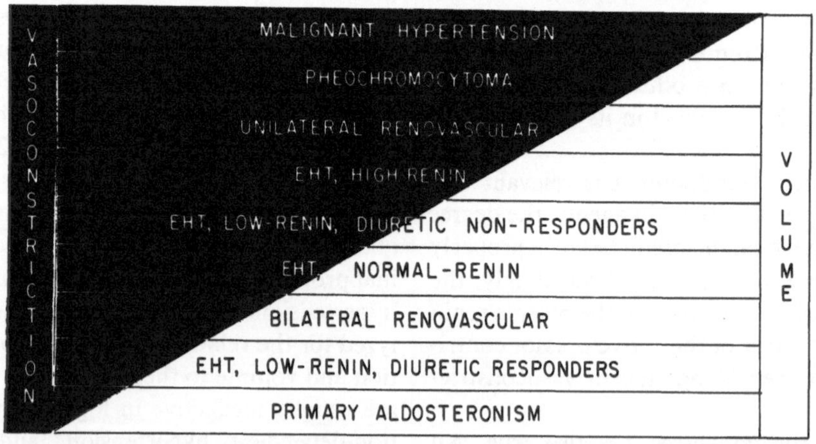

Fig. 5. Vasoconstriction–volume spectrum in hypertension. [Laragh et al. (33)]

More research is needed to define fully the accompanying physiologic differences among patients within the various renin subgroups. For example, we do know that volume is usually proportionally lower in hypertensive than in normotensive people (32), but we need to know conclusively if there are volume differences among equally hypertensive patients with differing renin profiles. The available data are in keeping with what the vasoconstriction-volume model predicts, that low-renin patients are relatively hemodiluted and volume-expanded (34, 35). Thus, patients with

A Flow Sheet for Diagnosis and Treatment of Hypertension

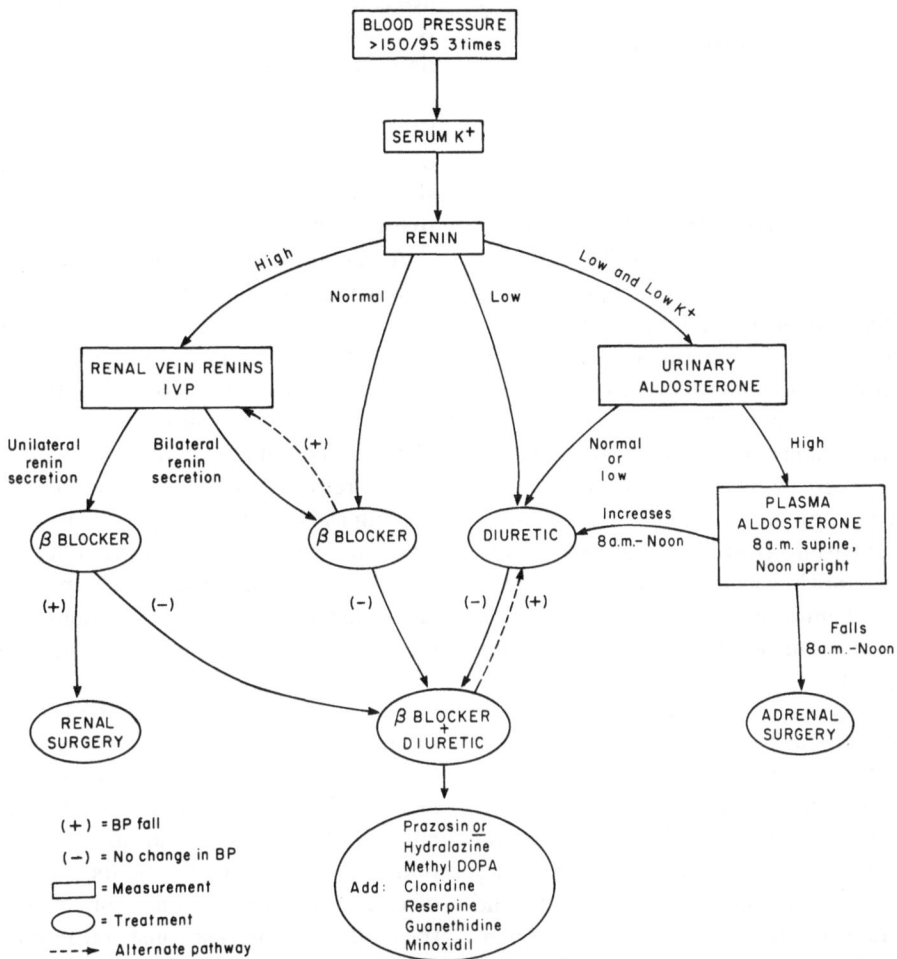

Fig. 6. Flow sheet for complete diagnosis and treatment of hypertension. Low-renin patients with hypokalemia (serum K+ <3.5) are evaluated for adrenocortical disease. Normokalemic low renin patients receive a diuretic first. The medium and high-renin patients are started on a beta-blocker or newer antirenin drugs such as a converting enzyme inhibitor. Whenever either course is only partly corrective, the antirenin agent is combined with a diuretic. Altogether this normalizes some 85% of patients. For the residual resistant group, other less palatable drugs are superimposed in traditional trial by error fashion as indicated. Also unlike so-called "stepped care," drug subtraction and dose reduction is performed whenever pressure is normalized, to achieve the fewest drugs in the smallest dose. Those medium or high-renin patients with a good response to a beta-blocker or captopril alone based on other clinical features too, are evaluated for surgically curable renovascular hypertension. Only if the renal vein renin study reveals hypersecretion with ischemia is angiography done for considering either angioplasty or surgery. When renin profiling is not available this basic approach can be partially applied, albeit more slowly, by serially evaluating the responses to antirenin or antivolume therapy, but renin profiling remains essential to diagnose curable forms. [Redrawn from Laragh et al. (34).]

low-renin hypertension have relatively lower blood urea, hematocrit, and hemoglobin values (13), and in all reported studies from the world over (32) their total blood volume and extracellular fluid volume are almost without exception as high or higher than those of the normal-renin patients. Low-renin patients also have a large central blood volume (33). And the converses are also true: when hypervolemia is present in hypertensive patients, renin values are considerably reduced. Moreover, high renin patients have the lowest plasma volumes (32, 36) (see also Session 13).

APPLICATIONS FOR DIAGNOSIS AND TREATMENT

Five major clinical applications of the renin-sodium profile emerge: (a) the definitive diagnosis of surgically curable renovascular hypertension; (b) the definitive diagnosis of adrenocortical hypertension; (c) acquisition of baseline information for planning simpler, more specific, and predictable therapy; (d) evaluation of the pace, severity, and prognosis of the underlying disorder, and (e) identification of patients whose hypertension cannot be explained by our current state of knowledge. These five applications from the matrix of an overall plan for diagnosis and treatment (34, 37, 38). The plan also defines an optional procedure for empiric use when the renin profile is not readily available (Fig. 6).

The proposed system differs fundamentally in concept from such previous approaches as "stepped care," which advise a single additive recipe system be used indiscriminately for all essential hypertension, without systematic drug substitution or dose reduction such trial and error approaches are workable but less efficient. In contrast, the new system identifies those large subgroups of people in whom long-term monotherapy with either an anti-vasoconstriction or anti-volume drug will be entirely effective by itself. Among the advantages of this approach is that for major fractions of all hypertensive patients it enables long-term therapy with one drug instead of two, or two instead of three or more. With it, the right type of drug can be selected to contain the pathophysiological lesion; i.e., anti-volume therapy with a diuretic for patients with low renin levels or anti-renin therapy with a beta-blocker (or newer anti-renin drug) in patients with high and normal renin levels (Fig. 6). The new algorithm, by aiding in

selection of patients for pyelography and arteriography, also reduces the need for those invasive procedures while providing the fullest possible evaluation for curable forms.

SUMMARY

Research of the past 20 years has revealed the renin-angiotensin-aldosterone axis for regulating arterial blood pressure and electrolyte balance. It is a control system that responds predictably to deformations in blood pressure or sodium balance. Characteristic derangements of the system have been shown to be involved in the pathogenesis of malignant hypertension, renovascular hypertension, primary aldosteronism, and oral contraceptive hypertension.

A research series using pharmacologic probes to block the renin system (beta-receptor blockers, saralasin, teprotide, and captopril) shows that essential hypertension is a spectrum in which absolute or relative overactivity of the renin system participates in the maintenance of the hypertension of most patients. The plasma renin level reflects the degree of renin-mediated vasoconstriction supporting the blood pressure and the urinary sodium value indicates the appropriateness of the renin level to the volume status. The presence of renin-vasoconstriction can also be related to attendant reductions in body fluid volumes and to hemoconcentration.

Renin-sodium profiling, together with determination of serum potassium levels, has become the basic approach for screening and for definitive diagnosis of the surgically curable forms of renovascular and adrenocortical hypertension. For the remaining majority of patients with various forms of essential hypertension, renin profiling, used in the context of the vasoconstriction-volume analytical model, helps expose the participation of vasoconstriction and volume factors and thereby guides simpler, more specific, and more predictable treatments using either antirenin or antivolume agents. The vasoconstriction-volume analysis also provides useful baseline information about the pace, severity, and prognosis of the disease in individual patients. Furthermore, it sets apart those unusual patients whose hypertension does not fit the model. In them other vasoconstrictors such as norepinephrine, vasopressin, or prostaglandins may prove to have a pressor role.

For medical practice the new knowledge defines

potentialities for even more specific physiologic corrections, and it has already enabled long-term treatment with one drug instead of two for major subgroups. Anti-renin monotherapy has the attraction of lowering blood pressure while actually improving blood flow to vital organs.

The research described may help explain why patients with similar degrees of hypertension differ so much not only in their pharmacologic responses, but also in their clinical course and the susceptibility to cardiovascular damage. With such understanding and the companion pharmacologic advances to do something specific about it, we seem to be nearing final solutions.

REFERENCES

1. Vaughan ED Jr, Laragh JH (1975) New concepts of the renin system and of vasoconstriction-volume mechanisms: Diagnosis and treatment of renovascular and renal hypertension. Urol Clin North Am 2: 237–257

2. Laragh JH, Ulick S, Januszewicz V, Demin QB, Kelly WG, Lieberman S (1960) Aldosterone secretion and primary and malignant hypertension. J Clin Invest 39: 1091–1106

3. Laragh JH, Angers M, Kelly WG, Lieberman S (1960) Hypotensive agents and pressor substances: The effect of epinephrine, norepinephrine, angiotensin II and others on the secretory rate of aldosterone in man. JAMA 174: 234–240

4. Laragh JH (1960) The role of aldosterone in man: Evidence for regulation of electrolyte balance and arterial pressure by renal-adrenal system which may be involved in malignant hypertension. JAMA 174: 293–295

5. Laragh JH, Sealey JE (1973) The renin-angiotensin-aldosterone hormonal system and regulation of sodium, potassium, and blood pressure homeostasis. In: Orloff J, Berliner RW (eds) American Physiological Society (Handbook of physiology—renal physiology). Waverly Press, Baltimore, pp 831–908

6. Sealey JE, Laragh JH (1974) A proposed cybernetic system for sodium and potassium homeostasis: Coordination of aldosterone and intrarenal physical factors. Kidney Int 6: 281–290

7. Bühler FR, Laragh JH, Baer L, Vaughan ED Jr, Brunner HR (1972) Propranolol inhibition of renin secretion: A specific approach to diagnosis and treatment of renin-dependent hypertensive diseases. N Engl J Med 287: 1209–1214

8. Laragh JH, Baer L, Brunner HR, Bühler FR, Sealey JE, Vaughan ED Jr (1972) Renin, angiotensin and aldosterone system in pathogenesis and management of hypertensive vascular disease. Am J Med 52: 633–652

9. Sealey JE, Laragh JH (1977) How to do a plasma renin assay. Cardiovasc Med 2: 1079–1092

10. Sealey JE, Laragh JH (1975) "Prorenin" in human plasma? Methodological and physiological implications. Circ Res 36, 37(Suppl I): I-10–I-16

11. Ryan MP, Weinberger MH (1980) Effect of sulphydryl reagents on the enzymatic activity of human renin: Implications for renin assay. Clin Chim Acta 106: 135–143

12. Laragh JH, Sealey JE, Ledingham JGG, Newton MA (1967) Oral contraceptives: Renin, aldosterone and high blood pressure. JAMA 201: 918–922

13. Ames RP, Borkowski AJ, Sicinski AM, Laragh JH (1965) Prolonged infusions of angiotensin II and norepinephrine and blood pressure, electrolyte balance, aldosterone and cortisol secretion in normal man and in cirrhosis with ascites. J Clin Invest 44: 1171–1186

14. Brunner HR, Laragh JH, Baer L, Newton MA, Goodwin FT, Krakoff LR, Bard RH, Bühler FR (1972) Essential hypertension: Renin and aldosterone, heart attack and stroke. N Engl J Med 286: 441–449

15. Brunner HR, Sealey JE, Laragh JH (1973) Renin as a risk factor in essential hypertension: More evidence. Am J Med 55: 295–302

16. Orjavik OS, Aas M, Fauchold P, et al (1975) Renin secreting tumors with severe hypertension. Acta Med Scand 197: 329–336

17. Perera GN, Haelig AW (1952) Clinical characteristics of hypertension associated with unilateral renal disease. Circulation 6: 349

18. Davis BA, Crook JE, Vestal RE, Oates JA (1979) Prevalence of renovascular hypertension in patients with grade III or IV hypertensive retinopathy. N Engl J Med 301: 1273–1276

19. Gavras H, Brunner HR, Laragh JH (1974) Renin and aldosterone and the pathogenesis of hypertensive vascular damage. Prog Cardiovasc Dis 17: 39–49

20. Laragh JH (1978) Renin as a predictor of hypertensive complications: Discussion. Ann NY Acad Sci 304: 165–177

21. Keim HJ, Drayer JIM, Case DB, Lopez-Ovejero JA, Wallace JM, Laragh JH (1976) A role for renin in rebound hypertension and encephalopathy after infusion of sar^1-ala^8-angiotensin II. N Engl J Med 295: 1175–1177

22. Laragh JH (1978) The renin system in high blood pressure, from disbelief to reality: Converting enzyme blockade for analysis and treatment. Prog Cardiovasc Dis 21: 159–166

22a. Amery A, Lijnen P, Fagard R, Reybrouck T (1976) Plasma renin activity vs. concentration. N Engl J Med 295: 1198C

23. Brunner HR, Gavras H, Laragh JH (1973) Angiotensin II blockade in man by sar^1-ala^8-angiotensin II for understanding and treatment of high blood pressure. Lancet 2: 1045–1048

24. Case DB, Wallace JM, Keim HJ, Sealey JE, Laragh JH (1976) Usefulness and limitations of saralasin, a partial competitive agonist of angiotensin II for evaluating the renin and sodium factors in hypertensive patients. Am J Med 60: 825–836

25. Case DB, Wallace JM, Keim HJ, Weber MA,

Drayer JIM, White RP, Sealey JE, Laragh JH (1976) Estimating renin participation in hypertension: Superiority of converting enzyme inhibitor over saralasin. Am J Med 61: 790–796

26. Gavras H, Brunner HR, Laragh JH, Sealey JE, Gavras I, Vukovitch RA (1974) An angiotensin converting enzyme inhibitor to identify and treat vasoconstriction and volume factors in hypertensive patients. New Engl J Med 291: 817–821

27. Case DB, Wallace JM, Keim HJ, Weber MA, Sealey JE, Laragh JH (1977) Possible role of renin in hypertension as suggested by renin-sodium profiling and inhibition of converting enzyme. N Engl J Med 296: 641–646

28. Case DB, Atlas SA, Laragh JH, Sealey JE, Sullivan PA, McKinstry DN (1978) Clinical experience with blockade of the renin-angiotensin-aldosterone system by an oral converting enzyme inhibitor (SQ 14,225, captopril) in hypertensive patients. Prog Cardiovasc Dis 21: 195–206

29. Brunner HR, Gavras H, Laragh JH, Keenan R (1974) Hypertension in man: Exposure of the renin and sodium components using angiotensin II blockade. Circ Res 34, 35(Suppl. I): I-35–I-45

30. Brunner HR, Kirshman JD, Sealey JE, Laragh JH (1971) Hypertension of renal origin: Evidence for two different mechanisms. Science 174: 1344–1346

31. Gavras H, Brunner HR, Vaughan ED Jr, Laragh JH (1973) Angiotensin-sodium interaction in blood pressure maintenance of renal hypertensive and normotensive rats. Science 180: 1369–1372

32. Laragh JH (1973) Vasoconstriction-volume analysis for understanding and treating hypertension: The use of renin and aldosterone profiles. Am J Med 55: 261–274

33. Tarazi RC, Dustan HP (1972) Beta adrenergic blockade in hypertension. Am J Cardiol 29: 633

34. Laragh JH, Letcher RL, Pickering TG (1979) Renin profiling for modern diagnosis and treatment of hypertension. JAMA 241: 151–156

35. Esler M, Randall O, Bennett J, et al (1976) Suppression of sympathetic nervous function in low-renin essential hypertension. Lancet 2: 115–118

36. Weidmann P, Hirsch D, Beretta-Piccol C, et al (1977) Interrelations among blood pressure, blood volume, plasma renin activity and urinary catecholamines in benign essential hypertension. Am J Med 62: 209–218

37. Laragh JH (1976) Modern system for treating high blood pressure based on renin profiling and vasoconstriction volume analysis: A primary role for beta blocking drugs such as propranolol. Am J Med 61: 797–810

38. Laragh JH, Sealey JE (1977) Renin-sodium profiling: Why, how and when in clinical practice. Cardiovasc Med 2: 1053–1075

Artifacts in the Diagnosis of Essential Hypertension

J. J. Brown, A. F. Lever, R. Fraser, J. I. S. Robertson, P. A. Mason, D. G. Beevers,
C. Beretta-Piccoli, A. M. M. Cumming, D. L. Davies, J. J. Morton, P. L. Padfield,
and J. Young

MILL'S DISEASE AMONG THOSE WHO CLASSIFY HYPERTENSION

Apart from increased arterial pressure, essential hypertension is a disease characterized by negative features. Diagnosis is reached by excluding conditions with positive features, Conn's syndrome, renal artery stenosis, pheochromocytoma, and others. Essential hypertension remains as a disease with a name but no shape. As such, it is vulnerable to errors of classification:

> The tendency has always been strong to believe that whatever receives a name must be an entity or being, having an independent existence of its own: and if no real entity answering to the name could be found, men did not for that reason suppose that none existed, but imagined that it was something peculiarly abstruse and mysterious, too high to be an object of sense.
>
> —*J. S. Mill.*

We suspect that the tendency recognized by John Stewart Mill is common among doctors. We refer to the tendency as "Mill's disease." Its basic fault is not in the giving of a name, but in the belief that whatever receives a name must be an entity. A classic example from our own field is the separation of normotension and hypertension, the fault being not so much the use of the term "hypertension," but the belief that it is an entity separable from "normotension" (1). Another example is the separation of normal-renin and low-renin hypertension (2). Renin is certainly sometimes subnormal in essential hypertension (3) and low-renin hypertension is a fair description of that finding, but it is also implied that low-renin hypertension is an entity separable from essential hypertension with normal renin. There is little evidence for this, in our view (2).

NONTUMOROUS PRIMARY HYPERALDOSTERONISM: ANOTHER NONENTITY?

We suspect that nontumorous primary hyperaldosteronism may be another nonentity and an example of Mill's disease among those (including ourselves at one time) who considered it otherwise. Tumorous and nontumorous primary hyperaldosteronism are usually considered variants of the same condition and are separated from essential hypertension by high aldosterone in the presence of low or low–normal renin. The tumorous variant, Conn's syndrome, is an undoubted entity: excess aldosterone released from the tumor causing significant sodium retention and potassium depletion. Sodium retention suppresses renin, and the concentration of renin or angiotensin II in plasma correlates negatively with the concentration of aldosterone (4).

Patients with nontumorous hyperaldosteronism, sometimes referred to as "idiopathic hyperaldosteronism" (5), or more suspiciously as "pseudo-primary hyperaldosteronism" (6), show few of these features. There is no significant decrease of exchangeable sodium or of exchangeable potassium in our experience (4, 7). Contrasting with Conn's syndrome, the relationship between the plasma concentration of angiotensin II and aldosterone is positive (4), which suggests that aldosterone is high because angiotensin II is high, not as in Conn's syndrome, that aldosterone is high because its oversecretion is primary, with renin and angiotensin II reduced as a result. On this evidence, the oversecretion of aldosterone in the nontumorous form of the disease does not seem to be primary. This is strongly supported by studies in which angiotensin II is infused with measure-

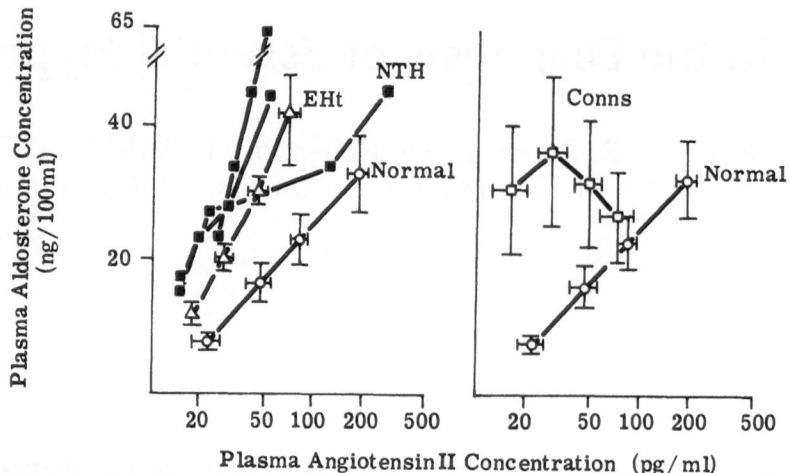

Fig. 1. Response of plasma aldosterone concentration to infusion of angiotensin II intravenously at three of the following rates: 0.5, 1.0, 2.0, and 4.0 ng/kg/min. Each rate was given for 1 h, plasma angiotensin II concentration before and during infusion on abscissa. Normal subjects, Conn's syndrome, and essential hypertension (EHt) shown as groups with mean values ± 1 SEM. Patients with nontumorous hyperaldosteronism (NTH) are shown individually.

ments of plasma aldosterone related to concurrent plasma concentrations of angiotensin II before and during infusion. Figure 1 shows results in tumorous and nontumorous hyperaldosteronism, in essential hypertension, and in normal subjects. The aldosterone response in the nontumorous form is abnormally enhanced as it is in essential hypertension. In Conn's syndrome, it is subnormal.

It has long been recognized that Conn's syndrome can be separated easily from nontumorous hyperaldosteronism using biochemical, clinical, and statistical methods. The separation may have been easy because the diseases compared are fundamentally different. If nontumorous hyperaldosteronism is not a variant of Conn's syndrome, what is it? We suggest that it belongs to the disease,

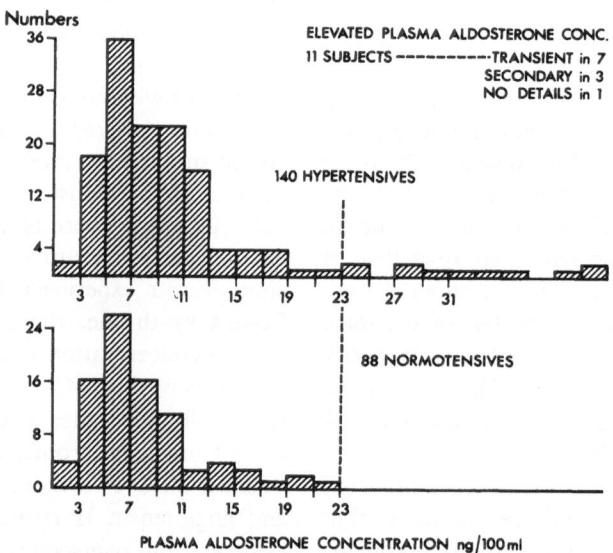

Fig. 2. Frequency distribution of plasma aldosterone measurements in 140 hypertensive and 88 age-matched normal subjects. Eleven hypertensives had aldosterone above the upper limit of normal.

or group of diseases, called essential hypertension and that aldosterone has a wider distribution in essential hypertension than it does in normal subjects, possibly because its response to stimuli such as angiotensin (Fig. 1 and refs. 8 and 9) and ACTH (10) is enhanced. Figure 2 shows data from an unselected population of hypertensive patients and their age-matched normal controls. The frequency distribution of plasma aldosterone is wider than normal in hypertensives, all of whom would otherwise be regarded as having essential hypertension.

Thus, high aldosterone may justify the name hyperaldosteronism, but the name does not *necessarily* justify the status of entity. It is hardly surprising that aldosterone is usually normal in essential hypertension if all cases with supranormal values are given a different name.

Table 1 shows the main features of essential hypertension, nontumorous hyperaldosteronism, and Conn's syndrome. It can be seen that in all respects essential hypertension and nontumorous hyperaldosteronism are similar, but both are different from Conn's syndrome. We have discussed this evidence in more detail elsewhere (4, 9). Baer and his colleagues (11) make the point that low-renin hypertension and nontumorous hyperaldosteronism are indistinguishable. This, coupled with evidence that low-renin hypertension and essential hypertension with normal renin are different aspects of the same disease rather than different diseases, makes the general point that all three conditions have been arbitrarily and wrongly separated from each other.

SUMMARY

Essential hypertension is particularly vulnerable to errors of classification because it is not an entity qualitatively different from normal. Its subdivision into low-renin hypertension and normal-renin hypertension is an artifact, in our view, as there is nothing to suggest that low-renin hypertension is qualitatively distinct.

It is customary to subdivide primary hyperaldosteronism into tumorous and nontumorous forms. The first, Conn's syndrome, is an entity with a distinct tumor. We suggest that the second represents the upper end of the range of aldosterone in essential hypertension and that it is wrongly classified as a variant of Conn's syndrome. Unlike Conn's syndrome, but like essential hypertension, it shows an abnormally increased response of aldosterone to infused angiotensin, near-normal exchangeable sodium and exchangeable potassium, and a decrease of renin with age. The nodular and hyperplastic changes seen in the adrenal cortex are quite distinct from the tumor of Conn's syndrome, but indistinguishable from the changes seen in essential hypertension.

REFERENCES

1. Pickering GW (1978) Normotension and hypertension: The mysterious viability of the false. Am J Med 65: 561–563
2. Padfield PL, Beevers DG, Brown JJ, Davies DL,

Table 1. Primary hyperaldosteronism.

Feature	Conn's syndrome	Nontumorous hyperaldosteronism	Essential hypertension	Source
Pathology	Tumor	Usually nodules	Often nodules	Dobbie (1969) J Pathol 99: 1 Grim (1974) J Clin Endocrinol Metab 39: 247 Neville (1978) Invest Cell Pathol 1: 99
Exchangeable Na	↑	Insignificantly different from normal (N)	N	Davies et al. (1979) J Endocrinol 81: 79P–91P
Exchangeable K	↓	N	N	Davies et al. (1979) Clin Sci 57: 69S–75S
Response of aldosterone to angiotensin II	↓	↑	↑	Wisgerhof, Brown (1978) J Clin Invest 61: 1456 Fig. 2 (this paper)

Lever AF, Robertson JIS, Schalekamp MAD, Tree M (1975) Is low-renin hypertension a stage in the development of essential hypertension or a diagnostic entity? Lancer 1: 548–564

3. Kaplan NM, Lieberman E (1978) Clinical hypertension. Williams & Wilkins, Baltimore, Md

4. Davies DL, Beevers DG, Brown JJ, Cumming AMM, Fraser R, Lever AF, Mason PA, Morton JJ, Padfield PL, Robertson JIS, Titterington M, Tree M (1979) Aldosterone and its stimuli in normal and hypertensive man: Are essential hypertension and primary hyperaldosteronism without tumour different parts of the same condition? J Endocrinol 81: 79P–91P

5. Liddle GW (1967) Secondary aldosteronism and reduced plasma renin in hypertensive disease. Trans Assoc Am Physicians 80: 168–182

6. Baer L, Sommers SC, Krakoff LR, Newton MA, Laragh JH (1970) Pseudo-primary aldosteronism: An entity distinct from true primary hyperaldosteronism. Circ Res 27 (Suppl I): 203–216

7. Davies DL, McElroy K, Atkinson AB, Brown JJ, Cumming AMM, Fraser R, Leckie BJ, Lever AF, Mackay A, Morton JJ, Robertson JIS (1979) Relationship in different forms of hypertension in man. Clin Sci 57: 69S–75S

8. Wisgerhof M, Brown RD (1978) Increased adrenal sensitivity to angiotensin II in low renin essential hypertension. J Clin Invest 61: 1456–1462

9. Mason PA, Beevers DG, Beretta-Piccoli C, Brown JJ, Cumming AMM, Davies DL, Fraser R, Lever AF, Morton JJ, Padfield PL, Young J (1981) Mill's disease amongst hypertension research workers. In: Sambhi M (ed) The fundamental fault in hypertension. Elsevier, Amsterdam

10. Honda M, Nowaczynski W, Guthrie GP, Messeri FN, Tolis G, Kuchel O, Genest J (1977) Response of several adrenal steroids to ACTH stimulation in essential hypertension. J Clin Endocrinol Metab 44: 264–272

11. Baer L, Brunner HR, Buhler F, Laragh JH (1972) Pseudoprimary aldosteronism, a variant of low renin essential hypertension. In: Genest J, Koiw E (eds) Hypertension 72. Springer, Berlin, pp 459–472

Low-Renin Essential Hypertension: Diminution of Aldosterone Suppression?

Thomas A. Wilson and Robert M. Carey

Renin profiling of hypertensive patients has led to the identification of a subgroup of patients with low-basal plasma renin activity (PRA) that does not increase in response to various maneuvers known to stimulate PRA in normal individuals. A small percentage of these individuals subsequently is found to have primary aldosteronism or glucocorticoid-suppressible hypertension, but the majority have normal plasma aldosterone concentrations. Despite differences in the methods of ascertainment of PRA and the stimuli applied to induce renin release, as well as difficulties in obtaining controls that are appropriately matched for age, sex, and race (1, 2), most investigators have identified suppressed PRA in 17%–46% of patients with essential hypertension (3). Yet, despite its prevalence, the pathophysiology of low-renin essential hypertension (LREH) remains obscure. In this paper, we will attempt to summarize what is known about LREH, particularly with respect to adrenal function, and propose a hypothesis of the pathophysiology involved.

It is likely that patients with LREH represent a heterogeneous group as a number of different mechanisms could result in suppressed PRA and hypertension (1, 3). Research directed at the etiology of LREH has focused on four main postulates: a) that mechanisms of renin release are defective; b) that expanded extracellular fluid volume (ECFV) results in hypertension and suppressed PRA; c) that mineralocorticoids other than aldosterone are responsible for sodium retention and the expanded ECFV; and d) that control mechanisms of aldosterone secretion are altered.

By definition, PRA in patients with LREH increases insignificantly in response to upright posture, sodium depletion, and furosemide administration with or without sodium depletion (4–7). Such a blunted response is more likely to occur in older individuals, blacks, women, and

diabetics (1, 7). It has been argued that this blunted response represents one end of the normal spectrum in the hypertensive population rather than a separate clinical entity (8). A constellation of other abnormal responses, however, suggests that LREH has a separate pathophysiology and may, therefore, represent a distinct clinical entity or group of entities.

Although basal levels of plasma catecholamines appear to be normal in patients with LREH, the expected rise in plasma norepinephrine in response to upright posture may be blunted (9). PRA and cyclic AMP responses to insulin-induced hypoglycemia are also reduced (10). Both observations suggest a defect in catecholamine release. However, PRA responses to infused norepinephrine, isoprenaline, and theophylline are reduced as well (9, 11). Furthermore, following diuretic therapy, PRA does eventually increase in patients with LREH (12, 13). These observations suggest that defects in catecholamine and PRA release may be secondary to other factors rather than primarily due to a defect in function of the juxtaglomerular apparatus, as has been suggested (14).

Based on the theory that an expanded ECFV would result in hypertension and suppressed PRA, various groups have examined sodium and fluid homeostasis in LREH. Provocative, but often conflicting, data have evolved. Woods et al. (15) found increased exchangeable sodium in patients with LREH when compared to patients with normal-renin essential hypertension, but not when compared to normotensive controls. Julius and Esler (16) described an increased central blood volume in patients with LREH on an uncontrolled diet, although total blood volume was normal. Others, however, have found no evidence of an expanded ECFV, plasma volume, or increased exchangeable sodium in LREH (17, 18). Such conflicting evidence may reflect the limitations in techniques used to measure sodium and fluid homeostasis directly. Indirect evidence, however, supports the concept that patients with LREH have an expanded ECFV. When sodium loaded, patients with LREH demonstrate enhanced natriuresis, similar to patients with primary aldosteronism who are volume expanded (19, 20). In addition, there is general agreement that, when compared to hypertensive patients with normal or high PRA, patients with LREH demonstrate a significantly greater fall in blood pressure in response to diuretic therapy, suggesting that an expanded fluid volume plays an integral role in maintaining the hypertensive state (4, 6, 13, 21).

Considerable attention, therefore, has been focused on the role of adrenal mineralocorticoids other than aldosterone in LREH. Evidence for and against increased mineralocorticoid activity has been summarized elsewhere (3). Again, there is little consensus in the findings with investigators having described increased excretion or plasma concentrations of DOC, 18-hydroxy-DOC, 16α,18-dihydroxy-DOC, DHEAS, and 16β-hydroxy-DHEA (3), while others have refuted these findings (3, 22–24). Utilizing a rat kidney radioreceptor assay, Baxter et al. (25) have reported no evidence for increased mineralocorticoid activity in plasma from patients with LREH. The general absence of hypokalemia in these patients supports this contention.

Despite the conflicting data on mineralocorticoid activity in LREH, the following lines of evidence suggest that abnormalities of adrenal function are at least in part responsible for maintenance of the hypertensive state:

1) Inhibition of adrenal steroidogenesis with aminoglutethimide or WIN 24,540 consistently reduces blood pressure in patients with LREH when compared to hypertensive patients with normal or high PRA (15, 24, 26). Although metyrapone does not have such an effect (26), one might not expect it to reduce blood pressure due to the accumulation of DOC, a potent mineralocorticoid in its own right.

2) Treatment with spironolactone results in a pronounced fall in blood pressure, whereas triamterene, a potassium-sparing diuretic that does not antagonize aldosterone, does not (12).

3) Patients with LREH demonstrate an enhanced aldosterone response to angiotensin II (12,

27, 28), while the pressor response does not differ from that of normal individuals (29).

4) When closely scrutinized by adrenal scintigraphy, selective adrenal vein sampling for aldosterone, and/or surgery, a high proportion of patients with LREH are found to have hyperplasia or adenomatous hyperplasia of the zona glomerulosa (30–32). Indeed, it has been suggested that LREH is simply an early or mild form of primary aldosteronism (33).

A consistent finding in the majority of patients with LREH is that plasma aldosterone concentrations and excretion rates are normal in the face of suppressed PRA and angiotensin II levels (5, 12, 24, 34, 35). This finding suggests either that aldosterone secretion is autonomous or that control mechanisms other than the renin–angiotensin system are responsible for maintaining aldosterone secretion. Other known stimuli for aldosterone secretion are ACTH and potassium. Serotonin has also been demonstrated to stimulate aldosterone secretion in vivo (36) and directly in vitro (37). There is, however, no evidence for excessive ACTH secretion in LREH, as 17-hydroxycorticosteroid excretion is normal (4) and dexamethasone administration does not reduce the blood pressure in most patients (38). Likewise, although a few patients with LREH have hypokalemia (39), most are normokalemic, and none are hyperkalemic. Therefore, neither ACTH nor potassium appear to play a major role in maintaining aldosterone secretion in LREH. Recently, cyproheptadine, a serotonin and histamine antagonist, has been shown to diminish plasma concentration of aldosterone in patients with bilateral hyperplasia of the zona glomerulosa (40). What role serotonin may have in maintaining aldosterone concentrations in the presence of suppressed PRA in patients with LREH is unknown.

An alternative possibility is that a normal inhibitor of aldosterone secretion is deficient. Recent data from this laboratory suggest that in normal subjects in a sodium-replete state, aldosterone secretion may be under "tonic" dopaminergic inhibition. Following the administration of metoclopramide, a dopamine antagonist, plasma aldosterone concentration increases in the absence of any alterations in PRA, cortisol, or potassium. Aldosterone responses to angiotensin II remain intact, although at a higher level (41). Conversely,

McKenna et al. (42) have shown that in a bovine adrenal cell suspension, aldosterone responses to angiotensin II are diminished in the presence of dopamine. We speculate that if dopaminergic activity were deficient, aldosterone secretion might occur at an inappropriately high level relative to the suppressed PRA—analogous to the situation in LREH. Inappropriately elevated aldosterone might result in sodium retention and increased intravascular volume, causing increased blood pressure and suppression of renin secretion (Fig. 1). Diminished dopaminergic inhibition might also explain the enhanced aldosterone responses described in patients with LREH when infused with angiotensin II (12, 27, 28). However, it must be stressed that the potential physiologic role of dopaminergic mechanisms in the control of aldosterone secretion remains to be elucidated through future investigations.

Dopamine may have a physiologic role in regulating sodium homeostasis by direct effects on the kidney, as well as indirectly through its effects on aldosterone secretion. It is known that infusions of dopamine induce natriuresis (43). Conversely, in normal subjects, plasma dopamine concentrations fall in response to sodium depletion (44), and dopamine excretion falls in response to upright posture (45). Both sodium depletion and upright posture induce sodium retention. What role diminished dopaminergic activity may have in reducing sodium excretion in response to these stimuli is unknown. One might speculate, however, that if dopaminergic activity were diminished in the kidney, sodium retention might ensue. Thus, if the pathophysiology of LREH involves decreased dopaminergic activity, sodium retention might occur both by direct effects on the kidney as well as indirectly via increased aldosterone secretion (Fig.

1). Both mechanisms would serve to increase intravascular volume and blood pressure.

Dopamine modulates sympathetic tone as well. Dopamine acts peripherally at presynaptic receptors to inhibit release of neurotransmitters from sympathetic nerve terminals (46), and bromocriptine, a dopamine agonist active in the central nervous system, reduces CSF and plasma concentrations of norepinephrine (47, 48). Were dopaminergic tone generally diminished, an increase in peripheral sympathetic tone might be expected. On the contrary, normal or diminished plasma concentrations of norepinephrine and epinephrine have been described in patients with LREH (5, 12, 49). There is evidence, however, that considerable heterogeneity of dopamine receptors exists among different organ systems, particularly between vascular and CNS receptors (46). Recent data from this laboratory demonstrate that while bromocriptine blocks the hyperprolactinemic response to metoclopramide in man, it does not affect the rise in plasma aldosterone concentrations. Dopamine, however, blocks both the pituitary and adrenal responses (50). Similarly, in the canine renal artery, there is a dissociation between the effects of dopamine itself and various agents that are known to serve as dopamine agonists in the central nervous system (51). Thus, a defect in dopaminergic mechanisms peculiar to the adrenal and/or kidney might have profound effects on regulation of blood pressure without necessarily altering sympathetic tone or pituitary prolactin release.

SUMMARY

Although the pathophysiology of LREH is not known, indirect evidence suggests that the hyper-

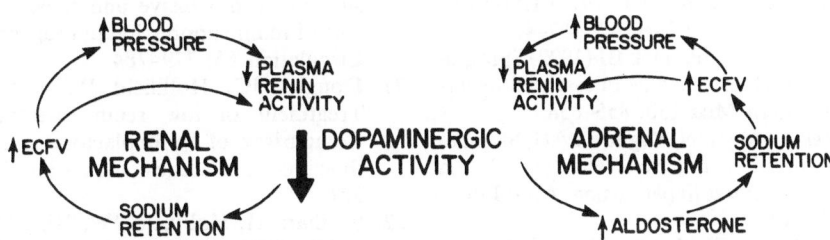

Fig. 1. Possible renal and adrenal mechanisms by which decreased dopaminergic activity could lead to expansion of the ECFV and hypertension with suppressed PRA.

tensive state may be mediated by a mineralocorticoid-induced hypervolemia. Attempts to identify a responsible mineralocorticoid, however, have not yielded consistent results. Aldosterone itself may be implicated since plasma aldosterone concentrations are not reduced as would otherwise be expected in the presence of ECFV expansion. Since plasma concentrations of aldosterone are maintained in the normal range despite the presence of suppressed PRA, mechanisms controlling aldosterone release other than the renin–angiotensin system may be involved. Recent studies suggest that dopamine may be an inhibitor of aldosterone secretion. We speculate that diminished dopaminergic activity at the level of the adrenal cortex and the kidney may be a mechanism that contributes to the pathogenesis of LREH in some patients.

ACKNOWLEDGMENTS

This work was supported by the Hypertension Research Training Grant IT32HL–07355 from the National Institutes of Health. R. M. Carey is an Established Investigator of the American Heart Association.

REFERENCES

1. Dunn MH, Tannen RL (1974) Low renin hypertension. Kidney Int 5: 317–325
2. Noth RH (1978) Interpretation of plasma renin activity. Arch Intern Med 138: 528–529
3. Kaplan NM (1978) Clinical hypertension. Williams & Wilkins, Baltimore, Md, pp 287–304
4. Carey RM, Douglas JG, Schweikert JR, Liddle GW (1972) The syndrome of essential hypertension and suppressed plasma renin activity: Normalization of blood pressure with spironolactone. Arch Intern Med 130: 849–854
5. Crane MG, Harris JJ, Johns VJ (1972) Hyporeninemic hypertension. Am J Med 52: 457–466
6. Adlin EV, Marks AD, Channick BJ (1972) Spironolactone and hydrochlorothiazide in essential hypertension. Arch Intern Med 130: 855–858
7. McDonald RH, Corder CN, Vagnucci AH, Shuman J (1978) The multiple functions affecting plasma renin activity in essential hypertension. Arch Intern Med 138: 557–561
8. Padfield PL, Brown JJ, Lever AF, Schalekamp MAD, Beevers DG, Davies DL, Robertson JIS, Tree M, Titterington M (1975) Is low renin hypertension a stage in the development of essential hypertension of a diagnostic entity? Lancet 1: 548–550
9. Esler M, Zweifler A, Randall O, Julius S, DeQuattro V (1978) The determinants of plasma renin activity in essential hypertension. Ann Intern Med 88: 746–752
10. Lowder SC, Humet P, Liddle GW (1976) Contrasting effects of hypoglycemia on plasma renin activity and cyclic adenosine 3'5' monophosphate (cyclic AMP) in essential hypertension. Circ Res 38: 105–108
11. Jose A, Crout JR, Kaplan NM (1970) Suppressed plasma renin activity in essential hypertension: Roles of plasma volume, blood pressure, and sympathetic nervous system. Ann Intern Med 72: 9–16
12. Mitchell JR, Taylor AH, Pool JL, Lake CR, Rollins DE, Bartter FC (1977) Renin-aldosterone profiling in hypertension. Ann Intern Med 87: 596
13. Vaughan ED, Laragh JH, Gavras I, Bühler FR, Gavras H, Brunner HR, Baer L (1974) The volume factor in low and normal renin essential hypertension: Its treatment with either spironolactone or chlorthalidone. In: Laragh JH (ed) Hypertension manual. Yorke Medical Group, New York, pp 851–871
14. Swales JO (1975) Low renin hypertension: Nephrosclerosis? Lancet 1: 75–77
15. Woods JW, Liddle GW, Stant EG, Michelakis AM, Brill AB (1969) Effect of an adrenal inhibitor in hypertensive patients with suppressed renin. Arch Intern Med 123: 366–370
16. Julius S, Esler M (1976) Increased central blood volume: A possible pathological factor in mild low-renin essential hypertension. Clin Sci Mol Med 51: 207S–210S
17. Lebel S, Schalekamp MA, Beevers DG, Brown JJ, Davies DL, Fraser R, Kremer D, Lever AF, Morton JJ, Robertson JIS, Tree M, Wilson A (1974) Sodium and renin-angiotensin system in essential hypertension and mineralocorticoid excess. Lancet 2: 308–310
18. Schalekamp MA, Lebel M, Beevers DG, Fraser R, Kolsters G, Birkenhäger WH (1974) Body fluid volume in low renin hypertension. Lancet 2: 310–311
19. Krakoff LR, Goodwin FJ, Baer L, Torres M, Laragh JH (1970) The role of renin in the exaggerated natriuresis of hypertension. Circulation 42: 335–345
20. Luft FC, Grim CE, Willis LR, Higgins JT, Weinberger MH (1977) Natriuretic response to saline infusion in normotensive and hypertensive man: The role of renin suppression in exaggerated natriuresis. Circulation 55: 779–784
21. Douglas JG, Hollifield JW, Liddle GW (1974) Treatment of low renin essential hypertension: Comparison of spironolactone and a hydrochlorothiazide-triamterene combination. JAMA 227: 518–521
22. Sekihara H, Hollifield JW, Island DP, Slaton PE, Liddle GW (1979) Evidence for heterogeneity of mineralocorticoids in urine of patients with low renin essential hypertension. J Clin Endocrinol Metab 48: 143–147

23. Tan SY, Mulrow PJ (1979) Low renin essential hypertension: Failure to demonstrate excess 11-deoxycorticosterone production. J Clin Endocrinol Metab 49: 790–793

24. Taylor AA, Mitchell JR, Bartter FC, Snodgrass WR, McMurty RJ, Gill JR, Franklin RB (1978) Effect of aminoglutethimide on blood pressure and steroid secretion in patients with low renin essential hypertension. J Clin Invest 62: 162–168

25. Baxter JD, Schambelan M, Matulich DT, Spinder BJ, Taylor AA, Bartter FC (1976) Aldosterone receptors and the evaluation of plasma mineralocorticoid activity in normal and hypertensive states. J Clin Invest 58: 579–589

26. Liddle GW, Hollifield JW, Slaton RE, Wilson HM (1976) Effects of various adrenal inhibitors in low renin essential hypertension. J Steroid Biochem 7: 937–940

27. Wisgerhof M, Brown RD (1978) Increased adrenal sensitivity to angiotensin II in low-renin essential hypertension. J Clin Invest 61: 1456–1462

28. Marks AD, Marks DB, Kanefsky TM, Adlin VE, Channick BJ (1979) Enhanced adrenal responsiveness to angiotensin II in patients with low renin essential hypertension. J Clin Endocrinol Metab 48: 266–270

29. Marks AD, Marks DB, Kim YM, Moctezuma J, Adlin EV, Channick BJ (1978) The pressor responses to angiotensin II in patients with low renin essential hypertension. Circ Res 42: 864–869

30. Rifai A, Beierwaltes WH, Freitas JE, Grekin R (1978) Adrenal scintigraphy in low renin essential hypertension. Clin Nucl Med 3: 282–286

31. Gunnells JC, McGuffin WL, Robinson RR, Grim CE, Wells S, Silver D, Glenn JF (1970) Hypertension, adrenal abnormalities and alterations in plasma renin activity. Ann Intern Med 73: 901–911

32. Grim CE, Esterly JA, Lungo DL, Keitzer WF (1974) "Inappropriate" production of aldosterone associated with adrenal hyperplasia (abstr). Endocrinology 94(Suppl): A243

33. Grim CE (1975) Low renin "essential" hypertension: A variant of classic aldosteronism? Arch Intern Med 135: 347–350

34. Genest J, Nowaczynski W, Kuchel O, Messerli F, Boucher R, Rojo-Ortega M (1975) Mineralocorticoid activity in patients in the early benign phase of essential hypertension. J Steroid Biochem 6: 755–760

35. Beevers DG, Morton JJ, Nelson CS, Padfield PL, Tittenington M, Tree M (1977) Angiotensin II in essential hypertension. Br Med J 1: 415

36. Mantero F, Opocher G, Armanini D, Boscaro M, Edwards CRW (1979) Effect of serotonin (5-HT) on plasma aldosterone in man (abstr). Acta Endocrinol [Suppl] (Copenh) 225S: 345

37. Haning R, Tait SAS, Tait JF (1970) In vitro effects of ACTH, angiotensins, serotonin and potassium on steroid output and conversion of corticosterone to aldosterone by isolated adrenal cells. Endocrinology 87: 1147–1167

38. Liddle GW (1975) Is hypertension essential? Trans Assoc Am Physicians 88: 55–69

39. Collins RD, Weinberger MH, Dowdy AJ, Nokes GW, Gonzales CM, Luetscher JA (1970) Abnormally sustained aldosterone secretion during salt loading in patients with various forms of benign hypertension: Relation to plasma renin activity. J Clin Invest 49: 1415–1426

40. Gross MD, Gniadek TC, Grekin RJ (1980) Inhibition of aldosterone secretion by cyproheptadine in primary aldosteronism due to bilateral hyperplasia. Clin Res 28: 260A

41. Carey RM, Thorner MO, Ortt EM (1979) Effects of metoclopramide and bromocriptine on the renin-angiotensin-aldosterone system in man: Dopaminergic control of aldosterone. J Clin Invest 63: 727–735

42. McKenna TJ, Island DP, Nicholson WE, Liddle GW (1979) Dopamine inhibits angiotensin-stimulated aldosterone biosynthesis in bovine adrenal cells. J Clin Invest 64: 787–791

43. Goldberg LI (1972) Cardiovascular and renal actions of dopamine: Potential clinical applications. Pharmacol Rev 24: 1–27

44. Carey RM, VanLoon GR, Baines AD, Ortt EM (submitted) Plasma and urinary dopamine during dietary sodium depletion in man: Evidence for decreased dopaminergic activity

45. Cuche JC, Kuchel O, Barbeau A, Boucher R, Genest J (1972) Relationship between the adrenergic nervous system and renin during adaptation to upright posture: A possible role for 3,4 dihydroxyphenylethylamine (dopamine). Clin Sci 43: 481–491

46. Goldberg LI, Volkman PH, Kohli JD (1978) A comparison of the vascular dopamine receptor with other dopamine receptors. Annu Rev Pharmacol Toxicol 18: 57–79

47. Ziegler MG, Lake CR, Williams AC, Teychenne PF, Shoulson I, Steinsland O (1979) Bromocriptine inhibits norepinephrine release. Clin Pharmacol Ther 25: 137–142

48. Kollock R, Kobayashi K, DeQuattro V (1981) Evidence in primary hypertension. Hypertension (in press)

49. Esler M, Zweifler A, Randall O, Julius S, Bennett J, Rydelek P, Cohen E, DeQuattro V (1976) Suppression of sympathetic nervous functions in low-renin essential hypertension. Lancet 2: 115–118

50. Carey RM, Thorner MO, Orth EM (1981) Dopaminergic inhibition of metoclopramide-induced aldosterone secretion in man: Dissociation of responses to dopamine and bromocriptine. J Clin Invest (in press)

51. Volkman PH, Goldberg LI (1976) Lack of correlation between inhibition of prolactin release and stimulation of dopaminergic renal vasodilation. Pharm 18: 130

Identifying Renin Participation in Hypertensive Patients

David H. P. Streeten, Gunnar H. Anderson, Jr., Frederick S. Sunderlin, Jr., Joseph S. Mallov, and Jay Springer

Theoretically, it might be possible to determine whether or not excessive renin activity is involved in the pathogenesis of human hypertension by ascertaining whether a) plasma renin activity (PRA) is elevated or b) inhibition of renin release or angiotensin II (AII) formation or antagonism of the action of AII overcomes the hypertension. The reliability of these procedures will be briefly examined in the purest clinical form of angiotensin-mediated hypertension, viz., that resulting from renovascular stenosis.

MEASUREMENTS OF PRA

Interpretation of the normality of PRA is fraught with many difficulties, since PRA is influenced by age, sex, Na balance, K balance, posture, and time of day, as well as by the activity of various hormones including estrogens, glucocorticoids, catecholamines, and probably others. Extremely high levels of PRA are often seen in patients who are normotensive or who have hypertension that is not caused by the elevations of PRA, while "normal" levels of PRA may be inappropriate to the state of volume expansion in some patients and may thus cause hypertension through excessive action of AII. It is not surprising to find from an analysis of the literature, therefore, that in patients with renovascular stenosis whose hypertension has been shown subsequently to be overcome by surgical correction of the renal ischemia, PRA levels has been "elevated" in only 35%–72% (mean 63%) of patients (Table 1) (1–18). There is, thus, overwhelming evidence that even when renal vein renin ratios and surgical correctibility of the hypertension strongly imply renin-induced hypertension, peripheral PRA levels are reliable markers of this type of hypertension in only about

two-thirds of the patients. There is no reason to believe that in other, less obviously renin-dependent, types of hypertension, peripheral PRA measurements would be any more reliable.

INHIBITION OF RENIN RELEASE OR OF A II FORMATION OR ACTIVITY

Beta-blocking drugs undoubtedly lower PRA and plasma AII concentrations. It is reasonable to believe that beta-blockers lower BP by this mechanism in patients whose hypertension results from excessive AII activity. However, these drugs may also lower BP by mechanisms entirely distinct from their renin-lowering effects. For this reason, it is not valid to conclude that the hypotensive action of beta-blockers in patients necessarily indicates angiotensin dependency of the patients' hypertension. Similarly, inhibitors of angiotensin-converting enzyme, such as captopril, are known to be capable of lowering BP not only by lowering plasma AII concentrations, but also by raising plasma bradykinin levels and probably by other mechanisms, even in nephrectomized patients (19). Their hypotensive actions, therefore, cannot necessarily be taken to indicate angiotensin dependency. On the other hand, although the agonistic action of such AII antagonists as saralasin may limit the depressor effects of this drug, there is no known mechanism, other than antagonism of endogenous AII, whereby saralasin can lower BP. For this reason, one would expect, *a priori*, that the extent to which saralasin lowered BP would accurately reflect the extent of AII dependency of the hypertension under the conditions prevailing at the time of such observations. Evidence from the literature supports this conclusion, since patients with renovascular hypertension, whose hypertension has

Table 1. Renovascular hypertension "cured" by surgery:* Percentages of positive tests reported in literature.

Authors	IVP	Peripheral PRA	Saralasin test
Gunnells (1)		69	
Hussain (2)		35	
Tucker (3)		67	
Vaughan (4)		72	
Stockigt (5)	81	67	
Bianchi (6)		55	
Marks (7)		70	94
Grim (8)	78	66	52
Poutasse (9)		63	81
Kaufman (10)	70	61	91
Streeten (11)		68	
Baer (12)			100
Wilson (13)			88
Lifschitz (14)			100
Krakoff (15)	80		75
Streeten (16)			88
Maxwell (17)	83		
Foster (18)	69		
Mean(%)	76.9	63.0	85.6

* Cured signifies a fall in diastolic BP to below 90 mmHg, without medical treatment, after surgical correction of the renovascular stenosis.

been corrected by surgery, showed a preoperative saralasin-induced fall in BP greater than that seen in similarly treated normotensive subjects in 52%–100% (mean 85.6%) of the patients (Table 1).

Although one group (8) has reported that an abnormal rapid-sequence intravenous urogram (IVP) was more effective than a positive saralasin test in screening for renovascular hypertension, the evidence from most authors (Table 1) shows that the IVP is abnormal in only 69%–83% (mean 76.9%) of such patients.

Our own recent data are in substantial agreement with the above results from the literature. In 2,000-referred hypertensive patients, 30 are known to have become normotensive after surgery for unilateral renin-producing renal lesions. Among these 30 patients, peripheral PRA was elevated in 70%, the rapid-sequence IVP was abnormal in 83%, and the saralasin test was positive in 90% (Fig. 1). The renin status in 125 of the same series of patients whose abnormal IVP was associated with a negative saralasin test has been analyzed. In these 125 patients, the prevalences of high (6%), normal (65%), and low (29%) peripheral PRA levels were very similar to the corre-

sponding prevalences (11%, 59%, and 30%, respectively) in 900 hypertensives who did not undergo pyelography and in whom angiotensin dependency was unlikely because of negative saralasin tests and, frequently, normal renin vein renin ratios (16). Thus, the abnormal IVP alone did not appear to increase the yield of angiotensinogenic hypertensives when the saralasin test was negative in these hypertensive patients.

Saralasin testing is, thus, apparently the most reliable method of screening for renovascular hypertension. It is also highly effective—and better than peripheral PRA levels or the IVP—in finding types of angiotensinogenic hypertension other than renovascular hypertension. In our experience, these types include renal parenchymal diseases, hydronephrosis, and Cushing's syndrome (16), as well as terminal renal failure, malignant hypertension, aortic coarctation, segmental renal infarction, traumatic perinephric hemorrhage, renal tumors, and congenital renal disorders of some types. In almost all of these instances where the lesion was

Observations in 30 Surgically "Cured" Patients with Renovascular Hypertension

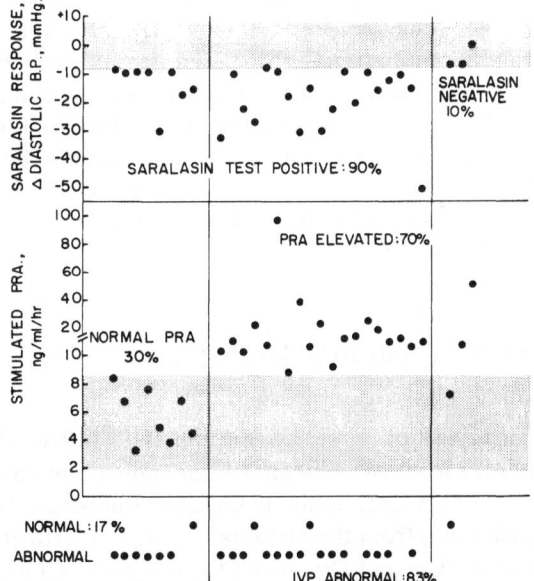

Fig. 1. Results of saralasin test, peripheral PRA, and rapid-sequence IVP in 30 patients with unilateral renal arterial stenosis associated with hypertension, renal vein PRA ratios >1.5, and a fall in BP after subsequent surgery to normal (diastolic <90 mmHg) without medications. The shaded areas depict the normal ranges of saralasin responses and PRA levels after intravenous furosemide and standing 2 h.

unilateral, elevated renal vein renin ratios supported the implication that hypertension was renin dependent. Although false negative results of saralasin tests undoubtedly do occur in these patients with an estimated frequency of approximately 12% (16), the evidence generally indicates that the saralasin test is the best method of identifying renin participation in the pathogenesis of human hypertension.

SUMMARY

The reliability of peripheral PRA, IVP, and the hypotensive response to saralasin administration has been compared in patients with renal arterial stenosis whose blood pressure subsequently fell to normal without the need for medications after surgical correction of the responsible lesion. In several series of such patients described in the literature (a) and in 30 patients of our own (b), the percentages of positive results of these tests were—peripheral PRA: (a) 63%, (b) 70%; IVP: (a) 77%, (b) 83%; and saralasin test: (a) 86%, (b) 90%. In this relatively "pure" type, and probably in other types, of angiotensin-dependent hypertension (segmental renal arterial obstruction, renal parenchymal disorders, aortic coarctation, Cushing's syndrome, etc.), a positive (i.e., depressor) response to saralasin administration under standardized conditions appears at present to be the most effective method of identifying renin participation in hypertension.

ACKNOWLEDGMENTS

Supported by Research Grants (HL 14076, HL 19428) from the National Heart and Lung Institute, a Graduate Training Grant in Endocrinology (AM7146) from the National Institue of Arthritis, Metabolism and Digestive Diseases, and a Clinical Research Center Grant (RR229) from the Division of Research Facilities and Resources, USPHS.

REFERENCES

1. Gunnells JC, McGuffin WL, Johnsrude I, Robinson RR (1969) Peripheral and renal venous plasma renin activity in hypertension. Ann Intern Med 71: 555–575
2. Hussain RA, Gifford RW, Stewart BH, Meaney TF, McCormick LJ, Vidt DG, Humphrey DC (1973) Differential renal venous renin activity in diagnosis of renovascular hypertension. Am J Cardiol 32: 707–715
3. Tucker RM, Strong CG, Brennan LA, Sheps SG, Brown RD, Weinshilboum RM (1978) Renovascular hypertension: Relationship of surgical curability to renin-angiotensin activity. Mayo Clin Proc 53: 373–377
4. Vaughan ED, Bühler FR, Laragh JH, Sealey JE, Baer L, Bard RH (1973) Renovascular hypertension: Renin measurements to indicate hypersecretion and contralateral suppression, estimate renal plasma flow, and score for surgical curability. Am J Med 55: 402–414
5. Stockigt JR, Collins RD, Noakes CA, Schambelan M, Biglieri EG (1972) Renal-vein renin in various forms of renal hypertension. Lancet 1: 1194–1198
6. Bianchi G, Campolo L, Vegeto A, Pietra V, Piazza U (1970) The value of plasma renin concentration per se, and in relation to plasma and extracellular fluid volume in diagnosis and prognosis of human renovascular hypertension. Clin Sci 39: 559–576
7. Marks LS, Maxwell MH, Kaufman JJ (1977) Renin, sodium, and vasodepressor response to saralasin in renovascular and essential hypertension. Ann Intern Med 87: 176–182
8. Grim CE, Luft FC, Weinberger MH, Grim CM (1979) Sensitivity and specificity of screening tests for renal vascular hypertension. Ann Intern Med 91: 617–622
9. Poutasse EF, Gonzalez-Serva L, Wendelken JR, Franz JP (1980) Saralasin test as a diagnostic and prognostic aid in renovascular hypertensive patients subjected to renal operation. J Urol 123: 306–310
10. Kaufman JJ (1980) Editorial comment. J Urol 123: 310
11. Streeten DHP, Anderson GH Jr, Bredenberg CE, Randall P (1978) The diagnosis and treatment of renovascular hypertension. Clin Invest Med 1: 155–161
12. Baer L, Parra-Carrillo JZ, Radichevich I, Williams GS (1977) Detection of renovascular hypertension with angiotensin II blockade. Ann Intern Med 86: 257–260
13. Wilson HM, Wilson JP, Slaton PE, Foster JH, Liddle GW, Hollifield JW (1977) Saralasin infusion in the recognition of renovascular hypertension. Ann Intern Med 87: 36–42
14. Lifschitz MD, Kirschenbaum MA, Rosenblatt SG, Gibney R (1978) Effect of saralasin in hypertension patients on chronic hemodialysis. Ann Intern Med 88: 23–27
15. Krakoff LR, Ribeiro AB, Gorkin JN, Felton KR (1980) Saralasin infusion in screening patients for renovascular hypertension. Am J Cardiol 45: 609–613
16. Streeten DHP, Anderson GH Jr (1979) Outpatient experience with saralasin. Kidney Int 15: S-44–S-52

17. Maxwell MH, Bleifer KH, Franklin SS, Varady PD (1972) Cooperative study of renovascular hypertension: Demographic analysis of the study. JAMA 220: 1195–1204

18. Foster JH, Oates JA (1975) Recognition and management of renovascular hypertension. Hosp Pract 61–70

19. Man in 't Veld A, Schicht IM, Derkx FHM, de Bruyn JHB, Schalekamp MADH (1980) Effects of an angiotensin-converting enzyme inhibitor (captopril) on blood pressure in anephric subjects. Br Med J, 1: 288–290

Renin–Angiotensin–Aldosterone System in the Maintenance of Blood Pressure

G. A. MacGregor, N. D. Markandu, and J. E. Roulston

It is not clear how far the renin–angiotensin–aldosterone system maintains blood pressure in normotensive subjects on a "normal" sodium intake (1) (see also Niarchos and Pickering, p 567). There is, therefore, controversy over how important this system is in the maintenance of blood pressure in essential hypertension (2). All drugs that inhibit or block the renin–angiotensin system have other actions, making it difficult to draw conclusions from the use of only one of these agents. In this study, we have compared the effect on blood pressure in normotensive and hypertensive subjects of two inhibitors of the renin–angiotensin–aldosterone system, saralasin and captopril.

METHODS

Unselected patients with essential hypertension, whose diastolic pressure after a 1–2 month period of observation was between 100 and 120 mmHg, and normal male subjects, whose diastolic pressure was less than 80 mmHg after a 1–2 month observation period, were included in the study. All subjects gave their informed consent. The majority of patients had not had previous antihypertensive therapy. In those who had had previous therapy, this was stopped at least 1 month before if they were on a beta-adrenoreceptor blocker, and at least 3 months before if they were on a diuretic. Patients were excluded if they were taking any other drug, including the oral contraceptive pill, or had evidence of renal failure, heart failure, or cerebrovascular disease. It was not possible to age or sex match the controls with the hypertensive subjects. The mean age of the controls was 22 years (range 21–26), all males. Mean age of the hypertensives was 47 years (range 21–63), approximately equal numbers of males and females. All blood pressures were measured by nurses using semiautomatic ultrasound sphygmomanometers (Ateriosonde 1217) (3). The mean value of five readings at 1–2-min intervals, supine, sitting, and standing, were taken as the blood pressure in that position. Blood pressure measurements were made at the same time of day, in the same room, by the same nurse. All studies were done as outpatients in both the normal and hypertensive subjects. Plasma renin activity was measured by radioimmunoassay (4). All measurements were made after the subject had been sitting upright for 10 min, between 10:00 A.M. and noon.

For studies with saralasin, patients and normal subjects ate either their usual diet or their usual diet with a supplement of 200 mEq sodium (given as 20 slow sodium (CIBA),) or a low-sodium diet (10mEq/day). Normal subjects on captopril were studied on sodium balance of 120 mEq sodium/day, (normal) 350 mEq/day, (high) or 10 mEq/day, (low). Patients who were studied with captopril ate their usual diet.

Saralasin was infused by using an incremental infusion: 0.05 μg/min/kg for 20 min, 0.25μg/min/kg for 20 min, and then 1.25 μg/min/kg for 20 min. Patients and normals were infused sitting upright with a one hour control period before, and after, infusion. Blood pressure was measured every 1–3 min on an Arteriosonde. The saralasin infusion was done either on the normal diet, after 5 days on a high-salt diet, or after 5 days of low-sodium diet. Percentage change in blood pressure was calculated from the change in mean blood pressure in the 20 min before infusion and the last 10 min at the highest rate of infusion.

Captopril (25 mg three times a day), was given to patients for 1 week, then increased to 50 mg T.I.D. in week 2, 100 mg T.I.D. in week 3, and in week 4 the dose was 150 mg three times a day.

If the supine diastolic pressure was less than 85 mmHg, the dose of captopril was not increased, but kept to the same amount for that week. All patients were studied on their normal diet as outpatients. It was not possible to treat the normals in the same way. They were given three doses of 25 mg for 1 day, increasing to three doses of 50 mg for day 2, 100 mg T.I.D. for the next 2 days, and a morning dose of 100 mg on day 5. There was a control period of a week before starting captopril in the normals, when they were on a fixed sodium intake of a normal-, high- or low-sodium diet, and a control period of a week after stopping captopril. The normal subjects pursued their usual activities throughout the study. Blood pressure change in the patients was calculated from the mean supine blood pressure on the day of starting treatment with captopril, and on week 4 of the treatment at the maximum dose. Blood pressure change in the normals was calculated from the mean supine blood pressure on the day of starting captopril and day 5 of treatment.

Percentage change in mean blood pressure was calculated from the change in mean blood pressure calculated as the diastolic plus one-third of the pulse pressure.

RESULTS

SARALASIN

Forty-four patients were studied on the low-sodium diet, four on their normal diet. There was a highly significant correlation in these patients between the logarithm of the plasma renin activity measured before infusion and the percentage change in mean sitting blood pressure with saralasin: $r = 0.88$, $p < 0.001$ (Fig. 1). Seventeen normals were studied, five on a high-sodium diet, one on a normal diet, and ten on a low-sodium diet. There was a highly significant correlation between the logarithm of the initial plasma renin activity and percentage change in mean sitting blood pressure with saralasin: $r = 0.85$, $p < 0.001$ (Fig. 1). There was no significant difference in the slope or elevation of the two regression lines (Fig. 1).

CAPTOPRIL

Captopril was given to 36 hypertensive subjects on their normal diet. There was a significant correlation between the logarithm of the initial plasma renin activity before treatment and the percentage

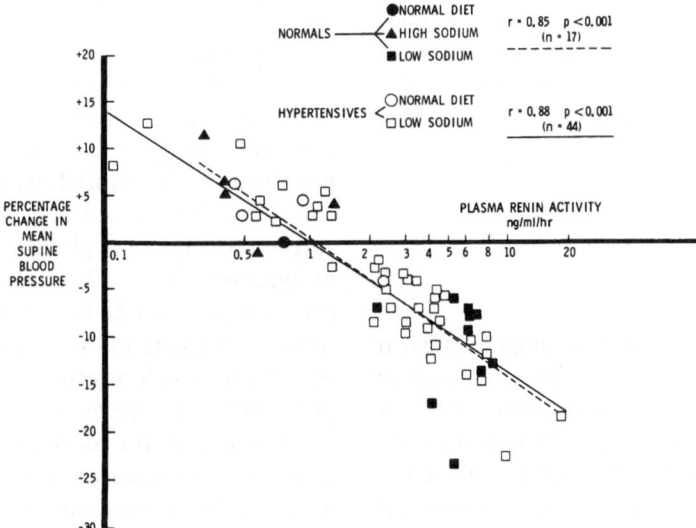

Fig. 1. Percentage change in mean sitting blood pressure with saralasin against log initial plasma renin activity.

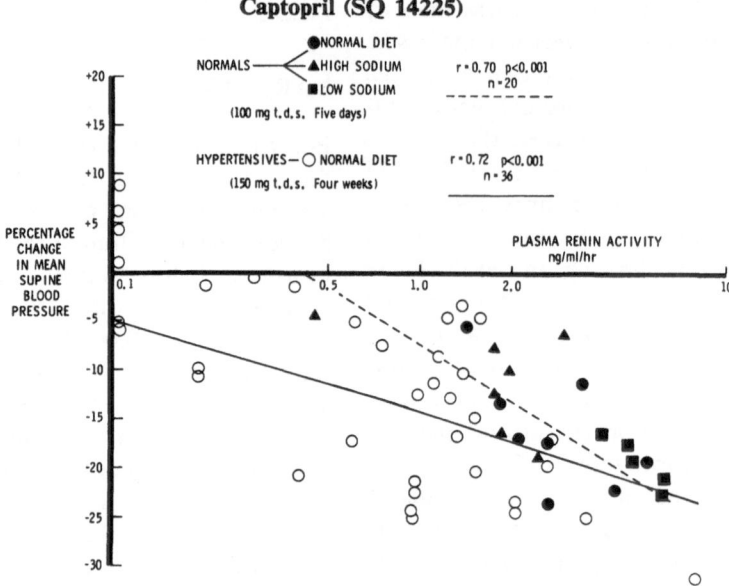

Fig. 2. Percentage change in mean supine blood pressure with captopril against log initial plasma renin activity.

change in mean supine blood pressure on week 4 of treatment: $r = 0.72$, $p < 0.001$ (Fig. 2). Twenty normals were studied with captopril given for 5 days, eight on their normal diet, seven on a high-sodium diet, and five on a low-sodium diet. There was a significant correlation between the logarithm of the initial plasma renin activity and percentage change in mean supine blood pressure ($r = 0.71$, $p < 0.001$) with captopril (Fig. 2). There was no significant difference between the regression lines, but the residual variance was such that they are not strictly comparable. This is due to the higher plasma renin activity in the normal subjects (Fig. 2).

DISCUSSION

Saralasin caused the same percentage change in blood pressure for a given plasma renin activity in the normotensive and hypertensive subjects. The results showed that when plasma renin activity was above 2–3 ng/ml/h, angiotensin II was maintaining blood pressure to some extent in both normotensive and hypertensive subjects. Saralasin, however, is a potent agonist (5–8) and, when given as a short-term infusion, blocks only the immediate effects of circulating angiotensin II. Both of these

factors will tend to underestimate the participation of the renin–angiotensin–aldosterone system in the control of blood pressure.

Captopril lowered blood pressure in normotensive subjects on all three sodium intakes. The percentage fall in blood pressure was similar to that seen in the patients with essential hypertension. Captopril is a potent inhibitor of angiotensin-converting enzyme, leading to a fall in circulating angiotensin II in hypertensive (9, 10) and normotensive subjects (11). As converting enzyme is also partially responsible for the breakdown of bradykinin, there could be an increase in bradykinin with captopril, but this has not been shown in patients with essential hypertension (12). Significant correlations between the fall in blood pressure and the fall in angiotensin II have been shown in hypertensive (9, 10) and normotensive subjects (11). Angiotensin II has other actions besides direct vasoconstriction of the arterioles, and these, plus the fall in aldosterone that occurs with captopril, could also have a blood pressure-lowering effect. If part of the mechanism whereby captopril lowers blood pressure is through the fall in angiotensin II that occurs, our results demonstrate that the renin–angiotensin system is a normal mechanism for the maintenance of blood pressure. The results with captopril and saralasin in the patients with essential hypertension demonstrate that the renin–angiotensin system plays no greater role in the maintenance of blood pressure in essential hypertension than it does in normotensive subjects for a given value of plasma renin activity.

SUMMARY

Saralasin and captopril changed blood pressure in normotensive as well as hypertensive subjects. The percentage change in blood pressure with these two drugs for a given plasma renin activity was similar in normotensive and hypertensive subjects. This suggests that when the renin–angiotensin system is maintaining blood pressure, it maintains the blood pressure to the same extent in percentage terms in normotensive and hypertensive subjects for a given plasma renin activity.

Saralasin has marked agonist activity, and underestimates the participation of the renin–angiotensin–aldosterone system in the maintenance of blood pressure. The fall in blood pressure that occurred with captopril in normal subjects on their normal-sodium intake suggests that the renin–angiotensin–aldosterone system maintains blood pressure in normal subjects on their normal-sodium intake. Our results suggest that the renin–angiotensin–aldosterone system plays no greater role in maintaining blood pressure in patients with essential hypertension than normotensive subjects for a given plasma renin activity.

ACKNOWLEDGMENTS

These studies were supported by the Medical Research Council, the Wellcome Trust, and the National Kidney Research Fund.

REFERENCES

1. Haber E (1976) The role of renin in normal and pathological cardiovascular homeostasis. Circulation 54: 849–861
2. Case DB, Wallace JM, Keim HJ, Weber MA, Sealey JE, Laragh JH (1977) Possible role of renin in hypertension as suggested by renin-sodium profiling and inhibition of converting enzyme. New Engl J Med 296: 641–646
3. George CF, Lewis PJ, Petrie A (1975) Clinical experience with use of ultrasound sphygmomanometer. Br Heart J 37: 804–807
4. Roulston JE, MacGregor GA (1978) Measurement of plasma renin activity by radioimmunoassay after prolonged cold storage. Clin Chim Acta 88: 45–48
5. MacGregor GA, Dawes PM (1976) Agonist and antagonist effects of Sar-Ala-angiotensin II in salt-loaded and salt-depleted man. Br J Clin Pharmacol 3: 483–487
6. Hollenberg NK, Williams GH, Taub KJ, Isikawa I, Brown C, Adams DF (1977) Renal vascular response to interruption of the renin-angiotensin system in normal man. Kidney Int 12: 285–293
7. Anderson GH, Streeten DHP, Dalakos ThG (1977) Pressor response to 1-Sar-8-Ala-angiotensin II (saralasin) in hypertensive subjects. Circ Res 40: 243–250
8. Case DB, Wallace JM, Keim HJ, Weber MA, Drayer JIM, White RP, Sealey JE, Laragh JH (1976) Estimating renin participation in hypertension: Superiority of converting enzyme inhibitor over saralasin. Am J Med 61: 790–796
9. Fagard P, Amery A, Lijnen P, Reybrouck T (1979) Haemodynamic effects of captopril in hypertensive patients: Comparison with saralasin. Clin Sci 57: 131S–134S
10. Atkinson AB, Brown JJ, Fraser R, Leckie B, Lever AF, Morton JJ, Robertson JIS (1979) Captopril in hypertension with renal artery stenosis and in intractable hypertension; acute and chronic changes in circulating concentrations of renin, angiotensins I and II and aldosterone, and in body composition. Clin Sci 57: 139S–143S
11. MacGregor GA, Markandu ND, Roulston JE, Jones JC, Morton JJ (in press) The renin angiotensin aldosterone system in the maintenance of blood pressure, aldosterone secretion and sodium balance in normotensive subjects. Clin Sci
12. Matthews PG, McGrath BP, Johnston CI (1979) Hormonal changes with long-term converting-enzyme inhibition by captopril in essential hypertension. Clin Sci 57: 135S–138S

DISCUSSION

Dr. Folkow (Göteborg, Sweden): I would like to take up a point made by Dr. Laragh when he discussed catecholamine versus renin-angiotensin control. First, it should be stressed that the minor concentrations of catecholamines present in the bloodstream are essentially subthreshold to virtually all cardiovascular smooth muscle. What really matters are the catecholamine concentrations released at the nerve endings, which at the peak of release, create such a high concentration in the junction gaps as to virtually saturate the alpha-receptors. When released locally in tonic sympathetic discharge, the transmitter, therefore, entirely dominates the effector cells, and do so as long as the fibers are active. Second, the angiotensin levels that raise blood pressure were studied in man some year ago by Drs. Johnsson, Henning, and Ablad in Göteborg [Johnsson, Henning, and Ablad (1965) Life Sci 4: 1549–1554], and they showed convincingly that these angiotensin concentrations elicit their pressor and constrictor responses by way of *centrally* activating the autonomic nervous system. Thus, when they regionally blocked the vasoconstrictor fibers, the regional constrictive effect of angiotensin vanished, and they had to increase angiotensin concentrations tenfold or more to get a *direct* smooth muscle constriction. Furthermore, if circulation in one forearm was stopped by a cuff, and the angiotensin was again intravenously infused in the other arm, there was a neurogenically mediated vasoconstriction in the excluded forearm, showing up as a venous pressure rise. So, actually, when Dr. Laragh gets sustained pressure rises by prolonged angiotensin infusions, he really tests the excellent capacity of the adrenergic nerve fibers to keep up a prolonged vasoconstriction.

Dr. Laragh (New York): In answer to your first question, you must understand that I am well aware that norepinephrine is probably not a hormone of the circulation and that it is actually mediated at transmitter sites at the nerve endings. That is a given. On the other hand, all we could do with our experiment was to infuse and see what would happen when we introduced norepinephrine activity in the bloodstream. Now, I don't think there is reason to believe that norepinephrine is going to act differently at the nerve ending when you give it intravenously than when locally released except for a possible distributional problem. It is still the same molecule, and all I was trying to show is the best we can do is give it intravenously. When we did so, it didn't fit the model of a circulating or generalized released hormone that might cause chronic hypertension because it induced natriuresis, and because in time there is a progressively increasing resistance to its pressor action even when doses are increased. One of the reasons we did this experiment is because so many investigators, including a number in this room, have spent their lives measuring plasma norepinephrine and trying to relate it to hypertension;

so, whether or not you or I believe in circulating blood levels, others do. We were trying to produce sustained hypernorepinephrinemia and succeeded, but we still couldn't produce sustained hypertension. That doesn't mean to say if you want to follow your reasoning that it could do it if it were instead released at nerve endings like acetylcholine or other local transmitters. But I think that we can conclude that a) circulating norepinephrine is not a reasonable vector and b) that sustained accumulation at nerve endings still might be a vector of chronic hypertension but our study gives this second possibility no support.

Now as to your other question about angiotensin acting via the central and automatic nervous system, I have no quarrel. I wouldn't argue with the fact that angiotensin may induce its vasoconstriction in some part by coordinating with the sympathetic nervous system. However, in fact, it still is the *vector,* because when we erase it, the blood pressure goes down every time and I don't see how you can argue with that. In other words, we can infuse angiotensin and raise the blood pressure, block its action with saralasin or its formation with captopril or its secretion with propranolol, and the blood pressure routinely falls by exactly the extent to which we block the system. Thus, I have no argument that its final mediation might involve the adrenergic system perhaps by the pathways you suggest. It could act via the head; you can route it anywhere you want, but the fact is that when angiotensin is deleted, the blood pressure falls commensurately. So, in this way angiotensin II is actually the vector of the protracted vasocontriction. You can't beat that argument.

Dr. Birkenhager (Rotterdam, The Netherlands): I have trouble finding anything to agree with in the papers by Drs. Laragh and Carey. I can only pick out a few points earlier in the session. Dr. Carey used a few arguments for a mysterious volume expansion in low-renin hypertension. These arguments were: first, the phenomenon of hypernatriuresis and, second, the good response to diuretics. Now, as far as hypernatriuresis is concerned, I can tell you that this is more the result of abnormal renal hemodynamics than of any volume disturbance; with respect to the response to diuretics, I think that you can translate that very easily as a phenomenon related to the unresponsiveness of the vessel wall rather than volume expansion. If you look at patients in whom plasma volume is actually in the upper range, they are not more responsive to diuretics than those who have normal or even reduced blood volumes. Furthermore, I would like to remark that both Drs. Laragh and Carey failed to take into account that low-renin hypertension is a feature of older hypertensives; I cannot see how you can fit the occurrence of low renin in older patients with any particular genesis of hypertension.

Dr. Carey (Charlottesville, Va.): Most investigators have shown that the normalization of blood pressure that accompanies diuretic therapy in low-renin essential hypertension is associated with diuresis, natriuresis, and weight loss. This response is much more impressive in low-renin hypertensives than in normal- or high-renin hypertensives, and is excellent indirect evidence that low-renin essential hypertension is a volume type of hypertension.

What evidence do you have Dr. Birkenhager that the excessive natriuresis in response to diuretics in low-renin essential hypertension in response to sodium loading is related to abnormal renal hemodynamics or redistribution of renal blood flow?

Dr. Birkenhager: Well, as a matter of fact, we think we have, and this has been published in Clinical Science in the early 1970s [Schalekamp, Krauss, Schalekamp-Kuyken et al. (1971) Clin Sci 41: 219–231].

Dr. T. G. Pickering (New York): Dr. Lever, the Cleveland group has described an aldosterone-stimulating peptide that could conceivably play a role in the patient with pseudoprimary aldosteronism. Do you have any comments about that?

Dr. Lever (Glasgow, Scotland): No, I don't, because we haven't measured it ourselves. I suggest that it is not necessary to look for another aldosterone-stimulating agent because the agent we already have (angiotensin II) produces a pronounced response of aldosterone.

Mr. Chairman, could I say something about the nature of low-renin hypertension. My earlier thesis was that the response of aldosterone to angiotensin II is enhanced in essential hypertension and even more enhanced in the nontumorous form of primary hyperaldosteronism, and that this was responsible for their artifactual separation because it leads to occasional aldosterone values outside the normal range. This, in itself, is not a qualitative difference.

The response of aldosterone to angiotensin II is also enhanced in low-renin hypertension as has

been shown by Wisgerhof and Brown and by ourselves. A consequence of this is that renin and angiotensin II are low relative to the aldosterone level. This relationship sometimes leads to subnormal plasma concentrations of renin and angiotensin II. Patients having subnormal concentrations are labeled "low-renin hypertension," and this is a perfectly fair description. I do not deny that such patients exist, nor do I object to the name. My objection is to the very common assumption that the name describes a state that is qualitatively different from essential hypertension. The abnormality it shows (low renin in relation to aldosterone) is present in this condition from which it is separated. This abnormality is demonstrated in Fig. 1, which plots concurrent plasma concentrations of angiotensin II and aldosterone in patients with essential hypertension and low-renin hypertension, all untreated. Compared with normal subjects (regression with steeper slope), most patients

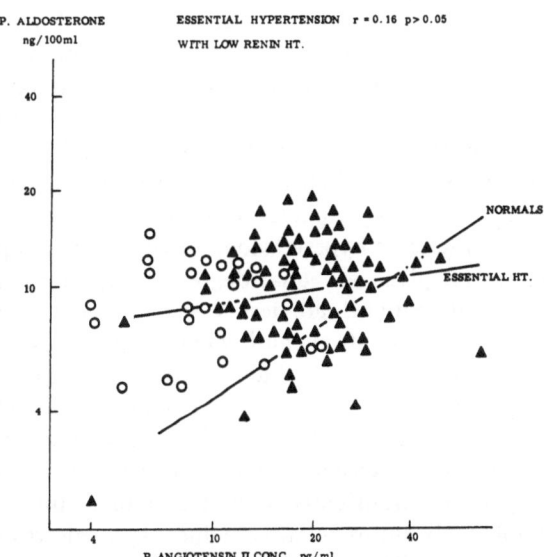

Fig. 1. Relationships between the plasma concentration of angiotensin II and aldosterone in essential hypertension with normal renin (▲) and low renin (○). The steeper regression is for data in normal subjects. Most patients with essential hypertension and low-renin hypertension have aldosterone values that are high relative to angiotensin II. Low-renin hypertension is defined arbitrarily as having a plasma concentration of total renin less than 38 μU/ml. Given the correlation of renin and angiotensin II, this is equivalent to a plasma angiotensin II concentration of approximately 9 pg/ml. [Davies et al. (1979) J Endocrinol 81: 79P–91P]

with essential hypertension and all with low-renin hypertension have an angiotensin II that is low relatively to aldosterone. Thus, low-renin hypertension is at the end of a continuous distribution.

Dr. Amery (Leuven, Belgium) (Chairman): Staying with the low-renin essential hypertensive patients could we ask what evidence is there of decreased vasoconstriction in these patients?

Dr. MacGregor (London, England): Experiments with either saralasin or captopril show that angiotensin II plays less of a role in maintaining blood pressure in low-renin patients as compared to normotensive subjects. This implies that some other mechanism is involved in narrowing their arterioles. While I agree with Dr. Lever that renin is normally distributed, low-renin hypertensives are, nevertheless, abnormal as the renin is below the normal range. Height is normally distributed, but giants and dwarfs exist!

Dr. Amery: Are there any hemodynamic studies showing this decreased vasoconstriction?

Dr. Laragh: Dr. Amery, I know what you are driving at. First, I think that we would all agree with what Dr. MacGregor says—that low-renin patients have little or no renin-induced vasoconstriction. What you are saying is that there is still vasoconstriction in them. Everybody who has hypertension is probably vasoconstricted because their calculated peripheral resistance, which is how we characterize hypertension, nearly always is up. However, given an equal degree of hypertension low-renin patients are less vasoconstricted than high-renin patients. I think what happens in low-renin states is what Arthur Guyton and his group have shown in the volume overload dog model. Thus, they give volume overload to a dog and produce hypertension in which the cardiac output may be up transiently at first and then, due to whole-body autoregulation, induces systemic vasoconstriction. Hence, there is a degree of vasoconstriction in low-renin hypertension albeit less than in medium- and high-renin states for an equal degree of hypertension. The dog model shows that this can happen. Now what I think is the relevant issue is the fact that low-renin patients are *less* vasoconstricted than high-renin, perhaps because of the vasoconstriction of autoregulation that Guyton has studied, but they don't have any added renin factor. The way you would prove that is to take two groups of people with equal degrees of hypertension and measure their cardiac output and resistance. This study has never been properly done. It simply requires comparing renin subgroups with equal degrees of hypertension. But there is a large body of corroborative data to support the idea that equally hypertensive low-renin patients have a better flow than high-renin patients, thus, when anyone has measured blood or extracellular fluid volumes in low-renin patients, it is either overtly high or on the high side of normal. Moreover, when anyone has measured it in high-renin states, the volumes are instead much lower. We have reviewed all of these published studies [Laragh JH, Letcher RL, and Pickering TG (1979) JAMA 241: 151–156]. So I think the implication is that while there may be some key studies missing, the low-renin state is one in which there is relatively better flow, higher volumes, and less vasoconstriction that occurs in an equally hypertensive high-renin patient. This is probably related to their better prognosis and greater longevity even when their blood pressures are comparatively higher. It may also explain why the low-renin patients give the best response to diuretics.

Dr. Amery: Are there any further comments related to that particular question, Dr. Seldin?

Dr. Seldin (Dallas, Tex.): Essential hypertension seems to embrace a variety of different entities. On one end of the spectrum is low-renin essential hypertension, a disorder that responds well to diuretics and is associated with a rise in plasma renin as extracellular volume is reduced. Salt retention, giving rise to steady-state volume over expansion, seems to be the causal factor initiating this hypertensive process. On the other end of the spectrum is high-renin hypertension, a disorder that responds well to antirenin agents such as propranolol. However, the high renins are strikingly resistant to suppression by volume expansion induced by salt loads.

Because of the marked differences in these two entities, Dr. Laragh has proposed that essential hypertension is heterogeneous, constituting a clinical label encompassing a number of different disease entities.

Another interpretation of these entities within the category of essential hypertension is also possible. The common thread running through all essential hypertension appears to be an inappropriately high volume for any given level of renin–angiotensin. The key feature may not be the absolute level of renin–angiotensin or aldosterone, but rather the inappropriate relationship of renin–angiotensin to volume. It is thus possible that renin–angiotensin, though low in absolute terms, may be inappropriately high relative to volume. By the same token, a normal or even slightly shrunken effective extracellular volume may be inappropriately expanded relative to very high values for renin–angiotensin. On this view, essential hypertension might be regarded as a disturbance in the "set" of the relationship between renin–angiotensin and volume such that the system is reset at a high value. And the differences among various types of essential hypertensive patients—high, normal, or low renin—could then simply represent a broad spectrum of variations of a single disease process. The variations might be attributable to differences among patients in: a) salt intake; b) sympathetic nervous system activity (as this is influenced by smoking, stress, etc.); and c) the development of autonomy of juxtaglomerular or zona glomerulosa activity, as this is influenced by the duration and intensity of the process.

Consider pseudoprimary hyperaldosteronism. This hypertension is associated with low renin and bilateral nodular adrenalhyperplasia. Since ordinary salt loads do not appear to suppress aldosterone in these patients, the disorder has been regarded as a primary disturbance, different from essential hypertension, in which there is disruption of the relationship between volume and renin on the one hand and aldosterone secretion on the other. This disorder might be conceived as a special disease entity in which autonomous oversecretion of aldosterone is the causal factor. On the other hand, it is possible, as Dr. Lever proposes, that the syndrome is simply one end of essential hypertension, in which prolonged stimulation of the zona glomerulosa has led to some degree of autonomous aldosterone oversecretion. In support of this hypothesis is the recent report of R.D. Gordon from Australia [Gordon RD, Jackson RV (1980) Lancet 1: 1422] demonstrating a fall in aldosterone levels if salt and 9α-fluorohydrocortisone were given for a sufficiently long period of time. Dr. Laragh has reported on one patient, followed for many years, in whom a high-renin hypertension gradually changed to low renin [Baer L, Sommers SC, Krakoff LR, et al. (1970) Circ Res 26&27: I203I–I220]. No other cases like this, to my knowledge, have been reported, so that this may not be the usual mechanism. But, as Dr. Lever's data indicate, some other feature of the process of essential hypertension may be responsible for chronic stimulation of the juxtaglomerular apparatus, lead-

ing to nodular hyperplasia. Other endocrine glands seem to acquire autonomy with chronic stimulation: Witness the hyperparathyroidism that develops in some patients with chronic renal failure.

Similarly, resistance of patients with high-renin hypertension to suppression of their renin levels by salt loads does not necessarily mean a unique disease. Were volume expanded in them for a sufficiently long period of time, as perhaps might be induced by administration of 9α-fluorohydrocortisone plus salt, renin might eventually fall.

That the patterns of volume, renin–angiotensin–aldosterone, are not fixed, but rather reset, is also suggested by the observation that in low-renin hypertension, plasma renin can be elevated by diuretic-induced volume contraction.

All of this suggests the possibility that the same basic disturbance may express itself with different levels of renin–angiotensin, aldosterone, and volume, but with the common quality of an inappropriately high product of renin–angiotensin and volume. In this model, essential hypertension might be viewed as a single disorder reflected in a spectrum of abnormal products within which the values for any component are reciprocally interconvertible. On the other hand, it is also conceivable, as Dr. Laragh argues, that the stability of the various patterns over long periods of time means that there are different primary lesions impinging on different sites of the volume, renin–angiotensin, and aldosterone cascade. The resolution of this issue will require identification of the causal factors initiating the hypertensive process as well as an elucidation of the mechanisms responsible for interconversion of the various elements generating the elevated blood pressure.

Dr. MacGregor: I wouldn't disagree with that; the only thing I would ask you is how you are going to measure the volume accurately enough to be able to prove what you are saying? Unfortunately, we can't measure volume, or effective volume, accurately to show that. But as you say in the normals: When they are on a low-salt diet, they have renin and so I would agree with what you are saying, but I don't think that we can actually prove it as yet.

Dr. Laragh: Dr. Seldin always brings forth very interesting ideas. I would say though, I don't know whether he means all hypertension is a single disease or whether low renin and pseudoprimary or idiopathic aldosteronism with low renin levels collectively define a single disease. I do agree that all hypertension is a spectrum of abnormal or inappropriate relationships between vasoconstriction (usually due to renin) and extracellular and vascular volume as determined by the sodium balance. This is the basis for our vasoconstriction-volume hypothetical model. The problem is that the abnormal spectrum we are seeing in hypertension is much broader than occurs in normotensives. Certainly as you move out to the extremes you have to go a long way to say that an overtly low-renin patient has the same pathogenesis and pathophysiology as the high-renin patient, but I am willing to debate that. The compensated states just differ too much from each other pathophysiologically as well as in drug responsiveness, not to mention natural history.

Dr. Case (New York): I would like to make a comment and then ask a question. There is a discrepancy between Dr. Streeten's interpretation and our own with respect to saralasin responses. Whereas he finds that the depressor responses to saralasin are "positive" in 86% of renovascular hypertension, we find that the reactive renin level measured during saralasin infusion is "positive" in greater than 98% [Case DB, Atlas SA, Laragh JH (1979) Clin Sci Mol Med 57: 313S–316S]. The same is true for converting enzyme inhibitors [Case DB, Laragh JH (1979) Annals Int Med 91: 153–160]. In addition, the evaluation of only the depressor response identifies many "false positives" whereas positive reactive renin responses in patients without renal ischemia are quite unusual. Maxwell and his colleagues have data which agree with ours [Maxwell MS, Veriday P, Zawada ET et al. (1978) Clin Sci Mol Med 55: 297s–299s]. For these reasons we prefer to use the response to captopril instead, as I will present later on.

I would also like to ask Dr. Carey a question. Has he given centrally acting dopamine agonists or peripheral dopamine to low-renin hypertensives on a long term basis?

Dr. Carey: No, as far as I am aware this has not been done as yet.

Dr. Januszewicz (Warsaw, Poland): Dr. Carey, may I ask you whether you have measured dopamine in patients with hypertension caused by aldosterone excess? We have found in patients with primary aldosteronism an increased dopamine plasma level and increased urinary excretion of dopamine. It is noteworthy that in patients with primary aldosteronism, in contrast to patients with essential hypertension, a decrease of plasma dopamine was observed after standing.

Dr. Carey: I have not measured dopamine in any hypertensive patients. I think that the people here should be aware though that there are methodologic difficulties in the measurement of plasma dopamine concentrations by means of the radioenzymatic method. Not all assays may, in fact, be measuring dopamine.

Dr. Streeten (Syracuse, New York): May I make one comment on Dr. Lever's talk. It seems to me that what Dr. Lever has shown is that the patients with what I would still call primary aldosteronism without tumor can respond to angiotensin II infusion. This does not prove that their elevated spontaneous levels of aldosterone production are due to stimulation by angiotensin II. In fact, if Dr. Lever has studied the aldosterone secretion in response to ACTH rather than to angiotensin II, he might have drawn the conclusion that primary aldosteronism associated with adenoma was not primary, because patients with such adenomas respond very well to ACTH, just as patients with nonadenomatous hyperplasia respond to angiotensin II. So I don't believe that it is valid, because the adrenal zona glomerulosa responds in these patients to angiotensin II, to conclude that angiotensin II necessarily has anything to do with their excessive aldosterone production.

Session 8
The Control of Renin Release

Chairman: D. W. Seldin

Position Paper: The Control of Renin Release

A. Zanchetti, A. Stella, G. Leonetti, and G. Mancia

Great efforts have been devoted to dissecting the various mechanisms controlling renin release in order to demonstrate that each of them can be independently involved in regulation of renin secretion. Without denying the importance of this approach, more attention will be paid in this report to the interrelationships between the individual mechanisms; indeed, in the intact organism under natural conditions the various stimuli influencing juxtaglomerular activity will most often involve more than a single mechanism of control.

Davis and Freeman (1) have classified mechanisms regulating renin secretion as: a) intrarenal (including both the renal vascular receptor in the afferent arteriole sensitive to local changes in perfusing pressure and the receptor in the macula densa of the distal tubule sensitive to changes in tubular sodium and/or chloride load or concentration); b) sympathetic (including the renal nerves as well as catecholamines); and c) humoral (including vasopressin, angiotensin II, and prostaglandins).

INTRARENAL MECHANISMS

VASCULAR RECEPTOR

Evidence favoring the existence of an afferent arteriolar receptor was provided by Davis and his associates in the nonfiltering kidney model. These data will not be discussed here in detail. Suffice it to say that renin release in response to hemorrhage, suprarenal aortic stenosis, and thoracic caval constriction was found to occur after the renal vascular receptor had been isolated in vivo from the other regulating mechanisms (sodium chloride excretion, nervous influences, circulating catecholamines) (1). This finding indicates that the renal

vascular receptor alone can account for renin release following these stimuli. This does not mean, however, that the other mechanisms, when not artifically impaired, do not contribute or might alone be responsible for renin release if the vascular receptor is inactivated. There is evidence that this is true, as in instance, for hemorrhage. Witty et al. (2) have shown that after papaverine has rendered the vascular receptor nonfunctional, hemorrhage can still release renin from a denervated kidney, a response that is presumably mediated through the sole remaining mechanism, the macula densa. Furthermore, it has also been shown that following a small nonhypotensive hemorrhage, the increase in renin is mediated by renal sympathetic activity (see below).

However, there are still uncertainties about the identity of the vascular receptor. For lack of other suitable candidates, the receptor has been identified with the juxtaglomerular cell itself, though there is no crucial evidence for this assumption. The vascular receptor has long been defined as a "baroreceptor" or "stretch receptor" in line with the conception brought forth by Tobian et al. (3) and supported by the work of Skinner et al. (4). More recently, it has been maintained (5) that renin release is related to autoregulated dilatation of the renal arterioles, but several investigators have shown that when the lower limit of the autoregulatory range is reached, there must still be tone in the renal vessels since infusion of papaverine can further lead to large increases in renal blood flow (1). Furthermore, renin release can be induced during decreases in renal perfusion pressure accompanied by either renal vasodilatation, as during aortic stenosis, or vasoconstriction, as after hemorrhage or salt depletion (1).

Presumably, the degree of stretch is influenced by concomitant intrarenal and extrarenal factors that affect the tone of the afferent arteriole, and that might not be faithfully gauged by what we calculate as renal vascular resistance. It might be interesting to speculate what might be the influence of sympathetic constriction of the afferent arteriole on the vascular receptor. For instance, stretch receptors in the carotid sinus are known to give a stronger response to a pressure transient when stiffness of the sinus wall is increased by cervical sympathetic stimulation. This response is due to the arrangement of the carotid sinus stretch receptors in series with the contracting elements (6). If in the afferent arteriole the sensing coincides with the contracting elements, or are disposed in parallel, contraction of the afferent arteriole would reduce the stretch and increase renin release. The same would occur if sympathetically induced contraction were prevalent in the more proximal portion of the afferent arteriole, while juxtaglomerular cells seem to be prevalent in the most distal end of the arteriole: Distally, perfusing pressure would be decreased and the juxtaglomerular cells unloaded and stimulated to release renin. However, recent observations by my group (7) have shown

identical degrees of autoregulatory vasodilatation in the innervated and the contralateral denervated kidney when renal perfusion pressure is reduced during suprarenal aortic constriction (Fig. 1), a finding which makes it unlikely that sympathetic tone alters the compliance of the afferent arterioles to changes in renal perfusion pressure.

The role of calcium in the contraction of afferent arteriolar smooth muscle and in inhibition of renin release has recently been stressed (8–10). In particular, Vandongen and Peart (8) have elaborated the interesting hypothesis that inhibition of renin secretion is related to smooth muscle activity by the involvement of a calcium-dependent process similar to that involved in contraction: Activation of renin release by vasodilators would result from blockade of this calcium-dependent process. It is interesting, under these circumstances, that in hypertensive patients administration of the calcium antagonist agent, verapamil, in doses significantly reducing blood pressure, does not induce the expected increase in plasma renin activity (11). These clinical observations, of course, are not mentioned to deny any important role for calcium in renin release, but only to caution against an unwarranted extrapolation of experimental data to a clinical context.

Macula Densa

Evidence on the macula densa has been extensively reviewed by Davis and Freemen (1) and will be briefly discussed here. The issue about the role of receptors in the macula densa is bewildered by the paucity of crucially supportive data and by conflicting interpretations of those available. The real nature of the stimulus leading to renin release has long been disputed, the stimulus being increased sodium concentration according to Thurau et al. (12) and decreased load or intracellular concentration according to Vander (13). It must be recognized, however, that the conflict between the two interpretations might have been unduly stressed. Indeed, Thurau's concept of an intrarenal feedback mechanism refers to macula densa control of the intrarenal effects of renin (i.e., local generation of angiotensin II to regulate glomerular filtration rate), not to macula densa regulation of renin release into the systemic circulation. For the latter function, the load hypothesis has further been supported by recent experiments (14), and appears now to be the most likely.

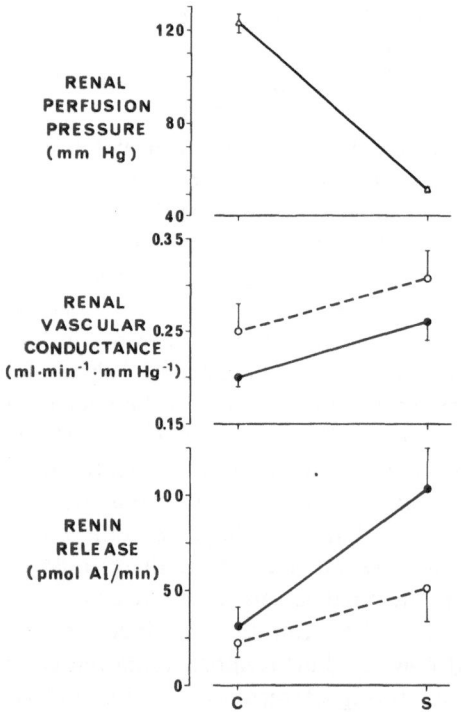

Fig. 1. Changes in renal vascular resistance and in renin release in the innervated kidney (●————●) and in the contralateral innervated kidney (○————○) when renal perfusion pressure is lowered by an aortic snare. [Stella et al. (7)]

The classical hypothesis that sodium is sensed by the macula densa has recently been debated, however. The evidence that chloride, rather than sodium, is actively transported in the thick ascending limb of the loop of Henle has suggested a role for chloride in mediating changes in renin secretion. Evidence is available now that both sodium and chloride can be involved: Stephens et al. (15) have shown that renin secretion can be decreased by infusion of sodium salts with anions other than chloride; Abboud et al. (16) have also been able to stimulate renin release by acute selective chloride depletion in the rat by peritoneal dialysis against 0.15 M $NaHCO_3$.

As to the relative importance of the macula densa in renin release in comparison with other known factors, Davis and Freeman (1) have rightly remarked that it remains to be established. They have also suggested that the macula densa may preferentially operate at low perfusion pressures.

SYMPATHOADRENERGIC MECHANISMS

Figure 2 summarizes some work of our group illustrating the sympathetic mechanism of activation of renin release, and the nature of the adrenergic receptors of the juxtaglomerular cells (17, 18). Electrical stimulation of the vasomotor center in the pons and medulla produces a sharp increase in renin release and a fall in renal blood flow to the innervated kidney, whereas no change in renin release and a slight passive increase in blood flow occur in the contralateral denervated kidney. Dissociation of vasomotor and renin-releasing effects of brainstem stimulation was obtained by intrarenal infusion of a very small amount of the alpha-adrenergic blocker, phenoxybenzamine: In these conditions, brainstem stimulation did not induce any vasomotor change on the injected side, but renin release occurred from both sides. It may be worth mentioning that because brainstem stimulation caused a conspicuous blood pressure rise, renin release from the phenoxybenzamine-treated kidney occurred in spite of a marked autoregulative vasoconstriction, a patent exception to the assumption that renin release and renal vasodilatation are necessarily associated. The lower part of the figure shows that renal vasoconstriction is preserved, but renin release abolished, by infusion of

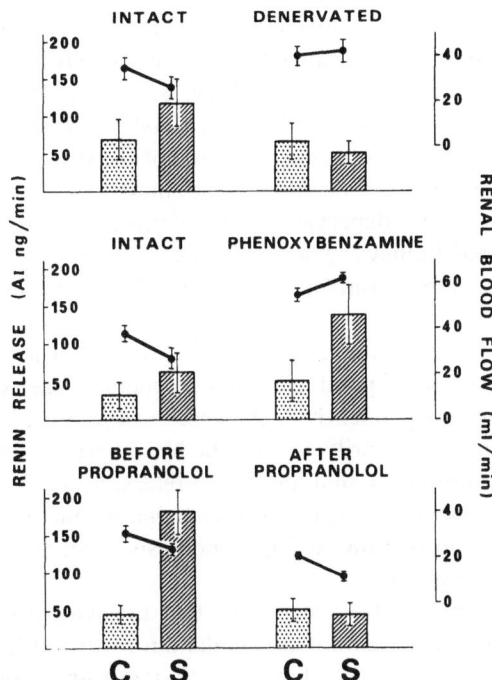

Fig. 2. Effect of electrical stimulation of the vasomotor center in the brainstem. Mean values ± SEM are shown for renin release *(histograms and bars, left ordinates)* and for renal blood flow *(filled circles, right ordinates)*. C, control; S, after a 5-min stimulation period. [Richardson et al. (17)]

the beta-adrenergic blocker, propranolol. Further evidence for a direct sympathetic action on juxtaglomerular cells independent of vascular and macula densa receptors comes from experiments in nonfiltering and papaverine-treated kidneys (1) and by low-frequency stimulation of renal nerves (see 18).

HUMORAL MECHANISMS

PROSTAGLANDINS

There has been mounting interest in prostaglandin–renin interactions. The well known renin-releasing action of prostaglandins PGI_2, PGD_2, and PGE_2 has been found to be independent of the macula densa and sympathetic tone, as it is preserved in denervated nonfiltering kidneys (19, 20). It appears, therefore, that these prostaglandins can modulate renin release via mediation of the intrarenal baroreceptor mechanism or via a direct stimulation of the juxtaglomerular cells. The latter hypothesis is the more likely, because it has recently been shown (21) that renal prostaglandin synthesis, by intrarenal infusion of the prostaglandin precursor arachidonic acid, increases renin release from denervated, nonfiltering papaverine-treated kidneys, where all other presently recognized renin control mechanisms had been abolished.

The latter observations seem to establish that the action of prostaglandins on renin release can occur independently of the vascular receptor; they are not necessarily against the hypothesis recently advanced (22) that the renin-releasing action of the vascular receptor is prostaglandin mediated, although this interesting hypothesis needs further confirmation.

It has also been suggested that the sympathetic influence on renin is prostaglandin mediated (23): There is evidence, however, that during hemorrhage, for instance, beta-adrenergic blockers and indomethacin have additive effects in blocking the increase in renin (24), and this indicates that the sympathetic influence is unlikely to be entirely prostaglandin mediated.

ANGIOTENSIN

The negative feedback action exerted by angiotensin II on renin release has been known for some time (13) and shown to be exerted directly on the juxtaglomerular cell or the vascular receptor (1). Renewed interest in this kind of control has been caused by the availability of angiotensin antagonists and converting enzyme inhibitors capable of interrupting the feedback system.

The exact site of the feedback action of angiotensin is still debated. Vandongen et al. (25) observed that the vasoconstrictor and renin-inhibitory activities of angiotensin are not interdependent since renin secretion remained suppressed after renal vasoconstriction was abolished by isoproterenol or glucagon. The fact that stimulation of renin release by isoproterenol and glucagon, which appears to involve different membrane receptors, is equally inhibited by angiotensin suggested to Vandongen et al. (25) a more distal site for the feedback action of angiotensin. An opposite view has been advanced by Pettinger and Mitchell (26), who observed that the increase in renin following interruption of the feedback by the angiotensin antagonist, saralasin, was suppressed by propranolol: They, therefore, suggested that the site for feedback inhibition is proximal to the beta-adrenergic receptor. Our recent experience with the converting enzyme inhibitor, captopril, does not favor this conclusion (27). Figure 3 shows that in a group of hypertensive patients tested with increasing doses of captopril (25–200 mg/day), there was a dose-related increase in plasma renin activity lasting several hours after captopril. When the same

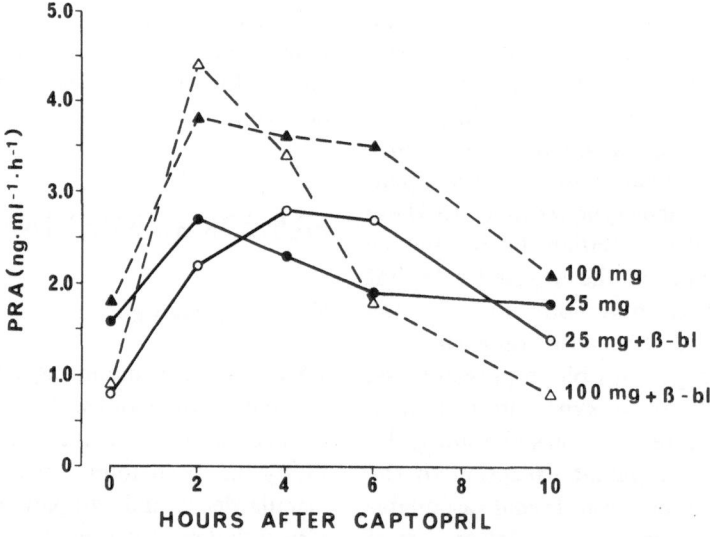

Fig. 3. Effect of two different doses of captopril (25 and 100 mg p.o.) before (● ▲) and after 1-week treatment with 160 mg/day propranolol (○). Means of observations in ten patients. [Leonetti et al. (27)]

doses of captopril were tested in the same subjects after a weeks' treatment with 160 mg/day propranolol, the increase of plasma renin in response to captopril was preserved, or was even more marked, though obviously starting from a considerably lower plasma renin level. The only additional influence of beta-adrenergic blockade was possibly a somewhat shorter duration of the renin-releasing effect of 100 mg captopril. Therefore, it does not seem likely that the negative feedback action of angiotensin is preferentially exerted on the neural mechanism of renin control, unless this mechanism is especially activated, as it was in Pettinger and Mitchell's patients concurrently treated with minoxidil.

INTERACTIONS BETWEEN THE VARIOUS MECHANISMS CONTROLLING RENIN RELEASE

In the intact organism, the various renin-releasing stimuli can seldom act in isolation on a single mechanism of control, and it is more likely that in most instances renin release results from an influence extended on multiple mechanisms.

HEMORRHAGE

We have already mentioned that hemorrhage can indeed stimulate a multiplicity of renin-controlling mechanisms, which can artificially be separated experimentally. Henrich et al. (24) have recently provided further support for this conclusion by showing that renin release induced by hemorrhage in the dog cannot be prevented by any of these single procedures alone, including beta-adrenergic blockade, renal prostaglandin inhibition with indomethacin, or control of renal perfusion pressure. However, renin release was prevented by combining beta-adrenergic blockade with either control of renal perfusion pressure or prostaglandin inhibition.

SUPRARENAL AORTIC STENOSIS AND LARGE DOSES OF FUROSEMIDE

The lower part of the Fig. 4 illustrates two conditions: infusion of large doses of furosemide and

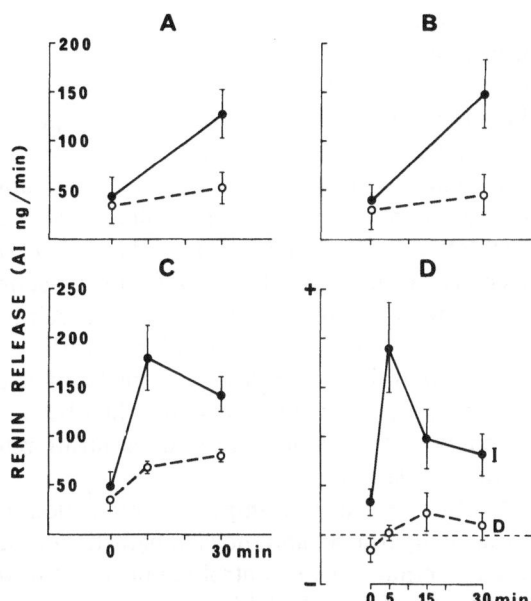

Fig. 4. Renin release of the innervated kidney (●———●) and the contralateral denervated kidney (○− − −○) in response to various stimuli: **A:** upright tilting; **B:** small dose of furosemide (0.75 mg/kg i.v.); **C:** large dose of furosemide (6.0 mg/kg i.v.); **D:** suprarenal aortic stenosis. Mean ± SEM. [Stella and Zanchetti (30)]

suprarenal aortic stenosis, in which renin release appears to result from the interaction of intrarenal and sympathoadrenergic mechanisms. Indeed, both stimuli can augment release of renin from a denervated kidney, but the release is much larger and prompter from the contralateral innervated kidney (18). It is interesting to discuss how this interaction may occur. It is unlikely that aortic constriction reflexly increases sympathetic activity directed to the kidney: The sinoaortic baroreceptors should be stimulated by the rise in arterial pressure above the aortic constriction, and this should reduce, rather than activate, sympathetic activity; the possibility that decreased renal perfusion pressure might deactivate renal arterial baroreceptors with reflex inhibitory functions similar to those of the sinoaortic reflexes has been disproved by experiments in which afferent renal nerve stimulation was found to induce pressor, rather than depressor, reflex responses and no change in renin release (28). It is likely, therefore, that the greater renin release from the innervated kidney when perfusion pressure is lowered results from a permissive facilitatory influence that tonic sympathetic activity exerts on intrarenal mechanisms, either on the vascular receptor or on the macula densa. This interpretation is supported by the observation that renin release can be potentiated when reduction in renal perfusion pressure is combined with beta-adrenoreceptor stimulation by isoproterenol or with low-voltage electrical stimulation of efferent renal nerve fibers (see 18). Recently, Thames and Di Bona (29) have shown that a much greater amount of renin is released when aortic constriction is combined with renal nerve stimuli that are ineffective alone to influence renin release; a similar potentiation had been observed when furosemide was infused during renal nerve stimulation.

Another possible example of interaction between sympathetic and nonsympathetic mechanisms of renin release control is illustrated in the upper part of Fig. 4. Tilting head-up and small doses of furosemide seem to release renin solely through reflex sympathetic activation as increased secretion occurs only from the innervated kidney, whereas, on the denervated side, there is no releasing effect, or even a suppression when adrenalectomy is also performed (30). There is reason to suppose, however, that during tilting the reduction of renal perfusion pressure may also play a role, which is a subsidiary and negligible one when pressure homeostasis is maintained during tilting and renal perfusion pressure is only slightly reduced, but the role may be a more substantial one when pressure homeostasis is impaired (31). Figure 5 illustrates that section of cardiopulmonary afferents by vagotomy does not disturb pressure homeostasis: The reduction of arterial pressure induced by tilting is as moderate as when the reflex was intact. However, reflex activation of juxtaglomerular cells is prevented by vagotomy, and innervated and denervated kidneys both have a similarly mild increase in renin during tilting. On the other hand, after sinoaortic denervation, cardiovascular adjustment to tilting is conspicuously impaired and blood pressure markedly falls in the upright posture (Fig. 6). In this condition, the increment of renin release from the innervated kidney is not impaired, but is rather augmented. The response, however, does not appear to be mediated through the vagi, as it is maintained after combined sinoaortic denervation and vagotomy. It is likely to be due to stimulation of intrarenal mechanism, by the conspicuous fall in renal perfusion pressure. The observation that only the innervated

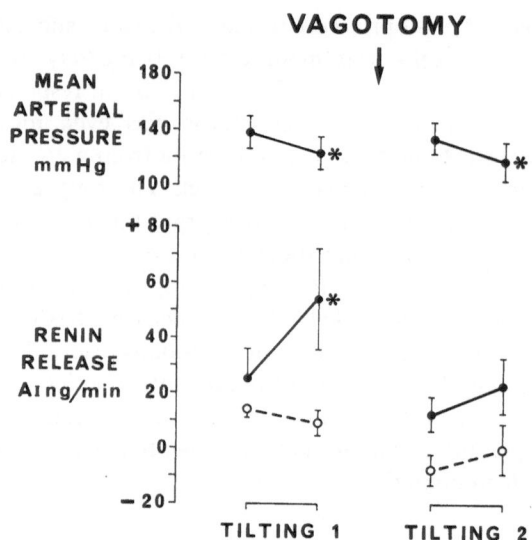

Fig. 5. Effects of two trials of tilting on mean arterial pressure *(top)* and renin release *(bottom)* in seven cats. Between the two trials, bilateral cervical vagotomy was performed. *Bottom:* ●——●, renin release from innervated kidneys; ○————○, renin release from denervated kidneys. [Stella et al. (32)]

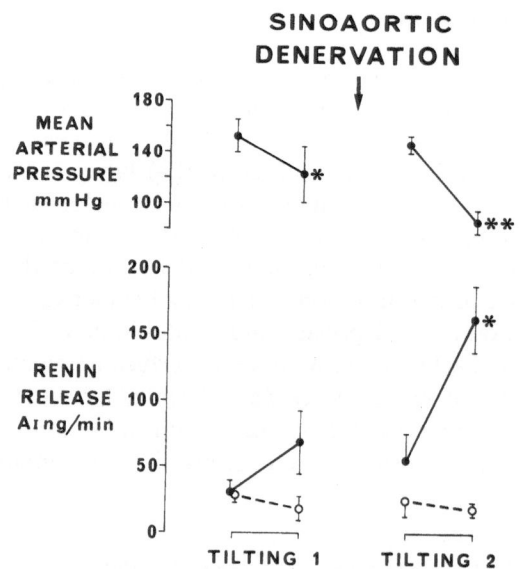

Fig. 6. Effects of two trials of tilting on mean arterial pressure *(top)* and renin release *(bottom)* in five cats. Between the two trials, sinoaortic denervation was performed. [Dampney et al. (31)]

kidney responds with an increment in renin release, even when tilting is associated with a large hypotension, confirms that only innervated juxtaglomerular cells can promptly and markedly respond to reduction in perfusion pressure (31).

The examples illustrated thus far are of mutual amplification between sympathetic and intrarenal mechanisms of renin release. Figure 7 illustrates a different type of interaction, by which intrarenal inhibition of renin release may obscure the excitatory response of juxtaglomerular cells to neural stimuli. Bilateral cervical vagotomy, by releasing renal sympathetic activity from the inhibitory influence of cardiopulmonary volume receptors, induces a transient, but large, increase in renin secretion from innervated (but not denervated) kidneys. This response is clear in moderately fluid-depleted animals, but it is totally prevented by even moderate fluid expansion. Fluid expansion should further stimulate cardiopulmonary volume receptors and enhance the effect of vagotomy; the opposite response observed is likely to be due to an antagonizing action of the increase in body fluid

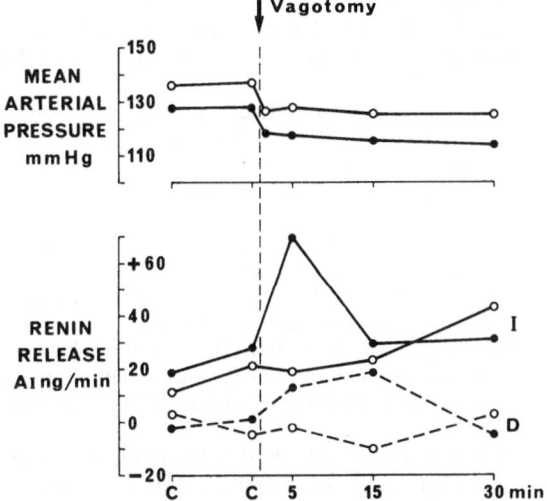

Fig. 7. Effects of bilateral cervical vagotomy on mean arterial pressure *(top)* and renin release *(bottom)* in a group of six moderately fluid-depleted cats (●) and in a group of five moderately fluid-depleted cats (○). *Bottom:* ●————●, renin release from the innervated kidney; ○————○, renin release from the denervated kidney. The first and second Cs *(below)* indicate control measurements 15 min and immediately before vagotomy; the numbers indicate time in minutes after vagotomy. Mean and standard error of the mean are represented. [Stella et al. (32)]

volume and in the sodium load on the vascular receptor or the macula densa (32).

We also have evidence in man about possible interactions between the various mechanisms of renin control. In a group of six essential hypertensive patients, we have studied changes in the renal vein–arterial difference in renin produced by stimulation or deactivation of carotid sinus baroreceptors. Manipulation of carotid sinus reflexes was performed by means of a variable pressure neck chamber, which causes either an increase or a decrease in carotid sinus transmural pressure and, therefore, stimulates or deactivates the baroreceptors. Figure 8 shows that baroreceptor deactivation induced a definite rise in mean arterial pressure and in heart rate, but caused only a very slight and nonsignificant increase in renin release. Likewise, baroreceptor stimulation produced hypotension but no decrease in renin release (33).

These observations suggest that in man, as in the experimental animal, the carotid sinus plays only a minor or complementary role in reflex regulation of renin release. Alternative explanations, however, should also be considered. Indeed, the reflex rise in arterial pressure induced by baroreceptor deactivation might partly counteract some reflex increase in renin secretion by stretching the renal vascular receptor; and the reverse might occur when carotid sinus baroreceptor stimulation induces hypotension and counteracts a possible reduction in renal nerve activity by unloading the vascular receptor.

That something of this kind is more than a remote possibility is suggested by observations we have recently performed in patients with renovascular hypertension due to unilateral renal artery stenosis, in whom there was high release of renin from one kidney and suppressed release from the contralateral one. In these patients, deactivation of the carotid sinus baroreceptors very moderately increased venous–arterial difference in renin, but the increase was somewhat greater on the stenosed than on the contralateral side. Stimulation of the baroreceptors, however, produced some unexpected results: It was followed, rather than by no change or by a decrease, by an increase in renal vein–arterial difference in renin, again more marked on the side with renal artery stenosis. Though several interpretations can be advanced to explain this unexpected observation, the most likely one, and the one in line with the kind of multiple interactions discussed so far, is that the

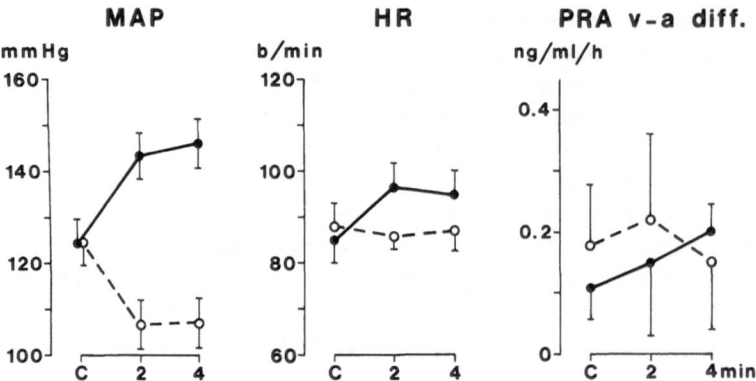

Fig. 8. Effects of reduced (●———●) and increased (○– – –○) carotid transmural pressure (by means of the neck pressure chamber) on mean arterial pressure (MAP), heart rate (HR), and renal vein–arterial difference in plasma renin activity (PRA v–a diff.) in six hypertensive patients (N = 6). [Mancia et al. (33)]

simultaneous reflex reduction in arterial pressure, though averaging only 13 mmHg, might have caused a more critical pressure fall through the stenosed renal artery, and the reflex inhibition of renin release might have been overwhelmed by unload of the intrarenal vascular receptor (34).

SUMMARY

Investigation on both experimental animals and man indicate that under most conditions influencing renin release in either direction, intra- and extrarenal mechanisms of control interact with mutual facilitation and, sometimes, with mutual inhibition. In particular, sympathetic innervation of juxtaglomerular cells can exert a direct stimulating action on renin release, but it also exerts an important permissive role in order to amplify and possibly accelerate response to stimuli directly affecting the intrarenal receptors. On the other hand, the response of juxtaglomerular cells to sympathetic stimuli is strongly influenced by concomitant activation or inactivation of intrarenal receptor mechanisms. As all body functions, control of renin release is an integrated function and cannot be properly understood without taking into account all possible interactions.

REFERENCES

1. Davis JO, Freeman RH (1976) Mechanisms regulating renin release. Physiol Rev 56: 1–56

2. Witty RT, Davis JO, Johnson JA, Prewitt RL (1971) Effects of papaverine and hemorrhage on renin secretion in the nonfiltering kidney. Am J Physiol 221: 1666–1671

3. Tobian L, Tomboulian A, Janecek J (1959) The effect of high perfusion pressures on the granulation of juxtaglomerular cells in an isolated kidney. J Clin Invest 38: 605–610

4. Skinner SL, McCubbin JW, Page IH (1964) Control of renin secretion. Circ Res 15: 64–76

5. Eide I, Löyning E, Kül F (1973) Evidence for hemodynamic autoregulation of renin release. Circ Res 32: 237–245

6. Peveler RC, Bergel DH, Brooks DE, Robinson JL, Sleight P, Worley J (1981) Modulation of baroreceptor firing by efferent sympathetic nerve stimulation in the dog. In: Proceedings of the Oxford baroreceptor workshop (in press)

7. Stella A, Calaresu F, Zanchetti A (1976) Neural factors contributing to renin release during reduction in renal perfusion pressure and blood flow in cats. Clin Sci Mol Med 51: 453–461

8. Vandongen R, Peart WS (1974) The inhibition of renin secretion by alpha-adrenergic stimulation in the isolated rat kidney. Clin Sci Mol Med 47: 471–479

9. Park CS, Malvin RL (1978) Calcium in the control of renin release. Am J Physiol 251: F22–F25

10. Fray JCS, Park CS (1972) Influence of potassium, sodium, perfusion pressure, and isoprenaline on renin release induced by acute calcium deprivation. J Physiol 292: 363–372

11. Leonetti G, Sala C, Bianchini C, Terzoli L, Zanchetti A (in press) Antihypertensive and renal effects of oral administration of verapamil. Eur J Clin Invest

12. Thurau K, Schnermann J, Nagel W, Horster M, Wohl M (1967) Composition of tubular fluid in the macula densa segment as a factor regulating the function of the juxtaglomerular apparatus. Circ Res 20, 21(Suppl II): 79–90

13. Vander AJ (1967) Control of renin release. Physiol Rev 47: 359–382
14. Churchill PC, Churchill MC, McDonald FD (1979) Effects of saline and mannitol on renin and distal tubule Na in rats. Circ Res 45: 786–792
15. Stephens GA, Davis JO, Freeman RH, Watkins BE (1978) Effects of sodium and potassium salts with anions other than chloride on renin secretion in the dog. Am J Physiol 234: F10–F15
16. Abboud HE, Luke RG, Galla JH, Kotchen TA (1979) Stimulation of renin by acute selective chloride depletion in the rat. Circ Res 44: 815–821
17. Richardson D, Stella A, Leonetti G, Bartorelli A, Zanchetti A (1974) Mechanisms of renal release of renin by electrical stimulation of the brainstem in the cat. Circ Res 34: 425–434
18. Zanchetti A, Stella A, Leonetti G, Morganti A, Terzoli L (1980) Control of renin release: Experimental evidence and clinical implications. In: Laragh JH (ed) Topics in Hypertension. Yorke Medical Books, New York, pp 122–158
19. Seymour AA, Davis JO, Freeman RH, De Forrest JM, Rowe BP, Williams GM (1979) Renin release from filtering and nonfiltering kidneys stimulated by PGI_2 and PGD_2. Am J Physiol 237(4): F285–F290
20. Gerber JG, Keller RT, Nies AS (1979) Prostaglandins and renin release: The effect of PGI_2, PGE_2, and 13,14-dihydro PGE_2 on the baroreceptor mechanism of renin release in the dog. Circ Res 44: 796–799
21. Seymour AA, Zehr JE (1979) Influence of renal prostaglandin synthesis on renin control mechanisms in the dog. Circ Res 45: 13–25
22. Data JL, Gerber JG, Grump WJ, Fröhlich JC, Hollifield JW, Nies AS (1978) The prostaglandins system: A role in canine baroreceptor control of renin release. Circ Res 42: 454–458
23. Campbell WB, Graham RM, Jackson EK (1979) Role of renal prostaglandins in sympathetically mediated renin release in the rat. J Clin Invest 64: 448–456
24. Henrich WL, Schrier RW, Berl T (1979) Mechanisms of renin secretion during hemorrhage in the dog. J Clin Invest 64: 1–7
25. Vandongen R, Peart WS, Boyd GW (1974) Effect of angiotensin II and its nonpressor derivatives on renin secretion Am J Physiol 226: 277–282
26. Pettinger WA, Mitchell HC (1975) Renin release, saralasin and the vasodilator-beta-blocker drug interaction in man. N Engl J Med 292: 1214–1217
27. Leonetti G, Bianchini C, Terzoli L, Zanchetti A (in preparation) Captopril beta-blocker interaction in hypertensive patients.
28. Calaresu FR, Stella A, Zanchetti A (1976) Haemodynamic responses and renin release during stimulation of afferent renal nerves in the cat. J Physiol 255: 687–700
29. Thames MD, Di Bona GF (1979) Renal nerves modulate the secretion of renin mediated by non-neural mechanisms. Circ Res 44: 645–652
30. Stella A, Zanchetti A (1977) Effects of renal denervation on renin release in response to tilting and furosemide. Am J Physiol 232: H500–H507
31. Dampney RAL, Stella A, Golin R, Zanchetti A (1979) Vagal and sinoaortic reflexes in postural control of circulation and renin release. Am J Physiol 237: H146–H152
32. Stella A, Dampney RAL, Golin R, Zanchetti A (1978) Afferent vagal control of renin release in the anesthetized cat. Circ Res 43: I107–I111
33. Mancia G, Leonetti G, Terzoli L, Zanchetti A (1978) Reflex control of renin release in essential hypertension. Clin Sci Mol Med 54: 217–222
34. Mancia G, Ferrari A, Leonetti G, Gregorini L, Terzoli L, Bianchini C, Zanchetti A (in preparation) Carotid sinus reflex control of renin release in hypertensive subjects with high renin secretion.

Humoral Mechanisms of Renin Release

Alexander G. Logan and Alice Chatzilias

The important pathways involved in regulating renin release from the juxtaglomerular (JG) cells are illustrated in Fig. 1. While the role of the three main receptor pathways in mediating renin secretion has been extensively investigated, in comparison there is relatively little information about the sequence of biochemical and physiologic events that translate the signal from the receptor into a change in renin release. Useful models for in vitro studies of JG cell function are currently not available and studies on cellular mechanisms involved in renin release have relied on the use of intact tissue. Accordingly, evidence favoring certain mechanisms must be considered circumstantial and confirmation awaits the development of improved techniques.

Despite this qualification, a series of observations has been made which allows one to formulate a hypothesis on cellular events concerned in renin release. In this paper, these observations will be reviewed, and a general scheme of those mechanisms involved in beta-adrenergic-mediated renin secretion will be presented.

Stimulation of intrarenal beta-adrenergic receptors leads to an increase in renin secretion (1–4). This effect is presumed to be mediated by activation of adenyl cyclase and the formation of cyclic adenosine monophosphate (cyclic AMP). Support for this assumption is provided by the many observations that cyclic AMP, dibutyryl cyclic AMP analog, or inhibitors of phosphodiesterase such as theophylline stimulate renin secretion (5–7). Further, albeit, indirect evidence is the observation that in isolated smooth muscle cells, the beta-adrenergic receptor agonist, isoproterenol, causes a rise in cyclic AMP levels (8). Thus, it would be reasonable to conclude that the intracellular mediator of beta-adrenergic receptor stimulation is the adenylate cyclase–cyclic AMP system.

An important role for Ca^{2+} in the regulation of renin release was described by Vandongen and Peart (9) in 1974 and confirmed by Fray (10) in 1977. In Fray's study, the basal renin concentration in the perfusate in the absence of extracellular Ca^{2+} was approximately fivefold higher than when the concentration of Ca^{2+} in the perfusate was 7.5 mM. This observation contrasted sharply from the many that secretory tissue requires extracellular Ca^{2+} to release their packaged secretions (11). We found that the intrarenal arterial infusion of norepinephrine in pressor doses inhibited renin release (12). However, during Ca^{2+}-free perfusion, the pressor effect of norepinephrine was abolished and the renin-secreting potential of this agent was unmasked. It was presumed that norepinephrine stimulated renin secretion in this situation by activating beta-adrenergic receptors on the JG cell. We also assessed the effect of blocking the slow inward Ca^{2+} current on smooth muscle tone and renin release during the intrarenal arterial infusion of norepinephrine (12). In these experiments, either verapamil or manganese chloride was used and neither agent alone stimulated renin secretion. The norepinephrine-induced reduction in perfusate flow was attenuated or abolished and as in the Ca^{2+}-free perfusion experiments, the inhibitory effect on renin release was removed. These observations suggested that extracellular Ca^{2+} and net Ca^{2+} influx are not prerequisites for renin secretion. In addition, there appears to be a close relationship between net Ca^{2+} entry into cells and inhibition of renin release.

Experimental evidence has been accumulating to suggest that the prostaglandin (PG) system is involved in the control of renin release (13). Arachidonic acid is the PG precursor substance of prostacyclin (PGI_2) and PGE_2. PGI_2 is generated by the endothelial cells of the vascular tissue, whereas PGE_2 is synthesized in the renal medulla. The physiologic actions of PGI_2 and PGE_2 appear

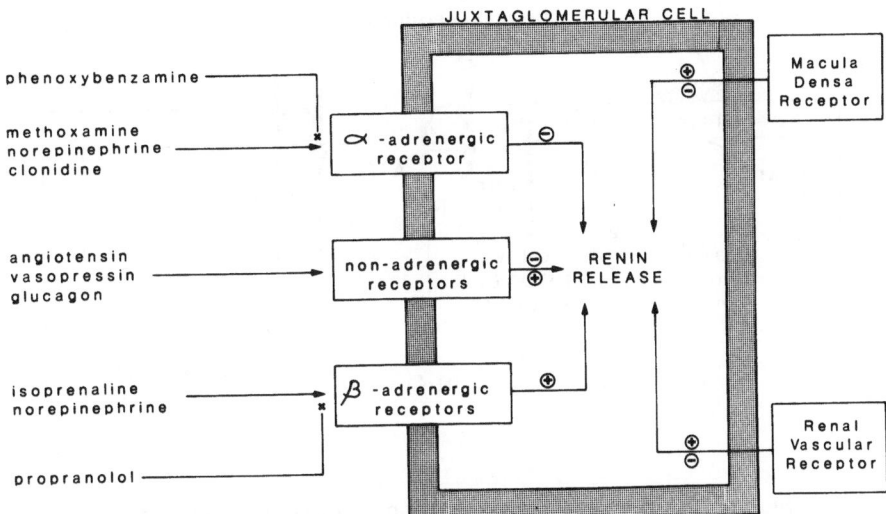

Fig. 1. Renal JG cell and its relationship to the three main receptor pathways involved in the regulation of renin release.

to be mediated through the adenylate cyclase–cyclic AMP system (14). We and others have observed an increase in renin secretion during the intrarenal arterial infusion of PGI_2 and PGE_2 (15–17). We found that PGE_2 was more effective in inducing a change in renin level than PGI_2.

Considerable evidence has accumulated to suggest that renin release evoked by activation of intrarenal stretch and macula densa receptors is PG mediated (18–20). On the other hand, renin secretion induced by direct stimulation of the JG cells may not be dependent on the PG system (15, 18). In the isolated rat kidney model, indomethacin was ineffective in attenuating isoproterenol-evoked renin release (15). Furthermore, similar results were obtained when meclofenamate was used as an alternative inhibitor of PG synthesis. Our observations are consistent with many, although not all, studies on this point (18, 21). We concluded that renal PGs do not appear to play an important role in mediating renin secretion induced by direct stimulation of beta-adrenergic receptors located on JG cells.

Changes in extracellular Na^+ concentration and transmembrane Na^+ gradient also appear to be important in the control of renin release (22–24), and may, in addition, play a role in mediating renin secretion induced by beta-adrenergic receptor agonists. A model for isoproterenol action of JG cells is shown schematically in Fig. 2. Stimulation of beta-adrenergic receptor leads to an in-

crease in intracellular cyclic AMP concentration. This, in turn, activates cyclic AMP-dependent protein kinase which could stimulate the cell membrane Na^+,K^+-ATPase. This enzyme system is involved in maintaining the appropriate concentration of cations across the cell membrane and appears to regulate intracellular ion activity (25). An increase in activity of this enzyme will cause extrusion of intracellular Na^+ and a net rise in intracellular K^+ level. Another mechanism regulating the concentration gradient of ions across cell membranes is the Na–Ca exchange (26). Entry of Na^+ into the cells is coupled to exit of Ca^{2+}. A rise in intracellular Na^+ concentration will lead to a rise in intracellular Ca^{2+} concentration.

The effect of isoproterenol on the influx and efflux of K^+ and Na^+ in isolated smooth muscle cells has recently been examined (8). K^+ influx and Na^+ efflux are increased in the presence of isoproterenol. These changes presumably are mediated by an increase in the activity of the Na^+,K^+-ATPase induced by isoproterenol.

It has been observed that ouabain, an inhibitor of Na^+,K^+-ATPase, inhibited renin release (23). In addition, reduction in extracellular Na^+ concentration inhibited the secretion of renin even with constant osmolality (22). These results suggested renin secretion was directly related to the transmembrane Na^+ gradient.

We recently completed some experiments to examine the effect of change in extracellular sodium

Juxtaglomerular Cell

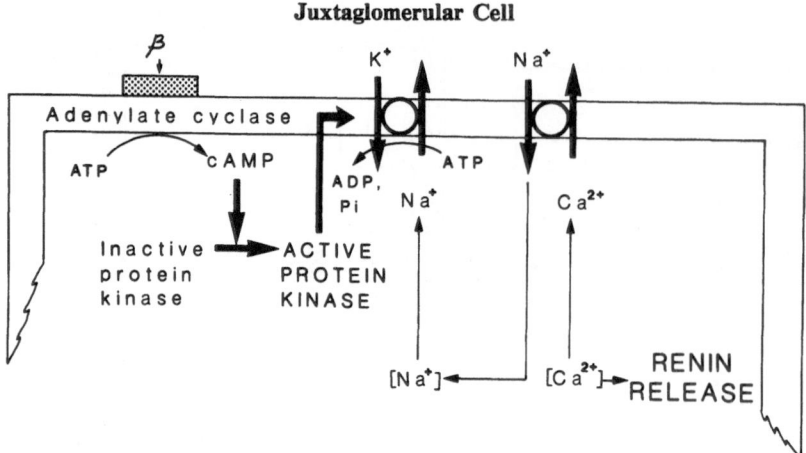

Fig. 2. Beta-adrenergic-mediated renin release from the JG cell.

and of ouabain on isoproterenol-induced renin release. When tetramethylammonium chloride was used as NaCl replacement, isoproterenol-induced renin secretion was abolished, even when manganese was added to the perfusate to block net Ca^{2+} influx. In another set of experiments, ouabain attenuated the rise in renin secretion evoked by isoproterenol. However, in contrast to the Na^+-free perfusion experiments, manganese blocked the inhibitory action of ouabain. It would, therefore, appear that isoproterenol stimulates renin secretion by increasing the transmembrane Na^+ gradient, which enhances the activity of the Na–K pump. Ouabain and zero extracellular Na^+ reduce the gradient and inhibit renin release. Inhibition of the Na–K pump by ouabain should enhance rat Ca^{2+} influx by causing some depolarization of the cell membrane. It was presumed that manganese blocked this movement and, by doing so, abolished the inhibitory effect of ouabain on renin release. In the Na^+-free experiments, on the other hand, despite the presence of manganese, isoproterenol failed to stimulate renin secretion, suggesting that the putative rise in free intracellular Ca^{2+} ion concentration was from some intracellular site.

In summary, the action of isoproterenol on renin release appears to be mediated through the changes in the adenylate cyclase–cyclic AMP system and transmembrane Na^+ gradient. On the other hand, isoproterenol-induced renin secretion does not depend on extracellular Ca^{2+}, net Ca^{2+} influx, and the PG system.

SUMMARY

The mechanism of beta-adrenergic-induced renin secretion is reviewed. The action of isoproterenol on renin release appears to be mediated through changes in the adenylate cyclase–cyclic AMP system and transmembrane Na^+ gradient. On the other hand, its effect does not depend on extracellular Ca^{2+}, net Ca^{2+} influx, and the PG system.

REFERENCES

1. Davis JO, Freeman RH (1976) Mechanisms regulating renin release. Physiol Rev 56: 1–56
2. Reid IA, Morris BJ, Ganong WF (1978) The renin-angiotensin system. Annu Rev Physiol 40: 377–410
3. Peart WS (1978) Renin release. Gen Pharmacacol 9: 65–72
4. Barajas L (1979) Anatomy of the juxtaglomerular apparatus. Am J Physiol 237: F333–F343
5. Winer N, Chokshi DS, Walkenhorst WG (1971) Effect of cyclic AMP, sympathomimetic amines and adrenergic receptor antagonists on renin secretion. Circ Res 29: 239–248
6. Winer N, Chokshi DS, Yoon MS, Freedman AD (1969) Adrenergic receptor mediation of renin secretion. J Clin Endocrinol Metab 29: 1168–1175
7. Nolly HL, Reid IA, Ganong WF (1974) Effect of theophylline and adrenergic blocking drugs on the renin response to norepinephrine. Circ Res 35: 575–579
8. Scheid CR, Honeyman TW, Fay FS (1979) Mecha-

nism of β-adrenergic relaxation of smooth muscle. Nature 277: 32–36

9. Vandongen R, Peart WS (1974) Calcium dependence of the inhibitory effect of angiotensin on renin secretion in the isolated perfused kidney of the rat. Br J Pharmacol 50: 125–129

10. Fray JCS (1977) Stimulation of renin release in perfused kidney by low calcium and high magnesium. Am J Physiol: 232: F377–F382

11. Rubin RP (1970) The role of calcium in the release of neurotransmitter substances and hormones. Pharmacol Rev 22: 389–428

12. Logan AG, Chatzilias A (1980) The role of calcium in the control of renin release from the isolated rat kidney. Can J Physiol Pharmacol 58: 60–66

13. Dunn MJ, Hood VL (1977) Prostaglandins and the kidney. Am J Physiol 233: F169–F184

14. Herman CA, Zenser TV, Davis BB (1979) Comparison of the effects of prostaglandin I_2 and prostaglandin E_2 stimulation of the rat kidney adenylate cyclase-cyclic AMP systems. Biochim Biophys Acta 582: 496–503

15. Logan AG, Chatzilias A (1978) The role of prostaglandins on renin release in the isolated perfused rat kidney. Kidney Int 14: 697

16. Gerber JG, Keller RT, Nies AS (1979) Prostaglandins and renin release: The effect of PGI_2, PGE_2, and 13,14-dihydro PGE_2 on the baroreceptor mechanism of renin release in the dog. Circ Res 44: 796-799

17. Seymour AA, Davis JO, Freeman RH, DeForrest JM, Rowe BP, Williams GM (1979) Renin release from filtering and nonfiltering kidneys stimulated by PGI_2 and PGD_2. Am J Physiol 237: F285–F290

18. Berl T, Henrich WL, Erickson AL, Schrier RW (1979) Prostaglandins in the beta-adrenergic and baroreceptor-mediated secretion of renin. Am J Physiol 236: F472-F477

19. Blackshear JL, Spielman WS, Knox FG, Romero JC (1979) Dissociation of renin release and renal vasodilation by prostaglandin synthesis inhibitors. Am J Physiol 237: F20–F24

20. Henrich WL, Schrier RW, Berl T (1979) Mechanisms of renin secretion during hemorrhage in the dog. J Clin Invest 64: 1–7

21. Campbell WB, Graham RM, Jackson EK (1979) Role of renal prostaglandins in sympathetically mediated renin release in the rat. J Clin Invest 64: 448–456

22. Capponi AM, Vallotton MB (1976) Renin release by rat kidney slices incubated in vitro: Role of sodium and of α- and β-adrenergic receptors, and effect of vincristine. Circ Res 39: 200–203

23. Churchill PC, McDonald FD (1974) Effect of ouabain on renin secretion in anaesthetized dogs. J Physiol (Lond) 242: 635–646

24. Churchill PC, McDonald FD, Churchill MC (1979) Phenytoin stimulates renin secretion from rat kidney slices. J Pharmacol Exp Ther 211: 615–619

25. Schwartz A (1976) Cell membrane Na^+,K^+-ATPase and sarcoplasmic reticulum: Possible regulators of intracellular ion activity. Fed Proc 35: 1279–1282

26. Lang S, Blaustein (1980) The role of the sodium pump in the control of vascular tone in the rat. Circ Res 46: 463–470

Intrarenal Renin–Angiotensin–Sodium Interdependent Renal Vasoconstriction Mechanism Controlling Postclamp Renal Artery Pressure and Renin Release in Chronic One-Kidney, One-Clip Goldblatt Hypertensive Dog

Martha G. Stoddard, Kenneth M. Baker, and Carlos R. Ayers

This work on renovascular hypertension was initiated in an attempt to answer several questions. First, why does plasma renin activity return to normal levels within 24–48 h after producing one-kidney, one-clip Goldblatt hypertension in the dog? Second, why do some patients maintain normal plasma renin activity and blood pressure despite developing severe renovascular occlusion?

We began to study these questions by developing a conscious dog model so that we could study renal function and plasma renin activity in the conscious unstressed state. Teflon catheters were placed in the inferior vena cava, aorta, and left renal artery so that pressures could be measured, blood samples obtained, and infusions made. A snare around the left renal artery enabled us to produce a gradient in the conscious unstressed condition (Fig. 1).

The first series of experiments evaluated renal function and hemodynamics after renal artery constriction. We found that, after producing an initial gradient of 35 mmHg, the aortic pressure began to increase within 5 min. Within the first hour, after an initial period of renal vasodilatation, renal vasoconstriction occurred. Renal artery pressure distal to the clamp began to increase and progressed so that by the end of the first 24 h, the renal artery pressure had returned to control levels and the aortic pressure was 35 mmHg above the control levels. This renal vasoconstriction reduced renal blood flow by approximately one-third as measured by [133]Xenon washout technique (1). Clearances of ^{3}H-PAH and ^{14}C-insulin demonstrated decreases in renal plasma flow and glomerular filtration. The fall in PAH clearance was proportionally greater, consistent with an increase in filtration fraction (2).

When we initiated these studies, it was felt that the mean arterial pressure, an indicator of blood volume, was the important regulator of renin release. The hypothesis that renal arteriolar vasoconstriction increased intrarenal pressure, thus suppressing renin release, was tested by infusing small doses of vasodilators into the renal artery,

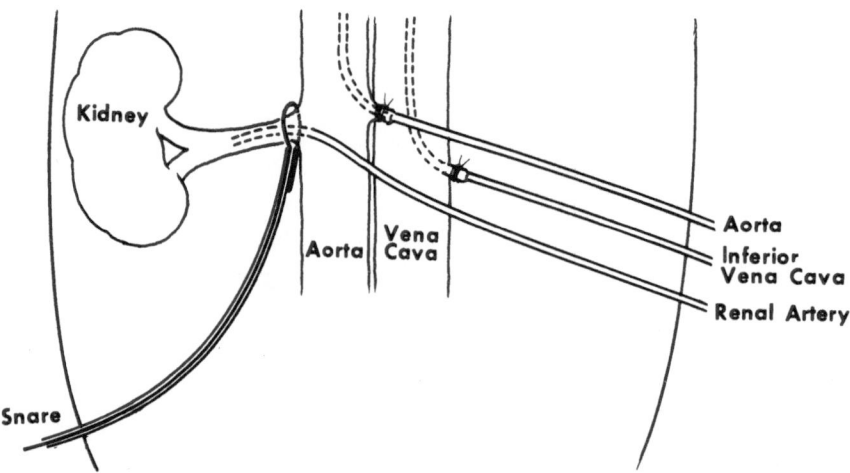

Fig. 1. Catheter and snare placement in the one-kidney, one-clip conscious dog model.

sufficient to produce a decrease in renal artery pressure distal to the renal artery occlusion without decreasing systemic pressure. Dopamine, acetylcholine, nitroprusside, and hydralazine all vasodilated the renal vasculature, decreased renal artery pressure, and markedly stimulated renin release (2). Another observation made in renovascular hypertension during renal vasodilatation with these drugs was a decrease in intrarenal pressure often sufficient to decrease filtration pressure to the point of cessation of urine flow. The same dose of these drugs when given into the renal artery of normal dogs on a low- and normal-salt diet produced an increase in renal blood flow, no change in renal artery pressure and less renin release, suggesting that the difference in stimulus for renin release was the change in intrarenal pressure.

We hypothesized that, after an initial period of renal vasodilatation, described by others as autoregulation and suggested to be mediated at least in part by prostaglandins, vasoconstriction began, with the vasoconstriction intrarenal pressure increased to control levels, resulting in a decrease in renin release and preservation of glomerular filtration pressure. We felt that the vasoconstriction was mediated by the renin–angiotensin system, but it was not until blockers of the renin–angiotensin system became available that we could test this hypothesis. Both Sar[1]-Ala[8]-angiotensin II and the converting enzyme inhibitor, teprotide (SQ 20881), produced a decrease in intrarenal vascular resistance, as demonstrated by a decrease in renal artery pressure distal to the renal artery occlusion when these blockers were given in small enough doses not to effect mean aortic pressure. The infusion of these blockers of the renin–angiotensin system caused a marked increase in plasma renin activity (Fig. 2); in some dogs, the decrease in intrarenal pressure was associated with cessation of urine flow (3). These findings supported our hypothesis that the renal vasoconstriction and negative feedback mechanism on renin release in renovascular hypertension was mediated by angiotensin II. In normal dogs at different levels of dietary sodium intake, intrarenal blockade of the renin–angiotensin system for 30 min produced no change in renal artery pressure and approximately a twofold increase in plasma renin activity as compared to a four- to five-fold increase in plasma renin activity during intrarenal blockade of the system in renovascular hypertension (4).

Response to Intrarenal Blockade of Angiotensin II
Early One Kidney Goldblatt Hypertensive Dog,
Normal Sodium

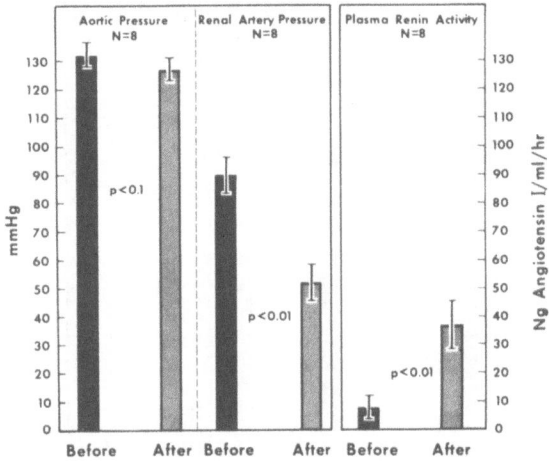

Fig. 2. Intrarenal infusion of teprotide (SQ 20881) produced a marked decrease in postclamp renal artery pressure and a marked increase in plasma renin activity during approximately the first 10 days after partial renal artery stenosis.

This finding suggests that the decrease in poststenotic renal artery pressure during blockade of the renin–angiotensin system is part of the stimulus for the increased renin release.

When a one-kidney, one-clip Goldblatt hyper-

Response to Intrarenal Blockade of Angiotensin II
Chronic One Kidney Goldblatt Hypertensive Dog,
Normal Sodium

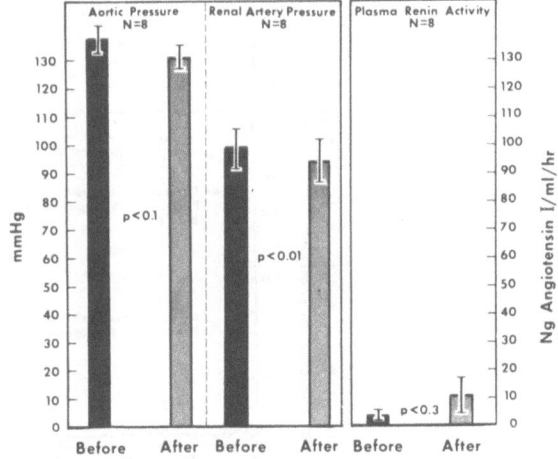

Fig. 3. After approximately 10 days, intrarenal blockade of the intrarenal renin–angiotensin system produced a small decrease in intrarenal pressure and no significant increase in plasma renin activity.

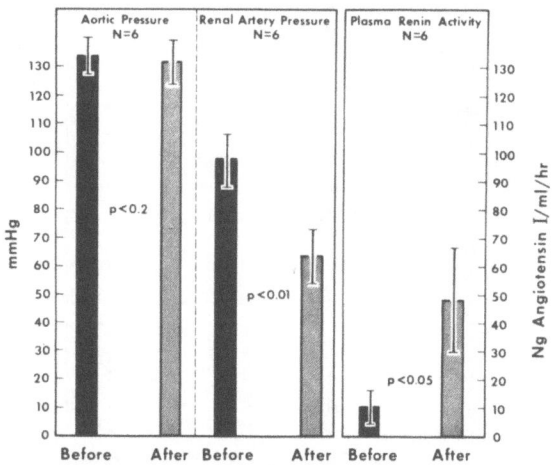

Response to Intrarenal Blockade of Angiotensin II
Chronic One Kidney Goldblatt Hypertensive Dog,
Low Sodium

Fig. 4. Approximately 5 days of a low-sodium intake will revert the dogs to a state so that intrarenal blockade of the renin–angiotensin system will again decrease intrarenal pressure and markedly increase plasma renin activity.

tension dog is followed, there is temporarily less and less renin released during intrarenal blockade of the renin–angiotensin system. After approximately 10 days, there is essentially no decrease in poststenotic renal artery pressure during intrarenal blockade of the renin–angiotensin system.

The quantity of renin released also decreases and approximates that seen in normal dogs on the same dietary sodium intake (Fig. 3), further supporting the hypothesis that poststenotic renal artery pressure is important in controlling renin release in renovascular hypertension (5). After the animals reach this point, a low-sodium intake (< 10 mEq/day for 5 days) will return them to a state where blockade of the renin–angiotensin system will again produce a marked decrease in poststenotic renal artery pressure and a large increment in plasma renin activity (Fig. 4). They can be transformed repeatedly from an angiotensin-dependent to a nonangiotensin-dependent intrarenal vasoconstriction by alternating sodium restriction and sodium loading (80 mEq/day sodium), demonstrating a sodium–angiotensin II-interdependent renal vasoconstriction controlling renin release and renal function (Fig. 5).

Just how sodium intake affects this intrarenal vasoconstriction is unclear. We thought that total body sodium might somehow control or influence the conversion of an angiotensin-dependent vasoconstriction to a sodium-dependent vasoconstriction. We tested this by studying this intrarenal mechanism in a two-kidney, one-clip dog model which would be expected to have less volume than the one-kidney model. We found that after partial renal artery occlusion, the plasma renin activity and mean arterial pressure increased in parallel,

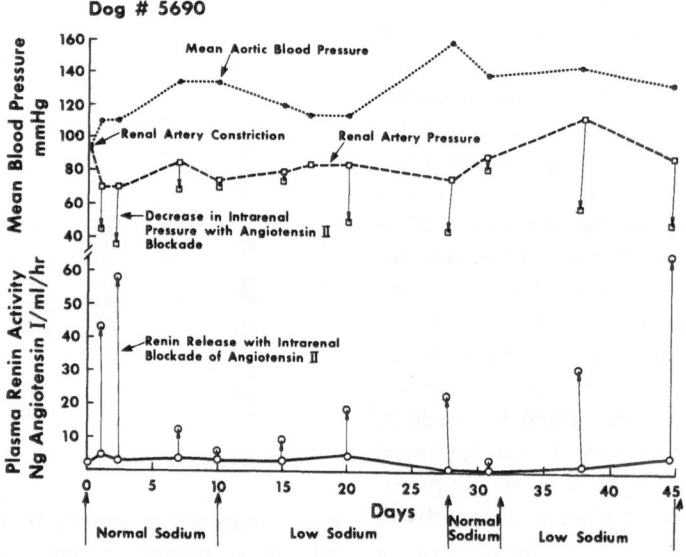

Fig. 5. Repeated transformation of an angiotensin-dependent to a nonangiotensin-dependent renal vasoconstriction mechanism controlling renin release in a dog followed for 45 days.

but that within 5–10 days both plasma renin activity and mean arterial blood pressure had returned to normal. The intrarenal pressure of the stenosed kidney and the plasma renin activity response to intrarenal blockade of the renin–angiotensin system were similar to the one-kidney, one-clip Goldblatt hypertension model, except it took on the average of 27 days instead of 10 days to reach the state of nonangiotensin II-dependent intrarenal vasoconstriction. This suggests that volume may be important in determining the rate of conversion to a nonangiotensin-dependent renal vasoconstriction.

The sodium–angiotensin-dependent negative feedback mechanism on renin release may be important in human hypertension. It could determine whether hypertension occurs after developing renal artery stenosis, and, when hypertension develops, it could dictate its severity. It could also be important in determining the amount of renin released and severity of hypertension in other renal diseases, especially those involving the renal vasculature, such as scleroderma. This mechanism could also be important in controlling renin release in essential hypertension, especially in those with nephrosclerosis.

SUMMARY

In one-kidney, one-clip Goldblatt hypertension, there is an initial increase in plasma renin activity followed by a return to control level within 24–48 h. This is paralleled by an initial decrease in postclip renal artery pressure, and then an increase in renal artery pressure to control level. The increase in postclip renal artery pressure is due to intrarenal vasoconstriction mediated by angiotensin II. The initial angiotensin II-dependent renal vasoconstriction becomes nonangiotensin dependent in approximately 10 days. The renal vasoconstriction can be repeatedly transformed from an angiotensin II-dependent to a nonangiotensin II-dependent state by alternating high- and low-dietary intake of sodium. These findings support the concept of an angiotensin II–sodium interdependent renal vasoconstriction negative feedback mechanism controlling renin release.

ACKNOWLEDGMENT

This work was supported in part by NHLBI Training Grant 5 T32HL07355 and NHLBI Research Grant R016044.

REFERENCES

1. Harris RH Jr, Ayers CR (1972) Renal hemodynamics and plasma renin activity after renal artery constriction in conscious dogs. Circ Res 31: 520–530
2. Ayers CR, Harris RH Jr, Lefer LG (1969) Control of renin release in experimental hypertension. Circ Res 24, 25(Suppl I): 103–112
3. Ayers CR, Vaughan ED Jr, Yancey MR, Bing KT, Johnson CC, Morton CL (1974) Effect of 1-sarcosine-8-alanine angiotensin II and converting enzyme inhibitor on renin release in dog acute renovascular hypertension. Circ Res 34, 35(Suppl I): 27–33
4. Kimbrough HM, Vaughan ED Jr, Carey RM, Ayers CR (1977) Effect of intrarenal angiotensin II on renal function in conscious dogs. Circ Res 40(2): 174–177
5. Ayers CR, Katholi RE, Vaughan ED Jr, Carey RM, Kimbrough HM, Yancey MR, Morton CL (1977) Intrarenal renin-angiotensin sodium interdependent mechanism controlling post clamp renal artery pressure and renin release in the conscious dog with chronic one-kidney Goldblatt hypertension. Circ Res 40(3): 238–242

Renin Responsiveness to Neural and Nonneural-Mediated Stimuli in the Renin Subgroups of Essential Hypertension

Alberto Morganti, Thomas G. Pickering, Jorge A. Lopez-Ovejero, and John H. Laragh

The mechanisms responsible for the differences in renin secretion among the renin subgroups of essential hypertension are controversial (1). None of the theories proposed to explain renin suppression in patients with low-renin hypertension has received general consent (2, 3); on the other hand, high-renin levels, which were originally attributed to severe vascular damage of the kidneys (4), are often present even in young patients with mild, uncomplicated, essential hypertension (5). Also, the hypothesis of Esler et al. (5, 6) that the high- and low-renin levels of renin may reflect, respectively, a hyper- and hypoadrenergic activity, has been recently denied by other investigators (7, 8).

To examine the alternative possibility that the renin subgroups might instead differ specifically in the sensitivity of the juxtaglomerular apparatus to adrenergic stimulation, we evaluated plasma catecholamines and renin responses to neural (head-up tilt) and nonneural (dietary sodium restriction) stimuli in a group of patients preclassified as having high, normal, and low renin.

MATERIALS AND METHODS

Forty-three hospitalized patients with established uncomplicated essential hypertension, aged 16–64 were entered into this study. After discontinuation of all the antihypertensive medications, they were admitted to the metabolic ward where they received a constant diet containing 100 mEq sodium and 60 mEq potassium/day. While in balance on this diet, the renin status was defined as high in 15, normal in 21, and low in 7 patients (4). The morning after renin profiling the patients were put supine for 60 min, after which a sequence of baseline sphygmomanometric arterial pressure and heart rate measurements were recorded and baseline blood samples for plasma renin activity, plasma norepinephrine, and epinephrine determinations were collected. The patients were then tilted to the 65°-head-up position and blood samples collected again after 15 and 30 min of tilt; blood pressure and heart rate were measured every 2 min during tilt. In 18 patients (6 high, 7 normal, and 5 low renin), sodium intake was then reduced to 10 mEq/day, and after 4–5 days on this diet, blood pressure, heart rate, plasma catecholamines, and renin activity were again measured in the supine position.

Plasma catecholamines were determined by radioimmunoassay according to Passon and Peuler (9), and plasma renin activity by radioimmunoassay according to Sealey and Laragh (10). Statistical significance was tested by Student's t-test for unpaired and paired data. Correlation coefficients have been calculated by Pearson's test.

RESULTS

High-renin patients were younger than those with normal and low renin (33.4 ± 2.6 versus 45.2 ± 2.2 and 50.8 ± 2.0 years) and had a shorter duration of hypertension (5.3 ± 1.3 versus 8.1 ± 1.6 and 16.4 ± 2.8 years). In the supine position, mean blood pressure was similar (high 117 ± 5, normal 128 ± 4, low 125 ± 12 mmHg) as well as heart rate, plasma norepinephrine, and epinephrine (Fig. 1). In contrast, plasma renin activity was always different ($p < 0.01$ at least).

RESPONSE TO HEAD-UP TILT ON 100 mEq SODIUM INTAKE

During tilt, six patients with high renin and one with normal renin fainted, and their data were

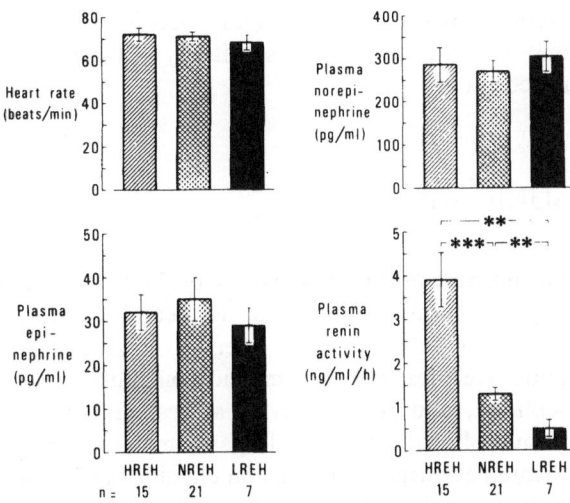

Fig. 1. Mean values of heart rate, plasma catecholamines, and renin activity in patients with high (HREH), normal (NREH), and low (LREH) renin essential hypertension in the supine position. Results represent mean ± SEM. * Statistical significance of the differences among the subgroups: *$p < 0.05$; **$p < 0.01$; ***$p < 0.001$.

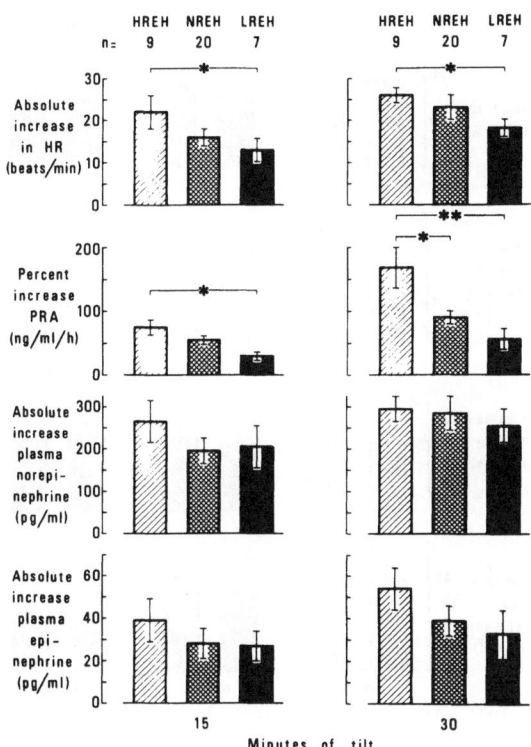

Fig. 2. Effects of 15 *(left panel)* and 30 *(right panel)* min of 65°-head-up tilt on heart rate, plasma renin activity, and plasma catecholamines in the three subgroups while in balance on 100-mEq sodium intake. Data from patients who fainted during tilt (see text) have been excluded. Abbreviations and statistical significance as in Fig. 1.

excluded from the analysis. A similar slight increase in diastolic blood pressure was observed during tilt in all the subgroups, whereas systolic blood pressure had a slight decrease only in normal- and low-renin patients. Heart rate response was greater in the high-renin group (Fig. 2), whereas the increases in norepinephrine and epinephrine were similar and correlated to each other ($p < 0.01$).

The tilt-induced absolute increments in renin were different among the subgroups at 15 and 30 min of tilt (high 3.1 ± 1.1 and 6.1 ± 2.2, normal 0.6 ± 0.1 and 1.2 ± 0.2, low 0.17 ± 0.05 and 0.26 ± 0.07 ng/ml/h, $p < 0.01$ for all); these increases in renin were different between high- and low-renin patients, even when expressed as percent of supine values (Fig. 2).

The absolute increments of renin during tilt were directly correlated with those of norepinephrine within the normal-renin group ($p < 0.01$) and inversely correlated with age in the overall population ($p < 0.01$).

RESPONSE TO SODIUM RESTRICTION

The three subgroups responded to sodium restriction with similar decrements in body weight and

with a slight decrease in supine blood pressure; heart rate increased slightly in the high-renin group, while plasma catecholamines were always unchanged (Fig. 3).

The increments in renin were, in absolute values, greater in high- than in low-renin patients (5.0 ± 1.2 versus 1.2 ± 0.4 ng/ml/h) but smaller, although not significantly, when expressed in percent of the values observed before sodium restriction (97 ± 24 versus 257 ± 106%). No correlation was found between age and the increments in renin.

DISCUSSION

Our data show that the renin responsiveness to similar increases in sympathetic activity elicited by head-up tilt is significantly greater in high- than

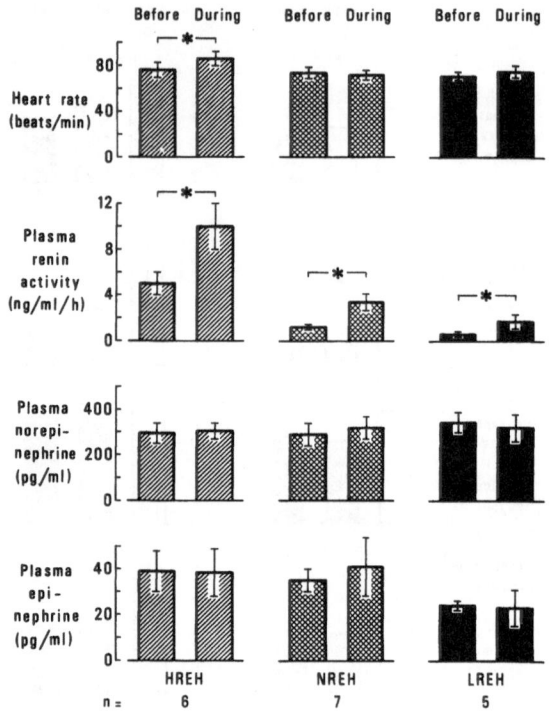

Fig. 3. Mean values of supine heart rate, plasma renin activity, and plasma catecholamines in the three subgroups before *(left column of each panel)* and during *(right column)* dietary sodium restriction. Abbreviations and statistical significance as in Fig. 1.

in low-renin patients, whereas that to sodium depletion is similar or, if anything, greater in the low-renin subgroup.

Our previous work has shown that the renin response to this degree of tilt is, in patients with essential hypertension, entirely under neural control (11); in contrast, the renin responses to dietary sodium restriction seem mediated through non-neural mechanisms since, in this study, they were not associated with increments in plasma catecholamines and, as previously shown by Bravo et al. (12), cannot be prevented by prior beta-adrenergic blockade.

Thus, the differences in renin responses to tilt cannot be attributed to a generalized hyper-and hyposensitivity of the high- and low-renin subgroups to any type of stimulus related, for instance, to an unspecific factor such as age, but rather to specific differences in renin responsiveness to sympathetic stimulation. Since the renin response to the tilt-induced neural stimulus is mediated through the juxtaglomerular beta-adrenoreceptors, we suggest that the differences in renin se-

cretion between the high- and low-renin subgroups may reflect differences in sensitivity of these adrenoreceptors.

SUMMARY

The purpose of this study was to evaluate the renin responsiveness to neural and nonneural stimuli in the renin subgroups of essential hypertension. Thus, we measured plasma norepinephrine, epinephrine, and renin activity at rest and during 30 min of head-up tilt in 43 patients with uncomplicated essential hypertension classified as having high, normal, and low renin while on a sodium intake of 100 mEq/day; in addition, we repeated the same measurements, at rest, in 18 patients after dietary sodium restriction.

On 100-mEq sodium intake, supine plasma catecholamines concentrations were similar, whereas plasma renin activity was always different among the subgroups. Head-up tilt caused similar increments in norepinephrine and epinephrine but significantly greater percent renin responses in high-than in low-renin patients. In contrast, dietary sodium restriction caused similar percent increments in supine renin without inducing changes in plasma catecholamines.

We conclude that the high- and low-renin subgroups have specific differences in renin responsiveness to neural stimulation.

ACKNOWLEDGMENT

We are indebted to Patricia Sulivan for her excellent nursing assistance.

REFERENCES

1. Mitchell JR, Taylor AA, Pool JL, Lake CR, Rollins DE, Bartter FC (1977) NIH conference: Renin-aldosterone profiling in hypertension. Ann Intern Med 87: 596–612
2. Dunn MJ, Tannen RL (1974) Low renin hypertension. Kid Int 5: 317–325
3. Ganguly A, Weinberger M (1979) Low renin hypertension: A current review of definitions and controversies. Am Heart J 98: 642–652

4. Brunner HR, Laragh JH, Baer L, Newton MA, Goodwin FT, Krakoff LR, Bard HR, Bühler FR (1972) Essential hypertension: Renin and aldosterone, heart attack and stroke. New Engl J Med 286: 441–449

5. Esler M, Julius J, Zweigler A, Randall O, Harburg E, Gardiner H, DeQuattro V (1977) Mild high-renin essential hypertension. New Engl J Med 296: 405–411

6. Esler M, Randall O, Bennet J, Zweigler A, Julius S, Rydeleck P (1976) Suppression of sympathetic nervous function in low renin essential hypertension. Lancet 2: 115–118

7. Taylor AA, Pool JL, Lake RC, Ziegler MG, Rosen AA, Rollins DE, Mitchell JR (1978) Plasma norepinephrine concentrations: No differences among normal volunteers and low, high or normal renin hypertensive patients. Life Sci 22: 1499–1510

8. Bühler FR, Bertel O, Kiowski DW (1978) Plasma noradrenaline and adrenaline and β-adrenoreceptor responsiveness in renin subgroups of essential hypertension. Clin Sci Mol Med 55: 57S–60S

9. Passon PG, Peuler JD (1973) A simplified radiometric assay for plasma norepinephrine and epinephrine. Ann Biochem 51: 618–631

10. Sealey JE, Laragh JH (1977) How to do a plasma renin assay. Cardiovasc Med 2: 1079–1092

11. Morganti A, Lopez-Ovejero JA, Pickering TG, Laragh JH (1979) The role of the sympathetic nervous system in mediating the renin response to head up tilt and their possible synergism in defending blood pressure against postural changes during sodium deprivation. Am J Cardiol 43: 600–604

12. Bravo EL, Tarazi RC, Dustan HP (1974) On the mechanism of suppressed plasma renin activity during beta-adrenergic blockade with propranolol. J Lab Clin Med 83: 119–128

Alpha- and Beta-Adrenoreceptors and Renin Release

U. Kopp, M. Aurell, I-M. Nilsson, M. Sjölander, and B. Åblad

There is considerable evidence that three primary mechanisms are involved in the control of renin release from the juxtaglomerular granular cells (1, 2): the direct sympathetic nervous control mediated by beta-adrenoreceptors on the juxtaglomerular granular cells, the baroreceptor, and the macula densa mechanisms. The latter two mechanisms are influenced indirectly by renal sympathetic nerve activity which, by causing alpha-adrenoreceptor-mediated vasoconstriction, produces a reduction in renal blood flow (RBF) and glomerular filtration rate.

The present study aimed at exploring the relative contribution of alpha- and beta-adrenoreceptors to the renin release produced by graded levels of renal nerve stimulation (RNS) in the anesthetized dog. Pharmacologic antagonists used were metoprolol, a beta-1-selective adrenoreceptor antagonist, *dl*-propranolol, a nonselective beta-adrenoreceptor antagonist, *d*-propranolol, which has the same membrane-stabilizing properties as *dl*-propranolol, but almost completely lacks its beta-blocking activity, and phenoxybenzamine (POB), an alpha-adrenoreceptor antagonist.

In each experiment, two 10-min periods of RNS at the same frequency were used, separated by an interval of 40 min, during which the blocking agents were administered. Low-level RNS, defined as that frequency which reduced RBF less than 5% (requiring frequencies between 0.5 and 1 Hz), resulted in renin release that was reduced by metoprolol (0.5 mg/kg i.v.) and by *dl*-propranolol (0.5 mg/kg i.v.) by 81% ± 12% and 87% ± 8% ($p < 0.01$), respectively. *d*-Propranolol, in the same dose, did not significantly affect the renin-release response to RNS. High-level RNS, defined by the frequency-reducing RBF by 50% (requiring frequencies between 2 and 3 Hz), resulted in renin release that was reduced only by 34% ± 11% by metoprolol (0.5 mg/kg). The dose of 2.0 mg/kg i.v. of metoprolol did not reduce the renin release further. The renal vasoconstrictor response to RNS was not affected by the drug. *dl*-Propranolol (0.5 mg/kg i.v.) produced the same reduction in renin release as metoprolol. Intrarenal administration of POB (0.6 μg/kg/min for 30 min) almost completely blocked the vasoconstrictor response to RNS and reduced the renin-release response by 50% ± 7% ($p < 0.01$). The combination of metoprolol (2.0 mg/g i.v.) and POB (0.6 μg/kg/min i.a.) resulted in an almost total abolition of the renal vasoconstrictor response and a 94% ± 4% inhibition of the renin-release response to RNS ($p < 0.01$).

Our interpretation of these results is shown in Fig. 1. RNS, at a frequency less than 1 Hz, which barely reduced RBF, results in renin release that is mainly mediated by beta-adrenoreceptors. These observations are in agreement with the results of the study of Taher et al. (3), which showed that *dl*-propranolol blocked the renin-release response to low-level RNS. Our study further indicates that the beta-adrenoreceptors involved are of the beta$_1$-subtype. Stimulation of the renal nerves at a higher frequency results in a more pronounced vasoconstriction and renin release, which is only partly mediated by beta-adrenoreceptors. The remaining portion of the renin release derives from alpha-adrenoreceptor-mediated renal vasoconstriction, which can be expected to activate the renin release via the baroreceptor and the macula densa mechanism.

In an additional study, we have examined the role of prostaglandins in the renin-release response to graded levels of RNS. Low-level RNS, which produced only minimal renal vasoconstriction, resulted in a renin release unaffected by prostaglandin synthesis inhibition (PSI) with indomethacin or diclofenac sodium (5 mg/kg i.v.). In contrast, high-level RNS resulted in renin release which was

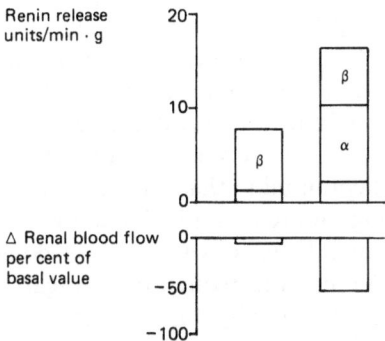

Fig. 1. Effects of low- and high-renal nerve stimulation (6). Left column: low level; right column: high level renal nerve stimulation.

inhibited by indomethacin or diclofenac sodium by $31\% \pm 8\%$ ($p < 0.01$). The vasoconstrictor response to RNS was not altered by the drugs. A combination of indomethacin or diclofenac sodium (5 mg/kg i.v.) plus metoprolol (0.5 mg/kg i.v.) resulted in a further reduction of the renin-release response. The reduction produced was $61\% \pm 7\%$ ($p < 0.01$).

These observations suggest that renal prostaglandins are not involved in beta-adrenoreceptor-mediated renin release. This finding supports results of other studies which have shown that prostaglandins are not involved in isoproterenol-induced renin release (4, 5). Our results indicate, however, that prostaglandins are involved in the renin release following alpha-adrenergic vasoconstriction.

In conclusion, our findings indicate an important role for a neuronally controlled beta₁-adrenoreceptor mechanism in the regulation of renin release. In addition, the present findings show that renal sympathetic nerves induce renin release through an alpha-adrenoreceptor mechanism at levels of discharge that produce more marked renal vasoconstriction. The chain of effect involves includes a significant prostaglandin release.

SUMMARY

The relative contribution of alpha- and beta-adrenoreceptors to the renin release produced by graded levels of RNS was studied in the anesthetized dog. Two different ranges of RNS were used: low-level RNS, defined by the frequency (0.5–1 Hz) producing 5% reduction of RBF; and high-level RNS, defined by the frequency (2–3 Hz) producing 50% reduction of RBF. The pharmacologic antagonists used were metoprolol, a beta₁-adrenoreceptor antagonist, dl-propranolol, a nonselective beta-adrenoreceptor antagonist, and POB, an alpha-adrenoreceptor antagonist. The renin-release response to RNS was evaluated before and after blockade.

Low level RNS resulted in renin release, which was reduced by metoprolol (0.5 mg/kg i.v.) and by propranolol (0.5 mg/kg i.v.) by $81\% \pm 12\%$ and $87\% \pm 8\%$, respectively. High level RNS resulted in renin release, which was reduced by metoprolol (0.5 mg/kg i.v.) by $34\% \pm 11\%$, POB (0.6 μg/kg/min i.a.) by $50\% \pm 7\%$. The vasoconstrictor response to RNS was unaffected by metoprolol but abolished by POB.

Taken together, the results indicate that the renin-release response to low-level RNS is almost completely mediated by beta₁-adrenoreceptors, while the renin-release response to high-level RNS is only partly mediated by beta₁-adrenoreceptors. The remaining portion derives from alpha-adrenoreceptor-mediated vasoconstriction.

REFERENCES

1. Davis JO, Freeman RH (1976) Mechanisms regulating renin release. Physiol Rev 56: 1–56
2. Reid IA, Morris BJ, Cianong WF (1978) The renin-angiotensin system. Annu Rev Physiol 40: 377–410
3. Taher MS, McLain LG, McDonald KM, Schrier RW (1976) Effect of beta-adrenergic blockade of renin response to renal nerve stimulation. J Clin Invest 57: 459–465
4. Berl T, Heinrich WL, Eriksson AL, Schrier RW (1979) Prostaglandins in the beta-adrenergic and baroreceptor mediated secretion of renin. Am J Physiol 236(5): F472–F477
5. Fröhlich JC, Hollifield JW, Oates JA (1976) Effects of indomethacin on isoproterenol-induced renin release. Clin Res 24: 9A
6. Kopp U (1980) Mechanisms involved in the neural control of renin release. Doctoral dissertation. University of Göteborg, pp 1–68

DISCUSSION

Dr. Frolich (Stüttgart, West Germany): I would like to make a brief comment concerning the renin–prostaglandin interaction. The data on beta-stimulation of renin release confirmed what we found in man, namely, that isoproterenol-induced renin release cannot be blocked by indomethacin. I would like to point out, however, that Pettinger's group has shown that in the intact rats isoproterenol-induced renin release can be blocked by indomethacin. I would also like to make a comment concerning Dr. Logan's paper on the effectivity of PGE_2 to cause renin release in the isolated perfused kidney. PGE_2 is a vasodilator and, as such, would be expected to cause renin release. In the dog, infusion of doses of prostacyclin and PGE_2, which had similar hemodynamic effects, showed that prostacyclin was much more powerful in releasing renin; in our studies using kidney slices in vitro, we could not show any affect of PGE_2 on renin release in contrast to PGI_2, which was as powerful as isoproterenol in causing renin release.

Dr. Logan (Toronto, Canada): In our preparation (isolated perfused rat kidney model), there was no change in perfusate flow either with PGI_2 or PGE_2. We, therefore, didn't feel that the effect was mediated through a differential vasodilatory effect. There are conflicting reports about PGE_2 stimulating renin release. Some reports, like yours, show that it doesn't stimulate, while other studies have confirmed our results.

Dr. Ayers (Charlottesville, Va.): I would like to comment on one project that we have done, that is, stimulation of intrarenal receptor with methoxamine. We found that with alpha$_1$-receptor stimulation of a magnitude that will decrease renal blood flow by approximately 50% or more, a marked increase in renin release is obtained, which can be blocked with indomethacin, so I think that the observation of Dr. Kopp's that renal nerve stimulation of renin through the alpha-adrenergic receptor is correct.

Dr. Bühler (Basel, Switzerland): I was pleased to see Dr. Morganti's data which confirm our reports finding normal, but not low-catecholamine concentrations, as well as blunted heart rate responses in the low-renin patients that we find to be paralleled by reduced isoproterenol sensitivity. I now wonder whether you might not consider the postulate of a generalized defect in beta-adrenoreceptor-mediated responses in those low-renin patients which relate to the heart, kidney, and the peripheral circulation. Such a defect may help explain the hyporesponsive renin and some of the hemodynamic characteristics of low-renin essential hypertension.

Dr. Morganti (Milan, Italy): I did not discuss this point because of time. I believe that the smaller increments in heart rate during tilt in low-renin patients might also reflect decreased sensitivity of the cardiac beta-adrenoreceptors. However, it must be kept in mind that the increments in heart rate during tilt are partially due to the withdrawal of parasympathetic activity, since we do not know whether or not the reduction in vagal tone was similar among the subgroups. We must be cautious in attributing the differences in heart rate response to tilt only to differences in cardiac beta-adrenoreceptor responsiveness.

Dr. Antonaccio (Princeton, New Jersey): Dr. Kopp, you claimed that the increase in renin release due to low-frequency stimulation was beta$_1$-mediated and this was based on the inhibition by metroprolol. Did you in fact show that metoprolol in the dose that you used did block selectively beta$_1$-receptors?

Dr. Kopp (Göteborg, Sweden): The dose of 0.5 mg/kg that we used has been found to be a good inhibitor of beta$_1$-adrenoreceptors in anesthetized animals.

Dr. Korner (Prahran, Australia): I would like to comment on Dr. Zanchetti's data where he showed that after renal denervation, the response to lowering renal perfusion pressure became blunted. In our laboratory, we have used a somewhat different kind of denervation. In the conscious adrenalectomized dog, large doses of guanethidine are given for many days, reducing cardiac catecholamines to less than 1%, and blunting their tyramine response to less than 5%. In these, we found exactly the opposite of Dr. Zanchetti. We got twice as great a rise in plasma renin activity for a given drop in perfusion pressure. They also had a greater rise in blood pressure. We concluded that normally when the various baroreceptor systems were intact, the rise in blood pressure that occurred in renal artery stenosis by stimulating the baroreceptors exerted a neural feedback on further renin release and also moderated the rise in blood pressure in the intact dog.

Dr. Zanchetti (Milan, Italy): I know your data, and we discussed them in Melbourne recently. I think that one should keep in mind several possible differences. First, what was observed in our experiments was a result of acute denervation, and we cannot extrapolate the results of acute to chronic denervation, particularly after chronic denervation supersensitivity to circulating catecholamines is known to develop. I think, however, the results of acute denervation are pertinent to show what may be the effect of a temporary suppression of sympathetic activity. A blunted response to the intrarenal stimuli after renal denervation does not mean, of course, that there is no response, and it is well known that the acute denervated kidney can also release renin in response to a decrease in perfusion pressure or to diuretics. Another important difference between your experiments and ours is that in your animals treated with guanethidine, circulatory homeostasis was lost, whereas this was obviously preserved in our animals with denervation limited to one kidney. When general homeostasis is lost, a large number of hardly controllable phenomena may happen, obscuring the results. Finally, a species difference is not a likely explanation, as some of our results in the cat have been confirmed by M. Thamer and G. DiBona in the dog.

I would like to comment on your data, Dr. Kopp. I think that they fit rather well in our way of thinking, although at first glance, some of your data may not seem to be entirely consistent with what we observed with phenoxybenzamine. If you remember, I showed in Fig. 2 [Position Paper, Session 8] that intrarenal phenoxybenzamine didn't decrease the renin response to stimulation of the vasomotor center. If any, the response was potentiated. I think there was a difference between our experiments, and this leads to the question for you. When one stimulates the vasomotor center rather than the renal nerve, even when the stimulus is strong, the decrease in renal blood flow is not sustained: There is a marked decrease during the first minute or so and then it starts to build up again and goes back to say 80% of prestimulus values. This might be the cause as to why we didn't see any reduction in renal release with phenoxybenzamine, because the effect of our stimulus on renal blood flow was similar to your mild stimulus. And then my question comes at this stage. We probably saw some increase, rather than decrease, in release after alpha-blockade, and there have been various suggestions in the literature that alpha-receptor may be indeed inhibitory to renin release. Have you ever tested phenoxybenzamine with or without beta-blockers on the renin response to the mild stimulus. This might help us in understanding the possible inhibitory role of alpha-receptors.

Dr. Kopp: No, unfortunately, we haven't done that, but I think that is a very interesting question.

Dr. Ayers: I think that the difference in the two observations of Drs. Zanchetti and Kopp can be explained. I think that Dr. Zanchetti is blocking the alpha$_2$-receptor (presynaptic) with an increase in plasma renin, and I think Dr. Kopp is stimulating renin release during severe renal nerve stimulation by stimulating prostaglandin synthesis through alpha$_1$-adrenergic receptor stimulation. This can be blocked with indomethacin. Thus, it appears that alpha$_2$-adrenergic receptor (presynaptic) stimulation suppresses norepinephrine and renin release, and alpha$_1$-adrenergic receptor stimulation, strong enough to reduce renal blood flow by approximately 50%, stimulates renin release through the prostaglandin system.

Dr. Birkenhager (Rotterdam, The Netherlands): I Would like to report quite briefly on what we have done together with Dr. Vandongen. We were able in the isolated rat kidney preparation to suppress the renin-stimulatory effect of a beta-agonist by giving at the same time an alpha-agonist. During the alpha-agonist, we observed renal vasoconstriction, and this could be an explanation of the inhibitory effect. But inhibition of renin release due to the alpha-agonist was still there when we inhibited renal vasoconstriction using hydralazine. So I would like to suggest giving that kind of substance during your high-level stimulation. [Vandongen R, Strang KD, Poessé MH et al. (1979) Circ Res 45: 435]

Dr. Zanchetti: I think that the role of the alpha-receptors can be seen both ways. There might be alpha-receptors directly inhibiting renin release as in your work with Vandongen, and then alpha-receptors mediating vasoconstriction and then stimulating renin release, as Dr. Kopp showed, because the constricting element in the afferent arteriole, as I mentioned in my presentation are probably proximal to the juxtaglomerular cells, which are more distally located in the afferent arteriole; thus, alpha-mediated constriction can unload the stretch receptor and release renin.

Dr. Birkenhager: Could there also be a species difference?

Dr. Zanchetti: That is always a too simple, and, therefore, bad way of explaining things: It should be kept as a last resource.

Session 9
Extravascular and Plasma Prorenin and Renin

Chairman: E. G. Erdös

Position Paper: Extravascular and Plasma Prorenin and Renin

Jean E. Sealey, Steven A. Atlas, and John H. Laragh

The renal enzyme renin is almost unique among blood proteolytic enzymes in that it circulates in active form until it is removed from the circulation by the liver. Thus, unlike most other blood proteases, renin does not have an intrinsic circulating inhibitor. Renin, therefore, has the characteristics of a true, albeit indirect, hormone whose target organs are the arterioles and adrenal cortex. Renin acts enzymatically in the blood to cleave the decapeptide angiotensin I from its circulating substrate. Angiotensin I remains largely inactive until it is enzymatically converted (predominantly in the pulmonary vascular bed) into the octapeptide angiotensin II, in preparation for delivery to the arterial circulation. Angiotensin II is the physiologically active hormone of the renin system; it vasoconstricts the arterioles and stimulates aldosterone biosynthesis, in these ways helping to maintain arterial pressure. Changes in arterial pressure, in turn, are detected by the kidneys which respond by adjusting the secretory rate of renin. Thus, renin is part of a cybernetic control system that participates in the maintenance of circulatory homeostasis (1).

Until recently, the preceding paragraph adequately described the functioning of the renin–angiotensin system. There were reports of renin in the submaxillary gland of the mouse (2) and in the uterus of pregnant animals (3); some had reported renin-like activity in the plasma of nephrectomized human subjects (4), but for the most part, circulating renin was considered to be of renal origin (1). Also, since there was no compelling evidence for the participation of activators or inhibitors of renin, circulating renin was generally assumed to be fully active. This point of view has to be reconsidered with the discovery that close to 90% of circulating renin is in fact inactive and that this inactive renin continues to be present in the circulation, although at subnormal levels, following chronic bilateral nephrectomy (5). Very high concentrations of inactive renin are present in amniotic fluid (6) and in the blood and tumor extracts of patients with Wilms' tumor (7). Also, as described by other authors in this session, there are new reports that renin is present in other tissues such as the vascular bed (8), brain (9, 10), and smooth muscle cells (11), even in animals that were previously nephrectomized. Therefore, there is now considerable evidence that renin can be synthesized at sites other than the kidney.

Many of these extrarenal sources of renin are considered in detail by other authors in this session (8–10). The purpose of this particular communication is to summarize current knowledge concerning the biochemical and physiologic characteristics of inactive plasma renin, often termed "prorenin," and to consider the possible biochemical and physiologic relationship of this substance to the renin–angiotension–aldosterone system. A more extensive review can be found elsewhere (5).

For convenience, the term prorenin will be used to describe inactive plasma renin, although the reader should be aware that there is, as yet, no definitive evidence that it is a true precursor of active renin. Plasma prorenin is completely inactive (12, 13). Detection of prorenin usually requires conversion to active renin, which is then quantitated by enzymatic assay. Thus, the prorenin concentration is calculated from the total renin measurement (following activation) minus the endogenous active renin (Table 1). Plasma prorenin can also be detected, at least qualitatively, by direct radioimmunoassay of renin (14) since available antibodies to active renin bind both active and inactive renin forms. Thus, even the direct RIA re-

Table 1. Detection and quantitation of plasma prorenin.

1. Completely inactive
2. Detected following conversion to active renin, or by direct RIA. Both techniques measure total renin (i.e., the sum of active plus inactive renin)
3. Prorenin is quantitated as follows: Prorenin = total renin − active renin
4. Prorenin, on average, comprises 86% of total renin in normal subjects

quires that active renin must be measured and subtracted from total renin, a source of considerable error.

TECHNIQUES FOR ACTIVATION OF PLASMA PRORENIN

Plasma prorenin, like inactive renin from amniotic fluid, can be activated by limited proteolysis with trypsin or pepsin (Table 2) (15, 16). These unrelated endopeptidases preferentially cleave peptide bonds containing entirely different aminoacyl residues, suggesting that exposure of the active site can be accomplished by cleavage at more than one bond. Both enzymes can also destroy renin if they are present in excess, but available evidence suggests that the concentration that will destroy renin is greater than the concentration required to activate prorenin (5, 17). The potency of trypsin and pepsin is markedly affected by inhibitors and other competing substrates, making it necessary to define the optimal concentration of enzyme needed to activate each sample. Lack of recognition of the wide range of enzyme sometimes required to activate prorenin in different samples explains some of the discrepancies in the literature concerning the elution characteristics of prorenin following chromatography (5). Pepsin has the additional disadvantage that it can cleave angiotensin

Table 2. Techniques for activation of plasma prorenin in vitro.

1. Limited proteolysis with, e.g., trypsin, pepsin
2. Cryoactivation
3. Acid activation

I from renin substrate; therefore, its presence can invalidate the enzymatic assay for renin.

Other enzymes, such as urinary kallikrein (18), plasma kallikrein (13), plasmin (19), and cathepsin D (20), can activate prorenin under defined conditions (see below). When these serine proteases become widely available, they may be preferable to trypsin or pepsin for activating prorenin if they do not simultaneously destroy it.

There are two in vitro techniques for activating plasma prorenin that take advantage of the presence in plasma of precursors of proteases that can activate prorenin (Table 2). These techniques are termed "acid activation" (6) and "cryoactivation" (21). Because they require plasma co-factors, they are not useful for activating prorenin in any medium other than whole plasma or serum (e.g., chromatographic fractions) (5).

Acid activation is accomplished by dialysis of plasma to pH 3.3 and then to pH 7.4, each for 24 h at 4°C. A rather complicated series of events occurs during acid activation. In early studies it appeared that only partial activation of inactive renin occurred during dialysis to pH 3.3. Further activation by neutral serine proteases during the dialysis to pH 7.4 was required to complete the activation process (22, 23) (Fig. 1). However, recent studies by Hsueh (24) and B. Leckie (manuscript in preparation) have shown that activation may indeed be complete at pH 3.3, but it is reversible if the sample is subsequently warmed at a higher pH, a procedure that is an essential step in the renin assay. During the cold pH 7.4 dialysis step the action of neutral serine proteases seems to render the activation irreversible. Available evidence suggests that the second stage of activation is dependent on Hageman factor activation of prekallikrein, and kallikrein, in turn, cleaves the acidified prorenin (25–27) (Fig. 2). This cascade of proteolytic events is able to occur in acidified plasma because inhibitors of serine proteases are destroyed during pH 3.3 dialysis (23). Altogether then, acid activation appears to involve the reversible activation of prorenin at acid pH and subsequent cleavage by plasma kallikrein at alkaline pH, resulting in irreversible activation. Hageman factor and plasma inhibitors of serine protease act as co-factors in the activation process.

Cryoactivation of plasma prorenin resembles the alkaline phase of acid activation in that it is mediated by a neutral serine protease (22, 23), most likely plasma kallikrein (5). Cryoactivation is ac-

The Two Phases of "Acid" Activation of Plasma Prorenin
Alkaline Phase Activation Inhibited by SBTI

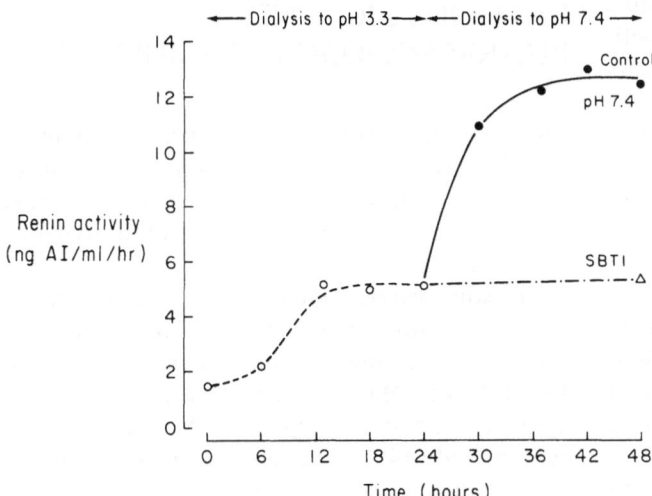

Fig. 1. Time-course and pH dependence of acid activation of inactive renin in human plasma; inhibition of alkaline (pH 7.4) phase by soybean trypsin inhibitor (SBTI).

Initiation of Prorenin Activation by Hageman
Factor-Dependent Conversion of Prekallikrein
to Kallikrein

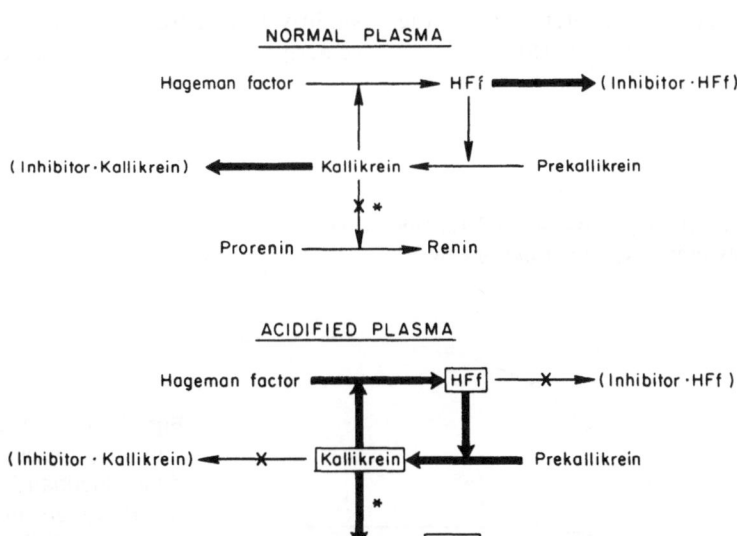

Fig. 2. *Upper panel:* Hageman factor-dependent activation of plasma prekallikrein and reciprocal activation of Hageman factor by kallikrein; inactivation of active enzymes by plasma inhibitors. *Lower panel:* Proposed cascade by which Hageman factor-dependent activation of prorenin occurs in acid-treated plasma. Heavy arrows indicate predominant pathway in each instance. *Kallikrein activation of prorenin may be direct or indirect. [Sealey et al. (25)]

250   J. E. Sealey et al.

complished by incubating plasma for 4 days at −4°C (Fig. 3) (28); it is inhibited by diisofluorophosphate (DFP) (22, 29) and by other inhibitors of neutral serine proteases (23). Interestingly, activation of plasma prorenin by trypsin also occurs optimally at temperatures below 0°C (16). The most likely explanation for this paradoxical effect of temperature on prorenin activation is that the efficacy of a plasma inhibitor of neutral serine proteases is decreased at low temperatures to a greater degree than the activity of the proteases themselves. Alternatively, cold may induce a conformational alteration of the prorenin molecule which facilitates its activation by plasma proteases. Similarly, it has been proposed that acidification of the prorenin molecule may facilitate its activation by kallikrein (13, 27).

Cryoactivation of plasma prorenin appears to take place in two phases. Close to one-third is activated over the first 2–3 days; then a plateau is reached that is followed by a second phase of activation, which starts after 6 days and takes up to 3 weeks to complete (30). After 3 weeks, the degree of activation caused by cold incubation is similar to that accomplished by limited trypsin proteolysis, or the combined phases of acid activation. When plasma is acid activated after various degrees of cryoactivation, the total degree of activation is always equal to that achieved by trypsin, suggesting that these three techniques affect the same source(s) of prorenin (Fig. 4) (5).

PRORENIN LEVELS IN PLASMA: ITS RESPONSE TO PHYSIOLOGIC, PATHOLOGIC, AND PHARMACOLOGIC STIMULI

The physiologic role of plasma prorenin is unresolved. However, plasma prorenin has been measured in a variety of circumstances, and the data provide a framework for evaluation of the dynamic potential of prorenin.

In a study carried out in a large group of normal subjects, it was found that the level of plasma prorenin following trypsin activation averaged 17.4 ± 19.1 (SD) ng/ml/h, while active renin averaged only 2.5 ± 1.7 ng/ml/h (5) (Table 3). On average, only 14% of the plasma renin is normally active, but there is a wide range of inactive renin levels among normal subjects. Hypertensives have a much wider range of active renin than normal subjects, which gives rise to the designation of low-, normal-, and high-renin hypertensive patients. Interestingly, however, the range of inactive renin is quite normal in hypertensive patients, and, within a particular renin subgroup, the range of prorenin values is much less variable than that found in normal subjects (5). High-renin patients do not have elevated levels of plasma prorenin. In contrast, low-renin patients generally have slightly low-prorenin levels. Thus, the proportion of active renin is only moderately reduced in low-

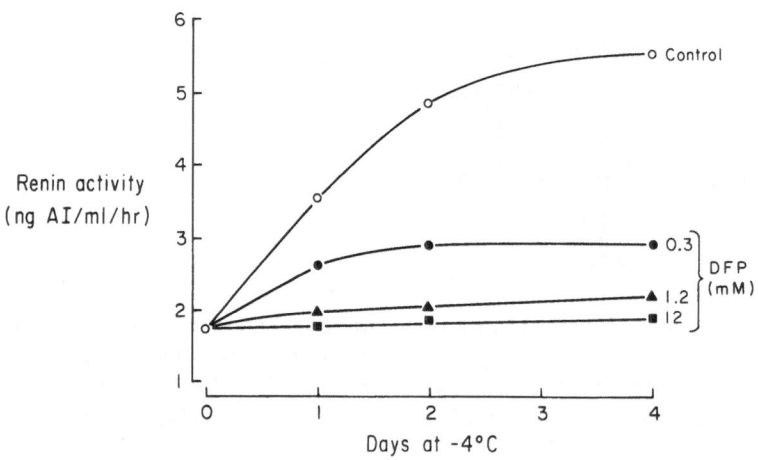

Time-Course of Cryoactivation and Its Inhibition by Diisopropylfluorophosphate

Fig. 3. Time-course of cryoactivation of prorenin in normal plasma during incubation at −4°C; inhibition of activation by diisopropylfluorophosphate (DFP).

**Effect of Prior Cryoactivation on Acid and Alkaline
Phases of Acid Activation**

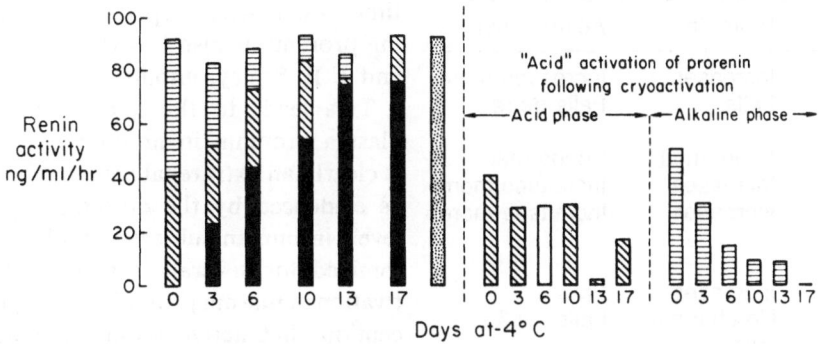

Days at-4°C

Fig. 4. Effect of prior cryoactivation on the acid and alkaline phases of acid activation of plasma prorenin. A pool of serum from pregnant women was cryoactivated from various times and then sequentially dialyzed to pH 3.3 and then to pH 7.4 for 24 h. An additional sample of serum was trypsin activated to quantitate the total prorenin concentration of the sample. The total degree of activation was quite similar in each sample, irrespective of whether the sample had been partially cryoactivated before acid activation was carried out *(left panel)*. ⊟, alkaline phase; ◩, acid phase; ■, cryoactivated; ▦, trypsin activated.

renin patients (7%) (Table 2) (5), while it is markedly elevated in the high-renin group (35%) (31).

Both active and inactive renin increase with sodium depletion (21) and diuretic therapy (31–34), and fall with sodium loading in hypertensive patients (Table 4). Patients with primary aldosteronism (5, 34), like those with low-renin essential hypertension, both of whom seem to have excess fluid volume as a basis for their hypertension, have

low levels of plasma prorenin (Table 3). Thus, increased sodium balance seems to suppress plasma prorenin in hypertensive subjects.

Plasma prorenin and active renin increase in hypertensive patients during long-term therapy with the oral converting enzyme inhibitor captopril (J. E. Sealey and A. Overlack, unpublished observations). However, like the effect of diuretics and other factors that alter plasma prorenin, the

Table 3. Plasma renin and prorenin measurements in normal subjects and in hypertensive and anephric patients.

Group	Active renin[b]	Prorenin	% Active
Normal subjects ($N = 114$)	2.5 (±1.6)	17.4 (±19.2)	14 (±10)
Essential hypertension[a]			
Low renin ($N = 8$)	0.7 (±0.3)	9.8* (±4.4)	7** (±4)
Normal renin ($N = 7$)	2.1 (±0.9)	18.6 (±5.5)	11*** (±3)
High renin ($N = 7$)	7.7 (±1.8)	16.2 (±8.0)	35*** (±10)
Hyporeninemic hyperaldosteronism ($N = 10$)	0.15 (±0.09)	3.3 (±2.0)	5 (±4)
Unilateral renovascular ($N = 7$)	17.5 (±12.6)	22.7 (±11.4)	42 (±19)
Anephric ($N = 8$)	< 0.15	5.7 (±4.1)	∼ 0

* $p < 0.05$; ** $p < 0.01$; *** $p < 0.001$.
When asterisk is next to data in low renin column it denotes the significance of the difference between low and normal renin groups; when asterisk is next to data in normal renin column it denotes significance of the difference between normal and high renin groups; when asterisk is next to data in high renin column it denotes the significance of the difference between low and high renin groups.
[a] UNaV over 50 mEq/day.
[b] Mean ± 1 SD (ng/ml/h).

Table 4. Prorenin response to physiologic, pharmacologic, and pathophysiologic stimuli.

Stimulus	Prorenin	Active renin
Sodium depletion	Increases	Increases more
Sodium loading	Falls	Falls more
Primary aldosteronism	Subnormal	Subnormal
Diuretics	Increases	Increases more
Captopril	Increases	Increases more
Beta-blockade		
Hypotensive response	Increases	Falls
No BP effect	No change/ falls	Falls
Pregnancy	Increases	Increases less
Nephrectomy	Falls	Absent

prorenin response to captopril lags several days behind that of active renin; the proportion of active renin in the circulation tends to rise, both initially and over the long term. Since the half-life of prorenin appears to be only about 2 h (34), other factors must be invoked to explain its slower response pattern. For instance, plasma prorenin may not be stored in large amounts, and changes in its plasma level may reflect an alteration in the rate of biosynthesis rather than in the rate of release of stored hormone.

Unlike diuretics or captopril, beta-blockers frequently cause opposite changes in active renin and prorenin in hypertensive patients (33, 35). Propranolol consistently lowers active renin, usually by at least 50%, but increases prorenin in many patients and causes no change or a slight decrease in others. The change in prorenin during beta-blockade has been shown to be inversely related to change in blood pressure; the greater the fall in systolic pressure with propranolol, the more prorenin increases and vice versa (33). In fact, when propranolol fails to affect blood pressure, the total renin in the circulation tends to fall. Thus, propranolol may act to suppress plasma renin both by lowering the proportion of active renin that is secreted and by diminishing the overall secretory rate.

Circulating prorenin increases by more than fivefold during pregnancy (36). The prorenin level reaches a maximum by 12 weeks, long before active renin (which also increases during pregnancy) has reached its peak. It is unclear whether prorenin is secreted from the fetoplacental unit during pregnancy, or from the kidney, or elsewhere. Whatever

the source, we have observed that whenever active renin is subnormal during pregnancy, as sometimes occurs when hypertension develops, circulating prorenin is also low (M. Wilson, B. Romney, and J. E. Sealey, unpublished observations).

This leads to the question of the source of plasma prorenin in nonpregnant subjects. There is clearly an extrarenal source of plasma prorenin, as evidenced by the detectable (but subnormal) levels in human subjects who have been nephrectomized for several years (32). Inadvertent activation of plasma prorenin led to the early misconception that active renin circulates in anephric subjects (4). The source of this extrarenal prorenin remains a mystery and may not be resolved until a suitable animal model of prorenin has been developed (37, 38). However, a key question is whether any of the circulating prorenin is of renal origin.

EVIDENCE THAT PLASMA PRORENIN IS SECRETED FROM THE KIDNEY

Measurements of plasma prorenin in renal venous effluents have provided inconsistent evidence that prorenin is secreted by the kidney (18, 34, 35, 39). A marked arteriovenous (A–V) increment in prorenin has been reported in some, but not all, patients with renovascular hypertension. On the other hand, other hypertensive patients show either no change or a decrement in prorenin across the kidney.

These studies do not rule out the kidney as a source of plasma prorenin, since the failure to consistently detect an A–V difference may be explained by several different factors: a) The clearance rate of prorenin may be slow, leading to a very low A–V difference that is difficult to detect accurately; b) prorenin may be both secreted and cleared from the circulation by the kidney; and c) calculation of the A–V difference in prorenin is very imprecise because the prorenin value itself is a calculated value. Active renin often represents a very high proportion of the total renin in renal vein samples, which further reduces the accuracy of the calculation.

Perhaps, more convincing physiologic evidence that prorenin may be of renal origin comes from the studies which show that prorenin usually falls after nephrectomy and increases after transplantation (34). Also, prorenin values are, on average, subnormal in anephric human subjects (32).

Until recently, the biochemical evidence that plasma prorenin is of renal origin was far from convincing, mainly because the characteristics of most large-molecular-weight forms of renal renin differ from those of inactive renin in plasma (5) (see below). However, a prorenin-like substance has now been identified in the effluent of isolated perfused human kidneys (40), and similar substances have been chromatographically detected in extracts from hog (41) and human kidney (40) (see below). It is of interest that the proportion of prorenin-like substance in human kidney was only 10% of the total renin, suggesting that prorenin may not be stored in the kidney to the same degree as active renin (40).

Altogether, the data suggest that plasma prorenin may be derived from both renal and extrarenal sources. The extrarenal source is unknown at present, and there is as yet no way of identifying what proportion of plasma prorenin is of renal origin.

BIOCHEMICAL CHARACTERIZATION OF PRORENIN

The literature is replete with reports of large-molecular-weight forms of renin, most of which have been identified in renal extracts (for review, see ref. 5). It is important to emphasize that the preceding discussion has dealt with a plasma substance that is totally inactive. Most large-molecular-weight forms of renal renin differ from plasma prorenin in that they have considerable intrinsic enzymatic activity. In a subsequent paper in this volume, Yamamoto and co-workers (42, 43) present evidence that certain of these large-molecular-weight renins may actually be formed after active renin is extracted from the storage granules. They appear to be the result of binding of active renin to another renal cortical protein. It is even possible that they are entirely in vitro artifacts and may not be normally present in vivo.

Preliminary biochemical characterization of plasma prorenin has been carried out by several groups. Its molecular weight has been characterized by gel filtration of whole plasma or of partially purified plasma fractions. Its size is reported to range between 60,000 and 40,000. This small dis-

crepancy in size can, in large part, be explained by the limitations of gel filtration and by the techniques used to activate and identify the prorenin peak. Obviously, estimation of molecular size in studies that used cryoactivation and acid activation cannot be accurate since the co-factors involved in these activation processes are unlikely to co-elute precisely with the prorenin peak (5, 17). Even activation by exogenous pepsin and trypsin is not precise since both enzymes can destroy renin when their proteolytic activity is very high, or submaximally activate at low levels, and their activity is determined not only by the amount of enzyme added, but also by the concentration of co-eluting plasma inhibitors and competing substrates. The range of reported apparent molecular weights of prorenin can, therefore, be explained by the fact that different activation techniques reveal different portions of the prorenin peak (5, 17).

Using precise activation techniques, the apparent molecular weight of human plasma prorenin by gel filtration is close to 57,000 (5, 13, 17, 44), while that of active renin is 48,000–a value higher than that of purified renal renin which consistently elutes around 40,000 (45). While there is precedent for a precursor being larger than the active enzyme, the reason why circulating active renin appears to be larger than active renal renin remains to be clarified. The molecular size of activated prorenin appears to range between that of unactivated prorenin and active plasma renin, but the limitations of the gel filtration technique do not allow precise identification.

Plasma prorenin elutes from anion exchange resins at a lower ionic strength than active renin (46, 49). Its binding properties to various affinity columns differ from those of active renin. It does not bind to the renin-binding acid-protease inhibitor pepstatin (50), but it does bind to antibodies against active renin (14). It also binds to Cibacron Blue–agarose, while active renin does not (Fig. 5) (5, 13, 39, 51, 52). Both moieties bind to concanavalin A–Sepharose, but prorenin is eluted by a lower concentration of α-methylmannoside (12). A large-molecular-weight trypsin-activable form of inactive renin has been recently identified in renal extracts that exhibits characteristics similar to those just described for plasma prorenin (39). Following activation both plasma and renal forms exhibit characteristics similar to those of active renin (53). Therefore, preliminary characterization

Separation of Active and Trypsin-Activable Renins in Human Plasma and Kidney on Cibacron Blue-Agarose

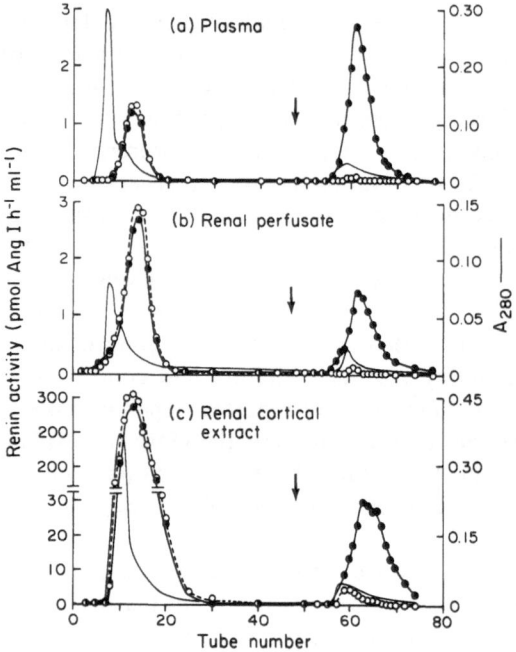

Fig. 5. Separation of active and trypsin activable renins from human plasma, the perfusate from a human kidney, and from an extract of human renal cortex, by affinity chromatography on Cibacron Blue F3G-A–agarose (Affi Gel Blue). [Atlas et al. (39)]

of plasma prorenin has permitted the identification of a similar prorenin-like substance in the kidney and has enabled investigators to discriminate it from other large-molecular-weight forms of renal renin.

SPECULATIONS CONCERNING THE ROLE OF PRORENIN

Although the definitive evidence that prorenin is indeed a precursor of renin has not yet been achieved, its known characteristics are consistent with its being so. A key question, then, is at what stage, or stages, in the biosynthetic pathway is prorenin converted to active renin. It is possible that renal prorenin is an intermediate in the intracellular biosynthesis of renin that finds its way into the circulation, but undergoes no further activation. If so, and if the major portion of circulating

prorenin is normally of renal origin, then plasma prorenin levels may reflect the rate of biosynthesis of active renin.

Alternatively, renal prorenin may be activated following release from its cell of synthesis, but prior to its secretion into the circulation. The observation that urinary kallikrein, a renal proteolytic enzyme, can activate prorenin has led to speculation that there might in fact be a coordinated link between the kallikrein–kinin system and the renin–angiotensin system, in which the simultaneous response of both kallikrein and renin results in increased systemic arterial pressure, via angiotensin-induced vasoconstriction, with concurrent protection of renal blood flow, via local effect of the kallikrein–kinin system (54). Recent preliminary data, demonstrating a possible protective effect of renal kallikrein during prolonged hemorrhage, provides evidence that the two systems might indeed function together as proposed (55).

Other investigators lean to the view that prorenin may be converted to active renin following its secretion into the circulation (56, 57). Both plasma kallikrein and plasmin are present in the blood as inactive precursors and both are capable of activating prorenin. Therefore, theoretically, renin might be formed whenever these enzymes are activated. In fact, a positive relationship has been observed between plasma prekallikrein and the active/total renin ratio (57). However, against this view is the observation that no activation of prorenin occurs in plasma in vitro at temperatures above 10°C (28), and anephric patients have no active plasma renin despite having significant levels of circulating prorenin (32). Also, all of the prekallikrein in plasma can be activated rapidly with the addition of kaolin in vitro, but no concurrent activation of prorenin occurs, unless the plasma has been previously acidified (58). Our own view is that if prorenin is normally activated after it is secreted into the circulation its activating enzyme is likely to be either membrane bound or sequestered from the circulation so that activation occurs at a particular tissue bed, rather than in the blood itself, in much the same way that angiotensin I is converted to angiotensin II as it passes through the lungs.

Research into the biochemistry and physiology of the renin system is currently one of the most lively areas of hypertension research. Further studies are needed to define the precise role of prorenin in the renin–angiotensin–aldosterone axis and to determine whether blockade of activation of prorenin provides a control point for regulation of the renin system in hypertensive patients.

SUMMARY

Close to 90% of the renin in normal human plasma is in the form of an inactive, prorenin-like substance. In vivo activation of prorenin to renin has yet to be demonstrated. However, prorenin can be activated in vitro by limited proteolysis with trypsin or pepsin. It can also be activated by acid activation and cryoactivation; these processes depend on a plasma neutral serine protease which, in the case of acid activation, has been identified as plasma kallikrein. Available evidence suggests that plasma prorenin is not normally activated in the blood in vivo.

The role of circulating prorenin is undefined. Its concentration is slightly low in patients with low-renin hypertension, in primary aldosteronism, and in anephric subjects. Prorenin values fall within the normal range in both normal- and high-renin hypertensive patients. Plasma prorenin levels fluctuate inversely with sodium balance, and during propranolol therapy prorenin changes inversely with blood pressure. Thus, prorenin appears to be physiologically related to active renin, but its concentration in plasma changes at a much slower rate.

Prorenin can be separated from active renin in a number of chromatographic systems and has been shown to be inactive. Using precise activation procedures following gel filtration, plasma prorenin has an apparent molecular weight of 57,000, while active plasma renin is 48,000, considerably larger than purified renal renin (40,000). A prorenin-like substance with similar characteristics to plasma prorenin has been identified in hog and human kidney, and in the perfusate from human kidneys. Therefore, plasma prorenin appears to be partly of renal origin. However, an extrarenal source of plasma prorenin also exists since it is present, although usually at subnormal levels, in the plasma of anephric subjects.

Future studies will be required to further define the biochemical and physiologic characteristics of prorenin and to determine whether it is merely a by-product of intracellular renin biosynthesis or, perhaps as well, a circulating precursor of active renin that is activated at a site distal to its source.

ACKNOWLEDGMENT

This work was supported by the National Heart, Lung and Blood Institute grants HL 21274, HL 18323-SCR, and HL 00570.

REFERENCES

1. Laragh JH, Sealey JE (1973) The renin-angiotensin-aldosterone hormonal system and regulation of sodium, potassium and blood pressure homeostasis. In: Orloff J, Berliner RW (eds) Handbook of physiology: Renal physiology (American Physiological Society). Waverly Press, Baltimore, Md, pp 831–908
2. Werle E, Vogel R, Goldel FL (1957) Ubër Blutdrucksteigerndes Prinzipin extracten aus Glandula submaxillaris der weissen Maus. Arch Exp Pathol Pharmakol 230: 236–244
3. Gross F, Turrian H (1964) A renin-like substance in the placenta and uterus of the rabbit. Lancet 1: 914–916
4. Capelli JP, Wesson LG, Aponte GE, Faraldo C, Jaffe E (1968) Characterization and source of a renin-like enzyme in anephric human. J Clin Endocrinol Metab 28: 221–230
5. Sealey JE, Atlas SA, Laragh JH (1980) Prorenin and other large molecular weight forms of renin. Endocrine Reviews 1: 365–391
6. Lumbers ER (1971) Activation of renin in human amniotic fluid by low pH. Enzymologia 40: 329–336
7. Day RP, Luetscher JA, Gonzales CM (1975) Occurrence of big renin in human plasma, amniotic fluid and kidney extracts. J Clin Endocrinol Metab 40: 1078–1084
8. Thurston H, Hurst BC, Bing RF, Swales JD (1981) Vascular renin. In: This volume, p 274
9. Ganten D, Speck G, Mann JFE, Unger Th (1981) Role of the brain renin-angiotensin system in central mechanism of blood pressure control. In: This volume, pp 268–273
10. Inagami T, Celio MR, Lau D, Clemens DL, Takii Y, Hirose S, Yokosawa H (1981) Brain renin. In: This volume, pp 265–267
11. Re R, Fallon JT, Dzau V, Quay S, Haber E (1979) Renin synthesis by arterial smooth muscle cells (abstr). Circulation 59, 60(Suppl II): 10
12. Atlas SA, Sealey JE, Laragh JH (1979) Chromatographic isolation of totally inactive plasma prorenin (abstr). Kidney Int 16: 791
13. Yokosawa N, Takahashi N, Inagami T, Page DL

(1979) Isolation of completely inactive plasma prorenin and its activation by kallikreins: A possible new link between renin and kallikrein. Biochim Biophys Acta 569: 211–219

14. Guyene TT, Galen FX, Devaux C, Corvol P, Ménard P (1980) Direct radioimmunoassay of human renin: Comparison with renin activity in plasma and amniotic fluid. Hypertension 2: 465–470

15. Morris BJ, Lumbers ER (1972) The activation of renin in human amniotic fluid by proteolytic enzymes. Biochim Biophys Acta 289: 385–391

16. Sealey JE, Atlas SA, Laragh JH, Oza NB, Ryan JW (1979) Activation of prorenin-like substance in human plasma by trypsin and by urinary kallikrein. Hypertension 1: 179–189

17. Atlas SA, Sealey JE, Laragh JH, Warekois TE (1979) Apparent molecular weight of inactive renin in human plasma (abstr) Clin Res 27: 466A

18. Sealey JE, Atlas SA, Laragh JH, Oza NB, Ryan RW (1978) Human urinary kallikrein converts inactive to active renin and is a possible physiological activator of renin. Nature 275: 144–145

19. Osmond DH, Lo EK, Loh AY, Zingg EA, Hedlin AH (1978) Kallikrein and plasmin as activators of inactive renin (letter). Lancet 2: 1375–1376

20. Morris BJ (1978) Activation of human inactive ("pro-") renin by cathepsin D and pepsin. J Clin Endocrinol Metab 46: 153–157

21. Sealey JE, Laragh JH (1975) Prorenin in human plasma? Methodological and physiological implications. Circ Res 36, 37(Suppl I): 10–16

22. Atlas SA, Sealey JE, Laragh JH (1978) "Acid-" and "cryo-" activated inactive plasma renin: Similarity of changes during β-blockade and evidence that neutral protease(s) participate in both activation procedures. Circ Res 42(Suppl I): 128–133

23. Atlas SA, Laragh JH, Sealey JE (1978) Activation of inactive plasma renin: Evidence that both cryo- and acid-activation work by liberating a neutral serine protease from endogenous inhibitors. Clin Sci Mol Med 55: 135S–138S

24. Hsueh WA, Carlson EJ (1981) Reversible activation of plasma inactive renin. In: Sambhi MP (ed) Heterogeneity of renin. Elsevier, New York

25. Sealey JE, Atlas SA, Laragh JH, Silverberg M, Kaplan AP (1979) Initiation of plasma prorenin activation by Hageman factor-dependent conversion of plasma prekallikrein to kallikrein. Proc Natl Acad Sci USA 76: 5914–5918

26. Derkx FHM, Bouma BN, Schalekamp MPA, Schalekamp MADH (1979) An intrinsic factor XII-prekallikrein-dependent pathway activates the human plasma renin-angiotensin system. Nature 280: 315–316

27. Hsueh WA, Carlson EJ, O'Connor D, Warren S (1980) Renin requires a structural alteration prior to activation by kallikrein. J Clin Endocrinol Metab 51: 942–944

28. Sealey JE, Moon C, Laragh JH, Alderman M (1976) Plasma prorenin: Cryoactivation and relationship

to renin substrate in normal subjects. Am J Med 61: 731–738

29. Osmond DH, Loh AY (1978) Protease as endogenous activator of inactive renin (letter). Lancet 1: 102

30. Pietro C, Egidio S, Domenico S (1979) Two fractions of cryoactivatable prorenin in human plasma (letter). Biochem Med 22: 264–265

31. Weinberger M, Aoi W, Grim C (1977) Dynamic responses of active and inactive renin in normal and hypertensive humans. Circ Res 41(Suppl II): 21–25

32. Sealey JE, Moon C, Laragh JH, Atlas SA (1977) Plasma prorenin in normal, hypertensive and anephric subjects and its effect on renin measurements. Circ Res 40(Suppl I): 41–45

33. Atlas SA, Sealey JE, Laragh JH, Moon C (1977) Plasma renin and "prorenin" in essential hypertension during sodium depletion, beta-blockade and reduced arterial pressure. Lancet 2: 785–789

34. Derkx FHM, Wenting GJ, Man In'T Veld AJ, Verhoeven RP, Schalekamp MADH (1978) Control of enzymatically inactive renin in man under various pathological conditions: Implications for the interpretation of renin measurements in peripheral and renal venous plasma. Clin Sci Mol Med 54: 529–538

35. Derkx FHM, van Gool JMG, Wenting GJ, Verhoeven RA, Man In'T Veld AJ, Schalekamp MADH (1976) Inactive renin in human plasma. Lancet 2: 496–499

36. Skinner SL, Cran EJ, Gibson R, Taylor R, Walters WAW, Catt KJ (1975) Angiotensins I and II, active and inactive renin, renin substrate, renin activity and angiotensinase in human liquor amnii and plasma. Am J Obstet Gynecol 121: 626–630

37. Gallagher JF, Laragh JH, Atlas SA, Sealey JE (1980) Effect of trypsin or acid treatment on dog plasma renin activity measurements. Endocrinology 107: 147–154

38. Nakane H, Nakane Y, Corvol P, Menard J (1979) Effect of acid, trypsin and cold treatment and of renin-plasma interaction on the activity of renin secreted by rat kidney. Clin Sci 57: 233–240

39. Birkenhager WH, DeLeeuw PW, Falke HE, Van Soust GAW (1978) Renin secretion by the human kidney. Clin Sci Mol Med 55: 147S–149S

40. Atlas SA, Laragh JH, Sealey JE, Hesson TE (1980) A prorenin-like substance in human plasma and kidney. Clin Sci 59: 29S–33S

41. Takii Y, Inagami T (1980) Evidence for a completely inactive renin zymogen in the kidney by affinity chromatographic isolation. Biochem Biophys Res Commun 94: 182–188

42. Yamamoto K, Ikemoto F, Takaori K, Kawamura M (1981) High-molecular-weight form of renal renin and renin-binding substance in the dog. In: This volume, pp 263–264

43. Funakawa S, Funae Y, Yamamoto K (1978) Conversion between renin and high-molecular-weight renin in the dog. Biochem J 176: 977–981

44. Takii Y, Takahashi N, Inagami T, Yokosawa N (1980) A new form of renin in normal human plasma: "Big renin" is a mixture of inactive prorenin and the new high molecular weight renin. Life Sci 26: 347–353

45. Corvol P, Devaux C, Galen FX, Soubrier F, Foote S, Ménard J (1981) Renin purification. In: This volume, pp 258–262

46. Shulkes AA, Gibson RR, Skinner SL (1978) The nature of inactive renin in plasma and amniotic fluid. Clin Sci Mol Med 55: 41–50

47. Day RP, Morris BJ (1979) Properties of inactive renin in human plasma. Clin Exp Pharmacol Physiol 6: 611–624

48. Derkx FHM, Tan-Tjiong HL, Man In'T Veld AJ, Schalekamp MPA, Schalekamp MADH (1979) Activation of inactive plasma renin by tissue kallikreins. J Clin Endocrinol Metab 49: 765–769

49. Boyd GW (1977) An inactive higher-molecular-weight renin in normal subjects and hypertensive patients. Lancet 1: 215–218

50. Corvol P, Devaux C, Ménard J (1973) Pepstatin, an inhibitor for renin purification by affinity chromatography. FEBS Lett 34: 189

51. Carlson EJ, Hsueh WA, Luetscher JA (1978) Separation of active and inactive renins in human plasma (abstr) Circulation 57, 58(Suppl II): 250

52. Johnson RL, Poisner AM, Crist RD (1979) Partial purification and chromatographic properties of inactive renin from human amniotic fluid. Biochem Pharmacol 28: 1791–1799

53. Atlas SA, Sealey JE, Hesson TE, Laragh JH (1981) Renin-like properties of activated inactive renin from human plasma and kidney. In: Sambhi MP (ed) Heterogeneity of renin. Elsevier, New York

54. Sealey JE, Atlas SA, Laragh JH (1978) Linking the kallikrein and renin systems via activation of inactive renin: New data and a hypothesis Am J Med 65: 994–1000

55. Maier M, Starlinger M, Binder BR (1980) The effect of aprotinin on renal cortical blood flow during hemorrhagic hypotension (abstr). Fed Proc 39: 321

56. Derkx FHM, Bouma BN, Tan-Tjiong HL, Schalekamp MADH (1980) Activators of inactive renin ("prorenin") in human plasma: Their connection in kinin formation, coagulation and fibrinolysis. Clin Sci 57: 89S–92S

57. Rumpf KW, Becker K, Kreusch U, Schmidt S, Vetter R, Scheler F (1980) Evidence for a role of plasma kallikrein in the activation of prorenin. Nature 283: 482–483

58. Blumberg AL, Sealey JE, Atlas SA, Laragh JH, Dharmgrongartama B, Kaplan AP (1981) Contact activation of human plasma prorenin in vitro J Lab Clin Med (in press)

Renin Purification

P. Corvol, C. Devaux, F. X. Galen, F. Soubrier, S. Foote, and J. Ménard

The first complete purification of renin (EC 3.4.99.19) has only been achieved during this last decade. The instability of the unpurified enzyme and its extremely low concentration in kidney and biologic fluids explain the difficulties encountered during the course of the purification. The complete purification of renin is a mandatory step for our understanding of the renin–angiotensin system, allowing the production of highly specific renin antibodies and the study of the possible renin precursors, the active site of the enzyme, its structure, and the mechanisms of its inactivation.

In this review, we will describe the sources from which renin has been purified to the stage of homogeneity, the recent progress in the renin purification procedures, the main physicochemical properties of the pure enzymes, and the developments that can be anticipated from the availability of pure renin and highly specific antibodies.

RENIN SOURCES

KIDNEY

Renin has been completely purified from hog, rat and human kidney. In the case of human renin, there have been many problems such as procuring human cadaver kidneys, the relatively low concentration of renin, approximately 20 times less than in hog kidney, and the possible postmortem proteolytic degradation of the enzyme. To date the best source of human renin has been a renin-producing tumor that required only a 40-fold purification (1) compared to the 200,000–420,000-fold purification needed to obtain pure human renin from cadaver kidneys (2, 3). The physicochemical, enzymatic, and immunologic properties of the tumor renin were indistinguishable from those of

standard human Medical Research Council renal renin (1).

OTHER TISSUES AND BIOLOGIC FLUIDS

Besides the kidney, the presence of an angiotensin I-forming enzyme, similar to renin, has been reported in various tissues and biologic fluids. Renin-like enzymes have been purified from *submaxillary glands* obtained from adult male mice (4). Only a 40-fold purification was required, due to the extremely high-renin-like content of the tissue. Antibodies directed against this enzyme cross react with mouse kidney renin, showing the immunologic identity of both renal and salivary enzymes. Several laboratories have undertaken the task of purifying renin in brain, amniotic fluid, or plasma, but have not yet reported a purification to the stage of homogeneity. Such experiments are of crucial importance in order to establish the physicochemical properties of these renins compared to those of kidney renin. They will make possible the investigation of the biochemical relationships existing between "active" and "inactive" renin. The difficulties lie in the low-specific activity of the starting material (at least ten times less than in the kidney) and in the presence of proteolytic enzymes, such as cathepsin D in the brain, which can be difficult to separate from renin.

PURIFICATION PROCEDURES

As pointed out by Haber and Slater (5), it is remarkable that Haas et al. as reported in 1953 (6) achieved a 56,000-fold purification of hog kidney renin by means of salt and solvent precipitations, the only techniques of purification available at that time. In 1965 the same authors succeeded in obtaining a large amount of a partially purified human renin free from angiotensinases (7), and this was the same material that was used 13 years later for the complete purification of the enzyme (2). Several technical improvements have been accomplished that facilitate renin purification.

USE OF PROTEASE INHIBITORS

The kidney contains numerous proteases that can be activated, during the purification procedures, even at 4°C. Inagami and Murakami (8) have reported the usefulness of protease inactivators to minimize renin destruction and to prevent the generation of partially proteolysed renin forms. Purification can be successfully conducted without an acidification step, which avoids activation of acid proteases and possible changes in the renin structure.

AFFINITY CHROMATOGRAPHY

The most potent renin inhibitor for affinity chromatography is pepstatin. Corvol et al. (9) and Murakami et al. (10) independently reported the usefulness of pepstatin coupled to insolubilized matrix for hog renin purification. Sepharose hexamethylene-diamino-pepstatin was the most efficient of the several Sepharose–pepstatin derivatives tested by Devaux et al. (11) and allowed a 100–300-fold purification in a single step during hog, dog, rat, and human renin purification studies.

The synthesis of competitive inhibitors of renin by Poulsen et al. (12) has allowed the use of these peptides for renin affinity chromatography. Two compounds have been used: His-Pro-Phe-His-Leu$_D$-Leu-Val-Tyr and Pro-His-Pro-Phe-His-Leu-Phe-Val-Tyr. The former was used with success by Poulsen et al. (13) to purify hog renin and the latter for human renin (2, 3). Enzymes were released from the affinity gel using much milder conditions than for pepstatin affinity columns, suggesting a weaker affinity for renin. Other affinity columns proved to be helpful in the purification of renin, such as hemoglobin–Sepharose in separating renin from acid proteases (14). This column has been used in the purification of human kidney renin (2) and brain renin (15). Since renin is a glycoprotein, it can also be partially purified on concanavalin A–Sepharose (8). Recently, it has been reported that active and inactive renin mole-cules can be separated on a column of blue dextran–Sepharose (16). Such a method might be extremely useful for the complete purification of these two forms of the enzyme.

PHYSICOCHEMICAL, ENZYMATIC, AND IMMUNOLOGIC CHARACTERISTICS OF PURE RENINS

PHYSICOCHEMICAL PROPERTIES

All purified renins exhibited quite similar biochemical characteristics, as shown in Table 1. Molecular weights of the pure enzymes were found to be around 35,000–40,000 depending on the method used. All purified renins showed a charge microheterogeneity, revealed by isoelectric focusing or by ion-exchange chromatography. This microheterogeneity could be due to a difference in glycosylation of the protein, deamidation, or limited proteolysis during the purification (1). Renin gave a single band on SDS polyacrylamide gel electrophoresis, except in the case of tumoral human renin where, under this dissociating condition, Galen et al. (1) described the presence of two small renin fragments (20,000 and 25,000). Whether these two "small renins" had been generated during purification or were preexistent in the juxtaglomerular cell remains to be determined.

ENZYMATIC PROPERTIES

Few studies deal with the enzymatic properties of pure renin, in part because of the unavailability of pure angiotensinogen. Experiments performed on synthetic renin substrate, N-acetlytetradeca-peptide (17) or octapeptide substrates show a pH dependence of renin activity, and a K_m similar to that observed with less purified preparations (Table 1).

IMMUNOLOGIC PROPERTIES

The production of specific renin antibodies has been possible through the isolation of the pure enzyme. Antibodies have been raised against mouse submaxillary (18) and hog (19), human (20), and dog (21) renal renins. In contrast to pre-

Table 1. Biochemical and enzymatic properties of pure renins from various sources.

Characteristics	Mice submaxillary glands (4)	Hog kidney (8, 23)	Rat kidney (24, 25)	Human cadaver kidney (2, 3)	JG cell tumor (1)	Dog kidney (26)
Purification factor	40	70,000–133,000	3,000–30,000	200,000–420,000	40	600,000
Molecular weight	36,000–37,000	36,500	35,000–37,000	ND	38,000–42,000	36,000
Isoelectric points	5.40–5.62	5.2	5.05, 5.15, 5.22	ND	4.95, 5.10, 5.35, 5.55, 5.7	5.7
Amino acid composition	+	+	+	ND	–	+
Presence of glycoresidues	+	+	+	ND	+	ND
Specific activity (G/U/mg protein)	400 (22)	1,100–2,000	110	830	810–860	4,200
Optimum pH						
Synthetic substrate	ND	6.5	4.0–6.0	ND	6.5	ND
Natural substrate	ND	6.5	6.0–6.8	ND	5.5	ND
$K_m \times 10^{-6}$ M						
Synthetic substrate	ND	7.7–33	30–40	ND	6.8	ND
Natural substrate	ND	ND	ND	ND	ND	ND

ND, not determined; JG, juxtaglomerular.

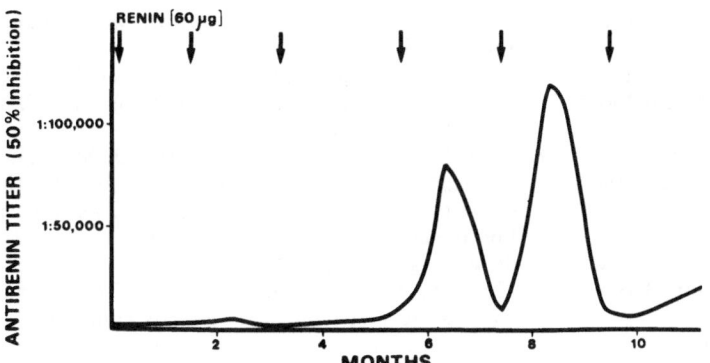

Fig. 1. Immunization schedule with pure human renin. The arrows indicate the time at which 60 μg renin were rejected. Renin titers were determined by their ability to inhibit 50% of the enzymatic activity of 50 μ Goldblatt Units.

vious reports concerning the poor immunogenicity of renin, high titers of renin antibodies have been obtained for human (Fig. 1), dog, and hog renin, although in the latter case, renin had to be either insolubilized or conjugated to tetanus toxoid (19). In the case of human renin, the antibody produced cross reacted with all isoforms of renin separated by isoelectric focusing (1). Both active and inactive renin from plasma or amniotic fluid were equally well inhibited by the same antibody dilution, suggesting that both renins share common antigenic determinants. No cross reaction was found with other renin species, and, similarly, hog renin antisera exhibited a low cross reactivity with renin from other species, suggesting specific antigenic sites for a given renin species.

Antirenin antibodies are presently used for different purposes:

1) Preparation of a renin-free human renin angiotensinogen by affinity chromatography on an antirenin immunoadsorbant gel.
2) Radioimmunoassay of renin in plasma, biologic fluids, and tissues.
3) Immunologic characterization of angiotensin-forming enzymes in brain and other tissues.
4) Immunofluorescence studies of renin in normal and pathologic kidneys, in brain, and in vascular walls.
5) In vivo investigation of the role of the renin–angiotensin system in physiologic and pathologic circumstances.
6) In vitro biosynthesis of renin.

SUMMARY

During this last decade, renin has been completely purified from hog, dog, rat, and human kidney. Several technical improvements have been accomplished that facilitate renin purification such as the application of affinity chromatography using protease and renin inhibitors such as pepstatin or renin substrate analogs. The physicochemical, enzymatic, and immunologic properties of these pure renins have been characterized, making possible the measurement of renin in plasma as a molecule, the localization of renin in the kidney, brain, and blood vessels, and the investigation of the role of the renin–angiotensin system in physiologic and pathologic circumstances.

REFERENCES

1. Galen FX, Devaux C, Guyenne T, Ménard J, Corvol P (1979) Multiple forms of human renin: Purification and characterization. J Biol Chem 254: 4848–4855
2. Yokosawa H, Inagami T, Haas E (1979) Purification of human renin. Biochem Biophys Res Commun 83: 306–312
3. Slater E, Cohn RC, Dzau JJ, Haber E (1978) Purification of human renal renin. Clin Sci Mol Med 55(Suppl. 4): 117S–119S
4. Cohen S, Taylor JM, Murakami K, Michelakis AM, Inagami T (1972) Isolation and characterization of renin-like enzymes from mouse submaxillary glands. Biochemistry 11: 4286–4293

5. Haber E, Slater E (1977) Purification of renin: A review. Circ Res 40(Suppl. I): 36–40
6. Haas E, Lamfrom H, Goldblatt H (1953) Isolation and purification of hog renin. Arch Biochem Biophys 42: 368–380
7. Haas E, Goldblatt H, Gipson E (1965) Extraction, purification and acetylation of human renin and the production of antirenin to human renin. Arch Biochem Biophys 110: 534–543
8. Inagami T, Murakami K (1977) Pure renin: Isolation from hog kidney and characterization. J Biol Chem 252: 2978–2983
9. Corvol P, Devaux C, Ménard J (1973) Pepstatin, an inhibitor for renin purification by affinity chromatography. FEBS Lett 34: 189–192
10. Murakami K, Inagami T, Michelakis AM, Cohen S (1973) An affinity column for renin. Biochem Biophys Res Commun 54: 482–487
11. Devaux C, Ménard J, Sicard P, Corvol P (1976) Partial characterization of hog renin purified by affinity chromatography. Eur J Biochem 64: 621–627
12. Poulsen K, Burton J, Haber E (1973) Competitive inhibitors of renin. Biochemistry 12: 3877–3882
13. Poulsen K, Burton J, Haber E (1975) Purification of hog renin by affinity chromatography using the synthetic competitive inhibitor (D-Leu⁶) octapeptide. Biochim Biophys Acta 400: 258–262
14. Chou HJ, Shaper JH, Gregerman RI (1978) Separation of human renal renin and pseudorenin by affinity chromatography on hemoglobin-Sepharose-2 B. Biochim Biophys Acta 524: 183–187
15. Philips MI, Weyhenmeyer J, Felix D, Ganten D, Hoffman WE (1979) Evidence for a brain renin-angiotensin system. Fed Proc 38: 2260–2266
16. Takii Y, Takahashi N, Inagami T, Yokosawa N (1980) A new form of renin in normal human plasma: "Big renin" is a mixture of inactive prorenin and the new active high molecular weight renin. Life Sci 26: 347–353
17. Galen FX, Devaux C, Grogg P, Ménard J, Corvol P (1978) Fluorimetric assay of renin. Biochim Biophys Acta 523: 485–493
18. Michelakis AM, Yoshida H, Merizie J, Murakami K, Inagami T (1974) A radioimmunoassay for the direct measurement of renin in mice and its application to submaxillary gland and kidney studies. Endocrinology 99: 1101–1105
19. Hirose S, Workman RJ, Inagami T (1979) Specific antibody to hog renal renin and its application to the direct radioimmunoassay of renin in various organs. Circ Res 45: 275–281
20. Galen FX, Guyenne TT, Devaux C, Auzan C, Corvol P, Ménard J (1979) Direct radio-immunoassay of human renin. J Clin Endocrinol Metab 48: 1041–1043
21. Dzan VJ, Kopelman RI, Barger AC, Haber E (1980) Renin specific antibody for study of cardiovascular homeostasis. Science 207: 1091–1093
22. Malling C, Poulsen K (1977) Direct measurement of high molecular weight forms of renin in plasma. Biochim Biophys Acta 491: 542–550
23. Corvol P, Devaux C, Ito T, Sicard P, Ducloux J, Ménard J (1977) Large scale purification of hog renin: Physico-chemical characterization. Circ Res 41: 616–622
24. Matoba T, Murakami K, Inagami T (1978) Rat renin: Purification and characterization. Biochim Biophys Acta 526: 560–571
25. Hackenthal E, Hackenthal R, Hilgenfeldt U (1978) Isorenin, pseudorenin cathepsin D and renin. Biochim Biophys Acta 522: 574–588
26. Dzau VJ, Slater EE, Haber E (1979) Complete purification of dog renal renin Biochemistry 18: 5224–5228

High-Molecular-Weight Form of Renal Renin and Renin-Binding Substance in the Dog

Kenjiro Yamamoto, Fumihiko Ikemoto, Kazuo Takaori, and Minoru Kawamura

A high-molecular-weight form of renin, has been reported to be detectable in kidney cortex (1), amniotic fluid (2), and plasma (3). However, little is known of its relevance in physiology and pathology, including the mechanism of formation.

Previously, we (4) reported the molecular weight of renin in the renal cortex homogenate of the dog to be approximately 40,000 daltons (low-molecular-weight form of renin). The addition of 5 mM sodium tetrathionate to the homogenate resulted in conversion of this renin to a high-molecular-weight form (molecular weight, 60,000), which was then reconverted to the low-molecular-weight form by the addition of 50 mM dithiothreitol. On the other hand, isolated renin granules were found to contain only the low-molecular-weight form of renin (4), and the addition of sodium tetrathionate to this renin did not convert it to the high-molecular-weight form unless a cytosol fraction (soluble fraction of the homogenate) of kidney cortex was added (5). These results clearly indicated that the molecular weight of the storage form of renin in the dog kidney is 40,000 daltons, and that the high-molecular-weight form of renin is a product of the 40,000 renin and a "renin-binding substance" that is a constituent of cytosol, presumably from the renal cortical cells. Interconversion of the two types of renin is attributed to an oxidation–reduction of sulfhydryl groups.

In this paper, we describe briefly our recent findings on the nature of the dog renin-binding substance that results in the conversion of the low-molecular-weight form of renin to the high-molecular-weight form.

The renin-binding substance is located in the cytosol fraction of kidney cortex, not in the kidney medulla or liver. The cytosol fraction of kidney cortex reacted with renin extracted from isolated renin granules in the presence of 5 mM sodium tetrathionate to form the high-molecular-weight form of renin, while those of renal medulla and liver did not. The renin-binding substance was nondialysable, heat unstable, and acid labile.

The molecular weight of renin-binding substance was evaluated. It was theoretically expected to be 20,000 daltons, calculated as the difference in molecular size between low- and high-molecular-weight forms of renin. The cytosol fraction (1 ml) from a 10% homogenate of kidney cortex was applied to a Sephadex G-200 column (1.6 × 90 cm) and eluted with phosphate buffer (pH 7.2) to separate the cytosol into four fractions: molecular weight range over 156,000 (I), 156,000–60,000 (II), 60,000–47,000 (III), and below 47,000 daltons (IV). A sufficient amount of renin extracted from isolated renin granules and 5 mM sodium tetrathionate were then mixed with each fraction, and the conversion of renin to the high-molecular-weight form was examined on a Sephadex G-100 column. The renin-binding substance was detected in fraction II, corresponding to the molecular weight region between 60,000 and 156,000 daltons. The possibility that the renin-binding substance might be an aggregated form was examined by applying it to a Sephadex G-75 column equilibrated with 4 M urea. The cortex of dog kidney was homogenized with two volumes of 6 M urea to give a final concentration of 4 M urea, and then the cytosol was prepared. Separation of this cytosol on Sephadex G-75 equilibrated with 4 M urea also resulted in demonstration of the renin-binding substance in a molecular weight region of over 60,000 daltons. These results indicate that the renin-binding substance is of quite high molecular weight, and may not be an aggregated form with weak binding. The reason for the unexpected higher molecular weight of the renin-binding substance remains unsolved, although it is possible that the extractable form is a complex of carrier protein and renin-binding substance.

Renal renin has been reported to be a glycoprotein. An affinity chromatography of the cytosol fraction using concanavalin A–Sepharose 4B was performed. The cytosol fraction (0.9 ml) was made from a 20% homogenate of dog kidney cortex. It was mixed with 0.1 ml of 10 mM $CaCl_2$ and then applied to a concanavalin A column (8.5 × 100 mm). The renin-binding substance passed through the column, being eluted with 0.05 M phosphate buffer containing 0.1 M NaCl (pH 7.4), while renin was retained in the column to be subsequently eluted with 0.5 M α-methyl-D-mannoside.

Binding of low-molecular-weight form of renin with the renin-binding substance proceeded in 1% Triton X-100, suggesting no involvement of lipids or lipoproteins in the binding reaction. Further, when the renal cortical homogenate was mixed with ten volumes of chloroform, the chloroform then discarded and 5 M sodium tetrathionate added to the aqueous phase, the low-molecular-weight form of renin was converted to the high-molecular-weight form as in experiments without chloroform. This result also strongly suggested no involvement of lipids in the conversion.

SUMMARY

The conversion of certain high- and low-molecular-weight forms of partially purified renal renin is reversible, involving oxidation–reduction of sulfhydryl groups. A renin-binding substance is required for conversion of the low-molecular-weight form of renin to the high-molecular-weight form. The renin-binding substance is located in the cytosol fraction of kidney cortex. It is heat unstable and acid labile. It seems to be neither a lipoprotein nor a glycoprotein. The molecular weight of the renin-binding substance is greater than the theoretically expected value of 20,000 daltons.

ACKNOWLEDGMENT

This work was financially supported by a grant from the Japan Ministry of Education.

REFERENCES

1. Boyd GW (1972) The nature of renal renin. In: Genest J, Koiw E (eds) Hypertension 72. Springer, Berlin/Heidelberg/New York, pp 161–169
2. Day RP, Luetscher JA, Gonzales CM (1975) Occurrence of big renin in human plasma, amniotic fluid and kidney extracts. J Clin Endocrinol Metab 40: 1078–1084
3. Day RP, Luetscher JA (1974) Big renin: A possible prohormone in kidney and plasma of a patient with Wilms' tumor. J Clin Endocrinol Metab 38: 923–926
4. Funakawa S, Funae Y, Yamamoto K (1978) Conversion between renin and high-molecular-weight renin in the dog. Biochem J 176: 977–981
5. Kawamura M, Ikemoto F, Yamamoto K (1979) Characteristics of a renin-binding substance for the conversion of renin into a higher-molecular-weight form in the dog. Clin Sci 57: 345–350

Brain Renin

T. Inagami, M. R. Celio, D. Lau, D. L. Clemens, Y. Takii, S. Hirose, and H. Yokosawa

The intraventricular or intracerebral administration of angiotensin II will elevate blood pressure directly and also elicit such indirect influences on blood pressure as thirst and the release of vasopressin and ACTH. Blood-borne angiotensinogen induces similar responses. The presence of angiotensinogen (1) and angiotensin I-converting enzyme in the brain suggests an independent renin-angiotensin system there. Ganton et al. (3) and Fisher-Ferraro et al. (4) have observed renin-like activity in brain extracts.

However, the persistent co-purification of both cathepsin D and renin in conventional chromatography (5) and the demonstration of low levels of angiotensin I-generating activity in purified cathepsin D (6) have led others to suggest that brain "isorenin" activity is a nonspecific action of cathepsin D and that the formation of angiotensin in the brain can be attributable to plasma renin instead (7).

EVIDENCE FOR BRAIN RENIN

To help resolve this, we devised an affinity column to separate cathepsin D and true renin. Casein–Sepharose gel at pH 3.5 sequestered cathepsin but not renin in rat and hog brain extracts, thus separating two angiotensin-generating peaks. The early peak did not have proteolytic activity and was inhibited by monospecific antibody, whereas the late peak, eluted by high NaCl concentration, was proteolytic but not sensitive to the antirenin antibody. The first peak is true renin and the second one is cathepsin.

Thus, we have provided unequivocal evidence for the existence of renin in extracts of the brain of nephrectomized and saline perfused rats (8, 9). Under ordinary assay conditions, however, the ca-

thepsin peak exhibited far greater renin-like activity than did that of true renin. This gives some support to the argument against endogenous brain renin since the renin-like activity observed in earlier experiments may have been predominantly that of cathepsin (9).

DISTRIBUTION OF RENIN IN THE BRAIN

The combination of casein–Sepharose affinity column and specific antirenin antibody provided a means for assessing true renin distinct from the contribution of the nonspecific action of cathepsin. Direct radioimmunoassay method was also employed for tissues containing sufficiently high concentration (10). Results obtained with hog brain are summarized in Table 1, which indicates high renin concentration in the pineal, adenohypophysis, and choroid plexus, although renin activity

Table 1. Regional distribution of renin in hog brain.

Region	Activity (ng AI/h/mg protein)	Concentration (ng/mg protein)
Pineal	332	1.96
Pituitary		
Anterior	33.8	0.39
Posterior	0.04	
Choroid plexus	22.3	
Hypothalamus	0.78	
Cerebellum	0.35	
Amygdaloid nucleus	0.35	
Kidney (cortex)	18,400.	

AI, angiotensin I.

in the neurohypophysis was negligible. Equally important is the widespread distribution of renin in every region of the brain. It is suggested that the renin–angiotensin system in the brain plays a hitherto unrecognized regulatory function.

RENIN-CONTAINING CELLS IN THE BRAIN

Since the brain consists of contiguous functional centers, determination of regional localization required identification of renin-containing cells. Purification of homogeneous renin from hog (11), rat (12) and human (13), kidney and from mouse submaxillary gland (14) permitted us to prepare monospecific antibodies to renin. Using these antibodies, renin-containing cells in rat and mouse brain were identified by the immunohistochemical method of Sternberger (15). Intense staining was observed both in glial and neuronal cells. The pineal, adenohypophysis, and choroid plexus were also renin positive.

Neuronal cells containing renin were pyramidal cells in the cortex, Purkinje cells in the cerebellum (Fig. 1a), neuronal cells in deep cerebellar nuclei, supraoptic nucleus, periventricular nucleus nuclear tractus solitarius, and in many more regions, particularly in the medulla oblongata (Fig. 1b). No staining was observed in the area postrema or subfornical organ.

Many small ovoid cells were intensely stained in the deep cerebellar region, the granular layer and white matter of the cerebellum, in the lamina terminalis and in the medulla oblongata. These cells were also stained by antigalactocerebroside antibodies on the same slide. Since this glycolipid is a specific marker of oligodendrocytes, these renin-containing cells were identified as oligodendroglial cells.

Small cells with morphology similar to astroglia were also renin positive in the thalamus, septum, hippocampus, dentate gyrus, and cerebral cortex.

The evidence for renin in glial cells provided evidence for hitherto unrecognized regulatory roles of glial cells. At present, it is not clear whether renin is synthesized in both glial and neuronal cells or in one type and taken up by another type of cell.

Many renin-positive glial cells are closely associated with small vessels in the brain. This indicates close interaction with the blood. Present findings that renin is found widely distributed outside of circumventricular regions indicate that angiotensin in the brain may have more general functions other than the hitherto recognized function associated with the circumventricular regions.

SUMMARY

Renin in the brain was separated from acid protease and identified as true renin in nephrectomized- and saline-perfused rats. Under ordinary assay conditions using homogenized brain extract, angiotensin I-generating activity mediated by true renin is much smaller than that mediated by acid proteases. However, the acid protease may not contribute to physiologic angiotensin generation. Renin is widely distributed in all regions of the

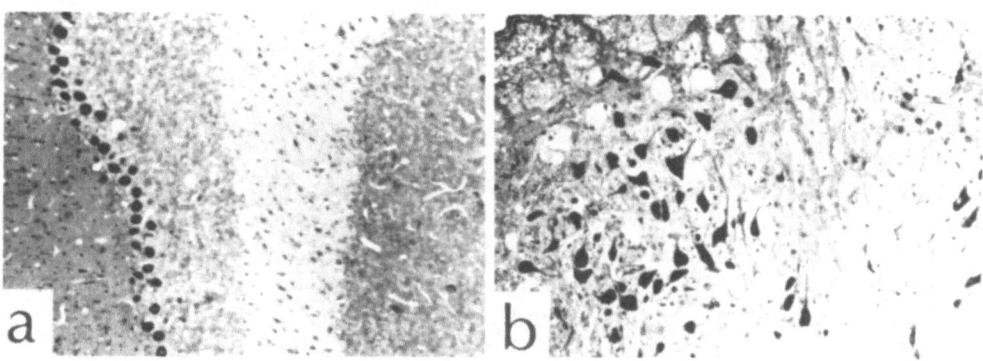

Fig. 1. Renin-containing cells in rat brain. **a:** Cerebellar Purkinje cells; **b:** neuronal cells in the medulla oblongata.

rat brain. Its concentration is particularly high in the pineal, adenohypophysis, and choroid plexus. Immunohistochemical studies show intracellular localization of renin both in glial and neuronal cells. Purkinje cells are stained very strongly. Intracellular localization indicates endogenous synthesis of renin in these cells. Perivascular tissues associated with oligodendrocytes are also stained, suggesting possible glial–vascular interaction and perivascular localization of renin.

REFERENCES

1. Printz MP, Lewicki JA (1977) Renin substrate in the CNS: Potential significance to central regulatory mechanism. In: Buckley JP, Ferrario CM (eds) Central action of angiotensin and related hormones. Pergamon, New York, pp 57–64
2. Yang HYT, Neff NH (1972) Distribution and properties of angiotensin converting enzyme of rat brain. J Neurochem 19: 2443–2450
3. Ganten D, Marquez-Julio A, Granger P, Hayduk K, Karsunky KP, Boucher RR, Genest J (1971) Renin in dog brain. Am J Physiol 221: 1733–1737
4. Fischer-Ferraro C, Nahmod VE, Goldstein DJ, Finkielman S (1971) Angiotensin and renin in rat and dog brain. J Exp Med 133: 353–361
5. Day RP, Reid IA (1976) Renin activity in dog brain: Enzymological similarity to cathepsin D. Endocrinology 99: 93–100
6. Hackanthal E, Hackenthal R, Hilgenfeld U (1978) Purification and partial characterization of rat brain acid protease (isorenin). Biochim Biophys Acta 522: 561–573
7. Reid IA (1977) Is there a brain renin-angiotensin system? Circ Res 41: 147–153
8. Hirose S, Yokosawa H, Inagami T (1978) Immunochemical identification of renin in rat brain and distinction from acid proteases. Nature 274: 392–393
9. Inagami T, Yokosawa H, Hirose S (1978) Definitive evidence for renin in rat brain by affinity chromatographic separation from protease. Clin Sci Mol Med 55: 121S–123S
10. Hirose S, Workman RJ, Inagami T (1979) Specific antibody to hog renal and renin and its application to the direct radioimmunoassay of renin in various organs. Circ Res 45: 275–281
11. Murakami K, Inagami T (1975) Isolation of pure and stable renin from hog kidney. Biochem Biophys Res Commun 62: 757–763
12. Matoba T, Murakami K, Inagami T (1978) Rat renin: Purification and characterization. Biochim Biophys Acta 526: 560–571
13. Yokosawa H, Inagami T, Haas E (1978) Purification of human renin. Biochem Biophys Res Commun 83: 306–312
14. Cohen S, Taylor JM, Murakami K, Michelakis AM, Inagami T (1972) Isolation and characterization of renin-like enzymes from mouse submaxillary glands. Biochemistry 11: 4286–4892
15. Sternberger LW (1974) Immunocytochemistry. Prentice-Hall, Englewood Cliffs, New Jersey, pp 129–171

Role of the Brain Renin–Angiotensin System in Central Mechanisms of Blood Pressure Control

D. Ganten, G. Speck, J. F. E. Mann, and Th. Unger

Selected aspects concerning the possible role of the brain renin–angiotensin system in central mechanisms of blood pressure control and recent advances in our laboratory on the biochemistry of brain renin will be discussed in this paper. For more detailed information on the brain renin–angiotensin system and for description of methods, the reader is referred to previous publications (1–21).

PURIFICATION OF BRAIN RENIN

The key enzyme for the generation of angiotensin from angiotensinogen is renin. We have, therefore, purified renin from human (5) and mouse brain (19) and tested its angiotensin-forming capacity in an in vivo enzyme assay (5, 6).

Human brains were obtained from the Department of Pathology not later than 24 h after death. Sephadex G-100 gel filtration after acetone extraction proved to be a powerful purification step, separating the bulk of protein and angiotensinase activity from renin. Renin (measured by angiotensin I generation from homologous angiotensinogen) and cathepsin D-like acid-protease activity (measured by its proteolytic activity with denatured hemoglobin substrate (1) eluted with the same volume; the enzyme pool from the Sephadex G-100 column was submitted to further purification, including affinity chromatography.

Separation of cathepsin D-like acid-protease activity from renin was achieved on pepstatin–Sepharose affinity chromatography; proteins and cathepsin D-like acid-protease activity eluted with phosphate buffers 0.02–0.1 M, pH 6.8, and 0.1–M acetate buffer, pH 5.2, containing 1–M NaCl. Renin was eluted with an increasing pH gradient 3.4–6.3 and a urea gradient 0–3 M in 0.1–M acetate buffer. The overall purification of renin from the acetone powder was 3,600-fold and the specific activity was 560 pmol angiotensin I/mg protein. The renin fraction was free of other enzyme activities (5).

Several extrarenal tissues of mice contained high concentrations of renin, and mouse brain proved to be a rich source for the enzyme. Gel chromatography of an acetone powder extract of brain and kidney from mice was performed on a Sephadex G-100 column similar to the purification of human brain renin. The enzymes were then further purified on different affinity chromatography systems using the acid-protease inhibitor pepstatin as well as hemoglobin, α-casein, and Cibacron Blue F3 GA as ligands on Sepharose or on agarose as a matrix (19).

The hemoglobin and casein affinity columns were developed with Theorell Stenhagen phosphate buffer at pH 3.5 and 8.5. On both systems, brain and kidney renin were not retained at pH 3.5, and they eluted with the void volumes (enzymes Hb-I and Ca-I). A second renin-like enzyme was eluted at pH 8.5 from both columns (enzymes Hb-II and Ca-II). From kidney, only the enzymes Hb-I and Ca-I corresponded to true renin. From brain, apart from the enzyme Ca-I, enzyme Ca-II was also similar to kidney renin and was inhibited by monospecific antibodies that were raised against pure mouse submaxillary gland renin (13). The separation of renin from cathepsin D-like activity was accomplished on Cibacron Blue affinity chromatography (19). Cathepsin D-like enzymes were eluted in the void volume, while renin from brain and kidney eluted with a 1–M NaCl gradient at pH 6.5. Brain and kidney renin had no angiotensinase activity, and the pH optimum of enzyme activity was in the neutral pH range (Fig. 1).

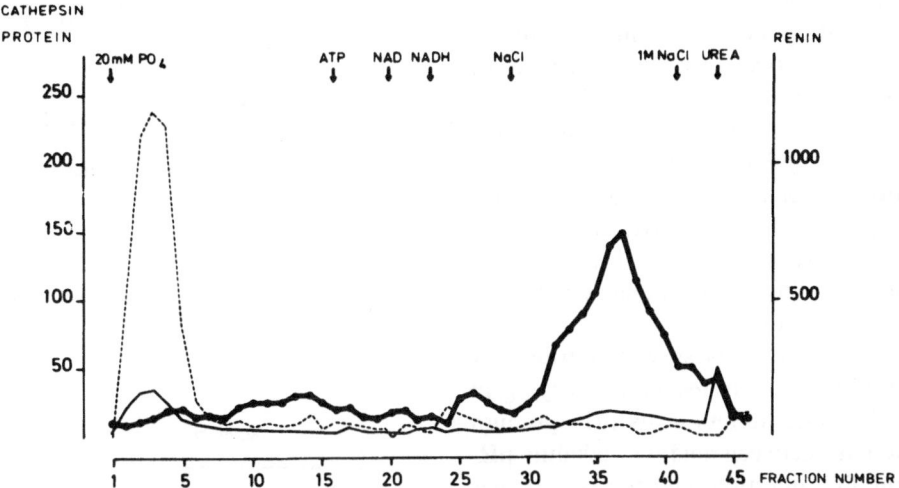

Fig. 1. Separation of mouse brain renin from cathepsin D-like activity on blue agarose column. This separation from cathepsin D-like acid protease activity was accomplished on Cibacron blue chromatography. Cathepsin D-like enzymes were not retained on the column when applied with 20-mM phosphate buffer pH 7.5. Brain renin resisted to nucleotide washings with ATP, NAO, and NAOH but eluted with a 1-M NaCl gradient. Mouse brain renin had no angiotensinase or nonspecific protease activity. The optimum of enzyme activity was in the neutral pH range. Mouse kidney renin was separated from cathepsin D-like enzyme activity in the same way. ●————●, Renin (pg angiotensin I/100 μl/h); – – – –, cathepsin (μ BSA (bovine serum albumin) Eq/100 μl/h; ————, protein μg BSA/100 μl.

IMMUNOHISTOCHEMICAL LOCALIZATION OF RENIN IN RAT AND MOUSE BRAIN

Brain and kidney renin from rat and mouse cross react with antibodies raised against pure mouse submaxillary gland renin (13). This fact allowed the immunocytochemical demonstration of renin-like material in mouse and rat brain (4). Two different histochemical techniques were used: a) For the peroxidase–antiperoxidase (PAP) staining, adult mice and rats were fixed by retrograde aortic perfusion with a solution of 0.25% glutaraldehyde in formaldehyde-picric acid. b) For the immunocytochemical fluorescence studies, adult male rats were treated with 75 μg intracerebroventricular (i.c.v.) colchicin, and 24 h later they were perfused with 4% formaldehyde solution.

Specificity of the antibody–antigen reaction was controlled a) by preabsorption of the antibody with pure renin, b) by lack of cross reactivity with ca-

thepsin D, and c) by use of preimmune serum (4). Essentially identical results were obtained with both immunohistochemical methods in rats and mice. Renin-like material was mainly localized in the following brain areas: nucleus paraventricularis, nucleus periventricularis, nucleus supraopticus, and a limited number of fibers in the posterior pituitary. Positive staining was also found in Purkinje cells and their dendrites in the cerebellar cortex and in some neurons of the midbrain in the vicinity of the vestibular nuclei (4).

IN VIVO ACTIVITY OF BRAIN RENIN

The evidence to date for the existence of an intrinsic renin–angiotensin system in the brain is based mainly on the fact that its components, renin, angiotensinogen, angiotensin I, angiotensin II, angiotensin II receptors, and angiotensinases, are present in brain tissue.

For a functional significance of the brain renin–angiotensin system, two questions need to be answered: 1) Do the components of this enzyme-peptide system interact in vivo, and is angiotensin being formed under physiologic conditions through hydrolysis of angiotensinogen by renin? and 2) Is the pharmacologic interference with the biosynthesis or with the action of endogenous brain angiotensin followed by a biologic effect on, for example, blood pressure?

Brain renin from various species, purified by different procedures and tested under varying in vitro assay conditions, differs in its pH optimum of enzyme activity between acid and alkaline pH. To answer the first question, and to test whether these enzymes can cleave angiotensin I from endogenous brain angiotensinogen under physiologic conditions, we have elaborated an "in vivo test" of enzyme activity. For this, a permanent cannula was implanted into the lateral brain ventricle of rats and purified renin from various sources was injected into the CSF. Due to the high angiotensinogen concentrations, angiotensin I will be locally formed if the enzyme is active. Angiotensin I will then be converted to angiotensin II by brain converting enzyme which is present in CSF, in the ependymal lining of the brain ventricles and in brain tissue (16). The in vivo activity of an enzyme preparation can thus be tested by its biochemical activity, that is, by the increase of CSF angiotensin I and angiotensin II and by the decrease of angiotensinogen concentration, all of which can be measured precisely after withdrawal of CSF at different time intervals following injection of the enzyme. The biologic effects on the newly generated brain angiotensin on drinking and on blood pressure can also be measured (Fig. 2).

We found that renin from human, rat, and mouse brain, from mouse submaxillary gland and from hog and mouse kidney, clearly exhibited biologic and biochemical activity in this in vivo enzyme activity test paradigm (5, 6, 16). This activity was indicated by increases of angiotensin I formation and simultaneous decrease of CSF angiotensinogen concentrations, as well as by drinking and blood pressure responses. The biologic responses could be inhibited by central angiotensin receptor blockade with saralasin (5–7).

IN VIVO ASSAY OF ENZYME ACTIVITY

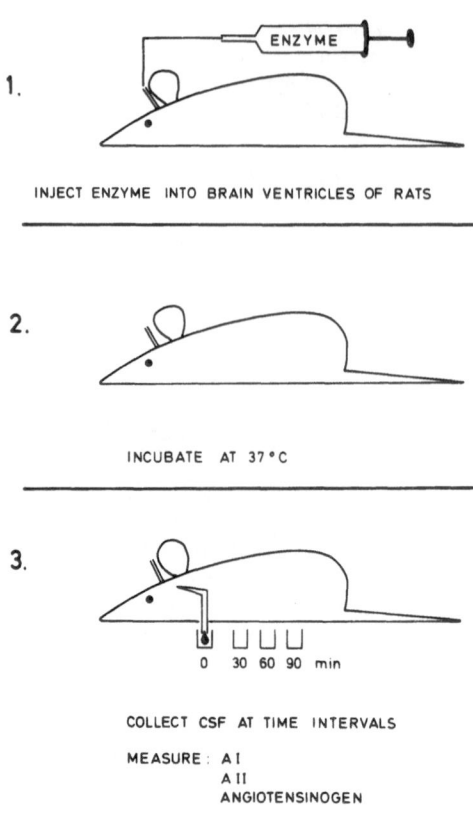

Fig. 2. In vivo assay of enzyme activity. *1.* Purified renin from kidney or extrarenal sources (brain, submaxillary gland) was injected into the brain ventricles of rats. *2.* Renin generates angiotensin I (AI) under in vivo conditions from CSF angiotensinogen. *3.* CSF is collected at time intervals from the fourth brain ventricle and renin–angiotensin parameters are measured in CSF. In separate experiments, the biologic effects (blood pressure, thirst) of stimulated brain angiotensin biosynthesis are measured. Brain renin has been found to generate angiotensin I under these conditions.

SIGNIFICANCE OF THE BRAIN RENIN–ANGIOTENSIN SYSTEM FOR BLOOD PRESSURE CONTROL

Pharmacologic interference with the brain renin–angiotensin system was chosen as an approach to answer the question of whether or not this system was involved in blood pressure regulation (8).

When the angiotensin II receptor blocker saralasin was given into the brain ventricles of spontaneously hypertensive rats of the stroke-prone strain (SHRSP), a significant and dose-dependent decrease of blood pressure was observed. This effect was not due to inhibition of plasma angiotensin, because the central blood pressure-lowering action of saralasin persisted after nephrectomy, and because intravenous administration of even higher doses of saralasin did not cause a decrease but, in contrast, an increase of blood pressure (Fig. 3). The latter can be explained by the low-plasma renin levels in SHRSP when tested at the age of 4–8 months (7, 14).

In separate experiments, saralasin was not injected but, instead, was continuously infused into

Effect of Longterm Angiotensin Blockade in the Brain of Spontaneously Hypertensive Rats *

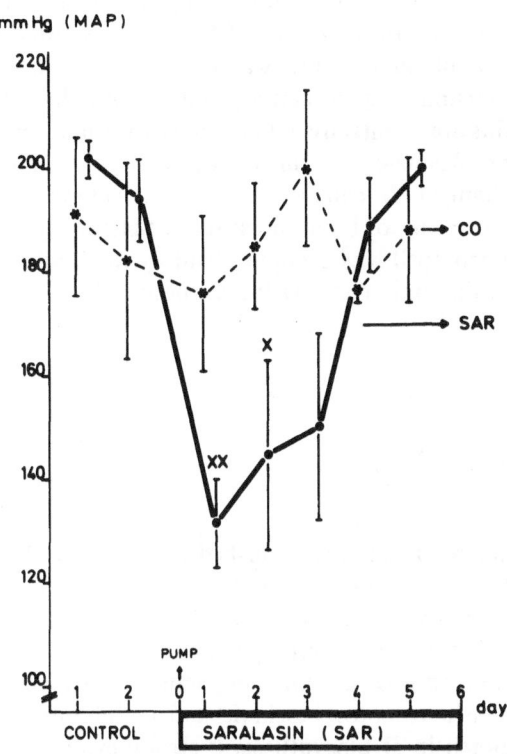

Fig. 4. Effect of long-term central angiotensin receptor blockade by saralasin (SAR) on mean arterial blood pressure (MAP) in SHRSP. Saralasin was administered into the brain ventricles continuously at 10 μg/h over 6 days by miniinfusion pumps. Note the MAP decrease in the SAR-infused rats with no change of MAP in the control saline (CO)-infused rats. X, $p < 0.05$; XX, $p, < 0.01$; *SHRSP, HD strain.

Effect of Central Angiotensin Blockade on Arterial Blood Pressure in Spontaneously Hypertensive Rats

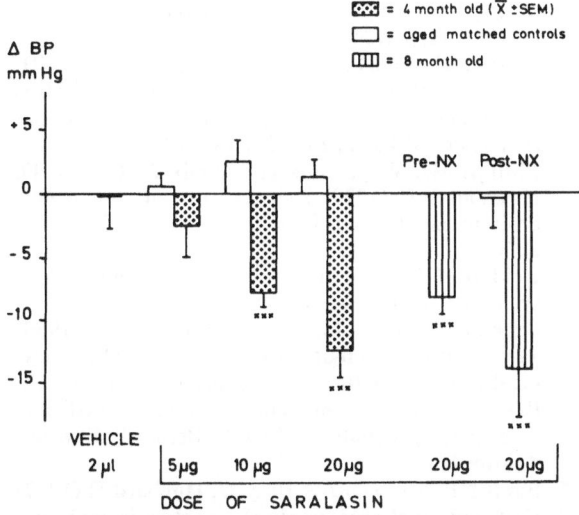

Fig. 3. Effects of central angiotensin receptor blockade by saralasin on blood pressure (Δ BP) in spontaneously hypertensive rats. Note the dose-dependent blood pressure decreases in these rats *(stippled columns)* even after nephrectomy [post-nephectomy (NX)]. Normotensive Wistar-Kyoto rats *(white columns)* showed slight increases of blood pressure following intraventricular saralasin. Saralasin given intravenously increased blood pressure in spontaneously hypertensive rats. $^{xxx}p < 0.01$.

the brain ventricles during 6 days at a rate of 10 μg/h using osmotic miniinfusion pumps. Blood pressure decreased to nearly normotensive levels in SHRSP (Fig. 4). In view of the increased renin activity in certain brain areas (16), but not in the plasma of SHRSP, these results are in harmony with the concept that the brain renin–angiotensin system participates in the maintenance of high blood pressure in these rats, and that the observed decrease of blood pressure is due to blockade of a stimulated brain renin–angiotensin system in SHRSP.

Recent results with the converting enzyme inhibitor captopril (SQ 14225) corroborate this conclusion (20). When 5 µg captopril were injected into the brain ventricles of SHRSP, a significant fall of blood pressure was observed. The brain-converting enzyme activity was blocked by 70% at this dose centrally, while, under the same conditions, plasma-converting enzyme activity remained unchanged. It can, therefore, be concluded that the lowering of blood pressure in SHRSP by central captopril was brought about by the inhibition of brain angiotensin II biosynthesis.

SUMMARY

Brain renin has been purified and it is localized in brain areas involved in blood pressure control. The enzyme is active under physiologic in vivo conditions, and its activity is stimulated in SHRSP. The blood pressure-lowering action of central angiotensin receptor blockade and of inhibition of angiotensin II biosynthesis is strong evidence for a participation of the brain renin–angiotensin system in central mechanisms of blood pressure control.

REFERENCES

1. Anson ML (1937) The estimation of cathepsin with hemoglobin and the partial purification of cathepsin. J Gen Physiol 20: 565–574
2. Daul CB, Heath RG, Garey RE (1975) Angiotensin-forming enzyme in human brain. Neuropharmacology 14: 75–80
3. Fischer-Ferraro C, Nahmod VE, Goldstein DJ, Finkielman S (1971) Angiotensin and renin in rat and dog brain. J Exp Med 133: 353–361
4. Fuxe K, Ganten D, Hökfelt T, Locatelli V, Poulsen K, Stock G, Rix E, Taugner R (1981) Renin-like immunocytochemical activity in the rat and mouse brain. Neurosci Lett (in press)
5. Ganten D, Speck G (in press) The brain renin-angiotensin system: A model for the synthesis of peptides in the brain. Biochem Pharmacol 27: 2379–2389
6. Ganten D, Stock G (1978) Humoral and neurohormonal aspects of blood pressure regulation: Focus on angiotensin. Klin. Wochenschr 56(Suppl I): 31–41
7. Ganten D, Fuxe K, Phillips MI, Mann JFE, Ganten U (1978) The brain isorenin-angiotensin system: Biochemistry, localization and possible role in drinking and blood pressure regulation. In: Ganong WF, Martini L (eds) Frontiers in neuroendocrinology, Vol 5. Raven Press, New York, pp 61–99
8. Ganten D, Unger Th, Rockhold R, Schaz K, Speck G (1979) Central peptidergic stimulation: Its possible contribution to blood pressure regulation. In: Albertini A, da Prada M, Peskar BA (eds) Radioimmunoassay of drugs and hormones in cardiovascular medicine. Elsevier, Amsterdam, pp 33–43
9. Haulica I, Hefco E, Rosca V, Branisteanu D, Petrescu GH, Stratone A, Coculescu M, Bordea I (1977) A renin-like activity in the human hypophysis. Rev Roum Med Endocrinol 15: 51–54
10. Inagami T, Yokosawa H, Hirose S (1978) Definitive evidence for renin in rat brain by affinity chromatographic separation from acid protease. Clin Sci Mol Med 55: 121S–123S
11. Kiprov D, Dimitrov T (1976) Renin activity in the prehypertensive and early hypertensive stage of spontaneously hypertensive rats. CR Acad Sci [Bulg] 29: 1543–1546
12. Osman MY, Smeby RR, Sen S (1979) Separation of dog brain renin-like activity from acid protease activity. Hypertension 1: 53–60
13. Poulsen K, Vuust J, Lykkegaard S, Nielsen AHOJ, Lund T (1979) Renin is synthesized as a 50,000 dalton single-chain polypeptide in cell-free translation systems. FEBS Lett 98: 135–138
14. Phillips MI, Weyhenmeyer J, Felix D, Ganten D, Hoffman WE (1979) Evidence for an endogenous brain renin–angiotensin system. Fed Proc 38: 2260–2266
15. Reid IA (1977) Is there a brain renin–angiotensin system? Circ Res 41: 147–153
16. Schelling P, Speck G, Unger Th, Ganten D (1980) The brain renin–angiotensin system: Biochemistry, localization and functional aspects. In: Parvez S, Parvez H (eds) Advances in experimental medicine: A centenary tribute to Claude Bernard. Elsevier, Amsterdam
17. Sirett NE, McLean AS, Bray JJ, Hubbard JI (1977) Distribution of angiotensin II receptors in rat brain. Brain Res 122: 299–312
18. Snyder SH (1978) Peptide neurotransmitter candidates in the brain: Focus on enkephalin, angiotensin II and neurotensin. In: Reichlin S, Baldessarini RJ, Martin JB (eds) Raven Press, New York, pp 233–244
19. Speck G, Under Th, Rettig R, Ganten D (1981) Purification, characterization and in vivo activity of mouse brain renin (in preparation)
20. Unger Th, Rockhold RW, Kaufmann-Bühler I, Hübner D, Schüll B, Speck G, Ganten D (1980)

Effects of converting-enzyme inhibitors on the brain. In: Horovitz ZP, Goldberg ME (eds) Proceedings of the symposium Angiotensin converting enzyme inhibitors: Mechanisms of action and clinical implications. Urban & Schwarzenberg, New York

21. Wallis CJ, Printz MP (1980) Adrenal regulation of regional brain angiotensinogen content. Endocrinology 106: 337–342

Vascular Renin

H. Thurston, B. C. Hurst, R. F. Bing, and J. D. Swales

Until recently, it has been generally assumed that renin maintains blood pressure by means of angiotensin II formed within the circulation. However, arterial wall extracts contain an enzyme that forms pressor substances from plasma (1, 2), and kinetic studies in the hog (3) and rat (4) indicate that the enzymatic activity is identical to renal renin. We have previously suggested that vascular renin generating angiotensin II was important in determining the pressor response to exogenous angiotensin II (5) and maintained the blood pressure in acute Goldblatt two-kidney hypertensive rats (6). In the rat, arterial wall renin activity changed in parallel with plasma renin after bilateral nephrectomy (7), but in the dog, renin activity was reported as persisting for 12 days after the kidneys were removed (8). However, a low-incubation pH was used in the latter study and, therefore, it is uncertain how far the persistent arterial activity merely reflects acid proteases rather than true renin. When rat arterial renin activity was measured using the rat renin pH optimum of 6.5, the levels rose with sodium depletion and fell with salt loading, but activity at pH 5.3 showed no consistent change (9). Aortic renin activity (pH 6.5) was markedly raised in acute Goldblatt two-kidney hypertensive rats, and although the arterial renin concentration fell with the duration of hypertension, the levels were still significantly above normal in the chronic phase of hypertension (Table 1). On the other hand, arterial wall renin levels were normal in DOCA salt and low in spontaneously hypertensive rats (Table 1). Thus, the presence of renin activity within the arterial wall in Goldblatt two-kidney hypertension was not the result of increased permeability because of raised arterial blood pressure.

However, all of these measurements show that arterial wall renin activity more or less reflects the plasma renin level, but do not in themselves provide convincing demonstration of arterial wall renin acting to maintain blood pressure (for discussion see ref. 10). Studies of changes in arterial wall and plasma renin after bilateral nephrectomy provide an opportunity to distinguish between the role of plasma and arterial renin. Thus, when both kidneys were removed from acute Goldblatt two-kidney, one-clip hypertensive rats, only a small

Table 1. Blood pressure and aortic and plasma renin in normal and hypertensive rats.

Rat group	N	Plasma renin (ng/ml/h)	Aortic renin (ng/h/100 mg)		Blood pressure (mmHg)
			pH 5.3	pH 6.5	
Normals	8	109.2 ± 13.17	2.56 ± 0.88	0.22 ± 0.13	103.1 ± 2.30
Acute Goldblatt two-kidney hypertension	11	619.3 ± 228.64	4.50 ± 0.58	3.24 ± 0.62	153.2 ± 3.58
Chronic Goldblatt two-kidney hypertension	8	225.9 ± 72.96	1.97 ± 0.53	0.80 ± 0.23	161.9 ± 7.90
Spontaneous hypertension	6	152.7 ± 5.19	0.89 ± 0.19	0.04 ± 0.02	163.3 ± 6.67
DOCA–salt hypertension	9	4.13 ± 1.11	3.97 ± 1.00	0.24 ± 0.11	158.9 ± 3.89

Mean values ± SEM.

fall in blood pressure occurred during the first hour, but plasma renin had fallen to a low level (11). Injection of the converting enzyme inhibitor teprotide (SQ 20881) produced a similar fall in blood pressure before (38.3 ± 8.1 mmHg) and 1 h following bilateral nephrectomy (38.0 ± 10.1 mmHg). Blood pressure had fallen by 32.1 ± 5.7 mmHg at 2 h, 6.3 ± 2.7 mmHg at 6 h, and +0.2 ± 2.1 mmHg at 24 h. Saralasin produced a similar fall in blood pressure in 1-h nephrectomized Goldblatt two-kidney hypertensive rats, and, moreover, the subsequent administration of teprotide produced no further fall in blood pressure, strongly suggesting that this effect was the result of blockade of the renin–angiotensin system. Aortic and plasma renin measurements showed there was virtually no change in arterial renin at 1 h with significant falls at 6 and 24 h, whereas plasma renin showed the major fall at 1 h (Fig. 1).

These observations clearly demonstrate that arterial wall renin persists after bilateral nephrec-

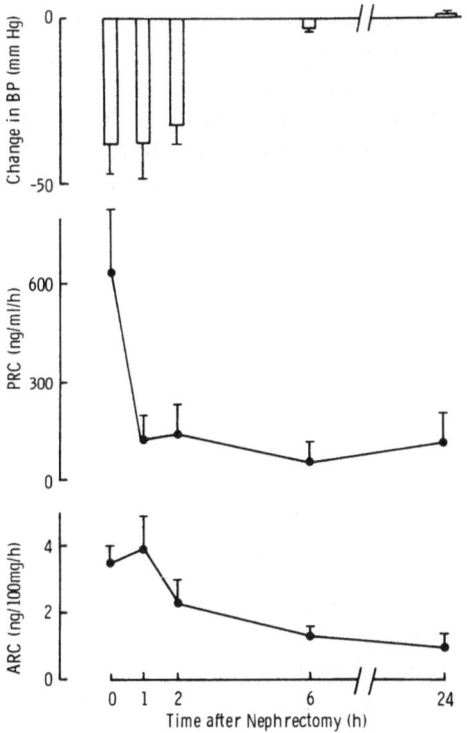

Fig. 1. Response of blood pressure to converting enzyme inhibitor and change in plasma (PRC) and aortic renin (ARC) concentrations in Goldblatt two-kidney hypertensive rats before and after bilateral nephrectomy.

tomy, falling slowly with a much longer half-life than in plasma. Taken with the response to converting enzyme inhibitor, these results indicate a major role for arterial wall renin in the maintenance of blood pressure in the Goldblatt two-kidney hypertensive rat. However, there was no evidence that arterial renin is of importance in DOCA salt or spontaneous hypertension.

In most situations, plasma renin measurement accurately reflects arterial wall renin activity, but since the half-life of vascular renin is considerably longer than renin in plasma (9), bilateral nephrectomy offers a method of distinguishing between the two.

SUMMARY

Aortic renin-like activity measured at an incubation pH of 6.5 changed in parallel with plasma renin, rising with salt restriction and falling with salt loading. Aortic renin was markedly elevated in Goldblatt two-kidney hypertensive rats, but normal in DOCA salt, and low in spontaneously hypertensive rats. Bilateral nephrectomy caused a rapid fall in plasma renin in Goldblatt two-kidney hypertensive rats, but aortic renin fell slowly for 24 h. These results suggest that vascular renin is of renal origin and has an important role to play in the blood pressure maintenance by the local generation of angiotensin II.

ACKNOWLEDGMENT

This research was supported by a grant from the National Kidney Research Fund.

REFERENCES

1. Jimenez-Diaz C, Barreda P, De La y Molina AF (1947) La regulaction quinica de la pression arterial. Rev Clin Esp 24: 417–419
2. Denger H (1956) Uber einen Reginartigen Wirkstoff in Arterienextraken. Arch Pharmakol Exp Pathol 2227: 481–487
3. Gould AB, Skeggs LT, Kahn JR (1964) Presence of renin activity in blood vessel walls. J Exp Med 119: 389–399
4. Darrett JD, Eggena P, Sambhi MP (1978) Partial characterization of aortic renin in the spontaneously

hypertensive rat and its interrelationship with plasma renin, blood pressure and sodium balance. Clin Sci Mol Med 55: 261–270

5. Swales JD, Thurston H (1973) Generation of angiotensin II at peripheral vascular level: Studies using angiotensin II antisera. Clin Sci Mol Med 45: 691–700

6. Thurston H, Swales JD (1974) Comparison of angiotensin II antagonist and antiserum infusion with nephrectomy in the rat with two-kidney Goldblatt hypertension. Cir Res 35: 325–329

7. Rosenthal J, Boucher R, Rojo-Ortega JM, Genest J (1969) Renin activity in aortic tissue of rats. Can J Physiol Pharmacol 47: 53–56

8. Hayduk K, Ganten D, Boucher R, Genest J (1972) Arterial and urinary renin activity. In: Genest J, Koiw E (eds) Hypertension 1972. Springer, Berlin, pp 435–443

9. Thurston H, Swales JD, Bing RF, Hurst BC, Marks ES (1979) Vascular renin-like activity and blood pressure maintenance in the rat. Hypertension 1: 643–649

10. Swales JD (1979) Arterial wall or plasma renin in hypertension? Clin Sci 56: 293–298

11. Thurston H, Swales JD (1977) Blood pressure response of nephrectomised hypertensive rats to converting enzyme inhibition: Evidence for persistent vascular renin activity. Clin Sci Mol Med 52: 299–304

DISCUSSION

Dr. Dzau (Boston, Mass.): We have also identified in the rat brain an enzyme with immunochemical properties similar to those of renal renin. We observed results similar to those of Drs. Inagami and Ganten when we fractionated rat brain extract with α-casein–Sepharose. In addition, we have successfully utilized antirenin antibody immunoaffinity chromatography and pepstatin–Sepharose chromatography to separate brain renin from acid and neutral proteases which were also capable of generating angiotensin I from substrate. Our immunohistochemical studies on brain tissue yielded similar results to those of Dr. Inagami's.

I will try to answer Dr. Ménard's question raised in his oral presentation about the differences in staining in the kidney and the brain. I think the difference is due to technique; that is, the localized staining he demonstrated in kidney slices was performed with the immunofluorescent method, whereas the brain immunohistochemical studies were done with the peroxidase antiperoxidase technique. As you know, the latter method is highly sensitive and may account for the apparent increased staining in the brain.

I would also like to address the question raised by Dr. Yamamoto's paper; that is, is renin synthesized first in a precursor form? As you know, despite the descriptions of an inactive plasma renin and big renin in kidney homogenate, there is as yet no evidence that these represent precursor forms. Dr. Carlson in our laboratory, utilizing our renin-specific antibody, performed pulse chase labeling experiments on intact canine glomeruli in suspension (see Figs. 1 and 2). Intact glomeruli were incubated with ^{35}S-methionine and then immunoprecipitated with renin-specific antibody and staphylococcal A protein. The complexes were dissociated by boiling in SDS, subjected to SDS gel electrophoresis and autoradiography. Figure 1 demonstrates the results after 4 h of ^{35}S-methionine incorporation. Two bands of immunoreactive proteins were synthesized by the glomeruli—one with molecular size of 55,000 daltons and the other 38,000. The former may be a precursor and the latter active renin. When a pulse chase experiment was performed, the 55,000 species appeared first in large quantities, but within 20 h most of the label appeared in the 38,000 species. Figure 2 is a densitometric profile of gels obtained at different time points of the chase. The above data strongly suggest that a precursor (prohormone) form of

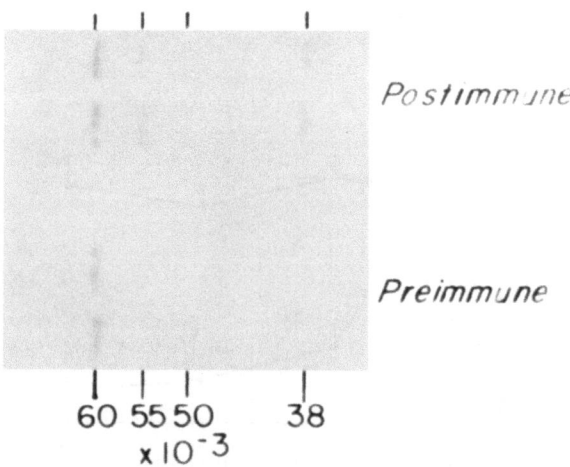

Fig. 1. Autoradiograph of SDS electrophoresis of ^{35}S-methionine incorporation into glomerular proteins that were precipitated with renin-specific antibody and staphylococcal A protein. This figure illustrates the results after 4 h of ^{35}S-methionine incorporation.

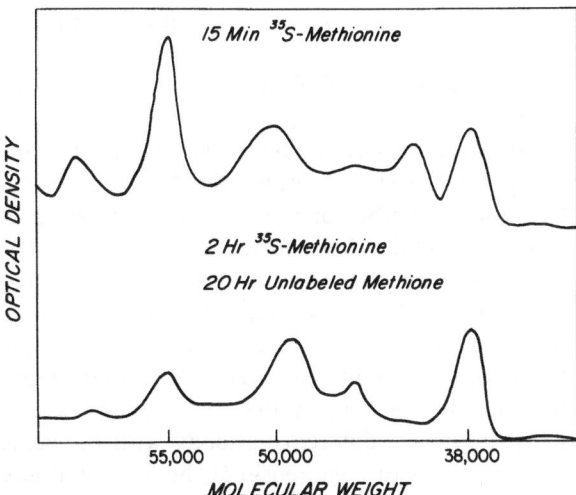

Fig. 2. Densitometric profile of SDS gels obtained during study described in Fig. 1.

55,000 is first biosynthesized and is converted to the active 38,000 form in the kidney.

Dr. Erdos (Dallas, Tex.): (Chairman) Dr. Sealey, what is the current concept about how urinary kallikrein gets in physical contact with the prorenin?

Dr. Sealey (New York): It is possible that kallikrein may activate prorenin inside the juxtaglomerular cells. It is also possible that prorenin passes into the renal interstitial fluid where kallikrein then converts it to active renin.

Dr. Erdos: We should take the following into consideration. Kallikrein was localized in the kidney by immunohistochemical techniques. But most of the kallikrein in the kidney is bound to plasma membranes where it reacts much less with antibody than soluble kallikrein. By using this technique, kallikrein was localized only on the luminal rim of the distal tubles. This makes it difficult to understand its role in renovascular resistance or its release into renal lymph and venous effluent. However, all of these actions could be explained if kallikrein is also located on the basolateral membranes of the distal tubular cells [Nishimura K, Alhenc-Gelas F, White A et al. (1980) Proc Natl Acad Sci 77: 4975–4978]

Dr. I. Reid (San Francisco, Cal.): One of the many problems with the brain renin–angiotensin system is proving that the different components in the brain do in fact interact to form angiotensin II. People have made attempts to measure angiotensin II in the brain, but many of these measurements have been complicated by problems of nonspecificity of bioassay procedures and tracer breakdown in radioimmunoassays. I would like to ask Dr. Inagami if he has tried to measure angiotensin II in the brain and, if so, what he finds?

Dr. Inagami (Nashville, Tenn.): We have not yet made serious attempts to determine the angiotensin distribution in various regions of the brain. It seems to be present at very low levels and variable results are obtained. Angiotensin in a CSF can be measured although, again, the level is very low. Whether we are measuring true angiotensin II or not has also been debated by Semple [Semple PF, Macrae WA (1980) Clin Sci Mol Med 58(2): 8]

Dr. Lumbers (Sydney, Australia): Most of the work on the extraction of high-molecular-weight forms of renin has been done using animal kidneys, and I personally have had a problem trying to find inactive plasma renin in any species other than human. Conversely, in the human, where inactive renin is present in plasma and the enzyme pathway for its activation seems to be worked out, the only reference I know that describes the molecular weight of renin from human kidney renin is that of Skinner, which suggests that it is a small-molecular-weight form [Shulkes AA, Gibson RR, Skinner SL (1978) Clin Sci Mol Med 55: 41–50]. I wonder if you could try and relate the existence of plasma prorenin to the existence of high-molecular-weight forms of renin in the kidney.

Dr. Inagami: We are closing in on this problem recently by a very careful approach to kidney renin extraction. We are trying to examine renin zymogen in human and pig kidney which we consider counterparts of the plasma prorenin. On the other hand, prorenin in the plasma of the nonhuman mammalian species seems to be species dependent. For example, in hog plasma, we can see considerable amounts of inactive renin. Dr. Mundy has long been working on inactive renin in rabbit plasma, although the concentration is very small. And then there are controversies as to whether the rat contains inactive renin. If one uses a large quantity of trypsin, one may observe artifacts.

Dr. Sealey: One of the difficulties is in identifying inactive forms of renin in the kidney. Because they have no enzymatic activity, they must be converted to active renin to be identified. The technique that has generally been used to activate is acidification.

This technique works well in whole plasma, because all of the co-factors required for acid activation are present in plasma. However, this does not appear to be true for kidney extracts. We find that when we acidify extracts of human kidneys, no activation of inactive renin occurs. If, instead, trypsin is used to activate, as in the studies that I presented earlier, inactive renin can indeed be detected in the kidney and in renal perfusates. The molecular weight is close to 57,000.

Dr. Lumbers: You have answered the question for the human, but I would emphasize that in other species there is little evidence for inactive renin in plasma. The levels of inactive renin in the rabbit are very small. In the dog, I think Dr. Sealey has shown that there is probably no inactive renin. In the rat, there are studies that show that there is destruction of renal perfusate renin by addition of plasma to the perfusate. So there doesn't even appear to be inactive renin there. And yet, there are species where there are high-molecular-weight forms. I wonder why the system isn't working for the plasma.

Dr. Sealey: Perhaps we don't know how to convert inactive to active renin in other species. If so, we would be unable to detect it in plasma.

Sir G. Pickering (Oxford, England): May I ask Dr. Inagami if he knows what those cells are in the brain that seem to contain renin. They look to me uncommonly like neuroglia, and that I find rather surprising because the cells Goormaghtigh described in the kidney, which hypertrophy when the renal artery is constricted, and which presumably is a source of renin, were described as modified smooth muscle cells.

Dr. Inagami: I think that several different types of cells contain renin. Cerebellar Purkinje cells are neuronal cells. There are also large neuronal cells in the cortex. Neuronal cells are stained in the brainstem, cerebellum, and hippocampus. And very small ovoid cells, of which I didn't show in my Fig. 1, can be counterstained by antigalactocerebroside antibody. Since galactocerebroside is a marker for oligodendrocytes, these small cells seem to be oligodendrocytes. It is rather puzzling that brain renin is distributed in several different types of cells.

Dr. Erdos: May I add that also in the human brain [Slater EE, Defendini R, Zimmerman EA (1980) Proc Natl Acad Sci 77: 5458–5460] you can find renin in all kinds of nerve cells widely distributed throughout, and including the Purkinje cells.

Sir G. Pickering: Well, I find that awfully hard to believe.

Dr. Lever (Glasgow, Scotland): Could I make two points. First, concerning Dr. Ian Reid's question about whether or not there is angiotensin II in the brain, Dr. Ian Morton from Glasgow has looked at brain tissue and can't find any angiotensin II at all. The second question is whether there is any angiotensin II in CSF. Dr. Peter Semple has looked for angiotensin II in CSF and indeed he can find some using one antibody. However, when he uses a different antibody with the same cross reaction to angiotensin II, he can't find any at all. This means that the material reacting with the first antibody is probably not angiotensin II. Next, he chromatographs the positive-reacting material, which moves in a position that is not angiotensin I, angiotensin II, or angiotensin III. All this is strong evidence that the material in CSF is a false positive. Could I finally say that seeing that immunofluorescence study from Dr. Ménard reminded me of something that I never believed before, that is, an observation by the prophet Goormaghtigh who, using very primitive staining techniques, noted that the positive staining material of the juxtaglomerular apparatus also spread into the interlobular arteries in renal artery stenosis. I wonder now, using these new improved techniques, whether it would be worth reappraising many of the things Goormaghtigh observed and seeing if renin is not demonstrable in some of the other sites in which he thought he had seen it.

Dr. Ganten (Heidelberg, West Germany): In our early studies in 1970, we showed that angiotensin is present in the brain. This was not due to radioimmunoassay artifact, as it appears to be the case in Glasgow. In our studies, angiotensin was also tested by bioassay. Also, there is positively no angiotensinase activity in our radioimmunoassay. I agree with Drs. Reid and Inagami that it is difficult to extract angiotensin from brain tissue. I also agree with the Glasgow group that angiotensin is frequently very low in CSF, and sometimes it is below the detection limit of the assay so that you don't always find it. This does not mean, however, that angiotensin II is not present in some instances in the CSF. There are several groups that have reported angiotensin II in CSF at or below plasma levels. There was no correlation between plasma and CSF angiotensin. The sequence of the peptide is not established, but the CSF peptide corresponded by all chemical criteria, including chromatography which separates angiotensin II from its fragments.

Dr. Ménard (Paris, France): I would like to make one comment about the sensitivity of the immunofluorescence techniques. Even with the IAP technique, there are still very few positives in juxtaglomerular cells. In the normal kidney, some cells in the juxtaglomerular apparatus are positive and some others are not. So, I am not convinced that the difference between the intensive staining of the brain and the weak staining of the kidney is explained by differences in technique sensitivities.

Dr. Erdos: In the kidney, renin may be in crystallized form in granules, so obviously it will react differently with the antibody than soluble renin, even in much lower concentration. This can explain why it cannot be detected in the kidney uniformly by immunohistochemical techniques.

Dr. Lever: May I return quickly to Dr. Ganten's point? Yes, of course, we have material reacting as angiotensin II in CSF. He has shown it and Hutchison has shown it. The trouble is that the "it" is not angiotensin II. That is my point.

Dr. Meyer (Paris, France): I have a question for Dr. Thurston. I am a little puzzled by your interpretation of maximal receptor occupancy, because, if this were the case, exogenous angiotensin II should not be pressor at all. And if it were the case, I suppose that it would also be the case before nephrectomy. In that case, that would bring a very important role to angiotensin II in maintaining blood pressure which I am prepared to admit. Another explanation could be an autoregulation of receptor sites by circulating angiotensin.

Dr. Thurston (Leicester, England): The pressor response to exogenous angiotensin II is reduced with sodium depletion when the angiotensin II levels are markedly raised. I said that many of the receptor sites were occupied, but some are still available to react to infused angiotensin II. Second, after the kidneys are removed, the angiotensin pressor response is temporarily reduced, probably due to excessive renin release with manipulation of the kidney causing a rise in angiotensin II levels. This is in keeping with the hypothesis I presented.

Dr. Dzau: Dr. Thurston, when you homogenize aorta and measure for renin activity, how can you

be sure you are not measuring other nonrenin proteolytic enzymes that are capable of generating angiotensin I?

Dr. Thurston: That is a very important point and I can't be absolutely certain. There are several enzymes in aortic homogenate, and more than one may be capable of generating angiotensin II at pH 6.5. For this reason, I have related the changes in the concentration of arterial wall renin to the fall in blood pressure with converting enzyme inhibitor and the angiotensin II pressor response.

Dr. Dzau: You are probably aware that we have recently examined the question of renin biosynthesis in smooth muscle cells in culture in collaboration with Drs. Re, Fallon, and Quay [Re R, Fallon JT, Dzau V, Quay S, Haber E (1979) Circulation 59/60 (Suppl II): 10]. About 30%–50% of the angiotensin I-generating activity in these cells was inhibitable by renin antibody. Immunofluorescent study revealed positive staining for renin in these cells. Furthermore, using radiolabeled amino acid incorporation and immunoprecipitation technique we can show biosynthesis of renin in those cells. This work also supports what Dr. Ménard showed in his presentation, that is, positive immunofluorescent staining of interlobular arteries in a severely stenotic kidney in the smooth muscle cells has the potential of producing renin under appropriate stimuli.

Dr. Ménard: I think that if Dr. Thurston used purified renin substrate instead of plasma as a substrate, he could find much more liberation of angiotensin I at pH 5.5. Enzymes other than renin are able to generate 10 times more angiotensin with pure rat renin substrate. This difference was also observed with pseudorenin (which is cathepsin D) in the kidney, and is due to the presence of protease inhibitors in plasma.

Dr. Thurston: I agree the activity measured at pH 5.3 represents a group of enzymes probably of local origin.

Dr. Ferrario (Cleveland, Oh.): At the Cleveland Clinic, we have also shown the existence of a brain neutral protease-forming angiotensin I. The work was done by Dr. Smeby who, like Dr. Inagami, believes that this is definite proof for presence of renin in brain. But we should be very careful in trying to equate brain renin with brain angiotensin on the one hand and peripheral angiotensin with its central actions on the other. It is known that peripheral angiotensin II can cross the blood–brain barrier at several points to effect increased central neurogenic activity. This action may have no bearing on the function of the endogenous brain renin system. Also there may, or may not, be angiotensin in brain tissue, but we think that this question will not be resolved until the amino acid sequence of angiotensin II in either CSF or in brain tissue is identified. There are differences in the amino acid sequence of angiotensin in different species; thus, there is no reason to believe that the angiotensin II in brain would have the same amino acid sequence than that found in plasma. Thus, we must really identify the amino acid sequence of the so-called angiotensin II polypeptide in the brain before we exclude a role for this peptide in brain function.

Session 10
The Sympathetic Nervous System and Hypertension

Chairman: W. Birkenhager

Position Paper: The Sympathetic Nervous System and Hypertension

Irwin J. Kopin, David S. Goldstein, and Giora Z. Feuerstein

The important role of the sympathetic nervous system in modulating cardiac output and peripheral resistance, which are the determinants of mean arterial pressure, has made attractive the notion that an abnormality in sympathetic neuronal function might contribute to the development or maintenance of high arterial pressure in patients with essential hypertension.

Norepinephrine, the neurotransmitter released from sympathetic nerve endings, and epinephrine, derived mainly from the adrenal medulla, are the physiologically active catecholamines found in plasma. Intravenously administered catecholamines are removed rapidly from the circulation either by metabolism (mainly o-methylation) or uptake into the tissues (specifically into sympathetic nerve endings) (1). Plasma levels of catecholamines must, therefore, be maintained by their continuous release; the actual levels depend on both the rate of their release and the rate of their removal. Rapid fluctuations in plasma catecholamines occur when any of a variety of environmental, emotional, or endogenous stimuli provoke a sympathetic response. Thus, pain, anxiety, exertion, hypoglycemia, hypoxia, hypotension from volume depletion, or arteriolar dilation evoke prompt increases in plasma norepinephrine, epinephrine, or both. These changes in plasma catecholamine levels mainly reflect altered rates of catecholamine release, but differences in the rates of removal of the catecholamines from the circulation may account for differences in catecholamines among patients or after administration of drugs (2, 3). Furthermore, the rate of entry of norepinephrine into the circulation depends not only on the level of sympathetic nerve activity (i.e., the impulse frequency), but on the amount of norepinephrine release per nerve impulse, the extent of its reuptake by the nerve ending, and the proportion that is metabolized in the tissues before reaching the circulation. Selective activation of portions of the sympathetic nervous system and alterations in blood flow sweeping the catecholamines out of the tissues may result in differences in catecholamine levels in venous blood derived from different parts of the circulation. For instance, peripheral vasoconstriction may be attended by selective increases in plasma norepinephrine levels in venous blood of an arm vein compared to those seen in plasma from mixed venous blood (4).

In spite of these caveats, measurement of plasma norepinephrine levels does appear to provide a fairly valid index of sympathetic nerve activity for comparison within a single individual (5, 6) or when large groups are compared (providing the groups have similar mean clearance rates for norepinephrine).

The next question is whether or not patients with essential hypertension, when viewed as a homogeneous group, have significantly increased levels of catecholamines. Numerous studies have provided data on plasma norepinephrine levels in hypertensive and normal subjects, but whether or not the patients with elevated blood pressure had higher catecholamine levels than the normotensive controls appears to have depended on the method used to assay the catecholamines, the relationship to age of the levels obtained in the normotensive groups, and the ages of the population studied (Table 1). There have been wide differences in the "normal"-plasma norepinephrine levels reported from various laboratories using older fluorimetric methods. When mean levels in reclining normal subjects were found to exceed 3 pmol/ml (approximately 0.5 µg/liter), it may safely be concluded the study was worthless. During the last 3 years, studies (7–11) have appeared from five different laboratories in which plasma norepinephrine levels were determined by methods based on the sensitive and reliable fluorimetric technique of Renzini et

Table 1. Plasma levels of norepinephrine[a] in normotensive and hypertensive patients.

Author (Ref.)	Normotensive (M)	Age-R[b]	Hypertensive (M)
Fluorimetric method			
Eide (7)	0.99 ± 0.18 (7)	Yes	1.42 ± 0.58 (7)[c]
Corea (8)	0.88 ± 0.07 (7)	?	1.10 ± 0.12 (31)[c]
Brecht (9)	0.76 [0.56–1.01](87)	No	1.19 [0.08–1.76](87)[c]
Philipp (10)	1.03 ± 0.05 (29)	?	1.27 ± 0.08 (29)[c]
Miura (11)	0.77 ± 0.11 (30)	No	1.11 ± 0.09 (92)[c]
COMT method			
Kobayashi (13)	1.33 ± 0.17 (21)	No	1.72 ± 0.11 (27)[c]
Geffen (14)	0.95 ± 0.24 (8)	?	2.36 ± 0.30 (20)[c]
Pedersen (15)	1.47 [0.47–4.44]	Yes	1.44 [0.47–2.50](19)
Franco-Morselli (16)	1.46 ± 0.33 (11)	?	1.60 ± 0.21 (19)
Weidmann (17)	1.00 ± 0.06 (90)	Yes	1.20 ± 0.09 (79)
Vlachakis (18)	1.19 ± 0.11 (11)	?	1.44 ± 0.07 (16)
Kiowski (19)	1.67 ± 0.12 (34)	?	1.71 ± 0.08 (44)
Bertel (20)	1.48 ± 0.16 (20)	Yes	1.56 ± 0.12 (24)
PNMT method			
Lake (21)	1.80 ± 0.12 (84)	Yes	2.01 ± 0.14 (67)
Sever (22)	2.38 ± 0.16 (44)	Yes	2.43 ± 0.15 (96)
Jones (23)	2.78 ± 0.18 (168)	Yes	2.49 ± 0.24 (31)
Taylor (24)	1.42 ± 0.36 (51)	?	1.54 ± 0.24 (26)
Cousineau (25)	1.34 ± 0.12 (28)	No	1.96 ± 0.25 (46)[c]
Hofman (26)	1.33 ± 0.17 (21)	Yes	1.72 ± 0.11 (27)[c]

[a] Results have been converted to pmol/ml in reclining subjects.
[b] Age correlation. Indicates that the report stated that there was (Yes) or was not (No) a correlation of plasma norepinephrine levels with age.
[c] Significantly greater than normotensive values.

al. (12). In all five, levels of norepinephrine were found to be significantly higher in hypertensive than normotensive subjects. In contrast, of 15 studies using a radioenzymatic method, only 4 reported significantly higher plasma norepinephrine in the hypertensive groups. One study (26) was limited to patients between the ages of 13 and 23, and the two others (13, 15) and studies in which fluorometric methods happen to have been used may have had problems with appropriate controls as discussed below.

The difficulty in defining appropriate controls may be illustrated by a study reported by Reid et al. (27) in which the mean-plasma norepinephrine in 32 hypertensive patients was found to be twice as high as that of 32 normotensive laboratory workers (3.39 ± 0.41 versus 1.58 ± 0.17 pmol/ml). A subsequent study from the same laboratory (23) compared plasma norepinephrine levels in 12 normotensive professional laboratory staff, 16 normotensive outpatients, and 152 normotensive nonmedical hospital personnel. The mean value for norepinephrine in plasma of the laboratory staff (1.42 ± 0.12 pmol/ml) was similar to that in the earlier study, but the mean levels in the normotensive outpatients (2.60 ± 0.41) and the nonmedical hospital staff (2.90 ± 0.16) were significantly higher, and not significantly different, from the hypertensives reported in that study (2.49 ± 0.24).

The selection of laboratory personnel or other relatively habituated individuals as older control subjects would result in lower mean-norepinephrine levels, smaller standard deviations, and the absence of a relationship of norepinephrine levels to age in the normotensive group (28). Comparison of the age distribution of norepinephrine levels in the study of Sever et al. (22) with that described by de Champlain and Cousineau (29) clearly shows omission from the latter study of older normotensive subjects with high-plasma norepinephrine levels. Of a total of 11 studies in which age was examined as a factor, all 6, which found no significant difference in norepinephrine levels between hypertensives and normals, reported a positive correlation with age, whereas only 1 of the 5 studies in which hypertensives were found to have significantly higher levels reported a positive age relationship ($\chi^2 = 7.51$, $p < 0.01$).

On the basis of this analysis of the data, one might reasonably conclude that when considered as a homogeneous group, hypertensive patients do not have a significantly elevated mean-plasma norepinephrine level.

The similar levels of plasma norepinephrine in hypertensives and normotensives do not necessarily mean that release of norepinephrine is the same in the two groups. If, as has been suggested (30), the rate of removal of norepinephrine from the circulation of hypertensives is retarded, then there might actually be a decrease in norepinephrine release.

The efficacy in treatment of hypertension with drugs that interfere with sympathetic nerve activation or diminish release of norepinephrine does not prove that the sympathetic system is responsible for the increased blood pressure, since these drugs also lower pressure in renovascular hypertensives and in normotensive subjects. Removal of a "normal" level of sympathetic activation in hypertensive patients would be expected to lower blood pressure.

The next question regards the possibility that there is a hyperadrenergic subgroup among young hypertensive patients. Of the studies (Table 1) in which there was no significant difference in plasma norepinephrine levels between hypertensive patients and normotensive controls, eight reported higher levels in the hypertensives. This may have been the result of inclusion of a few young patients with excessive plasma norepinephrine. Consistent with this hypothesis is the finding by Goldstein (31) that in a series of studies, the magnitude of differences in mean-plasma norepinephrine levels between hypertensive and normotensive groups varied inversely with the ages of the populations studies. In the present series, in eight of ten studies in which the mean age of the population was greater than 40, the mean-norepinephrine level in the hypertensives was not significantly different from that of the normotensives, whereas, in five of the seven studies using populations with a mean age under 40, there was a significant difference ($\chi^2 = 4.3$, $p < 0.05$). In addition, age-related increases in norepinephrine levels may be disrupted in the hypertensives because of young patients with high-norepinephrine levels (20, 22).

There appears to be reasonable agreement that among patients with high blood pressure, there is a subgroup with high levels of plasma catecholamines and hemodynamic changes usually associated with increased sympathetic activity (22, 32, 33). It does not appear likely that the hemodynamic changes are a result of increased plasma norepinephrine levels *per se*, since the levels are well below those known to produce hemodynamic effects. Thus, the increased levels reflect increased overflow of norepinephrine from the sympathetic nerve endings into the circulation. Increased overflow of norepinephrine may be a consequence of increased sympathetic nerve activation by the central nervous system, enhanced release of norepinephrine by the nerve endings, diminished reuptake, or decreased local inactivation. Most investigators appear to favor the view that increased sympathetic nerve activity is the cause of the elevated norepinephrine levels.

The significance of this observation is more controversial. The possibility that raised catecholamine levels can be a manifestation of an early phase in the development of hypertension is supported by the observations of Folkow et al. (34) in spontaneously hypertensive rats (SHR). In these animals, there appears to be a lowering of the threshold and enhancement of the cardiovascular responses to alerting or stressful stimuli. The plasma levels of norepinephrine in SHR resting quietly in these cages in similar to those of normotensive rats of the same (Wistar-Kyoto, WKY) strain, but under conditions of even mild disturbance, such as a transfer to the apparatus used for indirect measurement of blood pressure by tail plethysmography, SHR have greater increases in blood pressure and in plasma catecholamines (both epinephrine and norepinephrine than do WKY rats (35). Folkow et al. (34) suggested that genetically determined autonomic hyperactivity triggers episodes of blood pressure elevation, which eventually produces structural changes in the resistance blood vessels and sustained blood pressure elevation. While this may be an important factor, other genetic factors also appear to be of importance. Behavioral activation and increases in plasma norepinephrine levels under conditions of intermittent stress are greater in SHR and in stroke-prone SHR than in WKY rats, but WKY rats have greater sympathetic reactivity to stress than do Charles River, Sprague-Dawley, or several other normotensive strains of rats (36); they do not have higher blood pressures. The enhanced reactivity of SHR clearly is a response of the central nervous system, which presumably also activates the sympathetic nervous system to release norepinephrine;

but the possibility exists that there is also an abnormality in the peripheral sympathetic nervous system or in vascular reactivity. To examine this possibility, the central nervous system had to be eliminated as a variable. Gillespie and Muir (37) have described the use of the pithed rat to study the responses to stimulation of the sympathetic outflow in the absence of compensatory reflexes or central nervous system influences. In pithed rats, increases in plasma norepinephrine are directly proportional to the rate of stimulation; the rise in blood pressure is proportional to the logarithm of the increase in plasma norepinephrine (38). In pithed SHR, stimulation of the sympathetic outflow from the spinal cord elicits greater increases in blood pressure than in WKY rats (39). This increase occurs even in young rats (5–6 weeks of age), before there are any marked differences in blood pressure, as well as in older animals. There are no differences, however, in the stimulation-induced increases in plasma norepinephrine. This suggests that the pressor effect of norepinephrine released from the nerve endings is greater in SHR than WKY rats. Thus, there are at least two separate mechanisms that contribute to the greater elevation of blood pressure during stress of SHR: the central hyperresponsivity and the greater sensitivity of the vascular smooth muscle to neuronally released norepinephrine.

The responses of SHR to administered norepinephrine are greater than in WKY rats only when older animals are compared. The dose–response curves relating administered norepinephrine to elevation of blood pressure have similar thresholds, but higher maximal responses in older SHR. As Folkow noted, this difference in gain might be attributed to structural changes in the resistance blood vessels. In young (5–6-week-old) animals, however, the norepinephrine dose–pressor response curves are identical to SHR and WKY animals. The enhanced responses to sympathetic nerve stimulation, but not to administered norepinephrine, seemed paradoxical, but we have recently demonstrated that the pressor responses to administered norepinephrine are mediated by extrajunctional alpha$_1$-adrenoreceptors, whereas the responses to intrasynaptic, neuronally released norepinephrine are mediated by alpha$_1$-adrenoreceptors, and other genetically determined factors are required for the development of sustained hypertension in SHR (40).

If SHR provide a valid animal model for at least some forms of hyperadrenergic hypertension, then WKY rats may be a model of hyperadrenergic–nonhypertensive persons. As indicated earlier, during stress, WKY rats have greater increases in plasma catecholamines than do other strains of rats (35). In humans, high levels of plasma norepinephrine are not invariably attended by high blood pressure. Depressed normotensive patients, for instance, have higher levels of plasma norepinephrine than most hypertensive patients, but without elevated blood pressures (41), and normotensive patients with duodenal ulcer have elevated plasma norepinephrine (42).

Automatic responsivity varies among individuals (43, 44). The sources of these variations in sympathetic reactivity and norepinephrine sensitivity are probably quite complex, involving genetic, dietary, maturational, and other factors. The importance of habituation in determining autonomic reactivity to the situation in which blood is sampled is suggested by the low-norepinephrine levels reported in laboratory workers compared to outpatients or nonmedical personnel (23). With sufficient stress, a high proportion of young people have elevated blood pressures from increases in sympathetic activity. Jones et al. (45) found that in 48 male students, approximately 20 years of age, psychological stress of an oral examination in anatomy caused significant elevations in blood pressure (to a mean of 144/92, heart rate (to 103), and urinary excretion of epinephrine (+117%) and norepinephrine (+69%). It appears unlikely that over half of this group of students had labile hypertension. Thus, elevated blood pressure and high catecholamine secretion may be due to stress. The degree of stress or excitement in patients or volunteers may be difficult to evaluate and may be culturally conditioned as well as genetically influenced. It is possible that hyperadrenergic activity and attendant elevation of blood pressure for which the young patient is referred to a physician, where he also reacts, may only serve to identify excessively anxious or reactive young people. Presumably, not all young hyperadrenergic persons have sufficiently elevated pressures to warrant evaluation; and it is also possible that the extent of increase in blood pressure relative to the degree of sympathetic activation may provide an indication of those subjects who may have a genetically determined tendency to develop increases in blood pressure from any pressor stimulus. Some of these young people might have an increased probability of developing sustained hypertension, but only by prospective studies can the incidence of development of sustained hypertension in young hyperadrenergic individuals be estimated. An even more difficult question will be the determination if in these young hyperreactive persons prevention of the adrenergic reactions by therapeutic intervention will decrease significantly the development of sustained hypertension or diminish the incidence of the complications of blood pressure elevation. In young persons presenting elevated blood pressure and a hyperadrenergic state, there is at present insufficient information to establish definitively if: a) the combination is important in the pathogenesis of established hypertension; b) both are a manifestation of an interaction of the environment and a particular type of personality unrelated to the pathogenesis of hypertension; or c) the elevated blood pressure in response to the hyperadrenergic state is a physiologic marker indicating higher risk for the development of established hypertension from other causes.

SUMMARY

Most comparative studies of plasma norepinephrine in patients with essential hypertension and in normotensive controls have reported higher mean levels in the hypertensive group. However, only about half reported that these hypertensive–normotensive differences were statistically significant. Analysis of the data from these studies has identified the following factors that differentiate the positive from negative studies: a) Normotensive norepinephrine levels were significantly lower and less variable in positive studies; b) positive studies were associated with no significant age–plasma norepinephrine correlation, whereas negative studies showed this correlation; and c) in positive studies, the magnitude of the hypertensive–normotensive differences varied inversely with the ages of the study populations. Both the first and second factors can be explained by differences in the selection of normotensive controls. The third factor appears to derive from a preponderance of patients with elevated norepinephrine among the young hypertensives; this preponderance may also disrupt the age–norepinephrine correlation. The co-existence of elevated norepinephrine levels in young persons with elevated blood

pressure is not uncommon. It has not yet been established whether this observation means that: a) hyperadrenergic activity is involved in the pathogenesis of established hypertension; b) the elevated blood pressures and plasma norepinephrine are normal attendants of excessive anxiety or reactivity, independent of the development of hypertension; or c) the increased blood pressure associated with a hyperadrenergic state signifies a predisposition to established hypertension without a direct pathogenetic role for the hyperadrenergic state.

Animal models may provide insights into the pathogenesis of hypertension. During exposure to stress or alerting stimuli, both SHR and normotensive rats from the same WKY strain are hyperreactive relative to other rat strains. The SHR show greater reactivity than WKY strains. In addition, the SHR have greater pressor responses to norepinephrine released by sympathetic stimulation. Thus, both central nervous system hyperreactivity and peripheral hypersensitivity to neuronally released norepinephrine may contribute to the development of sustained hypertension in this animal model.

REFERENCES

1. Kopin IJ (1977) Catecholamine metabolism (and the biochemical assessment of sympathetic activity). Clin Endocrinol Metab 6: 525–549
2. FitzGerald GA, Hossmann V, Hamilton CA, Reid JL, Davies DS, Dollery CT (1979) Interindividual variation in kinetics of infused epinephrine. Clin Pharmacol Ther 26(6): 669–675
3. Ghione S, Palombo C, Pellegrini M, Fommei E, Pilo A, Donato, L (1978) The kinetics of plasma noradrenaline in normal and hypertensive subjects. Clin Sci Mol Med 55: 89S–92S
4. Kim YD, Lake CR, Lees DE, Schuette WH, Bull JM, Weise V, Kopin IJ (1981) Hemodynamic and plasma catecholamine responses to hyperthermic cancer therapy in humans. Am J Physiol (in press)
5. Mancia G, Leonetti G, Picotti GB, Ferrari A, Galva MD, Gregorini L, Parati G, Pomidossi G, Ravazzani C, Sala C, Zanchetti A (1979) Plasma catecholamines and blood pressure responses to the carotid baroreceptor reflex in essential hypertension. Clin Sci 57: 165S–167S
6. Andren L, Hansson L, Björkman M, Jonsson A, Borg KO (1979) Hemodynamic and hormonal changes induced by noise. Acta Med Scand [Suppl] 625: 13–18
7. Eide I, Kolloch R, DeQuattro V, Miano L, Dugger

R, van der Meulen J (1979) Raised cerebrospinal fluid norepinephrine in some patients with primary hypertension. Hypertension 1(3): 255–260

8. Corea L, Miele N, Bentivoglio M, Boschetti E, Agabiti-Rosei E, Muiesan G (1979) Acute and chronic effects of nifedipine of plasma renin activity and plasma adrenaline and noradrenaline in controls and hypertensive patients. Clin Sci 57: 115S–117S

9. Brecht HM, Schoeppe W (1978) Relation of plasma noradrenaline to blood pressure, age, sex and sodium balance in patients with stable essential hypertension and in normotensive subjects. Clin Sci Mol Med 55: 81S–83S

10. Philipp T, Distler A, Cordes U (1978) Sympathetic nervous system and blood-pressure control in essential hypertension. Lancet 2(8097): 959–963

11. Miura Y, Kobayashi K, Sakuma H, Tomioka H, Adachi M, Yoshinaga K (1978) Plasma norepinephrine levels and hemodynamics in young patients with essential hypertension. Jpn Circ J 42: 609–612

12. Renzini V, Brunori CA, Valori C (1970) A sensitive and specific method for determination of noradrenaline and adrenaline in human plasma. Clin Chim Acta 30: 587–594

13. Kobayashi K, Kolloch R, DeQuattro V, Miano L (1979) Increased plasma and urinary normetanephrine in young patients with primary hypertension. Clin Sci 57: 173S–176S

14. Geffen LB, Rush RA, Louis WJ, Doyle AE (1973) Plasma dopamine-β-hydroxylase and noradrenaline amounts in essential hypertension. Clin Sci 44: 617–620

15. Pedersen EG, Christensen NJ (1975) Catecholamines in plasma and urine in patients with essential hypertension determined by double-isotope derivative techniques. Acta Med Scand 198: 373–377

16. Franco-Morselli R, Elghoze JL, Joy E, DiGiuilio S, Meyer P (1977) Increased plasma adrenaline concentrations in benign essential hypertension. Br Med J 2: 1251–1254

17. Weidmann P, Beretta-Peccoli C, Ziegler WH, Keusch G, Gluck Z, Reubi FC (1978) Age versus urinary sodium for judging renin, aldosterone, and catecholamine levels: Studies in normal subjects and patients with essential hypertension. Kidney Int 14: 619–628

18. Vlachakis ND, Aledort L (1980) Hypertension and propranolol therapy: Effect on blood pressure, plasma catecholamines and platelet aggregation. Am J Cardiol 45: 321–325

19. Kiowski W, Van Brummelen P, Bühler FR (1979) Plasma noradrenaline correlates with α-adrenoreceptor-mediated vasoconstriction and blood pressure in patients with essential hypertension. Clin Sci 57: 177S–180S

20. Bertel O, Bühler FR, Lütold BE (1979) Decreased β-adrenoreceptor responsiveness as related to age, blood pressure, and plasma catecholamines. Hypertension 2: 130–138

21. Lake CR, Ziegler MG, Coleman MD, Kopin IJ (1977) Age-adjusted plasma norepinephrine levels are similar in normotensive and hypertensive subjects. New Engl J Med 296(4): 208–209

22. Sever PS, Osikowska B, Birch M, Tumbrodge RDG (1977) Plasma-noradrenaline is essential hypertension. Lancet 1(8021): 1078–1081

23. Jones DH, Hamilton CA, Reid JL (1978) Plasma noradrenaline, age and blood pressure: A population study. Clin Sci Mol Med 55: 73S–75S

24. Taylor AA, Pool JL, Lake CR, Ziegler MG, Rosen RA, Rollins DE, Mitchell JR (1978) Plasma norepinephrine concentrations: No differences among normal volunteers and low, high or normal renin hypertensive patients. Life Sci 22: 1499–1510

25. Cousineau D, de Champlain J, Lapointe L (1978) Circulating catecholamines and systolic time intervals in labile and sustained hypertension. Clin Sci Mol Med 55: 65S–68S

26. Hofman A, Boomsma F, Schalekamp MADH, Valkenburg HA, (1979) Raised blood pressure and plasma noradrenaline concentrations in teenagers and young adults selected from an open population. Br Med J 1: 1536–1538

27. Reid JL, Jones DH, Dargie HJ (1977) Plasma noradrenaline and hypertension. Postgrad Med J 53(Suppl. III): 40–42

28. Kopin IJ (1979) Plasma catecholamines in human and experimental hypertension. In: Meyer P, Schmitt H (eds) Nervous system and hypertension. John Wiley & Sons, New York, pp 267–276

29. de Champlain J, Cousineau D (1977) Lack of correlation between age and circulating catecholamines in hypertensive patients. New Engl J Med 297: 672

30. Ghione S, Palombo C, Pellegrini M, Fommei E, Pilo A, Donato L (1978) The kinetics of plasma noradrenaline in normal and hypertensive subjects. Clin Sci Mol Med 55: 89S–92S

31. Goldstein DS (1981) Plasma norepinephrine in essential hypertension: A study of the studies. Hypertension (in press)

32. de Champlain J, Farley L, Cousineau D, van Amerigen MR (1976) Circulating catecholamine levels in human and experimental hypertension. Circ Res 38(2): 109–114

33. Esler M, Julius S, Zweifler A, Randall O, Harburg E, Gardiner H, DeQuattro V (1977) Mild high-renin essential hypertension. N Engl J Med 296(8): 405–411

34. Folkow B, Hallback M, Lundgren Weiss L (1970) Structurally based increase of flow resistance in spontaneously hypertensive rats. Acta Physiol Scand 79: 373–378

35. Chiueh CC, Kopin IJ (1978) Hyper-responsivity of spontaneously hypertensive rat to indirect measurement of blood pressure. Am J. Physiol 234: H–690–H–695

36. McCarty R, Kopin IJ (1978) Sympatho-adrenal medullary activity and behavior during exposure to footshock stress: A comparison of seven rat strains. Physiol Behav 21: 567–572

37. Gillespie JS, Muir TC (1967) A method of stimulating the complete sympathetic outflow from the spi-

nal cord to blood vessels in the pithed rat. Br J Pharmacol Chemother 30: 78–87

38. Yamaguchi I, Kopin IJ (1979) Plasma catecholamine and blood pressure responses to sympathetic stimulation in pithed rats. Am J Physiol 237: H–305–H–310;

39. Yamaguchi I, Kopin IJ (1980) Blood pressure, plasma catecholamines, and sympathetic outflow in pithed SHR and WKY rats. Am J Physiol 238: H–365–H–372

40. Yamaguchi I, Kopin IJ (in press) Differential inhibition of α^1 and α^2-adrenoceptor-mediated pressor responses in pithed rats. J Pharmacol Exp Ther

41. Wyatt RJ, Portnoy B, Kupfer DJ, Snyder F, Engelman K, (1971) Resting plasma catecholamine concentrations in patients with depression and anxiety. Arch Gen Psychiatry 24: 65–70

42. Brandsborg O, Brandsborg M, Lovgreen NA, Christensen NJ (1978) Increased plasma noradrenaline and serum gastrin in patients with duodenal ulcer. Eur J Clin Invest 8: 11–14

43. Friedman M, Byers SO, Diamant J, Rosenman RH (1975) Plasma catecholamine response of coronary-prone subjects (type A) to a specific challenge. Metabolism 24(2): 205–210

44. Franhenhauser M, Patkai P (1965) Interindividual differences in catecholamine excretion during stress. Scand J Psychol 6: 117–123

45. Jones MT, Bridges PK, Leak D (1968) Relationship between the cardiovascular and sympathetic responses to the psychological stress of an examination. Clin Sci 35: 73–79

Effect of Posture, Isometric Hand-Grip Exercise, and Norepinephrine Infusion in Normal-Renin Hypertensive Patients

Lawrence R. Krakoff, Nicolas D. Vlachakis, and Milton Mendlowitz

The role of the sympathetic nervous system in the pathogenesis of clinical hypertension has remained unsettled and controversial. Development of methods for accurate and sensitive measurement of plasma catecholamine concentration offer promise in defining the role of noradrenergic and adrenomedullary function in this regard. Since the sympathetic nervous system plays a prominent role in rapid adjustment of the circulation to such perturbations as upright posture (1) or exercise (1, 2), quantification of the role of this system requires correlation between cardiovascular events and biochemical parameters. In comparing hypertensive to normotensive subjects, interpretation of the significance of levels of endogenous plasma catecholamines must be made in light of considerable evidence for vascular hyperresponsiveness to infused catecholamines in many hypertensive subjects (3, 4).

The studies to be described compare normotensive subjects and normal-renin hypertensive patients. The effects of upright posture, isometric hand-grip stress, and infusion of norepinephrine on systemic arterial pressure, heart rate, and the concentration of plasma norepinephrine and epinephrine were evaluated.

METHODS

Twelve normotensive volunteers and 11 hypertensive subjects were studied. None of the hypertensives had evidence for causes of secondary hypertension, which were excluded by urinalysis, serum electrolytes, serum urea nitrogen and creatinine, metanephrine excretion, and rapid-sequence intravenous urography. None of the subjects had evidence of left-ventricular enlargement, coronary heart disease, or cerebrovascular disease. All hypertensive patients were withdrawn from antihypertensive medication at least 2 weeks prior to study and allowed an unrestricted diet. Blood samples for ambulatory determinations of plasma renin activity (PRA) were determined on the day following a 24-h urine collection for sodium and potassium concentration. The normal range of PRA for subjects excreting 90–200 mEq sodium for 24 h is 1.3–7.0 ng/ml/h in our laboratory.

Prior to either the hand-grip or the infusion studies, patients were given instructions that allowed them a light breakfast, but no smoking on the day of the study. Subjects arrived at the laboratory at 9:00 AM where the procedure was explained and maximal hand-grip strength determined. They were then placed in a comfortable supine position. An indwelling venous catheter was placed in an antecubital vein in order to obtain samples without repeated venipuncture. Arterial pressure was monitored at 1-min intervals by the Roche Arteriosonde, and heart rate was recorded by electrocardiogram. After instrumentation was completed, patients were kept in the supine position for an additional 20 min, at which time a blood sample was obtained for plasma norepinephrine, epinephrine, and PRA. Subjects then assumed a position of quiet standing for 10 min and a second blood sample was obtained for plasma catecholamine concentrations and PRA. Isometric hand-grip exercise then immediately followed for 3 min by having subjects squeeze a partially inflated sphygmomanometer bag to two-thirds' maximal effort for this interval. At the end of this period, a third blood sample was obtained for measurement of plasma catecholamine concentration and PRA. Systemic blood pressure and heart rate were calculated from the last 2-min intervals in the supine and standing positions. Because of the short duration of isometric hand-grip exercise, heart rate and systemic arterial pressure during the last minute of exercise is reported. Mean arterial pressure (MAP) was calculated as one-third pulse pressure plus diastolic pressure.

Norepinephrine infusion studies were carried out with the patients in the supine position. All patients were studied between 9:00 and 10:00 AM. After placement of an intravenous infusion line and an intravenous catheter for blood sampling, arterial pressure and heart rate were monitored as above. Patients were kept supine for a 20-min control period, at which time a blood sample for catecholamine concentration was obtained. The infusion of norepinephrine (0.1 μg/kg/min) was started and maintained for 15 min, at which time a second blood sample for plasma catecholamine concentration was obtained. The arterial pressure and heart rate reponse during the final 5 min of the control period and of a norepinephrine infusion are reported. In five patients, blood samples were obtained after 5, 10, and 15 min infusion to assess stability of the induced changes in plasma catecholamine concentration and arterial pressure.

Plasma catecholamine concentrations were determined by radioassay, employing catechol-o-methyltransferase and thin layer chromatography to separate the o-methylated amines (5). PRA was determined by previously described methods (6, 7). Statistical comparisons were made by parametric testing employing the t-statistic, by nonparametric assessment with the Mann-Whitney test, or by regression analysis utilizing standard techniques (8) adapted for the Textronics 31 Desk Calculator. Results were considered significant if $p < 0.05$ or not significant if $p \geq 0.01$. In borderline situations, the calculated p value is given. When two groups were compared, there was complete agreement between the parametric assessment (unpaired t-test) and nonparametric test (Mann-Whitney).

RESULTS

The characteristics of the subjects who were studied are given in Table 1. Although the mean age of the hypertensives was lower than that of the normotensives, this difference was not statistically significant. Male–female ratios, ethnic distributions, and PRA levels were similar. In the hypertensive group, all of the PRA values fell within the normal range.

Table 1. Characteristics of subjects in study.

Characteristic	Normotensive	Hypertensive
Number	12	11
Age–year	52 ± 6	45 ± 6
Men/women	10/2	7/4
White/black	11/1	9/2
Ambulatory PRA (ng/ml/h)	4.1 ± 0.6	3.1 ± 0.3
Supine MAP (mmHg)	94 ± 2	113 ± 4*

Results expressed as mean $\pm$ SE.
* Compared to normotensive.

MAP, heart rate, and plasma catecholamine concentrations of both groups of subjects in the supine position, during quiet standing, and at the end of isometric hand-grip exercise are given in Fig. 1. The increments in blood pressure, heart rate, and plasma catecholamine concentration produced by these interventions are given in Table 2. Upright posture produced a significant increase in MAP in the hypertensives by paired t-test. How-

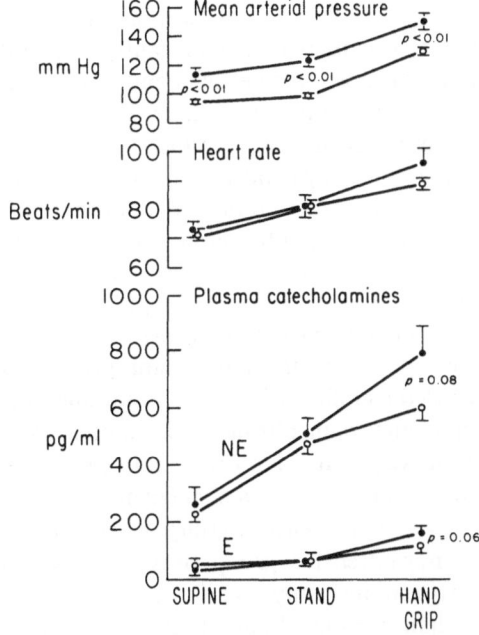

Fig. 1. Arterial pressure, heart rate, and plasma catecholamine concentration in the supine position, after quiet standing, and after isometric hand-grip exercise. NE, plasma norepinephrine; E, plasma epinephrine. Results are expressed as mean $\pm$ SE. p Values are given for comparison between groups. ○, Normotensive; ●, hypertensive.

Table 2. Changes in arterial pressure, heart rate, and plasma catecholamines between normotensive and hypertensive subjects.

Group	Supine to standing	p	Standing + handgrip	p
Δ MAP (mmHg)				
Normotensive	+4 ± 2	NS	+30 ± 3	<0.01
Hypertensive	+9 ± 2*	<0.01	+28 ± 2	<0.01
Δ Heart rate (beats/min)				
Normotensive	+10 ± 1	<0.01	+8 ± 2	<0.01
Hypertensive	+8 ± 2	<0.01	+15 ± 3*	<0.01
Δ Plasma norepinephrine (pg/ml)				
Normotensive	+252 ± 21	<0.01	+128 ± 24	<0.01
Hypertensive	+248 ± 37	<0.01	+287 ± 57**	<0.01
Δ Plasma epinephrine (pg/ml)				
Normotensive	+19 ± 5	<0.01	+42 ± 10	<0.01
Hypertensive	+24 ± 7	<0.01	+103 ± 19**	<0.01

* $0.05 < p < 0.1$ compared to normotensive; ** $p < 0.02$ compared to normotensive

ever, when this increase was compared to that observed in the normotensives, the difference was slightly below statistical significance ($p = 0.09$). Heart rate was increased significantly by standing in both groups. Isometric hand-grip exercise caused a significant, but similar, increase in the arterial pressure in both groups. The increase in heart rate caused by hand-grip exercise was greater in hypertensives when compared to normotensives. This difference was of borderline statistical significance ($p = 0.06$). Significant and similar increases in plasma norepinephrine and epinephrine were observed in both groups with assumption of the standing position. Isometric hand-grip exercise also caused significant increases in plasma norepinephrine and epinephrine in normotensive and hypertensive groups. However, both plasma catecholamines increased to a significantly greater extent in the hypertensive group when compared to the normotensive group. Regression analysis failed to establish any significant correlation between changes in MAP, heart rate, or plasma catecholamine concentration in either group when standing or with hand-grip exercise. The only significant change in PRA occurred in the normotensive group (+ 1.5 ± 0.6 ng/ml/h, $p < 0.05$) in going from the supine to standing position.

Figure 2 demonstrates the stability of the effect of norepinephrine infusion MAP and plasma nor-

epinephrine concentration. Following the beginning of the intravenous infusion of norepinephrine in these five subjects, MAP and plasma norepinephrine levels were quite similar after 5, 10, and 15 min.

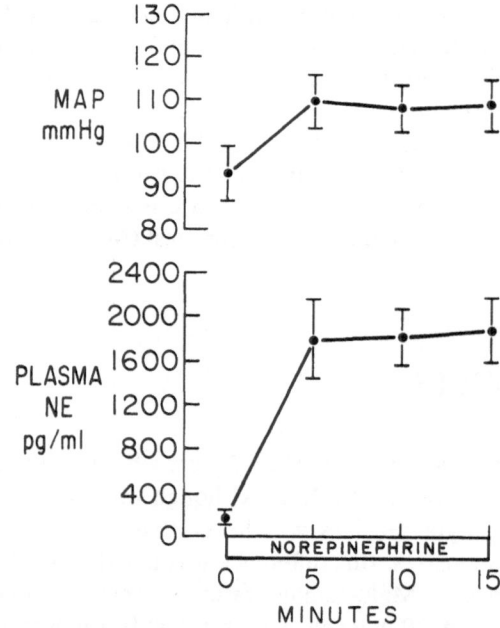

Fig. 2. Effect of the infusion of norepinephrine (0.1 μg/kg/min) on MAP in five normotensive subjects.

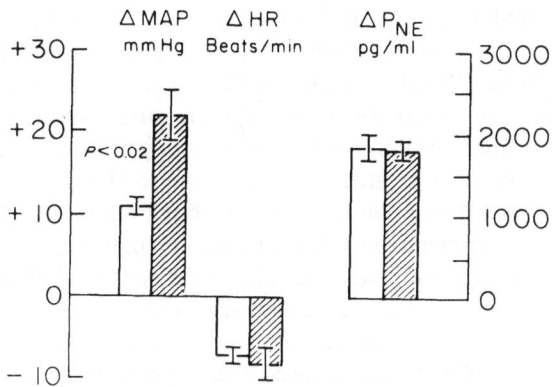

Fig. 3. Effect of the infusion of norepinephrine on arterial pressure, heart rate, and plasma norepinephrine concentration in 11 normotensive (□) and 8 hypertensive ▨ subjects. The changes in MAP (Δ MAP), heart rate (Δ HR), and plasma norepinephrine (Δ P_{NE}) are expressed as mean ±SE. The p value is for comparison between groups.

The effect of intravenous infusion of norepinephrine for 15 min on MAP, heart rate, and plasma norepinephrine in both groups of subjects is shown in Fig. 3. Norepinephrine infusion caused a significant increase ($p < 0.01$) in MAP and decrease in heart rate in both groups. As indicated in Fig. 3, the increase in MAP in the hypertensives was significantly greater than that observed in the normotensives. Prior to infusion, the plasma norepinephrine concentration was 228 ± 24 pg/ml in the normotensives and 320 ± 44 pg/ml in the hypertensives. The difference between the two groups was just above the level of significance ($p = 0.07$). The increase in the plasma norepinephrine observed during infusion was similar in both groups such that the achieved level of plasma norepinephrine was nearly identical in the two groups: 2,077 ± 163 pg/ml in the normotensive and 2,105 ± 130 pg/ml in the hypertensives.

DISCUSSION

Measurements of plasma catecholamine concentrations in patients with essential or primary hypertension have resulted in a variety of patterns. Several investigators have found elevations of total plasma catecholamine concentration or of plasma norepinephrine when blood samples were obtained in basal or unstimulated states (9–11). Such eleva-

tions of plasma catecholamines have been related to a high-renin state (12), increased heart rate (11), or left-ventricular enlargement (13). The significance of such observations has been challenged by a report that plasma norepinephrine concentration increases with age, and proper matching of normotensive and hypertensive subjects eliminates differences between these groups (14). Others have reported similar levels of plasma catecholamine concentrations in normal subjects and patients with either essential or renal hypertension (15). Correlation between the level of arterial pressure and plasma norepinephrine concentration has been observed in hypertensive patients without comparison to normal subjects (14). In this particular study, ganglionic blockade caused proportional reduction in both plasma norepinephrine and arterial pressure.

Assumption of upright posture activates autonomic reflexes which are reflected in increased concentrations of plasma catecholamines. Such changes are lacking in those with defective sympathetic reflexes (1). It has been suggested that some hypertensive patients have excessive reponses to the stimulus of the upright position (11, 17).

In the present study, normal-renin hypertensive subjects without evidence of cardiac disease were compared to normotensive subjects. Plasma norepinephrine and epinephrine concentrations were similar in the supine position. Quiet standing caused significant, but similar, increases in plasma catecholamine concentrations despite a tendency for a greater increase in arterial pressure in the hypertensives. A brief stress, isometric hand-grip exercise, caused a similar increase in arterial pressure in the two groups. However, this intervention produced a greater increase in heart rate in the hypertensives. The stress also provoked significantly greater elevations of both plasma catecholamines in the hypertensive subjects.

When norepinephrine was infused intravenously, hyperresponsiveness of arterial pressure was observed in the hypertensive group. This exaggerated response occurred in the presence of nearly identical increases of norepinephrine, so that the resultant levels of the catecholamine achieved during infusion were quite similar.

Increased arterial pressure or vascular responses to infused norepinephrine has been repeatedly observed in hypertensive patients (3, 4). In the past, such studies have not been coupled with sensitive and specific measurements of plasma catechol amines. Theoretically, reduced metabolism of circulating catecholamines could account for such observations and should be accompanied by increased concentrations of the amines in plasma as a result of reduced enzymatic metabolism by catechol-*o*-methyltransferase and monoamine oxidase (18). Previous studies have failed to indicate abnormalities in either of these enzymatic pathways in hypertensive patients (19, 20).

Alterations in sympathetic neural uptake of norepinephrine (18) might account for the increased responsiveness in hypertensives. The selective supersensitivity to norepinephrine observed after sympathectomy is due to reduced neural uptake (21), accounting for hyperresponsiveness to infused norepinephrine in neuropathy with efferent sympathetic denervation (22). One can speculate that reduced neural uptake, like reduced metabolism, should cause greater plasma norepinephrine concentration during infusion. Since the arterial pressure responsiveness of hypertensives is not accompanied by increased concentrations of norepinephrine during infusion, an enhanced vascular response is suggested. Whether this response is due to vascular hypertrophy of the hypertensive state (23) or to a specific alteration in the receptor–effector unit of the vascular wall, cannot be assessed in this study. Recent investigations have indicated that the threshold level for vascular response to norepinephrine is reduced in arterial pressure of DOC hypertensive pigs, and that this is not due to structural consequences of hypertension (24).

Despite the evidence for increased vascular responsiveness to infused norepinephrine in the normal-renin hypertensives, it is difficult to be certain that there is hyperresponsiveness to endogenously released catecholamines. Hand-grip exercise produced similar elevations of arterial pressure in the two groups, but greater increases in plasma norepinephrine in the hypertensives. The absolute increases in plasma norepinephrine produced by hand grip were small when compared to those observed during infusion of norepinephrine, despite the greater increases in MAP caused by hand grip. Furthermore, the increase in plasma norepinephrine during hand grip was well below the threshold level for increasing arterial pressure that has been observed in normal subjects (24). Finally, both standing and hand grip were associated with greater increases in norepinephrine than epinephrine, indicating that adrenal medullary release of

circulating catecholamines contributed a much smaller portion of the total change than overflow of neurally released amines (26). It is thus apparent that the increase in arterial pressure caused by the interventions (standing or hand-grip stress) observed in this study was not due to the increase in circulating catecholamines, but predominantly to norepinephrine released from sympathetic nerve terminals and inactivated by uptake or metabolism near these sites. Consequently, these changes in plasma catecholamines must represent a very small fraction of those released from sympathetic neurons. This may account for the lack of correlation between changes in arterial pressure or heart rate and plasma catecholamines caused by standing or hand grip in either the normotensive or hypertensive group. Without a more precise quantitation of norepinephrine, which is secreted from the sympathetic nerve terminals by such interventions as hand-grip stress, it may be difficult to assess cardiovascular responsiveness to endogenously released catecholamines. There is no evidence for reduced sympathetic function in the hypertensive patients we have studied as has been suggested in low-renin hypertensive patients (27). Our results suggest that normal sympathetic responses, coupled with enhanced vascular responsiveness to norepinephrine, are participating mechanisms in the established form of normal-renin essential hypertension. This may explain the effectiveness of antihypertensive agents such as prazosin, which possesses alpha-receptor-blocking activity (28) and the renewed interest in traditional alpha-receptor-blocking drugs in the management of clinical hypertension (29). Whether the greater plasma catecholamine responses to hand-grip stress observed in the hypertensives represents the residuum of a prior hyperadrenergic state (12) or is related to subclinical cardiac enlargement (13) must be settled by future studies.

SUMMARY

The effect of upright posture, isometric hand-grip exercise, and infusion of norepinephrine on systemic arterial pressure, heart rate, and plasma catecholamine concentration was studied in normotensive and normal-renin hypertensive subjects. Supine levels of plasma catecholamines were similar in the two groups as were the increases observed on quiet standing. Isometric hand-grip exercise caused similar increases in MAP in both groups. However, both plasma norepinephrine and epinephrine increased to a greater extent in hypertensives compared to normotensives. Infusion of norepinephrine caused a significantly greater increase in MAP in hypertensives. The achieved level of plasma norepinephrine during infusion was similar in both groups. The results indicate that hyperresponsiveness to norepinephrine in normal-renin hypertensives is probably not due to an abnormality in catecholamine metabolism or sympathetic neuronal uptake. The failure to document hyperresponsiveness to endogenously released catecholamines by quiet standing or hand-grip stress may be due to the small fraction of norepinephrine that reaches the circulation after release from sympathetic neurons. Normal sympathetic responses, coupled with vascular hyperresponsiveness to catecholamines, may participate in the pathogenesis of normal-renin essential hypertension.

ACKNOWLEDGMENT

This work was supported by grant HL-13595 and the Hypertension Division Fund.

REFERENCES

1. Ziegler MG, Lake CR, Kopin IJ (1976) Deficient sympathetic nervous response in familial dysautonia. New Engl J Med 294: 630–633
2. Kozlowski S, Brezinska Z, Nazar L, Kowalski W, Franczyk M (1973) Plasma catecholamines during sustained isometric exercise. Clin Sci Mol Med 45: 723–731
3. Goldenberg M, Pines KL, Baldwin EF, et al (1948) Hemodynamic response of man to norepinephrine and epinephrine and its relation to the problem of hypertension. Am J Med 5: 792
4. Mendlowitz M, Naftchi N (1958) Work of digital vasoconstriction produced by infused norepinephrine in primary hypertension. J App Physiol 13: 247
5. Vlachakis ND, Ribeiro AB, Krakoff LR (1978) Effect of saralasin upon plasma catecholamines in hypertensive patients. Am Heart J 95: 78–80
6. Krakoff LR (1973) Plasma renin substrate: Measurement by radioimmunoassay of angiotensin I concentration in syndromes associated with steroid excess. J Clin Endocrinol Metab 37: 110–118
7. Kodish ME, Katz FH (1974) Plasma renin concentration: Comparison of angiotensinase inhibitors and correlation with plasma renin activity and aldosterone. J Lab Clin Med 83: 705–715
8. Snedecor GW, Cochran WG (1967) Statistical methods. Iowa State University Press, Ames, Ia
9. Engelman K, Portnoy B (1970) A sensitive double isotope derivative assay for norepinephrine and epinephrine. Circ Res 26: 53–57
10. DeQuattro V, Chan S (1972) Raised plasma catecholamines in some patients with primary hypertension. Lancet 1: 806–809
11. de Champlain J, de Farley L, Cousineau D, van Ameringen MR (1976) Circulating catecholamine levels in human and experimental hypertension. Circ Res 38: 108–114
12. Esler M, Julius S, Zweifler A, et al (1977) Mild high-renin essential hypertension: Neurogenic human hypertension? New Engl J Med 296: 405–411
13. Cousineau D, Lapointe L, de Champlain J (1978) Circulating catecholamines and systolic time intervals in normotensive and hypertensive patients with and without left ventricular hypertrophy. Am Heart J 96: 227–234
14. Lake CR, Ziegler MG, Coleman MD, Kopin IJ (1977) Age-adjusted plasma norepinephrine levels are similar in normotensive and hypertensive subjects. New Engl J Med 296: 208–209
15. Christensen MS, Christensen NJ (1972) Plasma catecholamines in hypertension. Scand J Lab Clin Invest 30: 169–173
16. Louis WJ, Doyle AE, Anavekar S (1973) Plasma norepinephrine levels in essential hypertension. New Engl J Med 288: 599–601
17. Sever PS, Birch M, Osikowska B, Tunbridge RDG (1977) Plasmanoradrenaline in essential hypertension. Lancet 1: 1078–1081
18. Axelrod J, Weinshilboum R (1972) Catecholamines. New Engl J Med 287: 237–242
19. Sjoerdsma A (1961) Relationships between alterations in amine metabolism and blood pressure. Circ Res 9: 734–743
20. Wolf RL, Mendlowitz M, Roboz J, Gitlow SE (1975) Simultaneous urinary assays for the combined metanephrines and 3-methoxy,4-hydroxy phenylglycol in patients with pheochromocytoma and primary hypertension. New Engl J Med 237: 1459–1463
21. Krakoff, LR, Ginsburg SM (1973) Effect of chemical sympathectomy on pressor responses to norepinephrine, angiotensin and tyramine. Experientia 29: 995–997
22. Wilcox CS, Aminoff MJ (1976) Blood pressure responses to noradrenaline and dopamine infusions in Parkinson's disease and the Shy-Drager syndrome. Br J Clin Pharmacol 3: 207–214
23. Folkow B (1977) The haemodynamic consequences of adaptive structural changes of the resistance vessels in hypertension. Clin Sci 41: 1–12
24. Berccck K, Bohr D (1977) Structural and functional changes in vascular resistance and reactivity in the deoycorticosterone acetate (DOCA) hypertensive pig Circ Res 40(Suppl I): 146–152

25. Silverberg AB, Suresh DS, Haymond MW, Cryer PE (1978) Norepinephrine: Hormone and neurotransmitter in man. Am J Physiol 234(3): E252–E256

26. DeQuattro V, Margolin A, Stocks LO (1970) Pseudo-pheochromocytoma-adrenomedullary response to venography. J Clin Endocrinol Metab 30: 138–140

27. Esler M, Randall O, Bennett B, et al (1976) Suppression of sympathetic nervous function in low renin essential hypertension. Lancet 2: 115–118

28. Graham RM, Pettinger WA (1979) Prazosin. New Engl J Med 300: 232–236

29. Vlachakis MD, Mendlowitz M (1976) An approach to the treatment of essential hypertension. Am Heart J 92: 750–757

Interrelationships Between Plasma Norepinephrine and Blood Pressure Response to Norepinephrine in Normotension and Hypertension

A. Distler, Th. Philipp, B. Lüth, H. Zschiedrich, and U. Cordes

Slightly to moderately increased plasma norepinephrine levels thought to reflect increased sympathetic tone have been observed in a proportion of patients with essential hypertension (1–3). However, some authors have also reported on normal-plasma norepinephrine levels in essential hypertension (4, 5).

We have previously shown that an inverse correlation exists between plasma norepinephrine concentration during physical exercise and reactivity to exogenous norepinephrine in normotensive subjects (6). This relationship was invariably disturbed in age-matched patients with essential hypertension. In the patients with high-plasma norepinephrine levels, the pressor response to nor-epinephrine was not diminished appropriately, and, in the patients with normal- or low-norepinephrine, reactivity to norepinephrine was inappropriately increased. A multiple regression analysis revealed a highly significant correlation between the combination of both factors and the height of mean arterial blood pressure (Fig. 1), suggesting that sympathetic nervous activity and pressor response to norepinephrine together form an important determinant of arterial blood pressure level.

We are now interested in the *dynamic* interrelationships between sympathetic nervous activity and reactivity to norepinephrine. For this purpose, we studied patients who had undergone total thyroidectomy for thyroid cancer, and who were in hypo- and hyperthyroid state at different times. In addition, we studied hypertensive patients who were given the clonidine-like acting drug guanfacine.

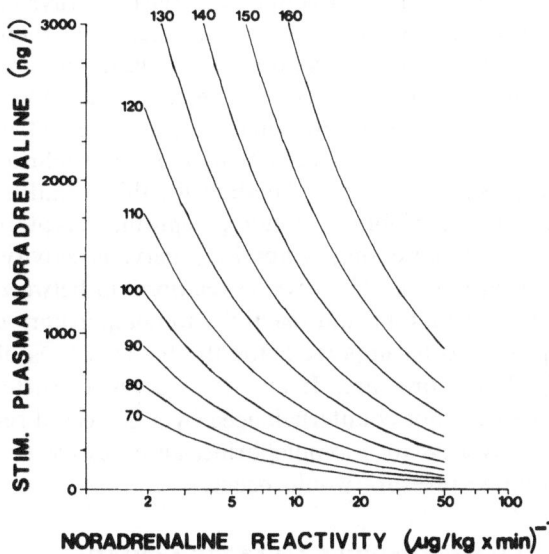

Fig. 1. Computer plot based on data from 29 normotensives and 29 patients with essential hypertension illustrating the dependency of mean arterial pressure (mmHg) on the combination of stimulated plasma norepinephrine (noradrenaline) concentration and reactivity to norepinephrine. [Philipp et al. (6)]

STUDIES IN HYPERTHYROID AND HYPOTHYROID STATE

PATIENTS AND METHODS

Eleven patients who had undergone total thyroidectomy for thyroid cancer were first studied while they were in a slightly hyperthyroid state resulting from high-dose substitution therapy with 200–350 μg thyroxine/day. The high doses of thyroxine were necessary to suppress thyroid-stimulating hormone release and to prevent a possible cancer spreading. A second study of the same patients was done after substitution therapy had been withdrawn for at least 4 weeks. This stop was necessary to accomplish the annual total body radioiodine scan. At that time, the patients were markedly

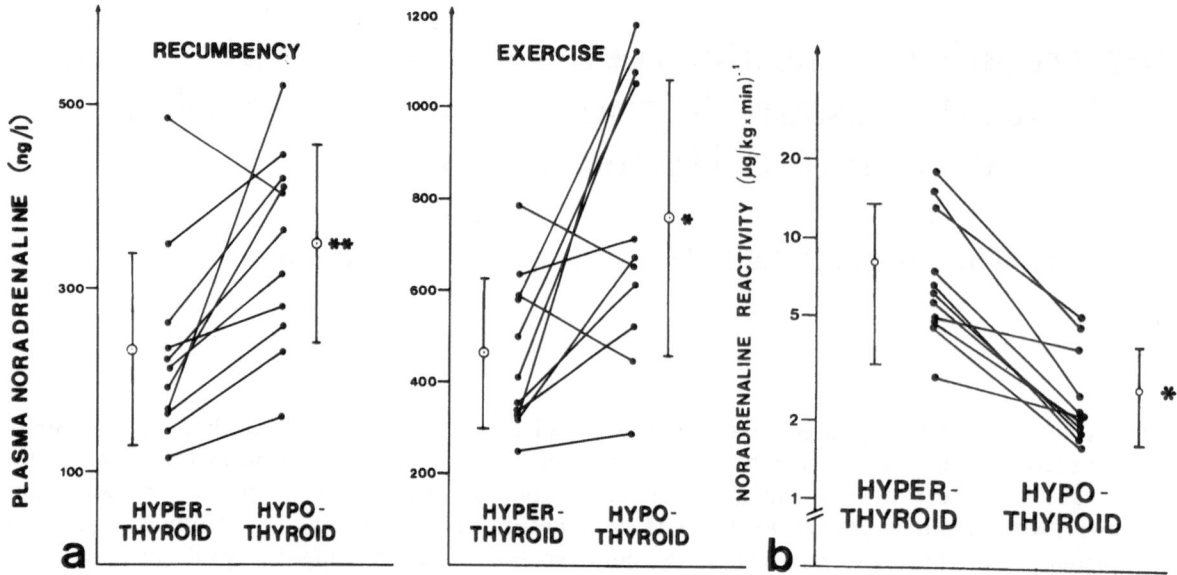

Fig. 2. a: Plasma norepinephrine concentration in 11 thyroidectomized patients in hyper- and hypothyroid state. *$p < 0.01$, **$p < 0.001$. **b:** Reactivity to exogenous norepinephrine in 11 thyroidectomized patients in hyper- and hypothyroid state. *$p < 0.001$.

hypothyroid as documented by very low-plasma levels of triiodothyronine and thyroxine.

As an index of sympathetic nervous activity, plasma norepinephrine concentration was measured at rest and after a standardized workload of 100 W for 2 min on a bicycle ergometer. Plasma norepinephrine was determined by the method of Renzini et al. (7). Reactivity to exogenous norepinephrine was estimated by determining so-called "pressor doses." Reactivity is expressed in terms of reciprocal values of the pressor doses as described previously (6).

RESULTS

Plasma norepinephrine was significantly higher during recumbency and following exercise in the hypo- than in the hyperthyroid state (Fig. 2a). Reactivity to norepinephrine was decreased in all patients in the hypothyroid state as compared to the hyperthyroid state (Fig. 2b).

Mean arterial blood pressure (diastolic pressure + one-third pulse pressure) was slightly increased (by 6 mmHg on the average) in the hypothyroid state as compared to the hyperthyroid state.

DISCUSSION

Confirming previous reports (8, 9), we found plasma norepinephrine concentration to be significantly higher in the hypo- than in the hyperthyroid state. The data seem to indicate again that there is an inverse relationship between plasma norepinephrine and reactivity to norepinephrine. When plasma norepinephrine increases, as observed in the hypothyroid state, reactivity to norepinephrine decreases. A likely explanation for this would be that the availability of norepinephrine receptors falls with increasing sympathetic nervous activity, and vice versa. The inverse relationship between sympathetic tone and reactivity to norepinephrine appears to be important for the homoeostasis of the blood pressure. If an increased sympathetic tone were not counterbalanced by a decreased responsiveness to norepinephrine, an excessive rise in blood pressure would occur.

STUDIES WITH GUANFACINE

PATIENTS AND METHODS

Seven male patients with essential hypertension WHO grade I–II (aged 19–42 years; mean age

33 years) were given guanfacine (3 mg daily p.o.), a clonidine-like acting drug (10, 11), for a period of 4 weeks. Plasma norepinephrine concentration was measured at rest and after stimulation by a 75%-maximum workload for 2 min on a bicycle ergometer before and after the fourth week of drug administration. Plasma norepinephrine was determined by the method of da Prada and Zürcher (12). Reactivity to exogenous norepinephrine was estimated as described above.

RESULTS AND DISCUSSION

Mean arterial pressure (diastolic + one-third pulse pressure) dropped from 120 ± 11.1 ($\pm$ SEM) to 107 ± 10.2 mmHg ($p < 0.01$); plasma norepinephrine concentration decreased from 205 ± 39 to 90 ± 24 ng/liter ($p < 0.05$) during rest and from 575 ± 162 to 269 ± 84 ng/liter ($p < 0.005$) following exercise. Reactivity to exogenous norepinephrine, however, did not increase significantly; the average reciprocal value of the pressor dose of norepinephrine was $[8.5 \pm 6.2\ \mu g/kg/min]^{-1}$ before and $[13.4 \pm 5.9\ \mu g/kg/min]^{-1}$ after the fourth week of guanfacine administration. Thus, the decrease in sympathetic outflow resulting from guanfacine treatment appears to produce a drop in blood pressure, since diminished outflow is not counterbalanced by an appropriate increase in reactivity to norepinephrine. The reason for the blunted increase in reactivity is unknown.

SUMMARY

To gain insight into the *dynamic* interrelationships between sympathetic tone and reactivity to norepinephrine we studied 11 patients who had undergone total thyroidectomy for thyroid cancer and who were in hypo- and hyperthyroid state at different times. Plasma norepinephrine was significantly higher during recumbency and following physical exercise in the hypo- than in the hyperthyroid state. Reactivity to exogenous norepinephrine was decreased in all patients in the hypothyroid state as compared to the hyperthyroid state. Mean arterial pressure was slightly increased (by 6 mmHg on the average) in the hypothyroid state as compared to the hyperthyroid state. The data obtained seem to indicate that an increase in plasma norepinephrine concentration (probably reflecting increased sympathetic tone) *normally* leads to a decrease in reactivity to norepinephrine, and vice versa. Therefore, when discussing the role of the sympathetic nervous system in essential hypertension, it is important to consider sympathetic tone in conjunction with its effectiveness (i.e., reactivity to norepinephrine). An increased sympathetic tone appears to contribute to high blood pressure only if reactivity to norepinephrine is *not* decreased.

Administration of the clonidine-like acting drug guanfacine (3 mg daily for 4 weeks) to seven patients with essential hypertension produced a significant fall in blood pressure and in resting, as well as stimulated plasma norepinephrine concentration. Reactivity to norepinephrine, however, did not change significantly. Thus, the decrease in sympathetic outflow resulting from administration of centrally acting drugs such as guanfacine appears to produce a drop in blood pressure, because diminished outflow is not counterbalanced by an appropriate increase in reactivity to norepinephrine.

REFERENCES

1. Engelman K, Portnoy B (1970) A sensitive double-isotope derivative assay for norepinephrine and epinephrine: Normal resting human plasma levels. Circ Res 26: 53
2. Louis WJ, Doyle AE, Anavekar SN, Johnston CI, Geffen LB, Rush R (1974) Plasma catecholamine, dopamine-beta-hydroxylase, and renin levels in essential hypertension. Circ Res 34, 35(Suppl I): 57
3. de Champlain J, Farley L, Cousineau D, van Ameringen MR (1976) Circulating catecholamine levels in human and experimental hypertension. Circ Res 38: 109
4. Pedersen EB, Christensen NJ (1975) Catecholamines in plasma and urine in patients with essential hypertension determined by double-isotope derivative techniques. Acta med Scand 198: 373
5. Lake CR, Ziegler MG, Coleman MD, Kopin IJ (1977) Age-adjusted norepinephrine levels are similar in normotensive and hypertensive subjects. New Engl J Med 296: 208
6. Philipp Th, Distler A, Cordes U (1978) Sympathetic nervous system and blood pressure control in essential hypertension. Lancet 2: 959
7. Renzini VC, Brunori CA, Valori C (1970) A sensitive and specific fluorimetric method for the determination of noradrenaline in human plasma. Clin Chim Acta 30: 587
8. Christensen NJ (1972) Increased levels of plasma noradrenaline in hypothyroidism. J Clin Endocrinol Metab 35: 359

9. Stoffer SS, Jiang N-S, Gorman CA, Pikler GM (1973) Plasma catecholamines in hypothyroidism and hyperthyroidism. J Clin Endocrinol Metab 36: 587

10. Scholtysyk G, Lauener H, Eichenberger E, Bürki H, Salzmann R, Müller-Schweinitzer E, Waite R (1975) Pharmacological actions of the antihypertensive agent N-amidino-2- (2, 6-dichlorophenyl) acetamide hydrochloride (BS 100–141). Arzneim Forsch 25: 1483

11. Distler A, Kirch W, Lüth B (1980) Antihypertensive effect of guanfacine: A double-blind cross-over trial compared with clonidine. Br J Clin Pharmacol 10: 495–535

12. da Prada M, Zürcher G (1976) Simultaneous radioenzymatic determination of plasma and tissue adrenaline, noradrenaline and dopamine within the femtomole range. Life Sci 19: 1161

Central Noradrenergic Mechanisms in Hypertension and in Postural Hypotension

Vincent DeQuattro, Patrick Sullivan, Andras Foti, Sarah Schoentgen, Rainer Kolloch, Gilda Versales, and Daniel Levine

Recently, we described evidence implicating the central sympathetic nervous system in the pathogenesis of primary hypertension (1, 2). We have also reviewed reports of enhanced peripheral sympathetic tone in primary hypertension (3). Earlier, Ziegler and his colleagues (4) described low-plasma norepinephrine and a blunted norepinephrine response to postural stress in patients with orthostatic hypotension. When these patients assume an upright posture, they have a hemodynamic state that is, in some respects, opposite to that of some patients with primary hypertension (5). Herein, we report the concentrations of norepinephrine, in both plasma and spinal fluid while supine and in plasma while standing, and the magnitude of changes after standing, in patients with either primary hypertension or postural hypotension and compare them with respective values of normotensive patients.

METHODS

Nineteen patients with mild primary hypertension aged 21–53 years, 37 ± 3 years (mean ± SEM), 11 normotensive patients aged 24–52 years (mean 35 ± 3), and 5 patients with idiopathic postural hypotension aged 46–79 (mean 59 ± 5) were the participants of this study. Results of 14 of these patients, 7 with primary hypertension and 7 with normal blood pressure, were reported previously (1). All patients with primary hypertension (a mean of three blood pressures on separate days of greater than 140/95 mmHg) underwent extensive diagnostic tests including timed intravenous pyelography to exclude patients with secondary hypertension or those with cardiovascular or renal sequelae. The normotensives had various minor neurologic disorders, such as headache, nerve root pain, Bell's palsy, or were recovered from more serious problems, such as seizure disorders and pseudotumor cerebri. One patient had associated Shy-Drager syndrome (6), two had postural hypotension and occasional supine hypertension, one patient with associated cyclic edema had previously been hypertensive, and one patient with a mild impairment of glucose tolerance was a diet-controlled diabetic. None of the patients were taking medication for at least 10 days before the study, and most had not taken any for at least the prior 3 weeks. After signing an informed consent approved by the Institutional Review Committee, the patients were admitted to the Clinical Research Center where they underwent a series of tests over a 4½-day period while on a constant 100-mEq Na^+, 80-mEq K^+ diet. Approximately one third of each group was admitted to the White Memorial Medical Center and was studied there. On the third hospital day, after fasting overnight, the patients stood erect for 1 h (two with postural hypotension could stand for only 5–10 min), and then they lay supine for 1 h. Blood samples were taken for norepinephrine and epinephrine at the end of each period. Spinal fluid was obtained in the left-lateral decubitus position after the blood was obtained. Norepinephrine and epinephrine were measured by a radioenzymatic assay (7).

RESULTS

POSTURAL HYPOTENSION

The concentrations of supine plasma norepinephrine of 4 of the 5 patients with postural hypotension were less than 120 ng/liter, whereas only 1 of the 11 patients with normal blood pressure had concentrations less than 120 ng/liter (Fig. 1). The

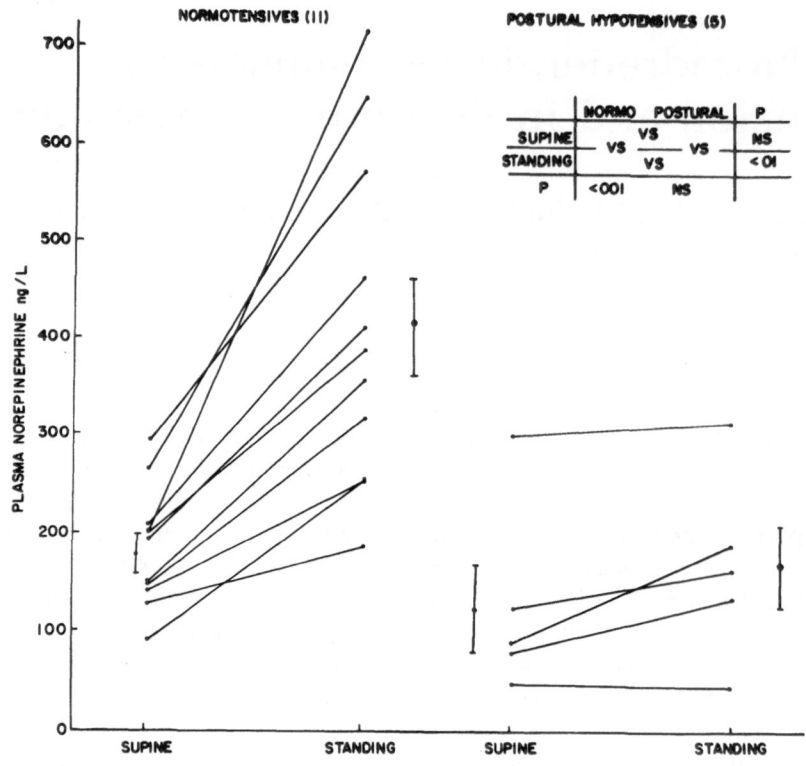

Fig. 1. Blunted plasma norepinephrine responses to standing in patients with postural hypotension. Values at margins are mean ± SEM.

standing norepinephrine values of the normotensives all exceeded 190 ng/liter, whereas only one patient with postural hypotension exceeded this value. The means of the norepinephrine content in plasma of normotensives while standing were over twofold greater than those of the patients with postural hypotension ($p < 0.01$) (Fig. 2). The mean percentage change in plasma norepinephrine after standing was threefold greater in the normotensive patients ($124\% \pm 16\%$ versus $44\% \pm 13\%$,

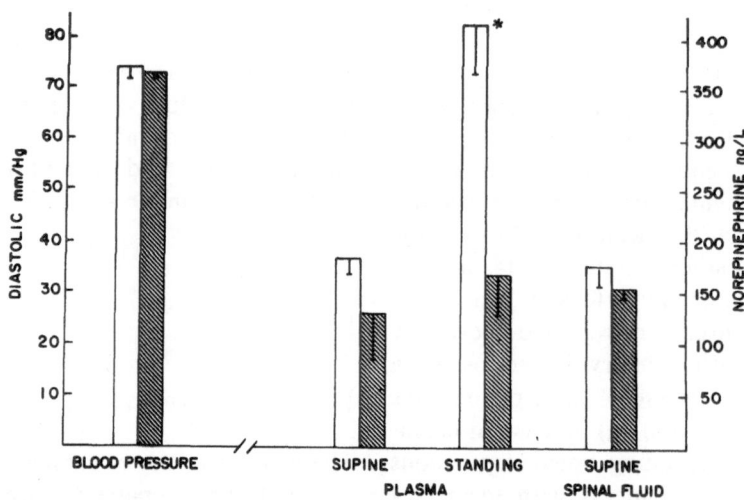

Fig. 2. Reduced sympathetic nerve function while standing in patients with postural hypotension. Values are mean ± SEM. ☐, Normotensives (11); ▨, postural hypotensives (5); *$p < 0.01$.

respectively, $p < 0.01$). The spinal fluid concentrations of norepinephrine were lower in patients with postural hypotension, but the differences were not significant.

PRIMARY HYPERTENSION

There was an increase of plasma norepinephrine of approximately twofold in the patients with primary hypertension. Three of the 19 patients had a blunted norepinephrine response to the postural stress.

The mean plasma concentrations of norepinephrine while standing were slightly, but not significantly, higher in the hypertensive group. The mean increment of norepinephrine after standing was twofold for both hypertensives and normotensives. However, both the mean concentrations of norepinephrine in plasma and spinal fluid while supine were 60% and 100% greater, $p < 0.01$, $p < 0.001$, respectively, in the patients with primary hypertension compared to the normotensives (Fig. 3).

DISCUSSION

Postural hypotension is a malady as diverse in its causes and its sequelae as is its hemodynamic opposite, primary hypertension. Zeigler and his colleagues (4) described two types of idiopathic orthostatic hypotension (IOH), classified according to whether they did (type II) or did not have (type I) diffuse neurologic signs of Shy-Drager associated with the hypotension. They found that type I patients had reduced plasma norepinephrine and a blunted norepinephrine response to standing. The type II patients had normal-plasma norepinephrine, but no increment with standing. Of the patients in our study, only one was diagnosed definitely as Shy-Drager. Her plasma norepinephrine levels were 79 ng/liter, and she had the lowest cerebrospinal fluid content of norepinephrine at 125 ng/liter. Of the remaining patients, the two with classical type I IOH also had low-norepinephrine concentration in plasma (49 and 91 ng/liter) and in spinal fluid (139 and 143 ng/liter). The oldest patient, aged 79, without neurologic sequelae, also had low-plasma and spinal norepinephrine and a blunted response. The patient with the highest supine plasma norepinephrine (Fig. 1) had mild glucose intolerance, but had some bizzare grimacing movements that could have been construed as a sign of a type II lesion. We conclude from our studies in this small group that some patients with IOH, both types I and II, have reduced central and peripheral noradrenergic tone. Further, most patients with IOH have a blunted noradrenergic response to postural stress.

Previously, we found evidence of enhanced peripheral sympathetic nervous tone in primary hypertension. Recently, we reviewed these findings

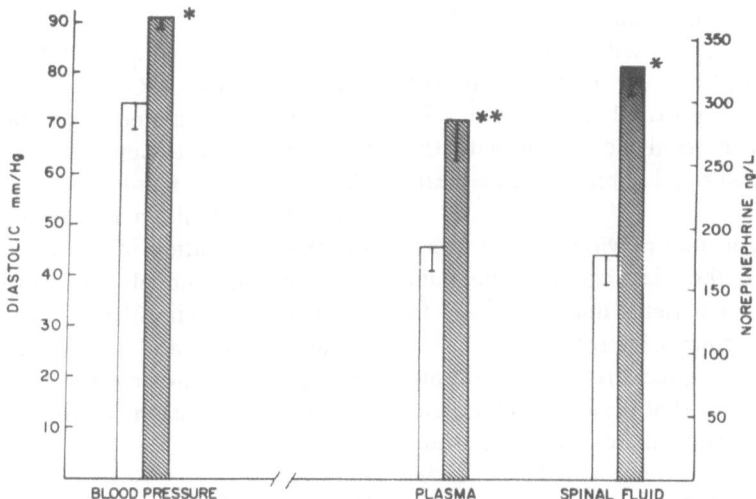

Fig. 3. Enhanced basal central and peripheral sympathetic tone in patients with primary hypertension. Values are mean ± SEM. ☐, Normotensives (11); ▨, primary hypertensives (19); $*p < 0.001$; $**p < 0.01$.

and also the work of several investigators who did not find any evidence in that regard (3). Although there were differences in methodology, we conclude that the major reasons for their not finding raised plasma norepinephrine in patients with primary hypertension were the age of the patients and the length of time that they were supine. The greatest prevalence rates of raised plasma norepinephrine seem to be in patients less than 40 years (2). Further, all of our studies have been performed with the patients supine 60 min, fasting overnight. Until recently, patients have come in to the Center for study as outpatients. However, those participating in the present study were all inpatients. Very few of the patients of normotensives in our studies have been black and most have had mild hypertension.

In many of our initial studies, the normotensive volunteers were laboratory or hospital personnel, but in the past 2–3 years both patients and normotensives have been recruited from in and outside the Medical Center. In some instances, there was a crossover in that medical personnel or students were classified as hypertensive patients, whereas patients with other problems served as normotensive controls (2, 8). It is indeed possible that either finding, elevated or lowered plasma norepinephrine, is not reliable evidence for enhanced or blunted sympathetic nervous system function, respectively. We assume that plasma norepinephrine is a measure of neuronal overflow from the synaptic cleft into the vascular compartment. Other factors such as turnover rate, metabolism, clearance, etc., might predominate in influencing the level of this marker. It is noteworthy, however, that plasma norepinephrine is not increased in the standing patient with postural hypotension, despite the reduction in renal blood flow with the likelihood for reduced renal norepinephrine clearance.

As we discussed in our previous report based on animal studies (9), the raised cerebrospinal fluid norepinephrine in our patients may be related to increased brain norepinephrine release (1).

The origin of the norepinephrine in spinal fluid is not known. It is likely that periventricular areas in the hypothalamus and midbrain are important contributing regions. We have standardized the protocol as to time of day, positional influence, and volume of spinal fluid withdrawn to mitigate against these factors on cerebrospinal fluid norepinephrine.

The findings of the present study indicate again that some patients with primary hypertension have enhanced central and peripheral noradrenergic tone in the basal state. However, when stimulated via postural stress, the level of plasma norepinephrine reached and the magnitude of increment were not different from values of the normotensives.

Our findings in the two "opposite" conditions suggest that central noradrenergic dysfunction is an important factor in the pathogenesis of primary hypertension as well as that of IOH.

SUMMARY

1) Some patients with idiopathic postural hypotension have low-plasma and spinal fluid concentrations of norepinephrine compared to values of normotensive patients. The former group also has blunted norepinephrine response to upright posture when compared with normotensives ($p < 0.01$).

2) Patients with primary hypertension had elevated concentrations of norepinephrine in plasma ($p < 0.01$) and in spinal fluid ($p < 0.001$) when compared with normotensive patients.

3) Central noradrenergic dysfunction appears to be an important factor in the pathogenesis of primary hypertension, as well in postural hypotension in man.

ACKNOWLEDGMENTS

This work was supported by NIH grants HL-24113 and CRC-RR-43.

We gratefully acknowledge the assistance of the Clinical Research Center nursing staff under the direction of Mrs. Hank Yagi, R.N., the technologic skills of Ms. Erlinda Lerias and Daantje Meijer, and the preparation of the manuscript by Ms. Jan Saito. We are indebted to Marian Fedak, M.D., and Bruce Dobkin, M.D., of the White Memorial Medical Center and UCLA Medical Center, respectively, for the referral of their patients with postural hypotension for these studies.

REFERENCES

1. Eide I, Kolloch R, DeQuattro V, Miano L, Dugger R, Van der Meulen J (1979) Raised cerebrospinal

fluid norepinephrine in some patients with primary hypertension. Hypertension 1: 255–260

2. Kolloch R, Kobayashi K, DeQuattaro V (1981) Dopaminergic control of sympathetic tone and blood pressure: Evidence in primary hypertension. Hypertension (in press)

3. DeQuattro V, Myers M (1979) the sympathetic nervous system and primary hypertension in man. In: DeGroot LJ et al (eds) Endocrinology, Vol 2. Grune & Stratton, New York, pp 1297–1305

4. Ziegler MG, Lake CR, Kopin IJ (1977) The sympathetic-nervous-system defect in primary orthostatic hypotension. N Engl J Med 296: 293–297

5. Campese V, DeQuattro V (1979) Orthostatic hypotension. In: DeGroot LJ et al (eds) Endocrinology, Vol 2. Grune & Stratton, New York, pp 1289–1295

6. Shy GM, Drager GA (1960) A neurological syndrome associated with orthostatic hypotension. AMA Arch Neurol 2: 41–57

7. Peuler J, Johnson G (1977) Simultaneous single isotope radioenzymatic assay of plasma norepinephrine, epinephrine and dopamine. Life Sci 21: 625–636

8. Kobayashi K, Kolloch R, De Quattro V, Miano L (1979) Increased plasma and urinary noremetanephrine in young patients with primary hypertension. Clin Sci [Suppl V] 57: 1735–1775

9. Ziegler MG, Lake CR, Wood JH, Ebert MH (1976) Circadian rhythm in cerebrospinal fluid noradrenaline of man and monkey. Nature 264: 656

Use of Circulating Catecholamines for the Detection of Autonomic Abnormalities in Human Hypertension

Jacques de Champlain

The search for autonomic dysfunctions in human hypertension has been a popular, but controversial, research topic for the last 50 years. A great variety of indirect and, sometimes, nonspecific hemodynamic, pharmacologic, and biochemical approaches have been used to obtain often contradictory results. In the last decade, the availability of highly sensitive and specific radioenzymatic techniques has permitted the more accurate measurement of circulating catecholamines (CA) in humans. Under standardized procedures, it has been possible to use those measures as a valid index of sympathetic activity (1).

Despite better uniformity of results in studies with radioenzymatic techniques, certain controversies have been raised over the years concerning mainly the interpretation of results. Earlier studies consistently reported elevated basal CA levels in essential hypertension (2–5). The observation by Lake and his co-workers (6), that circulating norpinephrine (NE) levels could be correlated with age, suggested a reappraisal of those earlier reports in which the groups of hypertensive patients were older than normotensive controls. Although a correlation between age and circulating CA was confirmed by some studies, such a correlation could not be demonstrated within the hypertensive population (1, 7–11). Moreover, recent studies carried in age-matched, labile or sustained hypertensive patients have confirmed the presence of elevated circulating CA or NE levels in approximately 30%–40% of hypertensive patients (12, 13). The finding of elevated levels in only one subgroup of hypertensive patients is not surprising considering that the populations of labile and sustained hypertensive patients are not homogeneous. Therefore, the search for a common and unique abnormality in hypertension is utopian. The most that can be achieved is to attempt to identify and characterize subgroups presenting common abnormalities within these populations. Although the measurement of circulating CA has focused attention mainly on the sympathetic system, it should be remembered that the release of NE from sympathetic fiber can be altered or modulated by various external factors such as acetylcholine, angiotensin or other hormones (14). Therefore, increases in circulating CA levels could very well reflect abnormalities occurring at the level of the parasympathetic system or at the circulating levels of certain hormones, as well as an increase in sympathetic fiber activity and/or an increased CA secretion by the adrenal medulla. Finally, it should also be remembered that an increase in sympathetic tone on the effector cells may not necessarily be associated with increased circulating CA levels, considering that it can be realized through increased postsynaptic receptor sensitivity or through an imbalance between the sensitivity of alpha- and beta-receptors (11).

ABNORMALITIES IN CIRCULATING CA LEVELS IN LABILE AND SUSTAINED HYPERTENSION

In our earlier studies, we proposed to subdivide the population of hypertensive patients into two subgroups on the basis of their basal circulating CA levels (1, 5, 12, 15). This subdivision has permitted us to uncover distinct clinical features characterizing each subgroup, despite the fact that either group had an identical average blood pressure. Hyperadrenergic patients (those with supine CA levels above normal range) demonstrated hyperkinetic cardiac functions such as an increased heart rate and a decreased preejection period compatible with an increased myocardial contractility. Since significant correlations were observed between circulating basal CA levels and heart rate or the preejection period within the whole hypertensive population (15), it was postulated that the hyperkinetic cardiac functions in this group of patients was probably linked to an increased sympathetic tone. In addition, the hyperadrenergic patients found to be characterized by an increased sympathetic reactivity (greater increase in circulating CA during change from supine to standing position), were also found to be better responders to treatment with beta-blockers (propranolol or metoprolol) (12). In contrast, normoadrenergic hypertensive patients (those with supine circulating CA levels within normal range) were found to have near normal heart rate and preejection periods (15). In addition, they were characterized by a normal sympathetic reactivity and responded poorly to treatment with beta-blockers (12). It was also of interest that beta-blockers had different effects on circulating basal and standing CA in these two subgroups of patients. In hyperadrenergic patients, the more efficient clinical effects were associated with a reduction in basal circulating levels and a normalization of the sympathetic reactivity. In normoadrenergic patients, the poor clinical response to beta-blockade was associated with an increase in basal circulating levels and an unchanged sympathetic reactivity (12). The mechanisms of action of beta-blockers on circulating CA levels in hyperadrenergic patients is compatible with the blockade of the presynaptic beta-mediated positive feedback mechanism localized on the peripheral sympathetic terminal fibers (16).

This classification of hypertensive patients may be useful for a better rationalization of the therapy of hypertensive patients. From our studies, it appears that hyperadrenergic patients are better responders to beta-blockade, while it was recently suggested that normoadrenergic patients would be more responsive to sodium restriction or diuretic treatment (17).

This classification remains crude, however, and may not take into consideration more subtle abnormalities in sympathetic functions. The availability of radioenzymatic techniques that allow for the differential determination of epinephrine (E) and NE levels has provided an approach that permits us to have a closer look at the function of the adrenal medulla, which contributes mainly to circulating E levels, versus the function of sympathetic fibers, which contribute mainly to circulating NE levels. Our more recent studies,

using the technique of Peuler and Johnson (18), have shown abnormalities in both circulating NE and E levels in human hypertension (Table 1). In both labile and sustained hypertensive patients, the supine and standing heart rate, blood pressure, and NE levels were significantly higher compared to normotensive subjects. The higher standing NE levels in labile hypertension suggested a greater sympathetic nerve reactivity in this group of patients. E levels were increased significantly only in the supine position in labile hypertension, but the reactivity of E to standing was normal in this group of patients. In stable hypertension, the increase in E levels on standing tended to be greater. These findings confirm our preliminary observations of increased supine E levels in patients with labile hypertension (12). Higher circulating E levels were also observed by others in labile or sustained hypertension (11, 17, 19).

In an attempt to refine the subclassification of hypertensive patients, we have separated the patients presenting NE or E levels above one standard deviation (high-NE or high-E subgroups) from the mean in normotensive subjects (Table 2). High-supine NE and E values were encountered in greater proportion in the labile hypertensive group. In sustained hypertension, the proportion of supine high NE was also important, but high E was found in much smaller proportion. High-standing NE values were found in greater proportion in labile hypertension, but high-standing E levels were found in greater proportion among patients with sustained hypertension. In this analysis, it was also of interest to note that there was little overlap between high-NE and high-E patients. These two parameters appear, therefore, to reflect two distinct functional mechanisms. For instance, high-supine NE patients demonstrated greater elevation of NE on standing, while high-supine E patients had a normal NE reactivity to postural change. This phenomenon was associated with a greater increase in mean arterial blood pressure on standing in high-NE subgroups. High-supine E subgroups had a higher basal heart rate than the high-supine NE groups.

This attempt to subclassify hypertensive patients on the basis of E and NE levels seems promising and could provide a better understanding of the various mechanisms of hypertension. From this standpoint, labile and sustained essential hypertension appear as two distinct pathologic entities. Without the concomitant evaluation of receptor

Table 1. Supine (20 min) and standing (10 min) circulating NE and E levels in labile and sustained hypertension.

Group	N	Age	Heart rate (beats/min)		Blood pressure (mmHg)		NE (pg/ml)	E (pg/ml)
					SBP	DBP		
Normotensive	35	29.4 ± 1.9	Supine	64.3 ± 1.2	112.0 ± 1.4	74.3 ± 1.4	169.1 ± 12.0	31.6 ± 4.0
			Standing	72.5 ± 1.7	108.4 ± 1.4	80.0 ± 1.5	360.0 ± 22.0	50.8 ± 6.9
Labile HT	40	29.5 ± 1.8	Supine	72.8 ± 2.1*	132.6 ± 1.4*	81.0 ± 1.4*	217.7 ± 13.3*	42.7 ± 3.8***
			Standing	79.9 ± 1.8*	131.3 ± 1.7*	88.7 ± 1.4*	463.4 ± 28.1*	57.3 ± 6.9
Sustained HT	27	40.7 ± 2.2*	Supine	76.9 ± 1.7*	150.3 ± 2.8*	100.0 ± 2.3*	211.7 ± 11.6**	30.7 ± 3.9
			Standing	82.0 ± 1.9*	149.9 ± 3.2*	104.8 ± 2.0*	434.1 ± 23.7***	59.3 ± 8.1

Results are expressed as the mean ± SE.
SBP, systolic blood pressure; DBP, diastolic blood pressure; HT, hypertension.
*$p < 0.01$, **$p < 0.02$, ***$p < 0.05$ versus values in normotensive subjects.

Table 2. Percent distribution of values above one standard deviation from the mean normal values.

Group	N	Supine		Standing	
		High NE	High E	High NE	High E
Normotensive	35	14.3	11.4	11.4	8.6
Labile HT	40	37.5	22.5	32.5	12.5
Sustained HT	27	29.6	7.4	22.2	14.8

sensitivity it is, however, difficult to understand the complete functional implications of these findings.

INTERPRETATION OF CIRCULATING CA LEVELS

So far, the finding of elevated circulating CA levels has been assumed to reflect a primary activation (peripheral or central) of the peripheral sympathetic system at the level of the fibers or the adrenal medulla. Although this may constitute a valid assumption in certain cases, it is possible that in others, the elevation of circulating CA levels might be a secondary manifestation of an abnormality occurring outside the sympathetic system. For instance, a close functional interaction has been observed between the parasympathetic and sympathetic components of the autonomic nervous system, characterized by an inhibitory predominance of the parasympathetic over sympathetic functions (20). Recent studies, in vivo, have suggested that the inhibitory influence of the parasympathetic system over cardiac sympathetic fibers is probably mediated through the activation of inhibitory presynaptic muscarinic receptors localized on cardiac sympathetic fibers (21, 22). It can, therefore, be postulated that a decrease in parasympathetic tone might be reflected by an elevation of basal circulating CA levels and/or by an enhanced sympathetic reactivity to postural change, to exercise, or to other stimuli. Since indications of a decreased parasympathetic tone have been documented in human (23–25) and in experimental hypertension (26), such a mechanism is plausible. In human hypertension, we have been able to obtain evidence supporting the presence of an abnormality in parasympathetic function, which might be reflected by an alteration in circulating

CA (J. de Champlain, R. A. Nadeau, and M. Lavallée, unpublished data). It was found that atropine could potentiate the increase in NE and E on postural change and isometric exercise in some patients, while atropine was not potentiating those responses in others. The potentiated group had a normal NE or E reactivity to standing and isometric exercise before atropine, while the nonpotentiated group was found to have increased NE reactivity to both form of stimuli before treatment. From these preliminary observations, it can be postulated that the parasympathetic tone is probably inhibited in the nonpotentiated group, and that the increased NE reactivity observed in these patients could be the consequence of the decreased parasympathetic tone. However, the possibility of a concomitant increase in sympathetic tone and a decrease in parasympathetic tone secondary to a dysfunction at the level of vasomotor centers or at baroreceptor sites cannot be excluded. These findings suggest that the measurement of circulating CA may also be useful for the evaluation of the parasympathetic component as well.

The interpretation of changes in circulating CA cannot be made without taking into consideration other circulating or local factors that might alter the liberation of CA from sympathetic fibers and from the adrenal medulla through presynaptic receptors (14). Moreover, the functional significance of circulating CA in hypertension can hardly be made without a closer look at the sensitivity of postsynaptic receptors.

CONCLUSIONS

Elevated circulating supine and standing NE and E levels have been observed in a significant number of patients presenting labile or sustained essential hypertension. These observations suggest the existence of an increased basal sympathetic tone and reactivity in important subgroups of these two populations. It is likely that these abnormalities reflect primary sympathetic dysfunctions in certain patients, while in others, they may constitute a secondary manifestation of a dysfunction occurring in the parasympathetic system or elsewhere. The better identification of these subgroups is important for the understanding of the clinical and physiopathologic significance of these abnormalities. The demonstration of an interaction between various hormones on the CA release from the adrenal medulla and the sympathetic nerves through presynaptic receptors supports the hypothesis that the sympathetic system could serve as a common pathway to a variety of etiologic factors in the development and maintenance of human hypertension. The possibility of alteration in the sensitivity of postsynaptic receptors, thus creating an imbalance between alpha- and beta-mediated functions, raises the possibility of sympathetic dysfunctions in the absence of elevated CA levels in hypertension. All this fragmented information constitutes only a first step, and it is only through patient, long-lasting, and probably, controversial studies that it will be possible to interpret, evaluate, and understand the role of these various autonomic abnormalities in the development, maintenance, and evolution of human hypertension. It is plausible that this approach could lead to a better rationalization of the therapy, to a more efficient prevention of cardiovascular complications, and to a better understanding of the mechanisms underlying that disease.

SUMMARY

Elevated supine CA or NE levels were reported in the blood of a significant proportion of patients suffering from essential sustained or labile hypertension by several groups of investigators. In our own studies, patients with elevated CA or NE levels were found to be characterized clinically by a higher heart rate, a faster preejection period, a greater sympathetic reactivity on postural changes, and by a better therapeutic response to beta-blockers. In addition, in more recent studies, it was found that a subgroup of labile hypertensive patients had higher E levels.

Although these findings suggest a hyperactivity of the sympathetic fibers or adrenal medulla in a significant proportion of patients with labile or sustained hypertension, these abnormalities in circulating CA levels could also reflect dysfunctions occurring outside the sympathetic system. In recent years, several presynaptic mechanisms have been described in the regulation or modulation of NE released by the sympathetic fibers. Among several mechanisms, the parasympathetic system has been found to inhibit the release of NE from sympathetic fibers by the action of acetylcholine on presynaptic muscarinic receptors. Since atropine was found to potentiate the increase in circulating NE in standing patients with a normal sympathetic reactivity while it did not potentiate the response in already hyperreactive patients, it is postulated that the parasympathetic tone is decreased in a group of hypertensive patients and that the state of sympathetic hyperactivity observed in these patients may be due to a reduced parasympathetic inhibition on the sympathetic fibers.

ACKNOWLEDGMENTS

The author is thankful for the efficient assistance of Ms. L. Farley, J. Le Guerrier, D. Papin, M. C. Renaud, and D. Miclette, and for the fruitful collaboration of Drs. R. Nadeau, G. Denis, D. Cousineau, L. Lapointe, and M. Lavallée in the realization of these studies. The author is also grateful for the financial support of the Medical Research Council of Canada and the Québec Heart Foundation.

REFERENCES

1. de Champlain J (1977) The sympathetic system in hypertension. Clin Endocrinol Metab 6: 633–655
2. Engelman K, Portnoy B, Sjoerdsma A (1970) Plasma catecholamine concentrations in patients with hypertension. Circ Res 26, 27(Suppl I): 141–146
3. Dequattro V, Chan S (1972) Raised plasma catecholamine in some patients with primary hypertension. Lancet 1: 806–809
4. Louis WJ, Doyle AE, Anavekar S (1973) Plasma norepinephrine levels in essential hypertension. New Engl J Med 288: 599–601
5. de Champlain J, Farley L, Cousineau D, van

Ameringen MR (1976) Circulating catecholamine levels in human and experimental hypertension. Circ Res 38: 109–114

6. Lake CR, Ziegler MG, Coleman MD, Koplin IJ (1977) Age-adjusted plasma norepinephrine levels are similar in normotensive and hypertensive subjects. New Engl J Med 296: 208–209

7. Cryer PE, Santiago JV, Shah S (1974) Measurement of norepinephrine and epinephrine in small volume of human plasma by a single isotope derivative method: Response to the upright posture. J Clin Endocrinol Metab 39: 1025–1029

8. Campese V, Myers MR, Dequattro V (1977) Plasma catecholamines and neurogenic hypertension. New Engl J Med 297: 53–54

9. Sever PS, Birch M, Osikowska B, Tunbridge (1977) Plasma noradrenaline in essential hypertension. Lancet 1: 1078–1081 RDG

10. Henry DP, Luft FC, Weinberger MH, Fineberg NS, Grim CE (1980) Norepinephrine in urine and plasma following provocative maneuvers in normal and hypertensive subjects. Hypertension 2: 20–28

11. Bertel O, Bühler FR, Kiowski W, Lutold BE (1980) Decreased beta-adrenoreceptor responsiveness as related to age, blood pressure and plasma catecholamines in patients with essential hypertension. Hypertension 2: 130–138

12. de Champlain J, Cousineau D, Lapointe L (1979) The significance of circulating catecholamines in the evolution and treatment of hypertension. In: Meyer P, Schmitt H (eds) Nervous system and hypertension. Wiley-Flammarian, New York, pp 277–286

13. DeQuattro V, Eide I, Kolloch R, Miano L, Campese V, van der Meulen J (1979) Peripheral and central markers of neurogenic tone in primary hypertension. In: Meyer P, Schmitt H (eds) Nervous system and hypertension. Wiley-Flammarian, pp 311–317

14. Langer SZ (1977) Presynaptic receptors and their role in the regulation of transmitter release. Br J Pharmacol 60: 481–497

15. Cousineau D, Lapointe L, de Champlain J (1978) Circulating catecholamines and systolic time intervals in normotensive and hypertensive patients with and without left ventricular hypertrophy. Am Heart J 96: 229–234

16. Yamaguchi N, de Champlain J, Nadeau RA (1977) Regulation of norepinephrine release from cardiac sympathetic fibers in the dog by presynaptic α and β-receptors. Circ Res 41: 108–117

17. Hong Tai Eng FW, Huber-Smith M, McCann DS (1980) The role of sympathetic activity in normal renin essential hypertension. Hypertension 2: 14–19

18. Peuler JD, Johnson GA (1977) Simultaneous single isotope radioenzymatic assay of norepinephrine, epinephrine and dopamine. Life Sci 21: 625–636

19. Franco-Morselli R, De Mendonca M, Beaudoin-Legros M, Guicheney P, Meyer P (1979) Plasma catecholamine in essential human hypertension and DOCA-salt hypertension of the rat. In: Meyer P, Schmitt H (eds) Nervous system and hypertension. Wiley-Flammaran, New York, pp 287–296

20. Levy MN, Ng M, Martin P, Zieske H (1966) Sympathetic and parasympathetic interactions upon the left ventricle of the dog. Circ Res 19: 5–10

21. Levy MN, Blattberg B (1976) Effect of vagal stimulation on the overflow of norepinephrine into the coronary sinus during cardiac sympathetic nerve stimulation. Circ Res 38: 81–85

22. Lavallée M, de Champlain J, Nadeau RA (1978) Muscarinic inhibition of endogenous myocardial catecholamine liberation in the dog. Can J Physiol Pharmacol 56: 642–649

23. Julius S, Pascual AV, London R (1971) Role of parasympathetic inhibition in the hyperkinetic type of borderline hypertension. Circulation 44: 413–418

24. Korner RI, Shaw J, Uther JB, West HJ, McRitchie RJ, Richards JG (1973) Autonomic and non-autonomic circulatory components in essential hypertension in man. Circulation 48: 107–117

25. Johnston LC (1980) The abnormal heart rate response to deep breath in borderline hypertension: A sign of autonomic nervous system dysfunction. Am Heart J 99: 487–493

26. Pfeffer MA, Pfeffer JM, Frohlich ED (1976) Autonomic inhibition in spontaneously hypertensive rats. In: Julius S, Esler MD (eds) The nervous system in arterial hypertension. Charles C Thomas, Springfield, Oh, pp 60–72

Sympathetic Nervous System, Catecholamine Receptors, and Hypertension

Robert J. Lefkowitz

This paper has three major goals. First, I would like to give a very brief overview of the current status of the classification of adrenergic receptors with the emphasis on evolving concepts of subclassification. Second, I would like to highlight several examples of the current state of the art in terms of measurement, by direct radioligand-binding techniques, not just of receptor number, but of receptor function. Finally, I would like to indicate how one can study receptor regulation in the adrenergic nervous system. Those who are directly involved in hypertension research should consider the use of direct-binding approaches in studying the adrenergic receptors as possibly providing new kinds of information that may be helpful in the various models and paradigms of hypertension (discussed in previous sessions).

The original classification of adrenergic receptors into two major types, alpha and beta, was proposed by Ahlquist (1) more than 30 years ago. His classification scheme was based on the relative potency series of agonists. For alpha-receptors, the series is: epinephrine > norepinephrine >> isoproterenol. For beta-receptors, the series is reversed: isoproterenol > epinephrine $\geq$ norepinephrine. There are two main subtypes of beta-adrenergic receptors, beta$_1$ and beta$_2$, differing in that for the beta$_1$-receptors epinephrine and norepinephrine are essentially equipotent, whereas epinephrine is much more potent than norepinephrine at beta$_2$ receptors (2). Most, if not all, beta-receptor-mediated effects seem to involve stimulation of the enzyme adenylate cyclase.

Even more recently, it has become clear that there are subtypes of alpha-receptors. The idea that has evolved over the past 5–10 years has been that the postsynaptic alpha-receptors mediating, for example, smooth muscle constriction are to be called alpha$_1$-receptors and have a characteristic antagonist potency series. In addition, however, there are presynaptic alpha-receptors that seem to have somewhat different relative potencies for agonists and antagonists. These "alpha$_2$"-receptors are allegedly located presynaptically and appear to mediate a feedback inhibition of norepinephrine release (3, 4).

In terms of drug specificity, the major characteristic of alpha$_1$-receptors is that prazosin is a much more potent antagonist than yohimbine, whereas for the alpha$_2$-receptors, yohimbine is a more potent antagonist than prazosin (5, 6). This seems to be the most valid basis at the moment I think for subclassifying these receptor subtypes. There are also some agonists that appear to have relative subtype selectivity. The terms pre- and postsynaptic alpha-receptors should probably be abandoned in favor of the more general terms alpha$_1$ and alpha$_2$ because, although the alpha$_1$-receptors seem to be located post-synaptically, there are examples of alpha$_2$-receptors located both pre- and postsynaptically (5). In general, alpha$_1$-receptors are excitatory, and the alpha$_2$-receptors inhibitory. The mechanism of action of alpha$_1$-receptors appears to involve changes in calcium flux, whereas alpha$_2$-receptors in a number of cases appear to be linked to inhibition of adenylate cyclase activity. Whether this will turn out to be their general mechanism of action, however, remains to be seen.

How can we study these different alpha-receptor subtypes by radioligand binding? There are a variety of radioligands available for study of alpha-receptors; one popular one is dihydroergocryptine. [^{3}H]Dihydroergocryptine is a nonsubtype selective alpha-adrenergic antagonist. It binds to the full population of alpha-receptors; that is, it binds to all alpha$_1$ and alpha$_2$-receptors in a given membrane preparation with equal affinity. One can then use subtype selective antagonists such as prazosin to construct competition curves. Figure 1 displays an example of this in three tissues: human platelets,

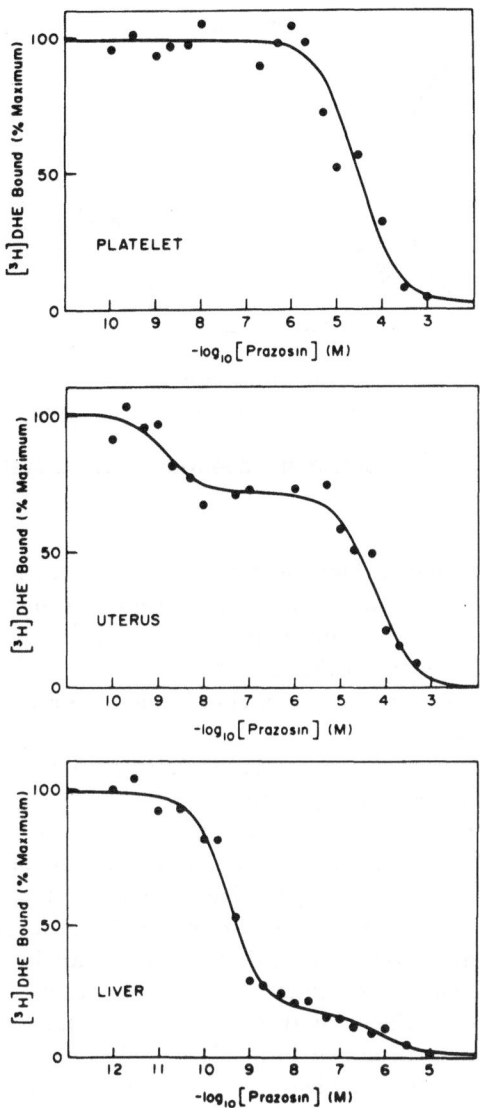

Fig. 1. Inhibition of [³H]dihydroergocryptine (DHE) binding to alpha-receptors in membranes derived from human platelet, rabbit uterus, and rat liver. [Hancock et al. (8)]

rabbit uterus, and rat liver. The datum points are real experimental points. The lines are computer-generated theoretical curves that best fit the datum points (6). The human platelet contains only one subtype of alpha-receptor as demonstrated by the fact that there is a homogeneous or uniphasic binding curve of very weak affinity. The EC_{50} for prazosin is about 10^{-5} M. This is typical for alpha$_2$-receptors (7). By contrast, in the liver, most of the receptors combined with prazosin with relatively high affinity and a smaller number with low

affinity. The liver has mostly alpha$_1$ and some alpha$_2$-receptors (8). In the uterus, there is also a mixture of sites binding prazosin with high and low affinity. The same kinds of analysis can be done for the beta-adrenergic receptor subtypes (9).

What about the assessment of receptor function or coupling by binding studies? This has been most extensively examined in the beta-adrenergic system of the frog erythrocyte (10, 11). These cells contain only beta$_2$-adrenergic receptors. Suppose one constructs competition curves using [³H]dihydroalprenolol as a radioligand and an antagonist like alprenolol or propranolol (Fig. 2A). This is a computer-modeled curve drawn according to the law of mass action, $H + R \rightleftarrows HR$, for hormone (H) receptor (R) interaction. It pro-

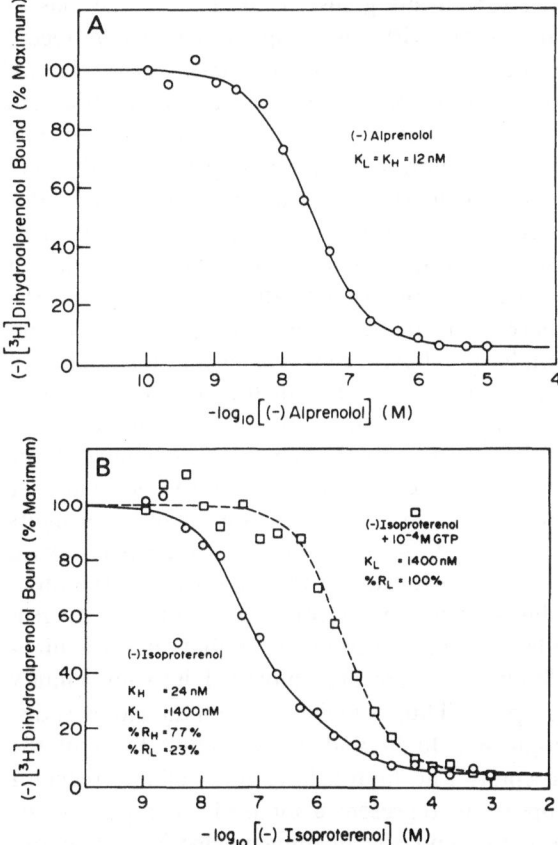

Fig. 2. Computer-modeled competition curves of **(A)** the antagonist alprenolol and **(B)** the agonist isoproterenol for [³H]dihydroalprenolol binding sites in frog erythrocyte membranes. K_H and K_L, high- and low-affinity dissociation constants; R_H and R_L, concentrations of high- and low-affinity state receptors. [Ken et al. (10)]

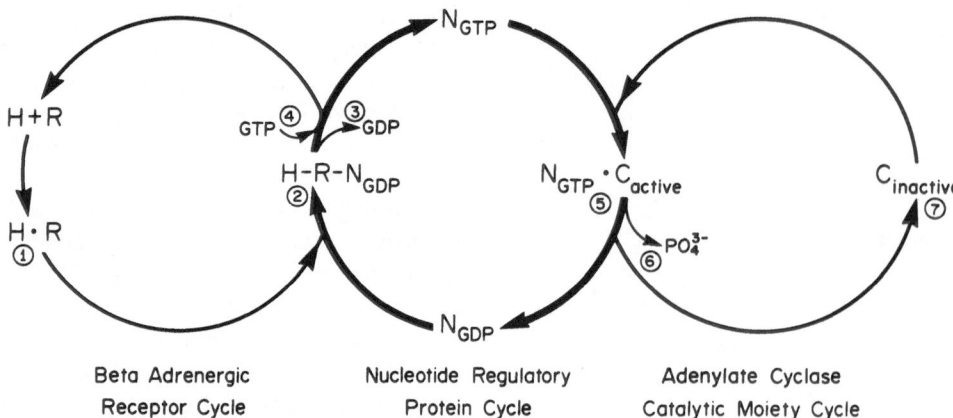

Fig. 3. Proposed model for the concerted functioning of the components of the adenylate cyclase system.

vides an excellent fit to the data and this is the case for all antagonists (10). The interactions of antagonists with pure populations of beta-receptors are explicable simply in terms of the law of mass action. Nonetheless, as shown in Fig. 2B, for all agonists tested, such as isoproterenol, one gets a shallow and complex displacement curve even though there is only one kind of receptor present (beta$_2$-receptors). In the presence of guanine nucleotides such as GTP, which are required for beta-adrenergic activation of the cyclase, the curve shifts to the right and becomes steep and uniphasic. Thus, even when only one kind of receptor is present, agonists such as isoproterenol still appear to distinguish two different affinity states of the receptor. By the computer modeling of these data, we have resolved them into one of higher and one of lower affinity, the affinity constants being about 24 and 1,400 nM, respectively, with about three-fourths of the sites being in the high-affinity form. In the presence of guanine nucleotides, a transition occurs such that all of the high-affinity receptors are converted into low-affinity receptors. Thus, agonists, but not antagonists, distinguish a high- and a low-affinity form of the receptor. The high-affinity form of this receptor appears to represent a molecular complex of the receptor, and the guanine nucleotide regulatory subunit of the adenylate cyclase system. In fact, the formation of this high-affinity state represents the coupling reaction of the receptor with the nucleotide site. This phenomenology appears to be similar for the inhibitory alpha$_2$-adrenergic receptors. Thus, if one examines norepinephrine competition with [^{3}H]dihydroergocryptine for the alpha$_2$-receptors in platelet membranes, again a shallow

curve due to high- and low-affinity states is observed. One also observes a transition in the presence of guanine nucleotides such that now all the receptors are in the low-affinity state.

Figure 3 shows a model to explain these various observations. The major point is that there appear to be at least three molecular subunits of the beta-adrenergic system: the receptor; the nucleotide regulatory protein; and the catalytic cyclase itself. Each of these three molecular components undergoes, we believe, a cycle of activation and deactivation (11, 12). The high-affinity complex of receptor and nucleotide protein that is formed only by agonists, and not by antagonists, seems to be an intermediate which, in turn, converts the nucleotide site into an active form. The nucleotide protein then leads to activation of the catalytic moiety. So, in essence, the high-affinity state of the receptor is an intermediate for activation of the cyclase. There are three intersecting cycles of activity.

Anything that modifies the ability to form the coupled high-affinity complex hormone receptor nucleotide (HRN) will obviously dampen hormone responsiveness. One can use these methods to investigate examples where catecholamine sensitivity is perturbed; a model case would be desensitization (13). We have read a great deal in this volume about situations in which responsiveness to one or another neurotransmitter is altered. This phenomenon can be studied in the frog erythrocyte. When frog erythrocytes are preincubated with isoproterenol, the ability of a beta-agonist to subsequently stimulate the adenylate cyclase becomes markedly attenuated with time. This is called desensitization. In this system, it is quite specific or "homologous." Other hormonal activators (such as PGE_1) retain normal sensitivity. We showed a number of years ago that this is associated with a fall in receptor number as assessed by dihydroalprenolol binding (3). If one performs the kind of detailed computer-assisted analyses I have discussed in terms of an agonist competition curve with [^{3}H]dihydroalprenolol binding to membranes derived from control cells and desensitized cells, one observes at least two major abnormalities (10). First, there is less [^{3}H]dihydroalprenolol binding after desensitization, because there has been a down regulation of the beta-adrenergic receptors. In addition, when one looks at the actual high- and low-affinity states as compared with the control situation, there is a marked reduction in the percentage of receptors that can form the high-affinity "coupled" state. So, in desensitization or tachyphylaxis, there are at least two alterations in the receptors. One is that there are less of them. The second is that those remaining are less capable of undergoing the transition to the HRN complex.

In summary, using ligand-binding studies, one can study with increasing degrees of refinement not only the numbers of alpha- and beta-adrenergic receptors present in tissues, but their functional status in terms of their ability to become coupled with other molecular components of the effector systems. Hopefully, using techniques such as these, one can begin to get at the molecular basis of altered neurotransmitter sensitivity in pathophysiologic situations such as, for example, hypertension.

SUMMARY

Alpha- and beta-adrenergic receptors can be studied by direct radioligand-binding techniques. These methods confirm the existence of two discrete subtypes (beta$_1$ and beta$_2$ and alpha$_1$ and alpha$_2$) of each receptor. Both subtypes of beta-receptors appear to stimulate adenylate cyclase, whereas the alpha$_2$-receptors inhibit the enzyme. The ambient level of catecholamines in contact with the beta-adrenergic receptors modulates both the number of the receptors and their coupling with other components of the adenylate cyclase system. Alterations such as these can be investigated by using receptor-binding methodology. Such techniques provide the opportunity to investigate possible receptor alterations in pathophysiologic states such as hypertension.

ACKNOWLEDGMENT

This work was supported by HEW grants HL-16037 and HL-20339. Dr. Robert Lefkowitz is an Investigator of the Howard Hughes Medical Institute.

REFERENCES

1. Ahlquist RP (1948) A study of the adrenotropic receptors. Am J Physiol 153: 586–600
2. Lands AM, Arnold A, McAuliff JP, Luduena FP, Brown TG Jr (1967) Differentiation of receptor systems activated by sympathomimetic amines. Nature 214: 597–598
3. Langer SZ (1974) Presynaptic regulation of catecholamine release. Biochem Pharmacol 23: 1793–1800
4. Starke K (1977) Regulation of noradrenaline release by presynaptic receptor systems. Rev Physiol Biochem Pharmacol 77: 1–124
5. Berthelsen S, Pettinger WA (1977) A functional basis for classification of alpha-adrenergic receptors. Life Sci 21: 595–606
6. Hoffman BB, De Lean A, Wood CL, Schocken DD, Lefkowitz RJ (1979) Life Sci 24: 1739–1745
7. Hoffman BB, Lefkowitz RJ (1980) Alpha-adrenergic receptor subtypes. New Engl J Med 302: 1390–1396
8. Hoffman BB, Lefkowitz RJ (1980) Heterogeneity of radioligand binding to alpha-adrenergic receptors: Analysis of guanine nucleotide regulation in relation to receptor subtypes. J Biol Chem 255: 4645–4652
9. Hancock A, De Lean A, Lefkowitz RJ (1979) Quantitative resolution of beta-adrenergic receptor subtypes by selective ligand binding: Application of a computerized model fitting technique. Mol Pharmacol 16: 1–9
10. Kent R, De Lean A, Lefkowitz RJ (1980) Quantitative analysis of beta-adrenergic receptor interactions: Resolution of high and low affinity states of the receptor by computer modelling of ligand binding data. Mol Pharmacol 17: 14–23
11. De Lean A, Stadel JM, Lefkowitz RJ (1980) A ternary complex model explains the agonist-specific binding properties of the adenylate-cyclase coupled beta-adrenergic receptor. J Biol Chem 255: 7108–7117
12. Stadel JM, De Lean A, Lefkowitz RJ (1980) Molecular mechanisms of coupling in hormone-receptor-adenylate cyclase systems. Adv Enzymol 51: 13
13. Lefkowitz RJ, Wessels M, Stadel J (1980) Hormones receptors and cyclic AMP: Their role in target cell refractoriness. In: Horecker B, Stadtman E (eds) Current topics in cellular regulation. Academic Press, Chicago

Changing Role of Beta- and Alpha-Adrenoreceptor-Mediated Cardiovascular Responses in the Transition from High-Cardiac Output into a High-Peripheral Resistance Phase in Essential Hypertension

Fritz R. Bühler, Wolfgang Kiowski, Regine Landmann, Peter van Brummelen, Wolfgang Amann, Peter Bolli, and Osmund Bertel

INTRODUCTION

The concept that the sympathetic nervous system might be implicated in essential hypertension was initially founded on the antihypertensive efficacy of anti-adrenergic drugs. Direct measurement of sympathetic nerve activity is difficult in man and, therefore, indirect estimates have been sought. Plasma norepinephrine concentrations reflect the rate of norepinephrine release from postganglionic adrenergic nerve terminals (1). Only 10%–20% of norepinephrine appears in the plasma and has no appreciable effect on adrenergic receptors (2). Plasma epinephrine reflects the rate of epinephrine release from the adrenal medulla and thus splanchnic preganglionic nerve activity. Epinephrine acts as a neurohormone on postjunctional adrenergic receptors, particularly those of the beta-type; it can also be taken up by adrenergic nerve endings, thereby enhancing, via prejunctional beta-adrenoreceptors, the rate of norepinephrine release (3).

Cardiovascular responses depend not only on the level of sympathetic activity but also the effector's ability to respond to a stimulus. Therefore, for assessing the role of the neuroeffector system, measurements of plasma catecholamine concentrations should be combined with stimulation or blockade of specific target organ responses. The effector response may also depend on the number and function of the receptor unit, which may be altered by prolonged hormonal activation (4).

To obtain a more comprehensive view of the sympathetic nervous system involvement in circulatory regulation, a series of experiments was designed for simultaneous assessment of plasma catecholamines and different physiologic and pharmacologic beta- and alpha-adrenoreceptor-mediated cardiovascular responses. Beta-adrenoreceptor density and affinity were quantified using mononuclear leukocytes as a relatively easy accessible model for receptor-binding studies.

SUBJECTS AND METHODS

SUBJECTS

Studies were performed on a total of 110 patients with mild to moderate uncomplicated essential hypertension and in 54 healthy normotensive subjects recruited mainly from sources outside the hospital. All subjects were divided into three age groups: less than 35, between 35 and 49, and older than 49 years. Secondary forms of hypertension were excluded and medication, if any, was withheld from patients for at least 6 weeks prior to the study. At the time of study, sitting diastolic blood pressure ≥ 100 mmHg in all patients. Normotensive controls on three occasions had a systolic blood pressure < 160 mmHg and < 90 mmHg. Informed consent was obtained. The studies were reviewed and approved by this institution's committee on the use of human subjects in clinical investigation.

PROTOCOL

Studies at rest: Blood pressure, heart rate, plasma renin activity, and plasma catecholamine concentrations were measured in all subjects after 30-min recumbent rest and after cannulas were placed. In 24 patients and 16 normal subjects blood pressures were measured intraarterially and, therefore, these subjects were not included in the analysis of data obtained at rest.

Beta-adrenoreceptor-mediated functions: In 51 patients and 38 normal subjects the cardiac response to intravenous bolus injections of isoproterenol was used to estimate the dose required to increase heart rate by 25 beats/min (chronotropic dose 25, CD25). These normal subjects were also exercised on a bicycle ergometer for 5 min each at 25%, 50%, and 75% of their previously determined maximal physical work capacity (PWCmax). Venous blood samples and measurements of heart rate and blood pressure were obtained after each step of exercise. Complete details of the protocol are published elsewhere (5).

Studies of the forearm circulation: In 24 hypertensive patients (aged 31–70 years) and 16 normotensive subjects (aged 30–65 years), 30 min after cannulating the left brachial artery for measurement of blood pressure, the beta-adrenoreceptor-stimulating agent isoproterenol was infused into the artery in doses of 0.12, 1.2, 4.0, and 12.0 ng/min/100 ml forearm tissue for 6 min each, and the increase in forearm blood flow above baseline value was measured after each step. The nonspecific vasodilator nitroprusside was infused at a rate of 0.5 μg/min/100 ml tissue for 3 min and the selective alpha$_1$-adrenoreceptor blocker prazosin at a rate of 0.5 μg/min/100 ml tissue over 10 min. None of the regional intraarterial infusions caused any systemic effects; thus, changes in blood flow directly represent changes in arteriolar resistance.

ANALYTICAL METHODS

Blood pressures at rest and during exercise were measured with a semiautomatic recorder (Physiometrics SR 1), with the exception of the 24 patients and 16 normal controls in whom pressure was measured intraarterially via a pressure transducer. Heart rate was derived from lead II of the ECG. Forearm blood flow was measured with venous occlusion plethysmography, using mercury in a Silastic strain gauge coupled to an electronically calibrated plethysmograph (Hokanson EC 10) (5–7). Plasma norepinephrine and epinephrine concentrations were measured radioenzymatically (9, 10) and plasma renin activity with radioimmunoassay (11). Infusions were made with a continuous flow pump.

To quantify beta-adrenoreceptor density, a radioreceptor assay with mononuclear leukocytes using (−) [3-H]-dihydroalprenolol (DHA) as a ligand was developed. Cells were isolated by density gradient centrifugation, lysed, homogenized and concentrated. A solution containing 2–3 mg/ml protein was incubated with 0.2–10 nM DHA for 16 min at 37°. An as yet unknown high-affinity beta-adrenoreceptor was characterized by rapid kinetics, saturability, and structural and stereospecificity (12).

Results are presented as the mean ± standard error of the mean as the index of dispersion. Student's t-test for paired and unpaired data and linear regression analysis were applied where appropriate.

RESULTS

HEMODYNAMIC DATA AND CATECHOLAMINES IN NORMOTENSIVE AND HYPERTENSIVE SUBJECTS OF DIFFERENT AGE

Resting and exercise data of the total study population and of the three age groups are summarized separately in Table 1. Patients and normal controls were well matched for age. Older hypertensive subjects had significantly higher resting blood pressures, and blood pressures during exercise tended to be higher in older normotensives and hypertensive patients alike.

Heart rate at rest was significantly higher in hypertensive than in normotensive subjects. This was most pronounced in younger controls, whereas in older hypertensive patients heart rate was not much different from normal subjects. Despite higher resting heart rates, exercise-induced tachycardia was significantly smaller in hypertensives mostly because of the decreased response in older hypertensives. A significant decrease in the heart rate response to exercise was also observed in the older normotensive subjects.

Plasma epinephrine concentrations were higher in hypertensive than in normal subjects at rest and during exercise (Fig. 1). This was so in all three age groups although the difference, while consistent, was not statistically significant during exercise (Fig. 2). As with reduced exercise tachy-

Table 1. Hemodynamic and biochemical data at rest and after exercise.

Rest vs Exercise	All Ages		<35 years		35–49 years		<49 years	
	NT	EHT	NT	EHT	NT	EHT	NT	EHT
Age (years)	38 ± 3	42 ± 1*	24 ± 1	27 ± 1	44 ± 2	43 ± 1	58 ± 2	56 ± 1
No. of subjects								
Rest	38	86	19	28	9	31	10	27
75% PWCmax	20	52	6	16	8	18	6	17
Systolic blood pressure (mmHg)								
Rest	120 ± 2	151 ± 3**	116 ± 3**	143 ± 4	122 ± 3**	149 ± 4	121 ± 5	163 ± 5**
75% PWCmax	192 ± 5	218 ± 5**	180 ± 4*	206 ± 7**	186 ± 6*	209 ± 8**	213 ± 10	242 ± 8
Diastolic blood pressure (mmHg)								
Rest	76 ± 2	96 ± 2**	68 ± 3	90 ± 2**	87 ± 2	98 ± 2	75 ± 5	99 ± 2**
75% PWCmax	89 ± 2	111 ± 2**	83 ± 4	105 ± 4**	90 ± 2	113 ± 2**	92 ± 4	115 ± 5*
Plasma epinephrine concentration (pg/ml)								
Rest	28 ± 3	58 ± 5**	27 ± 3	59 ± 10*	31 ± 6	63 ± 8*	28 ± 6	50 ± 6*
75% PWCmax	133 ± 11	159 ± 12	140 ± 18	182 ± 24	143 ± 16	167 ± 21	105 ± 22	125 ± 16
Plasma norepinephrine concentration (pg/ml)								
Rest	263 ± 18	270 ± 11	235 ± 24	252 ± 13*	288 ± 44	253 ± 19	289 ± 35	307 ± 21
75% PWCmax	1,229 ± 78	1,369 ± 83	1,273 ± 130	1,369 ± 134	1,166 ± 90	1,280 ± 146	1,211 ± 195	1,470 ± 156
Plasma renin activity (ng/ml/h)								
Rest	2.6 ± 0.3	2.6 ± 0.3	3.3 ± 0.7	3.1 ± 0.5**	2.5 ± 0.2	3.1 ± 0.6**	2.1 ± 0.3	1.5 ± 0.2
75% PWCmax	5.5 ± 0.6	6.6 ± 1.1	6.1 ± 1.1	9.8 ± 2.8*	4.8 ± 0.5	6.6 ± 1.4*	6.0 ± 1.6	3.1 ± 0.5*
Heart rate (beats/min)								
Rest	63 ± 1	70 ± 1**	61 ± 2	73 ± 3*	64 ± 2	71 ± 2	64 ± 2	67 ± 2
75% PWCmax	153 ± 4	151 ± 2	173 ± 5**	163 ± 3**	151 ± 2**	150 ± 2*	136 ± 3	140 ± 4
CD25 (µg isoproterenol/m²)								
Rest	180 ± 3	169 ± 2**	188 ± 2**	182 ± 2**	176 ± 5**	169 ± 2**	164 ± 4	157 ± 3
75% PWCmax	1.7 ± 0.3	3.4 ± 1.8**	1.3 ± 0.1**	2.0 ± 4**	1.2 ± 0.1*	2.2 ± 0.3**	2.8 ± 0.6	6.1 ± 1.2

NT, normotensive subjects; EHT, essential hypertensive subjects.
* $p < 0.05$ between <35, 35–49, and >49 years. ** $p < 0.01$ between the three age groups.

Plasma Adrenaline Concentrations in Normotensive and Hypertensive Subjects

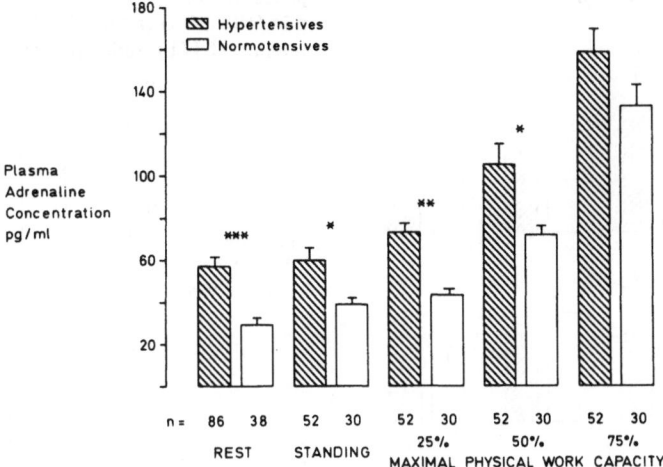

Fig. 1. Plasma epinephrine (adrenaline) concentrations in hypertensive (▧) compared with normotensive (▢) subjects are higher at rest and during sympathetic stimulation by ergometry. Mean ± SEM; *$p < 0.05$, **$p < 0.01$, ***$p < 0.001$.

cardia, there was reduced plasma epinephrine increase in older than younger subjects, normotensive and hypertensive alike. Plasma epinephrine at rest correlated with resting heart rate ($r = 0.33$, $p < 0.01$) and plasma renin activity ($r = 0.32$, $p < 0.01$) in hypertensive but not in normotensive subjects. Plasma norepinephrine concentrations at rest tended to be higher in older normotensive and hypertensive subjects but there was no significant group difference between normotensive and hypertensive subjects.

CARDIAC AND RENAL BETA-ADRENORECEPTOR-MEDIATED FUNCTIONS

The results of isoproterenol testing, maximal exercise heart rates, and exercise-stimulated plasma renin activity in the three age groups is shown in Fig. 3. CD25 increased with age in normotensive and, even more so, in hypertensive subjects. Maximal exercise heart rates as an index of response to endogenous beta-adrenergic stimulation de-

Plasma Adrenaline Concentrations in Normotensive and Hypertensive Subjects at Rest and During Ergometric Exercise

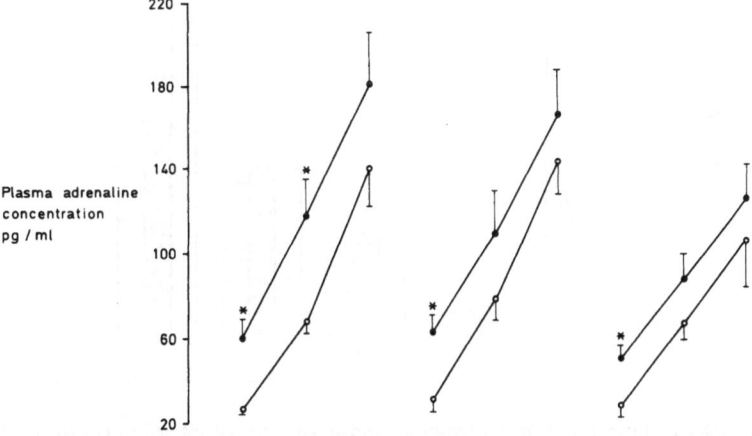

Fig. 2. Plasma epinephrine concentrations at rest and during ergometric exercise are higher in young, middle, and older age groups of hypertensive (●) than normotensive (○) subjects. Hypertensives: aged <35, $N = 17$; aged 35–49, $N = 18$; aged >49, $N = 16$. Normotensives: aged <35, $N = 15$; aged 35–49, $N = 9$; aged >49, $N = 6$. Mean ± SEM, *$p < 0.05$.

Comparison of Beta-Adrenoreceptor Mediated Functions in Three Age Groups of Normotensive and Hypertensive Subjects

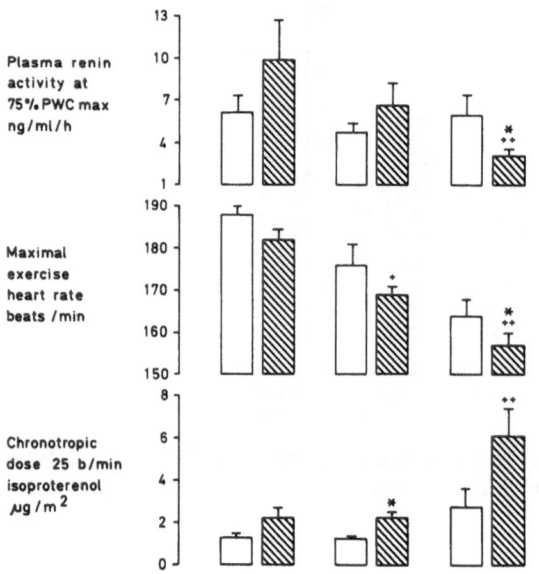

Fig. 3. Exercise-stimulated renin and heart rate responses decrease with older age, which tallies with the decreasing isoproterenol sensitivity. These age-related changes are enhanced in the older hypertensive patients. Hypertensives (◨): aged <35, $N = 17$; aged 35–49, $N = 18$; aged >49, $N = 16$. Normotensives (□): aged <35, $N = 15$; aged 35–49, $N = 9$; aged >49, $N = 6$. *$p < 0.05$ for differences between normotensive and hypertensive subjects; +$p < 0.05$ and ++$p < 0.01$ for differences between age groups.

Change in Forearm Blood Flow During Sodium Nitroprusside (0.6 μg/min/100 ml) and Prazosin (0.5 μg/min/100 ml) Infusions in Patients with Essential Hypertension (EHT) and Normotensive Subjects (NT)

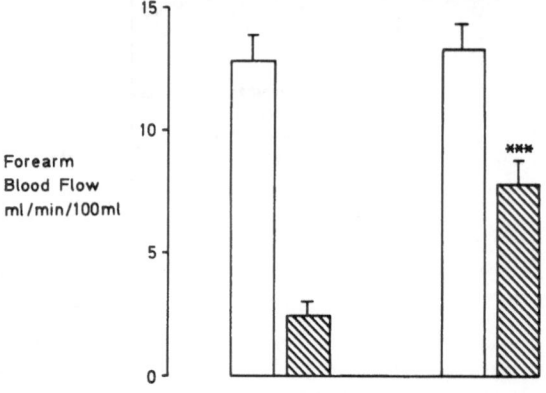

Fig. 5. Forearm blood flow during nonspecific vasodilator infusion of sodium nitroprusside (0.6 μg/min/100 ml) and during selective postjunctional alpha-adrenoreceptor blockade with prazosin (0.5 μg/min/100 ml) in normotensive (NT) subjects and patients with essential hypertension (EHT). The greater response to prazosin in patients suggests enhanced alpha-adrenoreceptor-mediated vasoconstriction in essential hypertension. Mean ± SEM; ***$p < 0.001$.

Change in Forearm Blood Flow with Increasing Dose of Isoproterenol in Normal, Mild and Severe Hypertensive Subjects

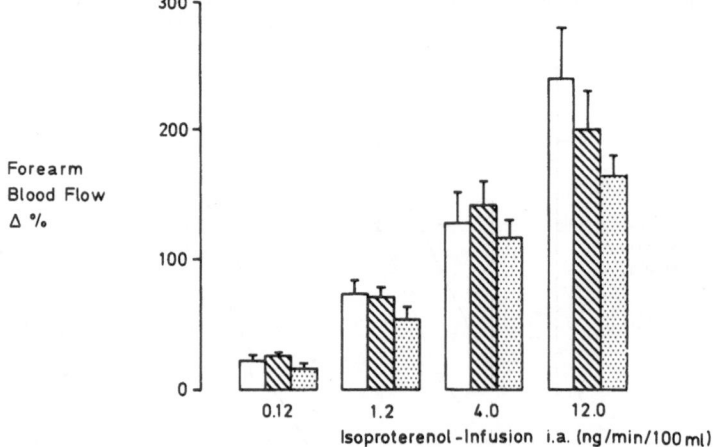

Fig. 4. Response of forearm blood flow to increasing doses of isoproterenol in normotensive and hypertensive subjects. Response is blunted in patients with higher blood pressures (mean intraarterial pressure > 120 mmHg). Normotensives (□): $N = 16$. Essential hypertension MBP < 120 (◨): $N = 12$. Essential hypertension MBP > 120 (▦): $N = 12$. Mean ± SEM.

creased significantly with age and, as with isoproterenol, were more reduced in hypertensive than normotensive subjects. Plasma renin activity during sympathetic exercise was significantly reduced in older hypertensives, but was approximately the same in all three normotensive age groups.

PERIPHERAL VASCULAR BETA- AND ALPHA-ADRENORECEPTOR-MEDIATED FUNCTIONS

The results of a brachial artery infusion of isoproterenol in a subset of 24 hypertensive and 16 normotensive subjects are shown in Fig. 4. The subsequent increment in forearm blood flow was not significantly different between hypertensive and normotensive subjects. However, the increment was smaller in patients with mean blood pressure above 120 mmHg than in patients below, particularly when compared with normotensive subjects. This difference was greatest at the highest infusion rate. The value of this test may be limited because systemic effects at higher doses of isoproterenol may obscure interpretation.

In contrast to a similar nonspecific dilator response to sodium nitroprusside, the increase in forearm blood flow following prazosin was significantly greater ($p < 0.001$) in hypertensive (56%) than in normotensive subjects (20%) (Fig. 5). In hypertensive, but not in normotensive, subjects plasma epinephrine concentrations and the increase in forearm blood flow during prazosin infusion were directly related (Fig. 6).

BETA-BLOCKER BINDING SITES ON MONONUCLEAR LEUKOCYTES

As depicted in Fig. 7, studies in 12 younger and 5 older normotensive subjects revealed no age differences with respect to binding capacity (57 ± 15 SD fmol/mg versus 68 ± 29), binding sites (1,948 ± 643/cell versus 1,829 ± 339), or the affinity constant measured at equilibrium (0.5 ± 0.2 nM for both). In contrast, plasma norepinephrine concentrations in the older subjects were higher and isoproterenol sensitivity reduced.

DISCUSSION

Increased activity of the sympathetic nervous system in the patients with established essential hypertension is suggested by on-average elevated plasma epinephrine concentration at rest and during standardized submaximal exercise. In approximately 25% of the patients, values of plasma epinephrine were higher than the upper limit measured in normotensive subjects. This confirms our earlier reports (4, 13) and agrees with studies made by Morselli et al. (14) and de Champlain et al. (15). The more sensitive radioenzymatic assays in the recent studies may partly explain why differences in plasma epinephrine were not found in earlier studies using double-isotope (16) or fluorimetric techniques (17).

In contrast, plasma norepinephrine concentrations did not differ between normotensive and hypertensive subjects, but did tend to increase with age, in agreement with other studies (4, 18–20). On the other hand, plasma epinephrine concentra-

**Relationship Between Plasma Adrenaline and Increase in
Forearm Blood Flow Following Postsynaptic Alpha Blockade**

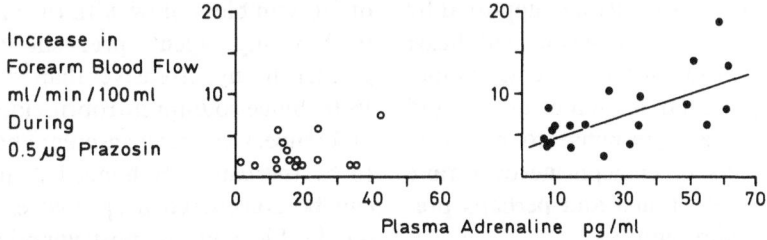

Fig. 6. Relationship between plasma epinephrine and the increase in forearm blood flow following postjunctional alpha-blockade with prazosin in patients with essential hypertension. Normotensive (○): $N = 16$; $r = 0.264$; $p = 0.35$. Essential hypertension (●): $N = 20$; $r = 0.634$; $p < 0.005$.

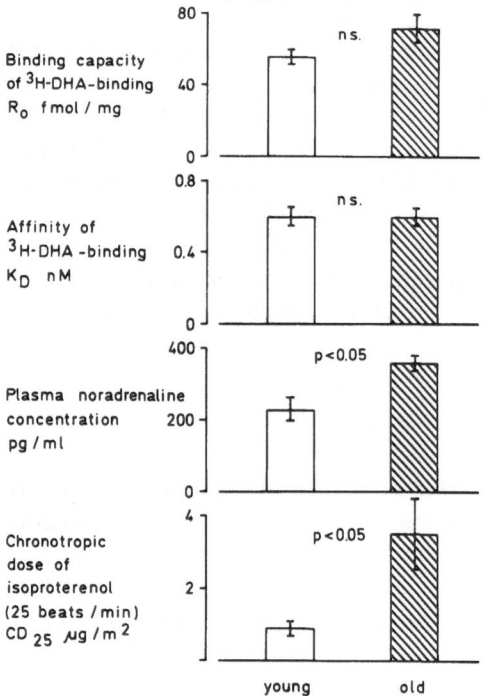

Beta-Adrenoceptor Binding, Isoproterenol Sensitivity and Plasma Noradrenaline

Fig. 7. Binding capacity and affinity of [³H]DHA on mononuclear leukocytes is similar in younger (18–40 years, $N = 14$) and older (53–65 years, $N = 8$) normotensive subjects. The reduced isoproterenol sensitivity in the presence of higher plasma epiconcentrations in the older subjects suggests a blunted beta-adrenoreceptor-mediated response, possibly due to a defect distal to the receptor.

tions did not change with age; but in each age group, values were higher in hypertensive than normotensive subjects. The consistently elevated plasma epinephrine concentrations can, therefore, be considered a better marker of overall sympathetic activity than plasma norepinephrine.

The concept of elevated sympathetic tone in such hypertensive patients is further supported by the relationship between epinephrine and heart rate as well as by their greater neurogenic component of peripheral vascular resistance as assessed by the-on-average greater response to prazosin. Conceivably an excess of epinephrine over time may desensitize postjunctional and perhaps prejunctional beta-adrenoreceptors.

Beta-adrenoreceptor-mediated cardiac, renal, and peripheral vascular responses to physiologic or pharmacologic stimulation were found to be

reduced with older age and higher pressure. Thus, exercise tachycardia and isoproterenol sensitivity were diminished in older subjects, particularly so in hypertensive patients, confirming other clinical studies (4, 21–24). Decreased isoproterenol sensitivity with elevated blood pressure has also been found in spontaneously hypertensive rats (25).

To the extent that renin is an index of a renal beta-adrenoreceptor-mediated response (26), renin measurement showed an age-related blunting of that response at rest in hypertensive and normotensive subjects both, but particularly in exercising older hypertensives, confirming previous studies (21, 27).

Reduced peripheral vascular response to isoproterenol with age was found recently by van Brummelen et al. (7). Similarly, the vasodilation produced by the beta-receptor stimulant metaproterenol was found to be reduced with older age in man (28) and in animals (29). While the difference between normotensive and hypertensive subjects did not reach significance in our study, the response to isoproterenol tended to be diminished in patients with the highest pressures, suggesting a pressure-related decrease of beta-receptor-mediated responses.

These changes may be due to a defect of the beta-adrenoreceptors secondary to age and perhaps blood pressure, possibly amplified in hypertensive patients because of sympathetic overactivation. In normal man, age was found to be associated with a decrease of the beta-adrenoreceptor-binding capacity of lymphocytes (30) and with blunted production of cyclic AMP; the latter also holds true in the older low-renin patients (31). However, our finding of similar receptor density in younger and older subjects favors an age-dependent defect in the beta-adrenoreceptor-effector unit distal to the receptor site.

In contrast to diminished beta-adrenoreceptor-mediated functions in hypertension, the increase in forearm blood flow with the alpha-adrenoreceptor-blocking agent prazosin was significantly greater in hypertensive than normotensive subjects. Since sodium nitroprusside induced no such difference, structural vascular changes are unlikely to be the cause. Enhanced response to prazosin can be considered a specific effect that depends on the blockade of postsynaptic alpha-adrenoreceptor-mediated vasoconstriction. Alpha-adrenoreceptor-mediated vascular resistance appears to remain unchanged with age.

The elevated plasma epinephrine concentrations in hypertensive patients suggest increased sympathetic activity, sustained in the older patients. With high pressure and older age, beta-adrenoreceptor-mediated cardiovascular functions tend to decrease, while alpha adrenoreceptor-mediated vasoconstriction is independent of age but greater in hypertensive patients. Therefore, it might be proposed that in an early developmental phase of hypertension, increased sympathetic activity via enhanced beta-adrenoreceptor-mediated responses accounts for the elevated heart rate and cardiac output as well as the stimulated renin-angiotensin-aldosterone system. Similarly, the intact beta-adrenoreceptor-mediated dilator force on peripheral vessels and renal and peripheral blood flow may explain the normal or even increased peripheral blood flow and the normal vascular resistance. Later, with sustained elevated sympathetic activity beta-adrenoreceptor-mediated functions are blunted, normalizing cardiac output and reducing renin secretion. Renal and peripheral vascular beta-responses are concomitantly diminished, contributing to a relative preponderance of alpha-adrenoreceptor-mediated vasoconstriction. This transition at the level of peripheral alpha- and beta-adrenergic receptor units may partly explain the long-known development from an early high-cardiac output into a later high-resistance form of hypertension.

in normal subjects. In hypertensives, this age-dependent decline tended to be enhanced. Decreased beta-adrenoreceptor-mediated functions but similar receptor density in the older subjects suggests a defect in enzymatic uncoupling systems distal to the receptor.

Beta-adrenoreceptor-mediated responses rendered defective by age and hypertension may contribute to development of unopposed alpha-adrenoreceptor-mediated vasoconstriction. This may help explain the change from an earlier high cardiac output and renin to a later high peripheral resistance phase of hypertension.

ACKNOWLEDGMENTS

This work was supported by Swiss National Scientific Funds no. 3.894.77, the Research Foundation of the University of Basel, and the Drs. C. and F. Demuth Swiss Medical Research Foundation.

We gratefully acknowledge the skillful technical assistance of Ms. D. Ellwanger, H. Fluri, D. Greter, S. Hänni, and M. Schnetz, as well as the editorial assistance of Dr. O. de Pinto and Ms. M. E. Guldimann.

SUMMARY

The sympathetic nervous system involvement in circulatory regulation was compared in 54 normotensive subjects and 110 age-matched patients with established essential hypertension. In essential hypertension, plasma epinephrine, regardless of age, was consistently higher and correlated with heart rate and the peripheral vasodilator response produced by postjunctional alpha-adrenoreceptor blockade with prazosin. The dilator response to prazosin was greater in hypertensive patients. Together, this suggests elevated sympathetic activity and enhanced alpha-adreno-receptor mediated vasoconstriction in essential hypertension.

Beta-adrenoreceptor-mediated tachycardia in response to exercise and intravenous isoproterenol, as well as the forearm vasodilator response to intraarterial isoproterenol, decreased with older age

REFERENCES

1. Robertson D, Johnson GA, Robertson RM, Nies AS, Shand DG, Oates JA (1979) Comparative assessment of stimuli that release neuronal and adrenomedullary catecholamines in man. Circulation 59: 637–643
2. Silverberg AB, Shah SD, Haymond MW, Cryer PE (1978) Norepinephrine: Hormone and neurotransmitter in man. Am J Physiol 234: E252
3. Rand MJ, Majewski H, McCulloch HW, Story DF (1978) An adrenaline-mediated positive feedback loop in sympathetic transmission and its possible role in hypertension. In: Proceedings of the IUPHAR satellite symposium on presynaptic receptors, Paris, 22–23 July
4. Lefkowitz RJ (1979) Direct binding studies of adrenergic receptors: Biochemical physiologic and clinical implications. Ann Intern Med 91: 450
5. Bertel O, Bühler FR, Kiowski W, Lütold BE (1980) Decreased beta adrenoreceptor responsiveness as related to age, blood pressure and plasma catecholamines in patients with essential hypertension. Hypertension 2: 130
6. Kiowski W, van Brummelen P, Bühler FR, Amann FW (1979) Plasma noradrenaline correlated with

blood pressure and alpha adrenoceptor-mediated vasoconstriction in essential hypertension. Clin Sci 57: 177S

7. van Brummelen P, Bühler FR, Kiowski W, Amann FW (1981) Age related decrease in cardiac and peripheral vascular responsiveness to isoproterenol (Submitted)

8. Amann FW, Bolli P, Kiowski W, Bühler FR (1981) Enhanced alpha adrenoreceptor-mediated vasoconstriction in essential hypertension (Submitted)

9. da Prada M, Zürcher G (1976) Simultaneous radioenzymatic determination of plasma and tissue adrenaline, noradrenaline and dopamine within the femtomole range. Life Sci 19: 1161

10. Lütold BE, Bühler FR, da Prada M (1976) Dynamik von Plasmakatecholaminen und Beta-Adrenozeptor-Funktionen: Anwendung einer neuen radioenzymatischen Mikromethode. Schweiz Med Wochenschr. 106: 1735

11. Sealey JE, Gerten-Banes J, Laragh JH (1972) The renin system: Variations in man measured by radioimmunoassay or bioassay. Kidney Int 1: 240

12. Landmann R, Bittinger H, Bühler FR, Dukor P (1980) High affinity beta adrenoceptor binding sites in human mononuclear leucocytes (abstr). In: European society for clinical investigation, annual meeting

13. Bühler FR, Kiowski W, van Brummelen P, Amann FW, Bertel O, Landmann R, Lütold BE, Bolli P (1980) Plasma catecholamines and cardiac, renal and peripheral vascular adrenoreceptor-mediated responses in different age groups of normal and hypertensive subjects. Clin Exp Hypertension 2: 409–426

14. Franco-Morselli R, Elghozi JL, Joly E, Diginilio S, Meyer P (1977) Increased plasma adrenaline concentrations in benign essential hypertension. Br Med J 2: 1251

15. de Champlain J (1981) Use of circulating catecholamines for the detection of autonomic abnormalities in human hypertension. In: This volume, pp 306–311

16. Louis WJ, Doyle AE, Anavekar SN (1973) Plasma norepinephrine levels in essential hypertension. New Engl J Med 296: 599

17. DeQuattro V, Chan S (1972) Raised plasma catecholamines in some patients with primary hypertension. Lancet 1: 806

18. Pedersen EB, Christensen NJ (1975) Catecholamines in plasma and urine in patients with essential hypertension determined by double-isotope derivative techniques. Acta Med Scand 198: 373

19. Lake CR, Ziegler NG, Coleman MD, Kopin IJ (1977) Age-adjusted plasma norepinephrine levels are similar in normotensive and hypertensive subjects. New Engl J Med 296: 208

20. Sever PS, Owikowska B, Birch M, Turnbridge RDG (1977) Plasma noradrenaline in essential hypertension. Lancet 1: 1078

21. Burkart F, Bühler FR, Pfisterer M, Lütold BE, Küng M (1976) Hemodynamic responses to exercise and acute beta-blockade in renin subtypes of essential hypertension. Clin Sci 51: 70

22. Åstrand PO, Rodahl K (1970) Textbook of work physiology. McGraw-Hill, New York

23. London GM, Safar ME, Weiss YA, Milliez PL (1976) Isoproterenol sensitivity and total body clearance of propranolol in hypertensive patients. J Clin Pharmacol 16: 174

24. McAllister RG, Love DW, Guthrie GP, Dominic JA, Kotchen TA (1979) Peripheral beta receptor responsiveness in patients with essential hypertension. Arch Intern Med 139: 879

25. Yamaguchi I, Kopin IJ (1980) Blood pressure, plasma catecholamines, and sympathetic outflow in pithed SHR and WKY rats. Am J Physiol 238: H365

26. Davis JO (1975) The use of blocking agents to define the functions of the renin-angiotensin system. Clin Sci 48: 3S

27. Bühler FR, Burkart F, Lütold BE, Küng M, Marbet G, Pfisterer M (1975) Antihypertensive beta-blocking action as related to renin and age: A pharmacological tool to identify pathogenetic mechanisms in essential hypertension. Am J Cardiol 36: 633

28. Strozzi C, Alboni P, Pereschi PL, Meduri P (1973) La riposta alla beta-stimolazione del circulo periferico nell'anziano. Acta Geront 23: 245

29. Fleisch JH (1980) Age-related changes in the sensitivity of blood vessels to drugs. Pharmacol Ther 8: 477

30. Schocken DD, Roth GS (1977) Reduced beta adrenergic receptor concentrations in ageing man. Nature 267: 856

31. Lowder SC, Hamet P, Liddle GW (1976) Contrasting effects of hypoglycemia on plasma renin activity and cyclic adenosine 3',5'-mono-phosphate (cyclic AMP) in low renin and normal renin essential hypertension. Circ Res 38(2): 105–108

DISCUSSION

Dr. Folkow (Göteborg, Sweden): I don't think it is surprising that there is so much controversy concerning plasma norepinephrine (NE) levels in early essential hypertension, because the neurogenic pattern then in action is a very specific one, reflecting a very mild defense reaction. Sympathetic nerve activity is increased to the heart, kidneys, and gastrointestinal tract, but is, if anything, slightly inhibited in skeletal muscle. The liver will clear almost all transmitter overflow coming from the important splanchnic area. What remains is the increased NE spillover from heart, kidneys, and some other tissue, while that from skeletal muscle may even be reduced. As a net effect, one may expect only *minor* shifts in mixed blood NE levels, despite the fact that hemodynamically a most important neurogenic pressor response is going on. I think this is illustrated nicely in a recent study by Hjemdal et al. [Hjemdahl P, Eliasson K (1979) Clin Sci 57 189S] in Stockholm on normotensive subjects. First, they tilted them and, of course, an increase in plasma NE levels ensued, because in this situation there occurs a generalized reflex increase in sympathetic discharge. Then, they exposed the same subjects to forced mental arithmetic which induces a mild defense reaction, precisely the type of autonomic pattern seen in early primary hypertension. Blood pressure then increased some 25%, heart rate increased some 30%, but there was no real increase in plasma NE levels, presumably because there was now no increase in sympathetic discharge to skeletal muscle, but rather a reduced discharge to this large tissue mass. I think this is the major dilemma in judging catecholamine levels in plasma in essential hypertension: A most important sympathetic activity pattern is present, but only poorly showing up in plasma NE levels.

Dr. DeQuattro (Los Angeles, Cal.): Dr. Folkow is right. We don't know where that sympathetic nerve activity is coming from in antecubital vein blood, but in human hypertension you can detect changes clinically in sympathetic function in terms of pallor, sweating, flushing, piloerection, etc. Thus, peripheral manifestations of sympathetic function that we see clinically may also be related to plasma NE from the periphery.

Dr. Eliahou (Tel Hashomer, Israel): To think that if you are to become hypertensive, you are born with a different number of beta-adrenergic receptors is most exciting. We followed Dr. Lefkowitz's work on a dozen essential hypertension patients and a dozen normotensives. There was no real difference in the number of beta-adrenergic receptor-binding sites in the two groups. The problem is that the number of beta-adrenergic receptors changes by autoregulation. Furthermore, in vivo, we don't have access to organs other than the leukocytes. I would like to ask Dr. Lefkowitz if he has overcome these points and if he has developed different methods, or micromethods, for the determination of binding sites.

Dr. Lefkowitz (Durham, N.C.): As you know, hypertension has not been a major thrust of our own investigation. We have worked with various animal models. I just came back from the clinical meetings last week where a group of clinical phar-

macologists at Vanderbilt had done just the kind of studies you are talking about [Nadeau JH, et al. (1980) Clin Res 28: 240A]. They took a group of patients and used the kind of methods that we've developed for studying beta-receptors on white blood cells. They sodium depleted the patients and showed that, depending on the level of sodium depletion, there were concurrent increases in plasma catecholamines; they were able to show a very nice inverse correlation between the level of circulating catecholamines and the beta-receptor number, suggesting that over the physiologic range of circulating catecholamine levels, there is a down regulation of the receptors. Thus, as catecholamine levels go up and down or (e.g., as thyroid hormone levels go up and down), the level of receptors might change so as to modulate responsiveness, and, conceivably, failures of normal compensatory mechanisms might lead to physiologic alterations. Again that's largely been speculative in terms of human physiology, although the recent data from the Vanderbilt group suggest that many of the same kind of mechanisms we've studied over the last few years in animal models are operative in humans and can be studied in circulating cells.

Dr. Bühler (Basel, Switzerland): In fact, Dr. Landmann in our group developed a model for quantifying high-affinity binding sites on mononuclear leukocytes (Fig. 7, Bühler et al., this volume, p 322). However, in contrast to Drs. Schocken and Roth's publication 2 years ago, we were unable to confirm an age-related decrease in beta-receptor-binding sites (ref 30, Bühler et al., this volume, p 324). Therefore, it may well be that the observed defect in beta-receptor-mediated effector response is the result of a defect distal to the receptor.

Dr. Hollenberg (Boston, Mass.): Dr. Kopin, was the thrust of your argument that one could dismiss the increased plasma catecholamines in young hypertensives because this was an alarm reaction?

Dr. Kopin (Bethesda, Md.): No, the question is if you do find an increase in catecholamines in the young person, what does this mean? There are three possibilities and I don't think that we can distinguish them at this time. One is that it's an intrinsic part of the pathogenesis of disease, and that the disease would not occur if there were normal adrenergic activity; the second is that the rise in blood pressure attending an adrenergic response is indicative of hyperresponsivity to pressor agents, which reflects a tendency to develop sustained hypertension by other mechanisms—some heritable, some environmental—in the future; and third, that the relationships are not of significance—the hyperadrenergic state as accompanied by a normal pressor response, reflecting an alarm reaction in a sensitive, aggressive, or anxious individual. This is not predictive of future development of established hypertension. I believe that perhaps individuals in each of these categories may be identified in the future. The research questions to be asked are clearly different than those addressed thus far.

Dr. J. Reid (Glasgow, Scotland): I have some difficulty in understanding the meaning of cerebrospinal fluid (CSF) NE. My concern is not only because these results disagree with our own findings measuring CSF MHPG in hypertensives, but I really am struck by the amazing coincidence of the one-to-one quantitative relationship between CSF NE and mixed venous and arterial NE. Is it possible that at least some of the CSF NE is derived from the brain perivascular space, from peripheral sympathetic nerve endings innervating cerebral blood vessels?

Dr. DeQuattro: I'm not as amazed about the CSF NE contents being similar to plasma levels as I'm amazed that the rat plasma NE are similar to those in humans. But there is really no answer for that coincidence. You found normal MHPG in hypertension. However, MHPG may be a different marker from NE. There is a difference in the pheochromocytoma patients from all of the other patients we studied. They were treated with alpha-blocking drugs, and in one case α-methyltyrosine; in another, the patient was treated with dilantin because we didn't think the patient had pheochromocytoma. Thus, it is possible that the drug treatment elevated their CSF NE levels above those they would have been if the patients weren't treated.

Dr. J. Reid: The blood CSF barrier is what you were testing with the pheochromocytoma patients.

It is quite a different thing to propose that the same barrier exists between nerve endings innervating brain vessels.

Dr. Meyer (Paris, France): I would like to make a brief comment about the localization of alpha$_1$ and alpha$_2$ sites. Dr. Lefkowitz was wise enough to warn us about the presynaptic and postsynaptic localization of these sites. I must say that it seems to be the same in the central nervous system. In the rat, after a complete section of the noradrenergic bundle and after 6-hydroxydopamine injection which lowers markedly the endogenous content of NE, we could find only a reduction of 20% of the alpha$_2$ binding sites. It seems, therefore, that either membranes of nerve endings are not affected by these treatments or another possibility is that these receptors may be located on nonadrenergic neurons.

Dr. Lefkowitz: I think these data are very interesting. We have unpublished data of our own on the peripheral nervous system which are exactly the same. That is, we cannot get a diminution in alpha$_2$-receptor binding in tissues like the uterus whether we surgically denervate or treat with 6-hydroxydopamine. So, I suspect many of these sites may, in fact, be postsynaptic.

Dr. Morganti (Milan, Italy): I have two questions for Dr. Bühler. First, did you observe age-related differences in forearm blood flow responses to prazosin in patients with essential hypertension? Second, are the increments in plasma renin activity in younger and older patients during exercise significantly different, even when considered in percent of the resting levels?

Dr. Bühler: First, there is no age effect in terms of prazosin-induced alpha-mediated dilatation. The other answer is "yes." Even though you express it in terms of percent, there is a smaller increment, at least at the highest exercise level, in the older patients; in fact, this also holds true for the low-renin hypertensives who are generally older patients.

Session 11
The Brain, Centrally Acting Drugs, the Renin System and Blood Pressure Regulation

Chairman: D. Ganten

Position Paper: The Brain, Centrally Acting Drugs, the Renin System and Blood Pressure Regulation

Ian A. Reid

It is now clear that the central nervous system and the renin–angiotensin system play important roles in the regulation of arterial pressure. It is also clear that there are important interactions between these two systems, the brain influencing the secretion of renin by the kidneys and angiotensin, in turn, acting on the brain to produce various cardiovascular and endocrine effects.

The purpose of this chapter is to review some of the mechanisms by which the central nervous system regulates blood pressure with emphasis on its role in the regulation of renin secretion by the kidneys, to describe recent progress concerning the central cardiovascular, dipsogenic and endocrine effects of angiotensin II, and to discuss how the various blood pressure control systems are affected by the centrally acting antihypertensive agent clonidine.

EFFERENT PATHWAYS BY WHICH THE CENTRAL NERVOUS SYSTEM REGULATES BLOOD PRESSURE

The pathways by which the central nervous system regulates blood pressure can be classified as neural and humoral. Neural control is exerted via the autonomic nervous system, which regulates cardiac output by way of the sympathetic and vagal innervation of the heart, and regulates total peripheral resistance by way of the sympathetic nervous system. Disorders of autonomic function can cause hypertension, as discussed elsewhere in this volume.

The hormones that are involved in the central nervous system control of blood pressure include corticotropin (ACTH), vasopressin, renin and angiotensin II, epinephrine and norepinephrine, the thyroid hormones, and a number of others. The present discussion will be limited to ACTH, vasopressin, and the renin–angiotensin system.

ACTH

ACTH affects blood pressure indirectly by regulating the secretion of various glucocorticoid and mineralocorticoid steroid hormones by the adrenal cortex. These steroids, in turn, influence blood pressure regulation via their effects on water and electrolyte excretion, vascular reactivity, and angiotensinogen production. Administration of ACTH elevates arterial pressure in experimental animals, and excessive secretion of ACTH can cause hypertension in humans (1).

VASOPRESSIN

Vasopressin is best known for its role in the regulation of water excretion. However, it also constricts vascular smooth muscle, and there is increasing evidence that, through this action, vasopressin plays an important role in blood pressure regulation. Elevations in plasma vasopressin concentration within the range observed in hypotensive and nonhypotensive hemorrhage increase blood pressure (2), and animals that have no circulating vasopressin, or that have been treated with vasopressin antagonists, have a reduced ability to regulate blood pressure during hypovolemia (3). Recent evidence indicates that vasopressin may play an important role in various forms of experimental hypertension (4).

RENIN-ANGIOTENSIN SYSTEM

The role of the renin–angiotensin system in the physiologic regulation of blood pressure and in various forms of hypertension is now well established. The major determinant of the activity of the renin–angiotensin system is the rate at which renin is secreted by the kidneys. This, in turn, is regulated by several mechanisms, one involving the central nervous system. The control of renin secretion by the central nervous system is, in part, mediated via the renal sympathetic nerves and, in part, by circulating catecholamines and vasopressin (5).

The effects on renin secretion of norepinephrine released locally by the renal nerves are complex. There is evidence, much of it indirect, that norepinephrine can stimulate renin secretion by a direct action on the juxtaglomerular cells. This effect is thought to be mediated via the stimulation of beta-adrenoreceptors and may involve the activation of adenylate cyclase and the formation of cyclic AMP (5). There is also evidence that alpha-adrenoreceptors are involved in the neural regulation of renin secretion. For example, it has been reported that the increases in renin secretion produced by carotid occlusion, hemorrhage, and renal nerve stimulation may be blocked by alpha-adrenoreceptor antagonists (5, 6). Exactly how alpha-stimulation increases renin secretion is not known, but likely possibilities include afferent arteriolar constriction with resultant activation of the renovascular receptor and decreased delivery of sodium chloride to the macula densa. In some situations, alpha-adrenoreceptor stimulation may actually inhibit the secretion of renin (5). However, the physiologic significance of this inhibitory effect remains uncertain, particularly because high doses of alpha-agonists are required to elicit it.

Circulating catecholamines may also increase renin secretion by the mechanisms just described for locally released norepinephrine. However, there is evidence that circulating catecholamines can increase renin secretion by stimulation of extrarenal beta-adrenoreceptors. This was first shown by Reid and associates (7) who demonstrated that low doses of isoproterenol, which failed to increase renin secretion when infused into the renal artery, markedly increased renin release when infused intravenously. Similar observations have recently been made for epinephrine and norepinephrine by Johnson and associates (8). The data of Johnson et al. also suggest that the stimulation of renin secretion by insulin-induced hypoglycemia may be largely mediated via these extrarenal beta-adrenoreceptors. The exact location of the extrarenal beta-adrenoreceptors, the

pathways by which they influence renin secretion, and their physiologic significance remain to be determined.

Less is known about the central pathways that are involved in the control of renin secretion. It is known that electrical stimulation of the medulla, pons, midbrain, and posterior hypothalamus increases renin secretion, while anterior hypothalamic stimulation causes suppression of renin release (5). There is also little information available concerning the neurotransmitters involved. Elevation of brain catecholamine levels by administration of a combination of L-dopa and carbidopa suppresses renin secretion, suggesting an inhibitory role for central catecholaminergic pathways (9). Data obtained with clonidine (see below) are consistent with this finding. More recent evidence indicates that central serotonergic neurons exert an excitatory effect on renin secretion (10). Characterization of these central pathways will be an important step in elucidating the mechanisms by which the central nervous system regulates renin secretion.

The sympathetic nervous system is not the only pathway by which the central nervous system influences renin secretion. It has been known for some time that administration of exogenous vasopressin inhibits renin secretion, and there is evidence that endogenous vasopressin can produce the same effect. The concentration of vasopressin required to inhibit renin secretion has been established and shown to be within the range observed during water deprivation (2). It is, therefore, likely that this effect of vasopressin is physiologically important. The mechanism by which vasopressin inhibits renin secretion has not been determined. It does not appear to involve vasoconstriction, since an analog of vasopressin that lacks vasoconstrictor activity inhibits renin secretion as effectively as vasopressin (11). A direct action on the juxtaglomerular cells seems a likely possibility, but further investigation is required.

Following release into the blood, renin catalyzes the formation of angiotensin I which is rapidly converted to the active peptide angiotensin II. Angiotensin II, in turn, increases blood pressure by a number of mechanisms, including direct arteriolar constriction, stimulation of aldosterone secretion, and a variety of effects mediated via the central nervous system. The actions of angiotensin II on the central nervous system are considered next.

ACTIONS OF ANGIOTENSIN II ON THE BRAIN

The actions of angiotensin II mediated via the central nervous system include elevation of arterial blood pressure, stimulation of drinking, and increased secretion of vasopressin and ACTH (12–14). These actions have been investigated in detail in several laboratories and a considerable amount of information has been obtained. Nevertheless, interpretation of these results in physiologic terms is often difficult. Many of the experiments have been performed in anesthetized animals in which cardiovascular and endocrine function are markedly altered. Very high doses of angiotensin have frequently been administered and several routes of administration have been used. In experiments where angiotensin was administered by the intravenous route, the systemic effects of the peptide may have interfered with some of its central actions.

This section summarizes the results of a recent investigation in this laboratory (15, 16), which was designed to further evaluate the physiologic significance of the central cardiovascular, dipsogenic, and endocrine effects of angiotensin. In these experiments, angiotensin was administered via the vertebral or carotid arteries of chronically prepared, conscious dogs. This approach was chosen so that the systemic effects of the peptide would be minimized; in addition, it was anticipated that comparison of the effects of intravertebral and intracarotid administration would provide information concerning the location of central sites of action of angiotensin.

Angiotensin was infused either into both carotid or both vertebral arteries. In most experiments, the doses tested were 0.1, 0.33, and 1.0 ng/kg/min infused into each artery (i.e., a total of 0.2, 0.66, and 2.0 ng/kg/min/animal). These doses had no effects on any of the measured variables when administered intravenously. In some experiments, the effects of intracarotid and intravertebral infusion of a higher dose of angiotensin II (2.5 ng/kg/min) were also tested. For the purposes of comparison, an additional series of experiments was performed in which angiotensin II was infused intravenously in doses of 2, 5, 10, and 20 ng/kg/min.

The effects on blood pressure of intravertebral and intracarotid infusion of angiotensin II at 0.1,

0.33, and 1.0 ng/kg/min are summarized in Fig. 1. All intravertebral doses produced statistically significant increases in blood pressure, the highest dose increasing mean arterial pressure by an average of 18.2 ± 3.0 mmHg ($p < 0.001$). Intracarotid infusion of the two higher doses of angiotensin also increased blood pressure significantly, but by a smaller amount, the largest increase averaging 9.1 ± 1.9 mmHg ($p < 0.001$). The increases in blood pressure produced by the intravertebral infusions of angiotensin II were accompanied by increases in heart rate; in marked contrast, heart rate was unchanged during the intracarotid infusions (15, 16).

There is now considerable evidence that the increase in blood pressure produced by intravertebral angiotensin II is mediated by the area postrema, a circumventricular organ located in the medulla oblongata (12). It seems reasonable to assume that the increases in blood pressure and heart rate produced by intravertebral infusion of angiotensin in the present experiments were mediated by this area. However, it is unlikely that the increase in blood pressure produced by intracarotid angiotensin was mediated by the area postrema. Most evidence indicates that the carotid arteries do not perfuse the medulla or other hindbrain regions, and this was confirmed in the present studies using the microsphere technique (16). It, therefore, seems likely that the blood pressure response to intracarotid angiotensin was mediated via a more rostral site or sites, the exact location of which remains to be determined. Possible sites include

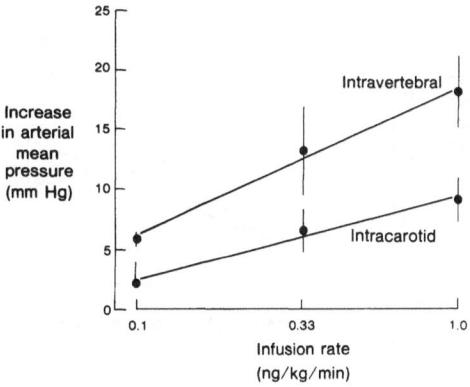

Fig. 1. Effects of intravertebral and intracarotid infusion of angiotensin II on mean arterial pressure in conscious dogs. [Data from Reid et al. (15) and Reid (16)]

the subfornical organ and the anteroventral region of the third ventricle, both of which have recently been implicated as possible central sites of action of angiotensin II on blood pressure.

It is known that carotid blood flow is higher than vertebral blood flow and, for this reason, the dose–response curves shown in Fig. 1 are somewhat misleading. In order to take this factor into account, measurements of right-carotid and right-vertebral blood flow were made in four conscious dogs. Right-carotid flow averaged 175 ± 21 ml/min and right-vertebral flow averaged 74 ± 12 ml/min. Using these values, and ignoring the problems of distribution, destruction, etc., the increases in the concentration of angiotensin II in the cerebral circulation resulting from the three intracarotid doses were estimated to be 29, 94, and 286 pg/ml, and for the vertebral infusions 68, 223, and 676 pg/ml. The basal plasma angiotensin II concentration in these animals averaged 15 pg/ml. In Fig. 2, the changes in blood pressure are replotted against the calculated increases in carotid or vertebral angiotensin II concentration. The curves are not significantly different, thus indicating similar sensitivities for the carotid and vertebral responses. It can also be seen from these curves that significant increases in blood pressure occur with increases in angiotensin II concentration of 100 pg/ml or less. These data thus provide additional evidence that the central cardiovascular actions of angiotensin represent physiologically significant actions of the peptide.

The efferent pathways by which centrally administered angiotensin II increased blood pressure were not investigated in these experiments. However, elevations in cardiac output and/or total peripheral resistance have been observed following central administration of angiotensin (12), and it is likely that such changes were responsible for the responses observed in the present study.

The effects of angiotensin on water intake are summarized in Fig. 3. Intracarotid angiotensin stimulated drinking in a dose-related manner. In marked contrast, intravertebral angiotensin had no effect on water intake. Figure 3 also demonstrates that intravenous angiotensin increases drinking, although not quite as effectively as intracarotid angiotensin. These results show that drinking can be stimulated by elevations in plasma angiotensin II within the physiologic range and thus add to a growing body of evidence that angiotensin II is involved in the physiologic regulation of water intake (14).

The effects of intracarotid and intravertebral infusion of angiotensin II on plasma vasopressin concentration (measured by radioimmunoassay) and plasma corticosteroid concentration (used as an index of ACTH secretion) are summarized in Figs. 4 and 5. It can be seen that the three lower doses of angiotensin II had little or no effect on either plasma vasopressin or corticosteroid concentrations. The highest intracarotid dose of angiotensin II (2.5 ng/kg/min: estimated increase in plasma angiotensin II concentration = 715 pg/ml) pro-

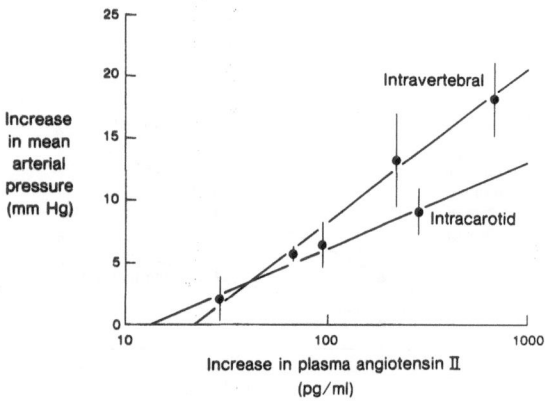

Fig. 2. Effects of intravertebral and intracarotid infusion of angiotensin II on mean arterial pressure, plotted as a function of the calculated increase in angiotensin II concentration in the cerebral circulation.

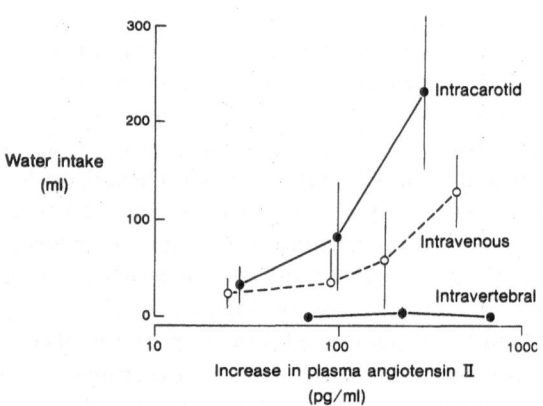

Fig. 3. Comparison of the effects of intravertebral, intracarotid, and intravenous infusion of angiotensin II on water intake. [Data from Reid et al. (15) and unpublished observations]

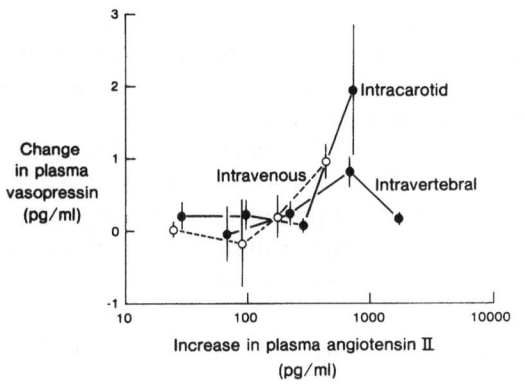

Fig. 4. Comparison of the effects of intravertebral, intracarotid, and intravenous infusion of angiotensin II on plasma vasopressin concentration. [Data from (15) and unpublished observations]

duced significant increases in plasma vasopressin and corticosteroid concentrations; intravertebral angiotensin was ineffective. The effects of intravenous angiotensin on plasma vasopressin and corticosteroid concentrations are also shown in Figs. 4 and 5. Only the highest dose of angiotensin (20 ng/kg/min), which increased plasma angiotensin II concentration by 435 pg/ml, increased plasma vasopressin and corticosteroid levels. These results confirm other reports that angiotensin II can increase vasopressin and ACTH secretion. However, they show that very high concentrations are required to produce this effect, and it is, therefore, unlikely that angiotensin II plays a significant role in the physiologic regulation of vasopressin or ACTH secretion.

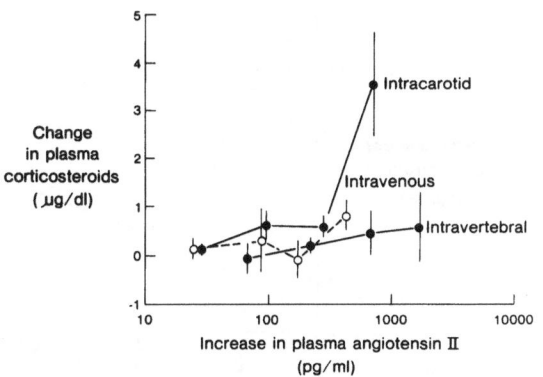

Fig. 5. Comparison of the effects of intravertebral, intracarotid, and intravenous infusion of angiotensin II on plasma corticosteroid concentration. [Data from (15) and unpublished observations]

In summary, these experiments confirm and extend previous observations that circulating angiotensin II can act on the central nervous system to elevate blood pressure, stimulate drinking, and increase the secretion of vasopressin and ACTH. Furthermore, the data suggest that the central pressor and dipsogenic actions of angiotensin represent physiologically important mechanisms by which the renin–angiotensin system participates in cardiovascular regulation. On the other hand, it is unlikely that the renin–angiotensin system plays a significant role in the regulation of vasopressin or ACTH secretion.

NEUROENDOCRINE EFFECTS OF CLONIDINE

Considerable research has been directed toward elucidating the mechanism of the antihypertensive action of clonidine. There is little doubt that the hypotensive effect of the drug largely results from an action on the central nervous system to decrease sympathetic activity and increase vagal tone, thus resulting in decreased total peripheral resistance and cardiac output (17). Clonidine also acts centrally to inhibit the secretion of a number of hormones, including renin, vasopressin, and ACTH. As discussed earlier in this chapter, the renin–angiotensin system, vasopressin, and ACTH are involved in the regulation of blood pressure, and it is, therefore, possible that the inhibition of the secretion of these hormones contributes to the antihypertensive action of clonidine. This section summarizes recent progress concerning the effects of clonidine on the secretion of renin, vasopressin, and ACTH.

RENIN

The inhibitory action of clonidine on renin secretion was first observed in hypertensive patients by Hökfelt and associates (18). This observation was subsequently confirmed by other investigators and extended to different species (19). In the initial studies, many of the mechanisms known to regulate the secretion of renin could be ruled out as possible mediators of the inhibition of renin secretion. These included the renovascular receptor and the macula densa, as well as alterations in the circulating level of angiotensin II, vasopressin, and potassium (18, 19). On the other hand, three lines of evidence indicated that the inhibition of renin secretion was secondary to the decrease in sympathetic activity produced by the drug. First, the suppression of renin secretion by clonidine is associated with diminished sympathetic activity as indicated by decreases in urinary norepinephrine and epinephrine excretion (18), renal nerve activity (20), and renovascular resistance (21). Second, the suppression of renin secretion by clonidine in dogs can be prevented by renal denervation (19), by ganglion blockade with pentolinium (22), and by spinal cord transection (23). Third, the stimulation of renin secretion that occurs in response to activation of the sympathetic nervous system by carotid sinus hypotension (24) or hemorrhage (25) is prevented by clonidine.

As mentioned earlier, the decrease in sympathetic activity produced by clonidine results from an action of the drug in the central nervous system. It now seems clear that the inhibition of renin secretion is also centrally mediated. For example, renin secretion is suppressed by injection of low doses of clonidine into the third cerebral ventricle or cisterna magna of dogs (19). Centrally administered clonidine also prevents the stimulation of renin secretion by carotid occlusion and hemorrhage (24, 25). Finally, intravenous administration of oxymetazoline, an imidazoline derivative that is closely related to clonidine but does not cross the blood–brain barrier, stimulates rather than inhibits the secretion of renin (22). Taken together, these observations indicate that the inhibitory action of clonidine on renin secretion results from an action of the drug in the central nervous system to decrease renal sympathetic neural activity.

Little information concerning the nature of the central receptors that mediate the renin-lowering action of clonidine is available. It is known that clonidine stimulates peripheral vascular alpha-adrenoreceptors, and that this action is responsible for the acute rise in blood pressure that is observed when the drug is administered intravenously. There is also evidence that some of the central effects of clonidine, including bradycardia and hypotension (17) as well as inhibition of ACTH secretion (see below), are mediated via stimulation of alpha-adrenoreceptors. The possibility that the central effect of clonidine on renin secretion is also mediated by alpha-adrenoreceptors has been investigated in this laboratory, but negative results have been obtained. In dogs, administration of phentol-

amine or piperoxane, either intravenously or directly into the third cerebral ventricle, failed to prevent the suppression of renin secretion produced by intravenous clonidine (26). In another study (27), centrally administered phenoxybenzamine also failed to prevent the suppression of renin secretion. Further pharmacologic characterization of the receptors that mediate the inhibition of renin secretion by clonidine is, therefore, required.

Vasopressin and ACTH

It has been known for some time that clonidine increases urine flow when administered intravenously in dogs or rats (28, 29). This increase is accompanied by a decrease in urinary osmolality and an increase in free water clearance and does not occur in hypophysectomized dogs receiving a vasopressin infusion (28). On the basis of these observations, it was proposed that clonidine inhibits vasopressin secretion. This has now been confirmed by direct radioimmunoassay of plasma vasopressin in both dogs and rats. In these animals, there is a prompt fall in plasma vasopressin levels following intravenous administration of clonidine (29, 30) (Fig. 6).

The mechanism of the inhibitory effect of clonidine on vasopressin secretion has not been established. In the initial studies, it was proposed that the inhibition might simply be a consequence of the acute hypertensive response to intravenous clonidine (28). However, subsequent studies showed this not to be the case. For example, suppression of vasopression secretion in dogs is not signifi-

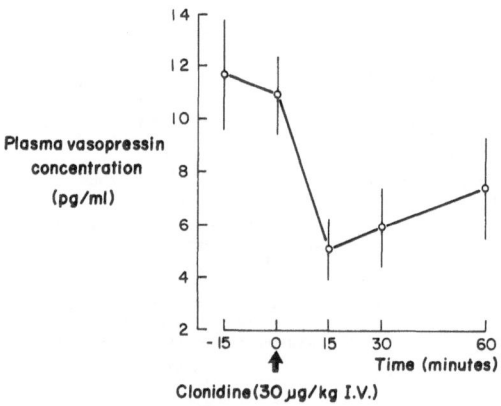

Fig. 6. Effect of intravenous clonidine on plasma vasopressin concentration in anesthetized dogs. [Data from Reid et al. (30)]

cantly altered when the pressor action of clonidine is prevented by intravenous administration of alpha-adrenoreceptor antagonists (30). Under these conditions, marked decreases in vasopressin secretion occur together with large falls in blood pressure. In rats, clonidine suppresses plasma vasopressin levels, even when it is administered in doses that do not increase blood pressure (29).

It has been reported that direct application of catecholamines to supraoptic neurosecretory cells decreases the electrical activity of these cells. In addition, elevation of brain catecholamine levels by administration of a combination of L-dopa and carbidopa produces marked inhibition of vasopressin secretion (31). On the basis of these observations, together with the other central actions of clonidine, it seems reasonable to propose that clonidine inhibits vasopressin secretion by an action on the brain, possibly a direct inhibitory effect on supraoptic neurosecretory cells. Further studies are required to test this possibility.

Clonidine also inhibits ACTH secretion when administered either intravenously or intraventricularly (32). This response appears to result from stimulation of central alpha-adrenoreceptors and is abolished by intraventricular administration of a small dose of phenoxybenzamine (32).

In summary, clonidine not only markedly alters the activity of the autonomic nervous system, but also inhibits the secretion of several hormones, including renin, vasopressin, and ACTH. As described earlier, these hormones play important roles in blood pressure regulation, and it seems likely that the endocrine effects of clonidine may contribute to its antihypertensive action. Further investigation is required to determine the extent of this contribution.

SUMMARY

1) The central nervous system regulates blood pressure by way of the autonomic nervous system and by way of a number of hormones, including renin, vasopressin, and ACTH.

2) The central nervous system control of renin secretion is mediated primarily by way of the renal sympathetic nerves and circulating catecholamines; vasopressin may also play an inhibitory role in some situations.

3) Circulating angiotensin II, formed by the re-nal renin–angiotensin system, acts on the brain to produce a variety of effects, including elevation of arterial pressure, stimulation of drinking, and increased secretion of vasopressin and ACTH. The central cardiovascular and dipsogenic effects of angiotensin appear to be physiologically important, but it is unlikely that angiotensin plays a significant role in the control of vasopressin or ACTH secretion.

4) The antihypertensive agent clonidine inhibits the secretion of renin, vasopressin, and ACTH. The inhibition of the secretion of renin, ACTH, and probably vasopressin results from actions of clonidine on the central nervous system. These inhibitory effects may contribute to the hypotensive action of this drug.

ACKNOWLEDGMENTS

This chapter contains the results of previously unpublished work that was supported by USPHS grant AM-06704. I. A. Reid is the recipient of Research Career Development Award HL-00104.

REFERENCES

1. Scoggins BA, Butkus A, Coghlan JP, Denton DA, Fan JSK, Humphrey TJ, Whidworth JA (1978) Adrenocorticotropic hormone-induced hypertension in sheep: A model for the study of the effect of steroid hormones on blood pressure. Circ Res 43(Suppl I): I76–I81
2. Malayan SA, Ramsay DJ, Keil LC, Reid IA (1978) Effects of vasopressin on plasma renin activity, blood pressure, heart rate and plasma 17–OH corticosteroid concentration in conscious dogs (abstr). Physiologist 21: 75
3. Cowley AW Jr, Switzer SJ, Guin MM (1980) Evidence and quantification of the vasopressin arterial pressure control system in the dog. Circ Res 45: 58–67
4. Möhring J, Kintz J, Schoun J (1979) Studies on the role of vasopressin in blood pressure control of spontaneously hypertensive rats with established hypertension (SHR, stroke-prone strain). J Cardiovasc Pharmacol 1: 593–608
5. Reid IA, Morris BJ, Ganong WF (1978) The renin–angiotensin system. Annu Rev Physiol 40: 377–410
6. Powis DA, Donald DE (1979) Involvement of renal α and β-adrenoceptors in release of renin by carotid baroreflex. Am J Physiol 236: H580–H585
7. Reid IA, Schrier RW, Earley LE (1972) An effect

of extrarenal beta adrenergic stimulation on the release of renin. J Clin Invest 51: 1861–1869

8. Johnson MD, Shier DN, Barger AC (1979) Circulating catecholamines and control of plasma renin activity in conscious dogs. Am J Physiol 236: H463–H470

9. Blair ML, Reid IA, Ganong WF (1977) Effect of L-dopa on plasma renin activity with and without inhibition of extracerebral dopa decarboxylase in dogs. J Pharmacol Exp Ther 202: 209–215

10. Zimmermann H, Ganong WF (1980) Pharmacological evidence that stimulation of central serotonergic pathways increases renin secretion. Neuroendocrinology 30: 101–107

11. Malayan SA, Reid IA (1979) Mechanism of the effects of vasopressin on renin secretion and sodium excretion (abstr). Fed Proc 38: 967

12. Ferrario CM, Gildenberg PL, McCubbin JW (1972) Cardiovascular effects of angiotensin mediated by the central nervous system. Circ Res 30: 257–262

13. Share L (1979) Interrelations between vasopressin and the renin–angiotensin system. Fed Proc 38: 2267–2271

14. Simpson JB, Epstein AN, Camardo JS Jr (1978) Localization of receptors for the dispogenic action of angiotensin II in the subfornical organ of rats. J Comp Physiol Psychol 92: 581–608

15. Reid IA, Rudolf CD, Keil LC, Jones TT, Hale SD (1979) Analysis of the central actions of angiotensin II in the dog (abstr). Fed Proc 38: 882

16. Reid IA (1980) Central actions of circulating angiotensin II on blood pressure in conscious dogs. In: Abstracts, sixth international congress on endocrinology, p 571

17. Laubie M, Delbarre B, Bogaievsky D, Bogaievsky Y, Tsoucaris-Kupfer D, Senon D, Schmitt H, Schmitt H (1976) Pharmacological evidence for a central α-sympathomimetic mechanism controlling blood pressure and heart rate. Circ Res 38(Suppl II): II35–II41

18. Hökfelt B, Hedeland H, Dymling JF (1970) Studies on catecholamines, renin and aldosterone following Catapresan (2-(2,6-dichlor-phenylamine)-2-imidazoline hydrochloride) in hypertensive patients. Eur J Pharmacol 10: 389–397

19. Reid IA, MacDonald DM, Pachnis B, Ganong WF (1975) Studies concerning the mechanism of suppression of renin secretion by clonidine. J Pharmacol Exp Ther 192: 713–721

20. Haeusler G (1975) Cardiovascular regulation by central adrenergic mechanisms and its alteration by hypotensive drugs. Circ Res 36, 37(Suppl I): 223–232

21. Cohen IM, O'Connor DT, Preston RA, Stone RA (1979) Reduced renovascular resistance by clonidine. Clin Pharmacol Ther 26: 572–577

22. Nolan PL, Reid IA (1978) Mechanism of suppression of renin secretion by clonidine in the dog. Circ Res 42: 206–211

23. Ganong WF, Wise BL, Reid IA, Holland J, Kaplan S, Shackelford R, Boryczka AT (1978) Effect of spinal cord transsection on the endocrine and blood pressure responses to intravenous clonidine. Neuroendocrinology 25: 105–110

24. Reid IA, Jones A (1976) Effects of carotid occlusion and clonidine on renin secretion in anesthetized dogs. Clin Sci Mol Med 51: 109S–111S

25. Leavitt ML, Miller RE, Kotchen TA (1980) Suppression of stimulated plasma renin by clonidine in the dog. Hypertension 2: 187–191

26. Reid IA, Jones A (1976) Effect of α-adrenergic blockade on the inhibition of renin secretion by clonidine (abstr). Endocrinology 98: A551

27. Ganong WF (1977) The renin–angiotensin system and the central nervous system. Fed Proc 36: 1771–1775

28. Humphreys MH, Reid IA (1975) Suppression of antidiuretic hormone secretion by clonidine in the anesthetized dog. Kidney Int 7: 405–412

29. Roman RJ, Cowley AW Jr, Lechene C (1979) Water diuretic and natriuretic effect of clonidine in the rat. J Pharmacol Exp Ther 211: 385–393

30. Reid IA, Nolan PL, Wolf JA, Keil LC (1979) Suppression of vasopressin secretion by clonidine: Effects of α-adrenoceptor antagonists. Endocrinology 104: 1403–1406

31. Blair ML, Reid IA, Keil LC, Ganong WF (1979) Role of peripheral adrenoreceptors and vasopressin in the suppression of plasma renin activity by L-dopa in carbidopa-treated dogs. J Pharmacol Exp Ther 210: 368–372

32. Ganong WF, Kramer N, Salmon J, Reid IA, Lovinger R, Scapagnini U, Boryczka AT, Shackelford R (1976) Pharmacological evidence for inhibition of ACTH secretion by a central adrenergic system in the dog. Neuroscience 1: 167–174

Sodium and Central Nervous System Mechanisms

Carlos M. Ferrario, K. Bridget Brosnihan, and Robert R. Smeby

The conspicuous importance of the renin–angiotensin axis in the maintenance of normal arterial pressure is best demonstrated in situations where "effective" blood volume is reduced as in the case of dietary sodium depletion (1). It is, however, possible that the dominant role of angiotensin in the heightened vasoconstrictive state of sodium depletion overshadows concomitant abnormalities of other major control mechanisms. Because sodium restriction produces a rise of plasma norepinephrine (NE) (2–4), it is necessary to consider that high levels of angiotensin II may stimulate sympathetic activity. There is, however, some problem regarding the acceptance of a direct relationship between the renin–angiotensin and sympathetic control mechanisms in the sodium-restricted state. For example, Rocchini et al. (5) showed blunted sympathetic responses to carotid sinus hypotension in the dog, and markers of neuronal activity were depressed in the studies of Ljundqvist (6) and Sybertz and Peach (7). We thus wondered whether sodium depletion affects the interaction between angiotensin and the sympathetic nervous system in an unsuspected manner, namely, by preventing the expression of the neurogenic effects of angiotensin II on the cardiovascular system. To test this hypothesis, various experiments were carried out in both normal and sodium-depleted dogs; procedures entailed assessment of the response to carotid occlusion, measurements of plasma and cerebrospinal fluid (CSF) catecholamines, and, lastly, evaluation of the renin activity in brain regions to establish whether it changed in a manner consonant with the existence of a negative feedback between the kidney and the brain as previously proposed by Sen et al. (8).

METHODS

All experiments were carried out in male mongrel dogs weighing between 16 and 22 kg. Control data were obtained in dogs fed a standard laboratory diet providing an intake of 65 mEq Na^+/day. To effect a state of Na^+ imbalance, dogs were placed on a diet (prescription[R] H/D[R], Purina Lab) for 21–28 days which provided no more than 4 mEq Na^+/day. This regimen was completed by injection of a diuretic (furosemide, 80 mg/day for 3–5 days). The techniques employed to monitor hemodynamics and assess sympathetic reflexes are described elsewhere (19). Fractionated catecholamines and plasma renin activity (PRA) were measured by radioenzymatic (10) and radioimmunoassays, respectively. Renin activity in various regions of the saline-perfused brain was measured as the amount of angiotensin I generated from exogenous dog substrate at a pH of 6.5 (R. R. Smeby, unpublished method). Cathepsin D was determined in the same brain tissues by the method of Anson et al. (11).

RESULTS

SYMPATHETIC REFLEXES PRODUCED BY CAROTID OCCLUSION

Dietary sodium restriction, as carried out in the laboratory, did not affect the mean arterial pressure of α-chloralose-anesthetized dogs, but did cause significant reductions in cardiac output that were compensated for by increased peripheral resistance. Other characteristics of sodium-depleted dogs were hemoconcentration, marked rise in plasma renin activity (PRA) (15–24-fold increase compared to normal averages of 2.0 ± 0.4 ng/ml/h), slight hyponatremia, increased protein concentration, and unchanged serum creatinine and BUN. In normal anesthetized animals, a 1-min occlusion of the common carotid artery produced a 61 ± 5 mmHg rise in mean arterial pressure at the plateau of the pressor response, while heart rate increased by 46 ± 9 beats/min. Increases in both cardiac output (33%) and total peripheral resistance (67%) were responsible for the rise in pressure. In dogs maintained on a low-sodium diet, the cardiovascular response to carotid sinus hypotension differed significantly from that obtained in normal dogs (Fig. 1). In all cases, the pressor response was about half that obtained in normal animals (35 ± 3 mmHg), reflex tachycardia was absent, and cardiac output did not increase.

CHANGES IN SYMPATHETIC ACTIVITY DUE TO SODIUM DEPLETION

The observation of decreased baroreceptor responsiveness in sodium-depleted animals led to the search for more direct evidence of decreased central vasomotor sympathetic drive. This was accomplished by measuring sympathetic nerve discharges from postganglionic twigs of a left renal nerve in dogs anesthetized with morphine and pentobarbital. Takishita and Ferrario (12) found that

renal sympathetic neural firing was consistently less at any given level of arterial pressure in dogs on a low-sodium diet compared to normal. In addition, the *critical pressure* (point at which renal sympathetic neural firing was reduced to noise levels) was lower in sodium-depleted than in normal dogs (12).

CATECHOLAMINE SYSTEM IN SODIUM-DEPLETED DOGS

In order to assess whether reduced sympathetic discharges originated centrally, samples of CSF from the cisterna magna and plasma were simultaneously taken to assess differences in the peripheral and central levels of catecholaminergic activity. After sodium depletion, plasma NE rose from 127 ± 19 to 223 ± 28 pg/ml ($p < 0.01$), but epinephrine (EPI) and dopamine did not change significantly (111 ± 33 versus 193 ± 43 pg/ml and 90 ± 43 versus 50 ± 6 pg/ml, respectively). In CSF, NE increased from 87 ± 9 to 126 ± 14

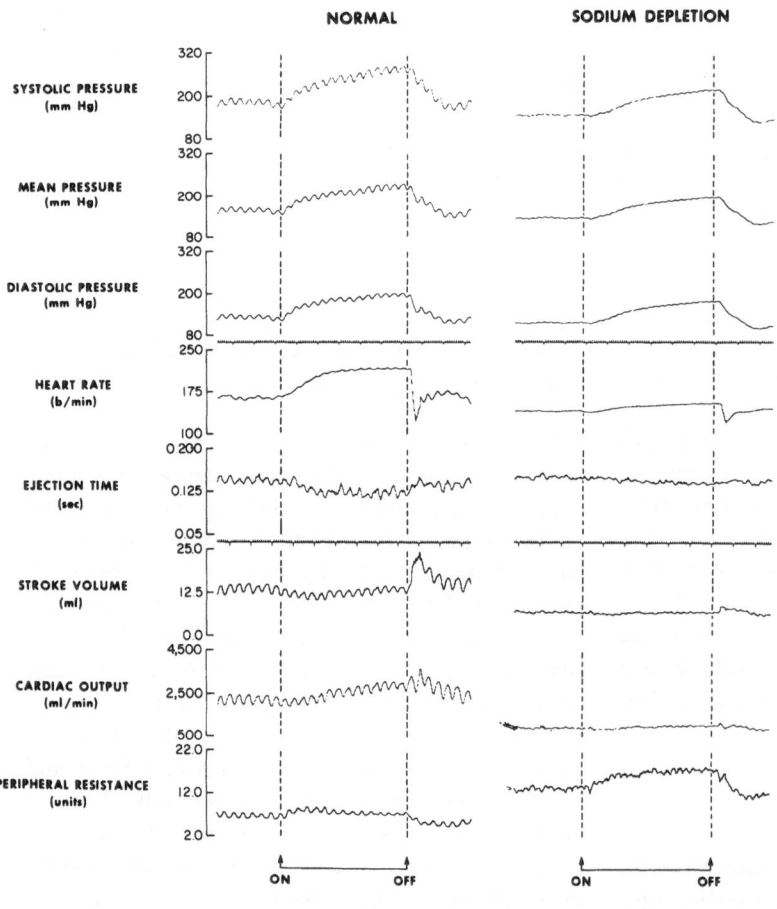

Fig. 1. Hemodynamic differences in the time-course of the cardiovascular response to occlusion of a sole-innervated carotid artery in a normal *(left panel)* compared to a sodium-depleted *(right panel)* dog. The reduced pressor response of salt-depleted dogs is associated with the absence of tachycardia and increased cardiac output.

pg/ml ($p < 0.05$), while EPI and dopamine levels remained unchanged (9 ± 3 versus 6 ± 1 pg/ml and 53 ± 10 versus 63 ± 25 pg/ml, respectively).

Because extravascular renin, particularly that which is endogenous to the brain, may be involved in blood pressure regulation, renin activity of the brainstem, cortex, cerebellum, and spinal cord were assayed in two groups of dogs. Renin activity was detected in all samples of brain tissue (Table 1), but the concentration was significantly less in the brainstem of sodium-depleted dogs in spite of the fact that these animals had an 18-fold increase in PRA. On the other hand, the concentration of Cathepsin D in the same tissues did not change (Table 1).

CONCLUDING REMARKS

Sodium depletion accomplished by a combination of diet and diuretics appears to produce significant alterations in the function of the automatic nervous system that do not conform to the usual understanding of the effect of increased levels of angiotensin II on sympathetic activity (13). Although it is certain that angiotensin II is capable of augmenting sympathetic activity at both peripheral and central sites (14), the state of the sodium balance appears to modify significantly the expression of the interplay between the renal pressor and sympathetic nervous systems. The present observations suggest that sodium depletion brings about a decrease in the rate of discharge from sympathetic nerves as indicated by the blunting of the pressor response that accompanies occlusion of a sole-innervated carotid artery and reduced efferent renal nerve activity. The concurrent increase in the levels of CSF NE may point to increased noradrenergic turnover, since Brosnihan et al. (15) showed a corresponding decrease in tissue NE concentration in the area postrema of sodium-depleted dogs.

Increasing evidence suggests that peptides generated in the brain are involved in cardiovascular function (15). The decrease in brain renin activity and the elevated CSF NE may reflect the CNS modulatory activity of angiotensin on adrenergic systems and, thus, may be a part of a neurohumoral feedback linking the renal pressor system with the central sympathetic nervous system as proposed by Ferrario and McCubbin (14). Further investigation of these factors may prove of great help in the analysis of the role of sodium in the control of cardiovascular function.

SUMMARY

We have examined the neuroendocrine alterations brought about by sodium depletion in the dog. The deficit in sodium balance persisted for 3 weeks as a result of the dogs eating a diet with a sodium intake of less than 4 mEq/day and given furosemide between the 18th and 21st day of the diet. Sodium depletion did not affect mean arterial pressure, but cardiac output was reduced and peripheral resistance rose. The concentration of NE rose in both plasma and CSF sampled at the level of the cisterna magna. The increase in neurotransmitter concentration was associated with marked hy-

Table 1. Effect of dietary sodium depletion on renin and cathepsin D activity in brain regions of the dog.

Region	Normal		Sodium depleted	
	Brain renin[a]	Cathepsin D[b]	Brain renin[a]	Cathepsin D[b]
Spinal cord	0.16 ± 0.04	0.08 ± 0.10	0.10 ± 0.01	0.78 ± 0.06
Cerebellum	0.22 ± 0.05	0.64 ± 0.10	0.12 ± 0.02	0.55 ± 0.03
Lower brainstem	0.25 ± 0.07	0.75 ± 0.09	$0.08 \pm 0.01^*$	0.62 ± 0.05
Upper brainstem	0.28 ± 0.08	0.76 ± 0.13	$0.09 \pm 0.02^*$	0.50 ± 0.03
Anterior cortex	0.27 ± 0.07	0.58 ± 0.08	0.09 ± 0.02	0.56 ± 0.05
Posterior cortex	0.25 ± 0.10	0.65 ± 0.07	0.08 ± 0.01	0.53 ± 0.04

Data are mean $\pm$ SE of ten normal and ten sodium-depleted dogs.
* $p < 0.05$, normal versus sodium depleted.
[a] Brain renin units = ng angiotensin I/h/mg protein.
[b] Cathepsin D units = mg tyrosine/0.5 h/mg protein.

perreninemia. However, the content of brain renin in samples obtained from both the upper and lower portions of the brainstem fell to about half that measured in control animals. It is concluded that sodium depletion alters the neurohumoral control of the dog's cardiovascular system at both central and peripheral sites. The lower concentration of brain renin activity, coupled with elevated levels of CSF NE, may reflect an important aspect of the modulatory activity of sodium affecting the interplay between the kidney renin–angiotensin and sympathetic nervous systems.

REFERENCES

1. Samuels A, Johnson G, Peuler A (1977) Physiologic effects of the renin angiotensin system on sympathetic nervous system activity in the conscious dog. In: Buckley J, Ferrario CM (eds) Central actions of angiotensin and related hormones. Pergamon, New York, pp 135–144
2. Romoff MS, Keusch G, Campese VM, Wang M, Friedler RM, Weidman P, Massry SG (1978) Effect of sodium intake on plasma catecholamines in normal subjects. J Clin Endocrinol Metab 48: 26–31
3. Nicholls MG, Kiowski W, Zweifler AJ, Julius S, Schork MA, Greenhouse J (1980) Plasma norepinephrine variations with dietary sodium intake. Hypertension 2: 29–32
4. Lake CR, Ziegler MG (1978) Effect of acute volume alterations on norepinephrine and dopamine β-hydroxylase in normotensive and hypertensive subjects. Circulation 57: 774–778
5. Rocchini AP, Cant JR, Barger AC (1977) Carotid sinus reflex in dogs with low to high sodium intake. Am J Physiol 233: H196–H202
6. Ljundqvist A (1975) The effect of angiotensin infusion, sodium loading, and sodium restriction on the renal and cardiac adrenergic nerves. Acta Pathol Microbiol Scand [A] 83: 661–668
7. Sybertz EJ, Peach MJ (1980) In vitro neurogenic and musculotropic responses to angiotensin peptides in normal and sodium-restricted rabbits. Circ Res 46 (in press)
8. Sen S, Ferrario CM, Bumpus FM (1974) Alteration in the feedback control of renin release by an angiotensin antagonist. Acta Physiol Lat Am 24: 529–532
9. Ferrario CM, McCubbin JW, Page IH (1969) Hemodynamic characteristics of chronic experimental neurogenic hypertension in unanesthetized dogs. Circ Res 24: 911–922
10. Peuler JD, Johnson GA (1977) Simultaneous single isotope radioenzymatic assay of plasma norepinephrine, epinephrine and dopamine. Life Sci 20: 625–636
11. Anson ML (1938) The estimation of pepsin, trypsin, papain, and cathepsin with hemoglobin. J Gen Physiol 22: 79–89
12. Takishita S, Ferrario CM (in press) Effects of chronic sodium depletion on renal sympathetic activity in the anesthetized dog (abstr). Physiologist
13. McCubbin JW, Page IH (1963) Neurogenic component of chronic renal hypertension. Science 139: 210–215
14. Ferrario CM, McCubbin JW (1974) Neurogenic factors in hypertension. Hosp Pract 9: 71–81
15. Brosnihan KB, Ferrario CM, Smeby RR, Saavedra JM (1980) Effects of sodium depletion on brain isorenin and catecholamines (abstr). Soc Neurosci (in press)
16. Ganten D, Hutchinson JS, Schelling P, Ganten U, Fischer H (1976) The iso-renin angiotensin systems in extrarenal tissue. Clin Exp Pharmacol Physiol 3: 103–126

Experimental Evidence in Support of a Central Neural Imbalance Hypothesis of Hypertension

Donald J. Reis

It has been proposed that imbalances within the central nervous system of control systems regulating the arterial pressure and favoring enhancement of sympathetic discharge will result in high blood pressure (1). To test the validity of the central neural imbalance hypothesis, studies have been undertaken in animals to demonstrate that experimentally produced disordered CNS function can result in abnormalities of blood pressure control similar to those of the human disease. The brain region selected as a target of inquiry is the intermediate one-third of the nucleus tractus solitarii (NTS), the area that serves as the principal site of termination of baroreceptor and other cardiopulmonary afferents (2–4).

ELECTROLYTIC LESIONS OF NTS: NTS HYPERTENSION

Destruction of NTS by placement of small bilateral electrolytic lesions will produce profound changes of blood pressure control, a syndrome called *NTS hypertension*. In rat (5–9), NTS lesions result in acute fulminating hypertension, fatal within 4–5 h. The rise in blood pressure is due to a massive increase in sympathetic vasomotor activity which is selective and differentiated and increases peripheral resistance two- to threefold. The increased resistance leads to ventricular overload, reduced cardiac output, left heart failure, pulmonary edema, and death. There is enhanced release of adrenal catecholamines, but with an intact sympathetic nervous system they do not contribute to the hypertension. Baroreceptor reflexes are abolished. The hypertension results in profound changes of cyclic nucleotide metabolism in blood vessels (9) similar to those seen in more chronic hypertensive models in the rat (10). Hypertension is abolished, or severely reduced, by numerous general anesthetics: ganglioplegics, alpha-blockers, and clonidine (11). It depends on the integrity of structures above the midbrain, possibly in the rostral basal hypothalamus (12).

In cat (13), NTS lesions result, after an initial acute phase, in the development of *chronic labile hypertension,* characterized by elevation in mean blood pressure, enhanced minute-to-minute variability of blood pressure (lability), exaggerated reactivity of the blood pressure in response to environmental stimuli or during naturalistic behaviors, enhanced conditionability of blood pressure by classic (Pavlovian) conditioning (14), and a fixed tachycardia. Baroreceptor reflexes are abolished or severely attenuated.

In dog, NTS lesions also produce chronic labile hypertension (15, 16) which, after many months, may evolve into fixed *sustained hypertension* (15). The hypertension is not associated with changes in peripheral renin or aldosterone (16). Baroreceptor and other cardiopulmonary reflexes are reduced or abolished.

IMPAIRMENT OF NEURO-CHEMICAL MECHANISMS IN NTS: LABILITY OF HYPERTENSION

Impairment of neurochemical systems projecting to or innervating NTS can also produce profound abnormalities of blood pressure control.

NORADRENERGIC INNERVATION

In rat, destruction of portions of the noradrenergic projections to NTS, either by local injection of the catecholamine neurotoxin 6-hydroxydopamine (6-OHDA) (17) or by electrolytically destroying the A2 catecholamine group of neurons located in the dorsal medulla (18) (which provides a large noradrenergic innervation of NTS), results in *chronic lability of blood pressure without hypertension* (18). Some exaggeration of blood pressure is seen during naturalistic behaviors. Baroreflexes may remain intact, blunted, or dissociated depending on the type of lesion (17–19). The effect appears selective for the noradrenergic innervation since lesions destroying the epinephrine-containing neurons of the C2 group, fail to produce hypertension (W. T. Talman and D. J. Reis, unpublished observations). Animals kept up to a year with A2 lesions maintain their lability of arterial pressure (19); however, they do not evolve into chronic hypertension, suggesting that lability *per se* will not necessarily evolve into hypertension.

Interference with glutamatergic transmission in NTS may also produce hypertension (20–23) because the finding relates to physiologic and biochemical observations, suggesting that the amino acid L-glutamate may be the neurotransmitter of baroreceptor afferents (20–23). The evidence for our conclusion is based on observations that in rat the local injection of low doses of L-glutamate (10^{-9}M) or its agonist kainic acid (10^{-11}) into NTS will simulate baroreflexes; and administration of doses sufficient to produce depolarization blockade of postsynaptic neurons, but less than those required for neurotoxicity, will block baroreflexes and result in fulminating hypertension with pulmonary edema. Similarly, the local administration of the glutamatergic antagonists glutamate diethylester (GDE) will also block baroreflexes and produce hypertension (22). These experiments raise the prospect that abnormalities in the transmission of glutamate in NTS, either as a consequence of reduced synthesis, storage, or release of the transmitter, or reduction in the efficacy of glutamate receptors, would favor the production of hypertension.

SUMMARY

1) Impaired neurotransmission in NTS, a brainstem region integrating major cardiovascular reflexes, can result in animals in abnormalities of blood pressure control with many features of human hypertension.

2) Such abnormalities, while varying with respect to species or the manner in which NTS function is disturbed, include the production of: a) fulminating neurogenic hypertension; b) chronic labile neurogenic hypertension; c) chronic sustained neurogenic hypertension; d) labile arterial pressure without hypertension; e) lability of arterial pressure; f) exaggerated reactivity of arterial pressure in response to behavioral emotional or environmental stimuli; g) enhanced conditionability of arterial pressure; and h) neurogenic hypertension lowered by drugs effective in treating hypertension in man (e.g., clonidine).

3) We conclude that an imbalance in neurotransmission in brain can result in hypertension.

REFERENCES

1. Reis DJ (in press) Experimental central neurogenic hypertension from brainstem dysfunction: Evidence for a central neural imbalance hypothesis of hypertension. In: Weiner H (ed) Brain, behavior, and bodily disease. Raven Press, New York
2. Miura M, Reis DJ (1969) Termination and secondary projections of carotid sinus nerve in the cat brain stem. Am J Physiol 217: 142–153
3. Seller H, Illert M (1969) The localization of the first synapse in the carotid sinus baroreceptor reflex pathway and its alteration of the afferent input. Pfluegers Arch 306: 1–19
4. Berger AJ (1979) Distribution of carotid sinus afferent nerve fibers to solitary tract nuclei of the cat using transganglionic transport of horseradish peroxidase. Neurosci Lett 14: 153–158
5. Doba N, Reis DJ (1973) Acute fulminating neurogenic hypertension produced by brainstem lesions in rat. Circ Res 32: 584–593
6. Doba N, Reis DJ (1974) Role of central and peripheral adrenergic mechanisms in neurogenic hypertension produced by brainstem lesions in rat. Circ Res 34: 293–301
7. Palkovitz M, DeJong W, Zandberg P, Versteeg DHG, van der Gugten J, Larenth C (1977) Central hypertension and nucleus tractus solitarii catecholamines after surgical lesions in the medulla oblongata in the rat. Brain Res 127: 127–131
8. Snyder DW, Doba N, Reis DJ (1978) Regional distribution of blood flow during arterial hypertension produced by lesions of the nucleus tractus solitarii in rat. Circ Res 42: 87–91
9. Amer MS, Doba N, Reis DJ (1975) Changes in cyclic nucleotide metabolism in aorta and heart of neurogenically hypertensive rats: Possible trigger

mechanisms of hypertension. Proc Natl Acad Sci USA 72: 2135–2139

10. Amer MS, Gomoll AW, Perhach JL Jr, Ferguson HC, McKinney GR (1974) Aberrations of cyclic nucleotide metabolism in the hearts and vessels of hypertensive rats. Proc Natl Acad Sci USA 71: 4930–4934

11. Rockhold RW, Caldwell RW (1979) Effects of lesions of the nucleus tractus solitarii on the cardiovascular actions of clonidine in conscious rats. Neuropharmacology 18: 347–354

12. Brody MJ, Fink GD, Buggy J, Haywood JR, Gordon FJ, Knuepfer M, Mow M, Mahoney L, Johnson AK (1979) Critical role of the anterior third ventricle (AV3V) region in development and maintenance of experimental hypertension. In: Meyer P, Schmitt H (eds) Nervous system and hypertension. Wiley-Flammarion, New York/Paris, pp 76–84

13. Nathan MA, Reis DJ (1977) Chronic labile hypertension produced by lesions of the nucleus tractus solitarii in the cat. Circ Res 40: 72–81

14. Nathan MA, Tucker LW, Severini WP, Reis DJ (1978) Enhancement of conditioned arterial pressure responses in cats after brainstem lesions. Science 201: 71–73

15. Schmitt H, Laubie M (1979) Destruction of the nucleus tractus solitarii in dogs: Acute effects on blood pressure and hemodynamics, chronic effects on blood pressure. Importance of the nucleus for effects of drugs. In: Meyer P, Schmitt H (eds) Nervous system and hypertension. Wiley-Flammarion, New York/Paris, pp 173–201

16. Carey RM, Dacey RG, Jane JA, Winn HR, Ayers CR, Tyson GW (1979) Production of sustained hypertension by lesions of the nucleus tractus solitarii of the American Foxhound. Hypertension 1: 246–254

17. Snyder DW, Nathan MA, Reis DJ (1978) Chronic lability of arterial pressure produced by selective destruction of the catecholamine innervation of the nucleus tractus solitarii in the rat. Circ Res 43: 662–671

18. Talman WT, Snyder DW, Reis DJ (in press) Labile arterial pressure produced by electrolytic lesions of A2 catecholamine neurons in rat. Circ Res

19. Talman WT, Alonso DR, Reis DJ (in press) Impairment of baroreceptor function and chronic lability of arterial pressure produced by lesions of A2 catecholamine neurons of rat brain: Failure to evolve into hypertension. In: Sleight P (ed) Baroreceptors and hypertension. Oxford University Press, Oxford

20. Reis DJ, Talman WT, Perrone M, Doba N, Kumada M (in press) L-glutamate as the neurotransmitter of baroreceptor afferents. In: Sleight P (ed) Baroreceptors and hypertension. Oxford University Press, Oxford

21. Talman WT, Perrone MH, Reis DJ (in press) L-glutamate: The neurotransmitter of primary baroreceptor afferent nerve fibers? Science

22. Talman WT, Perrone MH, Reis DJ (1980) Pharmacological evidence for L-glutamate as the neurotransmitter of primary baroreflex afferents (abstr). Soc Neurosci (in press)

23. Perrone MH, Talman WT, Reis DJ (in press) Biochemical evidence for the role of glutamate as a neurotransmitter of baroreceptor afferents (abstr). Soc Neurosci

Brain Centers for Pharmacologic Control of the Cardiovascular System

G. Haeusler

In contrast to many peripherally acting antihypertensive agents that have a well-defined site of action, the exact localization of the effects of centrally acting antihypertensives within the brain or spinal cord has not yet been achieved. One of the major centers for cardiovascular control is the bulbar nucleus of the solitary tract (NTS), which contains the first synapse of the baroreceptor reflex (1, 2). Its superficial location at the end of the fourth ventricle in immediate vicinity of the obex makes it easily accessible to various experimental interventions designed to localize drug actions. In the following study, three such interventions are described and their applicability illustrated using clonidine as an example.

METHODS

The experiments were carried out in 86 cats of either sex and a body weight of 2.4–3.2 kg. The animals were anesthetized with urethan (0.9 g/kg i.p.) and, after introduction of artificial respiration, immobilized with gallamine triethiodide (5 mg/kg i.v.). Blood pressure was recorded from the right femoral artery. The pulse waves triggered a cardiotachometer. Sympathetic nervous activity was recorded from the preganglionic splanchnic and a postganglionic renal nerve. The method of recording and quantification was described previously (3).

In the first method, to study transmission at the first synapse of the baroreceptor reflex, one carotid sinus nerve was stimulated with bipolar platinum electrodes, and a field potential was recorded from the ipsilateral NTS using glass micropipettes with a tip resistance of 1–2 megaΩ (Fig. 1). For the estimation of drug-induced changes of the amplitude of the field potentials, the potentials were averaged with a Datalab signal analyzer.

The second method involved cooling the NTS to approximately 8°C by placing thermodes (diameter 2 mm) on the exposed dorsal surface of the medulla oblongata, at a region corresponding to the underlying NTS. This procedure results in reversible interruption of transmission through the first synapse of the baroreceptor reflex. Spontaneous sympathetic nervous activity, blood pressure, and heart rate were monitored during 5- to 10-min periods of cooling.

In the third method, in debuffered cats, one carotid sinus nerve was stimulated electrically with supramaximal voltage at a frequency of 1 Hz. Each stimulus applied to the carotid sinus nerve produced a virtually total inhibition of spontaneous discharges for 400–500 ms in a renal sympathetic nerve. Cooling of the NTS to 13°–15°C shortened this silent period, indicating a partial impairment, but not total interruption, of transmission through the first synapse of the baroreceptor reflex. This experimental arrangement was chosen to allow recognition of both inhibitory as well as facilitatory drug effects on transmission at this synapse.

RESULTS AND DISCUSSION

EVOKED POTENTIALS IN THE NTS

The field potentials evoked in the NTS by electrical stimulation (frequency 1 Hz) of the carotid sinus nerves characteristically consisted of a negatively directed wave with an amplitude of 100–400 μV and a latency of 3–8 ms (Fig. 1). The configuration of the field potentials and their latencies varied somewhat depending on the location of the recording site within the NTS (Fig. 1).

Clonidine (10–100 μg/kg i.v.) caused a dose-dependent reduction in the amplitude of the field

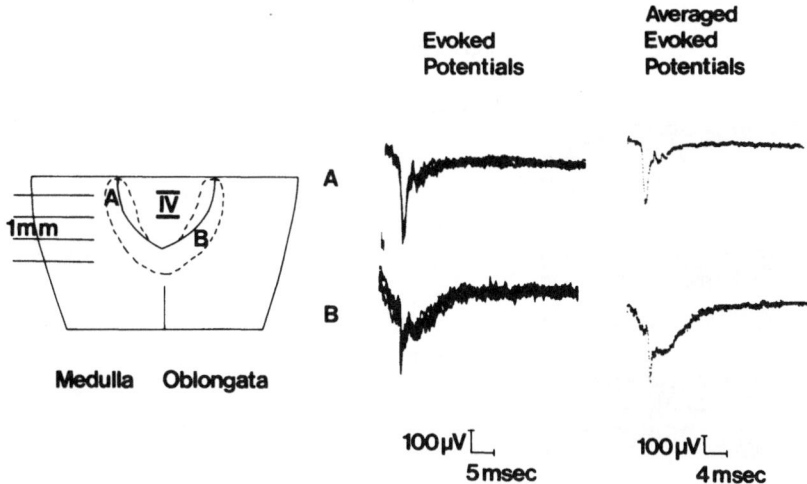

Fig. 1. Schematic representation of sites in the NTS at which field potentials were recorded in response to electrical stimulation of the ipsilateral carotid sinus nerve, and configuration of the field potentials observed in the rostral part *(A)* and the middle part *(B)* of the NTS. *Left Column:* tracings show 5 superimposed field potentials. *Right column:* tracings represent 16 potentials averaged by a signal analyzer [From Haeusler (6).]

potentials. The field potentials, however, never disappeared under the influence of clonidine; the maximal drug-induced reduction of the amplitude varied between 30% and 50%. The alpha-adrenoreceptor-blocking agents piperoxan and yohimbine antagonized the clonidine-induced reduction of the amplitude of the field potentials.

INTERRUPTION OF NEUROTRANSMISSION IN THE NTS BY COOLING

Reduction of the temperature of the NTS to 8°C caused an interruption of transmission through the first synapse of the baroreceptor reflex. This is evident from several observations: a) Cooling of the NTS increased spontaneous sympathetic nervous activity, blood pressure, and heart rate; b) the effect of electrical stimulation of the carotid sinus nerve on these parameters disappeared during cooling; and c) the effect of electrical stimulation of the posterior hypothalamus on blood pressure and sympathetic nervous activity was increased during cooling. The last effect results, in all probability, from a cooling-induced elimination of a restraining influence of the baroreceptor reflex on the excitatory effects of hypothalamic stimulation.

The decreases in spontaneous sympathetic nervous activity, blood pressure, and heart rate in-

duced by low doses of clonidine (3 and 10 μg/kg i.v.) were nearly entirely antagonized by cooling of the NTS. At a dose of 30 μg/kg i.v., only a partial antagonism was obtained by cooling. These results indicate that up to a dose of 10 μg/kg i.v., clonidine exerts its cardiovascular effects mainly at the level of the NTS; with higher doses, other parts of the central nervous system become increasingly involved.

IMPAIRMENT OF NEUROTRANSMISSION IN THE NTS BY COOLING

When the temperature of the thermodes used for cooling of the NTS was set to 12°–15°C, the silent period of 400–500 ms, which normally follows a single pulse applied to the carotid sinus nerve, was shortened to 100–200 ms, (Fig. 2), indicating impairment of transmission through the first synapse of the baroreceptor reflex. Clonidine (3 and 10μg/kg i.v.) prolonged this silent period both under normal conditions as well as during cooling.

In summary, both the influence of clonidine on evoked potentials recorded from the NTS and the antagonism of the cardiovascular effects of clonidine by cooling of the NTS allow localization of the action of clonidine to this medullary center. The improvement by clonidine of cooling-induced impairment of neurotransmission in the NTS lends

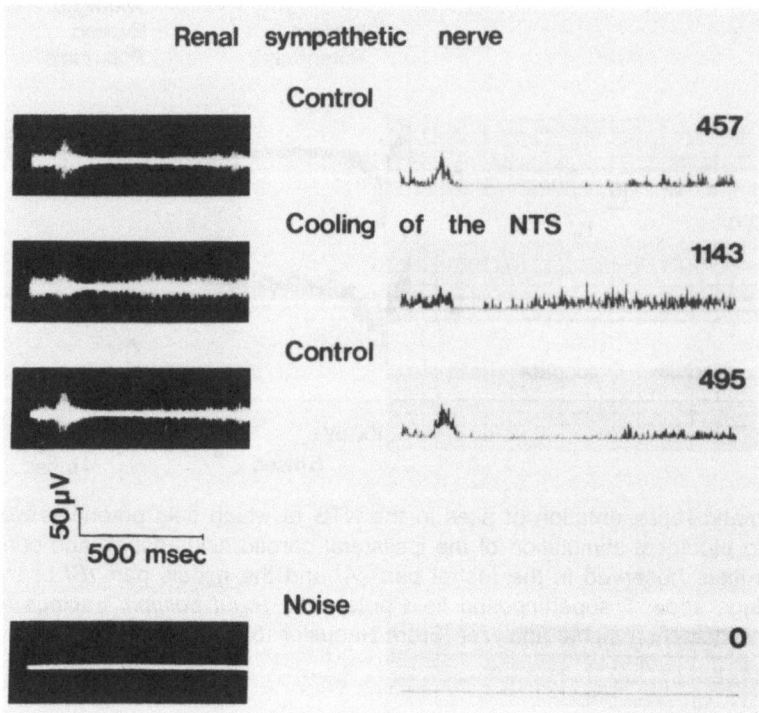

Fig. 2. The carotid sinus nerve of a debuffered cat was stimulated with 16 shocks at a rate of 1 Hz, producing an inhibition of spontaneous sympathetic nervous activity (postganglionic renal sympathetic nerve) for approximately 500 ms. The period of inhibition of the spontaneous activity was read from 16 superimposed tracings at a storage oscilloscope *(left panels)* and was also determined from the poststimulus time histogram *(right panels)* after feeding the nerve activity into a signal analyzer. The numbers on the poststimulus time histogram give the nerve activity in arbitrary units. Reduction of the temperature of the NTS to approximately 13°–15°C shortened the silent period of the sympathetic nerve to 125 ms, indicating impairment, but not interruption, of neurotransmission in the NTS. Note the reversibility of the cooling-induced changes.

credence to previous suggestions (4, 5) that clonidine facilitates transmission, or induces a central activation, of the baroreceptor reflex.

SUMMARY

The NTS, which contains the first synapse of the baroreceptor reflex, may be considered as one of the major centers for cardiovascular control. Three methods were used to study the effect of drugs on the NTS. The centrally acting antihypertensive clonidine was used as an example to illustrate the applicability of the methods, which involved: a) recording of drug-induced changes in NTS-field potentials evoked by electrical stimulation of the carotid sinus nerves; b) reversible interruption of synaptic transmission by cooling of the NTS with thermodes; and c) reversible partial impairment of transmission by graded reduction of the temperature of the NTS and monitoring the decline in the effectiveness of the baroreceptor reflex. The centrally acting antihypertensive clonidine reduced the amplitude of field potentials in the NTS. Cooling-induced interruption of transmission abolished the sympathoinhibitory effect of low doses of clonidine. Impairment of transmission through less intense cooling was partially antagonized by clonidine. It is concluded that clonidine facilitates transmission at the first synapse of the baroreceptor reflex.

REFERENCES

1. Miura M, Reis DJ (1969) Termination and secondary projections of carotid sinus nerve in the brain stem. Am J Physiol 217: 142–153
2. Seller H, Illert M (1969) Localization of the first synapse in the carotid sinus baroreceptor reflex pathway and its alteration of the afferent input. Pfluegers Arch 306: 1–19
3. Haeusler G (1976) Studies on the possible contribution of a peripheral presynaptic action of clonidine and dopamine to their vascular effects under in vivo conditions. Naunyn Schmiedebergs Arch Pharmacol 295: 191–202
4. Haeusler G (1973) Activation of the central pathway of the baroreceptor reflex, a possible mechanism of the hypotensive action of clonidine. Naunyn Schmiedebergs Arch Pharmacol 278: 231–246
5. Haeusler G (1974) Further similarities between the action of clonidine and a central activation of the baroreceptor reflex. Naunyn Schmiedebergs Arch Pharmacol 285: 1–14
6. Haeusler G (1979) Electrophysiological studies on the transmission through the first synapse of the baroreceptor reflex. In: Meyer P, Schmitt H (eds) Nervous system and hypertension: Perspectives in nephrology and hypertension. Wiley-Flammarion, New York/Paris, pp 209–218

Central and Peripheral Alpha-Adrenoreceptors and the Actions of Clonidine and Methyldopa

Carlene A. Hamilton and John L. Reid

Clonidine and methyldopa lower blood pressure in animals by an action on the brainstem to reduce efferent sympathetic activity (1–3). Clinical studies and the profile of side effects suggest that a similar site accounts for their antihypertensive effects in man (4).

The pharmacologic basis of the action of clonidine and methyldopa has been proposed to be mediated by stimulation of alpha-adrenoreceptors in the brain. Clonidine, like methylnorepinephrine, the decarboxylated, hydroxylated, active metabolite of methyldopa has alpha-receptor agonist properties (5, 6). However, both agents were atypical when compared with conventional alpha-agonists, and their central effects were antagonized by some, but not all, classic alpha-adrenoreceptor blockers (7). The paradox emerged whereby drugs blocking alpha-receptors lowered blood pressure, while drugs stimulating alpha-receptors also lowered blood pressure. A possible, but incomplete, explanation could be that the receptors were located in two different and distant sites—brain and peripheral vascular muscle—and the drugs had differential access to these sites. However, it is apparent that a more plausible and complex explanation lies in the heterogeneity of alpha-receptors.

Central alpha-receptors on which clonidine acts were noted both by classic pharmacologic methods and more recent radiologand-binding techniques to be similar to presynaptic alpha-receptors, which in the periphery inhibit neurotransmitter release (8, 9). Both differ from classic postsynaptic alpha-receptors (10). A preferred classification that makes no assumptions about anatomic location is $alpha_1$ for "classic" postsynaptic receptors and $alpha_2$ for receptors that may be presynaptic is some systems or tissues, and which are preferentially stimulated by clonidine and methylnorepinephrine (11). In several tissues, it is apparent that $alpha_2$-receptors are not presynaptically located (Table 1). These include platelets (12) and ganglion cells of the myenteric plexus in the gut (K. Starke, personal communication) and possibly in the brain. Recent studies in vitro and in vivo in several animal species have raised the possibility that receptors with similarities to $alpha_2$-receptors may be postjunctionally located on vascular smooth muscle (13–16). These findings are supported by the failure in several studies after surgical denervation or chemical sympathectomy with 6-hydroxydopamine (6-OHDA) to significantly alter the affinity for an apparent number of binding sites to ^3H-clonidine, a relatively selective $alpha_2$-receptor ligand, in peripheral tissues (16) (Table 2) or brain (17).

Recent pharmacologic studies have utilized drugs with a spectrum of alpha-receptor effects [antagonists including prazosin ($alpha_1$), phentolamine ($alpha_1$ and $alpha_2$), and yohimbine ($alpha_2$) and agonists including phenylephrine ($alpha_1$) norepinephrine ($alpha_1$ and $alpha_2$), methylnorepinephrine, guanabenz, and clonidine ($alpha_2$)]. Table 3 shows that in intact conscious rabbits, while phentolamine can antagonize phenylephrine and norepinephrine equally well, the $alpha_1$-selective blocker prazosin is more effective in blocking phenylephrine, while the $alpha_2$-selective blocker yohimbine preferentially antagonizes norepinephrine. Similar effects have been observed after the $alpha_2$-agonist clonidine and guanabenz, which exert a pressor response resistant to prazosin but antagonized by the mixed blocker phentolamine.

The full significance of the heterogeneity of alpha-receptors has not yet been established, nor has their distribution in different vessels and vascular beds. Preliminary experiments suggest, however, that the regulation of responsiveness and receptor–effector coupling to smooth muscle contraction may differ between $alpha_1$- and $alpha_2$-subtypes. There may also be differences in associa-

Table 1. Classification of drugs acting on alpha-adrenoreceptors.

Receptor	Location	Action	Agonist	Antagonist
Alpha-1	Smooth muscle (blood vessels, etc.)	Constriction	Phenylephrine Methoxamine	Prazosin Labetalol
	CNS	?		
	Platelets	?		
Alpha-2	Sympathetic nerve endings (presynaptic)	Reduce transmitter release	Clonidine	
	NS	Lowers blood pressure	Guanabenz Guanfacine	Yohimbine
			Methylnorepinephrine	
	Platelets	?Increase ADP aggregation		

Norepinephrine and epinephrine have nonselective actions on alpha$_1$- and alpha$_2$-receptors, and phentolamine and phenozybenzamine are nonselective antagonists.

tion with neuroeffector junctions and accessibility to circulating catecholamines.

The implication of multiple types and sites of alpha-receptor is clearly of relevance to the antihypertensive effects of clonidine and methyldopa, as these drugs are considered to act as alpha$_2$-agonists. A peripheral presynaptic action may be identifiable in animals (9) and under some conditions also in man (18), but it appears that the main site of antihypertensive effect is in the brainstem (4).

What of the precise location of action of centrally acting drugs? Several studies suggest that clonidine and methylnorepinephrine may act in or near the nucleus of the solitary tract in the brainstem (2). This nucleus, close to the obex, is the site of the primary synapse of many sensory neurons of the baroreceptor and chemoreceptor afferents. Clonidine modulates baroreflex activity to increase the sensitivity or gain of the baroreflex arc. Whether clonidine acts on an alpha$_2$-receptor on secondary neurons in the reflex arc or on modulatory interneurons is not known. Hökfelt et al. (19) presented immunohistofluorescent evidence for the existence of epinephrine-containing neurons in the brain which appear to innervate, among other regions, the noradrenergic cell bodies of the locus ceruleus and nucleus of the solitary tract and to inhibit the activity of these norepinephrine-containing fibers. There are reports of changes in epinephrine synthesis or turnover in brainstem areas of animals with spontaneous hypertension,

Table 2. Alpha-receptor-binding constants in heart and spleen membranes prepared from rabbit tissues with or without pretreatment with 6-OHDA 50 mg/kg intravenously 3–4 days before.

Animal group	Tissue	Ligand	K_D (nM)	B_{max} (fmol/mg protein)
Intact	Spleen	^{3}H-Prazosin	6.4 ± 1.5	152 ± 17
6-OHDA	Spleen	^{3}H-Prazosin	5.7 ± 1.7	184 ± 28
Intact	Heart	^{3}H-Phazosin	9.8 ± 4.4	80 ± 22
6-OHDA	Heart	^{3}H-Prazosin	11.9 ± 3.3	90 ± 15
Intact	Spleen	^{3}H-Clonidine	47 ± 17	171 ± 42
6-OHDA	Spleen	^{3}H-Clonidine	23 ± 4	146 ± 15
Intact	Heart	^{3}H-Clonidine	–	< 30
6-OHDA	Heart	^{3}H-Clonidine	–	< 40

K_D and B_{max} were determined by linear regression analysis of Scatchard plot data. Values given are the mean of six to eight experiments ± SD. There was no significant difference between intact and 6-OHDA-treated groups.

Table 3. Antagonism of the pressor response to intravenous phenylephrine and norepinephrine by alpha-antagonists in conscious rabbits.

Antagonist	Dose ratio phenylephrine	Dose ratio norepinephrine
Phentolamine		
1.0 mg/kg	5.2 ± 0.5	5.7 ± 0.8
5.0 mg/kg	12.0 ± 1.0	12.8 ± 1.0
Prazosin		
0.1 mg/kg	5.0 ± 0.6*	3.3 ± 0.6
0.5 mg/kg	10.5 ± 0.9*	6.3 ± 1.2
Yohimbine		
1.0 mg/kg	1.5 ± 0.2	2.8 ± 0.7*

The parallel shift of the pressor dose–response relationship is expressed as the dose ratio. The dose ratio to phenylephrine is compared with the dose ratio for norepinephrine using paired Wilcoxon test (*$p < 0.01$). Results expressed as mean $\pm$ SD ($N = 8$).
Source: Hamilton and Reid (16).

DOCA salt hypertension (20), and renovascular hypertension (21). Bolme et al. (22) have suggested that clonidine can reverse these effects and that it may act as an alpha$_2$-agonist on inhibitory receptors located on noradrenergic neurons which are usually activated by epinephrine. These receptors would thus be postjunctional with respect to the epinephrine-releasing neurons, although prejunctional to the noradrenergic neuron. If this were the case, it would be expected that destruction of noradrenergic neurons with central 6-OHDA would interfere with the hypotensive effect of clonidine. This finding was observed in early experiments (23), although not confirmed in studies utilizing other means of impairing central catecholamine transmission (1).

Methyldopa (through methylnorepinephrine) and clonidine appear to act predominantly by a sympathoinhibitory action in the brainstem. Both drugs act as alpha$_2$-agonists on receptors located in cardiovascular-regulating areas possibly modifying the consequences of an epinephrine neuron inhibitory modulation of efferent sympathetic outflow.

SUMMARY

Clonidine and methyldopa (through its metabolite methylnorepinephrine) lower blood pressure in animals and man by a sympathoinhibitory effect in the central nervous system probably at the level of the brainstem. The integrity of the baroreceptor afferents is not essential for this action, but efferent sympathetic pathways must be intact.

Methylnorepinephrine and clonidine act as alpha-adrenoreceptor agonists or stimulants and show a specificity for receptors of the alpha$_2$-subtype. These receptors are similar to presynaptic receptors on peripheral sympathetic nerve and are blocked by yohimbine and phentolamine, but not by prazosin. Alpha$_1$-receptor responses are blocked by prazosin (and phentolamine) and mimicked by phenylephrine or methoxamine. The alpha$_1$- and alpha$_2$-classification may be more useful than the terms pre- and postsynaptic, as alpha$_2$-receptor may be located postsynaptically in some tissues including the vascular neuroeffector junction. At brainstem cardioregulatory centers, clonidine and methylnorepinephrine may activate inhibitory alpha$_2$-receptors on noradrenergic or other neurons usually stimulated by endogenous brain epinephrine. These experimental actions and mechanisms of centrally acting drugs would be consistent with clinically observed effects on blood pressure, heart rate, and arousal.

ACKNOWLEDGMENTS

These studies were supported by the Medical Research Council of Great Britain. We are grateful to Mrs. Mary Wood for assisting in typing and preparation of this manuscript.

REFERENCES

1. Kobinger W (1975) Central cardiovascular actions of clonidine. In: Davies DS, Reid JL (eds) International symposium on central actions of drugs in regulation of blood pressure. Pitmans Medical, Tunbridge, Wells, UK, pp 181–193
2. Nijkamp FP, de Jong W (1977) Centrally induced hypotension by α methyldopa and α methylnoradrenaline in normotensive and renal hypertensive rats. Progr Brain Res 47: 349–368
3. Reid JL (1979) Central action of antihypertensive drugs. In: Melmon K (ed) Drup therapeutics: Concepts for physicians. Elsevier, New York, pp 135–150
4. Reid JL, Wing LMH, Mathias CJ, Frankel HJ, Neill E (1977) The central hypotensive effect of clonidine:

Studies in tetraplegic subjects. Clin Pharmacol Ther 21: 375–381

5. Kobinger W, Walland A (1967) Investigation into the mechanism of hypotensive effect of 2-(2,6-dichlorophenylamino)-2-imidazoline HCl. Eur J Pharmacol 2: 155–162

6. Schmitt H, Schmitt H (1969) Localization of the hypotensive effect of 2-(2-6-dichlorophenylamino)-2-imidazoline hydrochloride. Eur J Pharmacol 6: 8–12

7. Schmitt H, Schmitt H, Fenard S (1973) Action of α adrenergic blocking drugs on the sympathetic centres and their interactions with the central sympathoinhibitory effect of clonidine. Arzneim Forsch 23: 40–45

8. Starke K, Endo T, Taube HD (1975) Relative pre- and postsynaptic potencies of alpha adrenoceptor agonists in rabbit pulmonary artery. Naunyn Schmiedebergs Arch Pharmacol 291: 55–78

9. Langer SZ (1977) Presynaptic receptors and their role in the regulation of transmitter release. Br J Pharmacol 60: 481–498

10. Doxey JC (1977) Pre and postsynaptic effect of alpha agonists in the anococcygeus muscle of the pithed rat. Eur J Pharmacol 54: 185–189

11. Berthelsen S, Pettinger WA (1977) A functional basis for classification of α adrenergic receptors. Life Sci 21: 595–606

12. Grant JA, Scrutton MC (1979) Novel alpha₂ adrenoceptors primarily responsible for inducing human platelet aggregation. Nature 277: 659–661

13. Drew GM, Whiting SB (1979) Evidence for two distinct types of postsynaptic alpha adrenoceptor in vascular smooth muscle in vivo. Br J Pharmacol 67: 207–215

14. Docherty JR, McDonald A, McGrath JC (1979) Further subclassification of alpha adrenoceptors in the cardiovascular system, vas deferens and anococcygeus of the rat. Br J Pharmacol 67: 421–422P

15. Timmermans PB, Kwa HY, van Zwieten PA (1979) Possible subdivisions of post synaptic alpha receptors mediating pressor responses in the pithed rat. Naunyn Schmiedebergs Arch Pharmacol 310: 189–193

16. Hamilton CA, Reid JL (in press) A post synaptic location of α₂ adrenoceptors in vascular smooth muscle. Br J Pharmacol

17. U'Pritchard D, Snyder S (1979) Distinct alpha noradrenergic receptors differentiated by binding and physiological relationships. Life Sci 24: 79–88

18. Mathias CJ, Reid JL, Wing LMH, Frankel HL, Christensen NJ (1979) Antihypertensive effects of clonidine in tetraplegic subjects devoid of central sympathetic control. Clin Sci 57 (5): 4425–428

19. Hökfelt T, Fuxe K, Goldstein M, Johannson O (1974) Immunological evidence for the existence of adrenaline neurons in the rat brain. Brain Res 66: 235–251

20. Saavedra JA, Grobecker H, Axelrod J (1976) Adrenaline forming enzyme in brain stem: Elevation in genetic and experimental hypertension. Science 191: 483–484

21. Petty MA, Reid JL (1979) Catecholamine synthesizing enzyme in brain stem and hypothalamus during the development of renovascular hypertension. Brain Res 163: 277–288

22. Bolme P, Corrodi H, Fuxe K. Hökfelt T, Lindbrink P, Goldstein M (1974) Possible involvement of central adrenaline neurons in vasomotor and respiratory control. Eur J Pharmacol 28: 89–94

23. Dollery CT, Reid JL (1973) Central noradrenergic neurones and the cardiovascular actions of clonidine in the rabbit. Br J Pharmacol 47: 206–216

DISCUSSION

Dr. Cowley (Milwaukee, Wis.): I would like to make one brief comment. I continue to play the devil's advocate. This is directed more to Dr. Reis than other members of the panel. I question whether chronic denervation, either central denervation by NTS lesions or peripheral synoaortic denervation of the baroreceptors, results in a chronic sustained level of hypertension. I think it is still an appropriate question whether in fact this is a good model of hypertension, and I say this for the same reason I have said it in the past. Those of us who have looked at continuous 24-h mean arterial pressure (i.e., monitored pressures 24-h/day) and averaged up all these highs and lows come out with normal pressures. This has been done both in the dog model [Cowley AW Jr, Laird J-F, Guyton AC (1973) Circ Res 32: 564–576] and in the rat model now. Dr. R. Norman reported on the latter at the New Orleans meeting last week using the baroreceptor-denervated rat model. People who have not done 24-h recordings, including our own laboratory, will find elevated levels of pressure. I think that it's appropriate that if we are going to use the procedures that you describe for a model of chronic sustained hypertension that we at least do 24-h monitoring to establish whether it is indeed a true model of chronic hypertension.

Dr. Reis (New York): Cats with NTS lesions have, as Dr. M.A. Nathan and I demonstrated, an elevated arterial pressure during the night as well as during the day. However, the pressure is less labile. Drs. Carey in Virginia, Schmitt and Laubie in Paris, and Ferrario in Cleveland have all shown that in dog, NTS lesions can lead to chronic hypertension. Schmitt and Laubie in fact observed that the elevation is persistent, and after 3 or 4 months, dogs develop cardiovascular pathology. Another point relates to the fact that in human hypertensives, blood pressure is often at normal levels in sleep, and, hence, conceivably in borderline hypertensives, the pressure might not be elevated over 24 h, although they still have the disease. Thus, a 24-h-sustained elevation of blood pressure is not a valid criteria for drawing similarities between NTS hypertension in animals and the human disease.

Dr. Hollenberg (Boston, Mass.): The question for Dr. Ferrario deals with a rather confusing literature on dietary sodium and catecholamine handling. Lewis Landsburg has recently demonstrated that reduced caloric intake *per se* will sharply increase catecholamine turnover. In our laboratory, it has been very difficult to reduce sodium intake in animals and have them continue to eat. They will either reduce their intake or stop eating. Dr. Ferrario, your dogs weighed 17 kg and lost 2 kg, and I wonder if you would comment on the specificity of your observations. Is it really sodium?

Dr. Ferrario (Cleveland, Oh.): We have performed these studies for over 2 years. Our animals are subjected to a dietary sodium intake of 4 mEq/day and given furosemide in a dose of 40 mg on the 19th, 20th, and 21st day of the diet. Under those conditions, we get a very clear-cut and specific response. Of course, there are always variations, and some animals do fail to increase plasma renin activity or show hemoconcentration. When the criteria that I showed in my figure holds true, then all of these animals have the patterns as shown in the experiments. Moreover, their caloric intake is not reduced with respect to the control animals. They all eat the same amount.

Dr. Lumbers (Sydney, Australia): I just wanted to ask Dr. Ferrario a small point. I wondered if he considered that the high-circulating levels of angiotensin II could be responsible for the decreased sensitivity of the baroreflex that he showed? We have shown that the cardiac baroreflex is altered by high circulating levels of Angiotensin II (see Session 17). We get a decrease in cardiac baroreflex sensitivity. Clough et al. have shown that in the sodium-depleted dog administration of converting enzyme intravenously causes a shift in the position of the baroreflex curve. How-

ever, they could not show any enhancement or shift in the cardiac baroreflex with centrally administered converting enzyme inhibitor [Clough DP, Conway J, Hatton R, Scott KL (1979) J Physiol 295: 75–76].

Dr. Ferrario: Yes, I am very familiar with that work, having recently discussed it with Dr. Clough. First, I would like to say that we have repeated the baroreceptor reflex study in animals in which the high levels of circulating angiotensin II were blocked during the infusion of an angiotensin antagonist, and the response in sodium-depleted animals continued to be blunted. In regard to the apparent discrepancy between Dr. Clough's studies and ours, it is probably related to the fact that they used nitroglycerin and phenylephrine to determine the baroreceptor sensitivity curve. These two agents may not affect the activity of the vagal afferents in the same manner as the angiotensin or the converting enzyme inhibitors. We have shown previously that a part of the blunting of the barorecptor reflexes in sodium-depleted animals is due to an overactivity of vagal afferents. Thus, the effect of either agent on central venous pressure has to be taken into account when studying the baroreflex curve in relation to vagal afferents.

Dr. Meyer (Paris, France): I have a question for Dr. Reid. I fully agree with your conclusions brought about by beautiful experiments. However, I would like to get from you the explanation of the selectivity of the two postsynaptic receptor sites—alpha$_1$ and alpha$_2$—supposing that both are postsynaptic. I do not understand on which basis one would interact with neurogenic norepinephrine, while the other would do so with circulating norepinephrine.

Dr. J. Reid (Glasgow, Scotland): This suggestion comes from studies in pithed cats and rats in which the antagonism by selective alpha$_1$- and alpha$_2$-blockers was examined on the pressor responses to either nerve stimulation or pressor amine infusion. However, this point has not yet been finally established, and limited *in vitro* work would suggest that alpha$_2$-receptors that predominate in veins may be innervated.

Session 12
Hypertension Mechanisms in Experimental Animals and Their Relevance to Humans

Chairman: F. O. Simpson

Position Paper: Hypertension Mechanisms in Experimental Animals and Their Relevance to Humans

Louis Tobian

Sodium intake and Na balance play an important role in human essential hypertension. The evidence for this comes from various directions. Diets very low in Na content can lower the blood pressure of hypertension subjects (1). Such diets slightly reduce body Na. Thiazides, acting as natriuretic agents, also lower blood pressure, probably through the same mechanism. Such drugs also slightly reduce body Na. Moreover, a high-salt intake of 20 g daily can drown out the antihypertensive effect of these diuretic agents (2).

People living in remote areas all over the world often have a lifelong low intake of Na (less than 60 mEq/day) and completely avoid hypertension while on this low-Na regimen. A certain percentage of them would be susceptible to hypertension if they lived in the United States or Europe (3–10). In these population groups, the old men have the same level of blood pressure as the young men and so do not show the usual age-related rise in blood pressure seen in every highly acculturated society. A few primitive groups, one in the Solomon Islands, another in Iran, either cook their food in sea water (8) or eat salty foods and get their share of hypertension, even though they live in a low state of acculturation and are devoid of obesity. Samburu warriors are normotensive as they eat a low-Na diet on their farms, but a certain fraction become hypertensive when they are drafted into the army of Kenya and begin eating army rations containing 18 g NaCl daily (6).

The eating of less than 60 mEq Na/day is not an outlandish diet when one considers that this level of salt intake was part of the standard human diet for 3 million years up to around 1,000 years ago. The human race actually evolved on this low level of salt intake.

Very high intakes of Na as seen in the Akita prefecture of Japan (as high as 25–35 g NaCl/day) are associated with very high average blood pressures. In one report, 84% of adult males in this region had a systolic pressure above 140 mmHg, and the most common cause of death was stroke (11). This suggests that a very high-salt intake will increase the blood pressure in man.

Onesti found that feeding 300 mEq salt (NaCl) daily to the normotensive teenage children of hypertensive parents would produce a definite rise in blood pressure. A similar diet given to normotensive teenage children of normotensive parents produced no rise in blood pressure at all (G. Onesti, unpublished observation). The studies at Iowa revealed the same pattern: A daily 410 mEq NaCl diet raised the blood pressure in borderline hypertensives and caused no rise in blood pressure at all in normotensives (12, 13). Murray et al. (14) at Indiana found that 1,200 mEq NaCl daily will raise blood pressure even in normotensive subjects. Onesti et al. (15) also found that increasing body Na in dialysis patients raises blood pressure, usually by increasing peripheral vascular resistance. The Indiana group also noted that the normotensive children of hypertensive parents had a significantly delayed urinary excretion of a Na load (16). This sluggishness of natriuresis may partially explain why such children have a rise in blood pressure while eating 300 mEq salt/day.

ORIGINS OF HYPERTENSIVE STRAINS OF ANIMALS

Lewis Dahl et al. (17) were aware of many of these findings and sought to imitate them experimentally. They were aware that Meneely et al. (18) had fed diets containing 7%–10% NaCl to Sprague-Dawley rats, which brought on hypertension after several months of feeding. Dahl challenged rats with an 8%-NaCl diet and found which ones would have a rise in blood pressure and which ones would not. By selective breeding, he produced two strains of rats. One group, the "S" strain, was very sensitive to NaCl-induced hypertension and would get severely hypertensive when fed a diet with 8% NaCl. The other group, the "R" strain, is very resistant to NaCl hypertension and will usually have no rise in blood pressure whatsoever, when fed the same 8%-NaCl diet. However, when the two groups are on a low- (0.3%) NaCl diet, both groups have a blood pressure within the normal range.

GENETIC FACTORS

Having created these two strains of rats, Dahl came out with a working hypothesis to account for their characteristics, as well as those of human subjects. In formulating a hypothesis, one had to take into account that some people can eat 300 mEq NaCl/day and not become hypertensive, while others genetically susceptible to hypertension can eat 50 mEq/day and also not become hypertensive. Of course, if these same susceptible people eat 300 mEq/day, they will definitely become hypertensive. He felt that rats as well as humans could be divided into those genetically susceptible and those genetically resistant to hypertension. As long as both groups eat a low-Na diet, neither will become hypertensive. However, when both groups eat a high-Na diet, the susceptible group becomes hypertensive, while the resistant group remains normotensive. This working hypothesis can indeed account for much of what seems to occur in both humans and rats. So, as far as it goes, it is a satisfactory working hypothesis. Iwai et al. (19) found that the susceptible or "S" strain was also more susceptible to most other types of experimental hypertension, including two-kidney, one-clip Goldblatt hypertension and desoxycorticosterone hypertension. However, the "S" rat was equal to the "R" rat in susceptibility to one-kidney, one-clip Goldblatt hypertension. Iwai et al. (20) found that the "S" rat had relatively low-plasma renin activity on high- or low-NaCl diets. Thus, the hypertension in the "S" rat is a relatively low-renin hypertension. Ben-Ishay et al. (21) found that glomerular filtration rate (GFR) and renal blood flow were normal in the "S" rat on either high- or low-Na diets.

HUMORAL FACTORS

In parabiotic experiments, Dahl et al. (22) found evidence for a humoral factor produced by the kidney of the "S" rat which could travel into the body of the "R" rat and make it hypertensive. There were three main pieces of evidence supporting the presence of the humoral factor. First, when "S" and "R" rats were joined parabiotically, and both rats were fed a high-NaCl diet, the "R" rat became more hypertensive than the "S" rat during the first 12 weeks of salt feeding (22). This could be explained by a pressor substance passing from the "S" to "R" rat, but it could also be explained by higher volumes in the "R" rat as Floyer found when a similar type of experiment was done with one Goldblatt rat and one normal rat as parabiotic partners.

Second, when a one-kidney, one-clip Goldblatt "S" rat was joined to an "R" rat, it raised the blood pressure in the "R" rat. Conversely, when a one-kidney, one-clip Goldblatt "R" rat was joined to an "S" rat, it raised the pressure of the "S" rat very very little (19). As mentioned above, when the one-kidney, one-clip Goldblatt procedure was done on single, unjoined "S" and "R" rats, they developed hypertension to an equal degree. This gave evidence, according to Dahl, that the clipped "S" kidney put out two hormones, while the clipped "R" kidney put out only one. The extra hormone put out by the clipped "S" kidney could cross the parabiotic junction and raise the blood pressure of an "R" rat. However, it seemed to require the Goldblatt clipping procedure to bring forth this hormone from the "S" kidney.

The third experiment of Knudsen et al. (23) involved the parabiotic connection of rats with two kidneys to rats with no kidneys. When the pairs were on a very low-Na diet, an "S" rat with kidneys could somewhat raise the blood pressure of its "R" partner without kidneys. Conversely, an "R" rat with kidneys, could not raise the blood pressure of a parabiotic "S" rat without kidneys. This was further evidence of a pressor hormone coming only from "S" kidneys. Furthermore, when these pairs were on a higher salt diet, renoprival hypertension could only occur in an "S" rat without kidneys, but this hypertension was not transmitted to its parabiotic "R" partner with kidneys. This finding again pointed to the kidney as the source of the hypertensinogenic hormone (23).

It has also been shown that the "R" rat has special proteins in a pituitary cleft, while an "S" rat does not have such proteins. The "S" rat has been shown to make extra amounts of 18-hydroxy-desoxycorticosterone and slightly lesser amounts of corticosterone. However, in back–cross genetic experiments, this particular adrenal factor could amount for only one-eighth of the hypertension in the NaCl-fed "S" rat.

PATHOGENETIC MECHANISMS OF NaCl INDUCED HYPERTENSION

If we accept that relatively large NaCl intakes can increase blood pressure in genetically susceptible subjects, we are still not absolutely certain about the pathogenetic mechanism. Considering the many research observations, it seems likely that there are at least two links in the chain of causation of NaCl-induced hypertension. The first link would involve a transient accumulation of excess Na in the body; the second link is that an excess of body Na would lead to a rise in blood pressure. Both links need to be operative in order for NaCl-induced hypertension to occur.

To consider further the first link, the fact that susceptible humans and susceptible Dahl "S" rats remain normotensive if they are on a lifelong low-salt diet, provides evidence that at least a transient excess of body Na is necessary for NaCl-induced hypertension. Rats, pigs, and dogs given excess mineralocorticoid will also not develop a shred of hypertension if they consume a very low-Na diet. It is the one certain way to prevent mineralo-corticoid hypertension. Given the necessity for at least a transient excess of body Na, we still know that some humans and some rats can eat large amounts of salt and remain normotensive, while others on the same diet develop hypertension. One obvious hypothesis to account for the difference would be the existence of a delayed or sluggish excretion of Na in those genetically susceptible to hypertension. However, human hypertensives do not have an excess Na content in the body as a whole, though they do have an increased content of Na in the arterial walls (24). Similarly, Dahl "S" rats do not have excessive body Na levels

either on high- or low-Na diets. Moreover, when humans or rats with established hypertension are challenged with a Na load, they excrete the Na very expeditiously, actually a bit faster than the normotensive controls. Thus, they appear to have no problem in handling a Na challenge. However, there is one large consideration that perhaps makes this superficial conclusion invalid. The hypertensive kidney is perfused at an elevated pressure, while the normotensive kidney is perfused at a normal pressure. Selkurt (25) clearly showed in 1951 that high perfusion pressure in the renal artery greatly facilitates the urinary excretion of Na and urine volume. Thus, the intrinsic ability of kidneys to excrete Na cannot be validly compared when one kidney is perfused at high pressure and the other at normal pressure. To get at this perplexing question, we utilized isolated, blood-perfused kidneys from the two contrasting strains of Dahl rats, which are good models for human hypertension and normotension (26). Both strains had been eating a low-Na diet and, hence, had blood pressures within the normal range.

Figure 1 gives the urinary Na excretion/100 g isolated kidney/min at various inflow pressures. The top line shows the mean values of isolated kidneys from 23 hypertension-resistant "R" rats. As expected, the Na output markedly increases with each increment of inflow pressure. The bottom line gives the average values of isolated kidneys from 29 hypertension-prone "S" rats. These kidneys also show the pressure–natriuresis phenomenon with more Na excreted for each increment of inflow pressure. However, it is obvious that there is a striking difference between "S" and "R" kidneys. For instance, at a normotensive inflow pressure of 130 mmHg, the "R" kidneys excreted a mean of 146 μEq Na/min/100 g kidney, whereas at the same pressure the "S" kidneys averaged only 70 μEq. Thus, at 130-mmHg inflow pressure, the "S" kidneys from hypertension-prone rats excreted 52% less Na than comparable "R" kidneys. This difference was significant, with a p value less than 0.005. At 160-mmHg infusion pressure, we see the same phenomenon: The "R" kidneys averaged 416 μEq Na excretion, whereas the "S" kidneys averaged only 221. This is a 47% reduction of Na excretion in "S" kidneys, with a p value less than 0.001. At 100-mmHg inflow pressure, we see the same pattern, with the "R" kidneys excreting 30 μEq/min, while the "S" kidneys

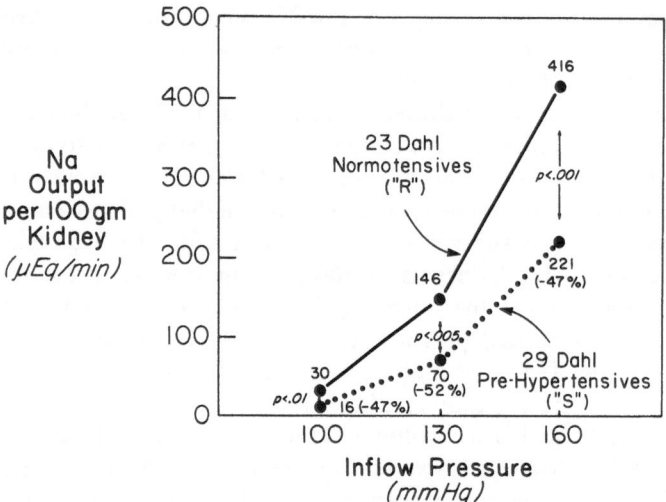

Fig. 1. Sodium excretion of isolated kidneys from "S" and "R" rats at varying inflow pressures. The distance between the large black dot (the mean value) and the tip of the arrowhead represents the standard error of the mean.

are excreting only 16. Hence, at 100-mmHg inflow pressure, the "S" kidneys excreted 47% less Na than the "R" kidneys, with a p value less than 0.01. When compared on an equal pressure basis, the "S" kidneys seem to have a very pronounced natriuretic handicap at all three inflow pressures. However, raising the inflow pressure can completely overcome this natriuretic handicap. For instance, the "S" kidneys perfused at 160 mmHg excrete about 50% more Na/min than the normotensive "R" kidneys perfused at a normal 130 mmHg.

One can consider that the pressure–natriuresis curve of the "S" rat has been shifted to the right. This amounts to a "resetting" of the curve so that

it takes a greater level of inflow pressure to bring about a given rate of natriuresis.

Figure 2 shows the urine flow rate at the various inflow pressures, expressed as mg urine/min/ 10 g kidney. Again, the differences were highly significant. At 130-mmHg inflow pressure, the "R" kidneys excreted 154 mg, while the "S" kidneys excreted only 84, a 45% reduction in flow rate in "S" kidneys. At 160-mmHg inflow pressure, the "R" kidneys averaged 303 mg urine/min, while the "S" kidneys averaged only 179, a 41% reduction in urine volume. At 100-mmHg inflow pressure, the "R" kidneys averaged 40 mg/min, while the "S" kidneys averaged 22, the "S" kidneys excreting 44% less urine volume. Here again, the

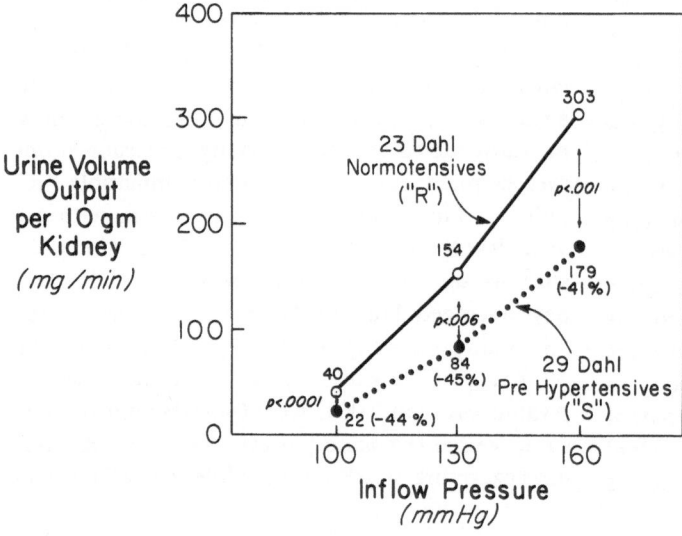

Fig. 2. Urinary volume output of isolated kidneys from "S" and "R" rats at varying inflow pressures. The distance between the large black dot (the mean value) and the tip of the arrowhead represents the standard error of the mean.

diuretic handicap of "S" kidneys can be completely overcome by increasing the inflow pressure. For instance, "S" kidneys perfused at 160 mmHg put out 16% more urine volume than "R" kidneys perfused at the normal 130 mmHg.

At a normal inflow pressure, the blood flow and GFR of the "S" and "R" rats were not significantly different. These studies indicate that the isolated kidneys from "S" rats excrete only half as much Na as kidneys from "R" rats, when the two contrasting strains are compared at equal levels of inflow pressure. Thus, the hypertension-prone "S" strain appears to have a resetting of the pressure–natriuresis curve, in that a higher inflow pressure is required to achieve a given Na excretion. This occurs even though the "S" kidney has no pathologic lesions. In either strain on a very low-Na intake, there would be virtually no tendency for Na retention and, hence, little stimulus for a rise in blood pressure beyond the normal range. However, when the "S" rats begin a high-Na intake, the resetting of the pressure–natriuresis curve could then conceivably become an important factor. If the relative rates of natriuresis of isolated "S" and "R" kidneys occurred in the intact rat during a high-Na intake, the "S" rat would tend to retain more Na than the "R" rat, and would tend to come into Na balance with an elevated body Na and extracellular volume. Such high-body Na and extracellular volumes frequently bring on a rise in blood pressure, as is commonly seen in hypertensions in renal parenchymal disease, mineralocorticoid excess, and in dialysis patients. If the arterial pressure did rise into the hypertensive range, the "S" kidney would then increase its rate of Na excretion through the mechanism of a pressure–natriuresis, and its natriuretic handicap would be overcome. With the raised arterial pressure, the kidney could then excrete Na rapidly enough to permit attainment of Na balance at a normal extracellular volume. The natriuretic handicap would then seem to disappear and renal excretory function would appear to be normal. Assuming such a resetting of the pressure–natriuresis curve for the intact, in vivo "S" kidney, the "S" rat would tend to become hypertensive when on a high-Na intake, which would in turn produce a pressure–natriuresis that would bring to normal its body Na content. If the accumulation of body Na did not induce the pressor response, as was observed in some of Onesti's patients, then Na balance would occur with a somewhat elevated level of body Na and a normal blood pressure. This would be a relatively unusual physiologic response.

The experiments of Iwai et al. (27) provide some evidence that there may, indeed, be an in vivo difference in pressure–natriuresis curves between "S" and "R" rats. When these two contrasting strains were fed in high-NaCl intake, the feeding of chlorothiazide significantly increased urinary Na excretion in "S" rats, but had no effect on Na excretion in "R" rats. Moreover, when the chlorothiazide was discontinued after some weeks, the Na excretion significantly dropped in "S" rats, while rising slightly in "R" rats. The findings could be interpreted as indicating that the "R" kidneys have a pressure–natriuresis curve favoring very rapid natriuresis at relatively low inflow pressures, such that adding chlorothiazide will not make an already rapid natriuretic capacity even more rapid. On the other hand, if there existed an in vivo resetting of the pressure–natriuresis curve in "S" rats favoring a slower rate of natriuresis, then adding chlorothiazide might have the effect of shifting the natriuresis curve of the "S" kidney to the left, thereby making Na excretion more rapid. The contrasting effect of thiazide on Na excretion in these two strains could be accounted for by this mechanism.

This formulation could conceivably account for much of the exquisite sensitivity to NaCl-induced hypertension in the Dahl "S" rat. It is pertinent to wonder whether the kidneys of patients with essential hypertension might also have a resetting of the pressure–natriuresis curve in favor of hypertension. Future studies will be needed to answer this question.

ACTION OF DIURETIC DRUGS

The hypothesis that an intrinsic shift in the pressure–natriuresis curve can lead to rat hypertension, or even human hypertension, certainly fits well with the action of diuretic drugs in reducing hypertensive pressure levels. Many diuretic agents are extremely effective in man in reducing high blood pressure. The same is true for the Dahl "S" rat. This would make physiologic sense. If a diuretic agent were given to an "S" rat, it would facilitate natriuresis and would tend to overcome the intrinsic defect in natriuresis that these rats have. In the presence of daily diuretic therapy, the body Na level would come into balance at a slightly lower than normal level. This should remove the previous Na stimulus leading to elevated pressure levels, and blood pressure should begin to drift toward normal levels. In the presence of a diuretic, an elevated pressure level would no longer be needed in "S" rats to facilitate natriuresis. Such a mechanism could explain the powerful antihypertensive action of diuretic agents.

In order to investigate the validity of this working hypothesis, we did a study in Dahl rats utilizing a thiazide diuretic, methyclothiazide (Fig. 3) (28). "S" and "R" rats weighing about 80 g were fed a diet containing 0.3% NaCl. Half of the rats in each strain were given the thiazide diuretic. Blood pressures were taken without anesthesia every week. The blood pressure of all four groups remained about the same until the tenth week of study. If the "S" rat tends to retain Na and becomes hypertensive on an 8.0%NaCl diet because of the shift in its pressure–natriuresis curve, then a thiazide diuretic should be able to prevent the Na retention, and the rise in blood pressure whould be averted. Where you see the vertical line in Fig. 3, all the rats began eating the 8.0%-NaCl diet, while half of them remained on thiazide.

As indicated in Fig. 3, the "R" rats, either on or off thiazide, had no tendency for a rise in blood pressure while taking the high-salt diet. Their blood pressures averaged 135 mmHg, after 9 weeks on the high-salt diet. On the other hand, the "S" rats not protected by the thiazide diuretic immediately began a stepwise week-by-week increase in blood pressure when they began eating the 8.0%-NaCl diet. Their average blood pressure had risen to 210 mmHg by the eighth week of the high-salt diet. In striking contrast to this rise, one notes that the "S" rats which were protected by the thiazide diuretic had virtually no rise in blood pressure when they commenced eating the high-salt diet. Their blood pressure line moves along parallel with that of the "R" rats and only about 5 mmHg above it. After 9 weeks of the high-salt diet, their blood pressures averaged 140 mmHg. Thus, treatment with the thiazide diuretic almost completely prevented the NaCl hypertension in the "S" rat. Apparently, the action of the thiazide to facilitate Na excretion overcomes the reduced rate of Na excretion in "S" kidneys and thereby prevents the tendency for an initial accumulation of body Na. Thus, there would be no Na stimulus for a rise in blood pressure, and pressure would remain at normal levels. Ordinary thiazide diuretics, including the methyclothiazide used here, do not have any direct action on arterioles and venules. Their action is mainly on the distal nephron to enhance Na excretion. The fact that they were effective in preventing NaCl-induced hypertension fits in with the hypothesis that a shift in the pressure–natriuresis curve in vivo is at least partially respon-

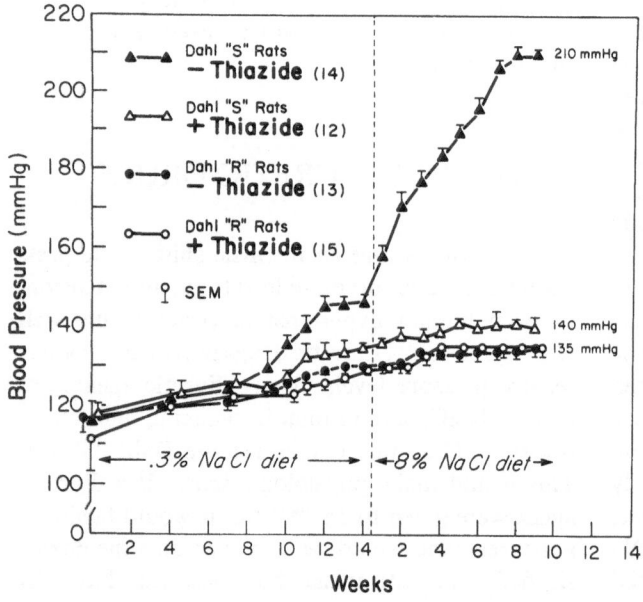

Fig. 3. Blood pressures of Dahl "S" and "R" rats as influenced by high and low levels of Na in the diet and by treatment with a thiazide diuretic agent.

sible for the great susceptibility to NaCl hypertension in the "S" rat. Moreover, since thiazide diuretics are such effective antihypertensive agents in humans, one might ask whether some type of aberration of natriuresis might not also be present in the kidneys of those with essential hypertension.

The shift of the pressure–natriuresis curve in the "S" rat could have several possible explanations. For instance, there is a 25%–32% reduction of plasma flow to the renal papilla of the "S" rat at any level of Na in the diet (29). This limitation of flow to the renal papilla might partially contribute to the reduced natriuresis, since any sizable Na challenge is always accompanied by a marked increase in papillary plasma flow. There is also the possibility that a humoral antinatriuretic agent could be contributing to the shift of the pressure–natriuresis curve in the "S" rat. Such a compound was searched for by allowing either "S" or "R" rats to perfuse normal isolated kidneys from normotensive Sprague-Dawley rats (28). There were 26 such perfusions utilizing "R" rats and 24 utilizing "S" rats. All these perfusing rats had been on a low-Na diet and, hence, had a blood pressure within the normal range. Moreover, the last kidney and adrenal had been removed from the perfusing rat 1 h before the perfusion to eliminate these organs as a source of a hormone. The isolated kidney had also been rendered strongly alpha-blocked with phenoxybenzamine to rule out alpha-adrenergic effects. In the 26 perfusions by "R" rats, Na excretion of the isolated kidneys averaged 164 μEq/min/100 g kidney. In the 24 perfusions by "S" rats, Na excretion averaged 84 μEq/min/100 g kidney. Since the isolated kidney was perfused at a constant pressure of 125 mmHg in these experiments, and since the hematocrits and colloid osmotic pressure in these perfusions were similar in "S" and "R" rats, one can conclude that the antinatriuretic result of perfusions with blood from "S" rats was caused by some circulating humoral effect. Additional perfusions were done utilizing normal Sprague-Dawley rats, and the hormonal effect on Na excretion of these rats resembled that of the "R" rats. Hence, it appears likely that there is either a circulating antinatriuretic humoral agent, or the lack of a circulating natriuretic agent, in the blood of "S" rats. When "S" blood circulates through these bioassay kidneys, it causes a 16% increase in renovascular resistance, relative to perfusions by "R" blood. It also causes a decrease in GFR of about the same magnitude. Both of these hemodynamic effects would be expected to increase the antinatriuretic effect of perfusions with "S" blood. However, when the four "S" perfusions with the highest renovascular resistance and the lowest GFR and the four "R" perfusions with the lowest renovascular resistance and the highest GFR were taken out of the comparison between these groups, the remaining rats had an equal level of renovascular resistance and GFR. The natriuresis of these selected kidneys could then be compared, with the hemodynamic factors apparently not playing a part. When this was done, it was still apparent that there was a humoral effect in "S" blood, which reduced Na excretion in the bioassay kidney by roughly 50%. Thus, there are circulating effects in the blood of "S" rats that independently cause a reduction in natriuresis as well as some renal vasoconstriction and some reduction of GFR. These various effects could easily contribute to the shift in the pressure–natriuresis curve of the "S" rat.

ADDITIONAL STUDIES

In further attempts to understand the NaCl-induced hypertension of Dahl "S" rats, we measured plasma flow to the renal papilla of Dahl "S" and "R" rats, as mentioned above, and found that it was about 25%–32% slower in "S" compared to "R" rats. This reduction in plasma flow to the renal papilla occurred at a time when the plasma flow to the kidney as a whole was not different between the "S" and "R" rats. Thus, we had a situation in which the vascular resistance in the kidney as a whole is somewhat elevated in the hypertensive "S" rat, but is disproportionately elevated to a still greater degree in the vessels supplying the renal papilla. Even when the blood pressure of the "S" rat on a low-sodium diet is within the normal range, one still finds a disproportionate increase in resistance to flow in the vessels supplying the papilla. This would suggest that these vessels in the "S" rat are especially sensitive to the hypertension process and show an increased resistance beyond that seen in most peripheral arterioles throughout the body. We also found that when almost any type of rat, an "S" or "R" or a Sprague-Dawley rat, begins eating a high-Na intake for a period of 5–7 days, there is a sharp increase in the plasma flow to the renal papilla.

It went up as much as 45% after 5 days of high-salt feeding in "R" rats. This increase in plasma flow to the renal papilla seems to be an integral part of the body's response to the challenge of a high-salt intake. Since the "S" rat seems to be unable to increase its flow to the renal papilla as much as the "R" rat, it would be unable to bring forth the maximum flow to the renal papilla in the face of a high-salt challenge, and this might somewhat limit its capacity for a brisk natriuresis. As mentioned above, such a limitation of natriuresis could encourage hypertension during a high-NaCl intake.

RELATIONSHIPS TO PROSTAGLADIN CONCENTRATION

The reduction in papillary flow in "S" rats is in striking parallel with changes in prostaglandin E_2 (PGE_2) concentration in quick-frozen renal papillas of "S" rats (30). Two principal findings emerged. First, the "S" rat, which is genetically susceptible to salt hypertension, had much lower PGE_2 levels than the "R" rat, which is resistant to salt hypertension. When both strains were normotensive in a low-salt diet, the PGE_2 in the "S" rat was 60% lower than that in the "R" rat. After either 4 or 11 weeks of a high-salt intake, with "S" rats hypertensive and "R" rats normotensive, the PGE_2 in the "S" papillas was half that in "R" papillas. All these differences were statistically significant.

The second main finding indicated that rats on the 4% high-salt diet for either 4 or 11 weeks, had about twice the papillary PGE_2 concentration as did control rats on the low-salt diet. This happened in both "S" and "R" rats, and the differences were significant. However, when the "S" rat more than doubled its papillary PGE_2 while on a high-salt diet, it s PGE_2 still rose up only to the level found in the "R" rat on a low-salt diet. Thus, on any of the diets, the "S" rat is always only half as high as the "R" rat in regard to PGE_2 level.

For several reasons, one can consider that the low papillary PGE_2 in "S" rats contributes to their inability to excrete Na rapidly. When either strain has a high-salt intake, the papillary PGE_2 doubles in concentraion. This would appear to be one of the many physiologic responses that permit the animal to meet the high-Na challenge. However, the "S" rat is unable to bring about the full rise in PGE_2 level. Lacking this, the capacity for rapid Na excretion may be compromised. Along this same line, Ferris has produced a low PGE_2 state in the rat kidney by reducing essential fatty acids in the diet. These rats have a diminished capacity to excrete a Na load and develop hypertension when fed a high-salt diet. (This material was presented at the annual meeting Council for High Blood Pressure Research, Cleveland Ohio, October, 1980.)

In Dahl rats, one notes a precise parallel between changes in papillary flow and changes in PGE_2 concentration. "S" rats have abnormally low flows and abnormally low PGE_2 concentrations at all levels of salt intake. A high intake of salt increases papillary flow and also increases papillary PGE_2. It may well be that PGE_2 is not a clear-cut vasodilator in the whole rat kidney, but our group and others have firm evidence that PGE_2 is a definite vasodilator for the circulation to the papilla. The low papillary flow in "S" rats is probably at least partially due to low PGE_2 levels. The high papillary flow after a high-salt diet is probably partially due to a high PGE_2 level.

Thus, the "S" rat has much less PGE_2 in the papilla, which may well contribute to its sluggish excretion of Na and its low papillary plasma flow. In either type of rat, a high-salt diet will double papillary PGE_2, but the "S" rat is always much lower than the "R" rat. This increase in PGE_2 may be part of the mechanism that increases urinary Na to match increased dietary Na. The "S" rat does not have this full increase of papillary PGE_2, which may limit its capacity for rapid Na excretion and thereby make it susceptible to salt hypertension.

The tendency to reduced natriuresis in the "S" rat may be also present in humans genetically susceptible to hypertension. As mentioned above, a study from Indiana found that normotensive children of hypertensive parents had an abnormally slow natriuresis after the challenge of a Na load (16). Black subjects, whose hypertension is often very responsive to diuretic therapy, have also demonstrated a relatively sluggish rate of natriuresis.

SODIUM AND ARTERIAL BLOOD PRESSURE

Now I will discuss the second link in the chain of causation: that an initial accumulation of body

Na leads to a rise in arterial pressure. We have clinical evidence for this second link in the chain. Subjects with disease of the renal parenchyma tend to retain Na as they come into Na balance, and they often develop hypertension. Patients with an adenoma that puts out too much aldosterone tend to retain Na, and they frequently become hypertensive. When dialysis patients retain Na, they usually become hypertensive. Onesti et al. (15) purposefully raised the level of body Na in the course of dialysis treatment and most subjects had a rise in pressure. When body Na was brought down to normal, blood pressure returned to normal. In these studies, when an increase in body Na raised blood pressure, in 60% of cases the rise in pressure was entirely due to an increase in peripheral resistance with no hint of even a transient increase of cardiac output. In 20% of cases, the rise in pressure was entirely due to a rise in cardiac output with no hint of an increase in peripheral resistance to subserve a whole-body autoregulation. In the last 20% of cases, the rise in body Na resulted from both an increase in peripheral resistance and an increase in cardiac output. The diseased kidneys had been removed in many of these dialysis patients, so kidneys were not necessary in these Na-induced blood pressure rises. This pressor response was not an invariable one. In six normotensive subjects with end-stage renal disease, raising body Na did not raise blood pressure at all. This probably explains why they remained normotensive as their kidneys were gradually being destroyed. Thus, Na accumulation in the body does not invariably raise blood pressure. In order to get Na-induced hypertension, this pressor response to Na accumulation must be present. Approximately one-fourth of dialysis patients fail to get a rise in blood pressure after Na loading.

NEUROGENIC MECHANISMS

The actual mechanism by which excess Na in the body leads to a rise in blood pressure is still not thoroughly understood. However, within the last 2 years, some new information has appeared. It has been known for some time that high-Na intakes make the circulation extra sensitive to the pressor actions of intravenous norepinephrine and angiotensin II. Conversely, Na deficits have the opposite effect and make the circulation hyposensitive to the pressor action of these compounds. Moreover, Takeshita and Mark (31) induced hypertension in the Dahl "S" rat by feeding a high-

salt diet. In the rats that became hypertensive, there was an increased vascular resistance in the hindquarters. When they acutely cut the sympathetic nerves to these hindquarters, they abolished half of this increase in vascular resistance. This suggests that at least half of the hypertensive response from high-salt feeding was being mediated through the sympathetic nerves. They also gave baby "S" rats 6-hydroxydopamine peripherally to destroy the peripheral sympathetic nervous system. In such rats, they were unable to induce hypertension by feeding a high-salt diet. These observations tend to implicate the participation of the sympathetic nervous system in the hypertension induced by high-salt feeding. Ikeda et al. (32) also found a state of hypersensitivity in CNS pressor reflexes in Dahl "S" rats, even when they were in a completely normotensive state. When rats are lightly anesthetized with pentobarbitol, hypertonic saline (2 μl) injected into the lateral brain ventricle will regularly elicit a transient rise in blood pressure. An even greater rise in blood pressure occurs when 500 ng of angiotensin II are injected into the lateral brain ventricle. When Dahl "S" and "R" rats are both normotensive on a low-Na diet, the pressor responses to angiotensin II are twice as large in "S" rats compared to "R" rats. Using hypertonic saline, "S" rats again have twice as large a rise in blood pressure. Dahl showed that feeding an equimolar amount of KCl could completely prevent NaCl-induced hypertension in "S" rats. To understand this, we utilized the CNS pressor effects of angiotensin and hypertonic saline. In this study, we provided half of the "S" and "R" rats with a 2%-KCl solution as a drinking fluid (30). The control "S" and "R" rats continued to drink tap water. All "S" and "R" rats were eating a low-salt diet and were, therefore, normotensive. In this study, the CNS pressor response to angiotensin in rats on tap water was again 2.5 times greater in "S" than "R" rats. However, 6 weeks of the KCl drink had a profound effect on the CNS pressor response to angiotensin II in "S" rats, reducing it by 44% and bringing it down almost to the level seen in "R" rats. This difference was significant with a p value of 0.01. The KCl drink almost completely normalized the CNS pressor response to angiotensin in "S" rats.

The CNS pressor responses to hypertonic saline were also elicited. Again in rats drinking tap water, the CNS pressor responses in "S" rats were more than three times greater than in "R" rats. Again, the KCl drink reduced the CNS pressor response in "S" rats by 44%, bringing it much closer to the response of "R" rats. The p value was less than 0.01.

The CNS pressor responses are clearly hyperactive in "S" rats, even when they are normotensive while eating a low-salt diet. The KCl drink profoundly lowered these hyperactive CNS pressor responses in the "S" rats, bringing then down almost to the level seen in "R" rats. This marked blunting of hyperactive CNS pressor responses in the "S" rats may explain a good part of the antihypertensive action of KCl in NaCl hypertension. The precise mechanism by which a high-salt intake causes increased activity of the sympathetic nervous system is not well understood at the present time.

In the experiments of Takeshita and Mark (31), an acute denervation of the hindquarters in the hypertensive salt-fed "S" rat caused the increased vascular resistance in the hindquarters to be cut in half. However, the other half of the increased vascular resistance was not abolished by cutting the sympathetic nerves. This suggested the possibility of a humoral vasoconstrictor agent contributing to the increased vascular resistance in the hypertensive hindquarters. Tobian et al. (33) searched for such a humoral agent, using the isolated denervated hindquarters of a salt-fed "R" rat as a bioassay organ. The bioassay hindquarters were perfused for 30 min at a constant flow with blood coming from either salt-fed "S" rats ($N = 14$) or from salt-fed "R" rats ($N = 14$). The blood would be pumped through the bioassay hindquarters and then pumped back to the perfusing rats. This study revealed that there was, indeed, either a circulating vasoconstrictor agent or the absence of a vasodilator agent in the blood of hypertensive "S" rats that was not present in the blood of normotensive "R" rats. When the blood from the hypertensive "S" rat was pumped through the bioassay hindquarters, the mean-peripheral vascular resistance went up 16% higher than when the hindquarters were perfused with the blood from normotensive "R" rats. This was a significant difference with a p value of 0.02. This result indicates that in addition to the participation of the sympathetic nerves causing vasoconstriction in the peripheral vascular bed, there is also a circulating vasoconstrictor humoral effect in salt-fed hypertensive "S" rats that also contributes to the increased vasoconstriction. This humoral effect is not present in normotensive "S" rats on a low-

Na diet. Further studies are required to learn more of the source and identity of this humoral vasoconstrictor effect. However, this pressor effect is not likely to be due to renin or angiotensin II, since "S" rats are known to have a low-renin type of hypertension, and the renin was 39% lower in "S" perfusions than in "R" perfusions.

In these studies of the Dahl "S" rats as a model for NaCl-induced hypertension, we do see evidence for the two links in the chain of causality mentioned above. The "S" rat has a shift in the pressure–natriuresis curve, leading to a diminished natriuresis for any given level of inflow pressure. If this state of renal function is joined to a high-salt intake, there would be every reason to expect a transient increase in body Na level. There is also reason to believe that such an increase in body Na triggers an increase in peripheral vascular resistance without a reduction of cardiac output, which would, of course, bring on an increased level of blood pressure. The increased peripheral vascular resistance is contributed to both by the sympathetic nervous system and possibly by circulating humoral vasoconstrictor agents. Essential hypertension in man shares many common features with the salt-induced hypertension of the "S" rat. However, it is still quite uncertain whether the causes for increased peripheral resistance in the "S" rat are the same causes that are operating in a patient with essential hypertension. To gain answers to this question, much further work will obviously need to be done.

While these Na connections with hypertension exist, there are certain types of hypertension that are quite refractory to drastic reductions of dietary Na. For instance, in our hands, either one-kidney or two-kidney Goldblatt hypertension in the rat is very resistant to either low-Na diets (34) or thiazide diuretic agents (35). The hypertension rolls merrily along when either thiazides or a low-Na diet are offered. Body Na is decreased by these maneuvers, but renin rises as a compensatory response and blood pressure does not decrease to any significant degree.

CONTRIBUTION OF RENIN

The same remarkable resistance to body Na reduction is also found in the Kyoto SHR. Several investigators have given such rats a low-Na diet and blood pressure did not go down. I still remain skeptical about this; possibly the diet was not started early enough and the hypertensive process had already set in irreversibly. To settle the matter we used Kyoto SHR from our own colony. They were given a stiff dose of methyclothiazide in the drinking water just at the start of weaning at 3 weeks of age. They also ate a 0.3% low-NaCl diet. The rats so treated were every bit as hypertensive as control Kyoto SHR on regular chow and receiving no added thiazide. Thus, this form of hypertension in the rat is indeed resistant to reductions in body Na. This makes one suspect that the renin contribution is very significant in these rats. The fact that they are so very sensitive to the antihypertensive effect of captopril would seem to bear out this supposition. Moreover, Hutchison and Doyle found that captopril introduced into the lateral brain ventricle of an SHR also decreased blood pressure markedly. Again, this tends to implicate the role of the renin system in the SHR. (This meterial was presented at the 6th International Congress of Hypertension, New Orleans, May 1980.)

This generalization carries over to human hypertension, in that hypertensive patients with very high-renin levels tend not to do well on treatment aimed just at reducing body Na. However, if the renin is neutralized by captopril or beta-blockers or saralasin, then body Na reduction will add further to the lowering of blood pressure.

SUMMARY

Certain types of hypertension have a definite link to NaCl in the diet and in the body. Human essential hypertension definitely fits into this category, as does the hypertension induced by feeding high-salt diets to susceptible rats. The rise in blood pressure in both cases is due primarily to an increase in general vasoconstriction of arterioles without any large drop in cardiac output. NaCl-induced hypertension appears to have two links in the chain of causation. The first link involves an initial, and often temporary, tendency to an excess of body Na. The second link is that the excess of body Na leads ultimately to an increase in peripheral resistance and arterial pressure.

In regard to the first link, the excess of body Na is most often brought about by a "normal" dietary intake of Na combined with a sluggish ability of the kidney to excrete it. It can also be brought about by a fairly normal kidney performance combined with a very large dietary intake of Na. Either of these processes can be averted by having very low amounts of salt in the diet or by combining normal dietary salt with natriuretic drugs such as thiazides.

In regard to the second link, it is becoming clear from studies on dialysis patients that about one-fourth of human subjects will not develop a rise in blood pressure and peripheral vasoconstriction, even though body Na is increased. There are studies that suggest that the central nervous system may be involved in this second link. Once the arterial pressure does increase through the mechanism of the second link, the rise in pressure facilitates natriuresis and may completely normalize the intrinsic slowness of natriuresis.

Genetic influences make some humans and some rats especially susceptible to NaCl-induced hypertension. These genetic features would likely involve both links, first, causing the kidney to have a slow rate of natriuresis and, second, causing the blood pressure to rise readily when the load of body Na is increased.

REFERENCES

1. Kempner W (1944) Treatment of kidney disease and hypertensive vascular disease with rice diet. NC Med J 5: 125
2. Winer BH (1961) The anti-hypertensive actions of benzothiadiazines. Circulation 23: 211
3. Maddocks I (1967) Blood pressures in Melanesians. Med J Aust 1: 1123
4. Lowenstein FW (1961) Blood pressure in relation to age and sex in the tropics and subtropics: A review of the literature and an investigation in two tribes of Brazil Indians. Lancet 1: 389
5. Kean BH (1944) The blood pressure of the Cuna Indians. Am J Trop Med 24: 341
6. Shaper AG (1972) Cardiovascular disease in the tropics: III. Blood pressure and hypertension. Br Med J 3: 805
7. Prior AM, Evans JG, Harvey HBP, Davidson F, Lindsey M (1968) Sodium intake and blood pressure in two Polynesian populations. N Engl J Med 279: 515
8. Page LB, Danion A, Moellering RC Jr (1974) Antecedents of cardiovascular diseases in six Solomon Islands societies. Circulation 49: 1132
9. Oliver WJ, Cohen EL, Neel JV (1975) Blood pressure, sodium intake and sodium related hormones in the Yanomamo Indians, a "no-salt" culture. Circulation 52: 146

10. Sinnet PF, Whyte HM (1973) Epidemiological studies in a total highland population, Tukisenta, New Guinea: Cardiovascular disease and relevant clinical, electrocardiographic, radiological and biochemical findings. J Chronic Dis 26: 265

11. Takahashi E, Sasaki N, Takeda J, et al (1957) The geographic distribution of cerebral hemorrhage and hypertension in Japan. Hum Biol 29: 139

12. Kirkendall W, Connor W, Abboud F, Rastogi S, Anderson T, Fry M (1972) Effect of dietary sodium on the blood pressure of normotensive man. In: Genest J (ed) International symposium on renin-angiotensin-aldosterone-sodium in hypertension. Springer, New York, p 360

13. Marl AL, Lawton WJ, Abboud FM, Fritz AE, Connor WE (1974) Effects of high and low sodium intake on blood pressure and vascular reactivity in borderline hypertensive subjects. Circulation 50(Suppl III): 107

14. Murray RH, Luft FC, Bloch R, Weyman AE (1978) Blood pressure responses to extremes of sodium intake in normal man. Proc Soc Exp Biol Med 159: 432

15. Onesti G, Kim KE, Greco JA, Del Guercio ET, Fernandes M, Schwartz C (1975) Blood pressure regulation in end-stage renal disease and anephric man. Circ Res 36(Suppl I): 145

16. Grim CE, Luft FC, Miller JZ, Brown PL, Gannon MA, Weinberger MH (1979) Effects of sodium loading and depletion in normotensive first-degree relatives of essential hypertensives. J Lab Clin Med 94(5): 764

17. Dahl L, Heine M, Tassinari L (1962) Effects of chronic excess salt ingestion: Evidence that genetic factors play an important role in susceptibility to experimental hypertension. J Exp Med 115: 1173

18. Meneely GR, Tucker RG, Darby WJ, et al (1953) Chronic sodium chloride toxicity in the albino rat: II. Occurrence of hypertension and of a syndrome of edema and renal failure. J Exp Med 98: 71

19. Iwai J, Knudsen KD, Dahl LK, Heine M, Leitl G (1969) Genetic influence on the development of renal hypertension in parabiotic rats: Evidence for a humoral factor. J Exp Med 129: 507

20. Iwai J, Dahl LK, Knudsen KD (1973) Genetic influences on the renin-angiotensin system: Low renin activities in hypertension-prone rats. Circ Res 32: 678

21. Ben-Ishay D, Knudsen KD, Dahl LK (1967) Renal function studies in the early stage of salt hypertension in rats. Proc Soc Exp Biol Med 125: 515

22. Dahl LK, Knudsen KD, Heine M, Leitl G (1967) Effects of chronic excess salt ingestion: Genetic influence on the development of salt hypertension in parabiotic rats: Evidence for a humoral factor. J Exp Med 126: 687

23. Knudsen KD, Iwai J, Heine M, Leitl G, Dahl LK (1969) Genetic influence on the development of renoprival hypertension in parabiotic rats. J Exp Med 130: 1353

24. Tobian L, Binion JT (1952) Tissue cations and water in arterial hypertension. Circulation 5: 754

25. Selkurt EE (1951) Effect of pulse pressure and mean arterial pressure modification on renal hemodynamics and electrolyte and water excretion. Circulation 4: 541

26. Tobian L, Lange J, Azar S, Iwai J, Koop D, Coffee K, Johnson MA (1978) Reduction of natriuretic capacity and renin release in isolated, blood-perfused kidneys of Dahl hypertension-prone rats. Circ Res 43:(Suppl I): 92

27. Iwai J, Ohanian EV, Dahl LK (1977) Influence of thiazide on salt hypertension. Circ Res 40(Suppl I): 131

28. Tobian L, Lange J, Iwai J, Hiller K, Johnson MA, Goossens P (1979) Prevention with thiazide of NaCl-induced hypertension in Dahl "S" rats: Evidence for a Na-retaining humoral agent in "S" rats. Hypertension 1: 316

29. Ganguli M, Tobian L, Dahl L (1976) Low renal papillary plasma flow in both Dahl and Kyoto rats with spontaneous hypertension. Circ Res 39: 337

30. Tobian L, Goto A, Ganguli M, Johnson M, Iwai J (1980) Three studies of NaCl hypertension. Clin Res 28: 550

31. Takeshita A, Mark A (1978) Neurogenic contribution to hindquarter vasoconstriction during high sodium intake in Dahl strain of genetically hypertensive rat. Circ Res 43(Suppl I): 87

32. Ikeda T, Tobian L, Iwai J, Goossens P (1978) Central nervous system pressor responses in rats susceptible and resistant to sodium hypertension. Clin Sci Mol Med 55: 225

33. Tobian L, Pumper M, Johnson S, Iwai J (in press) A humoral pressor agent in Dahl "S" rats with NaCl hypertension. Clin Sci Mol Med

34. Redleaf P, Tobian L (1958) Sodium restriction and reserpine administration in experimental renal hypertension. Circ Res 6: 3, 343–351

35. Tobian L, Coffee K (1964) Effect of thiazide drugs on renovascular hypertension in contrast to their effect on essential hypertension. Proc Soc Exp Biol Med 115: 196

Neurogenic Elements in Rat Primary Hypertension: Differences Between Spontaneously Hypertensive Rats and the Milan Hypertensive Strain

B. Folkow, M. Hallbäck-Nordlander, S. Lundin, S. E. Ricksten, and P. Thorén

The mistake is often made that the neurogenic contributions to primary hypertension imply a sustained and uniform sympathetic acceleration, more or less responsible for elevated resistance. Such misconceptions are, of course, bound to collide with experimental facts, and neurogenic influences are seldom rejected entirely, which certainly amounts to throwing the egg away with the shell.

Yet, it has been known for decades that central autonomic control generally acts via *differentiated* patterns. Here the "defense reaction" (DR) is best known (1–4), but this term is misleading in the sense that it is sometimes thought to mean the reaction only during severe stress. Actually, DR is more or less involved whenever individuals are mentally engaged, both in pleasant and unpleasant situations. For example DR is readily induced in humans by forced mental arithmetic (5) or competitive games.

DR is characterized by central inhibition of vagal tone, increased adrenergic activity to heart, capacitance vessels, and gastrointestinal and renal resistance vessels, including the renin-producing cells, while vasoconstrictor fiber discharge to skeletal muscle is inhibited where, instead, nervous and/or hormonal vasodilatation occurs (1, 3, 6). Cardiac output (CO) thus increases, favoring skeletal muscle, myocardium, and CNS, with restrictions elsewhere. As a result, systemic resistance (R) usually changes slightly, implying a substantial mean arterial pressure (MAP) elevation as CO rises, though a net R increase sometimes dominates. Despite the MAP elevation, heart rate (HR) always increases because the baroceptor-induced reflex bradycardia is centrally suppressed by DR. In all these respects, animals and humans respond almost identically.

Daily transient DR mechanisms may substantially elevate average MAP, particularly in predisposed humans and/or in a vivid psychosocial climate. This rise in pressure in turn, can trigger structural adaptation of resistance vessels, heart, and barostat mechanisms. In this way, DR may contribute to a gradual induction of chronic hypertension when the proper genetic predisposition is at hand (1, 2, 6). Moreover, as shown already by Brod's group (5), early human primary hypertension frequently displays a hemodynamic pattern strongly suggestive of a mild DR, where Lund-Johansen (7) recently illustrated the gradual shift of pattern toward that of established hypertension.

As an animal model for human primary hypertension, we have primarily used spontaneously hypertensive rats (SHR), in which neurohormonal cardiovascular influences are characterized as follows:

1) A clear-cut *central hyperreactivity* to environmental alerting stimuli, particularly in young "borderline hypertensive" SHR, this results in intensified and more prolonged neurogenic pressor and HR increases to such stimuli, as compared with controls (8, 9). The neurogenic drive on the heart is also modestly increased during rest.

2) CO is increased in young awake SHR, and also during rest central hemodynamics are neurogenically adjusted so as to mimic a mild DR. They further show accentuated DR with more powerful HR, CO, and MAP elevations in response to alerting stimuli. These accentuated DR influences during wakefulness fade during anesthesia and, particularly, after cardiac nerve blockade when the remaining MAP elevation is due to increased R (9).

3) Direct continuous recordings of splanchnic sympathetic activity and of MAP and HR in awake, freely moving SHR and (Wistar-Kyoto rats) WKR reveal more vivid variations in all these parameters in SHR as compared with WKR. It is apparent here how closely changes in HR and sympathetic discharge parallel each other (10). Further, single-fiber recordings from the sympa-

thetic renal supply in anesthetized SHR reveal a clear discharge elevation to this vascular bed (11). Again it is clear that SHR display a clear-cut central hyperreactivity with respect to sympathetic discharge, which is mainly responsible for the characteristically more vivid cardiovascular DR changes to environmental stimuli.

4) In sharp contrast to SHR, the Milan strain of hypertensive rat (MHS) shows *no* central hyperreactivity to environmental stimuli (12). Rather, in this mild variant of rat primary hypertension, autonomic cardiovascular control appears to reflexly *counteract* the triggering pressor influences, which here seem to be "volume dependent" and on a renal basis. This is in contrast to SHR, where total blood volume is, if anything, reduced, though it is "centralized" as a result of the increased sympathetic activity (13).

5) The importance of the inherited central hyperreactivity in SHR for hypertension induction becomes apparent when SHR are deprived of (for rats) ordinary psychosocial stimuli by relative isolation: Their hypertension is then attenuated, and so are the structural cardiovascular changes (14), illustrating the close relationship between genetic predisposition, environment, *and* early cardiovascular structural adaptation (1, 2). This latter element is a prerequisite for the creation of truly chronic hypertension.

Comparing these characteristics of SHR hypertension with both Brod's original data (5) and more recent analyses of borderline human hypertension (4), many close parallels show up. This is also the case with the interesting effects of mental "stress" in adolescents from families with and without predisposition for primary hypertension, which have recently been described by Falkner et al. (15). These genetically predisposed youngsters almost uniformly showed clear central autonomic hyperresponsiveness in response to forced mental arithmetic.

Considering the differentiated autonomic DR pattern displayed in these neurogenic human and rat variants of primary hypertension, a comment is appropriate concerning the attempts to trace sympathetic activity in human primary hypertension by either the direct neurography technique of Vallbo et al. (16) or by the widely used estimates of plasma norepinephrine (NE) levels. Unfortunately, only cutaneous and skeletal muscle sympathetic fibers are so far accessible for direct neurography in humans. Cutaneous vasoconstric-

tor fiber control is subordinated to the central temperature regulation and, therefore, only transiently involved in alerting responses. Further, in DR-like patterns, sympathetic activity to skeletal muscle should, if anything, *decrease* in both humans and animals, while activity should increase in cardiac, renal, or gastrointestinal sympathetic fibers.

Concerning plasma NE levels, an accentuated DR-like discharge pattern would give increased NE overflow in, for example, the gastrointestinal bed; but the liver passage almost completely clears this blood from NE overflow before it enters the general circulation. In the large skeletal muscle bed, one would expect, as mentioned, a reduced, or at least not an increased, NE. It is, therefore, doubtful whether the DR-like pattern involved in neurogenic variants of primary hypertension could, on the whole, be reliably reflected by plasma NE levels: Little would come from the gastrointestinal area, and perhaps even reduced amounts from skeletal muscle, tending to cancel out increased NE overflow from, for example, heart and kidneys. The NE levels would much better reflect changes in sympathetic discharge at tilting, for example, since then a considerable reflex vasoconstriction also occurs in skeletal muscle. In fact, a recent study in man clearly indicates this fact (17). As a further disturbing influence, changes in muscle blood flow at *constant* sympathetic discharge greatly influence the NE overflow fraction (18). At best, therefore, plasma NE levels are a very blunt indicator of sympathetic discharge, and may be entirely misleading when it comes to the particular pattern expected to prevail in neurogenic variants of primary hypertension.

SUMMARY

Central autonomic control generally acts via differentiated patterns such as DR, during which adrenergic activity increases in the heart, capacitance vessels, and gastrointestinal and renal resistance vessels, while it is inhibited in skeletal muscles. Plasma NE has been used extensively to evaluate the degree of sympathetic activation (e.g., during hypertension). However, such a different pattern of sympathetic nervous activation can hardly be traced by plasma NE levels, especially because NE released in the splanchnic vascular bed will be cleared in the liver. In contrast, a more generalized reflex sympathetic activation such as that during tilting will be adequately traced.

SHR display a clear-cut central hyperreactivity to altering stimuli. This hyperreactivity results in enhanced neurogenic pressure and increased HR, and in the young awake SHR, central hemodynamics are even at rest neurogenically adjusted so as to mimic a mild DR. Single-fiber recordings from the sympathetic renal supply of anesthetized SHR also reveal a clear discharge elevation in this vascular bed. In contrast, the MHS shows no such central hyperreactivity, and autonomic cardiovascular control appears here rather to reflexly counteract the triggering pressure influences, which in MHS seem to be volume dependent and on a renal basis.

ACKNOWLEDGMENT

This work was supported in part by grants 14X–00016 and 14X–4764, the Swedish Medical Research Council.

REFERENCES

1. Folkow B (1975) Central neurohormonal mechanisms in spontaneous hypertensive rats compared with human essential hypertension. Clin Sci Mol Med 48: 205S–214S
2. Folkow B (1978) Cardiovascular structural adaptation: Its role in the initiation and manitenance of primary hypertension. The fourth Volhard lecture. Clin Sci Mol Med 55(Suppl 4): 3–22
3. Folkow B, Neil E (1971) Circulation. Oxford University Press, Oxford.
4. Julius S, Esler MD (ed) (1976) The nervous system in arterial hypertension. Charles C Thomas, Springfield, Ill.
5. Brod J (1960) Haemodynamic response to stress and its bearing on the haemodynamic basis of essential hypertension. In: The pathogenesis of essential hypertension (Proceedings of the WHO-Czechoslov Cardiol Symposium). Prague-State Med Publ House, Prague, pp 256–264
6. Folkow B (1960) Haemodynamic responses to cortical and hypothalamic stimulation. In: The pathogenesis of essential hypertension (Proceedings of the WHO-Czechoslov Cardiol Symposium). Prague-State Med Publ House, Prague, pp 247–255, 265–266
7. Lund-Johansen P (1977) Hemodynamic alterations in hypertension—spontaneous changes and effects of drug therapy: A review. Acta Med Scand [Suppl] 603: 1–4
8. Hallbäck M, Folkow B (1974) Cardiovascular responses to acute mental 'stress' in spontaneously hypertensive rats. Acta Physiol Scand 90: 684–698
9. Hallbäck M, Lundin S (1979) Background of hypokinetic circulation in young SHR. In: Meyer P, Schmitt H (eds) Nervous system and hypertension. pp 256–260
10. Ricksten S-E, Thorén P (1979) Characteristics of the sympathetic nervous activity in awake normotensive and hypertensive rats. Acta Physiol Scand 105: 31A–32A
11. Thorén P, Ricksten S-E (1979) Recordings of renal and splanchnic sympathetic nervous activity in normotensive and spontaneously hypertensive rats. Clin Sci 57: 197S–199S
12. Hallbäck M, Jones JV, Bianchi G, Folkow B (1977) Cardiovascular control in the Milan strain of spontaneously hypertensive rats (MHS) at 'rest' and during acute mental 'stress.' Acta Physiol Scand 99: 208–216
13. Lundin S, Folkow B, Friberg P, Rippe B (in press) Central blood volume in spontaneously hypertensive rats and Wistar-Kyoto normotensive rats (Report to the VIIth scientific meeting of the international society of hypertension). Clin Sci
14. Hallbäck M (1975) Consequence of social isolation on blood pressure, cardiovascular reactivity and design in spontaneously hypertensive rats. Acta Physiol Scand 93: 455–465
15. Falkner B, Onesti G, Angelakos ET, Fernandes M, Longman C (1979) Cardiovascular response to mental stress in normal adolescents with hypertensive parents. Hypertension 1: 23–30
16. Vallbo AB, Hagbarth K-E, Torebjörk HE, Wallin BG (1979) Somatosensory, proprioceptive, and sympathetic activity in human peripheral nerves. Physiol Rev 59: 919–961
17. Hjemdahl P, Eliasson K (1979) Sympatho-adrenal and cardiovascular response to mental stress and orthostatic provocation in latent hypertension. Clin Sci 57: 189S–191S
18. Carlsson A, Folkow B, Häggendal J (1964) Some factors influencing the release of noradrenaline into the blood following sympathetic stimulation. Life Sci 3: 1335–1341

Hypertension and Stroke Mechanisms in Spontaneously Hypertensive Rats

Yukio Yamori, Akira Ooshima, Ryoichi Horie, Yasuo Nara, Masahiro Kihara, and Takehiro Igawa

SPONTANEOUSLY HYPERTENSIVE RAT MODELS FOR HUMAN ESSENTIAL HYPERTENSION

Since rats with spontaneous genetic hypertension were established, much progress has been made on the pathogenesis of hypertension. These models include genetically hypertensive rats of New Zealand strain (GH) 1958 (1), spontaneously hypertensive rats (SHR) 1963 (2), Lyon hypertensive strain (LH) 1973 (3), and Milan hypertensive strain (MH) 1974 (4). Dahl salt-sensitive (DS) rats 1962 (5) and Sabra hypertensive strain (SBH) 1972 (6) are rats that develop hypertension in response to excess sodium loading or DOCA-salt manipulation. These rats are now regarded as having somewhat different pathogenic factors from each other and can be utilized as models for essential hypertension in man, which is not a homogeneous disease entity, but rather primary hypertension probably caused by the different combination of etiologic factors. Among these models, SHR, which develop not only hypertension but also hypertensive complications, are superior to others that rarely develop cardiovascular diseases. Furthermore, stroke-prone SHR (SHRSP, 1974) (7) and arteriolipidosis-prone rats (ALR) 1977 (8), which were selectively bred from SHR, can develop cardiovascular diseases spontaneously or only by dietary manipulation, so that we can experimentally study not only the pathogenesis, but also the etiology and the prevention. Our studies have clarified that genetic predisposition and gene–environment interaction are important in the pathogenesis of these adult diseases. Therefore, there is a definite possibility that the predisposition of these diseases is detectable even at a young age, and that these cardiovascular diseases can be prevented by intervening pathogenic mechanisms through the control of environmental factors if prophylactic measures are started early enough (9).

PATHOGENESIS OF SPONTANEOUS HYPERTENSION

SHR develop moderate to severe hypertension spontaneously in 100% of the population and various hypertensive complications in a high incidence. Our genetic analysis clarified that this hypertension is transmitted to the offspring in an additive mode of inheritance consisting of at least three major genes (10), while environmental factors such as stress and salt loading accelerate hypertension and aggravate hypertensive complications (11). The hypertension mechanism in SHR is considered to consist of neurogenic and nonneurogenic factors, both of which contribute to the initiation and maintenance mechanisms (12–14). The deviation of central regulatory mechanisms of blood pressure (13, 14) increases sympathetic outflow to increase blood pressure, and the elevation of sympathetic tone itself and of blood pressure accelerate vascular noncollagenous and collagenous protein syntheses ("neurovascular linkage" and "adaptive metabolic changes"), which induce structural vascular changes to increase the peripheral vascular resistance and to stabilize hypertension (12–16). The cardiovascular response to hypertension, such as cardiac hypertrophy and accelerated vascular protein synthesis, is detected even in young SHRSP and stroke-resistant SHR (SHRSR) in comparison with the age-matched Wistar-Kyoto rats (WKY), so that genetic predisposition to cardiovascular hypertrophy may be primarily involved in the pathogenesis of hypertension closely interacting with neurogenic factors. Therefore, this predisposition (i.e., cardiac hypertrophy in early hypertension) may be utilized for the prediction of the further development of stable hypertension (17).

PATHOGENESIS OF STROKE AND OTHER COMPLICATIONS

SHRSP quickly develop severe hypertension (over 200 mmHg) at the age of 10–15 weeks and maintain the level until most of them (over 90%) die of stroke, while SHRSR gradually develop hypertension around 200 mmHg and less than 10% die of stroke. SHRSP show various symptoms of cerebrovascular lesions such as irritability, hyperkinesis, hypokinesis, and paralysis, and the average life-span in males and females is 9 and 13 months, respectively. At autopsy, both cerebral hemorrhage and infarction are observed in SHRSP. Cerebral lesions in the basal ganglia are especially similar to hypertensive cerebral lesions in man.

The hereditary mode of stroke has been analyzed by cross breeding between SHRSP and SHRSR; the mode is recessive and is controlled by at least two major gene loci, while severe hypertension is additively inherited by the almost similar number of major genes (9).

The pathogenic mechanisms of stroke in this model proved up to the present are summarized in Fig. 1. Under severe hypertension, regional cerebral blood flow is decreased. Thus, mild chronic ischemia increases vascular permeability and induces arterionecrosis. When microaneurysms formed at the necrotic arterial wall rupture, hemorrhage occurs. On the other hand, thrombosis at the necrotic arterial wall or within microaneurysms causes infarction. Therefore, stroke in this model is "arterio-necro-thrombogenic stroke" caused by hypertension, but not "atherothrombogenic stroke" caused by atherosclerosis (18, 19).

Our observations have repeatedly confirmed that a high-protein diet is effective for preventing stroke, and the experimental analyses have disclosed that this mechanism could be partly ascribed to the attenuation of the development of severe hypertension by some amino acids such as sulfoamino acids and tyrosine. These amino acids were proven to reduce blood pressure acting centrally (20). In particular, tyrosine administered peripherally and centrally increased the level of norepinephrine metabolite (MOPEG) in the brain when it reduced blood pressure. This finding, therefore, supports that the deviation of a noradrenergic mechanism is involved in the development of hypertension in these models (12–14), and suggests that high-protein intake may attenuate the

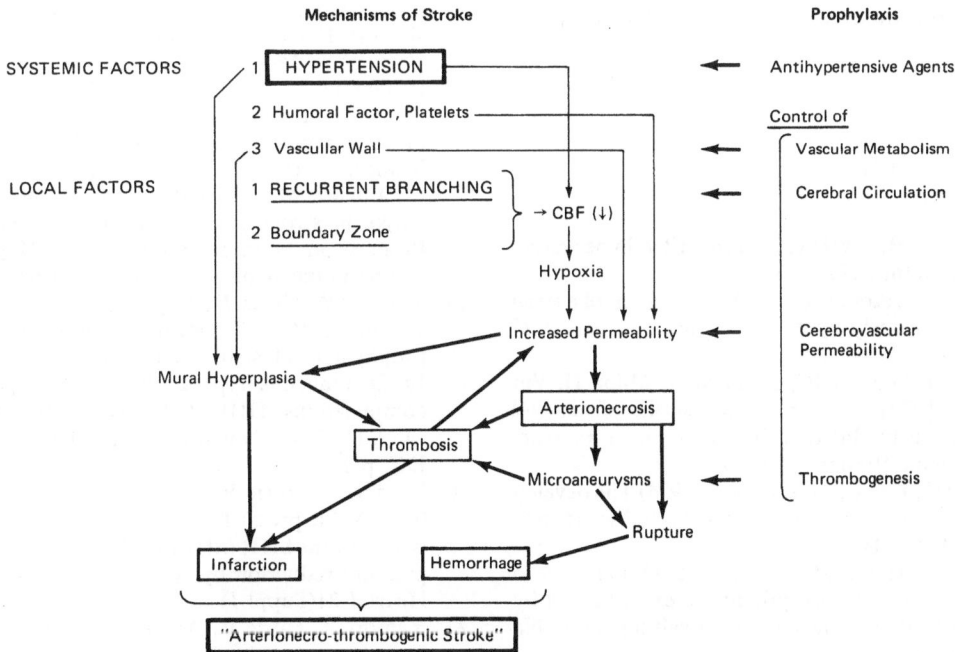

Fig. 1. Pathogenesis and prophylaxis of stroke.

development of severe hypertension by acting on the pathogenic mechanism of the central blood pressure regulation. Pathogenic factors of atherogenesis in ALR are hypertension and altered lipid metabolism (21). Hemodynamic derangement or rheologic stress caused by hypertension is one of the mechanisms of acute arterial fat deposition (i.e., the initial step of atherogenesis) (22). Another mechanism is reactive hypercholesterolemia, which seems to be induced by accelerated intestinal absorption of cholesterol, and also by a delay in cholesterol catabolism (23). We recently found the reduced HDL level that might be related to the marked fat deposition in arterial walls in ALR.

SUMMARY

Establishing animal models for hypertension, stroke and arterio- or atherosclerosis, has enabled us to study experimentally the pathogenesis of these cardiovascular diseases that are the most prevalent causes of death in man. Experimental analyses in these models have proved that increased peripheral resistance is the main contributing factor of hypertension, in which both neural and nonneural mechanisms are involved, and that the sustained hypertension interacting with other factors such as vascular permeability or lipidemia finally results in hypertensive vascular complications.

REFERENCES

1. Smirk FH, Hall WH (1958) Inherited hypertension in rats. Nature 182: 727
2. Okamoto K, Aoki K (1963) Development of a strain of spontaneously hypertensive rats. Jpn Circ J 27: 282
3. Dupont J, Dupont JC, Froment A, Milon H, Vincent M (1973) Selection of three strains of rats with spontaneously different levels of blood pressure. Biomedicine [Express] 19: 36
4. Bianchi G, Fox U, Imbasciati E (1974) The development of a new strain of spontaneously hypertensive rats. Life Sci 14: 339
5. Dahl LK, Heine M, Tassinari L (1962) Role of genetic factors in susceptibility to experimental hypertension due to chronic excess salt ingestion. Nature 194: 480
6. Ben-Ishay D, Saliternik R, Welner A (1972) Separation of two strains of rats with inbred dissimilar sensitivity to DOCA-salt hypertension. Experientia 28: 1321
7. Okamoto K, Yamori Y, Nagaoka A (1974) Establishment of the stroke-prone spontaneously hypertensive rats (SHR). Circ Res 34, 35(Suppl): 143
8. Yamori Y (1977) A selection of arteriolipidosis-prone rats (ALR). Jpn Heart J 18: 602
9. Yamori Y, Lovenberg W, Freis E (eds) (1979) Prophylactic approach to hypertensive diseases. Raven Press, New York
10. Tanase H, Suzuki Y, Ooshima A, Yamori Y, Okamoto K (1970) Genetic analysis of blood pressure in spontaneously hypertensive rats. Jpn Circ J 34: 1197
11. Yamori Y (1977) Hypertensive strains of rat. In: Inoue E, Nishimura H (eds) Gene-environment interaction in common diseases. University of Tokyo Press, Tokyo, p 151
12. Yamori Y (1976) Neural and non-neural mechanism in spontaneous hypertension. Clin Sci Mol Med 51: 431S
13. Yamori Y (1976) Interaction of neural and non-neural factors in the pathogenesis of spontaneous hypertension. In: Julius S, Esler M (eds) The nervous system in arterial hypertension. Charles C Thomas, Springfield, Ill., p 17
14. Yamori Y (1976) Neurogenic mechanism of spontaneous hypertension. In: Onesti G, Fernandez M, Kim KE (eds) Regulation of blood pressure by the central nervous system. Grune & Stratton, New York, p 65
15. Yamori Y (1976) Vascular protein metabolism in the pathogenesis of hypertension. Jpn Circ J 40: 879
16. Yamori Y, Nakada T, Lovenberg W (1976) Effect of antihypertensive therapy on lysine incorporation into vascular protein of the spontaneously hypertensive rat. Eur J Pharmacol 38: 349
17. Yamori Y, Mori C, Nishio T, Ooshima A, Horie R, Ohtaka M, Soeda T, Saito M, Abe K, Nara Y, Nakao Y, Kihara M (1979) Cardiac hypertrophy in early hypertension. Am J Cardiol 44: 964
18. Yamori Y, Horie R, Akiguchi I, Nara Y, Ohtaka M, Fukase M (1977) Pathogenetic mechanism of stroke in stroke-prone SHR. In: de Jong W (ed) Progress in brain research, vol 47: Hypertension and brain mechanisms. Elsevier, Amsterdam, p 219
19. Yamori Y, Horie R, Handa H, Ohtaka M, Nara Y, Fukase M (1977) Pathogenetic approach to the prophylaxis of stroke and atherogenesis in SHR. In: Spontaneous hypertension: Its pathogenesis and complications, DHEW Publication No (NIH) 77–1179, US Government Printing Office, Washington, DC, p 269
20. Yamori Y, Horie R, Nara Y, Fujiwara M, Lovenberg W (in press) Prophylactic trials for stroke in stroke-prone SHR (SHRSP): 5. Mechanism of blood pressure reduction by tyrosine administration. Jpn Heart J 21(Suppl I)
21. Yamori Y, Horie R, Akiguchi I, Ohtaka M, Nara Y, Fukase M (1976) New models of SHR for studies on stroke and atherogenesis. Clin Exp Pharmacol Physiol [Suppl] 3: 199

Pressor and Volume Effects of Vasopressin

A. W. Cowley, Jr., M. J. Smith, Jr., R. D. Manning, Jr., and T. E. Lohmeier

Vasopressin (AVP) acts on both the renal collecting ducts to promote the retention of water and on vascular smooth muscle as a vasoconstrictor. Recent studies concerning these two actions of vasopressin have expanded our understanding of the physiologic and possible pathophysiologic role of this hormone.

Contrary to previous beliefs, potent vasoconstrictor actions have now been demonstrated to occur in the dog at plasma levels associated with endogenous secretion rates (1). Plasma levels of AVP in conscious normally hydrated resting dogs average approximately 0.8 μU/ml. These levels fall to 0.2–0.3 μU/ml with water overhydration and rise to 8.0–10.0 μU/ml after 24 h water restriction. In the absence of compensatory autonomic reflex mechanisms, changes of plasma AVP within this range can raise arterial pressure 20–25 mmHg, as seen in Fig. 1. Since considerably greater levels of plasma AVP than this have been observed during hypovolemic states (80–150 μU/ml), a study was designed to quantitate the ability of endogenously released AVP to serve as a controller of arterial pressure during hemorrhage (1).

Mongrel dogs were studied in which the actions of the sympathetic nervous system and renin–angiotensin control system were abolished in order to prevent rapid offsetting effects of observed changes with AVP release. Sympathetic nerve activity was abolished with retrograde lumbar injection of the spinal cord with ethanol to the level of C1. Bilateral nephrectomy abolished the renin-angiotensin system. The ninth and tenth cranial nerves were left intact to mediate stretch-receptor afferent nerve activity from the cardiopulmonary and sinoaortic stretch-receptor areas. Arterial pressure was lowered rapidly to 50 mmHg by withdrawal of blood over a period of 1 min (Fig. 2). Arterial pressure returned to nearly 90 mmHg by the third minute after completion of the hemorrhage, and then stabilized at 85 mmHg over the next 30 min. This represented a steady-state fractional compensation of arterial pressure of 71% ± 3%. Compensation of arterial pressure was associated with a rise of plasma AVP from 19 ± 2 to 75 ± 9 μU/ml. With blood replacement, arterial pressure rose to 130 mmHg and gradually returned

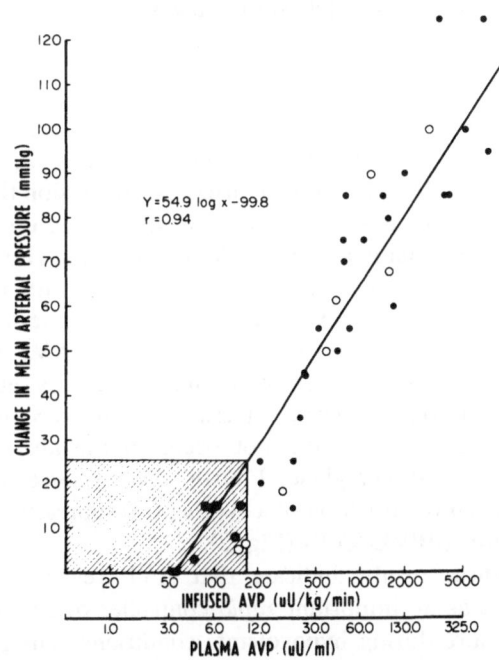

Fig. 1. AVP–arterial pressure dose–response curve obtained in spinal-areflexic-decapitated dogs. The graph summarizes the relationship between AVP infusion *(upper scale of abscissa)*, the corresponding changes of plasma AVP *(lower scale of abscissa)*, and the associated changes in mean arterial pressure obtained after 60-min infusion periods at each infusion rate. ● infused AVP vs change in mean arterial pressure (upper scale); ○ simultaneous determinations of plasma AVP during infusion of AVP as indicated on the upper scale. (1)

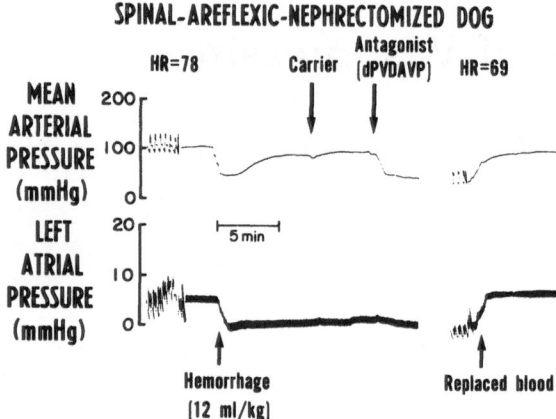

Fig. 2. Results of a hemorrhage in a spinal-areflexic-nephrectomized dog in which a rapid compensation of arterial pressure was obtained in 3–4 min after blood withdrawal. After recovery of arterial pressure, the competitive AVP inhibitor dPVDAVP (60 μg/kg) was injected, which resulted in a fall in arterial pressure to its precompensated state of 50 mmHg within 1 min after injection (1). dPVPAVP = [1-deaminopenicillamine, 4-valine]-8-D-arginine-vasopressin.

to normal over the next 30–40 min in association with a gradual decline of circulating levels of AVP.

Four observations supported the conclusion that pressure compensation was a result of the direct vasoconstrictor actions of AVP. First, the rise of arterial pressure was correlated closely with the rise of plasma AVP. Second, similar elevations of arterial pressure were observed with AVP infused to achieve levels of plasma AVP comparable to hemorrhage. Third, arterial pressure recovery after hemorrhage did not occur in the absence of the pituitary gland. Fourth, the response was blocked by injection of a synthetic vasopressin inhibitor (dPVDAVP) (Fig. 2).

These results indicate that AVP release can serve as an important *rapid* controller of arterial pressure during hypovolemic conditions. The experimentally determined strength of this control system as expressed by the calculated open-loop gain (−2.2) is greater than that which has been measured for either the renin–angiotensin system or the baroreceptor reflex control system. In support of these observations, recent studies by Montani et al. (2) in conscious instrumented dogs also indicate that the amount of AVP released with a hyperosmotic stimulus is sufficient to significantly increase total peripheral resistance. These

resistance changes were not associated with a rise of arterial pressure, however, unless the rapid-acting effects of the baroreceptor reflexes were removed.

Does this mean that AVP is important in determining the *long-term* level of arterial pressure? The answer to this is not yet clear. It appears that AVP is elevated in several animal models of hypertension including DOC-salt, Goldblatt, and SHR, especially in the malignant states (3–6). Similarly, it has been reported that AVP is elevated in benign and malignant essential hypertension in man (7, 8), but plasma levels appear to be only twice normal levels. The meaning of these observations is presently a matter or conjecture. Möhring et al. (4) and Crofton et al. (6) have suggested that these levels can make a significant contribution to hypertension since injection of AVP-specific antisera or a synthetic inhibitor resulted in a rapid fall of pressure to nearly normal levels in several rat models of severe hypertension in which plasma AVP was three to ten times normal.

Our own data indicate that a tenfold increase in plasma AVP can exert considerable pressor activity in the absence of the sympathetic nervous system or baroreceptor reflex control system. Whether this same degree of pressor activity is manifest in hypertension is unclear. Smith et al. (9) attempted to produce sustained hypertension with continuous infusion of AVP, which maintained plasma levels nearly ten times normal. Hypertension was not sustained beyond 2 weeks.

The most dramatic consequence of sustained elevated levels of AVP when water intake remained normal was the decrease of extracellular sodium concentration and osmolality which declined gradually to levels of 115 mEq/liter and 230 mosmol/kg by the 15th day of infusion. This large decrease could be attributed initially to renal fluid retention, but was chronically a result of net sodium loss. AVP appears in some manner to exert a strong effect on the regulation of renal sodium excretion.

Since AVP *per se* does not appear to be capable of sustaining hypertension, the question naturally arose as to whether elevated levels of AVP in the presence of high circulating levels of sodium-retaining hormones would result in an elevation of arterial pressure. Lohmeier and Cowley (10) infused angiotensin II (AII) in sufficient amounts to cause an initial sodium retention and a gradual elevation of arterial pressure to nearly 150 mmHg. After 2 weeks of continuous AII infusion, AVP was added to the infusate to raise plasma levels nearly tenfold. No changes of arterial pressure were noted during the 2-week period of combined angiotensin–AVP infusion, nor was there a measurable retention of water. Plasma sodium, however, was again decreased by the addition of AVP, but to a lesser extent. Similar results were obtained with combined infusions of aldosterone and AVP. Despite the inability of AVP to chronically raise the level of arterial pressure in these studies, a dramatic decrease of arterial pressure occurred during the first hour after stopping the AVP infusion, with no associated diuresis. This suggests that AVP was exerting chronic vasoconstrictor actions. This abrupt fall of arterial pressure to nearly normal levels is reminiscent of the observations by Möhring et al. (4) with a bolus injection of AVP–antiserum into malignant hypertensive rats. The important difference between the studies is that a sustained reduction of plasma AVP was achieved after termination of the AVP infusion, in the hypertensive dog model, in contrast to the short-acting antisera blockade. This appears to be an important difference because during the 24 h following termination of the AVP infusion in the present study, salt and water retention occurred and arterial pressure again rose to the same level of hypertension achieved with AII infusion alone. These observations suggest that AVP can exert sustained vasoconstrictor activity, but cannot chronically alter the ability of the kidney to maintain fluid homeostasis at a normal level of renal arterial perfusion pressure.

The only manner in which we have thus far been able to sustain hypertension with infusions of AVP has been in dogs with impaired renal function. Manning et al. (11) surgically reduced functional renal mass to one-third normal levels and infused AVP at levels similar to those used in previous studies. Arterial pressure in these experiments showed no signs of returning to normal following 2 weeks of AVP infusion.

In conclusion, results presently suggest that AVP can serve as a rapid controller of arterial pressure through its vasoconstrictor actions and can result in a temporary state of hypertension for several weeks as a result of its renal water-retaining effects. AVP does not appear to be capable of influencing the long-term level of arterial pressure, nor can it produce sustained changes in body fluid volumes except when renal excretory capacity is reduced. It is entirely possible, there-fore, that elevations of plasma AVP could importantly influence long-term levels of arterial pressure in certain situations associated with a functional reduction of renal mass.

SUMMARY

Evidence is presented which indicates that the short-term release of AVP can serve as an important rapid-acting controller of arterial pressure during hypovolemic states through its vasoconstrictor actions. The experimentally determined strength of the AVP–pressure control system (open-loop gain −2.2) was greater than that measured for either the renin–angiotensin system or arterial baroreceptor reflex systems. The role of AVP in the long-term control of arterial pressure and hypertension is less clear. Although plasma AVP may be elevated in a number of experimental models of hypertension and in essential hypertension, the significance of these observations is unclear. Chronic administration of AVP resulting in plasma levels ten times normal resulted in only a temporary state of hypertension for several weeks from renal retention of water. When administered with renal salt-retaining hormones (angiotensin or aldosterone), excess AVP did not increase the severity of hypertension. Sustained hypertensive actions were observed when excess AVP was administered to dogs with reduced excretory capacity. Available evidence, therefore, indicates that AVP participates in the rapid short-term control of arterial pressure and that AVP could contribute to hypertension in situations where functional renal mass is less than normal.

REFERENCES

1. Cowley AW Jr, Switzer SJ, Guinn MM (1980) Evidence and quantification of the vasopressin arterial pressure control system in the dog. Circ Res 46: 58–67
2. Montani J-P, Liard J-F, Schoun J, Möhring J (1981) Hemodynamic effects of exogenous and endogenous vasopressin at low plasma concentrations in conscious dogs. Hypertension (in press)
3. Möhring J, Möhring B, Peiki M, Haack D (1977) Vasopressor role of ADH in the pathogenesis of malignant DOC hypertension. Am J Physiol 232: F260–F269

4. Möhring J, Möhring B, Peiri M, Haack D (1978) Plasma vasopressin concentrations and effects of vasopressin antiserum on blood pressure in rats with malignant two kidney Goldblatt hypertension. Circ Res 42: 17–22

5. Crofton JT, Share L, Shade RE, Allen C, Tarnowski D (1978) Vasopressin in the rat with spontaneous hypertension. Am J Physiol 235: H361–H366

6. Crofton JT, Share L, Shade RE, Lee-Kuan W Jr, Manning M, Sawyer WH (1979) The importance of vasopressin in the development and maintenance of DOC-salt hypertension in the rat. Hypertension 1: 31–38

7. Khoklar AM, Slater JDH (1976) Increased renal excretion of arginine vasopressin during mild hydropenia in young men with mild essential benign hypertension. Clin Sci Mol Med 51: 691S–694S

8. Padfield PL, Brown JJ, Lever AF, Morton JJ, Robertson JIS (1976) Changes of vasopressin in hypertension: Cause or effect? Lancet 1: 1255–1257

9. Smith MJ Jr, Cowley AW Jr, Guyton AC, Manning RD Jr (1979) Acute and chronic effects of vasopressin on blood pressure, electrolytes, and fluid volume. Am J Physiol 237: F232–F240

10. Lohmeier TE, Cowley AW Jr (1978) Effects of vasopressin on high- and low-renin models of hypertension. Physiologist 21: 72

11. Manning RD, Guyton AC, Coleman TG, McCaa RE (1979) Hypertension in dogs during antidiuretic hormone and hypotonic saline infusion. Am J Physiol 236: H314–H322

DISCUSSION

Dr. Leonard T. Skeggs (Cleveland, Oh.): It has become abundantly clear, through the efforts of many investigators [Skeggs LT, Dorer FE, Kahn JR, Lentz KE, Levine M (1976) Am J Med 60: 737–748], that the renin–angiotensin system does not play a role in initiating or sustaining experimental one-kidney hypertension. This finding was distressing to me, since I had long been a true believer in the renin system as the cause of all forms of hypertension.

One of the tenets of my faith had been the work of Wakerlin and others [mentioned above] who had lowered the blood pressure of one-kidney hypertensive dogs by immunization with crude hog renin. Suddenly, it was obvious that this lowering of blood pressure was not due to renin, but to some other unknown antigenic substance that played an essential role in maintaining one-kidney hypertension. We decided to isolate the unknown antigen (antigen M).

We found that we could lower the blood pressure of rabbits with chronic one-kidney hypertension by direct immunization with hog kidney extracts (Fig. 1). Such rabbits do not lose weight and appear to be perfectly healthy. In many cases, their blood pressure can be maintained at low levels for days or weeks, providing the immunization is continued. Their blood pressures do not go below normal levels. No significant pathologic changes can be found in the kidneys of such rabbits that have been sacrificed [Skeggs LT, Kahn JR, Levine M, Dorer FE, Lentz KE (1975) Circ Res 37: 715–724].

The antigen that elicits the blood pressure-lowering antibody resembles renin in many of its chemical characteristics. It was very difficult to remove renin from our preparations. We finally succeeded by means of an antirenin affinity column, and thus demonstrated blood pressure lowering with an antigen that was completely free of renin [Skeggs LT, Kahn JR, Levine M, Dorer FE, Lentz KE (1976) Circ Res 39: 400–406].

We then recalled an experiment in which we had injected normal rabbits subcutaneously with crude hog renin in an effort to produce antirenin. The blood pressure of many of the rabbits inexplicably began to rise and remained elevated after the injections had been stopped. It seemed obvious to us that the rise in pressure was not due to renin.

In further work, we found that certain crude extracts of rabbit kidney did produce a rise in the blood pressure of young, normal rabbits (Fig. 2). Subcutaneous daily injection of the extracts yielded a delayed, moderate increase in blood pressure which persisted indefinitely. We were intrigued by the possibility that the agent causing the elevation in pressure might be antigen M, which elicits the blood pressure-lowering antibody in hypertensive rabbits [Skeggs LT, Kahn JR, Levine M, Dorer FE, Lentz KE (1977) Circ Res 40: 143–149].

In a burst of enthusiasm, we named the pressor substance "renopressin" and began work on its purification. I am sorry to report that after 36 experiments involving 55 preparations, we have made little progress. The lack of progress in this work may be due in part to the slowness and nonquantitative nature of the assay, it is partly due to the fact that the increase in pressure produced by active preparations is modest at most, which contributes to the difficulty of the assay. Finally, our lack of progress may be due to the elusive nature of the factor itself.

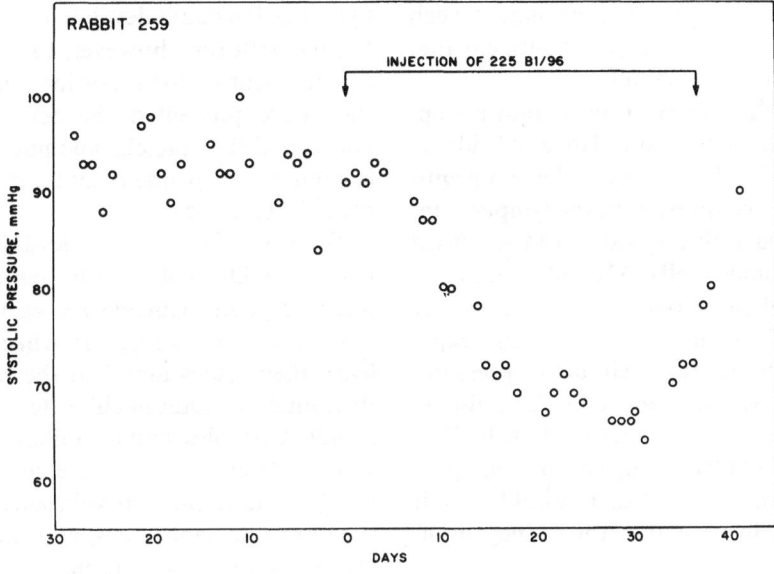

Fig. 1.

We believe we are correct in our finding, as yet unconfirmed by others, that certain crude, homologous kidney preparations do produce a persistent, moderate increase in the ear blood pressure of young (2.25–2.5 kg) male New Zealand rabbits. However, our inability to purify the responsible agent has convinced us that our initial enthusiasm was unwarranted and the assignment of the name renopressin was premature.

We have set aside the purification of renopressin and are concentrating our efforts on the purification of antigen M. It would seem that the purification of the latter substance would teach us the nature of renopressin if it is similar to antigen M and if it does indeed play a role in hypertension.

We have made substantial strides in our purification of antigen M. Our best preparations have been purified many fold by affinity chromatogra-

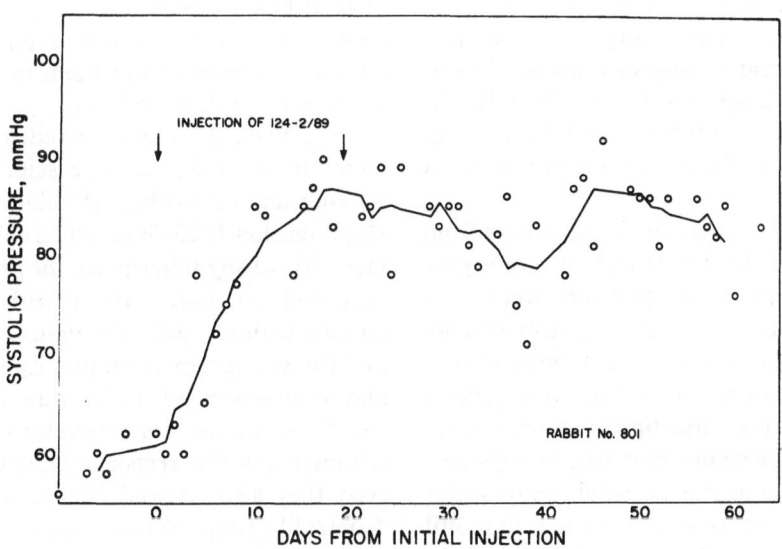

Fig. 2.

phy and isoelectric focusing. Unfortunately, such preparations still contain at least 12 antigens that cross react with immune serum.

We have recently embarked on an indirect approach. We are attempting to isolate a hybridoma that will produce the blood pressure-lowering antibody. In order to accomplish this, the lymphocytes of mice immunized with hog antigen M are fused with mouse myeloma cells. Hybrid clones are screened for antibodies that react with kidney antigens by the ELISA method. Promising preparations are then tested for their blood pressure-lowering effect in hypertensive rabbits. The discovery and production of such an antibody will allow us to isolate antigen M by affinity chromatography, or, when appropriately labeled, it would permit us to discover its locus within the kidney itself.

Dr. Dzau (Boston, Mass.): Dr. Skeggs' comments that renin does not play a role in initiation of experimental renovascular hypertension have left me a little confused. In my opinion, there is very convincing experimental evidence that renin is pathogenetic in the initiation of experimental renovascular hypertension, whereas the factor(s) responsible for the maintenance of hypertension is not characterized. In recent experiments that Dr. Haber et al [Dzau VJ, Kopelman RI, Barger AC, Haber E (1980) Science 207: 1091] conducted in one-kidney Goldblatt dog, purified renin-specific antibodies or Fab fragments to pure canine renin completely restored blood pressure to normal during the initiation phase of hypertension. Furthermore, recent experiments with peptide renin inhibitors performed by Drs. Cody and Burton in our laboratory also demonstrated similar effects at this stage [Burton J, Cody RJ Jr, Herd JA, Haber E (1980) Proc Natl Acad Sci in press] Dr. Skeggs, could you elaborate a little on your first statement?

Dr. Skeggs: I think there are some papers from Missouri by Dr. J. O. Davis and his colleagues in which they demonstrated that they were completely unable to block the development of one-kidney hypertension in dogs, and I think also in rats. Dr. Dzau, do you recall those two papers?

Dr. Dzau: Yes, these investigators infused saralasin or converting enzyme inhibitors to dogs during the acute phase of experimental renovascular hypertension. Hypertension did not develop until the fourth or fifth day of infusion of the blocking agents. They interpreted the data as evidence that

hypertension could develop in the absence of renin. I agree with this; however, the 4-day delay in the development of hypertension suggests to me that they have prevented the acute renin-dependent phase, and that the chronic phase of hypertension is nonrenin dependent and can develop in spite of renin blockade.

Sir George Pickering (Oxford, England): I would like to ask Dr. Tobian if he can tell me one single piece of good evidence for ascribing the rise in blood pressure that occurs when primitive people leave their tribes and join the police or army to their intake of sodium chloride. I have visited these primitive peoples, and the differences between their way of life and our own are absolutely enormous. I believe that these psychosocial differences are the most important ones, and these influences are also relevant to the studies reported by Folkow with his spontaneous hypertensive rats.

Dr. Tobian (Minneapolis, Minn.): Concerning those particular things you mentioned, there is no real proof. I think any of the population studies are in and of themselves no absolute proof of anything. There are a couple of studies where you had two comparable primitive groups. One of them cooks its food in sea water and the other does not. One gets its share of hypertension and the other does not. And they are about equally primitive. Dr. Lot Page described this. And I think Dr. Lowenstein studied a couple of Amazon tribes that seemed about equally primitive. One ate a low-salt diet and the other did not. The higher salt intake of one tribe induced a greater amount of high blood pressure. But, by themselves, these studies alone wouldn't provide any convincing evidence. You have to put them in the context of a whole lot of other evidence.

Dr. Folkow (Göteborg, Sweden): I have a comment on what Sir George said. Quite recently, Falkner and co-workers [Falkner B. et al. (1979) Hypertension 1: 23–30] studied children from families with strong inheritance for primary hypertension and compared them with children from families without such inheritance. It was then clear that the youngsters from predisposed families displayed exaggerated heart rate and pressor responses to the alerting stimulus of forced mental arithmetic, in this respect stimulating SHR. However, they also showed another difference in the "control" group. When both groups were given an extra 10 g NaCl/day, beyond what they normally use, those from hypertensive parents showed a modest pressure rise but the others hardly did. So there too, I think, the influence of both psychosocial and salt-intake "environmental" elements, superimposed on a genetic predisposition, seems to be illustrated in man. It might be so, however, that the salt effect is merely a secondary effect of a "primary" central neurohumoral effect on the renal handling of salt.

Dr. Meyer (Paris, France): A word to Dr. Tobian about our measurements of catecholamines in "R" and "S" strains of rats. After a 2-week sodium loading, there is a twofold increase in plasma catecholamines measured in "basal" condition both in "R" and "S" rats, but in reaction to a stressful condition (noise). In agreement with what you showed, plasma norepinephrine is remarkably higher in the "S" rats. I think this means that in addition to the genetic and environmental interaction, there may be a slight effect of sodium *per se.*

Dr. Tobian: I am thinking along those same lines. J. Iwai reported in New Orleans that the "S" rat has higher catecholamines in the hypothalamus, and it rises inordinately higher on high-salt diets. I don't know what higher catecholamines mean, but he did find that they were higher in "S" rats.

Dr. Logan (Toronto, Canada): Dr. Cowley, did you do sodium-balance studies in your 30-day vasopressin infusion experiments? Furthermore, did you give them sodium load to see if they had an exaggerated natriuresis?

Dr. Cowley (Milwaukee, Wis.): We did sodium-balance studies in all of these dogs, and they continued to progressively lose sodium for at least 2 weeks. As a matter of fact, the few that we have taken 3 or 4 weeks continued to be in a slight negative state of balance. It is very difficult to get them back into balance. They just start spilling sodium, and eventually they get back into balance; but, by 2–3 weeks, they are still slightly negative. We did not try to salt stimulate the animals or salt load them.

Dr. Boyd (Hobart, Australia): Dr. Skeggs, I too have puzzled for a long time about what it is that sustains the chronic phase of renal hypertension. I also took the view that it might be humoral and looked for other forms of renin and found them. But I am not sure that they answer the question about the nature of chronic hypertension even so, and it seems to me now that the maintenance phase of any hypertension may occur

almost independently of what initiated it. And the one factor common to all forms of chronic hypertension is the elevated blood pressure itself. Surely, after all this time, we have learned something from Dr. Folkow, namely, that hypertension when sustained will eventually lead, through structural arteriolar changes, to a maintenance of itself. Now as Dr. Folkow well knows, I don't happen to agree with him about the way in which these changes are mediated, but I think we should have learned by now that his general mechanism is very important. Because of it, it no longer seems to me necessary to postulate a very active continuing humoral drive in the chronic phase of renal or, indeed, of any other form of chronic hypertension.

Dr. Laragh (New York, N.Y.): Dr. Cowley, we gave vasopressin infusions to ourselves and to normal volunteers when Dr. Frank Goodwin was with us, first intravenously and then intramuscularly for up to a couple of weeks [Goodwin FJ, Ledingham JGG, Laragh JH (1970) Clin Sci 39: 641]. We didn't see any hypertension either. But we did observe rather impressive hyponatremia and some hypokalemia too together with lowered renin values. What I wonder is, what happened in your dog model to plasma or urine aldosterone and to plasma renin with continued vasopressin infusion?

Dr. Cowley: Unfortunately, we don't have aldosterone in the study that I showed you. We do have aldosterone from the study in which we reduced renal mass and then infused vasopressin too; those were running about half normal throughout the period of vasopressin infusion and the renins were suppressed to values under the technically measurable point.

Dr. Laragh: But you don't have it in the normal animal?

Dr. Cowley: No.

Dr. Laragh: I could answer the question that Dr. Logan asked. I think the answer is that it is known that in the presence of vasopressin and adequate water intake, you can have a tremendous rejection of saline in both humans and animals. Leaf et al. [Leaf A, Bartter FC, Santos RF, Wrong O (1953) J Clin Invest 32: 868] described the so-called vasopressin natriuresis some years ago and then Norman Levinsky and his group characterized it in the dog. The other question I want to ask Dr. Yamori is, are there differences in plasma renin levels in the stroke-prone SHR as opposed to other SHR?

Dr. Yamori (Izumo, Japan): It is very interesting

that the renin levels of the stroke-prone SHR are much increased at an advanced stage, maybe because of the kidney lesions. The renin levels become tremendously higher in symptomatic stroke-prone SHR and this begins well before the stroke occurs [Matsunaga M, Yamamoto J, Akira H et al. (1975) Jpn Circ J 39: 1305].

Dr. Laragh: So the stroke-prone SHR have tremendously higher renin than the nonstroke. This, to me, raises the possibility of renin involvement in pathogenesis of the stroke just as it seems to be involved in the encephalopathy of renal clip hypertension, so well described by Byrom [Byrom FB (1969) The Hypertensive Vascular Crisis. An experimental study. London, Heinemann].

Dr. Yamori: No significant increase is noted at a young age when stroke-prone SHR quickly develop severe hypertension, but after the age of 5 months, plasma concentration of renin, carefully determined on the blood obtained through indwelling catheters from nonstressed conscious stroke-prone SHR, becomes higher. In these stroke-prone SHR with high-plasma renin, arterial lesions such as arterionecrosis is noted in the kidney. Therefore, the increased level seems to be secondary, but may further aggravate cerebrovascular lesions. However, the higher renin levels clearly precede the onset of stroke. In contrast, some stroke-resistant substrains have "low-renin hypertension," showing a lower renin level when they develop spontaneous hypertension at a young age.

Session 13
Hypertension, Vasopressors, and the Susceptibility to Vascular Injury

Chairman: E. Muirhead

Position Paper: Hypertension, Vasoconstriction, and the Causation of Cardiovascular Injury: The Renin-Sodium Profile as an Indicator of Risk

John H. Laragh

It is recognized that for any hypertensive population there is a greater risk of premature illness and death from cardiovascular complications, in particular, heart attack and stroke. Notwithstanding, it is becoming increasingly evident that this risk is not equally distributed among people with similar elevations of blood pressure.

The clinical expression of this inequality in risk is exemplified by the well known observation that some patients with striking elevation of blood pressure enjoy uncomplicated longevity even though they disdain all therapy while some others with much less hypertension die prematurely. In the original Veterans Administration Study (1), it was evident that most of the subjects included in the untreated control group with severe diastolic hypertension survived the five-year trial period without serious problems. Other studies have shown that tobacco, obesity, hyperlipidemia, age, and target organ damage greatly enhance the risk of hypertension and conversely that their absence can greatly reduce it (2).

Because of the inability to pick out those who are at risk among similarly hypertensive people, we have been more or less forced to treat everybody to protect what may be a small minority (3).

The heterogeneity of natural history and prognosis among people with similar degrees of hypertension is in keeping with the concept that so-called essential hypertension represents a group of disorders involving different pathophysiologic mechanisms. This concept suggested by clinical and epidemiologic observations, has gained considerable support from biochemical, physiologic, and pharmacologic research. Over the past 20 years pathophysiologic differences have been identified which can be related to variations in drug response, clinical course, and susceptibility to lethal cardiovascular damage among patients with similar degrees of high blood pressure.

At the core of this development has been the exposure and definition of the renin-angiotensin-aldosterone hormonal system as a normal control mechanism for regulating blood pressure and sodium balance (4, 5) and the subsequent demonstration of a major participatory role for this system, not only in unusual forms of hypertension but also in most essential hypertension (6, 7). This research shows that patients with hypertension can be profitably analyzed and treated with reference to a biochemical profile called the renin-sodium profile (6, 8). A close correlation between the plasma renin activity value and its contribution to the blood pressure level has established that renin measurements are, in fact, a direct measure of renin-induced vasoconstriction (7). Renin measurements have taken on a clear physiologic relevance: when referenced to the urinary sodium excretion they allow an evaluation of the appropriateness or normalcy of the renin activity (i.e. the renin-sodium profile) (see also Session 7).

I propose that the presence or absence of renin system vasoconstrictor activity might provide an index of risk more physiologically oriented than are traditionally employed risk factors. In fact, earlier research on this question (6, 8, 9) convinced us that renin-sodium profiling, by revealing different mechanisms among hypertensive patients, might be a useful and clinically valuable indicator of prognosis and of variations in risk. Subsequent research has supported this.

In this discussion, I will first restate our hypothesis about plasma renin activity as a pathogenic factor in cardiovascular damage and an indicator of risk. I will then review the supporting evidence from collateral lines of research in animals and humans. I will next consider the classical "pressure hypothesis" and some of what is known about the relationship of blood pressure to cardiovascular injury. Finally, I will review a group of findings that relate basic physiologic differences to the presence or absence of renin activity. These differences suggest that low-renin patients have much better flow and tissue perfusion than do equally hypertensive high-renin patients. With this in hand I will attempt to synthesize the relevance of this information to the problem of vascular injury and propose what I think are frontier areas for future research.

RESTATEMENT OF THE HYPOTHESIS THAT RENIN-VASOCONSTRICTION IS A FACTOR IN VASCULAR INJURY IN HYPERTENSIVE PATIENTS

As a result of our research we have proposed (8) that:

> In untreated patients, a medium or high plasma renin level, assessed in relation to the 24-h urinary sodium excretion (i.e., the renin profile), defines a risk factor which directly or indirectly makes these patients more prone to develop a heart attack or a stroke than are equally hypertensive low-renin patients.

We did not conclude that renin-angiotensin itself necessarily causes strokes or heart attacks, but we do interpret our data to indicate that, for two patients with equal degrees of hypertension, the one with a greater degree of vasoconstriction as induced by angiotensin is more likely to develop cardiovascular damage (i.e. stroke or heart attack). While heart attacks and strokes may involve different primary pathophysiologic mechanisms, angiotensin probably works its harmful influences via the pathologic accompaniments of undue and protracted vasoconstriction, hemoconcentration, increased viscosity, tissue ischemia, and impaired microcirculatory flow (9).

This proposal was based at first on our largely retrospective study of 219 patients with essential hypertension in which we found highly significant differences in the frequency of heart attacks and strokes within three subgroups classified to their renin-sodium profiles (8). Thus, we observed no strokes or heart attacks in the first 59 consecutive low-renin hypertensive patients while, at the same

time there was an incidence of 11% and 14%, respectively among the 160 patients with either normal or high renin-sodium profiles.

These results were the more convincing because the low-renin patients were significantly *older* and actually had *higher* blood pressure levels than did the normal renin patients—two situations that in themselves are associated with increased incidence of heart attacks and strokes.

Since our first report, information has accumulated that gives greater strength to the conclusions (10, 11). More data has been collected relating to the degree, lability, and severity of low-renin hypertension. There was, for example, the outside possibility that our low-renin patients simply had hypertension of lesser duration or greater lability, or that they might have been more responsive to drug therapy. However, new evidence on these questions confirms that low-renin patients are truly *more* hypertensive than are normal-renin patients, are not more "labile," and can be at least as difficult to normalize with drugs. Moreover, while proof of this is hard to come by, they perhaps have had their hypertension for at least as long as the normal-renin patients, since most studies have verified that the low-renin patients as a group are significantly older than normal-renin subjects.

Our own continuing observations in over 600 hypertensive subjects confirm our initial impressions. In the first 100 consecutive low-renin patients we observed only one minor myocardial infarction. We are now beginning to see strokes in low-renin patients, but with a frequency approaching that of the other subgroups only at a significantly older age level.

For these reasons we remain convinced that low-renin patients are less prone to cardiovascular damage than are medium- or high-renin patients. We also believe the converse to be true: that high-renin patients have the worst prognosis. It is clear by now that malignant hypertension with its attendant vasculitis is caused by excess renin activity (4–6). It is also generally agreed that patients with renovascular hypertension have a poor prognosis; the disease often becomes malignant and is generally accompanied by greater vascular damage at a younger age (12, 13). Indeed, most investigators would probably agree that any clinical form of high-renin hypertension, including high-renin essential hypertension, has the greatest proclivity to cardiovascular complications and the poorest prognosis. However, high-renin hypertensive patients often have greater elevations of blood pressure, too, so that one could argue that more pressure and not renin is the culprit. The question of pressure's contribution is eliminated, however, when low-renin and medium-renin patients are compared, because medium-renin patients are equally or less hypertensive. Are they more at risk than low-renin patients? Our data indicates that they are.

In summarizing the proposal that plasma renin activity is a factor in vascular injury, I would stress once again that our group accepts and recognizes the body of evidence indicating that the higher the blood pressure, the greater the risk of cardiovascular damage. Our work was begun with this correlation firmly in mind. What we suggest is that for a given similar degree of hypertension the presence, as opposed to the absence, of excessive renin-vasoconstriction makes a difference pathophysiologically. Or, stated another way, a hypertensive subject with sustained vasoconstriction (most often due to renin activity) is worse off than is an equally hypertensive subject with less vasoconstriction and therefore comparatively better microcirculatory flow and tissue perfusion. The latter situation seems to obtain in low-renin essential hypertension.

Accordingly, our working hypothesis on this problem is based on the conception that all high blood pressure is not alike in mechanism and therefore in its propensity to cause vascular damage. I will come back to the pathophysiologic differences between low and high renin states in a later section. However, collectively, the data raise the pathophysiologic question, is hypertension with better flow less damaging (9)?

MINIMUM CRITERIA FOR TESTING THE RENIN-VASOCONSTRICTION-HYPOTHESIS FOR VASCULAR INJURY

In immediate reaction to our original study, a flurry of counterclaims appeared in which the relationship of renin levels to vascular injury was disputed. Indeed in one such report low-renin patients were the ones found ostensibly to be at significantly greater risk. The claims and counterclaims of these reports have been extensively analyzed elsewhere

(11). Most of the studies were flawed by serious methodologic problems involving inadequate renin assay methodology, lack of any reference to sodium balance, absence of normal controls, and failure to stop antihypertensive drugs.

However, acceptable laboratory methods are more available now, and it is possible to design more meaningful prospective studies. In this context then, what then are the minimum criteria for a valid test of the renin hypothesis?

First of all, patients should be "profiled" in the baseline untreated state or after they have been off all antihypertensive drugs for a minimum of 3 weeks. This is because most antihypertensive drugs affect plasma renin levels and/or sodium balance (6) and some of these drugs are only slowly eliminated after cessation of therapy.

Secondly, a renin method should be used that can tell low from normal values. It is our belief that the only reliable way to achieve this goal is to employ a method (14) which uses the acid pH optimum for renin during incubation of plasma and in which angiotensinase inhibition is complete to allow the incubation to be prolonged up to 18 h for greater sensitivity. Methods such as that of Haber et al. (15) that incubate without pH control for only 3 h and use BAL, which inhibits renin activity (16), instead of either DFP or PMSF are inadequate (see also Sessions 7 and 9).

Thirdly, to evaluate the appropriateness of the renin measurement the value must be indexed against the concurrent 24-h rate of sodium excretion used as an index of sodium balance (6, 8, 14) and compared with similarly indexed measurements in normotensive controls (see Session 7).

With these approaches in hand, an additional requirement is to compare the incidence of stroke and heart attack in relation to the renin profiles in patients of similar age ranges who have similar degrees of hypertension. Only in this way can a valid study of renin as a risk factor be made.

EVIDENCE SUPPORTING THE RENIN HYPOTHESIS

Nevertheless, a growing body of evidence implicates renin as a risk factor. A sizeable portion comes from animal studies indicating that an induced renin excess in relation to sodium balance can result in cardiovascular damage, particularly in the heart, brain, and kidneys. Space does not allow a comprehensive review of this evidence. It has been previously reviewed (6, 8, 17), but some salient and newer aspects of it are summarized in Table 1 (18–39).

Thus, there is a growing body of clinical evidence to relate plasma renin activity to vascular injury (Table 1). The case begins with studies showing that human malignant hypertension is caused by an abnormal renal-adrenal interaction causing excess renin and aldosterone secretion (4, 5). This condition is associated with diffuse vascular damage and fibrinoid change. Significantly, the entire syndrome can be reversed by specific antirenin therapy with propranolol (33), which suppresses renin secretion and thereby corrects the hypertension and the hyperaldosteronism and leads to healing of the vascular damage. The syndrome can also be reversed with other drugs that block the renin system, i.e., saralasin (40) which blocks the action of angiotensin II, and converting enzyme inhibitors which block its formation (34–36). The case for renin's culpability is also supported by numerous clinical studies showing that

Table 1. Experimental and clinical evidence for the vasculotoxic potential of renin system activity.

1. In animals, renin injections cause vascular damage in the heart, brain and kidneys (18, 19, 20).
    a. This is amplified by giving aldosterone (21, 22).
    b. It is prevented by sodium deprivation (19).
2. Aldosterone (or DOC) excess in animals lowers renin levels (23, 24) and causes vascular damage which develops at a slower rate (24, 25). This hypertension is amplified by renin or angiotensin administration (26, 27), is prevented by sodium deprivation (28, 29) and is partially corrected by vasopressin blockade (30, 31).
3. Stroke-prone SHR have markedly higher plasma renin levels which appear several months before the stroke (32).
4. In human malignant hypertension either total nephrectomy (5) or propranolol (33), or converting enzyme inhibitor treatment (7, 34–36) can reverse the syndrome and lead to healing of vascular lesions.
5. Human (12, 13) or animal (37) renovascular hypertension is often associated with vascular damage and malignant vasculitis.
6. Patients with renal artery graft closure (6) or with a renin-secreting tumor (38) have marked vascular damage affecting the brain, heart and kidneys.
7. Saralasin withdrawal in humans can be followed by rebound hyperreninemia, hypertension, acute encephalopathy, and coma (39).

total nephrectomy can reverse the malignant syndrome, normalize the blood pressure, and lead to healing of the vascular disease as shown by biopsy (6).

Complementing this research on malignant hypertension is the finding that patients with curable renovascular hypertension due to renin excess are also more prone to malignant vasculitis with vascular damage in the brain and heart (12, 13). Moreover, there is an increasing awareness that high-renin essential hypertension, too, seems associated with more vascular sequelae, a stormier course, and a shorter survival.

Many other clinical situations associated with high plasma renin levels are accompanied by striking vascular damage, stroke, or heart attack. These include patients with scleroderma (41), renal trauma, acute closure of a renal artery graft (6), or a renin-secreting tumor (38). After the use of the angiotensin II blocking agent, saralasin, as a diagnostic test, four patients with renal hypertension and hyperreninemia developed marked rebound hypertension with encephalopathy in two and coma in one (39). Since saralasin induced a marked increase in renin levels, it is likely that the rebound encephalopathic crisis was related to failure of hyperreninemia to subside following drug withdrawal.

Finally, in studies of patients with common untreated essential hypertension, evidence from yet another line of research has emerged that is relevant to the vascular injury problem (7, 34–36). This research has demonstrated that, contrary to an older opinion, renin-induces vasoconstriction which actively participates in maintaining all or part of the elevated blood pressure in about 70% of patients with essential hypertension (7, 34). This includes the high-renin and most normal-renin patients. At the same time a relative lack of renin-induced vasoconstriction in the 30% of patients with low-renin essential hypertension was shown. This proof of the active participation of renin in essential hypertension has evolved from a research series using pharmacological probes that block the renin system. All these agents produce parallel effects on blood pressure that are directly related to the pretreatment plasma renin level. The probes employed were the beta blocker, propranolol, which lowers renin secretion (33), then the angiotensin II receptor antagonist, saralasin (40). Finally, the converting enzyme inhibitors, first the nonapeptide, teprotide (7, 34–36), and more recently its orally active analog, captopril (35), were used to block the formation of angiotensin II (see also Session 7).

This research utilizing blockade of the renin system at different points also establishes that a properly measured plasma renin measurement can have explicit physiologic meaning because it reveals how much renin-induced vasoconstriction is involved in supporting the blood pressure. Accordingly, plasma renin measurements can be used to evaluate renin participation in the blood pressure of each patient and, when this value is referenced (i.e., "profiled") against sodium excretion, the appropriateness or normalcy of this participation can also be assessed. This information provides the physiological basis for the clinical use of renin-profiling to analyze pathophysiologic participation of the system in hypertension. At the same time it defines the lack of participation of renin-induced vasoconstriction in low-renin patients.

Altogether then, the evidence indicates that the gamut of high-renin forms of hypertension are associated with more cardiovascular damage. Our research also suggests that the more subtle excesses of plasma renin as they occur in essential hypertension might induce cardiovascular damage over a protracted period of time, in contrast to that which occurs more abruptly in the flagrant forms of hypertensive disease (see Table 1). This important issue obviously deserves more thought and study.

Until something better comes along, the existing evidence nominates the renin-sodium profile as a simple procedure for baseline definition of all patients, not only to rule out surgically curable renal or adrenal cortical causes, but to plan the strategy of drug treatment (42) (see also Session 7). Moreover, in terms of the present discussion, since the test accurately reflects renin-induced vasoconstriction, it is also a valid research tool for defining differences in hypertensive mechanisms and relating them to differences in clinical course and prognosis.

PRESSURE PER SE IN CARDIOVASCULAR DAMAGE: THE PRESSURE HYPOTHESIS AS OPPOSED TO THE RENIN HYPOTHESIS

An elevated pressure, if great enough, might damage any vascular structure. It is therefore not surprising that a large literature testifies to the fact that experimentally induced increases in blood pressure can disrupt a blood vessel (43). Moreover, there are data from certain human (44–46) and animal studies (17, 43, 47) indicating that the malignant phase of hypertension occurs or can be induced when the blood pressure increases beyond a critically high level. In this situation arteriolar necrosis develops, especially in those beds exposed to the high pressure, whereas the vasculature beyond the induced constriction is protected. It also appears that beyond a critically high pressure level "breakthrough" of autoregulation occurs (48) so that the resistance vessels are no longer able to constrict in response to the elevated blood pressure. Instead they give way, transmitting the high pressure load to the more distal and more fragile vasculature, where a blowout occurs.

Accordingly, published research in a number of animal models has described a good correlation between the height of blood pressure and the degree of vascular injury produced or observed. However, this does not necessarily mean that the high blood pressure *per se* is the critical or the only factor in causing vascular damage.

Moreover, it may not be appropriate to extrapolate to long-term situations in human subjects what has been observed mostly in acute or short-term animal studies. It is well known that chronic high blood pressure produces adaptive changes in the vascular wall, specifically, hypertrophy which reduces the lumen to wall ratio (49) and may substantially raise the breakthrough point for autoregulation. That this occurs has been suggested by research in hypertensive subjects (50) and experimental models (43).

Furthermore, many of the acute studies in animal models that have been used to support the pressure hypothesis have employed vasoconstrictor substances to induce the high pressure, usually renin-angiotensin or adrenergic agents. This type of study establishes that administration of vasoconstrictors can induce vascular damage correlated to the degree of hypertension. However, the issue rarely is addressed as to whether or not a similar degree of hypertension induced by volume expansion would produce commensurate vascular injury.

There is another, and perhaps even more important, criticism of the "pressure hypothesis." Many hypertensive patients and animal models exhibit and tolerate extremely high blood pressure levels without vascular damage. Moreover, the converse is also true, since marked vascular damage can occur in a variety of clinical and experimental situations at blood pressure levels well below what is thought to be critical. These compelling observations strongly suggest that factors in addition to an elevated blood pressure may be necessary to induce vascular damage.

Actually, a number of experiments suggest that vascular damage in hypertensive or in normotensive situations may be more closely related to the induction of hypovolemia, with compromised flow and ischemia of the tissues. This impression is supported by observations both in animals (51) and in humans (52) which indicate that malignant hypertension due to renin excess actually can be remitted by saline infusions. These infusions, even though they may raise the blood pressure, improve flow and relieve hypovolemia and ischemia. Recent studies have defined two animal models in which sustained hypertension is actually induced or maintained by sodium depletion (53) and is corrected by saline administration (54). This broadens the evidence suggesting that sodium depletion and consequent reduced flow can be critical factors for inducing vasoconstriction and hypertension.

Despite the association of high plasma renin levels with many hypertensive situations in the clinic and laboratory, most advocates of the "pressure hypothesis" refute a role for renin in vascular damage by citing two situations in which vascular damage occurs with renin either blocked or absent. However, both of these situations are ambiguous. For example, the first type of study shows that when the pressor actions of renin are offset by the concurrent administration of a vasodilator drug such as hydralazine vascular damage does not occur (55). But this really proves nothing, because at the same time the arterial pressure was also reduced, restoring adequate blood flow and creating an entirely different situation.

The second circumstance invoked to discredit the role of renin in vascular damage is the DOCA-salt hypertension model (23, 24). In this model vascular damage develops in association with massive sodium retention and a reactively low plasma renin level. However, it should be recognized that the vascular damage produced by DOC takes much longer to develop than does that induced by renin. In the final analysis, DOC damage is probably also associated with ischemia and reduced flow in consequence of slow edematous deterioration of the vascular wall (24). Actually,

it has been shown that onset of the malignant syndrome in DOCA-salt rats usually follows paroxysms of natriuresis (24) with resultant hypovolemia, high viscosity, lowered blood flow, and tissue ischemia. Furthermore, there is now good evidence that both the hypertension and the malignant syndrome of DOC-salt hypertension are sustained by abnormal vasoconstriction caused by excessive vasopressin release (30, 31).

Möhring and associates have further defined the key role of renin in the malignant vasculitis of experimental renovascular hypertension and have nicely demonstated the beneficial effect of sodium administration (51) in inducing remissions, presumably by restoring flow and suppressing renin. In this model, too, like the DOC model (24), onset of the malignant phase was preceded by natriuresis with hemoconcentration and by higher renin levels, while pressure levels remained unchanged. Accordingly, in both the DOC-salt and renin-induced renovascular models the findings suggest that sodium depletion with hypovolemia, reactive vasoconstriction, resultant poor flow, and tissue ischemia may be critical in precipitating vascular injury. Altogether, the data also show that severe vascular injury can occur in the absence of renin, as in the DOC model, but that very likely another vasoconstrictor agent, vasopressin, is critically involved instead.

These experiments and others indicate that renin is not necessary for vascular injury to develop in the presence of hypertension. However, before one can conclude that the cause is then purely pressure, it must be shown that other vasoconstrictor substances besides renin (e.g., vasopressin or catecholamine hormones) are not involved.

Meanwhile, the available evidence suggests that severe vasoconstriction, with its attendant adverse effects, even in the absence of any hypertension, may be a key prerequisite for inducing vascular damage. Such vasoconstriction leads to translocation of fluid from the vascular to the interstitial spaces, hypovolemia, hemoconcentration, higher blood viscosity, and finally to ischemia from reduced tissue flow particularly to the microcirculation. This helps explain the many clinical and experimental situations in which vascular damage occurs at pressure levels well below the so-called critical range. It might also explain results from numerous clinical trials in which successful antihypertensive therapy failed to protect from myocardial infarction (1, 56–63). In all such studies diuretic therapy was a part of the regimen (see also Session 1). Such therapy would be expected to lower pressure at the price of reducing effective volume and flow and inducing reactive renin-vasoconstriction. Conversely, protection from myocardial infarction has been regularly demonstrated in those clinical trials employing beta blockade alone (see Session 1); for example, the large Göteborg trial (64) involving 7,500 subjects. This form of drug therapy can be expected to suppress the vasoconstriction mediated by renin (33, 65). Accordingly, more research seems appropriate on the question of whether compromised *flow* or elevated pressure is the more critical determinant in causing cardiovascular damage.

PATHOPHYSIOLOGICAL DIFFERENCES BETWEEN LOW- AND HIGH-RENIN PATIENTS AND THEIR RELEVANCE TO DIFFERENCES IN CARDIOVASCULAR DAMAGE

In view of the possibly better prognosis proposed for low-renin as compared with high- and medium-renin patients, it is worth considering what might be the pathophysiological basis for this difference. As already indicated the presence of an inappropriate or absolutely increased plasma renin level is now known to be accompanied by sustained vasoconstriction due to angiotensin II (7). Conversely, in low-renin essential hypertension which appears significantly less prone to heart attack and stroke, there is little or no evidence for vasoconstriction due to renin activity while at the same time other evidence suggests that these patients are relatively more expanded with respect to sodium and volume. The latter evidence derives from a tabulation of all published space measurements presented in Table 2 (42), which shows that low-renin hypertensive patients exhibit the highest extracellular fluid and blood volumes and high-renin the lowest. The concept that low-renin patients have a relative volume excess is also supported by the gamut of clinical parameters indicating hemodilution and overfilling (9, 10, 66) and by numerous observations showing that low-renin patients are the most responsive to sodium-volume depletion therapy in terms of correction of their blood pressure (65).

What might be the pathophysiologic basis for the difference in prognosis of low-renin patients? The various parameters expressing proposed or known physiologic differences between equally hypertensive low- and high-renin patients are summarized in Table 3. Low-renin patients have increased peripheral resistance, to be sure, but the vasoconstriction which characterizes this form of hypertension is relatively less for a given degree of hypertension. That is to say that for a given degree of hypertension there is higher flow (i.e., higher cardiac output) and higher volume in low-renin patients. It is implied that greater vasoconstriction and greater increases in peripheral resistance, associated with renin activity, lead to poorer flow for a given level of hypertension and that this compromised flow to the microcirculation may well predispose to tissue ischemia and reduced ability to recover from vascular insult.

While more research is needed to define fully the suggested physiologic differences among patients within the various renin subgroups, many of the postulated differences shown in Table 3 have been demonstrated. Thus, patients with low-renin hypertension have evidence of hemodilution, exhibiting relatively lower blood urea, hematocrit, and hemoglobin values than medium- or high-renin patients (10). In a more recent computer analysis of 735 untreated patients with essential hypertension similar significant differences in hematocrit, hemoglobin, and total protein values were again observed (66). These data are in keeping with what the vasoconstriction-volume model predicts, i.e., that low-renin patients are relatively hemodiluted and volume expanded (see also Session 7).

In an analysis of a smaller subgroup of high- and low-renin patients studied under metabolic ward conditions, Brunner and his colleagues (10) demonstrated that, at three different levels of sodium intake, high-renin patients exhibit comparatively higher blood urea values than do either the normal- or low-renin patients. The data showed that at the high sodium intake BUN values of the high-renin patients never fell below 10 mg%. And for all three renin subgroups, BUN levels were inversely related to sodium intake, the lowest levels consistently seen during sodium loading and the highest during sodium depletion. It was noteworthy, however, that the low-renin patients exhibited, at all sodium intakes, the lowest mean urea levels; the difference during a normal sodium

Table 2. Body fluid volumes in essential hypertension.

	N	Low-renin group	N	Normal-renin group	p
A. Plasma volume					
1. Helmer et al. (1968) Circulation 38: 965	8	117%[a]	12	105%[a]	NS
2. Jose et al. (1970) Ann Intern Med 72: 9	5	1.53 L/M²	7	1.28 L/M²	>0.05
3. Woods et al. (1969) Arch Intern Med 123: 366	9	31 ml/kg	5	30 ml/kg	NS
4. Schalekamp et al. (1974) Lancet 2: 308	17	2.7 L/1.73 M²	38	2.65 L/1.73 M²	NS
5. Distler et al. (1975) Research on Steroids, North Holland-Elsevier	17	1.71 L/M²	17	1.57 L/M²	<0.025
6. Tarazi (1976) Circ Res 38 (Suppl II): II-73	13	33.4 ml/em+	26	26.2 ml/em[b]	<0.001
7. Weidmann et al. (1977) Am J Med 62: 209	15	110%[a]	48 (8)	102%[a] (92%) (high-renin patients)	<0.05 (<0.02)
B. Extracellular fluid volume					
1. Jose et al. (1969) Arch Intern Med 123: 141	11	9.6 L/M²	36	9.5 L/M²	NS
2. Jose et al. (1970) Ann Intern Med 72: 9	6	9.6 L/M²	7	7.7 L/M²	<0.01
3. Schalekamp et al. (1974) Lancet 2: 310	12	11.2 L/1.73 M²	29	11.1 L/1.73 M²	NS
C. Exchangeable sodium					
1. Woods et al. (1969) Arch Intern Med 123: 366	9	37.9 mEq/kg	5	32.3 mEq/kg	<0.05
2. Lebel et al. (1974) Lancet 2: 308	12	95%[a]	33	98%[a]	NS
3. Distler et al. (1975) Research on Steroids, North Holland-Elsevier	18	1609 mEq/M²	15	1549 mEq/M²	NS
4. Padfield et al. (1975) Lancet 1: 548	23	101%[a]	42	98%[a]	NS

[a] Figures given expressed as % normal control.
[b] Figure given is total blood volume calculated from plasma volume.

intake was statistically significant at the 5% level (Fig. 1).

In a recently completed study Drayer et al. (63) compared 27 age and sex matched untreated high- and low-renin patients with 27 normotensive people. They found that the low- and high-renin patients had similarly elevated systolic and diastolic blood pressures. However, the low-renin patients as a group had higher creatinine clearances and lower blood urea, uric acid, hemoglobin, hematocrit, and total protein values. These data describe once again the tendency toward hemodilution and volume expansion in low-renin patients as compared to high-renin patients, a tendency also reflected by a range of routine clinical measurements.

Complementing these observations are older findings that a high hemoglobin concentration is a risk factor for stroke: the incidence of cerebral infarction is doubled for men over 15 g and women over 14 g (67). A recent study shows that cerebral blood flow and alertness is inversely related to hematocrit and plasma viscosity, even for hematocrit and viscosity values within the normal range (68).

All available data from space measurements are in keeping with these impressions. As mentioned above a tabulation (42) of all reported studies from the world over (Table 2) reveals that the total blood volumes and extracellular fluid volumes of low-renin patients are, almost without exception, as high or higher than those of the normal-renin patients. Moreover, low-renin patients also have

Table 3. High blood pressure mechanisms.

Relatively Predominant Features

High renin (vasoconstricted)		Low renin (less vasoconstricted)

Arterioles

High renin (vasoconstricted)		Low renin (less vasoconstricted)
Higher	Peripheral resistance	High
High	Aldosterone	Low to high
Low	Plasma volume	High
Low	Cardiac output	High
High	Hematocrit	Low
High	Blood urea	Low
High	Blood viscosity	Low
Low	Tissue perfusion	High
Yes	Postural hypotension	No

Clinical Examples

High renin essential Renovascular and malignant		Low renin essential Primary aldosteronism

Vascular sequellae

High renin		Low renin
(+)	Stroke	(−)
(+)	Heart attack	(−)
(+)	Renal damage	(−)
(+)	Retinopathy–encelphalopathy	(−)

Treatments

No	Diuretics	Yes
Yes	Antirenin drugs	No
Yes	Direct vasodilators	±
Yes	Adrenergic blockers	±

Source: Laragh (9).

a larger central blood volume (69). And the converse is also true: When hypervolemia is present in hypertensive patients, renin values are considerably reduced. Moreover, high-renin patients in the one reported comparison study have the lowest plasma volumes (70).

In future space studies, account should be taken of the general relationship that plasma volumes tend to be lower in all hypertension (71). Moreover, patients with similar degrees of hypertension but different renin values should be compared while sodium balance is rigorously controlled. Great attention should also be paid to errors inherent in space measurement while also recognizing that the critical arterial volume is an unmeasurable fraction of total blood volume (see also Session 7).

A real problem with blood volume and other space measurements has been the lack of a meaningful reference standard. When these measure-

ments are related to height, weight, or surface area (Table 2), extremely broad normal ranges are found, leading to a large error in identifying possible abnormalities. More recently, a detailed study (72) has shown that this error can be greatly reduced when multiple samples are obtained and when the derived values for individuals are related instead to the degree of variation from ideal weight.

A CONCEPTUAL BASIS FOR FUTURE RESEARCH

Altogether, these findings indicate basic pathophysiologic differences between equally hypertensive low- and high-renin patients. In view of companion data suggesting attendant differences in susceptibility to vascular damage and in prognosis, the picture suggests that hypertension with more

MEAN BLOOD UREA NITROGENS
IN THE THREE RENIN SUBGROUPS

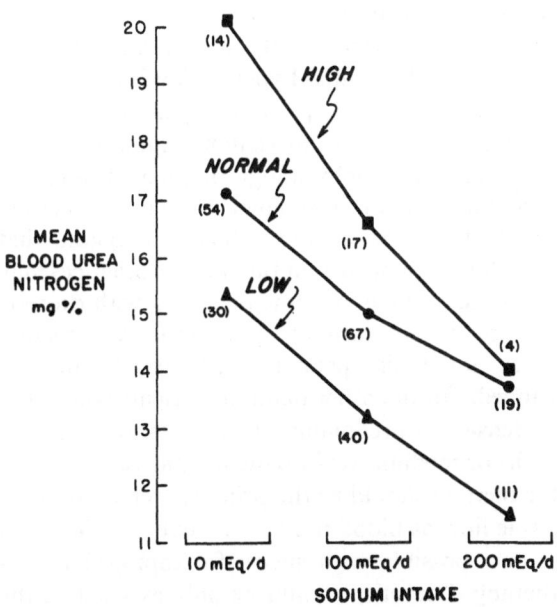

Fig. 1. Mean blood urea nitrogen levels of the low (▲) normal (●) and high (■) renin groups determined at constant dietary sodium intakes of 10,100 and 200 meq/day. Numbers in parenthesis represent the number of patients studied. Independent of sodium intake, low renin patients consistently exhibit the lowest blood urea nitrogen levels. [From Brunner et al. (10).]

vasoconstriction and compromised flow is a situation with increased risk. Conversely, the data suggest a minimal risk of vascular damage and premature death if hypertension is associated with adequate perfusion of the tissues and better microcirculatory flow. Accordingly, critical differences in *flow* amongst equally hypertensive patients may be the basis for critical differences in risk. Future research should be directed to test this hypothesis and define more precisely the basis for the adverse influence of renin-induced vasoconstriction or that of sustained vasoconstriction caused by other humoral agents.

That vasoconstrictor influences other than renin may also participate in essential hypertension is suggested by the finding that fully one third of patients with low-renin essential hypertension are not normalized by volume depletion. In this subset, it is possible that another vasoconstrictor influence, perhaps mediated in this case by the adrenergic nervous system with local release of norepinephrine, may be involved, suppressing renin secretion. Renin-sodium profiling places each patient in an analytical framework that makes the pursuit and further analysis of this hypothesis possible (see Section 7).

The data collected make it extremely unlikely that so-called essential hypertension is a single entity. This becomes especially apparent at the extremes of the vasoconstriction-volume spectrum where gross pathophysiologic differences and gross differences in pharmacologic response are easily demonstrated. Such information also suggests that a modification of current therapeutic practices may be in order. Thus, volume depletion with diuretic therapy seems entirely appropriate for treating those low-renin patients who are volume-expanded. On the other hand, in patients whose hypertension is predominantly vasoconstrictor (e.g., high- or medium-renin patients) antivasoconstrictor therapy should be the primary step to improve tissue flow as blood pressure is reduced. This goal is now possible with successful captopril monotherapy. Diuretics should be only avoided as the first step and added when it is clear that reactive sodium retention has superimposed an unwanted volume factor. Indeed, diuretic therapy as an initial step in the more vasoconstricted high- and medium-renin patients actually might have an adverse effect by further reducing already compromised volume and flow, thereby leading to reactive increases in renin-vasoconstriction.

It follows, too, from this analysis that it is proba-
bly inappropriate and premature to advise universal curtailment of dietary sodium for every patient with hypertension. This might produce undesirable hemoconcentration in patients who are already vasoconstricted (i.e., the medium- and high-renin patients). Directing primary treatment at the particular pathophysiologic mechanism, i.e., renin-vasoconstriction as opposed to sodium-volume depletion, makes long-term therapy simpler and more physiologic.

SUMMARY

Among hypertensive patients the greater risk of cardiovascular damage (i.e., heart attack, stroke and premature death) is not evenly distributed, nor is it necessarily related to the degree of hypertension. Accordingly, in the light of accumulating clinical and laboratory data we have reexamined the proposition that renin-sodium profiling of hypertensive patients identifies different pathophysiologic patterns that are related to differences in their clinical course and prognosis. More specifically, the question has been reexamined of why low-renin patients might live longer and suffer fewer heart attacks or strokes despite equal or even greater degrees of hypertension than exhibited by patients with medium-renin levels.

Accumulating evidence supports the thesis that an absolute or inappropriate excess of renin-induced vasoconstriction is a risk factor predisposing to cardiovascular damage. Clinical studies show that the various forms of high-renin hypertension have the most vascular damage and the poorest outlook. At the same time studies using a series of pharmacologic probes show that the plasma renin activity value directly reflects active vasoconstriction as a supporting factor in the high blood pressure of most essential hypertension (high- and medium-renin patients). In animal models, too, the degree of hypertension is not necessarily related to the degree of vascular damage, but injections of renin regularly induce cardiovascular damage modified by sodium balance; and stroke-prone genetically hypertensive rats have higher prestroke plasma renin levels.

Other research suggests a pathophysiologic basis for the differences in risk of cardiovascular damage of low as opposed to high renin patients. For equal degrees of hypertension, low-renin patients appear less vasoconstricted: they exhibit greater plasma and extracellular volumes, they are hemodiluted as suggested by a broad range of indices, and they respond best to diuretic therapy. All of this implies better tissue flow for a given level of hypertension.

Collectively, this analysis indicates that so-called essential hypertension is not homogeneous. A promising frontier for future research will involve further analysis of the spectrum of inappropriate vasoconstriction-volume interactions which composes essential hypertension. In view of the evidence that something besides pressure level is critically involved in vascular injury, we need to learn more about how vasoconstrictor substances induce vascular damage at both the biophysical and the metabolic level. Besides reducing flow, vasoconstrictors may promote vascular injury by changing the form of the pressure wave. Following papers will consider these questions.

Meanwhile, notwithstanding the possible adverse mechanical effects of a high pressure *per se*, the data suggest that a hypertensive condition associated with more vasoconstriction as occurs in high- and medium-renin patients (and which might also result from other unidentified vasoconstrictors) is more vasculotoxic than is a similar degree of hypertension in which arterial volume and tissue *flow* is better maintained (i.e., low-renin essential hypertension). Currently, angiotensin is the most well-defined long-term mediator of vasoconstriction, but the analytical approach will enable the evaluation of the participation of other pressor substances such as vasopressin or norepinephrine.

It follows that whenever vasoconstriction is the predominant factor, the ideal primary therapy should employ agents to block this vasoconstriction and thereby allow better tissue *flow*. Conversely, when volume excess is the predominant mechanism sodium deprivation or diuretic therapy becomes the rational first step.

REFERENCES

1. Veterans Administration Cooperative Study Group on Hypertensive Agents (1970) Effects of treatment on morbidity in hypertension. II. Results in patients with diastolic blood pressure averaging 90 through 114 mmHg. JAMA 213: 1143
2. Gordon T, Sorlie P, Kannel WB (1971) In: Kannel WB, T Gordon (eds) Framingham Study: An epidemiological investigation of cardiovascular disease. Section 27, U.S. Dept. Health, Education and Welfare. National Institutes of Health, Bethesda, Maryland
3. Alderman MH (1981) The variation in risk among hypertensive patients: Is broad scale therapy to help only a few justifiable? What pressure levels should be treated? In: This volume, p 9
4. Laragh JH, Angers M, Kelly WG, Lieberman S (1960) Hypotensive agents and pressor substances. The effect of epinephrine, norepinephrine, angiotensin II and others on the secretory rate of aldosterone in man. JAMA 174: 234–240
5. Laragh JH (1960) The role of aldosterone in man: Evidence for regulation of electrolyte balance and arterial pressure by renal-adrenal system which may be involved in malignant hypertension. JAMA 174: 293–295
6. Laragh JH, Baer L, Brunner HR, Bühler FR, Sealey JE, Vaughan ED Jr (1972) Renin, angiotensin and aldosterone system in pathogenesis and management of hypertensive vascular disease. Am J Med 52: 633–652
7. Case DB, Wallace JM, Keim HJ, Weber MA, Sealey JE, Laragh JH (1977) Possible role of renin in hypertension as suggested by renin-sodium profiling and inhibition of converting enzyme. N Engl J Med 296: 641–646
8. Brunner HR, Laragh JH, Baer L, Newton MA, Goodwin FT, Bard RH, Bühler FR (1972) Essential hypertension: Renin and aldosterone, heart attack and stroke. N Engl J Med 286: 441–446
9. Laragh JH (1973) Vasoconstriction-volume analysis for understanding and treating hypertension: The use of renin and aldosterone profiles. Am J Med 55: 261–274
10. Brunner HR, Sealey JE, Laragh JH (1973) Renin as a risk factor in essential hypertension: more evidence. Am J Med 55: 295–302
11. Laragh JH (1978) Renin as a predictor of hypertensive complications: Discussion. Annal NY Acad Sci 304: 165–177
12. Perera GN, Haelig AW (1952) Clinical characteristics of hypertension associated with unilateral renal disease. Circulation 6: 349
13. Davis BA, Crook JE, Vestal RE, Oates JA (1979) Prevalence of renovascular hypertension in patients with grade III or IV hypertensive retinopathy. N Engl J Med 301: 1273–1276
14. Sealey JE, Laragh JH (1977) How to do a plasma renin assay. Cardiovasc Med 2: 1079–1092
15. Haber E, Koerner T, Page LB, et al. (1969) Application of a radioimmunoassay for angiotensin I to the physiologic measurements of plasma renin activity in normal human subjects. J Clin Endocrinol Metab 29: 1349–1355
16. Ryan MP, Weinberger MH (1980) Effect of sulphydryl reagents on the enzymatic activity of human renin: implications for renin assay. Clin Chim Acta 106: 135–143
17. Gavras H, Brunner HR, Laragh JH (1974) Renin and aldosterone and the pathogenesis of hypertensive vascular damage. Prog Cardiovasc Dis 17: 39–49
18. Winternitz MC, Mylon E, Waters LL, et al. (1939–1940) Studies on the relation of the kidney to cardiovascular disease. Yale J Biol Med 12: 623

19. Masson GMC, Aoki K, Deodhar ShD (1966) Course of hypertension during prolonged treatment with heterologous renin. Experientia 22: 531

20. Gavras H, Brown JJ, Lever AF, et al. (1971) Acute renal failure, tubular necrosis and myocardial infarction induced in the rabbit by intravenous angiotensin II. Lancet 2: 19

21. Masson GMC, Corcoran AC, Page IH (1951) Experimental production of a syndrome resembling toxemia of pregnancy. J Lab Clin Med 38: 213

22. Masson GMC, Mikasa A, Yasuda H (1962) Experimental vascular disease elicited by aldosterone and renin. Endocrinology 71: 505

23. Goodwin FJ, Knowlton AI, Laragh JH (1969) Absence of renin suppression by deoxycorticosterone acetate in rats. Am J Physiol 216: 1476–1480

24. Gavras H, Brunner HR, Laragh JH, Vaughan ED Jr, Koss M, Cote LJ, Gavras I (1975) Malignant hypertension resulting from deoxycorticosterone acetate and salt excess. Circ Res 36: 300–309

25. Selye H, Hall CE, Rowley EM (1943) Malignant hypertension produced by treatment with desoxycorticosterone acetate and sodium chloride. Can Med Assoc J 49: 88–92

26. Masson GMC, Corcoran AC, Page IH (1952) Renal and vascular lesions elicited by "renin" in rats with desoxycorticosterone hypertension. Arch Pathol 53: 217–225

27. Masson GMC, Corcoran AC, Page IH, Del Greco F (1953) Angiotensin induction of vascular lesion in desoxycorticosterone treated rats. Proc Soc Exp Biol Med 84: 284–287

28. Mulinos MG, Spingarn CL, Lojkin ME (1941) Diabetes insipidus-like condition produced by small doses of desoxycorticosterone acetate in dogs. Am J Physiol 135: 102

29. Relman AS, Schwartz WB (1952) Effect of DOCA on electrolyte balance in normal man and its relation to sodium chloride intake. Yale J Biol Med 24: 540

30. Möhring J, Möhring B, Petri M, Haack D (1977) Vasopressor role in ADH in the pathogenesis of malignant DOC hypertension. Am J Physiol 232: F260–F269

31. Crofton JT, Share L, Shade RE, Lee-Kwon WJ, Manning M, Sawyer WH (1979) The importance of vasopressin in the development and maintenance of DOC-salt hypertension in the rat. Hypertension 1: 31–38

32. Matsunaga M, Yamamoto J, Akira H, Yamori Y, Ogino K, Okamoto K (1975) Plasma renin and hypertensive vascular complications: An observation in the stroke-prone spontaneously hypertensive rat. Jpn Circ J 39: 1305–1310

33. Bühler FR, Laragh JH, Baer L, Vaughan ED Jr, Brunner HR (1972) Propranolol inhibition of renin secretion. A specific approach to diagnosis and treatment of renin-dependent hypertensive disease. N Engl J Med 287: 1209–1214

34. Case DB, Wallace JM, Keim HJ, Weber MA, Drayer JIM, White RP, Sealey JE, Laragh JH (1976) Estimating renin participation in hypertension. Superiority of converting enzyme inhibitor over saralasin. Am J Med 61: 790–796

35. Case DB, Atlas SA, Laragh JH, Sealey JE, Sullivan PA, McKinstry DN (1978) Clinical experience with blockade of the renin-angiotensin-aldosterone system by an oral converting enzyme inhibitor (SQ 14,225, captopril) in hypertensive patients. Prog Cardiovasc Dis 21: 195–206

36. Gavras H, Brunner HR, Laragh JH, Sealey JE, Gavras I, Vukovitch RA (1974) An angiotensin converting enzyme inhibitor to identify and treat vasoconstrictor and volume factors in hypertensive patients. N Engl J Med 291: 817–821

37. Byrom FB (1963) The nature of malignancy in hypertensive disease. Evidence from the retina of the rat. Lancet i: 516–520

38. Orjavik OS, Aas M, Fauchold P, et al. (1975) Renin secreting tumors with severe hypertension. Acta Med Scand 197: 329–336

39. Keim HJ, Drayer JIM, Case DB, Lopez-Ovejero JA, Wallace JM, Laragh JH (1976) A role for renin in rebound hypertension and encephalopathy after infusion of Sar¹-ala⁸-angiotensin II. N Engl J Med 295: 1175–1177

40. Brunner HR, Gavras H, Laragh JH, Keenan R (1974) Hypertension in man. Exposure of the renin and sodium components using angiotensin II blockade. Circ Res 34 & 35: Suppl. I: I-35–I-45

41. Gavras H, Gavras I, Cannon PJ, Brunner HR, Laragh JH (1977) Is elevated plasma renin activity of prognostic significance in progressive systemic sclerosis? Archives Intern Med 137: 1554–1558

42. Laragh JH, Letcher RL, Pickering TG (1979) Renin profiling for modern diagnosis and treatment of hypertension. JAMA 241: 151–156

43. Byrom FB (1969) The hypertensive vascular crisis: An experimental study. William Heinemann Medical Books Ltd., London

44. Heptinstall RH (1953) Malignant hypertension: a study of fifty-one cases. J Pathol Bacteriol 65: 423–429

45. Garner A, Ashton N, Tripathi R, Kohner EM, Bulpitt CJ, Dollery CT (1975) Pathogenesis of hypertensive retinopathy. Br J Opthalmol 59: 3–44

46. Pickering G (1968) High blood pressure, 2nd Edition. Churchill, London

47. Okamoto K, Yamori Y, Nagaoka A (1974) Establishment of the stroke-prone spontaneously hypertensive rat (SHR). Circulation Res 34 & 35 (Suppl I): I-143–I-153

48. Lassen NA, Agnoli A (1972) Upper limit of autoregulation of cerebral blood flow on the pathogenesis of hypertensive encephalopathy. Scand J Clin Lab Invest 30: 113–116

49. Folkow B (1971) The haemodynamic consequences of adaptive structural changes of the resistance vessels in hypertension. Clin Sci Mol Med 41: 1–12

50. Strandgaard S. Olsen J, Skinhøj E, Lassen NA (1973) Autoregulation of brain circulation in severe arterial hypertension. Br Med J i: 507–510

51. Möhring J, Petri M, Szokol M, Haack D, Möhring B (1976) Effects of saline drinking on malignant course of renal hypertension in rats. Am J Physiol 230: 849–857

52. Kincaid-Smith P, Fang P, Laver MC (1973) A new

look at the treatment of severe hypertension. Clin Sci Mol Med 45 (1): 75–87

53. Romero JC, Holmes Dr, Strong CG (1977) The effect of high sodium intake and angiotensin antagonist in rabbits with severe and moderate hypertension induced by constriction of one renal artery. Circ Res 40 (Suppl I): I-17

54. Seymour AA, Davis JO, Freeman RH, DeForrest JM, Rowe BP, Stephens GA, Williams GM (1980) Hypertension produced by sodium depletion and unilateral nephrectomy: A new experimental model. Hypertension 2: 125–129

55. Goldby FS, Beilin LJ (1972) How an acute rise in arterial pressure damages arterioles. Electron microscopic changes during angiotensin infusion. Cardiovasc Res 6: 569–584

56. Stewart IMcDG (1971) Long-term observations on high blood pressure presenting in fit young men. Lancet i: 355

57. Robinson SK (1972) Coronary artery disease and antihypertensive drugs. J Clin Pharmacol 12: 123

58. Stewart, IMcDB (1976) Compared incidence of first myocardial infarction in hypertensive patients under treatment containing propranolol or excluding β-receptor blockade. Clin Sci Mol Med 51: 509S-511S

59. Jones JV, Dunn FG, Fife R, Lorimer AR, Kellett RG (1978) Benzothiadazine diuretics and death from myocardial infarction in hypertension. Clin Sci Mol Med 55: 315S–317S

60. Morgan T, Adam WR, Hodgson M, Gibberd RW Failure of therapy to improve prognosis in elderly males with hypertension. Med J Australia (in press).

61. Smith WMcF (1977) Treatment of mild hypertension: Results of a ten-year interaction trial. US-PHS Hospital Cooperative Study Group. Circ Res 40 (Suppl 1): 98–105

62. The Australian therapeutic trial in mild hypertension. Report by the Management Committee (1980) Lancet i: 1261–1267

63. Helgeland A (1980) Treatment of mild hypertension; a 5-year controlled drug trial: The Oslo Study. Am J Med 69: 725–732

64. Berglund G, Sannerstedt R, Andersson O, Wedel H, Wilhelmsen L, Hansson L, Sivertsson R, Wilkstrant J (1978) Coronary heart disease after treatment of hypertension. Lancet i: 1

65. Laragh JH (1978) The renin system in high blood pressure, from disbelief to reality: converting-enzyme blockade for analysis and treatment. Prog Cardiovasc Dis 21: 159–166

66. Drayer JIM, Weber MA, Sealey JE, Laragh JH (1981) Low and high renin essential hypertension: A comparison of clinical and biochemical characteristics. Am Heart J (in press)

67. Kannel WB, Gordon T, Wolf PA, McNamara P (1972) Hemoglobin and the risk of cerebral infarction: The Framingham Study. Stroke 3: 409–520

68. Willison JR, Thomas DJ, deBoulay GH, Marshall J, Paul EA, Pearson TC, Russel RWR, Symon L, Wetherly-Mein G (1980) Effect of high haematocrit on alertness. Lancet 846–848

69. Esler M, Randall O, Bennett J, et al. (1976) Suppression of sympathetic nervous function in low-renin essential hypertension. Lancet 2: 115–118

70. Weidmann P, Hirsch D, Beretta-Piccol C, et al. (1977) Interrelations among blood pressure, blood volume, plasma renin activity and urinary catecholamines in benign essential hypertension. Am J Med 62: 209–218

71. Tarazi RC, Dustan HP (1972) Beta adrenergic blockade in hypertension. Am J Cardiol 29: 633

72. Feldschuh J, Enson Y (1977) Prediction of the normal blood volume—Relation of blood volume to body habitus. Circulation 56: 4

Vascular Compliance and Pulsatile Flow as Determinants of Vascular Injury

Roger F. Palmer

Many suggestions implicating "hydrodynamic forces" as determinants of vascular injury have been made. Unresolved questions concerning the exact hydrodynamic mechanisms involved are reflected in the clinical observations typified by the distribution of atherosclerotic plaques at arterial bifurcation points, the predominant involvement of terminal arterioles in arterial hypertension, and the distribution of lesions in coarctation of the aorta and other obstructive arterial disorders, etc. Some experimental work has focused on such factors as "shear forces," "turbulence," and vascular "stress." It is the purpose of this presentation to introduce the nature of forces generated by pulsatile flow as determinants of arterial injury, and perhaps quantitatively more important determinants than others previously discussed.

BACKGROUND

Certain clinical and animal observations suggested the importance of pulsatile flow in the propagation of dissecting aneurysm of the aorta. Palmer et al. in 1965 (1) first reported on the use of negative inotropic agents in the clinical treatment of acute dissecting aneurysm of the aorta in humans. These clinical studies were buttressed by observations in domestic turkeys that are ordinarily hypertensive and susceptible to dissecting aneurysms of the aorta. Original observations by Ringer (2) and subsequent observations by Simpson et al. (3) concluded that negative inotropic agents were beneficial in reducing the incidence of dissecting aneurysm in these flocks and potential inotropic agents increased the incidence, especially in β-aminopropionitrile (β-APN)-treated animals that have a mortality rate of perhaps 50% from dissecting aneurysm.

A representative observation of such dramatic effects occurs when propranolol is administered to "turkeys at risk," that is, animals fed β-APN. When 0.3% propranolol is introduced into their feed at birth or later, there is complete protection from aortic rupture, even though there is no effect on blood pressure or pulse rate (Table 1). Recent catheterizations of dogs or turkeys fed low doses

Table 1. Incidence of aortic rupture, blood pressure, heart rate, and aortic tensile strength of turkeys fed β-APN and various levels of propranolol (Inderal).

| Treatment (32 birds/diet) | Mortality rate (%) | Blood pressure* | | Heat rate (beats/min) | Aortic tensile strength (g/mm^2) |
		Systolic (mmHg)	Diastolic (mmHg)		
None	0[b]†	179[a]	136[b]	300[a]	111.8[b]
β-APN	46.8[a]	176[a]	143[a]	330[a]	40.0[a]
β-APN + 0.1% propranolol	0	148[b]	115[b]	210[b]	70.5[ab]
β-APN + 0.03% propranolol	3.2[b]	173[a]	133[ab]	300[a]	60.5[ab]
β-APN + 0.01% propranolol	41.9[a]	183[a]	146[a]	300[a]	54.8[a]
β-APN + 0.003% propranolol	37.5[a]	186[a]	150[a]	330[a]	47.3[a]

* Averages for four turkeys per diet.

† Values with different superscripts are significantly different ($p < 0.05$), according to Duncan's Multiple Range Test.

of propranolol demonstrate alterations in the shape of the pulse wave (reduction in dP/dt_{max}) in both species at doses that do not effect measured systolic or diastolic blood pressure (C. T. Simpson, unpublished observations).

IN VITRO MODEL AORTAS

A simulated model for dissecting aneurysm was created by layering stained rubber cement on the interior of a segment of Tygon tubing (4). The rubber cement, when dried, adheres loosely to the Tygon tubing and can easily be separated by any forces that would be operative in the genesis or propagation of dissecting aneurysm. The "intimal tear" can be produced by a knife (Fig. 1), and the simulated aorta can be attached to a pump capable of producing pulsatile or nonpulsatile flow as shown in Fig. 2. The rubber cement inner layer of the "aorta" does not separate unless pulsatile flow is introduced (Table 2), regardless of the systolic or diastolic pressure produced by the pump. (The pressure in the tubing is controlled by a resistance clamp at the end of the tubing.) The rate of dissection per pulse is a function of the rate

of rise of the initial phase of the pulsatile flow pressure (dP/dt_{max}) (Fig. 3), and the dissection occurs both in the direction of flow and retrograde as in the human counterpart. An explanation for these observations is depicted in Fig. 4, where, under nonpulsatile flow conditions, a driving force (pressure gradient) does not exist over the susceptible area in which early separation of the rubber cement lining from the Tygon tubing occurs. However, under pulsatile flow conditions, a temporary pressure gradient exists both in the forward and in the retrograde susceptible segment. The pressure gradient ΔP_A is greater if the pressure profile is steepest (increased dP/dt_{max}). Such an analysis explains separation of the rubber cement lining in a direction opposite to flow. An explanation for how negative inotropic agents decrease mortality in turkeys is thus afforded. If such drugs decrease the steepness of the wave-form (decrease in dP/dt_{max}), then the pressure gradient over the susceptible area would be less, decreasing the forces that would tend to separate the layers as depicted in Fig. 4.

CALCULATION OF WAVE-FORM AVERAGE ENERGY

Symmetrical sound waves have been analyzed in terms of their average energy (5). It has been found that the energy *(E)* of a wave-form is the product of the following relationship:

$$E = k\frac{A^2}{T^2}$$

where A is the amplitude of the wave, T is the period of the wave or distance between troughs, and k is a constant. Derivation of the equation yields:

$$-dE = 2K\frac{A}{T^2}dA - 2K\frac{A^2}{T^3}dT$$

By substituting numerical values of physiologic parameters (e.g., A in mmHg and T in fractions of a second), a solution for energy changes can be made as depicted in Fig. 5. By holding one variable constant (either A or T), one can assess the relative contribution of each to the energy

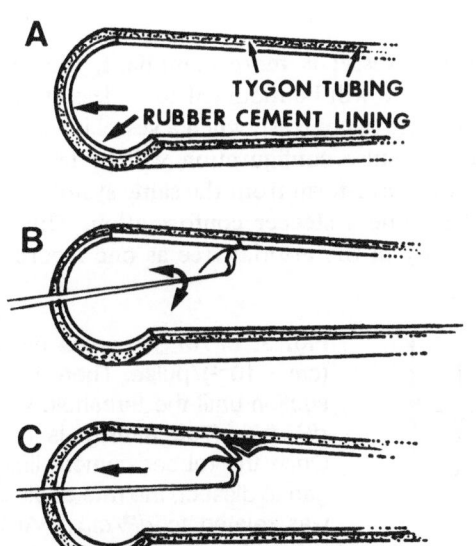

Fig. 1. Tygon tubing layered internally with rubber cement to create an "intimal lining" *(A)*. A small incision is made to represent an "intimal tear" *(B)*. The layer is gently separated to create an area of susceptibility where dissection may take place *(C)*.

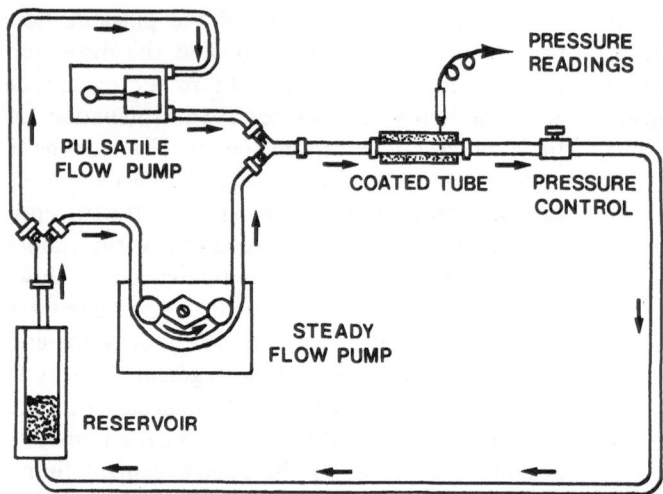

Fig. 2. Schematic drawing of apparatus used for subjecting the standard model of an aorta with the intimal tear to nonpulsatile and pulsatile flows. Pulsatile flow was generated by a Harvard pulsatile blood pump. Steady flow was produced by a Sarns pump. The pressure readings were measured by a Statham physiologic pressure transducer and recorded on a Grass polygraph. The pressure control consisted of a clamp which changed the resistance to flow by changing the diameter of the tube.

Table 2.

Flow	No. tubes	Avg. forward rate of dissection at constant rate (cm/min)	Range
Nonpulsatile	97	0.0	–
Pulsatile	97	1.87	(0.38–5.7)

change over the appropriate physiologic ranges of A or T.

It is apparent from the analysis that the energy change is affected to a much greater extent when T is varied. T corresponds to the steepness of the wave-form or loosely related to dP/dt_{max}. A simplistic conclusion to the aforementioned analysis would be that a decrease in the average energy of a wave-form is best accomplished by a decrease in the period of the wave or: steeper waves have more energy. If the steepness of a wave-form can be modulated to a less steep form, either by increasing vascular compliance or reducing the rate of ejection, less energy would have to be absorbed by the confining structures.

ROLE OF VASCULAR COMPLIANCE IN DETERMINING SHAPE OF PULSE WAVE

When a vessel is more compliant, the recorded pulse wave will be modified to a "less steep" conformation; in contrast, when a vessel is less compliant, the pulse configuration will be less damped and the wave-form from the same systolic ejection will assume a steeper conformation. This occurs normally in the arterial tree as one records from

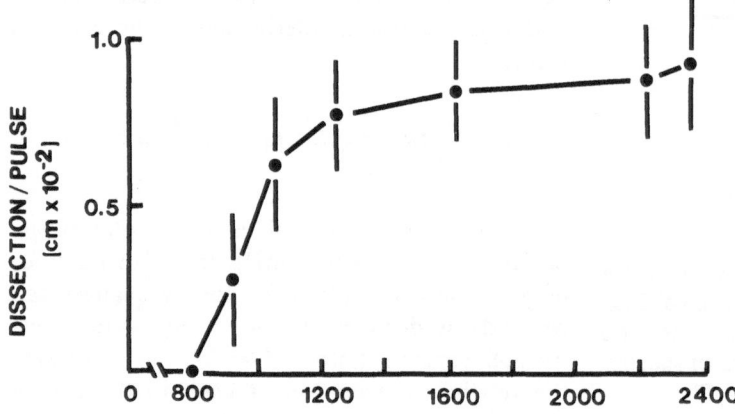

Fig. 3. dP/dt_{max} versus dissection (cm · 10^{-2})/pulse. There is no dissection until the threshold value for dP/dt_{max} (790 mmHg) is reached. Once the rubber cement lining began to dissect, the rate of dissection was related to dP/dt_{max}. At higher values for dP/dt_{max}, the rate of dissection reached a plateau, and there was a small change in dissection rate for large changes in dP/dt_{max}. Each point represents the mean rate of dissection for five experiments at the same dP/dt_{max}.

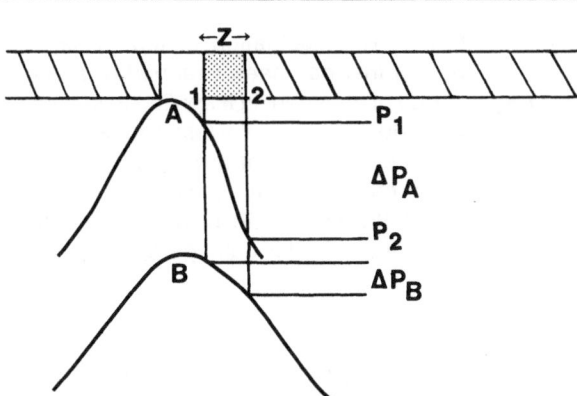

Fig. 4. Schematic representation of pressure curve in aorta: *A,* normal or increased pulse wave; *B,* modified or decreased pulse wave; *Z,* length of torn intima and media; P_1, pressure applied to aortic wall at point 1; P_2, pressure applied to aortic wall at point 2. Illustrates that if the pressure curve can be flattened as in *B,* the driving force ΔP_A will be less over the effective distance *Z.*

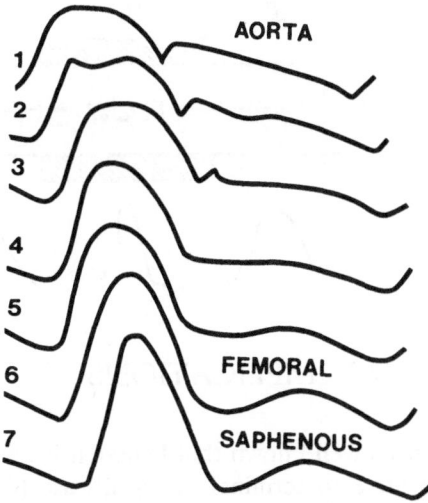

Fig. 6. Configuration of pulse waves in various portions of the arterial tree. As one examines the configuration, the pulse "steepness" increases as the vessel becomes less compliant.

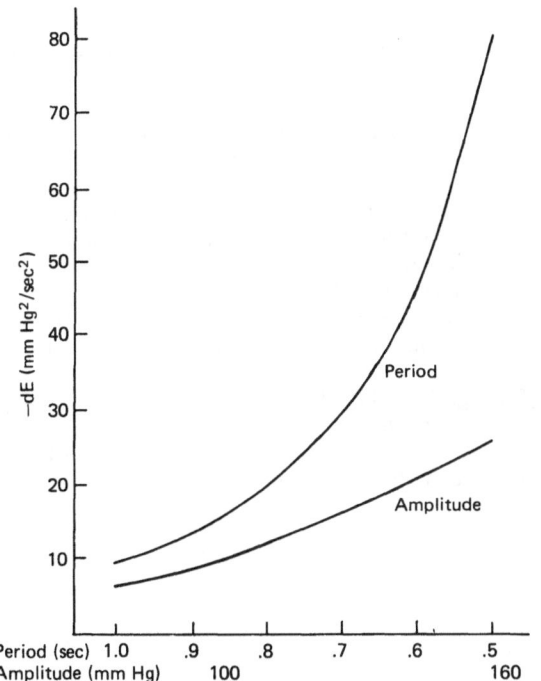

Fig. 5. Plot of the change in energy (mmHg²/s²) of an idealized wave when the amplitude (mmHg) is kept constant and the period (s) is varied *(upper curve),* and when the period is constant and the amplitude varied *(lower curve).* The period ranges 1–0.5 s, and the amplitude varies 100–160 mmHg. The change in energy of the system is negative.

a proximal portion (aorta) to a more distal portion (resistance vessels) (Fig. 6). It would be logical to assume that the less compliant vessel would absorb more energy from the prior analysis, and it is interesting to speculate that resistance vessels may suffer more damage because of their necessity to absorb more energy.

IMPLICATIONS AND FUTURE EXPERIMENTS

From the previously discussed observation and analysis, a general simplistic hypothesis can be formulated that would lend itself to experimental testing. This hypothesis can be generally stated: The less compliant a vessel, the more susceptible it is to hydrodynamic injury. Preliminary experiments indicate such to be the case. If an isolated portion of the femoral artery of a dog is wrapped to make it stiffer, or if a planchette of angiotensin II is applied to the isolated segment, the effect is to increase the steepness of the wave-form. The contralateral femoral artery is loosely wrapped so as not to influence the shape of the wave to serve as a control. In the wrapped segment, fragmentation of elastic tissue occurs and lipid deposition can be noted. Similar changes do not occur in either the proximal or distal segment (Fig. 7).

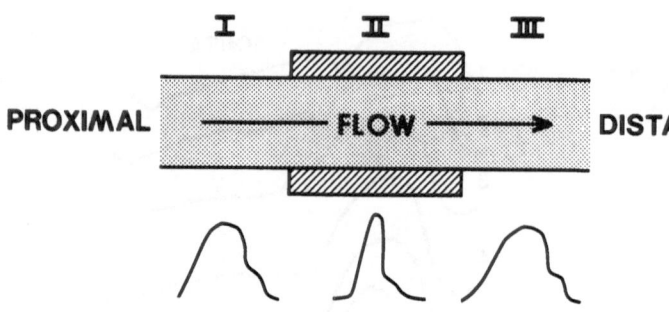

Fig. 7. Representation of femoral artery of dog that has been wrapped or a planchette of angiotensin II applied to segment II, rendering segment II less compliant. Beneath each segment are typical recorded pulse configurations. Only in segment II, where the pulse rate of rise is steepest, does any vascular damage occur.

CLINICAL IMPLICATIONS

It has been well known that hypertensive patients are sensitive to terminal artery disease (6). The terminal or resistances arterioles would be less compliant, creating a steeper, more energetic wave configuration. They would be responsible for receiving the brunt of the wave-form energy, and, therefore, suffer more injury. Reduction of either inotropic activity of the heart or the use of vasodilators should decrease the extent of injury, thereby decreasing vascular injury. Such experiments are in progress.

SUMMARY

A potential mechanism to explain vascular damage in hypertension and other clinical states is offered. The mechanism examined involves the nature of pulsatile flow, particularly the rate of rise of the pulse wave contour. Both experimental and theoretical observations are consistent with the conclusion that the more rapid the rate of intraarterial pressure (dP/dt_{max}), the more energy must be absorbed by the vascular wall and, consequently, the greater the potential degree of vascular damage.

Two factors contribute to the magnitude of the rate of rise; inotropic activity of the heart and compliance of the vessel (the rate of rise will be less in a more compliant vessel). These physical factors are discussed in clinical terms, particularly in the hypertensive state.

REFERENCES

1. Palmer RF, Seelman RC, Wheat MW Jr (1965) Pharmacologic approach to therapy of acute dissecting aneurysms of the aorta. Clin Res 13: 27
2. Ringer RK (1960) Aortic rupture, plasma cholesterol, and arteriosclerosis following Serpasil administration to turkeys. In: The second conference on the use of reserpine in poultry production (May 6, University of Minnesota, St Paul, Minn). CIBA, Summit, NJ, p 32
3. Simpson CT, Kling JM, Palmer RF (1968) Use of propranolol for protection of turkeys from development of aminopropionitrile-induced aortic ruptures. Angiology 19: 414
4. Prokop EK, Palmer RF, Wheat MW Jr (1970) Hydrodynamic forces in dissecting aneurysm. Circ Res 27: 121
5. Raleigh L (1945) The theory of sound, 1st American ed. Dover, New York
6. McDonald DA (1974) Blood flow in arteries. Williams & Wilkins, Baltimore, Md

Endothelial Injury in Hypertension

Stephen M. Schwartz and Donna M. Standaert

There are attractive reasons for considering the possibility that platelet mitogen released at sites of endothelial denudation accounts for the smooth muscle cell proliferation found in arteriosclerosis of hypertensive large and small arteries (1–3). The first question in this research is whether endothelial injury occurs. Endothelial injury is well documented in acute renal hypertension (4), and a number of studies have tried to identify a direct toxic effect of angiotensin II (5–8). This is supported by evidence that vasoactive agents are capable of opening cell junctions of postcapillary venular endothelium (9). This effect, however, is specific for these vessels and may relate to the incomplete junctional complexes seen only in the postcapillary venular endothelium (10). There have been reports that angiotensin II has a similar effect on the arterial endothelium. This effect is said to occur under conditions of normal or low blood pressure—thus suggesting a direct effect on endothelial contractility (7). We have confirmed the effect, but only see effects at doses sufficient to produce a marked elevation in pressure. Goldby and Beilin (5, 6) have similar data and were able to reproduce the effect by purely hemodynamic manipulation. Increased permeability to high-molecular weight plasma solutes has also been reported during the first few weeks of hypertension resulting from a variety of causes (4, 8, 11–15). There is no clear association with renin levels, and Gabiani and his collaborators (11) have suggested that the critical factor may be the plasma concentration of mineralocorticoids. In summary, injury does occur in acute hypertension. The effect may be purely hemodynamic, but the etiologic factors are poorly defined. As discussed below, evidence for endothelial injury in chronic hypertension is more limited.

Our work in acute hypertension is based on studies of endothelial cell turnover in the aortic endothelium of the rat. In the normal animal, the rate of turnover is very low, on the order of 1 cell/1,000/day (Fig. 1) (16). During acute renal hypertension, this rate increases by tenfold, as confirmed by Gabbiani and his coworkers (11). In contrast, we have been unable to find an increase in endothelial cell turnover either following acute hypertension induced by exposure to angiotensin II or evidence of loss of prelabeled endothelial cells when angiotensin was given following exposure of the animal to tritiated thymidine (Table 1). These data conflict with reports from Hladovec (17) that angiotensin II causes an increase in num-

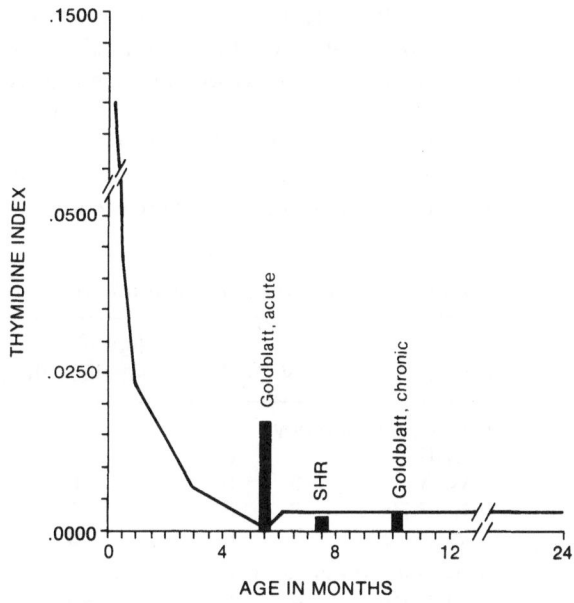

Fig. 1. Thymidine index as a function of age. Endothelial replication rates decrease with age to about 4 months, at which point thymidine index remains stable to 24 months. Superimposed on the curve are histograms for acute and chronic Goldblatt animals and SHR.

Table 1. Prelabeling experiment.*

Group	N	Thymidine index (%)
Controls	4	0.0022 ± 0.0005
Angiotensin II	4	0.0019 ± 0.0002

* Both groups given ³HTdR 24 h prior to infusion of either angiotensin II or saline.

ber of circulating endothelial cells. The significance of these data is made a bit more clear by some recent experiments in our laboratory on the response of the endothelium to removal of strips of endothelium only one- or two-cells wide. These strips are regenerated by cell spreading within 8 h, without cell replication. Thus, repair can occur by cell movement alone (18). Alternatively, our prelabeling study may label too few cells to allow detection of a small number of lost cells, or labeled cells may be lost at an equal frequency with the general population.

There is a second major open question about the animal models. The experiments discussed above studied changes occurring either during transient hypertensive episodes induced by vasoactive agents or during the first few weeks of onset of hypertension following experimental manipulation. These states may not represent reasonable models for the status of the endothelium in chronic, mild hypertension as seen in the majority of patients. This may be a very important issue given the current interest in the effects of mild hypertension on cardio- and cerebrovascular risk (19). The evidence, however, that there is endothe-

lial injury in chronic hypertension is unclear. In our studies of chronic two-kidney Goldblatt hypertension, we find no increase in replication (Fig. 1), nor is there a difference in replication between spontaneously hypertensive rats (SHR) and Wistar-Kyoto (WKY) rats (Table 2). Similarly, increased replication in acute hypertension with a return to normal values in chronic hypertension is seen in smooth muscle (20, 21). These data suggest that increased replication is an adaptive change associated with hemodynamic or humoral changes peculiar to acute hypertension. We may not, however, be secure in concluding that all chronic hypertension is free from accelerated endothelial turnover. As noted above, endothelial replication is the same in SHR and WKY rats. The usual caveat in this system is that the WKY rat may differ from the SHR in a number of alleles, independent of the presence of hypertension. We tried to side-step this dilemma by examining the effects of antihypertensive therapy on cell replication (Table 2). Antihypertensive therapy lowers replication in the SHR—although not in the WKY. It is unclear whether the treated SHR or the WKY represents a more reasonable control. Interestingly, the SHR released from therapy returns to the pretherapy replication rate, while the WKY actually overshoots. In summary, there are reasons to suspect that endothelial turnover is altered in genetic chronic hypertension in the rat. This is consistent with recent morphologic studies, which also show differences between the endothelium of the SHR and WKY systems (22, 23), although the effects of therapy have not yet been studied at the morphologic level.

Table 2. Spontaneous hypertension.

Strain	N	Sex	Age at sacrifice (mo.)	Duration of drug treatment (mo.)	Thymidine index (%)
I. Effects of therapy					
SHR	9	F	6	–	0.072 ± 0.008
WKY	5	F	6	–	0.060 ± 0.017
SHR Rx	8	F	6	4.5	0.027 ± 0.0038*
WKY Rx	7	F	6	4.5	0.088 ± 0.019
II. Effects of release from therapy					
SHR Rx	6	M	12	3	0.074 ± 0.016**
SHR RX/R	7	M	12	2[a]	0.220 ± 0.044**
WKY Rx	5	M	7	3	0.105 ± 0.012***
WKY Rx/R	7	M	7	2[a]	0.210 ± 0.038***

[a] Animals were released from treatment 1 month prior to sacrifice.
* Significantly different ($p < 0.05$) from all others in group I; ** $p \leq 0.001$; *** $p \leq 0.025$.

SUMMARY

A causal connection between hypertensive effects on endothelium and the increased risk of atherosclerosis is suggested by evidence for endothelial injury in hypertension and that this injury may be an initiating event in atherosclerosis. Endothelial injury, reflected by increased cell replication, occurs in renal hypertension of 3–5 weeks' duration. No increase in cell turnover is seen following a brief hypertensive episode induced by angiotensin II. Our studies of endothelial regeneration, however, show that the endothelium can repair transient, small areas of denudation by cell spreading without cell replication. Evidence of effects of chronic hypertension is more relevant; however, this evidence is unclear. Animals with chronic renal hypertension do not show elevated endothelial turnover, and turnover in WKY and SHR is the same. On the other hand, treatment with antihypertensive drugs lowers replication in SHR, but not in WKY rats. It is unclear whether the drug regimen may have a direct effect on endothelial replication in the hypertensive strain or whether the treated SHR represents a better normotensive control than WKY. If the latter is true, then the endothelium of SHR is subject to chronic injury, possibly explaining the subendothelial changes found in morphologic studies from other laboratories.

REFERENCES

1. Thorgeirsson G, Robertson AL (1978) The vascular endothelium: Pathobiologic significance. Am J Path 93: 804–848
2. Schwartz SM (1977) Hypertension, endothelial injury and atherosclerosis. Cardiovasc Med 2: 10: 991–1002
3. Ross R, Vogel A (1978) The platelet-derived growth factor. Cell 14: 203–210
4. Fernandez D, Crane WAJ (1970) New cell formation in rats with accelerated hypertension due to partial aortic constriction. J Pathol 100: 307–316
5. Goldby FS, Beilin LJ (1972) Relationship between arterial pressure and the permeability of arterioles to carbon particles in acute hypertension in the rat. Cardiovasc Res 6: 384–390
6. Goldby FS, Beilin LJ (1972) How an acute rise in arterial pressure damages arterioles: Electron microscopic changes during angiotensin infusion. Cardiovasc Res 6: 569–584
7. Robertson AL, Khairallah PA (1973) Arterial endothelial permeability and vascular disease: The "trap door" effect. Exp Mol Pathol 18: 241–260
8. Giese J (1973) Renin, angiotensin and hypertensive vascular damage: A review. Am J Med 55: 315–332
9. Majno G (1965) Ultrastructure of the vascular membrane. In: Hamilton WF, Dow P (eds) American Physiological Society—Handbook of physiology, Sect 2, Vol 3: Circulation. Williams & Wilkins, Baltimore, Md, pp 2293–2375
10. Simionescu N, Simionescu M, Palade GE (1978) Structural basis of permeability in sequential segments of the microvasculature of the diaphragm: I. Bipolar microvascular fields. Microvasc Res 15: 1–16
11. Gabbiani G, Elemer G, Guelpa C, Vallotton MB, Badonnel M-C, Hüttner J (1979) Morphologic and functional changes of the aortic intima during experimental hypertension. Am J Pathol 96: 399–423
12. Greditzer HG, Fischer VW (1978) A sequential ultrastructural study of different arteries in the hypertensive rat. Exp Mol Pathol 29: 12–28
13. Todd ME, Friedman SM (1972) The ultrastructure of peripheral arteries during development of DOCA hypertension in the rat. Z Zellforsch Mikrosk Anat 128: 538–554
14. Giacomelli F, Rooney J, Wiener J (1978) Cerebrovascular ultrastructure and permeability after carotid artery constriction in experimental hypertension. Exp Mol Pathol 28: 309–321
15. Suzuki K, Ookawara S, Ooneda G (1971) Increased permeability of the arteries in hypertensive rats: An electron microscopic study. Exp Mol Pathol 15: 198–208
16. Schwartz SM, Benditt EP (1977) Aortic endothelial cell replication: I. Effects of age and hypertension in the rat. Circ Res 41: 248–255
17. Hladovec J (1978) Circulating endothelial cells as a sign of vessel wall lesions. Physiol Bohemoslov 27: 140–144
18. Reidy MA, Schwartz SM (in press) Mechanism of endothelial repair after injury. Fed Proc
19. Hypertension Detection and Follow-up Program Cooperative group (1979) Five-year findings of the hypertension detection and follow-up program: I. Reduction in mortality of persons with high blood pressure, including mild hypertension. JAMA 242: 2562–2571
20. Wolinsky H (1970) Response of the rat aorta media to hypertension: Morphological and chemical studies. Circ Res 26: 507–522
21. Bevan RD (1976) An autoradiographic and pathologic study of cellular proliferation in rabbit arteries correlated with an increase in arterial pressure. Blood Vessels 13: 100–128
22. Limas C, Westrum B, Limas C (1980) The evolution of vascular changes in the spontaneously hypertensive rat. Am J Pathol 98: 357–385
23. Haudenschild CC, Prescott MF, Chobanian AV (1980) Effects of hypertension and its reversal in aortic intima lesions of the rat. Hypertension 2: 33–44

Hypertension-Induced Vascular Fibrosis and its Reversal by Antihypertensive Drugs

Sidney Udenfriend, George Cardinale, and Sydney Spector

It is generally accepted that neuronal and/or humoral (neurohumoral) factors play an important role in the initiation of hypertension and that the increase in blood pressure, if maintained for a length of time, results in a hypertrophy of the vasculature. The increased wall-to-lumen ratio in the vasculature leads to an increase in peripheral resistance. This initiates a cyclic process, for the increased peripheral resistance further aggravates the situation and blood pressure is elevated even more (1). Although there have been great advances in our understanding of both the etiology and therapy of hypertension, almost all of them concern the neuronal or humoral factors involved (i.e., renin, angiotensin, aldosterone, catecholamines, Na^+, etc.). However, the biochemical consequences in the vasculature due to elevated blood pressure have only recently begun to be studied.

Several years ago we began to utilize our existing methods for collagen biochemistry to determine whether the changes in elasticity and peripheral resistance were related to collagen. We soon discovered that we were not the first to ask that question. Wolinsky (2) had already shown a significant correlation between increased pressure and deposition of arterial collagen and elastin. Our subsequent studies (see below) in rats confirmed Wolinsky's findings and extended them to the dynamic state of collagen synthesis and degradation in isolated blood vessels, as well as to the levels of collagen-related enzymes. Those studies led to three important conclusions:

1) The increased blood pressure *per se* acts locally on the arterial bed (arteries and arterioles) to induce collagen biosynthesis (fibrogenesis) and hypertrophy.

2) Reducing the blood pressure to normal with antihypertensive drugs reduces fibrogenesis and hypertrophy.

3) Not only is collagen biosynthesis reduced by effective antihypertensive drug therapy, but if the normotensive state is maintained pharmacologically for a sufficient period of time, the fibrosis of the blood vessels may actually be reversed.

Some details of our animal experiments will be presented as well as relevant data from patient studies gathered from the literature to show that the vascular components of hypertension are, at certain stages, reversible by a limited period of treatment with antihypertensive drugs.

EXPERIMENTAL METHODS

Two animal models of hypertension were used, the spontaneously hypertensive rat (SHR) and the uninephrectomized DOCA-salt rat. Following the development of hypertension, blood vessels were isolated and subjected to several different assays indicative of collagen content and collagen biosynthesis. Four markers of collagen metabolism were monitored in minces or extracts of vascular tissues: prolyl hydroxylase activity; prolyl hydroxylase-related antigen; incorporation of ^{14}C-proline into collagen; and total tissue collagen based on hydroxyproline content. It should be noted that essentially all tissue hydroxyproline is present in collagen.

VARIATION OF ARTERIAL COLLAGEN SYNTHESIS WITH BLOOD PRESSURE

In both animal models, increased blood pressure was soon followed by a marked increase in collagen synthesis and deposition in the aorta and mesenteric artery (3). This was also true of brain and retinal microvessels (4). Changes in one of the collagen biosynthetic markers in blood vessels with increased blood pressure are shown in Table 1. Similar changes were observed in the other markers (5). When antihypertensive drugs were given prophylactically to prevent the increase in blood pressure, the increases in collagen biosynthesis were not observed. Furthermore, when antihypertensive drugs were given to animals that had been hypertensive for some time, arterial collagen biosynthesis was diminished concomitant with the fall in blood pressure (3). Information as to the nature of the pressure-induced biochemical lesion at the cellular level has been obtained by Ooshima (6) using immunohistochemical procedures to localize the enzyme prolyl hydroxylase in arteries.

In hypertension, only the arterial bed is subjected to the increased pressure. Since veins contain as large a proportion of collagen as arteries, it was of interest to compare collagen metabolism in the arterial versus the venous beds of hyperten-

Table 1. Prolyl hydroxylase activity of various blood vessels in DOCA-salt-treated rats and normotensive controls.

Model	Prolyl hydroxylase activity (cmp/mg DNA)
Brain microvessels	
Control	10,448 ± 490 (4)
DOCA-salt	14,437 ± 901* (4)
Pial artery	
Control	33,973 ± 2,218 (3)
DOCA-salt	45,794 ± 1,959** (3)
Basilar artery and circle	
of Willis Control	33,307 ± 2,116 (3)
DOCA-salt	44,573 ± 8,019 (3)
Testicular artery	
Control	14,917 ± 997 (5)
DOCA-salt	30,556 ± 1,767* (5)
Mesenteric artery	
Control	27,775 ± 3,123 (6)
DOCA-salt	54,269 ± 7,074* (6)
Aorta	
Control	10,912 ± 976 (10)
DOCA-salt	30,476 ± 3,507* (10)

For the smaller arteries, the values in parentheses represent the number of pools of tissue, each comprising four to ten rats. For the larger arteries, the values in parentheses signify the number of rats used. Enzyme activity is presented as ± SEM (*p < 0.01; **p < 0.05). Treated groups were compared to normotensive controls.
Source: Ooshima et al. (4).

Table 2. Arterial and venous collagen content in hypertensive rats compared to controls.

	Total collagen (mg/g tissue)	
Model	DOCA-salt	SHR
Aorta		
Control	97.4 ± 2.5	77.9 ± 1.0
Hypertensive	116.0 ± 2.1*	101.0 ± 5.9*
Mesenteric artery		
Control	80.8 ± 1.6	86.1 ± 3.3
Hypertensive	94.9 ± 2.2*	111.0 ± 5.8**
Vena cava		
Control	51.1 ± 2.8	71.5 ± 2.5
Hypertensive	57.3 ± 4.3	67.0 ± 1.7
Mesenteric vein		
Control	74.4	81.5
Hypertensive	73.1	83.8

Isolated vessels were homogenized and assayed for hydroxyproline, and their collagen content was calculated. Each value represents the mean ± SEM obtained from results in five rats (*p < 0.01; **p < 0.05). The values for the mesenteric vein could not be treated statistically for technical reasons.
Source: Iwatsuki et al. (7).

sive animals (7). As shown in Table 2, increased collagen metabolism is limited to the arterial bed. It was subsequently shown that when pressure is increased locally in the vascular bed by an experimental coarctation of the aorta, collagen deposition occurs in the area proximal to the constriction, where pressure is elevated (8). Distal to the constriction, pressure and collagen metabolism remain normal. Additional evidence of the direct effect of blood pressure on arterial collagen production has now been reported (9).

EFFECT OF AN INHIBITOR OF COLLAGEN CROSS-LINKING ON EXPERIMENTAL HYPERTENSION

The above studies demonstrated the effect of blood pressure on collagen synthesis. If the deposition of arterial collagen is a factor in raising blood pressure, then inhibition of collagen deposition should reduce blood pressure. To investigate this possibility, the specific inhibitor of collagen cross-linking, β-aminopropionitrile (β-APN) (10), was used (11). This compound has no acute effects on blood

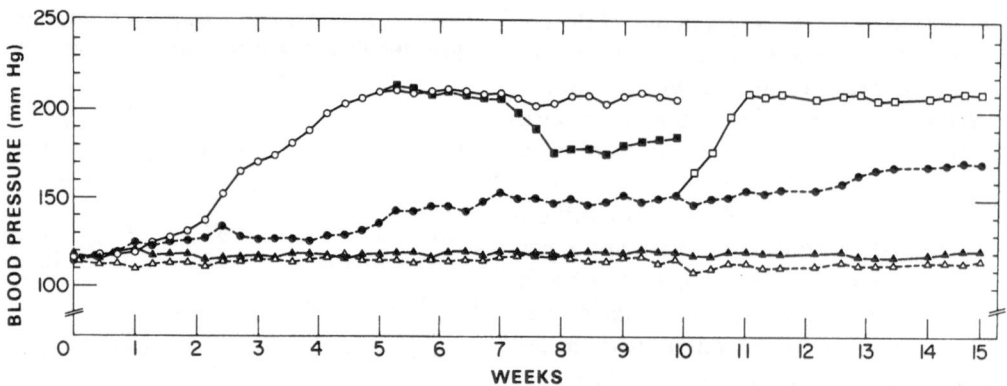

Fig. 1. Uninephrectomized male rats (12 weeks old) were given DOCA-salt (5 mg/kg) twice weekly and maintained on saline (O). After 5 weeks of DOCA-salt treatment. β-APN (100 mg/kg i.p.) was administered twice daily (■). Another group of rats was given the same dose of β-APN concomitant with the start of DOCA-salt treatment (●). After 10 weeks of the combined DOCA-salt treatment, the β-APN injections were stopped (□). Intact, normotensive rats (▲) and uninephrectomized normotensive rats given the standard dose of β-APN (△) served as controls. At 15 weeks, the remaining rats were killed and tissue collagen was measured. Each point represents the mean of values for at least three rats. [Iwatsuki et al. (11)]

pressure and, in adult animals, has little toxicity over the period of time used here. As can be seen in Fig. 1, β-APN blocked the severity of hypertension when given early and lowered the blood pressure in already hypertensive animals. When β-APN was discontinued, blood pressure gradually increased to pretreatment levels. The lowering of blood pressure by β-APN was paralleled by a reduction in arterial insoluble collagen content. These effects of β-APN were subsequently confirmed by Franklin and Morris (12) and Franklin (personal communication).

TURNOVER OF ARTERIAL COLLAGEN IN NORMAL AND HYPERTENSIVE RATS

Another way of monitoring changes in metabolism of a protein is by measuring its turnover. Collagen turnover was determined by administering a single dose of ^{14}C-proline to rats followed by large doses of unlabeled proline daily for several days to dilute the pool of free proline in the tissues to negligible levels and prevent relabeling (13). On the specified days, tissues were removed, hydroxyproline isolated, and specific activity determined. Under such experimental conditions, turnover can be assumed to be directly proportional to the rate of disappear-

ance of radioactivity from tissue hydroxyproline. The data in Fig. 2 are from DOCA-salt hypertensive rats and their controls. It can be seen that in normal animals, hydroxyproline (collagen) in arteries, skin, and tail tendon has a half-life of about 70 days. In hypertensive animals, the half-life of collagen in both the mesenteric artery and aorta was markedly reduced (16–20 days), but there were no changes in turnover of collagen in skin or tail tendon. Similar changes in collagen turnover were observed in the arterial bed of SHR as compared to their normotensive Wistar-Kyoto controls. The increased turnover of arterial collagen produced by hypertension is in agreement with the observed increases in collagen markers.

Since the turnover of a protein represents the balance of synthesis and degradation, it can be used to monitor the latter as well. The experiments with β-APN gave the first indication that vascular collagen is degradable. As shown in Fig. 1, when β-APN was administered to rats in which hypertension had been long established, a significant fall in blood pressure occurred. This took place over a period of about 3 weeks. In these rats, arterial fibrosis presumably had occurred and was a factor in maintaining the hypertension. The antihypertensive effect of β-APN, in this case, would best be explained by the continued degradation of arterial collagen following inhibition of its deposition.

Increased degradation of arterial collagen was

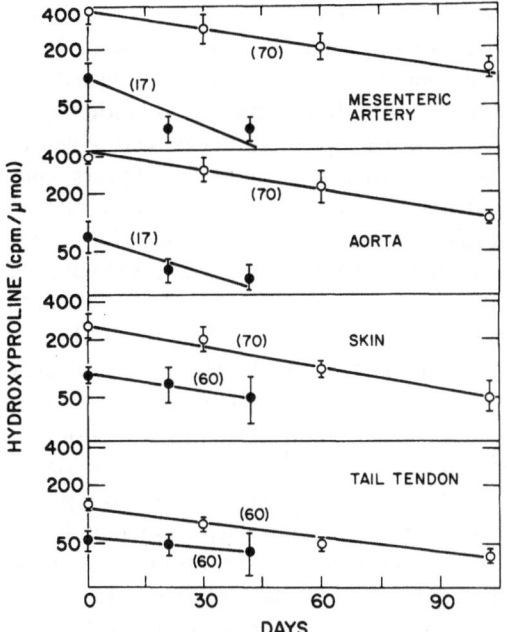

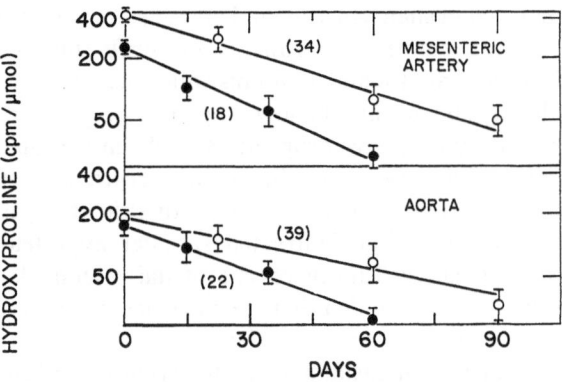

Fig. 3. Decay of tritiated hydroxyproline in arteries of untreated SHR and those treated with syrosingopine. Eight-week-old SHR were administered syrosingopine (650 μg/day p.o.) for 4 weeks. At this time, the blood pressure of the treated animals was normal and both groups were injected with 1 mCi L-[2,3-³H]proline, and the turnover measured as described in Fig. 2. ○, Treated, ●, hypertensive.

Fig. 2. Decay of tritiated hydroxyproline in several tissues of normotensive and hypertensive rats. Twelve-week-old normotensive and DOCA-salt hypertensive rats were injected with 1 mCi L-[2,3-³H]proline. During the next 12 days, all animals received 3 g unlabeled L-proline/day by subcutaneous injection. The rats were killed at the times indicated, and the specific activity of bound hydroxyproline was measured. Each point is the mean ± SD determined from three to five rats. The numbers in parentheses are the calculated half-lives in days for the various tissues. ○, Normotensive; ●, hypertensive. [Nissen et al. (13)]

and is responsible for a remodeling of "fibrotic" blood vessels.

DOCA-SALT RAT AS A MODEL OF PURE VASCULAR HYPERTENSION

It has long been known that when DOCA-salt is discontinued in uninephrectomized rats made hypertensive by the treatment, a large proportion of the animals remains hypertensive (14). Hypertension may continue in these animals for well over a year, although the original humoral factors (DOCA and salt) have been long gone and no other humoral factors have yet been detected to account for the sustained pressure. We have corroborated these findings on blood pressure and have found that arterial fibrosis is also maintained in such animals. Hollander (15) refers to this condition as hypertensive cardiovascular disease and reported that it is maintained indefinitely in rats treated for a relatively short time with DOCA-salt. In uninephrectomized rats treated with DOCA-salt for a limited time, the long-lasting residual hypertension may be maintained entirely through the vascular fibrosis and hypertrophy (i.e., "vascular hypertension"). We considered the possibility that the reversal of arterial fibrosis by antihypertensive therapy would be most readily

also deduced from the following turnover studies. SHR were treated with sufficient syrosingopine to lower blood pressure to normal and maintain it at that level for a time sufficient for markers of collagen biosynthesis to have returned to normal. As shown in Fig. 3, the half-life of arterial collagen in these, now, normotensive animals was indeed longer (ca. 36 days) compared to their still hypertensive counterparts. However, turnover was still far more rapid than in control normotensive animals (half-life ≈ 60–70 days) (see Fig. 2). The increased turnover of collagen in the absence of increased synthesis must be indicative of collagen degradation. Thus, the arterial fibrosis produced by hypertension appears to be reversible. Since collagen can only be degraded by collagenase, this specific enzyme most probably comes into play

detected in such experimental animals. As we were carrying out the experiments to verify this, we learned that Hollander and his colleagues (16) had already shown that the lowering of blood pressure by antihypertensive drugs for 8 weeks in vascular hypertensive rats brought about a regression of the hypertensive cardiovascular disease (fibrosis and hypertrophy). Untreated vascular hypertensive rats showed no regression of the vascular lesion. They concluded that chemical and structural changes in the cardiovascular system play an important role in sustaining the hypertension. More importantly, and in agreement with our metabolic and turnover studies, they concluded that hypertensive vascular disease is reversible. Recently, we have carried out similar studies in vascular hypertensive rats and corroborated the studies of Hollander and Colombo.

EVIDENCE THAT VASCULAR FIBROSIS MAY BE REVERSIBLE IN MAN

Our experiments and those of Hollander indicate that if the rate of synthesis of collagen and other arterial proteins of hypertensive animals can be returned to normal, then degradative processes (collagenase, others) will reverse the process of fibrosis and hypertrophy. In the animal models of hypertension that were used, we would assume that lowering the blood pressure for two to three half-lives (60–90 days) would be sufficient to reverse the fibrosis appreciably. Colombo et al. (16) administered antihypertensive drugs to their hypertensive rats for 56 days (ca. two half-lives) and observed a reversal of the arterial changes.

We wondered whether there were any human data that would enable us to extrapolate these findings to man. Discussions with Dr. Edward D. Freis led us to a number of published studies in which various antihypertensive drugs were given to hypertensive patients for more than 2 years, and then the drugs discontinued. A summary of some of the relevant studies is shown in Table 3 (17–21). We recognize that we may be overlooking some studies and also that in the studies included in this table the patients varied greatly in the severity of their hypertension, in the length of therapy, and in many other parameters. However, the conclusion drawn by all of the investigators is that a significant number of hypertensive patients (ca. 15%), after 2 years of successful antihypertensive therapy, remain normotensive indefinitely (over 2 years) when therapy is discontinued. Another way of summarizing the data of these studies is presented in Fig. 4. Some patients, following discontinuance of therapy, returned fairly rapidly to pretreatment hypertensive levels. However, most patients remained normotensive for several months and a large number for 6–12 months. We had the opportunity to follow one patient very carefully (Table 4). Hypertension appeared in this patient for the first time in 1968, and after some time approached a mean value of about 170/100. Over the next few years, various drugs were tried with varying degrees of success and side effects. In 1976, spironolactone was introduced and maintained the pressure at an average value of 125/80 for a period of 2 years. At that time, the findings in Table 3 became known to us and spironolactone was discontinued. In this patient, blood pressure remained at about 120/80 without drug for over 10 months and then gradually began to rise. Spironolactone was resumed successfully before pre-

Table 3. Modification of hypertension after long-term treatment with antihypertensive drugs.

Reference	Findings after discontinuation of therapy
Page and Dustan (17)	9 of 27 remained normotensive ½–5 years.
Dustan et al. (18)	Long remissions in patients with essential hypertension.
Perry et al. (19)	11 of 16 of essential hypertension in remission; 16 of 316 of severe hypertension in remission.
Thurm and Smith (20)	16 of 69 remained normotensive 1–3⅓ years.
Fries et al. (21)	15% remained normotensive at least 1 year.

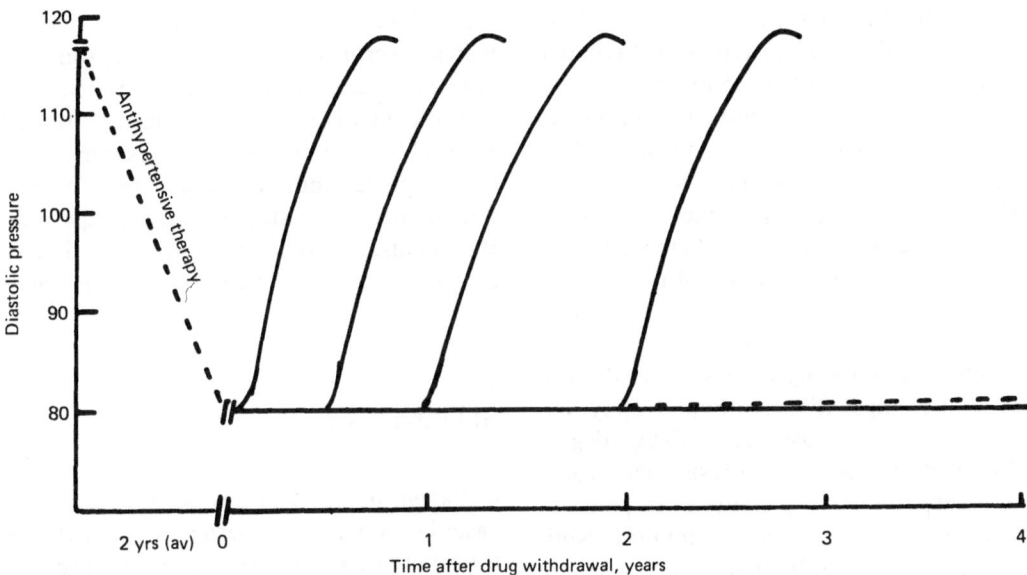

Fig. 4. Schematic presentation of changes in blood pressure in patients after discontinuing successful antihypertensive therapy.

treatment blood pressure levels were reached. These long-lasting effects are certainly not due to residual drug.

It has been suggested by some that the effects are due to an alteration of the baroreceptors during antihypertensive therapy (20). This may be true, but based on our experiments in rats we offer another explanation; namely, that the effects are due to a reversal of the arterial fibrosis and hypertro-

phy during the prolonged normotensive period of therapy. Some questions remain. For instance, why didn't all patients respond in the same way? Obviously, they did not have the same severity of hypertension, the duration and efficacy of therapy was not comparable, and the etiology of hypertension was different. Dr. Freis has indicated to us that if such studies were limited to moderate hypertensives (160/100), he would expect more than 15%

Table 4. Case history.

Period	Blood pressure (mmHg)		
	High	Average	Low
Untreated			
1969–1976	180/106	160/100	150/95
	170/110	–	–
	170/120	–	–
Spironolactone (75 mg)			
16 June 1976–			
25 March 1978	130/88	120/85	114/75
Discontinued all drugs			
26 March 1978–			
20 November 1978	135/94	125/86	110/82
25 November 1978	Spironolactone (75 mg) reinstituted when diastolic blood pressure was 95 mmHg on successive days.		

to require no further therapy after 2 years. How does one explain the gradual return to hypertension after a period as long as 6–15 months? Several factors may explain the variability. The most obvious reasons are differences in duration and severity of hypertension and duration and efficacy of treatment. However, it is quite possible that even if these factors were all comparable, there would still be large variations in the duration of response on discontinuing therapy. The etiology of the hypertension may be the important variable. The duration and intensity of the hypertension would lead to the arterial changes (fibrosis, hypertrophy, hypertensive vascular disease) of variable degree which, by increasing peripheral resistance, would further increase the blood pressure in response to the same degree of neurohumoral stimulus. Antihypertensive drugs generally lower blood pressure by neutralizing the neurohumoral factors. During the prolonged normotensive interval induced by therapy, the arterial changes would be reversed in some cases to normal. Recurrence of hypertension may then be related to the etiology of the specific hypertension. A patient with renal hypertension or pheochromocytoma would most likely have a rapid recurrence, since the neurohumoral factors would still be operative when antihypertensive therapy is stopped. Longer remissions might be expected in hypertension induced by stress or other neural factors. In such cases, it is possible that the original pressure-inducing events may never again occur, in which case the patient would be cured of his hypertension (i.e., a remission). Recurrence of hypertension after a prolonged remission might be considered a completely new event. It may be that these recurrences are in fact recapitulations of a patient's original onset of hypertension. If so, then remissions of hypertension brought on by 1 or 2 years of antihypertensive therapy may provide clinical investigators with patients who will soon go on to become hypertensive. Careful follow-up of such patients may provide important information on the origins of human hypertension.

From a practical standpoint, our studies raise the issue of whether hypertension, once discovered, must be treated for life. For many, this may be true; for many others, this is apparently not true. Even a period of 6 months to 1 year without drugs may be considered beneficial. Obviously, even the animal studies require further confirmation. The findings in patients are mere suggestions.

Nevertheless, the consequences of these findings warrant verification by large-scale, well-controlled clinical studies in man in conjunction with whatever biochemistry can be utilized. If hypertension is curable even in 15% of hypertensives, we are talking about millions of people. We must carry out the necessary studies and perhaps change our therapeutic approaches to hypertension so as to do away with a lifetime of needless therapy for so many patients.

SUMMARY

Collagen metabolism has been investigated in the vascular system of hypertensive rats. It was found that increased blood pressure acts directly on the arterial bed to induce collagen biosynthesis and fibrogenesis. Lowering the blood pressure with antihypertensive drugs reduces collagen formation. Not only is collagen biosynthesis reduced by effective antihypertensive drug therapy, but, if the normotensive state is maintained pharmacologically for a sufficient period of time, the fibrosis of the blood vessels may actually be reversed. There is indirect evidence that all the above may hold true for hypertensive patients.

REFERENCES

1. Folkow B, Hallbäck M, Lundgren Y, Sivertsson R, Weiss L (1973) Importance of adaptive changes in vascular design for establishment of primary hypertension, studied in man and in spontaneously hypertensive rats. Circ Res 32, 33(Suppl I): 2–16
2. Wolinsky H (1970) Response of the rat aortic media to hypertension. Circ Res 26: 507–521
3. Ooshima A, Fuller GC, Cardinale GJ, Spector S, Udenfriend S (1974) Increased collagen synthesis in blood vessels of hypertensive rats and its reversal by antihypertensive agents. Proc Natl Acad Sci USA 71(8): 3019–3023
4. Ooshima A, Fuller G, Cardinale G, Spector S, Udenfriend S (1975) Collagen biosynthesis in blood vessels of brain and other tissues of the hypertensive rat. Science 190: 898–900
5. Fuller GC, Ooshima A, Cardinale GJ, Spector S, Udenfriend S (1977) Hypertension-induced increase in vascular collagen synthesis. In: Spontaneous hypertension: Its pathogenesis and complications. DHEW Publication No (NIH) 77–1179, US Government Printing Office, Washington, DC, pp 61–69

6. Ooshima A (1978) Localization of prolyl hydroxylase by the immunoperoxidase method in cardiovascular tissues of hypertensive rats. Jpn Circ 42(8): 971–978

7. Iwatsuki K, Cardinale GJ, Spector S, Udenfriend S (1977) Hypertension: Increase of collagen biosynthesis in arteries but not in veins. Science 198: 403–405

8. Hume WR, Bevan JA (1978) Amino acid uptake in rabbit blood vessels two weeks after induction of hypertension by coarctation of the abdominal aorta. Cardiovasc Res 12: 106–113

9. Foidart JM, Rorive GL, Nusgens BV, Lapiere CM (1978) The relationship between blood pressure and aortic collagen metabolism in renal hypertensive rats. Clin Sci Mol Med 55: 27S–29S

10. Levene CI, Gross J (1959) Alterations in state of molecular aggregation of collagen induced in chick embryos by β-aminopropionitrile (Lathyrus factor). J Exp Med 110: 771–791

11. Iwatsuki K, Cardinale GJ, Spector S, Udenfriend S (1977) Reduction of blood pressure and vascular collagen in hypertensive rats by β-aminopropionitrile. Proc Natl Acad Sci USA 74(1): 360–362

12. Franklin TJ, Morris WP (1979) Inhibition of collagen deposition in aortae of hypertensive rats. In: Abstracts of the XIth international congress of biochemistry, Toronto, July, p 660

13. Nissen R, Cardinale GJ, Udenfriend S (1978) Increased turnover of arterial collagen in hypertensive rats. Proc Natl Acad Sci USA 75(1): 451–453

14. Friedman SM, Friedman CL, Nakashima M (1951) Sustained hypertension following the administration of desoxycorticosterone acetate. J Exp Med 93: 361–371

15. Hollander W (1973) Hypertension, antihypertensive drugs and atherosclerosis. Circulation 48: 1112–1127

16. Colombo MA, Nagraj S, Hollander W (1977) Reversibility of hypertensive disease induced by high salt intake and desoxycorticosterone (DOC). Circulation 55, 56(Suppl III): 241

17. Page IH Dustan HP (1962) Persistence of normal blood pressure after discontinuing treatment in hypertensive patients. Circulation 25(3): 433–436

18. Dustan HP, Page IH, Tarazi RC, Frohlich ED (1968) Arterial pressure responses to discontinuing antihypertensive drugs. Circulation 37: 370–379

19. Perry HM, Schroeder HA, Catanzaro FJ, Moore-Jones D, Camel GH (1966) Studies on the control of hypertension: VIII. Mortality, morbidity, and remissions during twelve years of intensive therapy. Circulation 33: 958–972

20. Thurm RH, Smith WM (1967) On resetting of "barostats" in hypertensive patients. JAMA 201(5): 85–88

21. Veterans Administration Cooperative Study Group on Antihypertensive Agents (1975) Return of elevated blood pressure after withdrawal of antihypertensive drugs. Circulation 51: 1107–1113

Hypertension, Vasopressors, and Susceptibility to Vascular Injury: Experimental and Clinical Studies

Haralambos Gavras, Irene Gavras, and Hans R. Brunner

The association of high blood pressure with vascular damage has long been recognized, and so has the fact that control of severe hypertension may lead to reversal of certain vascular changes (1). It is also recognized that hypertension of comparable magnitude and duration in different subjects may cause vascular lesions of different severity, suggesting that the mechanical effect is not sufficient to explain these lesions. Moreover, microvascular lesions similar to those of malignant hypertension (i.e., fibrinoid necrosis and hyalinization) have been observed in the absence of excessive blood pressure elevation (e.g., in progressive systemic sclerosis with renal involvement, Bartter's syndrome, and familial chloride diarrhea). A number of clinical and experimental studies lend support to the thesis that humoral factors such as blood viscosity, sodium kinetics, and vasoactive hormones may affect vascular pathology.

Experimentally, necrotizing arteriolar lesions were produced by injection of kidney extracts (2), semipurified renin, or synthetic angiotensin II (3), particularly if the animals had previously been nephrectomized or pretreated with mineralocorticoids (4). Goldblatt-type hypertension induced by renal artery constriction led to malignant hypertension with disruption of cerebral autoregulation, cerebral edema, and hypertensive encephalopathy (5). Infusion of pharmacologic amounts of angiotensin II produced a "vasomotor type" acute renal failure with extensive renal tubular necrosis, as well as widespread multifocal myocardial infarctions (6). Administration of 0.9% saline as drinking water to animals with two-kidney renovascular hypertension prevented or reversed malignant vascular changes, despite significantly higher blood pressure levels (7). This apparent paradox may be interpreted by two possible mechanisms: suppression of the renin–angiotensin system by fluid volume expansion and/or altered rheologic conditions following fluid retention and hemodilution.

Clinically, evidence of acute myocardial lesions was observed in patients shortly after they were exposed to excessive elevation of endogenous angiotensin II, permitting speculation about a cause and effect relationship between the two events (8). Hypertensive retinopathy grade III or IV Keith-Wagener, known to be the clinical hallmark of accelerated hypertension, is far more common in renovascular hypertension as well as other reversible forms associated with high plasma renin activity (PRA) (renal tumor, etc.), than it is in idiopathic hypertension or primary aldosteronism. And statistically, it has been suggested that the high-renin subgroup of essential hypertension may be more prone to cardiovascular complications than the low- and normal-renin subgroups (9).

Taken together, these findings lend support to the theory that it is the angiotensin-mediated vasoconstrictor effect, rather than the level of blood pressure, which determines the susceptibility to vascular damage.

However, malignant-phase hypertension with the same characteristic microvascular lesions (i.e., arteriolar necrosis with fibrinoid deposits) can be produced in mineralocorticoid-type hypertension without participation of the renin–angiotensin system (10). It was suggested that another vasoconstrictor agent, possibly vasopressin (11), may be involved, but its participation remains to be confirmed.

Other vasoconstrictor hormones, such as norepinephrine and epinephrine, should also be considered. Infusion of norepinephrine increased blood pressure (12) and produced microinfarcts in the myocardium indistinguishable from those produced by angiotensin (8). Epinephrine, on the other hand, may exert combined constrictor and dilator (alpha- and beta-adrenergic-mediated) effects, varying in intensity depending on the different sensitivity in the vasculature of different organs. Accordingly, adrenergic stimulation during the induction of acute experimental hypertension might possibly exert a protective, rather than detrimental, effect in certain vascular areas, namely, the coronary (13) and cerebral (14) circulation.

It is of particular interest that animals entering the malignant phase of hypertension, be it of renovascular or DOCA-salt origin (i.e., renin or sodium dependent), exhibit the same behavior (7, 10): paroxysms of excessive diuresis and natriuresis, characterized by weight loss, hemoconcentration, increased blood viscosity, and signs of microangiopathic hemolytic anemia, which also happen to be the clinical characteristics of human malignant-phase hypertension (15) regardless of origin or magnitude of blood pressure elevation. Actually, in both of the above experimental models, animals entering the malignant phase of hypertension tend to have lower blood pressure levels than their nonmalignant counterparts.

Based on information from the literature as well as our own experience, we tried to reconstruct, as follows, the sequence of events leading eventually to widespread injury: What both models have in common seems to be sudden mobilization and excretion of sodium and fluid. The ensuing hemoconcentration and increased blood viscosity leads to a state of hypercoagulability. Increased plasma viscosity impairs perfusion of the inner layers of the wall of small arterioles, which depend on diffusion of plasma nutrients for their metabolism, and, therefore, contribute to vascular wall damage. Anatomic alterations have also been induced already to these arterioles by the mechanical effect of high blood pressure as well as the constricting effect of vasopressor substances. They consist mostly in alternating localized areas of constrictions and dilatations, giving arterioles the characteristic "string-of-beads" appearance (16). The dilated areas exhibit increased permeability (17), permitting passage of plasma constituents through the contracted endothelial cells (18), a process termed "plasmatic vasculosis." The damaged vascular wall, together with the state of hypercoagulability, trigger off various degrees of disseminated intravascular coagulation with fibrin deposits, leading to microangiopathic hemolytic anemia. Microscopically, the microvascular lesions exhibit exudative, proliferative, and necrotizing components including deposits of amorphous fibrinoid material

within the lumen, thickening and edema of the media, and, if the subject survives long enough to permit the healing process to occur, intimal hyalinization and periadventitial fibrosis.

SUMMARY

In addition to the mechanical effect of high arterial blood pressure, a number of other factors determine the occurrence and severity of hypertensive vascular injury: vasoactive hormones, sodium kinetics, and changes in blood rheology. Thus, experimental data and clinical observations suggest that a stimulated renin–angiotensin system may enhance malignant vasculitis. Likewise, elevated norepinephrine and vasopressin were found to be associated with microvascular injury and malignant hypertension. Sudden loss of sodium often precedes malignant hypertension, whereas administration of saline may reverse it, despite further blood pressure rise. Hemoconcentration, with increased blood viscosity and hypercoagulability, may trigger off microangiopathic hemolytic anemia with fibrinoid deposits contributing to necrotizing microvascular lesions.

ACKNOWLEDGMENTS

This work was supported, in part, by USPHS grant 18318. H. Gavras is an Established Clinical Investigator of the American Heart Association.

REFERENCES

1. Pickering GW (1968) High blood pressure, 2nd ed. Churchill, London
2. Winternitz MC, Mylon E, Waters LL, Katzenstein R (1939–1940) Studies on the relation of the kidney to cardiovascular disease. Yale J Biol Med 12: 623
3. Giese J (1963) Pathogenesis of vascular disease caused by acute renal ischaemia. Acta Pathol Microbiol Scand 59: 417
4. Masson GMC, Mikasa A, Yasuda H (1962) Experimental vascular disease elicited by aldosterone and renin. Endocrinology 71: 505
5. Byrom FB (1954) The pathogenesis of hypertensive encephalopathy and its relation to the malignant phase of hypertension: Experimental evidence from the hypertensive rat. Lancet 2: 201
6. Gavras H, Brown JJ, Lever AF, MacAdam RF,

Robertson JIS (1971) Acute renal failure, tubular necrosis, and myocardial infarction induced in the rabbit by intravenous angiotensin II. Lancet 2: 19

7. Dauda G, Möhring J, Hofbauer KG, Homsy E, Miksche U, Orth H, Gross F (1973) The vicious circle in acute malignant hypertension of rats. Clin Sci Mol Med 45: 251S

8. Gavras H, Kremer D, Brown JJ, Gray B, Lever AF, MacAdam RF, Medina A, Morton JJ, Robertson JIS (1975) Angiotensin- and norepinephrine-induced myocardial lesions: Clinical and experimental studies in rabbits and man. Am Heart J 89: 321

9. Brunner HR, Laragh JH, Baer L, Newton MA, Goodwin FT, Krakoff LR, Bard RH, Bühler FR (1972) Essential hypertension: Renin and aldosterone, heart attack and stroke. New Engl J Med 286: 441

10. Gavras H, Brunner HR, Laragh JH, Vaughan ED, Koss M, Cote LJ, Gavras I (1975) Malignant hypertension resulting from deoxycorticosterone acetate and salt excess: The role of renin and sodium in vascular changes. Circ Res 36: 300

11. Möhring J, Möhring B, Petri M, Haak D (1977) Vasopressor role of ADH in the pathogenesis of malignant DOC hypertension. Am J Physiol 232: F260

12. Laragh JH, Angers M, Kelly WG, Lieberman S (1960) Hypotensive agents and pressor substances: The effect of epinephrine, norepinephrine, angiotensin II and others on the secretory rate of aldosterone in man. JAMA 174: 234

13. Gavras H, Liang C (in press) Acute renovascular hypertension in conscious dogs: Interaction of the renin-angiotensin system and sympathetic nervous system in systemic hemodynamics and regional blood flow responses. Circ Res

14. Heistad DD, Marcus MD (1979) Effect of sympathetic stimulation on permeability of the blood-brain barrier to albumin during acute hypertension in cats. Circ Res 45: 331

15. Gavras H, Brown WCB, Brown JJ, Lever AF, Linton AL, MacAdam RF, McNicol GP, Robertson JIS, Wardrop C (1971) Microangiopathic hemolytic anemia and the development of the malignant phase of hypertension. Circ Res 28, 29(Suppl II): 127

16. Byrom FB (1969) The hypertensive vascular crisis: An experimental study. Heinemann, London

17. Goldby FS, Beilin LJ (1973) The evolution and healing of arteriolar damage in renal clip hypertension in the rat: An electron microscope study. Clin Sci 44: 5P

18. Giese J (1961) Deposition of serum proteins in vascular walls during acute hypertension. Acta Pathol Microbiol Scand 53: 167

DISCUSSION

Dr. Shkvatasabaya (Moscow, Russia): First, I would like to thank Dr. Laragh for the invitation to participate in this excellent meeting which was very stimulating from many points of view. Second, I would like to show some figures. From the point of view of what we are discussing in this session, it seems important to have some clinical parameters that will give us the possibility to assess the changes in the cardiovascular system. We have used echocardiographic technique and have some experience using occlusive plethysmography which, I think, give quite essential information about the situation in the cardiovascular system. First, we got a close correlation ($r = 0.77$) between the mass of myocardium and mean arterial pressure (Fig. 1). Using occlusive plethysmography, we can get important information about the minimal resistance of arteries that can be assessed at maximal vasodilatation after 5-min occlusion of the extremities (so-called reactive hyperemia). Figure 2 demonstrates a close correlation ($r = 0.74$) between minimal vascular resistance and mean arterial pressure. We found very close correlations between minimal resistance and mass of myocardium ($r = 0.75$) (Fig. 3). I think these data are important since they permit us to assess hypertrophic changes in the cardiovascular system. I think these data could also be used as a basis for assessment of effectiveness of treatment and follow-up of the patient.

Dr. Tarazi (Cleveland, Oh.): Dr. Udenfriend, relating to the study with β-aminopropionitrile (β-APN), did you measure systolic pressure only, or both systolic and diastolic blood pressure? The reason for my question is the possibility that the alterations in aortic collagen that you determined

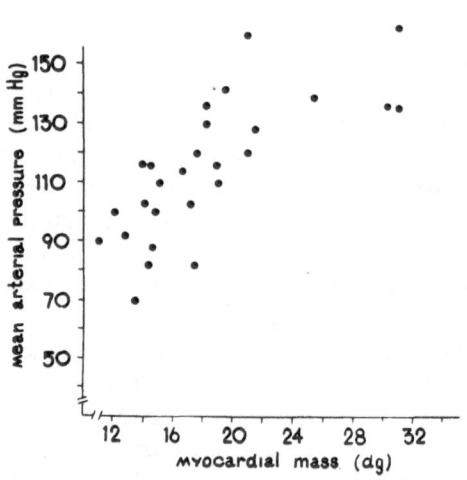

Fig. 1. $r = 0.77$.

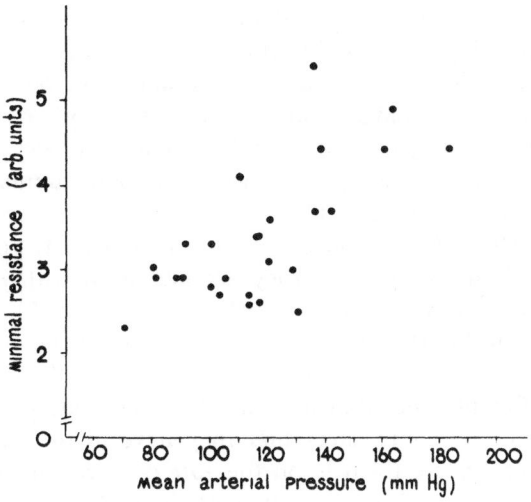

Fig. 2. r = 0.74.

could have an undue influence on systolic pressure levels. Reduction in aortic collagen content is expected to increase aortic compliance and, thus, reduce the pulse pressure.

Dr. Udenfriend (Nutley, New Jersey): We measured mean arterial pressure indirectly in most cases. At times, we used the direct method. I don't really understand your question. If collagen changes the blood pressure, then we are studying the effect of changes in collagen on blood pressure?

Dr. Tarazi: I mean that a reduction in aortic collagen might have led to an increase in aortic compliance; this, in turn, would reduce pulse pressure and possibly lower systolic pressure levels without necessarily reducing diastolic blood pressure.

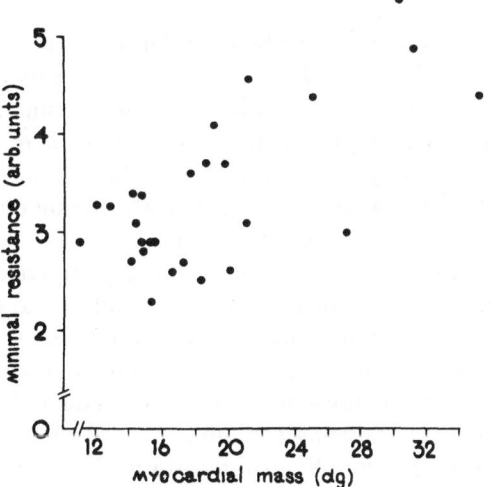

Fig. 3. r = 0.75.

Dr. Udenfriend: I do not remember if the effects were on both systolic and diastolic pressure.

Dr. Tarazi: Different antihypertensive drugs can have varying and sometimes discrepant effects on cardiac and vascular structural changes with little apparent relation to their effects on blood pressure. Thus, together with Drs. Sen and Bumpus [Sen S, Tarazi RC, Bumpus FM (1977) Cardiovasc Res 11: 427–433], we showed that hydralazine did not reduce cardiac weight in SHR while methyldopa did, although both drugs lowered arterial pressure equally. In a study with Dr. Yamori [Yamori Y, Tarazi RC, Ooshima A (1980) Clin Sci (ISH Suppl), in press], when he was in Cleveland, we again found that hydralazine lowered blood pressure in SHR while propranolol did not, yet aortic collagen was reduced by propranolol but not by hydralazine. Thus, not all antihypertensive treatments are the same as regards their impact on structural cardiovascular changes, and there are indeed, as Dr. Laragh pointed out, other factors besides pressure (such as activity of the adrenergic nervous system) that we believe to be very important in influencing the structural response to hypertension.

Dr. Boyd (Hobart, Australia): I want to see if we can establish some common ground here. It seems clear that structural arteriolar changes occur in all forms of chronic hypertension, so that the factor that causes them is unlikely to be humoral. On the other hand, we have heard that these changes do not always correlate with pressure *per se*, so the missing factor seems likely to be something that is only incidentally related to blood pressure. What I would like to suggest is that it may be a different sort of factor. First, there is a very close analogy between the histologic changes of large-vessel atherosclerosis and the structural arteriolar changes of chronic hypertension. And, since we know that one of the ways we can cause atherosclerosis experimentally is by injury to the arterial endothelium, it seems to me that the factor we are looking for is something that damages the arteriole. I would suggest that this could be a more profitable way to look at the stimulus than to regard it, as Dr. Folkow has, as some sort of physiologic process. Moreover, I think that the likely factor causing this damage is an increased arteriolar flow velocity which would occur when the arterioles constrict and the cardiac output is forced through their narrowed lumens, so placing a greatly increased shearing stress on their walls.

Dr. Gavras (Boston, Mass.): I think it is already well demonstrated that there is increased hemoconcentration and increased blood viscosity and hypercoagulability at the stage of onset of microvascular lesions [Gavras et al. (1971) Circ Res 28, 29 (Suppl II): 171]. Now the question is how to reconstruct the sequence of events and whether we can influence them somehow. I don't agree with your comment that the process begins with arteriolar injury.

Dr. Palmer (Miami, Fla.): I think everything that has been presented here has been consistent with my experiments that suggest that damage is related to the stiffness of the vessel. The stiffer the vessel is, the more susceptible it appears to be to injury. I think that we've looked at a number of different drugs and ruled out any kind of biochemical influence. The injury occurs, in my view, from the vessel being less compliant and stiffer, and I have in my paper offered an explanation as to why that occurs. I think that in the experiments of Dr. Udenfriend, narrowing of the vessel by a coarctation of the aorta causes the pulse wave to become very steep at that particular point where there is the narrowing. Proximally, the pulse wave becomes "stiff" and that's where the atherosclerosis occurs. I really feel that it is a mechanical factor that causes the injury, and all other phenomena are secondary to it. Vasoconstriction of arterioles produces the same effects on the large vessels proximal to the constriction. Conversely, beta-blockade actually causes the vessel to become more compliant, and the shape of pulse wave would be altered this influence regardless of the ambient pressure level.

Dr. Udenfriend: If you suggest that the fibroid vessel is less compliant, then I agree. I would compare the changes to a generalized fibrosis, not arteriosclerosis. I want to ask two questions of the previous discussants. If there are other factors involved in the changes in vascular wall, obviously the blood pressure is a necessary accompanying event. Dr. Laragh, when you spoke about the effects of renin, did you indicate whether renin affects veins as well as arteries? You used the general term vascular.

Dr. Laragh (New York): There is some debate about how much action angiotensin has on veins, but in the context of my discussion, I was only concerned with its action to vasoconstrict the arteriolar bed.

Dr. Udenfriend: Therefore, there may be some agreement in our finding. In other words, pressure is a primary event, but then other factors come into play. Secondarily, this would rule out veins. Dr. Palmer, is the turkey experiment the one in which you have obtained severe toxicity? Were there very young animals. In young animals, β-APN is lethal. You can't use it in young animals in the way that I did.

Dr. Palmer: You can do it either way. If you feed the birds when they are first born with β-APN, then they have a 50% mortality rate. Later on in life, they don't have that sort of thing. But it provides a very nice model to study all these different drugs that have no effect on blood pressure. The only effect that they have in the way that we use them is on the *rate* of development of pressure. Yet, regardless of the ambient pressure, it protects, and this is also true, regardless of the drug that one uses. It's not the pressure *per se* that protects; it's changing the rate of development of pressure that is crucial.

Dr. Muirhead (Memphis, Tenn.): I think in our jargon, acute vascular disease has always meant arterial, but maybe we should change that.

Dr. Birkenhager (Rotterdam, The Netherlands): I always enjoy listening to Dr. Laragh, especially when he is defending an untenable position. I could touch on many aspects of your paper, but I have to select one to which I took particular exception, and that's when you mixed up in your material retrospective and prospective observations on the relationship between renin status and cardiovascular events. We have carried out a different approach in that we took stock of the renin status in a number of patients and followed them up for 5 years in order to see what would happen to their cardiovascular status. It appeared that quite a few of the low-renin cases met with myocardial infarction or cerebrovascular accident, and what we observed then was that after patients had recovered from myocardial infarction, renin appeared to be higher than before. So, in a retrospective study, you have a chicken and egg problem if you include patients with a rising renin due to the cardiovascular event.

Dr. Laragh: First, may I accept your condolences, Dr. Birkenhager. Then I would like to extend to you my sincere sympathy for your lugubrious position because you are really the one who is in an indefensible position. You did all of your studies using a renin assay, which as we heard in Session 9 also measures the inactive plasma renin. Now we all know that the inactive renin moiety occurs in plasma in from 5 to 20 times the amount of active renin. Moreover, since prorenin varies from patient to patient the error introduced by the acid-activation step is inconsistent and unpredictable. Accordingly, with the method you employed, which activates inactive renin, there is no way in the world that you could have discerned the low-renin patients. If you discount the renin measurements, which I think you must, then I don't know what your study tells us.

May I also make another comment, because I enjoy your having come here to debate these issues face to face. This relates to your criticism of our group for doing a retrospective study. We made that same criticism ourselves, but I must tell you, Dr. Birkenhager, I believe that often a great deal has been learned from retrospective studies in this world, probably more than from prospective studies. Ideally, you should have both, but this is not easy or even possible now that withholding therapy is considered unfair to the patient. However, I don't think one can *a priori* criticize a study simply because it is partly retrospective. Moreover, our study actually was partially prospective [Brunner HR, Laragh JH, Baer L, et al. (1972) New Engl J Med 286: 441].

Dr. Birkenhager: I still think it is a basic problem that you try to derive a prognostic significance from certain kinds of data which are really occurring after the fact of the injury. As far as the renin assay is concerned, both our group and Amery's found in the steady-state a very close relationship between active and total renin, and so we should really be able to discriminate between low- and high-renin situations.

Dr. Laragh: This was discussed in Session 7. We would be glad to do the study again with you— that is, a double-blind exchange of samples. A patient who has a low-active renin level, after acid treatment, can be either low, high, or normal with the five- to ten-fold or more increment of active renin added after acid conversion. I don't believe there is any chance of your consistently telling low from high values using acid-activated plasmas. Moreover, if you believe the published data, Amery et al. have conceded that your method failed to reveal the well-known and easily demonstrable renin suppression of beta-blockade because of the acid-activation step [Amery A, Biller L, Boel A, et al. (1976) Lancet 2: 849].

Dr. Cohn (Minneapolis, Minn.): I don't want to argue with anyone, but I would like to submit for consideration what I think is an important study that Drs. C. Limas and C. Limas did in my laboratory last year. They took SHR and salt loaded one group and not the other, an intervention that did not change blood pressure significantly in these two groups of animals. They then looked at the vascular tissue and found marked vascular changes both in the small vessels and in the large arteries in the salt-loaded animals, and not in the non-salt-loaded animals. They were on, I think, 1%–2% salt in the drinking water. I think what this does is to raise the possibility that we must revise our concept of why salt raises blood pressure. It is entirely possible that the mechanism of salt hypertension is, in part, related to primary vascular damage, leading to a secondary rise in blood pressure. These data also provide support for another reason to restrict salt intake in hypertensive subjects.

Dr. Ganten (Heidelberg, West Germany): Dr. Schwartz, we have shown that angiotensin is a growth factor in its own right. For example, we have reported that angiotensin stimulated growth of fibroblasts in vitro and also increased proliferation of adrenal gland glomerulosa cells which were kept in cell culture. The Cleveland group has reported results on increased protein synthesis under the influence of angiotensin. My question, therefore, is: Does angiotensin have an effect on the turnover rate of the vascular endothelial cells?

Dr. Schwartz (Seattle, Wash.): We have looked for that. First, we repeated the work that was done by Abel Robertson some years ago (unpublished observations), and have shown accumulation of carbon under aortic endothelium with angiotensin. In our work, however, as in the work of Goldby and Beilin in the small vessels, the effects were entirely proportional to blood pressure [Goldby FS, Beilin LJ (1972) Cardiovasc Res 6: 384–390, 569–584]. There was no evidence that angiotensin directly caused an increase in permeability. Nonetheless, because it did cause an increase in entry of carbon, if only secondary to pressure, it seemed interesting to examine endothelial cell turnover. Animals were prelabeled with ^{3}HTdR to identify cells in areas of high turnover. One might expect, if angiotensin was toxic, that it would dislodge those replicating cells. In our hands, there was no change in disappearance of prelabeled cells, nor an increase in replication in subsequent days. At the time, I thought that was conclusive and I lost interest. Two developments changed my mind. The first results from recent studies by Michael Reidy of my laboratory on the response of the endothelium to loss of small numbers of cells [Reidy MA, Schwartz SM (in press) Lab Invest]. Dr. Reidy can mechanically remove individual endothelial cells. The cells around the denuded area respond simply by movement into the area without replicating. Thus, with a short period of angiotensin infusion, you might not expect to see any change in replication, even though, as has been suggested by Hladovec in Czechoslovakia, there may be cell detachment. Our attempts to demonstrate cell injury with angiotensin II in cell culture have also been negative. The only evidence for "injury" I am aware of is a report by Michael Gimbrone of an effect of angiotensin II on prostaglandin metabolism by cultured endothelial cells [Gimbrone MA, Jr, Alexander RN (1975) Science 189: 219–220]. The second development is some recent work from Joseph Wiener, reported at the Federation meetings [Skoza L, Giacomelli F, Wiener J (1979) Fed Proc 38: 3:5184]. Using renal hypertensive rats, he found endothelial damage despite protection by an arterial clip. If this holds up, it would be the most convincing data supporting a direct, humoral form of endothelial injury.

Dr. J. Myers (New South Wales, Australia): I'd like to ask Dr. Laragh whether there is any change in the plasma factor VIII coagulant activity according to renin groups? And, Dr. Udenfriend, would you agree that a study of intermittent therapy in patients with hypertension who are well controlled and could be well followed up could provide useful information as to whether this would be a useful therapeutic advance?

Dr. Laragh: To answer your question, I don't know. I think Dr. Gavras might know. In the meantime, I want to ask Dr. Palmer whether his data suggest that lowering the cardiac output and the rate of cardiac contraction in all of us would prevent vascular disease even in normotensive people? Does he believe this concept can be applicable to normotensive subjects?

Dr. Palmer: In the brief time allowed, I wasn't able to show you all of the material. The animals to which we give the negative inotropic agents do not develop any vascular disease, even though their blood pressure, as I showed you before, doesn't change very much at all. And my point is that the answer to your question would be, in my mind, yes. The other side of the evidence comes from work showing the difference between hydralazine and other agents. It fits with the concept very nicely, because hydralazine will increase car-

diac output, and it is a positive inotropic agent. Even though you lower the blood pressure to the same level, as with a negative inotropic agent, you see vast differences between the two types of agents, since hydralazine does not protect from vascular injury. The point is that it is not the level of blood pressure, but the way the blood is carried through the vessel, and I offered one explanation as to why that occurs. Certainly, on propranolol, the turkey does not develop aortic damage, even with extraordinary high levels of cholesterol. Also, when we give a little bit of propranolol to the turkey, it doesn't affect the absolute blood pressure level, but the bird does not develop vascular damage.

Dr. Gavras: There are two conditions in which you have normal blood pressure and very high-renin levels. These are Bartter's syndrome and the familial chloride diarrhea. In both, you clearly have vascular changes in the arteries, even though blood pressure is lower than normal sometimes. These microvascular changes cannot really be distinguished easily from the changes in malignant hypertension in the kidney.

Dr. Ames (New York): If you increase the lipid content of plasma in vivo or in vitro, do you get any change in endothelial turnover or collagen biosynthesis?

Dr. Schwartz: In vitro there are reports that an increase in low-density lipoprotein will cause endothelial injury. We have not been able to confirm this report. In vivo the evidence is confusing. There is one report in 1969, that hypercholesterolemia causes an increase in endothelial turnover. Later reports, in a somewhat different system, failed to show this increase.

Dr. Udenfriend: But in those reports, would they not have produced atherosclerotic lesions? In the latter case, there are localized lesions in collagen synthesis in arteries. These lesions differ from the hypertensive vascular fibrosis where collagen synthesis and deposition is increased uniformly along the vessel wall.

Dr. Laragh: To summarize some of what has been exchanged, I would say that it is clear that vascular damage to large or small vessels in both experimental and clinical situations is not necessarily directly related to the height of the blood pressure. Thus, while a high pressure may predispose, something besides the absolute blood pressure level seems to be critical.

Our own research has led us to believe that

flow is an important determinant; if you have adequate tissue flow, even very high pressures may produce little or no damage. Conversely, if you have intense vasoconstriction, hypovolemia, and tissure ischemia (as with a renin excess) even with less or no hypertension vascular damage is more likely.

Dr. Palmer's research shows too, in still another way, that the absolute pressure level is not necessarily a key determinant. His paper suggests that the steepness of the pressure wave may be a critical determinant. This wave-form is made steeper by vasoconstriction of arterioles as caused by angiotensin or sometimes norepinephrine. The steepness can be modified by negative inotropic agents or by agents that block arteriolar constriction when the latter is operative.

I think that traditionally we have all focused too much on the absolute pressure level because it is what we can quickly measure. In future research, we should think more about *flow* than pressure *per se* and more about the form of the pressure curve. These characteristics loom as likely more relevant to the vascular damage issue than the absolute level of blood pressure, and they may help us to understand the wide differences in risk that obtain among equally hypertensive experimental models or equally hypertensive patients.

Session 14
Antihypertensive Actions of Beta-Blockers

Chairman: J. Reid

Position Paper: Antihypertensive Actions of Beta-Blockers

Fritz R. Bühler

The depressor effect of beta-blockers in hypertensive patients was recognized in the mid-1960s (1–3) with great reserve. It was puzzling that these drugs lowered blood pressure in some but not all patients. Occasionally a rise was even seen. Their pharmacologic properties, particularly the vascular beta-2-adrenoreceptor blocking effect, resulting in vasconstriction and a subsequent rise in pressure, seemed to contradict the antihypertensive action.

Initially it was theorized that the antihypertensive efficacy of propranolol was due to a resetting of the baroreflex (1) due to diminished pulse pressure and rate of rise of intra-aortic pressure, probably resulting in increased baroreflex sensitivity and reduced sympathetic tone.

In the late 1960s the negative chronotropic and inotropic effects of beta-blockers led to their application in patients with hyperkinetic hypertension (4) and to the explanation that they reduced blood pressure because they reduced cardiac output.

In the early 1970s a marked renin-suppressive effect of propranolol was described in normotensive (6) and hypertensive humans (7, 8). This prompted two additional observations: the correlation between the antihypertensive effectiveness of propranolol and the patient's pretreatment renin activity (8, 9) and between the degree of renin suppression produced by long-term propranolol therapy and the attendant fall in blood pressure (8).

A central nervous system effect was suggested by animal studies in which propranolol was found to reduce central sympathetic nerve activity (10). More recently, blockade of prejunctional beta-adrenoreceptors and the subsequent reduction of norepinephrine release were proposed to contribute to the antihypertensive effect (11). Again, another theory postulated that changes distal to postjunctional beta₂-adrenoreceptor blockade causes the adenylate cyclase system to be more responsive to unknown vasodilating influences (12).

However, any explanation of the antihypertensive mode of action of beta-blockers must account for at least three basic findings:

1) Beta-blockers alone control blood pressure in the majority but not in all patients.
2) There is a time lag of hours or days between the administration of beta-adrenoreceptor blockade and the onset of the reduction in blood pressure.
3) The fall in pressure appears to be related to the reduction in peripheral vascular resistance.

In the present discussion, we put forward the concept that the degree of renin secretion before therapy predicts the patient's subsequent antihypertensive response to beta-blockers and that suppression of the renin–angiotensin system is the vector of the antihypertensive action, although other mechanisms subsequent to renin suppression may contribute.

RENIN AND AGE PREDICTING ANTIHYPERTENSIVE RESPONSE

The clinical experience that only about half of all hypertensive patients respond well to beta-blocker monotherapy (13–17) led to the search for a predictor of drug response.

Patients with essential hypertension were classified into approximately 20% with a high, 60% with a normal, and 20% with a low renin-sodium index (18, 19). The drug was most effective in patients with high renin, inconsistent in those with normal renin, and almost completely ineffective in those with low renin (8, 9). The observations have been extended in studies using various beta-blockers (16, 20–23) (Table 1). The response pattern initially found with propranolol was confirmed in these studies regardless of the ancillary pharmacologic properties of the beta-blockers used. In a total of 243 patients the beta-blockers achieved control (diastolic ≤ 95 mmHg) in 75% of high-renin patients, 65% of normal-renin patients, and only 10% of low-renin patients. The overall response rate of 58% agrees well with studies that did not identify "responders" or "nonresponders" on the basis of renin profiles (13–15).

Other investigators who adopted a similar approach to renin profiling confirmed our results, as summarized in Table 2 (24–44). Agreement appears to depend largely on methodology. Thus, most confirmatory studies used a plasma renin activity assay similar to ours. Also, as in our studies, the plasma was obtained with the patient in the upright position (while renin was being stimulated) and the renin measurement was related to sodium balance or sodium excretion rates. Most studies were large enough to provide a sizable number of patients with high and low plasma renin activity (see also Fig. 2). The type of beta-blocker used was not crucial.

Since age influences the state of renin secretion (16, 45), and since the renin level is related to the response to beta-blockers, a relationship may exist between the age of the patient and the antihypertensive effect of a beta-blocker. Such an age analysis is shown in Fig. 1, which includes the

243 patients treated with different beta-blockers presented in Table 1. Beta-blockers controlled three-fourths of patients under 40 years, half of those 40 to 59, and only a fifth of those over 60. This analysis confirms our first (8, 9) and subsequent reports (16, 20–23, 46) as well as studies by other authors (26, 31). A decreasing response to beta-blockers with age tallies with other investigations in which heart rate response both to beta-adrenoreceptor blockade with propranolol (47) and to stimulation with isoproterenol (48–51) were blunted with age.

The depressor response to beta-blockers was also thought to be related to pretreatment plasma catecholamine levels. In one study a relationship was found between the height of plasma norepinephrine, as measured during acute exhaustive ergometry, and the subsequent fall in blood pressure with atenolol therapy (38). However, using similar protocols, we and others have been unable to reproduce these results with atenolol, pindolol, propranolol, or oxprenolol (52, 53).

POWERFUL RENIN SUPPRESSION BY ALL BETA-BLOCKERS

In an endeavor to compare the renin-suppressive capacity of various beta-blockers, their effects on resting and exercise renin levels were measured. For the purpose of standardization, constant beta-blocker-induced reductions of exercise tachycardia

Table 1. Antihypertensive comparison of seven beta-blockers in patients with high-, normal, and low-renin essential hypertension.[a]

Beta-blocker (ref.)	Total	Responders[b] of renin groups		
		High	Normal	Low
Propranolol (16)	55/90	22/26	33/50	0/14
Oxprenolol (16, 20)	24/36	8/11	16/20	0/5
LL 21945 Sandoz (21)	24/35	5/7	18/24	1/4
LT 31200 Sandoz (22)	13/27	4/5	7/16	2/6
Pindolol (23)	10/25	3/6	7/14	0/5
Atenolol (16)	10/17	2/3	8/12	0/2
Metoprolol (16)	6/13	3/3	3/7	0/3
Total response	142/243 (58%)	47/61 (77%)	92/143 (64%)	3/39 (8%)

[a] Pretreatment diastolic pressure 100–130 mmHg.
[b] Responder, diastolic pressure ≤ 95 mmHg in beta-blocker monotherapy.

Table 2. Confirmation of a renin-related antihypertensive response of various beta-blockers.

Referencea	Beta-blocker	Renin indexb H	N	L	Antihypertensive response related to Pretreatment renin r	p	Fall in renin r	p
Hollifield et al. (24)	Propranolol	H	N	L	ND	ND	0.36	0.05
Karlberg et al. (25)	Propranolol	H	N	L	0.71	0.001		
Drayer et al. (26)	Propranolol	H	N	L	0.18	0.05	0.27	0.05
Drayer et al. (27)	Propranolol	H	N	L	0.43	0.001		
MacGregor et al. (28)	Propranolol	H	N	L	ND		ND	
Klumpp et al. (29)	Propranolol	H	N	L	ND			
Moore and Goodwin (30)	Propranolol	ND			ND		0.90	0.001
Stumpe et al. (31)	Propranolol/pindolol	ND			ND		0.79	0.001
Weidmann et al. (32)	Propranolol/bufuralol	H	N	L	0.44	0.05	0.53	0.005
Castenfors et al. (33)	Alprenolol	ND			ND		0.58	0.05
Meekers et al. (34)	Atenolol	H	N	L				
Balansard et al. (35)	Atenolol	ND			0.55	0.01	0.49	0.02
Zech et al. (36)	Atenolol	ND			0.48	0.05	ND	
Philipp et al. (37, 38)	Atenolol	ND			0.54	0.05		
Ménard et al. (39)	Acebutolol	H	N	L	0.50	0.001	ND	
Alhenc-Gélas et al. (40)	Acebutolol	ND			0.64	0.001	ND	
von Bahr et al. (41)	Metoprolol				0.61	0.05		
Tsukiyama et al. (42)	Metoprolol	H	N	L	ND		ND	
Karlberg et al. (43)	Metoprolol	H	N	L				
Weber et al. (44)	Metoprolol	ND			0.48	0.05	0.51	0.05

a excluding studies with author's involvement (refs. 7–9, 16, 20–23).
b H, high; N, normal; L, low; ND, not determined.

were selected. Beta-blocking drugs were tested 2 h after they had been given in doses ascertained in preceding studies to produce equivalent reductions in exercise tachycardia. Beta-blocker-induced reductions in plasma renin activity at rest and during exercise are indicated in percent of control values in Fig. 2; these findings are presented in greater detail elsewhere (41, 43, 54, 55). All beta-blocking drugs included in this comparison significantly suppressed upright plasma renin activity 30–60%. Resting recumbent values were also generally reduced, but the responses did not reach significance when oxprenolol, pindolol, and labetalol were used. Generally, better renin suppressibility was achieved with the cardioselective beta$_1$-type drugs.

Since the comparison was made at equipotent levels of efficacy with cardiac beta$_1$-type drugs, these data suggest that renin secretion, like heart rate, may predominantly depend on beta$_1$-type receptor function, the opposing alpha-receptor playing a minor role. Such indirect evidence conflicts with the concept that renin secretion is a function

of beta$_2$-type receptors (56) but supports the findings from other studies in which isoproterenol, but not the more specific beta$_2$-type receptor agonist salbutamol, was found to stimulate renin (57).

The problem, however, remains still unresolved, since one specific beta$_2$-antagonist, H35/25, was shown to be a most effective renin suppressor (58). Beta$_1$-type renin selectivity can be masked by intrinsic sympathomimetic activity. This agonistic effect appears to be even more important with non-cardioselective-blocking drugs such as oxprenolol, which lowered renin levels only slightly after a single dose but significantly when given over several days (20, 29, 46, 59). In this regard, pindolol appears to be an exception, since it reduced renin only in states of increased adrenergic nervous activity, whereas average basal renin levels remained unchanged, or in response to larger doses, even increased (60). On the other hand, d-propranolol, which has the quinidine-like but not the beta-adrenoreceptor-blocking properties of the clinically used racemate, dl-propranolol, cannot prevent renin stimulation by various maneuvers (58), sug-

Age-Dependent Antihypertensive Efficacy of Beta-Blocker Monotherapy in Essential Hypertension

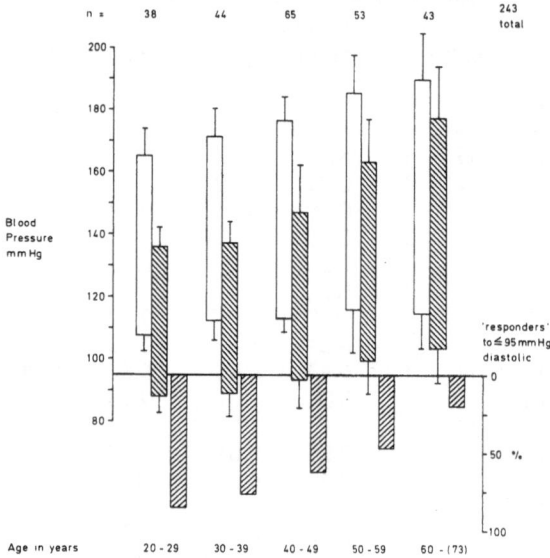

Fig 1. Pressure response to long-term monotherapy with beta-blockers in 243 patients with essential hypertension classified according to age. Pretreatment pressures *(white bars)*, beta-blocker-induced pressure responses, and percent of patients in each age group with diastolic pressure responses ≤ 95 mmHg *(hatched bars)* are shown.

gesting that this property has no effect on renin release.

Opinions still differ whether or not chronic therapy with particular beta-blocking drugs suppresses renin. In our experience a sustained renin-suppressive effect can be shown with all beta-blockers tested. Consequently, cardioselective blockers including atenolol and metoprolol (16), as well as noncardioselective blockers including oxprenolol (16), propranolol (8, 16), Sandoz LL 21945 (61), and most recently Sandoz LT 31200 (22) lower renin effectively. Our results agree with most other studies in which such beta-blocking agents as practolol (62), atenolol (63), oxprenolol (59, 64), timolol (65), alprenolol (33), bunolol (66), acebutolol (39), and nadolol (67) have been reported to lower renin. Other authors, however, maintain that some of these drugs do not suppress renin (68, 69). Pindolol, too, has been shown to reduce plasma renin activity after long-term administration, but its effect on renin remains controversial since some investigators (70, 71) have demonstrated a rise in renin.

Acute Blocker Induced Changes in Renin at Supine Rest and During Upright Exercise

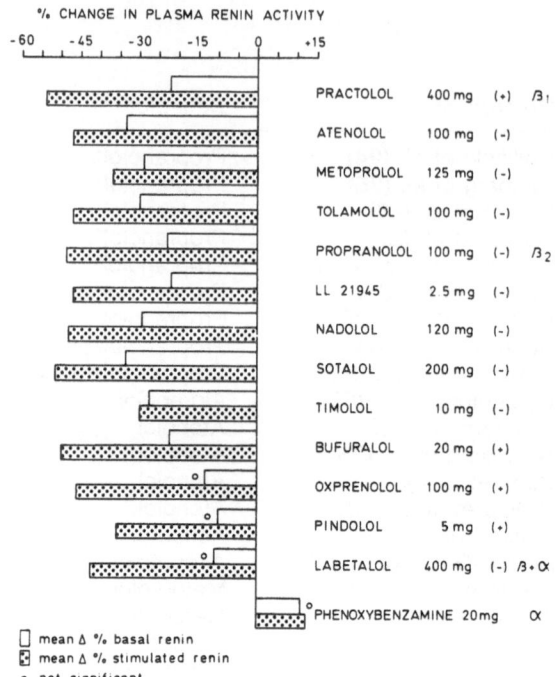

Fig. 2. Adrenergic blocker-induced percent changes in supine resting renin values *(dotted bars)* and in upright exercise-stimulated renin *(hatched bars)* compared in six normal subjects. Changes in resting renin did not reach significance with compounds exhibiting intrinsic sympathomimetic or alpha-adrenoreceptor-blocking properties. All beta-blockers significantly suppressed exercise-stimulated renin values.

BETA-BLOCKER EFFECTS ON ALDOSTERONE AND PLASMA POTASSIUM

As might be expected from a drug that suppresses renin release, inhibition of aldosterone secretion was found with metoprolol (72), nadolol (67), oxprenolol (20), penbutolol (73), and propranolol (8, 27). However, while renin suppression amounted to between 60% and 80%, the reduction of plasma aldosterone was smaller. This discrepancy can be explained by increased plasma potassium concentrations, which suppresses renin release but stimulates aldosterone secretion (74). Several beta-blockers, including propranolol (8), oxprenolol (20), metoprolol (75), *l*-bunolol (66), and nadolol (67), have been found to have a small, but significant, hyperkalemic effect. The effect is probably due to the reduction in aldosterone secretion subsequent to the reduced renin. This increase in the plasma potassium levels may in turn retard the fall in plasma aldosterone.

Whether this beta-blocker-induced rise in plasma potassium may help prevent the hypokalemia associated with diuretic drugs remains to be shown. It has also been suggested that the degree of aldosterone reduction is an important determinant for the antihypertensive response (27, 76).

FALL IN PRESSURE RELATED TO SUPPRESSION OF RENIN SYSTEM

Considering the predictive value of the pretreatment renin profile and the potent renin-suppressive capacity of all beta-blockers tested so far, there are at least four arguments in favor of an antirenin antihypertensive mechanism.

In an early study we found a correlation between the propranolol-induced fall in pressure and the reduction in renin activity (8). In Fig. 3 these early results with propranolol are combined with data from studies using metoprolol and oxprenolol. Plasma renin activity was always measured with the patient in a seated position before noon (i.e., under conditions of slight renin and sympathetic nervous system stimulation). A sizable number of

high- and low-renin patients were included. It is important to note that only studies using beta-blocker monotherapy and applying some renin stimulation have confirmed the original observation (Table 2).

A second argument is the observation that in patients with low renin the antihypertensive effect of beta-blockers was poor; in some patients even a rise in pressure was observed (9, 26). This may indicate that whenever a renin–angiotensin vasoconstrictor component is not available for suppression, a rise in pressure occurs due to unopposed alpha-adrenoreceptor-mediated vasoconstrictor mechanisms subsequent to beta-receptor blockade.

A third and convincing argument for an antirenin component in the antihypertensive action of beta-blockers is the parallel spectrum of response provided by specific angiotensin-blocking drugs, that is, saralasin and the converting enzyme inhibitors teprotide (SQ 20881) and captopril (SQ 14225). A direct relationship was observed between the renin type, the level of pretreatment renin, and the pressure response to the renin system-blocking drugs (77, 80). The antihypertensive efficacy of captopril when given alone is comparable to that obtained with beta-blocker monotherapy (28, 31).

Recent animal experiments further support the antirenin concept. Dogs made hypertensive by in-

Relationship Between Beta-Blocker Induced Pressure and Renin Response

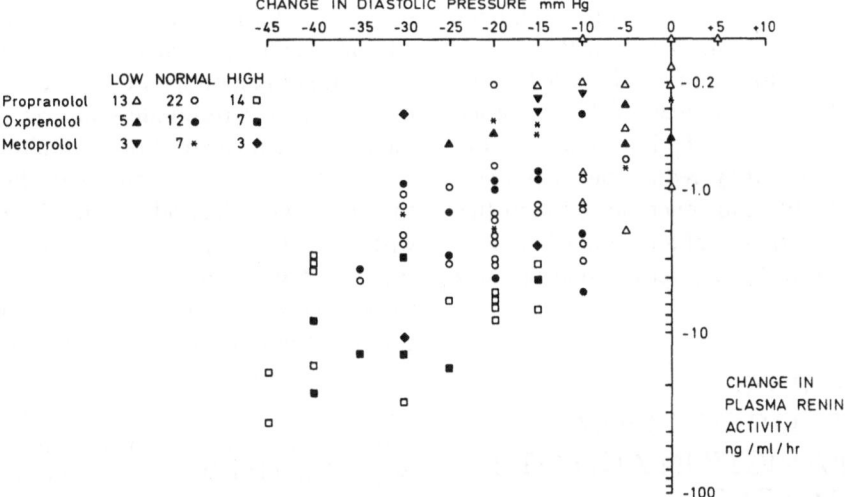

Fig. 3. Correlation between beta-blocker-induced changes in diastolic pressure and changes in plasma renin activity ($r = -0.59$, $p < 0.01$). Long-term monotherapy with 3 beta-blockers in 86 patients.

fusion of angiotensin II had undetectable renin levels and their blood pressure responded neither to captopril nor to propranolol. On the other hand, dogs with renal artery constriction and raised renin and angiotensin levels exhibited a similar fall in pressure with either captopril or propranolol (82, 83). Similar antihypertensive responses to captopril and propranolol have been described in spontaneously hypertensive rats; the effects of both drugs were related to pretreatment renin levels and were not demonstrable following nephrectomy (84).

Two observations, however, are not fully explained by the antirenin concept alone:

1) Renin suppression is observed almost immediately, although the fall in pressure occurs only after hours or days. This delay can probably be explained by a reflex increase in sympathetic activity and an attendant, unopposed, alpha-adrenoreceptor-mediated vasoconstriction temporarily maintaining the high pressure. The more gradual and sustained reduction of aldosterone (8) as a result of renin-angiotensin suppression, at least in part, may account for the delay. The antialdosterone effect of beta-blockers may explain the lack of the weight gain or sodium-volume retention (9, 76) that usually accompanies all other sympatholytic and vasodilating drugs. Reduced aldosterone secretion may also account for the diminution of plasma volume encountered during beta-blocker therapy (85).

2) Doses needed to inhibit renin release are usually many times smaller than those needed to lower pressure (86). This discrepancy, if true, is less well understood. Actually, in patients with a high renin there was some relationship between the dose of propranolol needed to reduce renin and that required to decrease blood pressure (9). This observation is supported by the finding that even low doses of propranolol may reduce blood pressure significantly (87). We and others have found that a small (25 mg daily) dose of atenolol, which lowers renin, may provide long-term blood pressure control (88, 89).

ROLE OF ALPHA-ADRENORECEPTOR-MEDIATED VASOCONSTRICTION AND OTHER NEURAL FACTORS

Elevated peripheral vascular resistance is a hallmark of established essential hypertension. It is determined to a great extent by neurogenic vasoconstriction mediated by postjunctional alpha-adrenoreceptors (49, 90). Two studies link the response to beta-blocker therapy to a diminution of alpha-adrenoreceptor-mediated vasoconstriction (see Figs. 4a, b and 5).

The hemodynamic response pattern during acute beta-blockade is characterized by an initial fall in cardiac output. However, pressure remains unchanged due to a reactive increase in peripheral resistance, which may be attributed to unopposed alpha-adrenoreceptor-mediated vasoconstriction. In the chronic setting, the antihypertensive response to beta-blockade is determined by a reduction in peripheral vascular resistance while cardiac output remains reduced (91). The contribution of alpha-adrenergic vasoconstriction was assessed by superimposing alpha-blockade with phentolamine after acute and chronic propranolol administration. The increase in peripheral vascular resistance during acute propranolol administration was completely countered by phentolamine in all patients (Fig. 4a, b). In the fourth week of propranolol therapy, alpha-adrenergic vasoconstriction was diminished in the "responders" (diastolic pressure $\leq$ 95 mmHg; Fig. 4a), but was practically unchanged in the "nonresponders" (Fig. 4b).

These systemic hemodynamic results corroborate observations on forearm blood flow obtained with the selective postjunctional alpha-blocker prazosin. In the fourth week of propranolol therapy in responders, the prazosin-induced increase in forearm blood flow was smaller than that obtained before propranolol (Fig. 5). Taken together, these two studies suggest a diminution of alpha-adrenoreceptor-mediated vasoconstriction in the propranolol responders. On the other hand, in the propranolol nonresponders, alpha-adrenoreceptor-mediated vasoconstriction may either be small to start with or is not reduced during propranolol therapy. These hemodynamic observations agree with several earlier reports relating the fall in pressure to a fall in peripheral vascular resistance (16, 91–94). However, they are at variance with other studies of long-term beta-blocker therapy (95).

There is almost unanimity over the acute and chronic decrease in cardiac output (56, 91–97), similar in magnitude in the 'responders' and 'non responders' (16). If cardiac output were a principal determinant for pressure response, a greater fall of blood pressure would be expected in hyperdynamic hypertension but this has not been found to be the case (98).

Hemodynamic Responses to Acute Alpha-Blockade (↑) Following Acute and Chronic Beta-Blockade in Responders

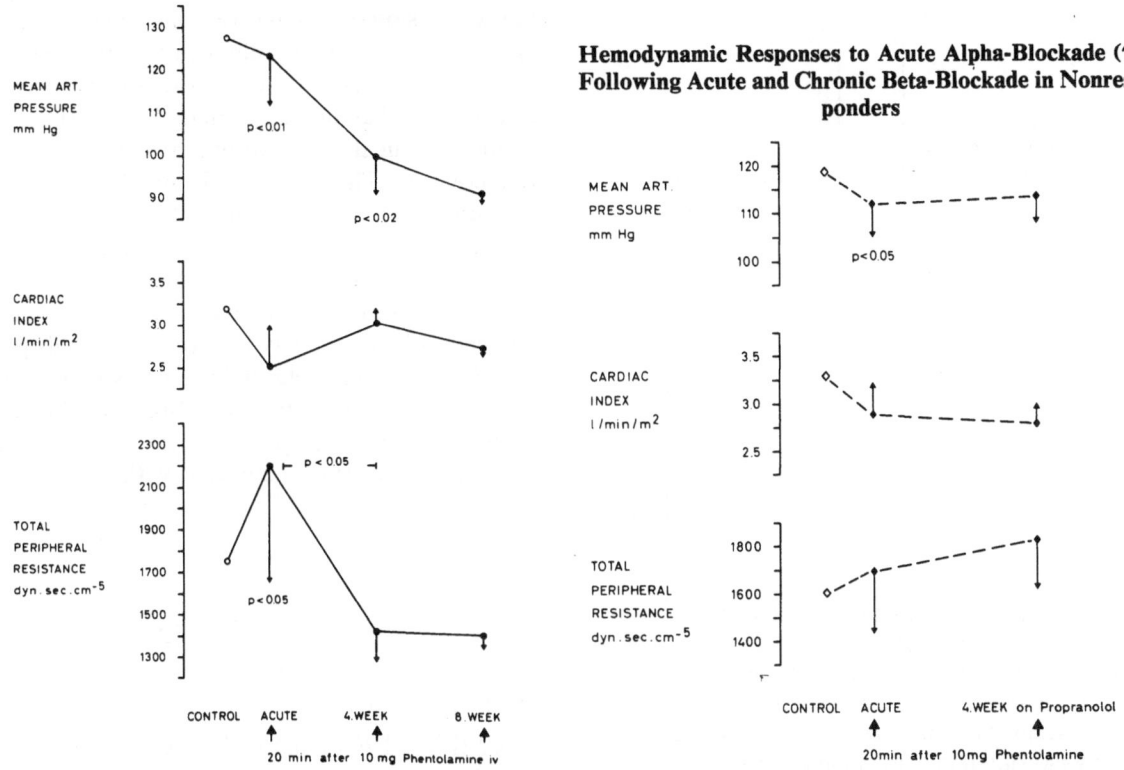

Hemodynamic Responses to Acute Alpha-Blockade (↑) Following Acute and Chronic Beta-Blockade in Nonresponders

Fig. 4. a: Hemodynamic variables before (○) and during acute and chronic propranolol administration (●) in four beta-blocker responders (———). Response to superimposed alpha-adrenoreceptor blockade with phentolamine decreases in the course of propranolol therapy *(arrows)*. **b:** Hemodynamic variables before (◇) and during acute and chronic propranolol administration (◇) in four beta-blocker nonresponders (– – –). Response to superimposed alpha-adrenoreceptor blockade with phentolamine remaining unchanged in the course of propranolol therapy *(arrows)*.

What then determines the decrease of alpha-adrenoreceptor-mediated vasoconstriction and the fall in peripheral vascular resistance? Several mechanisms resulting in decreased sympathetic nerve activity or in an alteration of the adrenergic receptor–effector system must be considered.

The search for a *possible central site* for the antihypertensive action of beta-blockers was prompted by the discovery of the central alpha-adrenoreceptor agonistic effect of clonidine, resulting in reduced nerve activity (99). Central beta-adrenoreceptor blockade was thought to result in unopposed central alpha-adrenoreceptor stimulation. The hypertensive effect of intraventricular administration of isoproterenol (100) suggests such a role for central beta-adrenoreceptors. This notion is supported by the finding that intraventricular administration of the *l*-isomers of beta-blockers reduces arterial pressure (99–101), and the verte-

bral artery infusion of propranolol diminishes impulse traffic in splanchnic nerves (10). However, this latter effect did not occur with practolol (10). The marked antihypertensive effectiveness of a number of beta-blockers that because of low lipid partition coefficients do not readily cross the blood–brain barrier—for example, sotalol (102), practolol, metoprolol, and atenolol (103)—does not support a central site of action. Even when given intraventricularly sotalol failed to lower blood pressure (104). The time lag between the administration of beta-blockers and the fall in blood pressure is also difficult to explain by a central site of action.

A baroreflex alteration by beta-receptor blockade is contradicted by the fact that beta-blockade does not affect the sensitivity of the baroreflex (65), although changes in pulse intervals at a reference pressure ("resetting") may occur. Such a resetting

Prazosin Induced Increase in Forearm Blood Flow Before and Following Antihypertensive Response to Propranolol

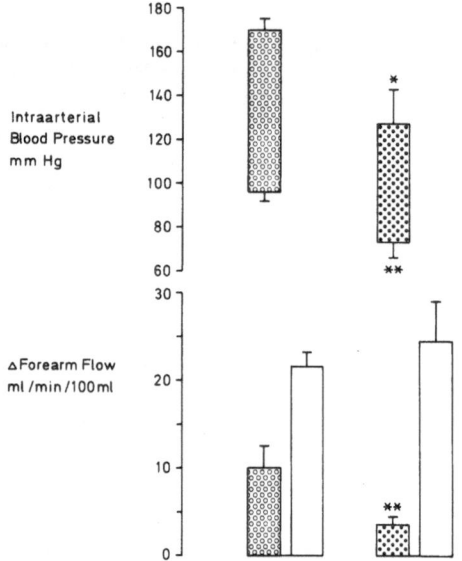

Fig. 5. Response in forearm blood flow to post junctional alpha-adrenoreceptor blockade with prazosin intraarterially (0.5 µg/min/100 ml tissue) *(lower panel, stippled bars)* is diminished in the fourth week of propranolol therapy, whereas response to nonspecific vasodilatation with sodium nitroprusside *(lower panel, white bars)* remains unchanged.

could be secondary to a decreased frequency of aortic distension as a result of cardiac beta-receptor blockade.

A prejunctional mechanism has been proposed because blockade of prejunctional beta-adrenoreceptors can result in decreased norepinephrine liberation at the sympathetic nerve endings (11). Whether or not this mechanism can achieve the pharmacotherapeutic effect is speculative, particularly since the inhibition operates only at a low-neural impulse traffic (105). In essential hypertension significant changes in resting plasma catecholamines were not observed (72, 73, 106–109), with one exception (110). This argues against a central or prejunctional neural action of beta-adrenoreceptor blockade, at least under these resting conditions. However, ergometric exercise may activate a central component, since stimulated plasma norepinephrine and epinephrine decrease in responders but not in nonresponders (109).

Postjunctional vascular beta₂-adrenoreceptor blockade has also been suggested in explaining the

antihypertensive effect of beta-blockade at the subcellular level (12). According to this theory, the adenyl cyclase complex, inhibited by beta-receptor blockade, slowly regains responsiveness to other agents (e.g., prostaglandins) normally mediating vasodilatation. Attractive as this theory may be, at present it has no experimental support.

Some clinical observations also argue against this concept. Thus, cardioselective beta-1-adrenoreceptor blockers (e.g., atenolol) reduce blood pressure comparably with other beta-blockers (46, 89, 94, 111) even when given in low doses (88, 89). The advent of selective vascular beta₂-adrenoreceptor blockers may help to unravel this problem. However, in preliminary studies with a drug having predominantly beta-2-receptor-blocking properties, the fall in pressure was significant and comparable to that achieved with propranolol (112).

SUPPRESSION OF RENIN-ANGIOTENSIN SYSTEM DETERMINING ANTIHYPERTENSIVE ACTION OF BETA-BLOCKERS

A pivotal role for renin-angiotensin suppression in the antihypertensive effect of beta-blockers is suggested by the following observations:

1) The positive correlation between the antihypertensive efficacy and the pretreatment renin levels;
2) The suppression of renin by all types of beta-blockers;
3) The correlation between the reduction in renin and the long-term fall in blood pressure and peripheral vascular resistance (113);
4) The similarity of pressure response to beta-blockers and to more selective inhibitors of the renin-angiotensin system.

The antihypertensive effect of beta-blockers resulting from suppression of the renin-angiotensin system can be explained by the following sequence of events. Initially, blockade of beta-adrenoreceptors immediately results in a reduced cardiac output and attendant baroreflex-mediated stimulation of sympathetic nerve activity (as reflected in a rise in plasma norepinephrine and epinephrine) and in an enhanced alpha-adrenoreceptor-mediated vasoconstriction. Thus, alpha-adrenoreceptor-mediated vasoconstriction may override the vasodilating effect of renin-angiotensin suppression regardless of the response to chronic beta-blocker therapy.

Within hours or days sympathetic nerve activity, as judged from plasma catecholamines, returns to normal. During chronic beta-blockade the key determinant for the vasodilatation is suppression of renin release with a decrease in angiotensin-mediated vasoconstriction. While cardiac output remains reduced, the initially elevated peripheral resistance returns to or below normal. This vasodilatation is due not only to a diminution of the direct angiotensinergic vasoconstriction, but also to additional factors. Thus, renin suppression is followed by a diminishing angiotensin effect on aldosterone secretion; this promotes sodium diuresis and reduces plasma volume. These effects may partly explain the delayed antihypertensive response. A diminution of angiotensin's central feedback stimulation of the sympathetic activity may also contribute to reduced alpha-adrenoreceptor-mediated vasoconstriction.

Consequently, lack of antihypertensive response to beta-blockers may be explained by a nonsuppressible or low pretreatment renin level or a failure of aldosterone secretion to fall. It may also be due to persistent alpha-adrenoreceptor-mediated vasoconstriction.

Suppression of the renin–angiotensin system as a consequence of beta-adrenoreceptor blockade is a more satisfactory explanation of the antihypertensive action of beta-blockers than any of the proposed alternatives. This does not imply that non renin factors are unimportant, but that they may not be critical.

SUMMARY

All beta-blockers suppress renin secretion. The antihypertensive response to monotherapy with beta-blockers can be predicted by the renin-sodium index, because control of diastolic blood pressure (≤ 95 mmHg) was achieved in about three-fourths of the patients with high renin, half with normal renin, but in only a few with low renin. Increasing age is associated with some decrease in renin as well as in the antihypertensive efficacy of beta-blocker monotherapy.

The relationship between the decrease in renin levels and the long-term reduction in blood pressure with beta-blockers as well as the similar renin-related blood pressure responses to the more selective inhibitors of the renin-angiotensin system indicates that renin suppression plays a pivotal role in the antihypertensive action of beta-blockers. Acute beta-adrenoreceptor blockade is followed by a baroreflex-mediated stimulation of sympathetic activity with enhanced alpha-adrenoreceptor-mediated vasoconstriction, which initially counters the vasodilating effect of renin suppression. Later, a fall in blood pressure occurs whenever the renin-angiotensin system is involved in the maintenance of the hypertension. This is probably largely due to reduced direct angiotensin-vasoconstriction. Concomitant reduction of aldosterone secretion, resulting in sodium diuresis and reduced plasma volume, may also contribute to the delayed onset of antihypertensive action of beta-blockers. Other less important factors may be decreased indirect angiotensin amplification of alpha-adrenoreceptor-mediated vasoconstriction, and possibly, diminished central sympathetic stimulation.

ACKNOWLEDGMENTS

This work was supported by special grants from the Swiss National Funds No. 3.894.77, Swiss Cardiology Foundation, Foundation for Teaching and Research of the University of Basel, and the Dr. C. and F. Demuth Swiss Medical Research Foundation.

The author is indebted to the editorial help of P. Bolli, M.D., L. Hulthen, M.D., O. de S. Pinto, M.D., and Mrs. M. E. Guldiman.

REFERENCES

1. Prichard BNC, Gillam PMS (1964) Use of propranolol in treatment of hypertension. Br Med J 2: 725
2. Schroeder G, Werkoe L (1964) Nethalide, a beta-adrenergic blocking agent. Clin Pharmacol Ther 5: 159
3. Prichard BNC, Gillam PMS (1966) Propranolol in hypertension. Am J Cardiol 18: 387

4. Frohlich ED, Dustan HP, Page IH (1966) Hyperdynamic beta-adrenergic circulatory state. Arch Intern Med 117: 614

5. Frohlich ED, Tarazi RC, Dustan HP, Page IH (1968) The paradox of beta-adrenergic blockade in hypertension. Circulation 37: 417

6. Michelakis AM, McAllister MG (1972) The effect of chronic adrenergic receptor blockade on plasma renin activity in man. J Clin Endocrinol Metab 34: 386

7. Bühler FR, Baer L, Vaughan ED Jr, Brunner HR, Laragh JH (1972) Inhibition of renin secretion by propranolol: A specific treatment for renal hypertension? (abstr). J Clin Invest 51: 17A

8. Bühler FR, Laragh JH, Baer L, Vaughan ED Jr, Brunner HR (1972) Propranolol inhibition of renin secretion: A specific approach to diagnosis and treatment of renin-dependent hypertensive diseases. New Engl J Med 287: 1209

9. Bühler FR, Laragh JH, Vaughan ED Jr, Brunner HR, Gavras H, Baer L (1973) The antihypertensive action of propranolol: Specific anti-renin responses in high and normal renin forms of essential, renal, renovascular and malignant hypertension. Am J Cardiol 32: 511

10. Lewis PJ, Haeusler G (1975) Reduction in sympathetic nervous activity as a mechanism of the hypotensive effect of propranolol. Nature 256: 440

11. Adler-Grashinski E, Langer SZ (1975) Possible role of a beta-adrenoceptor in the regulation of noradrenaline release by nerve stimulation through a positive feedback mechanism. Br J Pharmacol 53: 43

12. Amer MS (1976) Mechanism of action of beta-blockers in hypertension. J Biochem Pharmacol 26: 171

13. Prichard BNC, Gillam PMS (1969) Treatment of hypertension with propranolol. Br Med J 1: 7

14. Zacharias FJ, Cowen KJ, Prestt J, Vickers J, Wall BG (1972) Propranolol in hypertension: A study of long term therapy, 1964–1970. Am Heart J 83: 755

15. Hansson H, Hood B (1972) Propranolol in hypertension. Report on 158 patients treated up to one year. Klin Wochenschr 50: 364

16. Bühler FR, Burkart F, Lütold BE, Küng M, Marbet G, Pfisterer M (1975) Antihypertensive beta-blocking action as related to renin and age: A pharmacologic tool to identify pathogenetic mechanisms in essential hypertension. Am J Cardiol 36: 653

17. Veterans Administration Cooperative Study Group on Antihypertensive Agents (1977) Propranolol in the treatment of essential hypertension. JAMA 237: 2303–2310

18. Brunner HR, Laragh JH, Baer L, Newton MD, Goodwin FT, Krakoff LR, Bard RH, Bühler FR (1972) Essential hypertension: Renin and aldosterone, heart attack and stroke. New Engl J Med 286: 441

19. Bühler FR, Patel U, Marbet G (1974) Ambulante und stationäre Bestimmung des Renin-Natrium Index zur Unterteilung und gezielten Behandlung der essentiellen Hypertonie. Schweiz Med Wochenschr 104: 1802

20. Bühler FR, Lütold BE, Küng M, Koller FJ (1976) Once daily dosage beta-blockade: Antihypertensive efficacy of slow release oxprenolol as related to renin and age. Aust NZ J Med 6(Suppl III): 37

21. Bühler FR, Marbet G, Koller FJ, Küng M (1975) Single daily dose renin-suppressive and antihypertensive action of a new beta-adrenoceptor blocking agent (abstr). 9th Annual Meeting of the European Society for Clinical Investigation, Rotterdam, April 1975.

22. van Brummelen P, Bühler FR, Amann FW, Bolli P, Aellig W (1980) New long-acting non-cardioselective betablocker Sandoz LT 31200: Effects on blood pressure, plasma catecholamines, renin and cholesterin. In: Abstracts, seventh scientific meeting international society of hypertension, New Orleans p 138

23. Kiowski W, Bühler FR, Stumpe O (in press) Simplified antihypertensive therapy with slow release pindolol. Eur J Clin Pharmacol

24. Hollifield JW, Sherman K, Zwagg RV, Shand DG (1976) Proposed mechanisms of propranolol's antihypertensive effect in essential hypertension. New Engl J Med 295: 68

25. Karlberg BE, Kagedahl B, Tegler L, Tolagen K, Bergman B (1976) Controlled treatment of primary hypertension with propranolol and spironolactone. Am J Cardiol 27: 642

26. Drayer JIM, Keim HJ, Weger MA, Case DB, Laragh JH (1976) Unexpected pressor response to propranolol in essential hypertension. Am J Med 60: 897

27. Drayer JIM, Weber MD, Longworth DL, Laragh JH (1978) The possible importance of aldosterone as well as renin in the long term antihypertensive action of propranolol. Am J Med 64: 187

28. MacGregor GA, Markandu ND, Roulston JE (1979) Does the renin-angiotensin system maintain blood pressure in both hypertensive and normotensive subjects? A comparison of propranolol, saralasin and captopril. Clin Sci 57: 145A

29. Klumpp F, Braun B, Klaus D, Lemke R, Zehner J (1976) Die Behandlung der essentiellen Hypertonie mit Propranolol. Dtsch Med Wochenschr 101: 1482

30. Moore SB, Goodwin FJ (1976) Effect of beta-adrenergic blockade on plasma-renin activity and intractable hypertension in patients receiving regular dialysis treatment. Lancet 2: 67

31. Stumpe, KO, Kolloch R, Vetter H, Gramann W, Krück F, Ressel Ch, Higuchi M (1976) Acute and longterm studies of the mechanisms of action of betablocking drugs in lowering blood pressure. Am J Med 60: 853

32. Weidmann P, Beretta-Piccoli C, Ziegler W, Hirsch D, De Chatel R, Reubi FC (1976) Beziehungen zwischen Blutdruck, Blutvolumen, Plasma-Renin und Urin-Katecholaminen während Betablockade

bei essentieller Hypertonie. Klin Wochenschr 54: 765

33. Castenfors J, Castenfors H, Oro L (1973) Effect of alprenolol on blood pressure and plasma renin activity in hypertensive patients. Acta Med Scand 193: 189

34. Meekers J, Missotten A, Fagard R, Demyynck D, Harvengt C, Pas P, Billiet L, Amery A (1975) Predictive value of various parameters for the antihypertensive effect of the betablocker ICI 66.082. Arch Int Pharmacodyn Ther 2: 294

35. Balansard P, Chabrillat Y, Paulin R, Libes M, Gérard R (1977) Effect of atenolol, a new cardioselective betablocker on plasma renin activity in treatment of hypertension. Acta Cardiol (Brux) 32: 229

36. Zech P, Sassard J, Pozet N, McAinsh J, Legheand J (1977) Pharmacokinetic and pharmacodynamic studies on atenolol (ICI 66082) in hypertensive patients with renal impairment. Postgrad Med J 53(Suppl III): 134

37. Philipp T, Cordes U, Distler A (1977) Sympathikusaktivierbarkeit und blutdrucksenkende Wirkung einer Beta-Rezeptorenblockade bei essentieller Hypertonie. Dtsch Med Wochenschr 102: 569

38. Distler A, Keim HJ, Cordes U, Philipp T, Wolff HP (1978) Sympathetic responsiveness and antihypertensive effect of beta-receptor blockade in essential hypertension. Am J Med 64: 446

39. Ménard J, Bertagna X, N'Guyen PT, Degoulet P (1976) Rapid identification of patients with essential hypertension sensitive to acebutalol (a new cardio-selective betablocker). Am J Med 60: 886

40. Alhenc-Gélas F, Plouin PF, Ducrocq MG, Corvol P, Ménard J (1978) Comparison of the antihypertensive and hormonal effects of a cardioselective betablocker, acebutolol, and diuretics in essential hypertension. Am J Med 64: 1005

41. von Bahr C, Collste P, Frisk-Holmberg M, Haglund K, Jorfelt L, Orme M, Östman J, Sjöqvist F (1976) Plasma levels and effects of metoprolol on blood pressure, adrenergic beta receptor blockade and plasma renin activity in essential hypertension. Clin Pharmacol Ther 20: 130

42. Tsukiyama H, Otsuka K, Higuma K, Kitamura Y (1979) Paradoxical rise in blood pressure with various beta-adrenergic blocking agents. Jgakuno-Ayumi 108: 307

43. Karlberg BE, Nilsson O, Tolagen K, Nitelius E, Waern U (1979) Once-daily metoprolol in primary hypertension. Clin Pharmacol Ther 25: 399

44. Weber MA, Priest RT, Ricci BA, Eltorai MI, Brewer DD (1980) Low dose diuretic and beta-adrenoceptor blocker in essential hypertension. Clin Pharmacol Ther 28: 149

45. Brunner HR, Sealey JE, Laragh JH (1973) Renin subgroups in essential hypertension. Further analyses of their pathophysiological and epidemiological characteristics. Circ Res 22(Suppl I): 99

46. Bühler FR, Bertel O, Lütold BE (1978) Simplified and stratified antihypertensive therapy based on betablockers. Cardiovasc Med 3: 135

47. Conway J (1970) Effect of age on the response to propranolol. Int J Clin Pharmacol Ther Toxicol 4: 148–150

48. Bertel O, Bühler FR, Kiowski W, Lütold BE (1980) Decreased beta-adrenoreceptor responsiveness as related to age, blood pressure and plasma catecholamines in patients with essential hypertension. Hypertension 2: 130

49. Bühler FR, Kioski W, Landmann R, van Brummelen P, Amann W, Bolli P, Bertel O (1981) Changing role of beta and alpha-adrenoceptor-mediated cardiovascular responses in the transition from a high cardiac output into a high peripheral resistance phase in essential hypertension. In: This volume

50. Bühler FR, Kiowski W, van Brummelen P, Amann FW, Bertel O, Landmann R, Lütold BE, Bolli P (1980) Plasma catecholamines and cardiac, renal and peripheral vascular adrenoceptor-mediated responses in different age groups of normal and hypertensive subjects. Clin Exp Hypertension 2: 409

51. van Brummelen P, Bühler FR, Kiowski W, Amann FW (in press) Age-related decrease in cardiac and peripheral vascular responsiveness to isoproterenol: Studies in normal subjects. Clin Sci (in press)

52. Bühler FR, Kiowski W (1980) Plasma catecholamines, renin, age and antihypertensive response of man to betablockers. In: Bevan JA, et al (eds) Vascular neuroeffector mechanisms. Raven Press, New York p 376

53. Littler WA (1981) Catecholamines as predictors of drug response. In: This volume

54. Bühler FR, Marbet G, Patel U, Burkart F (1975) Renin suppressive potency of various betablockers at supine rest and during upright exercise. Clin Sci 48: 61

55. Kiowski W, Bühler FR, van Brummelen P, Küng M (1979) Blunting of exercise-induced tachycardia and renin release 24 hours after a single dose of sotalol. J Clin Pharmacol 19: 513

56. Amery A, Billiet L, Boel A, Fagard R, Reybrouck R, Willems J (1976) Mechanism of hypotensive effect during beta-adrenergic blockade in hypertensive patients: Hemodynamic and renin response to a new cardioselective agent: Tenormin or ICI 66,082. Am Heart J 91: 634

57. Davies R, Gesses DM, Slater JDH, et al (1975) The specificity of beta-adrenoceptors for the release of renin in man. In: Medical research society meeting, London

58. Weber MA, Stokes GS, Gain JM (1974) Comparison of the effects on renin release of beta-adrenergic antagonists with differing properties. J Clin Invest 54: 1413

59. Davies R, Payne NN, Slater JDH (1975) The effect of oxprenolol on renin release in man. In: Burley DM, Birdwood GFB, Fryer JH et al (eds) Hypertension—Its nature and treatment. CIBA Horsham, Horsham, England. p 169

434   F. R. Bühler

60. Stokes GS, Weber MA, Thornell IR (1974) Beta-blockers and plasma renin activity in hypertension. Br Med J 1: 60

61. Bühler FR, Marbet G, Koller FJ, Küng M (1975) Single daily dose renin-suppressive and antihypertensive action of a new beta-adrenoceptor blocking agent (abstr). 9th Annu Meet Eur Soc for Clinical Investigation, Rotterdam 1975

62. Esler MD, Nestel PJ (1973) Evaluation of practolol in hypertension: Effects on sympathetic nervous system and renin responsiveness. Br Heart J 35: 469

63. Åberg H (1974) Beta-receptors and renin release. New Engl J Med 290: 1026

64. Salvetti A, Arzilli F, Baccini C (1973) The effect of a betablocker on plasma renin activity of hypertensive patients. J Nucl Biol Med 17: 142

65. Simon G, Kiowski W, Julius S (1978) Antihypertensive and beta-adrenoceptor antagonist action of timolol. Clin Pharmacol Ther 23: 152

66. Gavras H, Gavras I, Brunner HR, Laragh JH (1977) Effect of a new beta-adrenergic blocker l-bunolol on blood pressure and on the renin-aldosterone system. J Clin Pharmacol 17: 350

67. Volicer L, Gavras H, Liang C, Tifft CP, Kershaw GR, Gavras I, Griffith DL, Salit M, Vukovich R, Brunner HR (1979) The effect of nadolol in the treatment of hypertension. J Clin Pharmacol 19:137–147

68. Amery A, Billiet L, Fagard R (1974) Beta-receptors and renin release. New Engl J Med 290: 284

69. George CG, Lewis PJ, Steiner JA, et al (1975) A comparison of propranolol and compound RO3–4787 (Bufuralol) in the treatment of arterial hypertension in man. Clin Sci 48: 65S

70. Stokes GS, Weber MA, Thornell IR (1974) Beta-blockers and plasma renin activity in hypertension. Br Med J 1: 60

71. Morgan TO, Roberts R, Carney SL, et al (1975) Beta-adrenergic receptor blocking drugs, hypertension and plasma renin. Br J Clin Pharmacol 2: 159

72. Hansson BG, Dymling JF, Hedeland H, Hulthén UL (1977) Long term treatment of moderate hypertension with the beta-1 receptor blocking agent metoprolol. Eur J Clin Pharmacol 11: 239

73. Hansson BG, Hökfelt B (1975) Long term treatment of moderate hypertension with penbutolol (Hoe 893d): I. Effects on blood pressure, pulse rate, catecholamines in blood and urine, plasma renin activity and urinary aldosterone under basal conditions and following exercise. Eur J Clin Pharmacol 9: 9

74. Brunner HR, Baer L, Sealey JE, Ledingham JGG, Laragh JH (1970) The influence of potassium administration and potassium deprivation on plasma renin in normal and hypertensive subjects. J Clin Invest 49: 2128

75. Waal-Manning H (1976) Hypertension: which betablocker? Drugs 12: 412

76. Bolli P, Bühler FR, Raeder EA, Amann FW, Meier M, Rogg H, Burckhardt D Safe abrupt withdrawal of long term betablockade with oxprenolol in hypertensive patients. Circulation (in press)

77. Brunner HR, Gavras H, Laragh JH, Keenan R (1974) Hypertension in man: Exposure of the renin and sodium components using angiotensin II blockade. Circ Res 34(Suppl I): 33

78. Streeten DHP, Anderson GH, Freiberg JM, et al (1975) Use of an angiotensin II antagonist (saralasin) in the recognition of 'angiotensinogenic' hypertension. New Engl J Med 292: 657

79. Gavras H, Brunner HR, Laragh JH, et al (1974) An angiotensin-converting enzyme inhibitor to identify and treat vasoconstrictor and volume factors in hypertensive patients. New Engl J Med 291: 817

80. Brunner HR, Gavras H, Waeber B, Kershaw G, Turini G, Vokovitch RA, McKistry D, Gavras I (1979) Oral angiotensin-converting enzyme inhibitor in longterm treatment of hypertensive patients. Ann Intern Med 90: 19

81. Case DB, Atlas SA, Laragh JH, et al (1978) Clinical experience with blockade of the renin-angiotensin-aldosterone system by an oral converting enzyme inhibitor (SQ 14225, captopril) in hypertensive patients. Prog Cardiovasc Dis 21: 195

82. Young DB, Diepstra GR (1978) Lack of antihypertensive effects of propranolol in experimental angiotensin II hypertension. Physiologist 21: 132

83. Young DB (1981) Comparison of a beta-blocker and converting enzyme inhibitor in two types of experimental hypertension. In: This volume

84. Chui PIS, Sommer EJA (1979) Effect of Na^+ restriction on blood pressure responses to beta-adrenoceptor blockade in spontaneously hypertensive rats (SHR) (abstr). Fed Proc 2370–2375

85. Sederberg-Olsen P, Ibsen H (1972) Plasma volume and extracellular fluid volume during long term treatment with propranolol in essential hypertension. Clin Sci 43: 165

86. Leonetti G, Mayer G, Morganti A, Terzoli L, Zanchetti A, Bianchetti A, Disalle E, Morselli PL, Chidsey CA (1975) Hypotensive and renin-suppressing activities of propranolol in hypertensive patients. Clin Sci Mol Med 48: 491

87. Davies R, Pickering TG, Morganti A, Laragh JH (in press) Blockade by low dose propranolol of cardiac and renal beta-receptors in normal subjects—Clues to its antihypertensive effects. Br Heart J

88. Douglas-Jones AP, Cruickshank JM (1976) Once-daily dosing with atenolol in patients with mild or moderate hypertension. Br Med J 1: 990

89. Bolli P, Hulthén L, Amann FW, Bühler FR (in preparation) Antihypertensive efficacy of atenolol and slow oxprenolol: A double blind crossover comparison.

90. Amann FW, Bühler FR, Bolli P, Kiowski W (in press) Enhanced alpha-adrenoceptor-mediated vasoconstriction in essential hypertension. Hypertension

91. Tarazi RC, Dustan HP (1972) Beta-adrenergic blockade in hypertension. Am J Cardiol 29: 633

92. Conway J (1974) In: Oliver M (ed) Progress in cardiology. Butterworth, London

93. Amery A, Billiet L, Boel A, Fagard R, Reybronk T, Willems J (1976) Mechanism of hypotensive effect during beta-adrenergic blockade in hypertensive patients. Am Heart J 91: 634

94. Pfisterer M, Burkart F, Bühler FR, Schweizer W (1976) Hämodynamische Veränderungen unter Metoprolol bei hypertensiven Patienten im Vergleich zu Propranolol. Schweiz Med Wochenschr 106: 1567

95. Lund-Johansen P, Ohm PJ (1976) Hemodynamic long term effects of beta-receptor-blocking agents in hypertension: A comparison between alprenolol, atenolol, metoprolol and timolol. Clin Sci Mol Med 51: 481S

96. Ferlinz J, Easthope JL, Hughes D, Siegel J, Tobis J, Aronow WS (1980) Antihypertensive and hemodynamic effects of oxprenolol vs. propranolol. Clin Pharmacol Ther 27: 733

97. Birkenhäger WH, Krauss XH, Schalekamp MADH, Klosters G, Kroon BJM (1971) Antihypertensive effects of propranolol. Folia Med Neerl 14: 67

98. Ibrahim MM, Tarazi RC, Dustan HP, et al (1975) Hyperkinetic heart in severe hypertension: A separate clinical hemodynamic entity. Am J Cardiol 35: 667

99. Reid JL, Lewis PJ, Myers MG, Dollery CT (1974) Cardiovascular effects of intracerebroventricular d-, l- and dl-propranolol in the conscious rabbit. J Pharmacol Exp Ther 188: 394

100. Day MD, Roach AG (1974) Central alpha- and beta-adrenoceptors modifying arterial blood pressure and heart rate in the conscious cat. Br J Pharmacol 51: 325

101. Day MD, Roach AG (1974) Cardiovascular effects of beta-adrenoceptor blocking agents after intracerebroventricular administration in conscious normotensive cats. Clin Exp Pharmacol Physiol 1: 333

102. Garvey HL, Ram N (1975) Comparative antihypertensive effects and tissue distribution of beta-adrenergic blocking drugs. J Pharmacol Exp Ther 194: 220

103. Regardh CG, Borg KO, Johnson G, Palma L (1974) Pharmacokinetic studies on the selective beta1-receptor antagonist metoprolol in man. J Pharmacokinet Biopharm 2: 347

104. Klevans LR, Kovacs JL, Kelly R (1976) Central effect of beta-adrenergic blocking agents on arterial blood pressure. J Pharmacol Exp Ther 196: 389

105. Celuch SM, Dubocovich ML, Langer SL (1978) Stimulation of presynaptic beta-adrenoceptors enhances (^{3}H)-noradrenaline release during nerve stimulation. Br J Pharmacol 63: 97

106. Pedersen EB, Christensen NJ (1975) Catecholamines in plasma and urine in patients with essential hypertension determined by double-isotope derivative techniques. Acta Med Scand 198: 373

107. Gierlichs HW, Planz G, Planz R, Stephany W, Rahn KH (1976) Der Einfluss des Beta-Rezeptorenblockers Propranolol auf die Katecholaminkonzentration im Plasma von Hypertonikern. Verh Dtsch Ges Inn Med 82: 1316

108. Franz IW, Lohmann FW, Koch G (1980) Differential effects of long-term cardioselective and nonselective beta-receptor blockade on plasma catecholamines during and after physical exercise in hypertensive patients. J Cardiovasc Pharmacol 2: 35

109. Bühler FR, Burkart F, Lütold BE, Bertel O, Pfisterer M (1977) Plasmakatecholamine und Hämodynamik im Verlauf der antihypertensiven Betablockade: Verschiedene Muster bei 'Propranolol-Responders' und 'Non Responders.' Schweiz Med Wochenschr 107: 1590

110. Brecht HM, Banthien F, Ernst W, Schoeppe W (1976) Increased plasma noradrenaline concentrations in essential hypertension and their decrease after long-term treatment with a beta-receptor-blocking agent (prindolol). Clin Sci Mol Med 51: 485S

111. Waal-Manning HJ (1976) The antihypertensive action of several beta-adrenoceptor blocking drugs. NZ Med J 83: 223

112. Amann FW, Hulthén L, Bühler FR (in preparation) Antihypertensive and renin suppressive effects of the selective beta2-adrenoceptor blocking agent LM 21009 (Sandoz)

113. Tarazi RC, Fouad FM, Bravo EL (1981) Total peripheral resistance and beta-adrenergic blockade. In: This volume

Comparison of a Beta-Blocker and Converting Enzyme Inhibitor in Two Types of Experimental Hypertension

David B. Young

In the last 3 years, two models of experimental hypertension have been developed in my laboratory that are useful in studying mechanisms of action of antihypertensive agents. The first is angiotensin II hypertension in the dog, produced by continuously infusing angiotensin II intravenously at a rate of 10 ng/kg/min. This infusion produces a stable hypertension with a mean arterial pressure of 130–140 mmHg, undetectable plasma renin activity (PRA), but levels of angiotensin II comparable to those found in moderate-to-severe sodium restriction or high-renin forms of hypertension (1, 2). The second model of hypertension is two-kidney, two-constrictor Goldblatt hypertension in the dog. In this laboratory, the renal artery constrictions are produced by ameroid constrictors (Three Point Products, Montreal) placed around the two renal arteries at 7-day intervals. The constrictors slowly compress the renal arteries, requiring 4–6 days to achieve maximum constriction. This results in a stable hypertension ranging between 140 and 160 mmHg with PRA between three to five times normal. The course of this form of hypertension in a group of seven dogs is shown in Fig. 1. Notice that arterial pressure (measured via an indwelling catheter) and PRA remained greatly elevated for at least 5 weeks after the second constrictor was placed on the renal artery.

These two models are similar in that both are highly dependent on angiotensin II. The important difference is that in the first, angiotensin II levels are fixed; in the second, the angiotensin II level is a function of the activity of the renin–angiotensin control system. These similarities and differ-

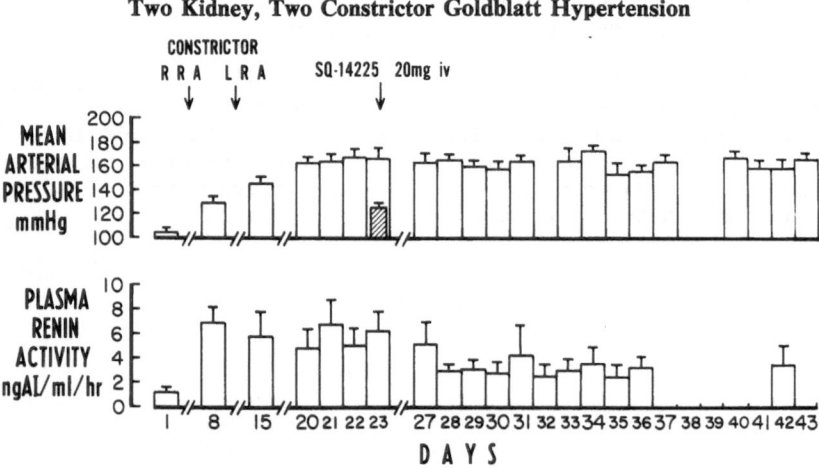

Fig. 1. Time-course of arterial pressure in two-kidney, two-constrictor Goldblatt hypertension as produced in this laboratory. Ameroid constrictors were placed on the right and left renal arteries on days 1 and 8. On day 23, a 20-mg bolus of captopril (SQ 14225) was given to assess the "renin dependence" of the model. The hatched bar is the mean arterial pressure recorded 20-min postinjection. Notice that arterial pressure and PRA remain markedly elevated for up to 6 weeks following placement of the second constrictor. Means and standard errors of the mean are indicated.

ences were used to assess the mechanisms by which the beta-blocker, propranolol, and the converting enzyme inhibitor, captopril, achieve their antihypertensive effects.

RESULTS

In Fig. 2, arterial pressure and PRA data are shown for a group of eight dogs with two-kidney, two-constrictor Goldblatt hypertension prepared in the same manner as those discussed above and shown in Fig. 1. Day 1 in Fig. 2 corresponds to day 27 in Fig. 1; therefore, all data shown were taken during the stable phase of the hypertension. Notice that on day 4 of Fig. 2, 20 mg captopril (SQ 14225) were given as an i.v. bolus. This resulted in a fall in arterial pressure of 18 mmHg from 144 ± 5 to 126 ± 5 mmHg ($p < 0.01$) in 20 min. After data collection was completed on day 5, propranolol was given to the dogs p.o., 240 mg/day: 120 mg at 8:00 AM and 120 mg at 4:00 PM. Notice that on the first day of propranolol treatment, arterial pressure fell from 137 ± 4 to 122 ± 6 mmHg ($p < 0.01$). PRA also fell dramatically on the first day of treatment, from 3.4 ± 1.2 to 2.0 ± 0.5 ng angiotensin I (AI)/ml/h

($p < 0.05$). Over the course of the 10 days of propranolol treatment, arterial pressure and PRA remained suppressed, the final values being 116 ± 4 mmHg and 1.4 ± 0.7 ng AI/ml/h, respectively. Captopril had no effect on arterial pressure on the final day of propranolol treatment.

Seven dogs with sustained angiotensin II hypertension were treated with the same dose of propranolol. These data are presented in Fig. 3. Notice that there was no change in arterial pressure in these animals whose PRA levels were undetectable.

In Fig. 4, data from a group of four dogs with stable angiotensin II hypertension are shown. On day 4, a 20-mg bolus of captopril was given, causing a fall from 130 ± 10 to 121 ± 7 mmHg. Each dog's arterial pressure fell to a similar degree over a 20-min period, suggesting that in spite of the small number of animals used, the effect was in fact significant, as well as being statistically significant ($p < 0.05$, paired-t). After completion of measurements on day 4, a continuous infusion of captopril was started at a rate of 400 mg/day. The group mean was 117 ± 8 mmHg after 24-h infusion, although one of the four animal's arterial pressure had returned to its previous level. On all succeeding days of combined angiotensin II and captopril infusion, arterial pressure remained at or above the control mean of 130 mmHg.

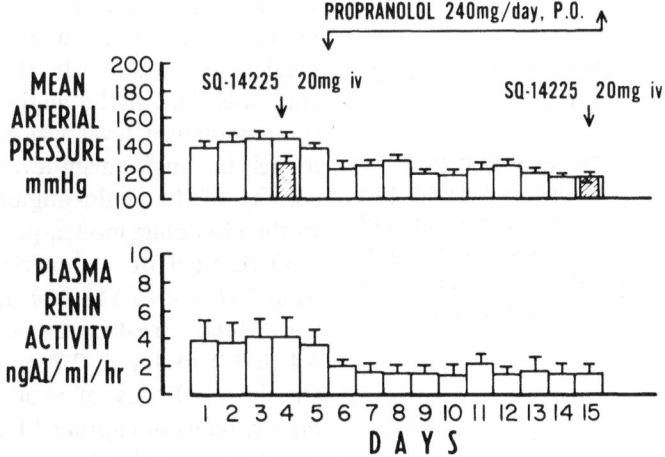

Two Kidney, Two Constrictor, Goldblatt Hypertension

Fig. 2. Mean arterial pressure and PRA data for a group of dogs prepared in the same manner as the group presented in Fig. 1. Day 1 of Fig. 2 corresponds to day 27 of Fig. 1. Captopril was given on day 4 as described in Fig. 1. After completion of data collection on day 5, propranolol treatment was begun and continued for 10 days. On the final day of treatment, a bolus of captopril was again given intravenously.

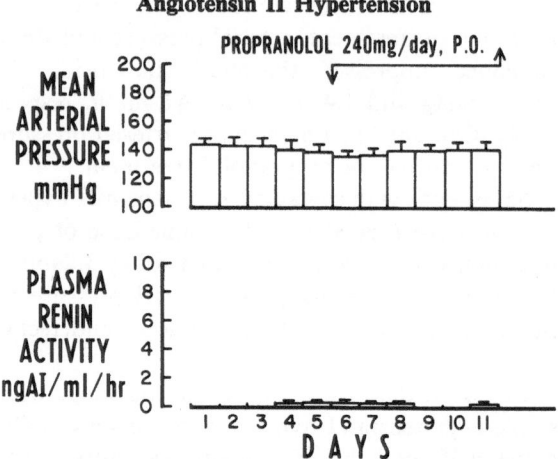

Fig. 3. Arterial pressure and PRA data for a group of dogs with angiotensin II hypertension treated with propranolol starting after completion of data collection on day 4. Notice that in this form of hypertension, arterial pressure was not affected by the same dose of propranolol given in the study presented in Fig. 2.

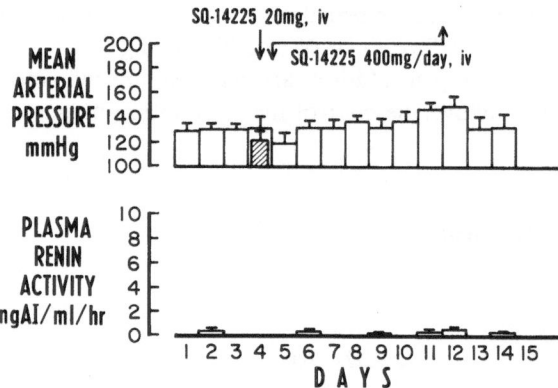

Fig. 4. Response of arterial pressure to captopril in angiotensin hypertension. An initial i.v. bolus produced a significant reduction of arterial pressure, although, after 48 h, arterial pressure returned to pretreatment levels. The hatched bar is the mean arterial pressure recorded 20-min post injection.

DISCUSSION

The results of the propranolol experiments presented here are consistent with the hypothesis that the primary antihypertensive action of the beta-blocker is suppression of angiotensin II levels. If propranolol achieved its effect via a central neural effect resulting in peripheral vasodilation, or via a negative inotropic effect, then one might have suspected arterial pressure to fall when propranolol was given to the dogs with angiotensin hypertension. The fact that arterial pressure levels were not affected by propranolol in the dogs with fixed angiotensin levels does not support the proposal that propranolol's antihypertensive action is mediated by a central neurogenic or cardiac mechanism.

The lack of long-term effect of captopril in the angiotensin hypertensive dogs is consistent with the hypothesis that converting enzyme inhibitors act by preventing formation of angiotensin II, not by potentiating the bradykinin system; however, the short-term response to the bolus of SQ 14225 may have been due to accumulation of kinins resulting from converting enzyme inhibition.

SUMMARY

Two experimental models of hypertension were used to assess the mechanisms of action of propranolol and the converting enzyme inhibitor captopril. The first model was two-clip, two-kidney Goldblatt hypertension in the dog, a highly renin-dependent form of hypertension. The second was angiotensin II infusion hypertension in the dog produced by infusing intravenously 10 ng/kg/min angiotensin II continuously for several weeks. The models were similar in that both were highly dependent on angiotensin II. The important difference was that in the angiotensin infusion model, the angiotensin level was fixed; in the Goldblatt model, the angiotensin level was a function of the activity of the renin–angiotensin control system. In the Goldblatt model, propranolol (240 mg/day p.o.) resulted in a reduction in arterial pressure from 137 ± 4 to 116 ± 4 mmHg ($p < 0.01$) over the 10-day treatment period. PRA fell from 3.4 ± 1.2 to 1.4 ± 0.7 ng AI/ml/h ($p < 0.01$). On the tenth day of propranolol treatment, 20-mg i.v. bolus of captopril had no effect on arterial blood pressure. In the angiotensin infusion model, neither propranolol (240 mg/day p.o.) nor captopril (400 mg/day i.v.) produced a sustained change in arterial pressure, although an initial 20-mg i.v. bolus of the converting enzyme inhibitor did reduce acutely arterial pressure from 130 ± 10 to 121 ± 7 mmHg ($p < 0.05$). These results are consistent with the hypotheses that propranolol's antihypertensive effect is mediated by suppression of the renin–angiotensin system, and that the long-term antihypertensive effect of captopril is the result of inhibition of formation of angiotensin II.

REFERENCES

1. Young DB, Murray RH, Bengis RG, Guyton AC (1977) Angiotensin II hypertension. Physiologist 20: 104
2. Young DB, Murray RH, Bengis RG, Markov AK (in press) Experimental angiotensin II hypertension. Am J Physiol

Pressor Effect of Beta-Adrenergic Blockade and Angiotensin II in Nephrectomized Rats

A. Iaina, D. Goldfarb, and H. Eliahou

An increase in blood pressure in approximately 11% of patients with essential hypertension was observed by Drayer et al. (1) following short-term therapy with the beta-blocker propranolol. The acute i.v. administration of propranolol in these patients did not decrease cardiac output, and in some of the figures presented a certain amount of increase could be seen (2). This clinical observation is obviously the end result of certain compensatory mechanisms. The readjustment of total peripheral resistance (TPR) to compensate for the decreased cardiac output (2) and an unopposed reactive alpha-sympathetic activity (1) were suggested as explanations for this phenomenon.

It is already known that following propranolol administration there is an increase in TPR (2–5). This increase is attributed to various compensatory mechanisms: sympathetic nervous system overstimulation as a consequence of the sudden decrease in cardiac output (4, 5), increased alpha-adrenergic activity that is left unhindered by the beta-adrenergic blockade, and lack of the beta-mediated vasodilatory effect on the blood vessels of skeletal muscles. It has also been shown that high-angiotensin II (AII) levels increase circulating catecholamines (CA) (5, 6). Therefore, the administration of a beta-adrenergic blocker, in the presence of high-AII concentration, with its attendant increase in CA, is expected to accentuate the rise in TPR and to result in a marked pressor effect.

The aim of this study was to verify the validity of the hypothesis that propranolol administration can indeed have a pressor effect in the presence of high AII levels. The experiments were performed in bilaterally nephrectomized rats under continuous background infusion of exogenous AII. The bilateral nephrectomy was performed in order to eliminate compensatory mechanisms associated with the renin–angiotensin system as well as other possible renal regulatory mechanisms.

MATERIALS AND METHODS

Female Charles-River rats, weighing between 250 and 300 g, obtained from a local commercial supplier (Yokneam, Israel), were used in all the experiments. In the first series of experiments, bilateral nephrectomy was performed 24 h prior to the actual experiment, in which the rats underwent anesthesia with intraperitoneal nembutal [3.5 mg/100 g body weight (BW)], tracheotomy, jugular vein cannulation for fluid administration with a constant infusion pump, and femoral artery cannulation for blood pressure measurements and drug administration. Blood pressure was monitored and recorded on a dual channel recorder (MG 92201 A module, MG Electronics, Rehovot, Israel) with the aid of a Stetham Transducer, Model P37 (Statham Instruments Inc., Oxnard, Cal.).

Every experiment lasted 40 min and was divided into four periods of 10 min each. Blood pressure measurements were taken at the end of the first 30 s, 2 min, and 10 min of each period. The basal blood pressure for further comparisons was that obtained at the end of the first 10-min period during which AII or saline alone were given. In the following 10-min periods, increasing doses of the same drug were administered. During the 40-min experiments, each rat received a total of 2 ml/100 g BW. Six groups of rats were studied:

Group A: This group received a continuous i.v. infusion of AII (Hypertensin, CIBA) in saline at 7 ng/min/100 g BW. The fluid was infused at the rate of 50 μl/min/100 g BW.

Group B: AII was administered as in group A, but at the rate of 36 μl/min/100 g BW. Starting from the 10th min and every 10 min thereafter, i.v. boluses of propranolol were administered in increasing amounts (dose 1: 0.06 mg/100 g BW; dose 2: 0.12 mg/100 g BW; dose 3: 0.36 mg/

100 g BW), all taken from a 1-mg/ml propranolol solution.

Group C: AII was administered as in group B, but with 5% glucose instead of propranolol in the same way and amount.

Group D: Propranolol and AII were administered as in group B. Different doses of phentolamine were added to propranolol (dose 1: 0.03 mg/100 g BW; dose 2: 0.06 mg/100 g BW; dose 3: 0.18 mg/100 g BW), all taken from a 1-mg/ml phentolamine solution. Care was taken to reduce the diluting volume of AII in order to maintain identical volumes per 40 min/100 g BW as in the other groups.

Group E: AII was administered as in group D, but with a 5%-glucose solution instead of propranolol.

Group F: as in group B, but saline alone was administered instead of AII. In a second series of experiments, bilateral nephrectomy and adrenalectomy were performed under intraperitoneal nembutal anesthesia. Two-hours later, while the rats were still under the initial anesthesia, the protocol of groups B and E from the first series of experiments were repeated; these are groups G and H, respectively.

Mean, standard error, and student's *t*-test were used for assessing significance (*p* < 0.05 was considered significant).

RESULTS OF BLOOD PRESSURE CHANGES AFTER EACH PERIOD

THIRTY-SECOND PERIODS

Propranolol: After propranolol administration in rats receiving saline, the blood pressure decreased (Fig. 1). The mean decrease in blood pressure was -3.3 ± 0.9 mmHg after the first dose, -6 ± 1.5 mmHg after the second dose, and -7.6 ± 3.9 mmHg after the third dose. In nephrectomized–adrenalectomized rats, the values were -10.7 ± 2.3, -14.9 ± 3.6, and -16.7 ± 5.0 mmHg, respectively, for the three different doses of propranolol.

Propranolol and AII: When similar doses of propranolol were administered in rats receiving a continuous infusion of AII, the mean decrease in blood pressure at the end of the 30-s periods was -7.7 ± 1.5, -11.6 ± 2.5, and -10.8 ± 4.4 mmHg, respectively. In the nephrectomized–adrenalectomized rats, the values were -21.0 ± 9.9, -21.9 ± 3.0, and -37.0 ± 5.5 mmHg, respectively.

Propranolol, phentolamine, and AII: Propranolol and phentolamine administration to nephrectomized rats receiving continuous infusion of AII was followed by a decrease in blood pressure. The mean decrease was -17.7 ± 1.9, -22.7 ± 3.7, and -37.3 ± 6.9 mmHg, respectively. This de-

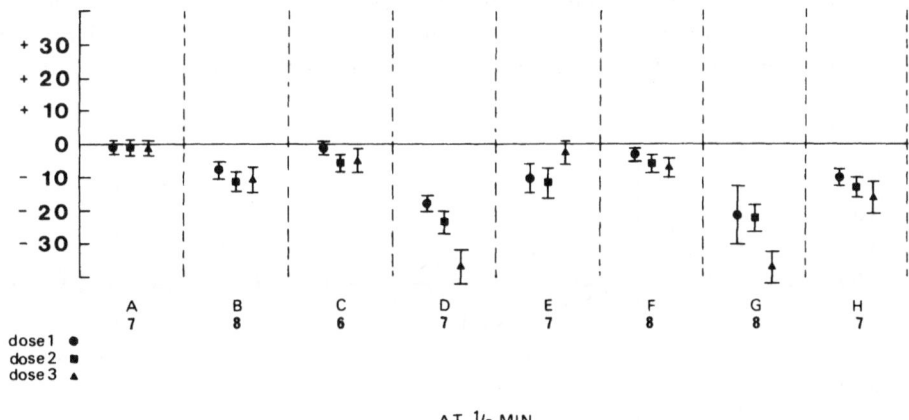

Fig. 1. Blood pressure changes in mmHg (mean ± SE), as compared with the control period (0), in the different experimental groups: measured at 30 s after administration of each dose. *Group A:* AII alone; *group B:* AII and propranolol; *group C:* AII and glucose; *group D:* AII, propranolol, and phentolamine; *group E:* AII, glucose, and phentolamine; *group F:* saline and propranolol; *group G:* AII and propranolol; *group H:* saline and propranolol. Groups A–F were all bilaterally nephrectomized rats, whereas groups G and H were nephrectomized–adrenalectomized rats. The numbers appearing under groups A–H represent the number of rats in each group.

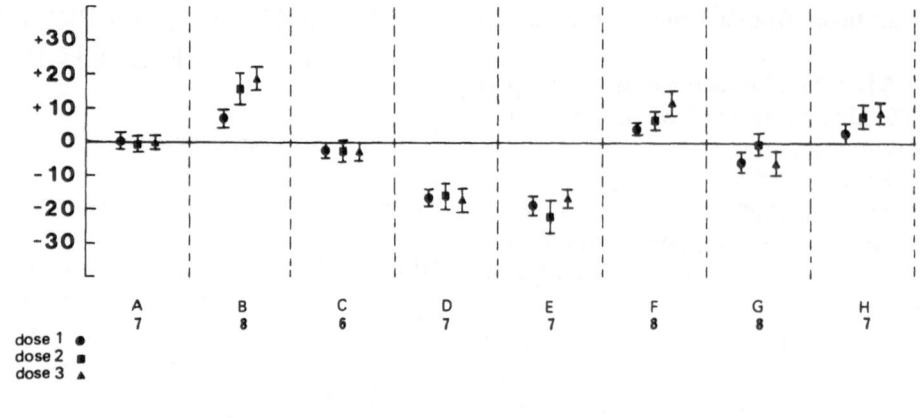

Fig. 2. Blood pressure changes in mmHg, measured at 2 min after administration of each dose. Description as in Fig. 1.

crease is significantly higher than that obtained in the first two groups receiving propranolol and propranolol with AII ($p < 0.01$), but not different from the nephrectomized–adrenalectomized rats.

Phentolamine: The changes in blood pressure at the end of the 30-s periods were similar to those in rats receiving propranolol alone, with a background infusion of AII.

TWO-MINUTE PERIODS

Propranolol: After propranolol administration in rats receiving saline, there was a certain amount of increase in blood pressure (Fig. 2). The mean of this increase was 4.0 ± 1.0 and 11.0 ± 4.5 mmHg for the three different doses, respectively.

In nephrectomized–adrenalectomized rats, the values were 3.1 ± 3.0, 8.3 ± 2.2, and 9.3 ± 2.6 mmHg, respectively. These values are significantly higher than those obtained in the control period ($p < 0.05$).

Propranolol and AII: With similar doses of propranolol in nephrectomized rats receiving a continuous infusion of AII, the mean increase in blood pressure was 7.3 ± 1.4, 14.0 ± 3.2, and 18.7 ± 4.3 mmHg, respectively. These values are significantly higher than those in the previous groups receiving propranolol without AII ($p < 0.05$). In adrenalectomized–nephrectomized rats receiving different doses of propranolol under the continuous infusion of AII, the blood pressure changes at the end of the 2-min periods were -6.0 ± 3.0,

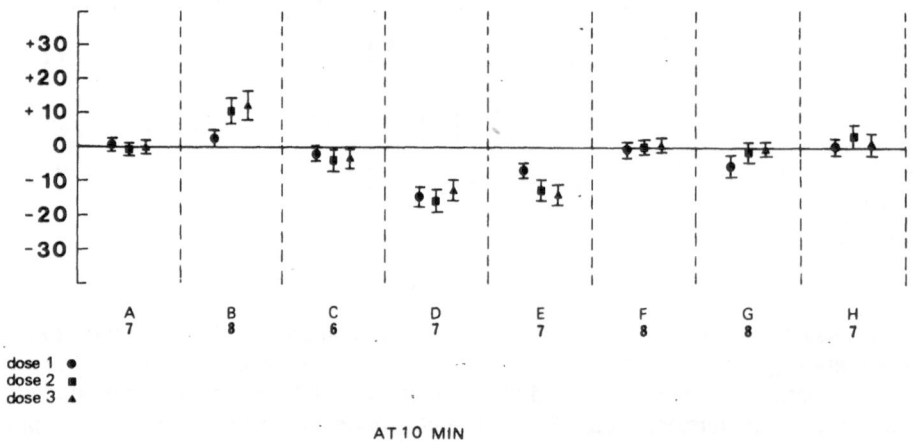

Fig. 3. Blood pressure changes in mmHg, measured at 10 min after administration of each dose. Description as in Fig. 1.

-0.5 ± 2.5, and -6.6 ± 3.3 mmHg, respectively.

Propranolol, phentolamine, and AII: When phentolamine was added to propranolol in nephrectomized rats receiving AII, the blood pressures remained significantly lower than those obtained at the control period. The mean decreases in blood pressures in this group were -15.7 ± 2.2, -4.7 ± 3.7, and -16.8 ± 2.8 mmHg, respectively.

TEN-MINUTE PERIODS

Blood pressure measurements at the end of most of the 10-min periods remained not significantly different from those obtained after the 2-min periods, although the mean values showed a tendency to return to pretreatment levels (Fig. 3). This tendency was more pronounced in the rats receiving propranolol alone, in which the blood pressure at the end of the 10-min periods returned almost to the control values.

DISCUSSION

Acute beta-adrenergic blockade, with intravenously administered boluses of propranolol in the presence of high-exogenous AII levels, resulted in a marked rise in mean arterial blood pressure following an initial short-lived drop. This pressor effect was present also, but to a lesser extent, in rats that did not receive the background AII infusion. The administration of glucose in equivalent volumes in place of propranolol was not followed by blood pressure changes, indicating that this was not due to changes in volume.

This agonistic pressor effect between AII and propranolol was completely abolished by alpha-adrenergic blockade with phentolamine. In rats with bilateral adrenalectomy in addition to bilateral nephrectomy, the administration of propranolol during the AII infusion resulted in the usual short-lived drop in blood pressure, which returned toward the basal levels within 2–10 min, but did not rise above it at any time.

The AII effect, in addition to its direct vasoconstrictive effect (7, 8), has a facilatatory-modulating role in the adrenergic neurotransmission (9). This role was demonstrated in the pre- and postsynaptic sites of the adrenergic nerve terminals and their synaptic gap. This results in the enhancement of the response to nerve stimulation as well as to the sympathetic amines (10). AII was also found to increase norepinephrine (NE) concentration in the synaptic cleft (11), most probably not by an inhibitory effect of reuptake (12). AII is known to increase the sympathetic outflow by an action on the central nervous system (13), adrenal medulla (14), and sympathetic ganglia (15), as a result of which the AII increases the NE levels, not only at the synaptic clefts, but also in the blood.

The beta-adrenergic blockade interrupts the effect of both the NE on the target organ and the neurotransmitter feedback loop (16). It follows, therefore, that beta-blockers are expected to diminish peripheral vasoconstriction. However, the acute (5) and chronic (6) administration of beta-adrenergic blockers resulted in elevated NE concentrations as a compensatory mechanism, probably due to the decrease in cardiac output, masking the expected opposite effect at the synaptic cleft and resulting in an increase in the TPR. Indeed, beta-adrenergic blockade was found to increase TPR (2, 3, 5, 17–20).

The rise in blood pressure following propranolol administration in the presence of high-AII levels is explained by the resulting high-blood NE levels stimulating alpha-adrenergic receptor activity and resulting in an increase in TPR. This is supported by the fact that concomitant alpha-adrenergic blockade was followed by the elimination of the propranolol–pressor effect as well as by the inability to return blood pressure to its basal level following its initial fall. The abolition of the propranolol-pressor effect was also observed in nephrectomized–adrenalectomized rats receiving background AII infusion. This could be logically explained by the lack of AII effect on NE release from the adrenal medulla. We can also speculate that the effect of AII administration on the central nervous system of bilaterally nephrectomized–adrenalectomized rats is accompanied by an increased NE release, which results in a high-central alpha-agonistic effect. This release can cause an important alpha-adrenoreceptor-mediated inhibition of adrenergic neurotransmission (9). It could be a good reason why in bilaterally nephrectomized–adrenalectomized rats, the administration of propranolol maintains its pressor effect in the complete absence of AII.

Parallels could be drawn between our experimental results and the unexpected pressor responses to propranolol in certain hypertensive patients

(1) who might, under certain circumstances, develop the necessary relationship between the sympathetic and the renin–angiotensin system for such a response.

SUMMARY

The acute administration of propranolol in bilaterally nephrectomized rats, with or without concomitant adrenalectomy, resulted in a rise in blood pressure after an initial short-lived drop. This effect was more pronounced in the nephrectomized rats during a continuous infusion of AII. The pressor effect of propranolol in bilaterally nephrectomized rats with AII infusion was abolished by alpha-adrenergic blockade with phentolamine or by bilateral adrenalectomy. The rise in blood pressure was attributed to propranolol's pressor effect by the increase in TPR through the unhindered alpha-adrenergic system during beta-adrenergic blockade, as well as by the stimulating AII effect on CA secretion and/or its modulatory role on adrenergic neurotransmission.

REFERENCES

1. Drayer JIM, Keim HJ, Weber MA, Case DB, Laragh JH (1976) Unexpected pressor response to propranolol in essential hypertension. Am J Med 60: 897–903
2. Hansson L, Zweifler AJ, Julius S, Hunyor SN (1974) Hemodynamic effects of acute and prolonged β-adrenergic blockade in essential hypertension. Acta Med Scand 196: 27–34
3. Ulrych M, Frohlich ED, Dustan HP, Page IH (1968) Immediate hemodynamic effects of β-adrenergic blockade with propranolol in normotensive and hypertensive man. Circulation 37: 411–416
4. Christensen NJ, Trap-Jensen J, Clausen J, Noer I, Kroisyaard AR, Larsen OA (1975) Effect of beta-adrenergic blockade on heart rate, hepatic blood flow and circulating noradrenaline at rest. Acta Physiol Scand 95: 62A–63A
5. Hansen JF, Hesse B, Christensen NJ (1978) Enhanced sympathetic nervous system activity after intravenous propranolol in ischemic heart disease: Plasma adrenalin splanchnic blood flow and mixed venous oxygen saturation at rest and during exercise. Eur J Clin Invest 8: 31–36
6. Esler M, Julius S, Zweifler A, Randall O, Harburg E, Gardiner H, DeQuattro V (1977) Mild high-renin essential hypertension: Neurogenic human hypertension? New Engl J Med 296: 405–411
7. Dyer DC (1970) The pharmacology of isolated sheep umbilical cord blood vessels. J Pharmacol Exp Ther 175: 565–570
8. Drimal J (1968) Effects of angiotensin II on coronary smooth muscle. Eur J Pharmacol 5: 56–62
9. Westfall TC (1977) Local regulation of adrenergic neurotransmission. Physiol Rev 57: 659–728
10. Johnson EM, Marshall GR, Needleman P (1974) Modification of responses to sympathetic nerve stimulation by the renin-angiotensin system in rats. Br J Pharmacol 51: 541–547
11. Zimmerman BG, Gomer SK, Liao JC (1972) Action of angiotensin on vascular adrenergic nerve endings: Facilitation of norepinephrine release. Fed Proc 31: 1344–1350
12. Hughes J, Roth RH (1971) Evidence that angiotensin enhances transmitter release during sympathetic nerve stimulation. Br J Pharmacol 41: 239–255
13. Buckley JP (1972) Actions of angiotensin on the central nervous system. Fed Proc 31: 1332–1337
14. Feldberg W, Lewis GP (1964) The action of peptides on the adrenal medulla: Release of adrenaline by bradykinin and angiotensin. J Physiol (Lond) 171: 98–108
15. Aiken JW, Reit E (1969) A comparison of the sensitivity to chemical stimuli of adrenergic and cholinergic neurons in the cat stellate ganglion. J Pharmacol Exp Ther 159: 211–223
16. Stjarne L, Brundin J (1975) Dual adrenoceptor-mediated control of noradrenaline secretion from human vasoconstrictor nerves: Facilitation by β-receptors and inhibition by α-receptors. Acta Physiol Scand 94: 139–141
17. Frohlich ED, Tarazi RC, Dustan HP, Page IH (1968) The paradox of β-adrenergic blockade in hypertension. Circulation 37: 417–423
18. Prichard BNC, Shinebourne E, Fleming J, Hamer J (1970) Hemodynamic studies in hypertensive patients treated by oral propranolol. Br Heart J 32: 236–240
19. Glover WE, Hutchison VJ (1965) The effect of beta-receptor antagonist (propranolol) on the cardiovascular response to intravenous infusion of noradrenaline in man (abstr). J Physiol 177: 59P
20. Achong MR, Piafsky KM, Ogilvie RI (1975) The effects of timolol (MK 950) and propranolol on peripheral vessels in man. Clin Pharmacol Ther 17: 228

Catecholamines as Predictors of Drug Response

W. A. Littler, R. D. S. Watson, and T. J. Stallard

Plasma levels of norepinephrine are a useful index of short-term changes in sympathetic activity (1, 2). We have measured plasma catecholamine levels and intraarterial blood pressure in hypertensive patients before and after beta-adrenoreceptor antagonism in order to determine how blood pressure and plasma catecholamines are altered by treatment.

PATIENTS AND METHODS

Seventeen hypertensive patients were studied (blood pressure >140/90 on at least three occasions as an outpatient). They had no evidence of an underlying cause of hypertension and there was no evidence of target-organ damage (Table 1).

Patients were studied before and after chronic administration of beta-adrenoreceptor antagonist administered once daily; after treatment, the last dose was taken at 8:00 AM on the day of investigation. In addition, observations were made in seven patients 3 h after the first dose. Ambulatory intra-arterial pressure was measured continuously over 24 h (3).

Patients were studied in an open hospital ward, and physical activity was standardized throughout the 24 h. Sodium intake was also standardized while in the hospital, patients receiving a diet containing 60 mEq sodium daily (2).

PLASMA CATECHOLAMINE SAMPLES

Blood samples were obtained from a forearm venous cannula without occlusion at least 30 min after cannulation. They were taken into cool-syringe heparinized tubes, centrifuged at 4°C and stored at −20°C within 30 min of sampling.

Samples from patients 1–6 were analyzed for norepinephrine by the method of Henry et al. (4), using bovine phenylethanolamine-N-methyltransferase.

Samples from patients 7–17 were analyzed for norepinephrine and epinephrine by the method of Peuler and Johnson (5), using catechol-o-methyltransferase; glutathione was added as an antioxidant.

Matched plasma samples were obtained before and after chronic treatment in patients 1–6 during standardized activities: a) sleep; b) supine rest (after 15 min); c) sitting (after 10 min); d) standing (after 10 min); e) walking; and f) cycling.

Resting specimens were obtained in nine patients (7–14 and 16) after lying supine for 40 min in a quiet room before and after chronic treatment (4 h after last dose).

In ten patients (7–16), samples were obtained during the last 30 s of upright bicycle exercise before and after chronic treatment; in seven patients (7–12 and 17), specimens were also obtained 3 h after acute oral administration of the first dose of beta-adrenoreceptor antagonist.

BICYCLE EXERCISE

Subjects performed upright bicycle exercise at constant load for 8 min on an ergometer; the load was determined from a previous exercise test to exhaustion as the load caused 85% of maximum heart rate.

RESULTS

Average duration of treatment was 16 ± 3 weeks (range: 8–52).

Table 1. Personal details of patients, mean blood pressures, and drugs used for treatment.

| Patient no. | Age (years) | Outpatient (mmHg) | | Mean blood pressure (mmHg) | | Treatment (mg/day)[c] |
		Pretreatment	After treatment	Ambulatory pretreatment	Ambulatory after chronic treatment	
1	42	143	131	142	105	P 320
2	44	142	130	121	109	A 400
3[a]	44	129	126	103	93	A 400
4[a]	23	130	117	100	99	A 400
5	48	125	118	101	96	A 400
6	52	134	113	102	92	P 160
7	44	118	117	90	77	ME 200
8	30	112	82	97	86	ME 200
9[a]	54	132	132	117	104	ME 200
10	27	119	98	99	80	P 240
11[a]	17	130	93	107	73	P 240
12	44	136	119	120	108	ME 200
13	32	116	99	96	92	P 240
14	42	118	103	92	78	ME 200
15	53	127	112	96	86	P 240
16	32	113	90	108	90	P 240
17[ab]	49	135	–	125	–	P 240
Mean ± SE	40 ± 3	127 ± 2	111 ± 4	107 ± 3	92 ± 3	

[a] Female patient.
[b] Observations made after acute treatment only.
[c] P, propranolol; A, acebutolol; ME, metoprolol.

BLOOD PRESSURE AND HEART RATE

Mean blood pressure during ambulatory recording decreased in every patient after chronic treatment from 106 ± 3 to 92 ± 3 mmHg ($p < 0.001$); mean heart rate decreased from 77 ± 3 to 60 ± 2 beats/min ($p < 0.001$).

Mean blood pressure and heart rate during exercise, and the responses to exercise, were significantly reduced after acute and chronic treatment; at 24 h after the last dose, exercise heart rate was significantly reduced from 152 ± 6 to 135 ± 6 beats/min ($p < 0.001$), but the reduction in exercise blood pressure at this time was not significant ($p > 0.01$).

PLASMA NOREPINEPHRINE AND BLOOD PRESSURE AND HEART RATE DURING A RANGE OF ACTIVITIES (PATIENTS 1–6)

We have previously reported a linear relationship between the logarithm of plasma norepinephrine and blood pressure and heart rate with increasing levels of physical activity prior to treatment in these patients (2). After treatment, mean-plasma norepinephrine levels tended to increase during each activity. Statistically significant increases were not observed during any activity. After treatment, the linear relationship between the logarithm of plasma norepinephrine and heart rate and blood pressure remained statistically significant in all patients, except patient 6, in whom only seven observations were made.

For patients as a group, there was a highly significant linear relationship between log-plasma norepinephrine and systolic blood pressure both before treatment ($r = 0.72$, $N = 81$, $p < 0.001$) and after chronic beta-adrenoreceptor antagonism ($r = 0.76$, $N = 67$, $p < 0.001$); the shift in position of the regression line upward and to the left was not statistically significant ($p > 0.01$).

PLASMA CATECHOLAMINES AT REST (PATIENTS 7–14 AND 16)

Resting-plasma norepinephrine was unchanged or increased in five of nine patients after chronic treatment; Fig (1) the mean levels before and after treatment were identical (0.42 ± 0.1 μg/liter). Resting-plasma epinephrine decreased in six of nine patients after treatment; the reduction in mean values from 0.08 ± 0.05 to 0.05 ± 0.02 μg/liter was not significant. Mean blood pressure decreased by 15% ± 2% in patients in whom resting-plasma norepinephrine decreased with treatment similar to the 14% ± 5% fall observed in patients in whom plasma norepinephrine was unchanged or increased after treatment. Similarly, for plasma epinephrine, mean pressure decreased by 14% ± 4% in patients in whom epinephrine decreased, and by 17% ± 2% in patients in whom it was unchanged or increased after treatment. There was no significant correlation between the percentage fall in pressure and the change in plasma norepinephrine ($r = 0.40$) or epinephrine ($r = 0.09$).

PLASMA CATECHOLAMINES DURING EXERCISE (PATIENTS 7–17)

After acute beta-adrenoreceptor antagonism, mean-plasma norepinephrine during exercise had increased significantly from 1.31 ± 0.18 μg/liter before treatment to 1.65 ± 0.23 μg/liter after treatment ($p < 0.02$); after chronic treatment, changes were inconsistent and the mean increase from 1.25 ± 0.19 μg/liter before treatment to 1.77 ± 0.36 μg/liter after treatment was not significant. Similarly, plasma epinephrine increased significantly from 0.19 ± 0.04 μg/liter before treatment to 0.30

± 0.05 μg/liter after treatment ($p < 0.05$); after chronic treatment, the increase was not significant.

There was no significant correlation between the fall in mean-ambulatory blood pressure after chronic treatment and the change in exercise-plasma norepinephrine ($r = -0.24$) or plasma epinephrine ($r = -0.12$).

RELATIONSHIP BETWEEN PRETREATMENT CATECHOLAMINE LEVELS AND FALL IN PRESSURE

There was no significant relationship between the fall in pressure and the pretreatment resting-plasma norepinephrine or epinephrine levels ($r = 0.06$ and -0.36, respectively); neither was there a significant relationship between exercise-plasma norepinephrine or epinephrine ($r = 0.11$ and 0.40, respectively), nor the ratio between exercise and resting norepinephrine and epinephrine ($r = 0.17$ and 0.34, respectively).

DISCUSSION

We selected patients without evidence of target-organ damage in order to standardize the study group and to minimize the influence of impaired renal and cardiac functions. The lower level of average waking pressure in comparison with average outpatient recordings in these patients is con-

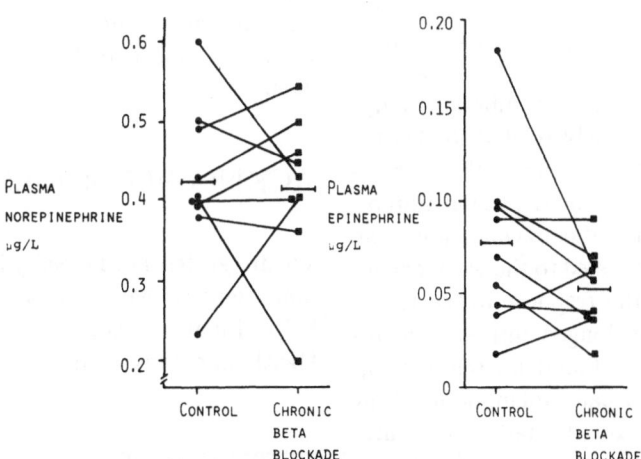

Fig. 1. Plasma norepinephrine and epinephrine after 40-min supine rest before (control) and after chronic beta-adrenoreceptor antagonism. Plasma catecholamines were measured by the method of Peuler and Johnson (5).

sistent with the observations of others that pressures are lower in the majority of patients on prolonged recording (6).

In untreated patients, we have previously reported a linear relationship between the logarithm of plasma norepinephrine and blood pressure and heart rate, physiologic measurements that reflect sympathetic activity (2). In the first six patients, we found a similar significant linear relationship between plasma norepinephrine and physiologic measurements of sympathetic activity after chronic beta-adrenoreceptor antagonism. This indicates that plasma norepinephrine remains an index of sympathetic activity despite the influence of chronic beta-adrenoreceptor antagonism.

In the remaining patients, resting-plasma norepinephrine levels were identical before and after chronic treatment. After acute treatment, plasma norepinephrine levels during exercise were significantly higher than control, which is in agreement with the observations of Irving et al. (7). After chronic treatment, variable changes were observed during exercise, and the small increase in plasma norepinephrine was not significant.

We were unable to confirm the observation of Bühler et al. (8) that plasma norepinephrine decreased with treatment in four propranolol-responsive patients, but not in four patients showing smaller falls in blood pressure. Although our patients were not selected in regard to responsiveness to treatment, these observations would suggest a relationship between the response to treatment and changes in plasma norepinephrine that we were unable to confirm.

Distler et al. (9) used the ratio between exercise and resting-plasma norepinephrine levels measured fluorometrically as an index of sympathetic responsiveness and observed that subsequent hypotensive response was closely related to this index. We have been unable to confirm these observations in our patients in whom plasma norepinephrine was measured radioenzymatically, the exercise workload was adjusted to the work capacity of the patients, and the response to treatment was determined from prolonged intraarterial recording. Furthermore, we found no relationship between the pretreatment catecholamine levels at rest or during exercise and the fall in pressure, and no relationship between the change in plasma catecholamine levels during treatment and the change in pressure.

Reduction in circulating plasma catecholamine levels after beta-adrenoreceptor antagonism would be consistent with a decrease in sympathetic activity mediated by either a central or a presynaptic mechanism. Our observations provide no evidence that the hypotensive response to beta-adrenoreceptor antagonism is associated with a reduction of plasma catecholamine levels. However, it may be simplistic to suggest that failure to demonstrate a reduction necessarily excludes either the central sympatholytic or presynaptic mechanisms, since plasma levels represent only the small fraction of the released norepinephrine that has escaped from local neuronal reuptake in metabolism, and regional variation in norepinephrine uptake and release in possible. Rather, we conclude that our observations do not support the hypothesis that central or presynaptic mechanisms are of predominant importance in determining the response to beta-adrenoreceptor antagonist in hypertension.

SUMMARY

Plasma catecholamines were measured before and after treatment with beta-adrenoreceptor antagonist in 17 hypertensive patients. Chronic treatment with beta-adrenoreceptor antagonists caused substantial reductions in heart rate and intraarterial blood pressure recorded continuously during ambulation. Chronic treatment caused no significant change in mean-resting-plasma norepinephrine and epinephrine. During exercise, plasma norepinephrine and epinephrine were significantly elevated above control after acute, but not after chronic, treatment. Pretreatment levels of plasma catecholamines did not help to predict the hypotensive response to beta-adrenoreceptor-blocking agents.

ACKNOWLEDGMENTS

We are grateful to Dr Sally Hill for technical assistance and to Miss Alison Strong for secretarial help. Financial support was provided by A.B. Hässle and May & Baker Limited.

REFERENCES

1. Lake CR, Ziegler MJ, Kopin IJ (1976) Use of plasma norepinephrine for evaluation of sympathetic neuronal function in man. Life Sci 18: 1315–1326

2. Watson RDS, Hamilton CA, Reid JL, Littler WA (1979) Changes in plasma norepinephrine, blood pressure and heart rate during physical activity in hypertensive man. Hypertension 1: 341–346

3. Littler WA, Honour AJ, Sleight P, Stott FD (1972) Continuous recording of direct arterial pressure and electrocardiogram in unrestricted man. Br Med J 3: 76–78

4. Henry DP, Starman BJ, Johnson DG, Williams RH (1975) A sensitive radioenzymatic assay for norepinephrine in plasma and tissues. Life Sci 16: 375–384

5. Peuler JD, Johnson GA (1977) Simultaneous single isotope radioenzymatic assay for norepinephrine, epinephrine and dopamine. Life Sci 21: 625–636

6. Kain HK, Hinman, AT, Sokolow M (1964) Arterial blood pressure measurements with a portable recorder in hypertensive patients. Circulation 30: 882–892

7. Irving MH, Britton BJ, Wood WG, Padgham C, Carruthers M (1974) Effects of beta adrenergic blockade on plasma catecholamines in exercise. Nature 248: 531–533

8. Bühler FR, Burkart F, Lütold BE, Bertel O, Pfisterer M (1977) Plasmakatecholaminen und Hamodynamik im Verlauf der antihypertensiven Betablockade: verschiedene Muster bei Propranolol—Responders und non-responders. Schweiz Med Wochenschr 106: 1735–1738

9. Distler A, Keim HJ, Cordes U, Philipp T, Wolff HP (1978) Sympathetic responsiveness and antihypertensive effect of beta receptor blockade in essential hypertension. Am J Med 64: 446–451

Renin Activity and the Response to Beta-Blockade

J. Ménard, P. F. Plouin, M. Thibonnier, F. Alhenc-Gélas,
P. Deqoulet, and P. Corvol

Biologic tests of the hypertension work-up are used for two different purposes: to determine diagnosis and treatment and to detect rare diseases. For all patients, it is useful to conduct initial tests of plasma creatinine and potassium, and, very often, of plasma glucose, cholesterol, and uric acid. A second group of tests is useful in some patients for detection of surgically curable causes of hypertension.

As regards plasma renin activity (PRA) measurements, these would fit into the first group of tests if they were demonstrated to constitute a completely reliable basis for the choice of therapy. Some investigators have reported that patients with low PRA are very responsive to diuretics (1), and patients with normal or high PRA are more responsive to beta-blockers (2). These observations form the basis of the vasoconstriction analysis for the understanding and treatment of hypertension (3). They imply that low-renin hypertension is the result of a more-or-less positive sodium balance, and that normal- and high-renin hypertension are partly, or completely, dependent on the renin–angiotensin system. According to this view, routine measurement of PRA might help to improve the choice of the initial monotherapy in hypertension. Moreover, the decrease in renin secretion induced by beta-blockers would participate in their antihypertensive effect, whereas an excessive renin response to diuretic therapy would limit the antihypertensive potential of this treatment. Nevertheless, the findings of Bühler et al. (2) have not been confirmed in some reports (see review, ref. 4) and the mechanism of the antihypertensive effects of beta-blockers is still controversial.

In this report, we will review our findings from 1974 to 1980. They consistently confirm that blood pressure induced by beta-blockers is significantly correlated to initial PRA. We shall then attempt to explain the divergent results obtained in the literature and discuss the practical and theoretical limitations of these findings.

CORRELATIONS BETWEEN PRA AND BLOOD PRESSURE RESPONSE TO BETA-BLOCKERS

The results of eight successive trials are summarized in Table 1 (5–12). In each study, PRA was measured by radioimmunoassay of angiotensin I after 1 h of ambulation (8:00–9:00 AM) on the third day in hospital with normal-sodium intake (100 mEq/day). Patients were given no antihypertensive drugs for 15 days before the investigation. All eight studies included subjects with low-, normal-, and high-renin levels. (Normal values in our laboratory were 0.7–3 ng/ml/h.)

The value of renin measurements in predicting the antihypertensive effects of beta-blockers was estimated in six hospital trials, after 2 days of treatment, and two conducted in the outpatient clinic for 4–6 weeks (6, 11). The very significant correlation observed between the fall in blood pressure measured on the third day of acebutolol administration and after 6 weeks of treatment has also been reported for other beta-blockers (12–15). No correlation was found between PRA and the fall in blood pressure within any of the subgroups of patients with low-, normal-, and high-renin levels, respectively.

Although highly significant, the correlations between PRA and the decrease in blood pressure after beta-blockade do not account for a sufficient variance to allow prediction of the efficacy of beta-blocker treatment in the individual patient. Besides the cost and technical difficulties involved in obtaining accurate measurements of renin from both the clinical and laboratory viewpoints, these fluc-

Table 1. Correlation between initial PRA and the fall in blood pressure induced by beta-blockers in eight successive studies.

Study	No. of subjects	r	p	Ref.
Systolic time intervals	31	0.580	0.001	5
Inpatient evaluation of acebutolol	44	0.498	0.001	6
Outpatient evaluation of acebutolol	30	0.639	0.001	7
Plasma norepinephrine	9	0.683	0.05	8
Saralasin test	24	0.620	0.001	9
Labetalol–acebutolol	16	0.739	0.001	10
Oxprenolol	22	0.740	0.001	11
Stepped-care treatment of hypertension	60	0.520	0.001	12

tuations from one individual to another greatly limit the practical interest of these correlations. Consequently, routine measurements of PRA are at present restricted to patients referred to hypertension clinics for special reasons.

TENTATIVE EXPLANATIONS FOR LACK OF CORRELATION BETWEEN PRA AND BLOOD PRESSURE RESPONSE TO BETA-BLOCKERS

It is hardly conceivable that so many divergent results can be recorded in the medical literature for a correlation between two parameters that are apparently easy to measure.

The lack of predictive value of renin measurement is easy to explain in many studies by such factors as the acidification of plasma and the measurement of total renin (16), the absence of stimulation of renin secretion in the upright posture (17), the failure to include patients with high-renin levels (18, 19), and the inclusion of patients taking diuretics (20).

Another explanation is the variability of the PRA measured on two different occasions in the same patient. For instance, in 100 hypertensive hospitalized patients, PRA was measured in the upright posture on the first and third days in hospital (Fig. 1), and the mean PRA values for each of these 2 days were respectively, 1.39 ± 1.06 and 1.47 ± 1.10 ng/ml/h. The correlation between these two measurements is even more significant ($r = 0.793$) than that between the two measurements of 24-h natriuresis ($r = 0.413$). Although PRA values for patients can be classified into three

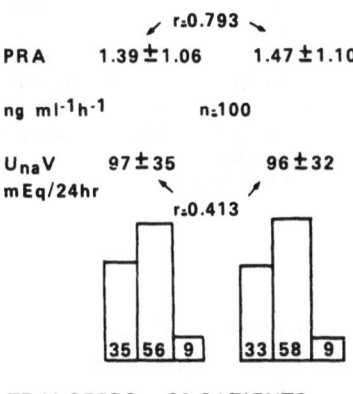

Fig. 1. Renin subgroups in 100 hypertensive patients: Classification at days 1 and 3 in the hospital.

groups compared to control normotensive subjects, 28 of 100 patients did not remain in the same group when PRA was measured twice, even though the percentage of low-, normal-, and high-renin patients remained identical. These fluctuations around a "cutoff" point obviously also apply to blood pressure measurements. Individual sensitivity to beta-blockade is far from being the main component of the overall hypotensive response to beta-blockers. These drugs have a moderate antihypertensive effect on most patients, and clear demonstration of the differences observed from one individual to the other is difficult.

We performed variance analysis of blood pressure measurements during a 2-day treatment of 50 hospitalized patients with acebutolol. Blood pressure was measured four times before and four times after acebutolol absorption. Systolic blood pressure in recumbency decreased from 168 ± 17 to 145 ± 16 mmHg, and diastolic blood pressure

Table 2. Variance analysis of blood pressure measurements in 50 patients four times before and after treatment.

Source of variation[a]	Sums of squares	Degrees of freedom	Mean squares	"F" value
Diastolic blood pressure				
P	25,509	49	521	13.0[b]
T	13,654	1	13,654	341[b]
PT	10,391	49	212	5.3[b]
R	525	3	175	–
Error	12,001	297	40	–
Systolic blood pressure				
P	83,229	49	1,701	18.3[b]
T	43,326	1	43,326	466[b]
PT	23,490	49	479	5.2[b]
R	400	3	133	–
Error	27,608	297	93	–

[a] P, patient factor; T, treatment factor; R, reproducibility factor; PT, patient–treatment interaction.
[b] Significance.

from 106 ± 9 to 94 ± 10 mmHg. As shown in Table 2, only 13.2% of the total variability (sum of the square of the variance analysis) of systolic blood pressure measurements and 16.6% of diastolic measurements depended on differences among individuals in the antihypertensive effects of beta-blockers.

ANTIRENIN EFFECT OF BETA-BLOCKERS: ITS PARTICIPATION IN THEIR ANTIHYPERTENSIVE PROPERTY

Administration of beta-blockers to patients with malignant hypertension or stenosis of the renal artery reduced blood pressure within a few hours (13, 21), and this fall was accompanied by a rapid decline in PRA. These clinical observations are certainly the best evidence indicating that one way in which beta-blockers exert hypotensive effects is by inhibiting the renin–angiotensin system. This concept is strengthened by the positive correlation observed in large groups of essential hypertensive patients between the circulating level of renin and its decline under treatment on the one hand, and

the fall in blood pressure on the other. Nevertheless, the concept has two limitations. First, the fall in renin secretion induced by beta-blockers is far from accounting for complete elimination of the renin–angiotensin system; neither is there any evidence in intrarenal blockade with its consequent effects on renal hemodynamics and tubular sodium reabsorption. For this reason, other blockers of the renin–angiotensin system will have to be found (22). Second, the renin level might indicate some disorder that does not primarily involve the renin–angiotensin system. Thus, in a small group of selected hypertensive patients, we found that the fall in blood pressure induced by beta-blocker treatment correlated just as well with plasma norepinephrine measured after 5 min in the upright posture as with PRA (8), which has also been observed in other studies, where plasma norepinephrine was measured during exercise (23). Similarly, in ten severely hypertensive patients, Thibonnier et al. (24) have observed that the fall in blood pressure induced by the acute blockade of converting enzyme with captopril (1 mg/kg) correlated with both initial PRA and initial plasma vasopressin. The antivasopressin effect of this blockade of the renin–angiotensin system might, therefore, partly account for its hypotensive action, just as well as its antiangiotensin effect.

SUMMARY

In eight successive trials, performed between 1974 and 1980, a highly significant correlation between the fall in blood pressure induced by beta-blockers and the initial level of PRA was consistently observed. Renin measurement was performed in the upright posture, after 3 days in hospital, under a diet containing 100 mEq sodium daily.

The variability of PRA and blood pressure measured on different occasions in the same patient explains why such correlations are useful in describing a phenomenon in a group of low-, normal-, and high-renin patients, but have a limited value in allowing prediction of the efficacy of beta-adrenoreceptor blocking drug treatment in the individual patient.

REFERENCES

1. Vaughan ED Jr, Laragh JR, Gavras I, Bühler FR, Gavras H, Brunner HR, Baer L (1973) Volume factor in low and normal renin essential hypertension: Treatment with either spironolactone or chlorthalidone. Am J Cardiol 32: 523
2. Bühler FR, Laragh JH, Baer L, Vaughan ED Jr, Brunner HR (1972) Propranolol inhibition of renin secretion: A specific approach to diagnosis and treatment of renin-dependent hypertensive diseases. New Engl J Med 287: 1209
3. Laragh JH (1976) Modern system for treating high blood pressure based on renin profiling and vasoconstriction-volume analysis: A primary role for beta-blocking drugs such as propranolol. Am J Med 61: 797
4. Birkenhäger WH, De Leeuw PW, Wester A, Kh TL, Vandongen R, Falke HE (1977) Therapeutic effects of beta-adenoceptor blocking agents in hypertension. In: Advances in internal medicine and pediatrics. Springer, Berlin/Heidelberg, p 117
5. Ducrocq MB, Degoulet P, Charpentier A, Corvol P, Ménard J (1975) Le test à l'acébutolol dans l'hypertension artérielle modérée: Action sur les intervalles de temps systoliques. Nouv Presse Med [Suppl] 4(46): 3268
6. Ménard J, Bertagna X, N'Guyene PT, Degoulet P, Corvol P (1976) Rapid identification of patients with essential hypertension sensitive to acebutolol. Am J Med 60: 886
7. Alhenc-Gélas F, Plouin PF, Ducrocq MB, Corvol P, Ménard J (1978) Comparison of the antihypertensive and hormonal effects of a cardioselective beta-blocker, acebutolol, and diuretics in essential hypertension. Am J Med 64: 1005
8. Plouin PF, Comoy E, Bohuon C, Corvol P, Ménard J (1979) Activité rénine et noradrénaline plasmatiques au cours du traitement antihypertenseur par l'acebutolol. Nouv Presse Med 8: 1905
9. Kreft C, Ménard J, Corvol P (1979) Value of renin measurement, saralasin test and acebutolol treatment in hypertension. Kidney Int 15: 176
10. Thibonnier M, Lardoux MD, Corvol P (in press) Comparative trial of labetalol and acebutolol, alone or associated with dihydralazine, in treatment of essential hypertension. Br J Clin Pharmacol
11. Thibonner M, Lardoux MD, Corvol P (1980) Comparative trial of labetolol acebutolol alone or assoc. in dihydralazine in treatment of essential hypertension. Rr J Clin Pharmacol 9: 561–567
12. Plouin PF, Alhenc-Gélas F, Degoulet P, Corvol P, Ménard J (in press) Importance and limitation of PRA measurement for the choice of initial medication in "stepped-care" treatment of hypertension. Cardiovasc Rev Rep
13. Bühler FR, Burkart F, Lütold BE, Küng M, Marbet G, Pfisterer M (1975) Antihypertensive beta-blocking action as related to renin and age. A pharmacological tool to identify pathogenetic mechanism in essential hypertension. Am J Cardiol 36: 653
14. Lehtonen A (1976) Atenolol in hypertension. Acta Ther 2: 125
15. Collste P, Haglund K (1979) Time-course of blood pressure decrease during initiation of antihypertensive treatment with metoprolol. In: Program VI scientific meeting of the ISH Göteborg, June 11–13, p 126
16. Meekers J, Missotten A, Fagard R, Demuynck D, Harvengt C, Pas P, Billiet L, Amery A (1975) Predictive value of various parameters for the antihypertensive effect of the beta-blocker ICI 66,082. Arch Int Pharmacodyn Ther 213: 294
17. Hansson L (1973) Beta-adrenergic blockade in essential hypertension: Effects of propranolol on hemodynamic parameters and plasma renin activity. Acta Med Scand [Suppl] 194: 550
18. Woods JW, Pittman AW, Pulliam CC (1976) Renin profiling in the treatment of hypertension. N Engl J Med 294: 1137
19. Stokes GS, Weber MA, Thornell IR (1974) Beta-blockers and plasma renin activity in hypertension. Br Med J 1: 60
20. Bravo EL, Tarazi RC, Dustan HP (1975) Beta-adrenergic blockade in diuretic-treated patients with essential hypertension. N Engl J Med 292: 66
21. Plouin PF, Ménard J, Corvol P, Milliez P (1978) Incidence des bêta-bloquants sur l'activité rénine plasmatique: Point actuel. Nouv Presse Med 7: 2769
22. Ménard J, Corvol P (1980) L'inhibition du système rénine-angiotensine: Un progrès majeur. Nouv Presse Med 11: 709
23. Distler A, Keim HJ, Cordes U, Philipp T, Wolff HP (1978) Sympathetic responsiveness and antihypertensive effect of beta-receptor blockade in essential hypertension. Am J Med 64: 446
24. Thibonnier M, Soto ME, Ménard J, Corvol P, Aldigier JC, Elkik F, Milliez P (1981) Role of vasopressin in the antihypertensive effect of captopril in severe hypertension. (Submitted for publication)

Total Peripheral Resistance and Beta-Adrenergic Blockade

Robert C. Tarazi, Fetnat M. Fouad, and Emmanuel L. Bravo

The hemodynamic hallmark of hypertension is an increased systemic vascular resistance, hence, the particular importance of the action of antihypertensive agents on that functional index. The long-term effect of beta-adrenergic blockade on total peripheral resistance (TPR) is currently in dispute; reports that beta-blockers leave this index unchanged, or even raise it further (1, 2), contrast with others describing a reduction of resistance below pretreatment levels (3–5). This controversy is important both in theory and in practice, because, in practice, it must influence our choice of antihypertensive therapy and, in theory, it relates to some fundamental principles in analysis of hemodynamic data (6).

HEMODYNAMIC PATTERNS AND INTERPRETATION

There is much more to hemodynamic investigations than a determination of cardiac output and calculation of TPR (6). The translation of biologic data into a hydrodynamic formula ($\Delta P = F \times R$) can be helpful only if the limitations inherent in that exercise are clearly recognized (7). To state that arterial pressure is the product of cardiac output and TPR, is mathematically correct; it is important, however, to take into account the complexity of often divergent functions that this calculated value (TPR) covers. Even with this proviso, it is an oversimplification to deduce from that premise that the reduction of blood pressure must be *either* by a lowering of output *or* by a vasodilation. Such a view fails to take into account the mutual interaction between variations in output and changes in TPR as well as the multiple factors that can influence the hemodynamic response to a drug (8) (Table 1).

Table 1. Factors influencing hemodynamic response to neural-blocking drugs

Drug
  Site of action (central, peripheral)
  Possible agonistic effect
Pretreatment factors
  Hemodynamic setting (level of neurogenic activity, age, physical fitness)
  Cardiac status
Factors during long-term therapy
  Duration of treatment
  Hemodynamic side effects
    Fluid retention
    Influence on cardiac performance
  Compensatory mechanisms and humoral responses
  Structural readaptation

In the case of beta-blockade, these factors include the type of beta-blocker used (9–11), the preblockade hemodynamic setting (8, 9), the duration of therapy (3, 9), the level of physical activity or adrenergic drive, and the age of the subject (12, 13). Under these conditions, it is *not* possible to dismiss the beta-blockers summarily as agents that lower blood pressure but increase peripheral resistance (2).

HEMODYNAMIC RESPONSES TO LONG-TERM BETA-BLOCKADE

The pattern of hemodynamic responses to beta-blockade and their evolution with therapy covers a wide spectrum (for review, see ref. 14) (Fig. 1). These patterns are not mere mathematical combinations; their biologic importance was underlined by the observations of Guazzi et al. (4) regarding cardiac performance during propranolol therapy.

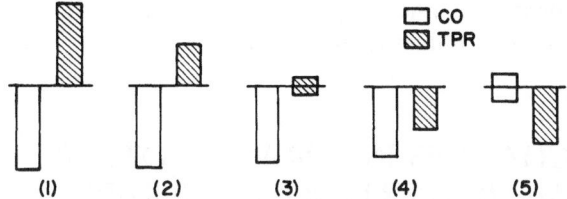

Fig. 1. The pattern of hemodynamic findings during beta-adrenergic blockade can vary along a wide spectrum from reduction in output (CO) and full compensatory rise in TPR (pattern 1) to reduction in TPR with normal CO (pattern 5). Pattern 1 occurs following i.v. propranolol and in nonresponders to the drug [Tarazi et al. (3)]; factors determining the pattern found during long-term treatment with beta-blockers are listed in Table 1.

The left-ventricular filling pressure (estimated from pulmonary wedge records) in their patients varied in relation to changes in TPR. Among patients whose blood pressure was reduced by propranolol, the pulmonary wedge pressure increased in those with lowered output and increased TPR (patterns 2–3), whereas it was reduced in those with unchanged output and lowered resistance (pattern 5).

The predominance of TPR in determining blood pressure response to beta-blockers is widely agreed upon (1–6). It is indicated by the significant correlations found between changes in resistance and blood pressure response, in contrast to the lack of correlation between changes in cardiac output and changes in blood pressure (Fig. 2). These results were obtained with both cardioselective [practolol (10) and metoprolol (9, 15)] and noncardioselective [propranolol (16) and timolol (5)] beta-blockers. Of particular relevance to this discussion is the wide spectrum of changes in TPR shown in Fig. 2, indicating the wide variety of hemodynamic patterns during beta-blockade.

A common error must be guarded against in consideration of hemodynamic patterns, and that is the all-too-frequent tendency to view them as static combinations that define, once and for all, response of a patient or of a group of patients to beta-blockade. On the contrary, it is quite possible, indeed probable, that patients will change from one pattern to the other with duration of therapy or conditions of the study (16). Thus, a gradual reduction of TPR during beta-blocking therapy with a return of cardiac output to or toward normal, has been described by many investigators (14). Because of the multitude of factors involved, it is not really possible to decide at the present time in man whether the type of beta-blocker used has a major influence on the hemodynamic pattern observed (9, 10). Moreover, under stress, patients change their hemodynamic profile from pattern 4 or 5 to pattern 1, as was described by Tarazi and Dustan (16) for office hypertension and by

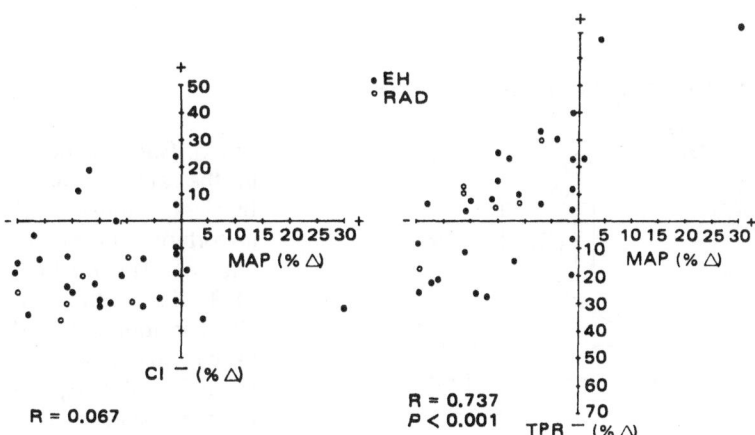

Fig. 2. Relationship between change in mean arterial pressure (MAP, *abscissa*) and change in cardiac index (CI, *ordinate of left panel*) and in TPR *(ordinate of right panel)* during oral propranolol therapy in 33 hypertensive patients. Changes are expressed as percent of control. EH, essential hypertension; RAD, renal arterial disease associated with hypertension. [Tarazi and Dustan (16), with permission of the Editors of the American Journal of Cardiology]

Nicotero et al. (17) and Ulrych (18) for painful stimuli or mental work.

PLASMA RENIN ACTIVITY AND HEMODYNAMIC RESPONSES

There was no correlation in our experience between plasma renin activity (determined with the patient resting supine for at least 30 min) and blood pressure response to either propranolol (3, 16), metoprolol (15), or practolol (10). However, this lack of correlation does not in our opinion negate a possible role for renin suppression in the blood response to beta-blockade. Thus, we found an intriguing correlation between changes in plasma renin activity and variations in TPR during chronic propranolol therapy. In two separate studies, one involving propranolol alone (3) and the other the addition of propranolol to chronic diuretic therapy (10), the alterations in TPR correlated with changes in plasma renin activity ($r = 0.528$, $p < 0.02$ and $r = 0.593$, $p < 0.05$, respectively). It must be pointed out, however, that no such correlation was found following intravenous propranolol; plasma renin activity was suppressed while TPR increased. Considering the number of factors that regulate arterial pressure, as well as the complex mechanisms regulating renin release, it is not surprising that the two do not always correlate. Variations in plasma renin accounted for only 28%–35% of changes in TPR in the studies just

CHANGES IN TPR WITH OTHER ANTIHYPERTENSIVE THERAPY

Apart from vasodilators that influence vascular resistance directly, most antihypertensive drugs lead to a complex pattern of hemodynamic responses. In fact, the evolution of TPR during long-term beta-blockade is strikingly similar to that observed with diverse drugs such as diuretics (19, 20), guanethidine (21), methyldopa (21), and lofexidine (22). Underlying the long-term effect of all is a common thread, namely, an initial reduction in output followed sometime later by a reduction in TPR with a greater or lesser degree of normalization of cardiac output. Each drug, to be sure, colors this pattern differently according to its specific action. Thus, there is no reflex compensatory increase in TPR to the initial reduction in output produced by guanethidine (23), whereas diuretics allow a partial rise in systemic resistance (24, 25). The rise in resistance following intravenous propranolol is fully compensatory so that blood pressure is not reduced (26). However, sometime later, with all these drugs, cardiac output was seen to return toward normal and TPR to come down.

This commonality of pattern suggests the influence of other factors besides the specific effect of each drug. A persistent reduction in blood pressure

mentioned, and there are other factors beside TPR that can influence arterial pressure.

FACTORS in ANTIHYPERTENSIVE EFFECT of β - ADRENERGIC BLOCKADE

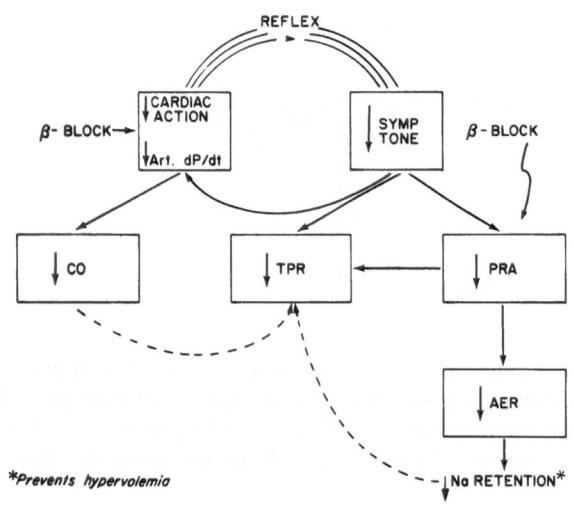

Fig. 3. Some of the many factors involved in the antihypertensive effect of beta-blocking agents may assume overriding importance in some individual circumstances. The dashed line joining CO to TPR refers to the autoregulation hypothesis. The reduced tendency to sodium retention might be a factor in progressive reduction of TPR; it was also suggested as a possible mechanism for the infrequency of false tolerance to the antihypertensive effects of beta-blockers. [Tarazi (14), with permission of the Editors of Excerpta Medica.]

must lead to readaptation of *both* functional and structural mechanisms. A reduction in sympathetic tone, whatever its mechanism of control, reflex or resetting of baroceptors (14), as well as a blunting of renin response (27), will help lower TPR. As important for long-term hemodynamic changes are structural readaptations of the cardiovascular system; these are helped by drugs that reduce effective sympathetic drive either centrally or peripherally (28, 29). The reversal of vascular (29) as well as cardiac (30) hypertrophy will help "normalize" the circulation. In that reversal, both blood pressure and nonpressure-related factors play important roles.

SUMMARY

The hemodynamic patterns underlying arterial pressure responses to beta-adrenergic blockers demonstrate a wide spectrum of findings that cannot be forced under the single category of "lower output and increased resistance." Differences in responses of peripheral resistance to beta-blockade depend on many factors such as duration of therapy, hemodynamic setting before blockade, circumstances of the study, and possibly on the type of drug used. The biologic importance of these differences was underlined by the influence of TPR changes on pulmonary wedge pressure and by their correlation with the level of plasma renin activity. It would appear, therefore, that recognition of gradation in responses of TPR and of differences among patients allows a more accurate evaluation of beta-blockade in hypertension than aggregation of all data into a single average value.

ACKNOWLEDGMENT

This work was supported in part by grants from the National Heart, Lung and Blood Institute (HL-6835) and the Whitaker Foundation.

REFERENCES

1. Frohlich ED (1978) Concepts of pressor mechanisms in hypertension evolved through clinical experience with beta-adrenergic receptor blocking drugs. In: Braunwald E (ed) Beta-adrenergic blockade: A new era in cardiovascular medicine. Excerpta Medica/Elsevier, Amsterdam, pp 225–235
2. Lund-Johansen P (1979) Hemodynamic consequences of long-term beta-blocker therapy: A 5-year follow-up study of atenolol. J Cardiovasc Pharmacol 1: 487–495
3. Tarazi RC, Dustan HP (1976) Hemodynamic effects of propranolol in hypertension. Postgrad Med J 52(Suppl IV): 92–100
4. Guazzi M, Polese A, Fiorentini C, Olivari MR, Magrini F, Bartorelli C (1976) Cardiac function in the treatment of arterial hypertension with propranolol. Clin Sci Mol Med 51: 555S–561S
5. Franciosa JA, Freis ED, Conway J (1973) Antihypertensive and hemodynamic properties of the new beta-adrenergic blocking agent timolol. Circulation 48: 118–124
6. Tarazi RC, Fouad FM (1978) Hemodynamic characteristics in hypertension. Herz 3: 245–251
7. Dustan HP, Tarazi RC, Hinshaw LB (1976) Mechanism controlling arterial pressure. In: Frohlich ED (ed) Pathophysiology, 2nd ed. Lippincott, Philadelphia, Pa, pp 49–82
8. Tarazi RC (1978) Therapy for multifactorial hypertension. Ann Intern Med 88: 705–706
9. Sannerstedt R (1972) Haemodynamic effects of adrenergic β-receptor-blocking agents in arterial hypertension. In: Berglund G, Hansson L, Werko L (eds) Pathophysiology and management of arterial hypertension. Molndal, Lindgren, pp 194–200
10. Niarchos AP, Tarazi RC (1976) Hemodynamic effects of β-adrenergic blocking agents in hypertension. In: Onesti G, Fernandes M, Kim KE (eds) Regulation of blood pressure by the central nervous system. Grune & Stratton, New York, pp 397–409
11. Hansson L (1973) Beta-adrenergic blockade in essential hypertension: Effects of propranolol on hemodynamic parameters and plasma renin activity. Acta Med Scand 550(Suppl I): 1–40
12. Conway J, Wheeler R, Sannerstedt R (1971) Sympathetic nervous activity during exercise in relation to age. Cardiovasc Res 5: 577–581
13. Ibrahim MM, Tarazi RC, Dustan HP, Bravo EL (1974) Cardioadrenergic factor in essential hypertension. Am Heart J 88: 724–732
14. Tarazi RC (1978) Antihypertensive effect of beta-blockade: Relation of its hemodynamic component to other mechanisms. In: Braunwald E (ed) Beta-adrenergic blockade: A new era in cardiovascular medicine. Excerpta Medica/Elsevier, Amsterdam, pp 210–224
15. Fouad FM, Tarazi RC, Bravo EL (1980) Cardiac, hemodynamic and humoral effects of a cardioselective beta-blocker (abstr). Clin Pharmacol Therr 27(2): 254
16. Tarazi RC, Dustan HP (1972) Beta-adrenergic blockade in hypertension: Practical and theoretical implications of long-term hemodynamic variation. Am J Cardiol 29: 633–640
17. Nicotero JA, Beamer V, Moutsos SE, Shapiro AP

(1968) Effects of propranolol on pressor responses to noxious stimuli in hypertensive patients. Am J Cardiol 22: 657–666

18. Ulrych M (1969) Changes of general haemodynamics during stressful mental arithmetic and nonstressing quiet conversation on modification of the latter by beta-adrenergic blockade. Clin Sci 36: 453–461

19. Conway J, Lauwers P (1960) Hemodynamic and hypotensive effects of long-term therapy with chlorothiazide. Circulation 21: 21–27

20. Villarreal H, Exaire JE, Revollo A, Soni J (1962) Effects of chlorothiazide on systemic hemodynamics in essential hypertension. Circulation 26: 405–407

21. Chamberlain DA, Howard J (1964) Guanethidine and methyldopa, a hemodynamic study. Br Heart J 26: 528–536

22. Fouad FM, Vidt DG, Tarazi RC, Bravo EL (1980) Acute hemodynamic effects of a new central adrenergic blocker (lofexidine) (abstr). Clin Pharmacol Ther 27(2): 254

23. Cohn JN, Liptak TE, Freis ED (1963) Hemodynamic effects of guanethidine in man. Circ Res 12: 298–316

24. Dustan HP, Cumming GR, Corcoran AC, Page IH (1959) A mechanism of chlorothiazide-enhanced effectiveness of antihypertensive ganglioplegic drugs. Circulation 20: 360–365

25. Frohlich ED, Schnaper HW, Wilson IM, Freis ED (1960) Hemodynamic alterations in hypertensive patients due to chlorothiazide. N Engl J Med 262: 1261–1263

26. Ulrych M, Frohlich ED, Dustan HP, Page IH (1968) Immediate hemodynamic effects of beta-adrenergic blockade with propranolol in normotensive and hypertensive man. Circulation 37: 411–416

27. Bühler FR, Laragh JH, Vaughan ED, Brunner HR, Gavras H, Baer L (1973) Antihypertensive action of propranolol: Specific antirenin responses in high and normal renin forms of essential, renal, renovascular and malignant hypertension. Am J Cardiol 32: 511–522

28. Tarazi RC, Sen S (1979) Catecholamines and cardiac hypertrophy. In: Catecholamines and the heart (Royal Society of Medicine: International congress and symposium series no 8). Academic Press and Royal Society of Medicine, London, pp 47–57

29. Yamori Y, Nakada T, Lovenberg W (1976) Effect of antihypertensive therapy on lysine incorporation into vascular protein of the spontaneously hypertensive rat. Eur J Pharmacol 38: 349–355

30. Sen S, Tarazi RC, Khairallah PA, Bumpus FM (1974) Cardiac hypertrophy in spontaneously hypertensive rats. Circ Res 35: 775–782

Mechanisms of Beta-Blockade Hypotension

Thomas G. Pickering

Although there are now many different beta-blocking drugs available that vary in some of their individual properties, certain generalizations can be made about their effects in hypertensive patients (1): a) all are more-or-less equally effective in lowering blood pressure, but not in all patients; b) all lower stimulated plasma renin activity; and c) all lower cardiac output. Properties such as cardioselectivity and penetration of the central nervous system are probably of minor importance, since each of these may or may not be features of different drugs that have similar effects on blood pressure.

At the present time, three different theories to explain the hypotensive effect of beta-blockers are popular: a) blockade of beta receptors in the heart is responsible, leading to a decreased cardiac output; b) blockade of beta-receptors in the kidney, leading to a decreased renin release; and c) blockade of beta-receptors in the brain, leading to a decreased sympathetic outflow. Each of these theories will be briefly discussed.

CARDIAC OUTPUT THEORY

Bradycardia and a reduced cardiac output are nearly universal findings in patients treated with beta-blockers, but only approximately 60% of patients show a fall of blood pressure (2). On this basis Tarazi and Dustan (3) divided hypertensive patients given propranolol into responders and nonresponders. The initial effect in all patients was a decrease of cardiac output offset by an increase of peripheral resistance, so that blood pressure did not change. In the responders, the subsequent fall of blood pressure occurred in parallel with a fall of peripheral resistance to pretreatment levels, whereas, in the nonresponders, both pressure and resistance remained high. Thus, what distinguished the two groups was what happened to peripheral resistance, not cardiac output, which remained low in all patients.

Much has been written about patients with a so-called high-cardiac output form of hypertension. It might be expected that such patients would respond particularly well to beta-blockers if reduction of cardiac output were the principal mechanism by which they lower blood pressure; but, in fact, this does not seem to be the case (4). We must, therefore, look to other mechanisms to explain why beta-blockers lower blood pressure, although the reduction of the pressor response to dynamic exercise can be explained by the reduction of cardiac output (5). Unlike the delayed effect on the resting blood pressure, this effect is immediately apparent.

NEURAL MECHANISMS

Two different neural mechanisms have been proposed to explain beta-blockade hypotension. First, beta-blockers act directly on the central nervous system, and, second, they act via the sinoaortic baroreceptors. In both cases, the net result would be a reduction of central sympathetic outflow. Most of the evidence favoring a central mechanism comes from animal rather than human studies, and two major objections to the central theory in man are, first, that beta-blocking drugs (e.g., atenolol) which do not readily enter the central nervous system are no less effective hypotensive agents than those which do (6), and, second, that most drugs which produce a centrally mediated decrease of sympathetic nervous activity (e.g., clonidine and methyldopa) lower plasma norepinephrine levels; this is not the case with beta-blockers

(5). It has also been claimed that propranolol may enhance the sensitivity of baroreceptor afferents (7), but this has not been substantiated.

RENIN THEORY

The original impetus for the renin theory came from Bühler et al.'s observation (8) that patients with high-plasma renin activity respond better to beta-blocking drugs than those with low renin. Since then, this observation has been confirmed by numerous other groups (9, 10), but has remained controversial because some workers have failed to show it (11). There are, however, many reasons for this failure, such as patient selection (if all the patients have similar renin levels, it will not be seen), and variations in the methods of measuring renin, etc., none of which invalidate the basic observation. Further support for the theory has come from the less controversial finding that captopril also lowers blood pressure more effectively in high-renin patients (12), and in a comparison of captopril and propranolol, we have found that patients who respond well to one drug also respond well to the other (D. B. Case, T. G. Pickering, P. A. Sullivan, and J. H. Laragh, unpublished observations). The animal experiments quoted elsewhere in this volume also support this theory.

MECHANISM OF DELAYED HYPOTENSIVE EFFECT

One of the problems faced by all the theories is that although both cardiac output and plasma renin activity are reduced within an hour or so following the acute administration of a beta-blocker, the fall of blood pressure takes much longer, except for the immediate effect on the pressure during exercise (mentioned above). In hemodynamic terms, this is due to peripheral vasoconstriction, which seems paradoxical in the face of declining concentrations of angiotensin. It cannot be attributed solely to the blockade of the beta$_2$-vasodilator vascular receptors, because it also occurs after a cardioselective beta$_1$-blocking

drug is given (1). We have observed that plasma norepinephrine levels tend to rise after intravenous propranolol administration, leading us to suggest that the vasoconstriction may be initiated as a sympathetic baroreceptor reflex mediated by the alpha-adrenergic system (5, 13) (Fig. 1). Support for this view comes from the observation of Struyker-Boudier et al. (14), who showed that propranolol has no immediate hypotensive effect in spontaneously hypertensive rats, unless the baroreceptors are denervated. It is the nature of baroreceptor reflexes to reset over a prolonged period of time, and a gradual reduction of the reflexly increased sympathetic constrictor tone would allow the blood pressure to fall in those patients whose blood pressure is renin dependent. In keeping with this, we have found that plasma norepinephrine levels return to normal in patients treated with propranolol for

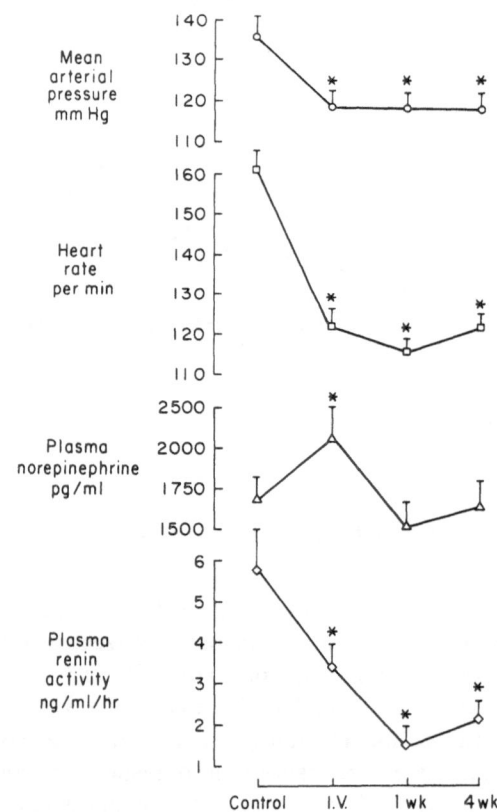

Fig. 1. Effects of propranolol on blood pressure, heart rate, plasma norepinephrine and plasma renin activity during exercise. There is an initial increase of norepinephrine following i.v. propranolol, but this is not apparent after 1 and 4 weeks of oral treatment.

a week or longer, by which time the full hypotensive effect is apparent. Furthermore, we have also found that renin release is suppressed to a greater extent by long-term than by acute propranolol treatment (5).

In conclusion, there is no reason to suppose that beta-blockers lower blood pressure by any mechanism other than sympathetic beta-adrenergic blockade. The role of the sympathetic nervous system in beta-blockade hypotension is complex: First, beta-blockers inhibit that component of renin secretion which is modulated neurally via the beta-adrenergic receptors; second, the alpha-adrenergic system may temporarily oppose the renin-lowering effects of blockade of the beta-receptors; and third, the reduction of cardiac output contributes to the blood pressure lowering during dynamic exercise. Of the three theories discussed, the renin theory of beta-blockade hypotension is the only one that can adequately account for why some hypertensive patients respond well to beta-blockade, while others do not, and to predict who these patients will be. It is now well supported by both animal and human data, and has gained added strength from the findings that more specific means of blocking the renin–angiotensin system, such as converting enzyme inhibition, will also lower blood pressure in patients with high- or normal-renin hypertension.

SUMMARY

Three theories have been proposed to explain beta-blockade hypotension: a) via blockade of cardiac beta-receptors, leading to a diminished cardiac output; b) via blockade of receptors in the central nervous system, leading to a diminution of central sympathetic outflow; and c) via blockade of renal beta-receptors, leading to a diminished renin release. The first mechanism is important during exercise, but cannot account for the effects at rest, because cardiac output is depressed in all patients; but not all show a fall of blood pressure. Direct evidence for a central mechanism is lacking in man, and most centrally acting drugs lower plasma catecholamines; but beta-blockers do not. The renin theory has support from both animal and human data. The delay in the hypotensive effect can be explained by a transient reflexly mediated increase in sympathetic vasoconstrictor tone.

REFERENCES

1. Pickering TG, Laragh JH (1980) Mechanisms of beta blockade hypotension: The evidence points to renin suppression. In: Hunt JC, et al (eds) Hypertension update. Health Learning Systems, Bloomfield, NJ, p 247
2. Veterans Administration Cooperative Study Group (1977) Propranolol in the treatment of essential hypertension. JAMA 237: 2303
3. Tarazi RC, Dustan HP (1972) Beta blockade in hypertension. Am J Cardiol 29: 633
4. Ibrahim MM, Tarazi RC, Dustan HP, et al (1975) Hyperkinetic heart in severe hypertension: A separate clinical hemodynamic entity. Am J Cardiol 35: 667
5. Pickering TG, Raine, AEG, Levitt M, et al (1979) Immediate and delayed hypotensive effects of propranolol at rest and during exercise. Trans Assoc Am Physicians 92: 277
6. Davidson C, Thadani U, Singleton W, et al (1976) Comparison of antihypertensive activity of beta-blocking drugs during chronic treatment. Br Med J 2: 7
7. Angell James JE, Bobik A (1979) Preventative treatment for hypertension and arterial baroreceptor function. In: Yamori Y, et al (eds) Prophylactic approach to hypertensive diseases. Raven Press, New York, p 259
8. Bühler FR, Laragh JH, Baer L, et al (1972) Propranolol inhibition of renin secretion: A specific approach to diagnosis and treatment of renin-dependent hypertensive disease. New Engl J Med 287: 1209
9. Castenfors JH, Johnsson H, Örö L (1973) Effect of alprenolol on blood pressure and plasma renin activity in hypertensive patients. Acta Med Scand 193: 189
10. Karlberg BE, Kagedal B, Tegler L (1976) Controlled treatment of primary hypertension with propranolol and spironolactone: A crossover study with special reference to initial plasma renin activity. Am J Cardiol 37: 642
11. Hansson L, Zweifler AJ (1974) The effect of propranolol on plasma renin activity and blood pressure in mild essential hypertension. Acta Med Scand 195: 397
12. Case DB, Atlas SA, Laragh JH, et al (1978) Clinical experience with blockade of the renin-angiotensin-aldosterone system by an oral converting-enzyme inhibitor (SQ 14225, captopril) in hypertensive patients. Prog Cardiovasc Dis 21: 195
13. Morganti A, Pickering TG, Lopez-Ovejero J, Laragh JH (1979) Contrasting effects of acute beta blockade with propranolol on plasma catecholamines and renin in essential hypertension: A possible basis for the delayed antihypertensive effect. Am Heart J 98: 490
14. Struyker-Boudier HAJ, Smits JF, Van Essen H (1979) The role of the baroreceptor reflex in the cardiovascular effect of propranolol in the conscious spontaneously hypertensive rat. Clin Sci 56: 163

Aldosterone: Possible Roles in Sustaining Essential Hypertension and in Determining Response to Antihypertensive Treatment

Michael A. Weber, Ralph E. Purdy, and Diana E. Hurlbut

KNOWN ACTIONS OF ALDOSTERONE

A clear role for aldosterone in sustaining hypertension was first described with the syndrome of primary aldosteronism, a condition in which this mineralocorticoid hormone is secreted autonomously by adenomatous or hyperplastic adrenal glands. It has been presumed that this form of hypertension is sustained by aldosterone-mediated sodium and water retention, but there has been no consistent evidence for volume expansion. And, although spironolactone, a specific antagonist of aldosterone's mineralocorticoid action, normally corrects the metabolic abnormalities of primary aldosteronism, it does not restore blood pressure to normal levels in all cases.

Secretion of aldosterone is regulated chiefly by changes in potassium (1) and sodium (2) homeostasis, and is also influenced by ACTH (3). The most important factor in governing aldosterone, however, is the renin–angiotensin system (4). Thus, unlike primary aldosteronism, where high-aldosterone levels are associated with suppressed plasma renin activity, the levels of aldosterone in most patients with essential hypertension tend to parallel those of renin. Because of this relationship, antihypertensive medications such as beta-blockers or clonidine that suppress renin release usually also decrease aldosterone. The aldosterone-lowering properties of these drugs might be critical in their effectiveness, for the counter productive volume accumulation that occurs with other types of nondiuretic antihypertensive drugs appears to be avoided by the reduction of aldosterone's mineralocorticoid activity. Indeed, there is good evidence that plasma volume remains constant (5, 6) or is even decreased (7) during beta-blocker monotherapy of hypertension.

DOES ALDOSTERONE HAVE PERIPHERAL VASCULAR EFFECTS?

Beyond the benefits of avoiding volume retention, it has been suggested that changes in aldosterone production might, in addition, influence the response to antihypertensive treatment by effects that are independent of volume balance. Thus, in studies with beta-blockers (8, 9), clonidine (10), and captopril (11), patients responding best to treatment were found to have significantly greater aldosterone decrements than nonresponders; whereas in studies with the diuretic agents triamterene (12) and chlorthalidone (13), the responders were those patients in whom aldosterone rose least during treatment. Interestingly, the changes in aldosterone were overall more closely linked to treatment response than were either control renin values or treatment-induced changes in renin. Clinical measures of volume status, including serum and urinary sodium and potassium levels and body weight, did not differ between responder and nonresponder patients, suggesting the involvement of non volume-related mechanisms.

There has been speculation concerning the manner in which aldosterone might be involved in sustaining blood pressure through actions in the peripheral vascular circulation. It has been shown that aldosterone receptors may exist in the arterial circulation, and that the stimulation of these receptors can produce pressor effects that appear to be independent of changes in total body sodium or potassium homeostasis (14). Application of aldosterone directly to the carotid sinus can also produce a pressor response in the rabbit (15). In other studies with vascular tissue, aldosterone has been shown to facilitate movement of sodium from the intracellular to the extracellular space (16), an action that might lead to the increased intracellular concentration of potassium that appears to make vascular tissue more responsive to pressor stimuli (17). Several mechanisms by which aldosterone and other mineralocorticoids can sustain blood pressure through enhancement of adrenergic factors recently have been reviewed (18).

PRELIMINARY STUDIES OF ALDOSTERONE'S VASCULAR EFFECTS

In preliminary studies, we have examined the possibility that aldosterone might exhibit pressor properties through inhibition of extraneuronal uptake of norepinephrine (19). In this investigation, we have employed the isolated perfused rabbit ear artery, an in vitro preparation characterized by spontaneous neurotransmitter release that allows a resting state of contraction to be sustained. Experiments were performed on 3-mm vessel rings suspended in O_2/CO_2 (95/5%) gassed krebs–bicarbonate solution at 37°C.

When we added aldosterone alone to the tissue bath, there was little or no contractile response. But if the tissue was first exposed to the blocker of neuronal reuptake of norepinephrine, desmethylimipramine (DMI), aldosterone then produced a potent contraction. This indicates that aldosterone is most likely to exhibit its pressor properties when endogenous norepinephrine has first diffused into the proximity of the receptors that mediate vasoconstriction. There was a clear dose–response relationship for the contractile effects of aldosterone, showing that this phenomenon is concentration dependent and suggesting that it might have physiologic importance. If the arterial tissue was pretreated with the alpha-blocker phentolamine, no contractile effect occurred with the administration of aldosterone. Similarly, the later addition of either phentolamine or prazosin could completely reverse the pressor effects of aldosterone. Thus, we have so far concluded that aldosterone might exhibit vasoconstrictor properties through its inhibition of norepinephrine uptake in the vascular tissues, an action that allows a local accumulation of norepinephrine which, in turn, produces vasoconstriction by activation of alpha-adrenergic receptors.

Clearly, much work is needed to further eluci-

date the participation of aldosterone in peripheral vascular mechanisms, and to determine whether these actions of aldosterone (and of other adrenocorticoid hormones) are clinically relevant in sustaining hypertension and in determining the responsiveness of essential hypertension to treatment.

SUMMARY

Although the role of aldosterone in sustaining the elevated blood pressure levels in the syndrome of primary aldosteronism is well documented, its involvement in essential hypertension mechanisms is more speculative. It is believed, however, that decreased aldosterone production secondary to the renin inhibition produced by antihypertensive agents such as the beta-blockers and clonidine might be key in preventing reactive volume retention during treatment. But there is also evidence that aldosterone may sustain blood pressure by pressor actions in the peripheral vasculature that are independent of its effects on volume. In preliminary in vitro studies in the rabbit ear artery, we have found that aldosterone produces a concentration-dependent contractile effect that is related to its inhibition of extraneuronal uptake of norepinephrine. The relevance of this alpha-receptor-mediated vasoconstriction to clinical hypertension has yet to be elucidated.

REFERENCES

1. Davis JO, Urquhart J, Higgins JT Jr (1963) Effects of alteration of plasma sodium and potassium concentration in aldosterone secretion. J Clin Invest 42: 597–609
2. Blair West JR, Coghlan JP, Denton DA, Goding RR, Wintour M, Wright RD (1965) Effect of variations of plasma sodium concentration on the adrenal response to angiotensin II. Circ Res 17: 386–393
3. McCaa RE, Read VH, Bower JD, McCaa CS, Guyton C (1971) Adrenal cortical response to hemodialysis, ACTH and angiotensin II in anephric man. Circulation 44(Suppl II): 67
4. Laragh JH, Angers M, Kelly WG, Lieberman S (1960) Hypotensive agents and pressor substances. JAMA 174: 234–240
5. Ibsen H, Sederberg-Olsen P (1973) Changes in glomerular filtration rate during long-term treat-

ment with propranolol in patients with arterial hypertension. Clin Sci 44: 129–134

6. Dreslinski GR, Aristimuno GG, Messerli FH, Suarez DH, Frohlich ED (1979) Effects of beta blockade with acebutolol on hypertension, hemodynamics, and fluid volume. Clin Pharmacol Ther 26: 562–565

7. Tarazi RC, Frohlich ED, Dustan HP (1971) Plasma volume changes with long-term beta-adrenergic blockade. Am Heart J 82: 770–776

8. Weber MA, Lopez-Ovejero JA, Drayer JIM, Case DB, Laragh JH (1977) Renin reactivity as a determinant of responsiveness to antihypertensive treatment. Arch Intern Med 137: 284–289

9. Drayer JIM, Weber MA, Longworth DL, Laragh JH (1978) The possible importance of aldosterone as well as renin in the long-term antihypertensive action of propranolol. Am J Med 64: 187–192

10. Weber MA, Case DB, Baer L, Sealey JE, Drayer JIM, Lopez-Overjero JA, Laragh JH (1976) Suppression of renin and aldosterone in the antihypertensive action of clonidine. Am J Cardiol 38: 825–830

11. Atlas SA, Case DB, Sealey JE, Laragh JH, McKinstry DN (1979) Interruption of the renin-angiotensin system in hypertensive patients by captopril induces sustained reduction in aldosterone secretion, potassium retention and natriuresis. Hypertension 1: 274–280

12. Keim HJ, Drayer JIM, Thurston H, Laragh JH (1976) Triamterene-induced changes in aldosterone and renin values in essential hypertension. Arch Intern Med 136: 645–648

13. Weber MA, Drayer JIM, Rev A, Laragh JH (1977) Disparate patterns of aldosterone response during diuretic treatment of hypertension. Ann Intern Med 87: 558–563

14. Kornel L. Kanamarlapudi N, Baum R, Chen C, Travers T (1975) Mineralocorticoid receptors in blood vessels. Rush Presb–St Luke's Med Bull 14: 3

15. Burstyn PG, Horrobin DF (1970) Possible mechanism of action for aldosterone-induced hypertension. Lancet 1: 973–976

16. Llaurado JG (1970) Some effects of aldosterone on sodium transport rate constants in isolated arterial wall: Studies with computer simulation and analysis. Endocrinology 87: 517–526

17. Demura H, Fukuchi S, Takahashi H, Goto K (1965) The vascular reactivity to vasoactive substances and the electrolyte contents in arterial walls. Tohoku J Exp Med 86: 366–379

18. Rosenthal J (1979) An appraisal of the role of aldosterone and the sympathetic nervous system in essential hypertension. Horm Metab Res 11: 379–382

19. Weber NA, Purdy RE, Hurlbut DE (1980): Contractile effects of aldosterone in the isolated rabbit ear artery. The Pharmacologist 22: 194

DISCUSSION

Dr. Peter Chiu (Bloomfield, New Jersey): We have studied propranolol as an antihypertensive drug using spontaneously hypertensive rats (SHR) 17–22 weeks old. The animals included low-sodium, normal-sodium, and high-sodium groups. The experiments were conducted under Inactin anesthesia (Fig. 1). The blood pressure responses to intravenous propranolol are summarized in the upper graphs. As indicated by the solid line, the low-sodium SHR consistently responded to propranolol with a marked drop in mean arterial pressure. The dosage used was 1 mg/kg plus a sustaining infusion at a rate of 1 mg/kg. The blood pressure changes were modest in normal-sodium rats and were variable in high-sodium rats. Additional experiments revealed that moderate pressor responses to propranolol were frequent in this latter group (Fig. 2). The plasma renin activity (PRA) in ng/ml/h measured before propranolol was 48 in low-sodium rats, 16 in normal-sodium, and 1.5 in high-sodium SHR. The lower left trace illustrates the typical depressor response to intravenous propranolol in low-sodium SHR. As shown in the same figure, in a separate experiment, following captopril pretreatment, which itself caused a drop in pressure, propranolol had little further effect. Conversely, propranolol pretreatment also inhibited the antihypertensive action of captopril. The blood pressure reduction by propranolol was abolished following bilateral nephrectomy in low-sodium SHR (Fig. 3). As shown in the upper tracing, instead, propranolol produced marked and sustained *pressor* responses. The solid line represents 1-h postnephrectomy, and the broken line represents 20-hour post nephrectomy. In both conditions propranolol could invoke pressor responses in low-sodium SHR. We conclude that in SHR anesthetized with Inactin, the antihypertensive actions of intravenous propranolol is related closely to the pretreatment PRA and to the sodium status, and that propranolol causes *pressor*, instead of depressor, responses in the absence of renin following bilateral nephrectomy in low-sodium SHR (Fig. 4).

Dr. Ganten (Heidelberg, West Germany): I would like to comment on the possible site and the mode of action of beta-adrenoreceptor blockers, namely sotalol, and *l*- and *d*-propranolol into the brain ventricles of rats. We have observed that blood pressure increased acutely following all three

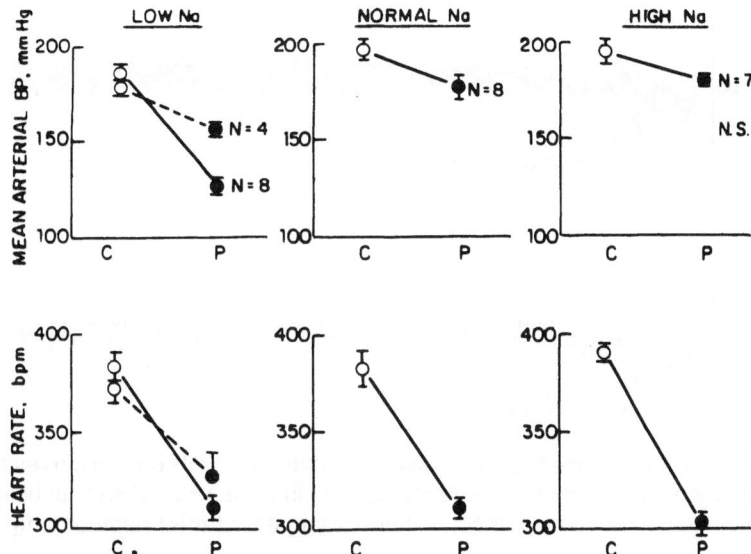

Fig. 1. Blood pressure and heart rate responses to intravenous propranolol in anesthetized SHR of low-, normal-, and high-sodium status. ○ and ●, values before (C) and after (P) propranolol, respectively; ———, propranolol 1 mg/kg plus 1 mg/kg/h; ———, propranolol 0.1 mg/kg plus 0.1 mg/kg/h. All changes are statistically significant ($p<0.05$; t-test for paired comparison) except where N.S. (not significant) is indicated.

blockers, including *d*-propranolol which reportedly has no beta-blocking activity but only membrane-stabilizing, local anesthetic effects. After 24-h administration of these drugs, we tested central effects of two peptides (i.e., angiotensin and leucine–enkephalin on blood pressure and heart rate). The effects of leucine–enkephalin and angiotensin on blood pressure and heart rate were markedly decreased by prior beta-adrenoreceptor blockade. These were clearly central effects, because at this time there was absolutely no peripheral beta-adrenoreceptor-blocking activity. In our opinion, this indicates that some of the blood pressure-lowering action of beta-blockers could be

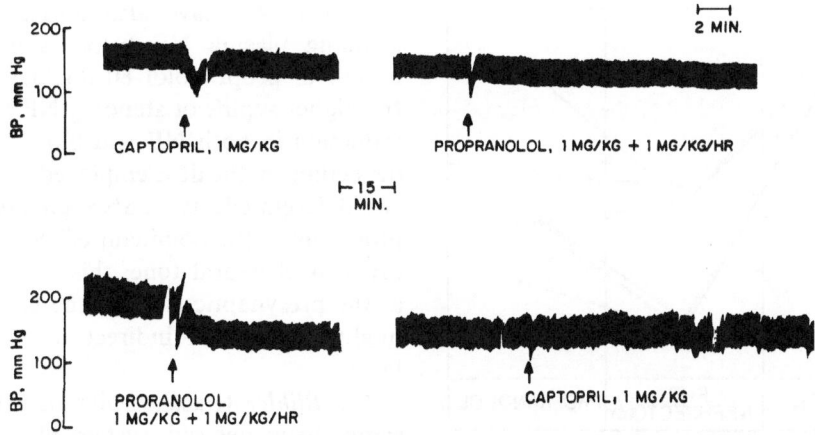

Fig. 2. Effect of intravenous captopril and propranolol on arterial pressure (BP) in anesthetized SHR on sodium restriction. *Upper graph:* propranolol, when preceded by captopril, caused little or no fall in BP. *Lower graph:* in a separate animal, BP decreased rapidly in response to propranolol, and captopril had no further effect. Part of the trace (15 min) was not shown.

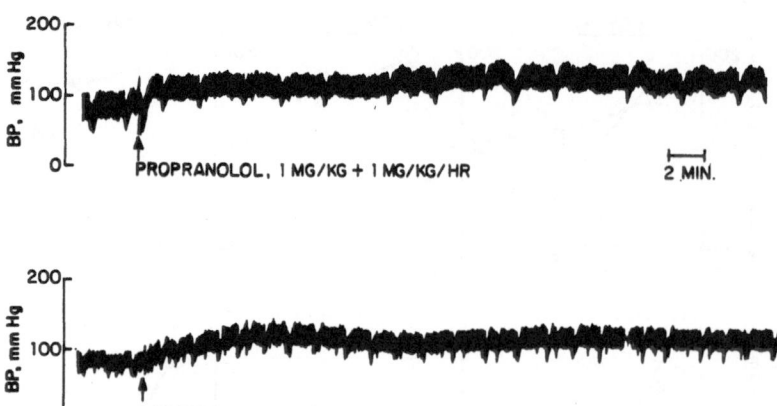

Fig. 3. Postnephrectomy BP response to propranolol and captopril in SHR on sodium restriction. Intravenous propranolol or captopril provoked a marked pressor response in low-sodium SHR with bilateral nephrectomy. The acute hypotensive response seen in intact animals disappeared after nephrectomy.

brought about by inhibition of central pressor peptides. This effect may be a direct action, but more probably beta-blockers interfere with brain peptide action at the level of a secondary neuron, since it is known that the central peptides do stimulate serotoninergic and catecholaminergic pathways.

Dr. DeQuattro (Los Angeles, Cal.): Our findings are in contradistinction to those of Drs. Littler, T. G. Pickering, and also to Dr. Reid, since he works with Dr. Littler. However, they are similar to those of Dr. Bühler, although his interpretation is different from ours. We have data that indicate

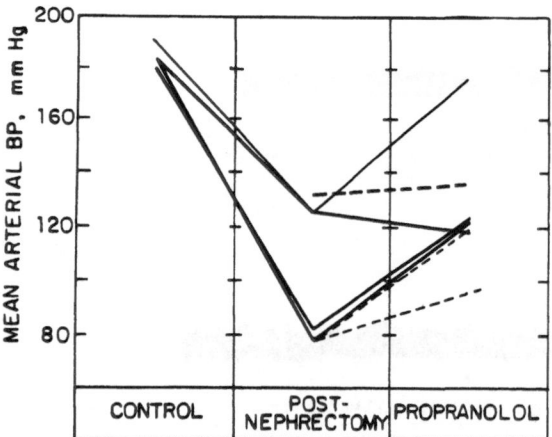

Fig. 4. Postnephrectomy BP response to intravenous propranolol in SHR on sodium restriction. ——, Acute nephrectomy (*N* = 4); ——, 20-h postnephrectomy (*N* = 3).

that hypertensives with higher plasma norepinephrine (NE) are more sensitive to propranolol therapy when that therapy is associated with propranolol blood levels of 30 ng/ml. When doses were administered, which achieved plasma levels of 30/ng/ml, no enhanced blood pressure reduction was seen in the higher NE patients [Esler M, Zweifler A, Randall O, DeQuattro V (1977) Clin Pharmacol Ther 22(3): 299–308]. In hypertensives not segregated into high or low NE, there was a mild but not significant reduction of basal NE after doses of 40 and 80 mg/day for periods of 1 month. When the doses were increased to 360 mg/day, plasma NE was increased [Esler M, Julius S, Zweifler A, Randal O, Harburg E, Gardiner H, DeQuattro V (1977) N Engl J Med 296: 405–411]. We have also measured supine and standing plasma NE before and again after 1 month of propranolol 80 mg/day. Patients with the higher supine or standing NE had the greatest reduction in both NE and blood pressure. Thus, depending on the dose employed, we have observed two different effects on SNS function. At low-dose propranolol, the dominant effect seems to be suppression of neural tone; this could be central or at the presynaptic site. At the higher dose, there might be direct or indirect activation of NE release.

Dr. Bühler (Basel, Switzerland): Clearly, the sympathetic nervous system plays a role in the antihypertensive mode of action of beta-blockers. Acute beta-receptor blockade is followed by reactive increase in sympathetic tone and alpha-receptor-mediated vasoconstriction, which diminishes in those patients whose pressure responds to chronic beta-blocker therapy. However, the important point is that no other real difference has been shown between patients who respond and those who do not respond to antihypertensive beta-blocker therapy, except for the PRA. In addition, the similarity between beta-blockade and the antihypertensive effectiveness of saralasin, and particularly captopril, strongly supports an important antirenin mechanism in the beta-blocker's antihypertensive mode of action.

Dr. DeQuattro: The point I am trying to make is that you don't have to put renin or angiotensin in the system. It could be directly through suppression of sympathetic nerve function.

Dr. J. Reid (Glasgow, Scotland): There is a lot of dispute on that point. A large number of studies have failed to show a consistent fall in plasma NE in responders to beta-blockers.

Dr. DeQuattro: The plasma NE in those patients may not have been lowered because of the large doses used. Dr. Littler used 240 mg as a single dose, and I am not sure what doses Dr. T. G. Pickering used in his exercise studies. Exercise responses might be different from those obtained in the basal state.

Dr. J. Reid: I think the real problem here is that there have been people with the highest levels. There is going to be a regression to the mean with the repeat studies in those who started with high pressures and high NE. One would have to be careful with controls, including placebo treatment, to be certain of a drug effect and not a habituation effect.

Dr. Korner (Melbourne, Australia): I would agree with Dr. DeQuattro that plasma concentrations are important. I would like report on a study we did about the mechanisms causing the hypotension in rabbits. Our conclusions were rather similar to Fritz Bühler's. In our first experiment published about 2 years ago, we studied renal baroreflex curves in anesthetized rabbits in which we looked at the relationship between blood pressure and renal sympathetic efferent activity using the same kind preparation that Dr. Haeusler showed us earlier. We found that if the plasma concentrations of propranolol were very high, you could shift the curve so that you have less sympathetic activity for a given blood pressure. More recently, we studied this in conscious rabbits. In addition, we tried to correlate plasma levels with the hemodynamic responses of conscious rabbits. We found that we got maximum cardiac beta-blockade at quite low-plasma concentrations, something in the order of approximately 20 ng/ml. But, we only really got significant falls in blood pressure and total peripheral resistance (TPR) over the 3-h period of the experiment when the plasma concentrations were well above 150 ng/ml. Our view is that you get peripheral beta-blockade to physiologic sympathetic stimulation at quite low concentrations of propranolol. However, you require high levels to obtain the central effect, and, when you finally get it, it permits, in a sense, the peripheral (cardiac) effects to become manifest.

Dr. Tarazi (Cleveland, Oh.): In reference to the comments about the central effects of propranolol, I wonder how they would apply to the effects of beta-blockers that do not cross the blood–brain barrier?

Dr. DeQuattro: That is an obvious question. Are we saying that propranolol works one way and the other beta-blockers another? There are two alternative explanations: The beta-blockers may suppress sympathetic tone presynaptically by blocking the epinephrine modulation of the presynaptic receptor. The drug might also get past the blood–brain barrier in relatively small amounts and yet be cumulative with time. That is why, I believe, that even with low-dose propranolol therapy, there may be enough concentration in brain to produce central inhibition obviating higher doses and other effects.

Dr. Tarazi: May I suggest still another possibility? It is conceivable that the level of sympathetic activity could be reduced reflexly by beta-adrenergic blockers. To the extent that afferent information from the arterial system and the heart can modulate central neurogenic control mechanisms, a reduction in the speed of cardiac contractions or in its velocity of ejection or in the steepness of the pulse, may all play a role in toning down the general level of sympathetic activity. This could be one of many ways by which beta-blockers, even when cardioselective, could still have a depressor effect on peripheral resistance. This hypothesis has the advantage that it restores, in the overall picture of beta-blockade, its all important effects on the heart.

Dr. Littler (Birmingham, England): Can I just establish from Dr. Reid when he is talking about low-dose therapy, is this given as once-daily therapy?

Dr. J. Reid: When one is talking about penetration of drug into the CNS, one really has to make the measurements, not extrapolate from single-dose studies in small mammals.

Dr. Korner: We have done some measurements with atenolol and what we found is that it does, in fact, get into the brain. It does it in about $\frac{1}{25}$ the amount penetrated by propranolol. This raises the question of whether this is enough to account for a central effect. We do not know the answer to that question, but it certainly gets into the brain to some extent.

Dr. Birkenhäger (Rotterdam, The Netherlands): I would like to confirm both Dr. Bühler's data and his explanation. As my colleague reported at the recent meetings in New Orleans, (7th meeting International Society Hypertension) we took a slightly different approach in that we looked at the renal circulation, particularly at the outer cortical area. In the responders to propranolol, we found some sign of outer cortical vasodilatation together with a reduction in renal NE release, while in the nonresponders we saw marked vasoconstriction in the outer cortical area together with an elevation of NE secretion. The second pattern apparently reflects alpha-receptor stimulation, confirming what Dr. Bühler has said.

Commenting on Dr. Littler's paper, I would like to remark that we were also unable to predict the response to either beta- or alpha-blockade on the basis of control plasma NE levels.

Dr. Logan (Toronto, Canada): Dr. Tarazi, I was interested in your Fig. about the change in protein synthesis with beta-blockade therapy without a fall in blood pressure. From a theoretical point of view, it is possibly worrisome that you may lose the protective effect of changes in the walls of blood vessels to hypertension by decreasing protein synthesis in the continued presence of very high blood pressure. Was the incidence of stroke increased in stroke-prone SHR on beta-blocker therapy that had no reduction in blood pressure?

Dr. Tarazi: These studies, done in collaboration with Dr. Yamori, were short-term experiments; the rats were sacrificed after 7–10 days in order to determine changes in cardiac and aortic weight and any alteration in cardiovascular protein synthesis. Your point, however, is well taken; if the thickness of arterial or cardiac walls can be reduced while systemic pressure remains high, the stress on these walls will necessarily increase. Obvious long-term studies are urgently needed to determine whether this dissociation between pressure

level and cardiovascular structural changes persists, and if it does, what would be its ultimate effects.

Dr. Morganti (Milan, Italy): Dr. Weber, I wonder whether the changes in potassium *per se*, regardless of the changes in aldosterone, might have a role in determining different contractile responses. Is there a way of dissecting out these two factors in your in vitro model?

Dr. Weber (Irvine, Cal.): We have not yet had the opportunity to study the effects of potassium concentration changes *per se* on arterial contractility in our tissue bath medium. However, it is known from previous studies that increases in smooth muscle intracellular potassium concentrations will enhance sensitivity to pressor substances such as NE. It is also quite possible that aldosterone facilitates such a shift of potassium into cells in exchange for sodium. Our clinical studies with the renin–aldosterone axis were relatively long term and did not allow precise monitoring of potassium homeostasis. But, overall, the actions postulated for aldosterone in the peripheral vasculature did not appear to be related to changes in plasma or urine measurements of potassium.

Dr. MacGregor (London, England): Dr. Pickering, if the renin–angiotensin system is maintaining our blood pressure, it seems obvious that beta-blockers must partly work through the fall in angiotensin II; however, if it does not, then I do not see how it can. Working on that basis, we have given normal subjects propranolol. There was a significant correlation between the fall in blood pressure and initial PRA, and the percentage fall was the same in hypertensives for a given PRA. I wonder if studies in normal subjects who can be controlled much better than patients might reveal some of the answers to some of the problems being discussed.

Dr. T. G. Pickering: We did give propranolol to normal subjects and we did find a decrease of pressure in small doses of 5 mg three times a day. This dose was sufficient to suppress plasma renin [Davies R, Pickering TG, Morganti A, Wilson M, Laragh H (1979) Br Heart J 41: 331–335].

Dr. Young (Jackson, Miss.): I have also given propranolol to normal dog subjects, and, as you would expect, if the normal dog subject is sodium depleted and has raised its renin level, there is quite a marked fall in arterial pressure with propranolol.

Dr. Bühler: To summarize, I think we can say

that beta-blockers might theoretically lower blood pressure in a number of ways. However, from much research, by far the best correlation that emerges is that showing the degree of blood pressure reduction related to the height of the preexisting PRA. The studies reported by Drs. Young, Eliahou, Ménard, and Pickering support this thesis in different ways. Moreover, the absence of beta-blockade hypotensive action in anephric or low-renin animal models or humans provides evidence too that renin suppression is a major key for mediating the blood pressure drop. This, of course, should not deter us from looking further into the means of this mediation and into other possible contributory action. So far, the possible role of the sympathetic nervous system and of the catecholamines remains perhaps of some promise, but undefined.

Session 15A
Differential Features of Beta-Adrenoreceptor Blocking Drugs for Therapy

Chairman: D. Shand

Position Paper: Differential Features of Beta-Adrenoreceptor Blocking Drugs for Therapy

Denis G. McDevitt

More than 30 years ago, in studying the effects of six sympathomimetic amines on a variety of effector systems, Ahlquist (1) classified adrenoreceptors into two distinct types: alpha-receptors, whose stimulation produces excitatory responses, and beta-receptors, whose activation results in inhibitory responses plus cardiac stimulation. Beta-receptors have been further classified into $beta_1$-receptors (which occur chiefly in the heart) and $beta_2$-receptors (which occur elsewhere) (2). The distribution of adrenoreceptors is shown in Table

Table 1. Distribution of adrenoreceptors.

System	Receptor type	Effects of stimulation
Heart	$beta_1$	Increased rate of sinoatrial node discharge
	$beta_1$	Increased cardiac contractility
	$beta_1$	Increased conduction velocity in atria, AV node, and ventricles
	$beta_1$	Increased ventricular automaticity
Blood vessels	alpha	Constriction of arterioles and venules
	$beta_2$	Dilatation of arterioles, especially in skeletal muscle
Lungs	$beta_2$	Dilatation of bronchi
Gastrointestinal tract	alpha, beta	Inhibition of peristalsis
Fat cells	beta	Lipolysis
Pancreas (islets of Langerhans)	alpha	Decreased insulin release
	beta	Increased insulin release
Liver	beta	Glygogenolysis, gluconeogenesis
Kidney	beta	Increased renin release

1, although it now appears that more than one type of beta-receptor may be present both in the heart and in the lung (3).

Since the discovery of dichloroisoproterenol (4), drugs have been available that selectively inhibit responses mediated by beta-adrenoreceptors. These drugs are designated beta-adrenoreceptor blocking drugs, and they have become widely used in the treatment of a number of common diseases including angina pectoris, hypertension, cardiac dysrhythmias, myocardial infarction, hyperthyroidism, anxiety neurosis, and migraine. Because of their large potential in the management of common diseases, particularly ischemic heart disease and hypertension, a succession of new beta-adrenoreceptor blocking drugs has been developed and marketed by different pharmaceutical companies. As a result, the prescribing physician may be faced with a choice between as many as 11 different agents (Table 2), depending on the country in which he works: Each drug is promoted by its manufacturer as having advantages over its competitors, and these claims often appear to be in conflict with one another. This chapter will attempt to examine and summarize some of the differences between the available beta-adrenoreceptor antagonists.

CLINICAL PHARMACODYNAMIC PROPERTIES

BETA-ADRENORECEPTOR BLOCKADE

All beta-adrenoreceptor blocking drugs competitively inhibit the effects of catecholamines at beta-adrenoreceptor sites (5). This means that in the presence of the antagonists, a higher concentration of agonist will be required to produce the same

Table 2. Beta-adrenoreceptor blocking drugs.

| Drug | | Potency |
Generic name	Proprietary name	ratio[a] (propranolol-1)
Acebutolol	Sectral	0.3
Alprenolol	Aptin	0.3
Atenolol	Tenormin	1
Metoprolol	Lopressor, Betaloc	1
Nadolol	Corgard	—
Oxprenolol	Trasicor	0.5–1
Pindolol	Visken	6
Practolol	Eraldin	0.3
Propranolol	Inderal	1
Sotalol	Beta-Cardone, Sotacor	0.3
Timolol	Blocardren	6

[a] Inhibition of isoproterenol tachycardia.

Table 3. Properties of beta-adrenoreceptor blocking drugs.

Drug	Membrane stabilizing activity	Partial agonist activity	Cardio-selectivity
Acebutolol	+	+	±
Alprenolol	+	+	−
Atenolol	−	−	+
Metoprolol	+	−	+
Nadolol	−	−	−
Oxprenolol	+	+	−
Pindolol	+	++	−
Practolol	−	+	+
Propranolol	+	−	−
Sotalol	−	−	−
Timolol	−	−	−

effect or, in pharmacologic parlance, that the dose–response curve is shifted to the right. What may vary between the different drugs is their potency, i.e., the amount that the isoproterenol dose–response curves are shifted to the right in the presence of equal doses of each drug. If we use propranolol as the standard drug, it can be seen from Table 2 that pindolol and timolol are more potent, and that acebutolol, alprenolol, practolol, and sotalol less potent. Since these differences can be compensated for by adjustment in dose size, and since a patient is not disadvantaged by the quantity of active drug in an individual tablet, variable potency does not appear to be a factor of clinical significance.

Besides their capacity to block beta-adrenoreceptors competitively, some of these drugs have additional properties. They may have membrane stabilizing activity and partial agonist activity, cardioselectivity, or both. Claims for the relative advantages or disadvantages of these properties, singly or in combination, have caused an enormous amount of confusion and misunderstanding during the last decade.

MEMBRANE STABILIZING ACTIVITY

The term membrane stabilizing activity includes quinidinelike effect and local anesthetic activity and refers to properties that some beta-adrenoreceptor antagonists have been shown to exhibit in animals (6) (Table 3). They reduce the rate of rise of the action potential of cardiac cells without affecting the overall duration of the spike or the resting potential. For some time, it was believed that this property was important in the effectiveness of these drugs in treating cardiac arrhythmias and angina pectoris in man. However, in vitro experiments with human cardiac muscle subsequently demonstrated that membrane stabilizing activity was only exerted by propranolol at a concentration of 10 mg/liter (7), about 100 times greater than that required to block an exercise tachycardia or to suppress ventricular ectopic beats. It would appear that membrane stabilizing activity is unimportant in the clinical efficacy of these drugs, a fact confirmed by the ineffectiveness of d-propranolol (which has membrane stabilizing activity but almost no beta-adrenoreceptor blocking activity) and by the effectiveness of drugs such as sotalol and practolol, which have no membrane activity.

PARTIAL AGONIST ACTIVITY

Several beta-adrenoreceptor blocking drugs can be shown to produce a tachycardia in animals depleted of their norepinephrine stores by pretreatment with reserpine or syrosingopine (Table 3). This partial agonist activity has not been easy to demonstrate in man, but it has been shown that the flattening of the dose–response curve to severe exercise that occurs with single doses of some beta-adrenoreceptor antagonists is attributable to this property (8). The partial agonist activity of beta-adrenoreceptor blocking drugs differs from that of epinephrine or isoproterenol in that the maximum response that can be obtained is less, although the affinity for the receptor site is high.

Antagonists with partial agonist activity may produce less reduction in resting heart rate than do drugs without this property. Hence if resting bradycardia is a clinical problem, a drug with partial agonist activity may be preferred. Similarly, the clinical implication of the flat dose–response curves in the presence of partial agonist activity is that, where the desired therapeutic effect is due to beta-adrenoreceptor blockade, there is little point in increasing the dose of a drug with this property beyond modest levels (e.g., 200 mg with oxprenolol). If the required end point has not been achieved with this type of dose, then either another drug should be added, or the patient should be switched to a beta-adrenoreceptor antagonist that does not have partial agonist activity. However, it has not yet been shown that these differences with single doses are carried over into chronic administration and steady state.

Various clinical benefits have been claimed for drugs with partial agonist activity. On theoretical grounds, it has been postulated that drugs that have this property are less likely to induce cardiac insufficiency than are those devoid of this property, since the former will diminish the force of contraction of the heart muscle to a lesser extent (9). However, Gibson (10), in surveying the available literature for the effects of beta-adrenoreceptor blocking drugs on heart rate and cardiac output both at rest and on exercise, has shown that the greater the drop in heart rate, whether due to a larger dose of the drug or to a higher initial heart rate, the greater the reduction in cardiac output. This is true both for normal subjects and for patients with heart disease and is not modified in nonselective drugs by partial agonist activity. Recently, the hemodynamic effects of oxprenolol (with partial agonist activity) and propranolol were not shown to differ significantly in hypertensive patients with respect to heart rate, blood pressure, cardiac output, stroke volume, and systemic vascular resistance (11). This area is still under investigation, but currently there is no good evidence to support the belief that drugs with partial agonist activity are safer. All beta-adrenoreceptor blocking drugs are likely to be harmful in patients whose cardiac function is dependent on sympathetic drive.

Similarly, it has been claimed that drugs with partial agonist activity behave in patients with obstructive airways disease as though they were cardioselective (12, 13). Some of the studies on which this claim are based contain inadequate methodology (14), for it is necessary to distinguish between the effects of beta-adrenoreceptor antagonists on resting respiratory function and their effects on respiratory function at a time when the cardiac effects of sympathetic stress are adequately blocked. Drugs with partial agonist activity may affect resting respiratory function in some patients with bronchial asthma and will block the beneficial effects of inhaled bronchodilator drugs (15). Thus although there may be some grounds for the belief that drugs with partial agonist activity are preferable to nonselective drugs without this property, the suggestion that these drugs are as good as or better than cardioselective drugs must be regarded as unproved. It is necessary to use all these drugs cautiously in patients with obstructive airways disease, recognizing that an individual patient may suffer a deterioration of respiratory function with any beta-adrenoreceptor antagonist.

Claims have also been made for the benefits of drugs with partial agonist activity in patients predisposed to Raynaud's phenomenon or ischemic limb disease. This was the conclusion of one uncontrolled, retrospective study in hypertensive patients that compared the effects of propranolol, oxprenolol, and atenolol (16). Further carefully designed prospective studies are required to test this hypothesis. Meantime, patients likely to be at risk from this type of side effect should only be given beta-adrenoreceptor antagonists when absolutely essential, and then individual patient preference should be assessed starting with a drug with partial agonist activity or cardioselectivity.

CARDIOSELECTIVITY

The division of beta$_1$-receptors in the heart and beta$_2$-receptors elsewhere raised the possibility that antagonist drugs might be found that selectively blocked cardiac receptors, but that left respiratory receptors unoccupied. The theoretical benefits of this to patients with obstructive airways disease were clearly seen, since early experience had shown that propranolol produced severe bronchospasm in some patients with bronchial asthma (17).

Practolol was the first drug that appeared to

fulfill these criteria for cardioselectivity in animals, and early experience confirmed that blockade in man was selective (18). However, several problems have clouded this area, not the least of which is an understanding of what cardioselectivity is. It has often been equated with drug effects on resting respiratory function, rather than with the selective blockade of the cardiac effects of a sympathetic stimulus while the respiratory effects remain unhindered (14). Difficulties in the development of adequate techniques for measuring cardioselectivity have not helped. Several drugs since practolol, including atenolol and metoprolol, have been shown to be cardioselective in man (Table 3). In others, notably acebutolol, evidence has been less clear cut. Another problem associated with cardioselectivity is that it is a dose-related phenomenon, tending to disappear at higher doses (19): Again, because of the difficulty in making accurate and repeated measurements of cardioselectivity in the same subject or patient, this dose dependency has been inadequately delineated, and the upper limits of cardioselective dosage for atenolol and metoprolol are not known.

The advantages of cardioselective beta-adrenoreceptor antagonists are therefore not as clearly defined as might be expected:

1. In patients with bronchial asthma or obstructive airways disease, cardioselective drugs would be expected to cause fewer respiratory side effects and, therefore, to be the drugs of choice. This is generally the case, but in individual patients, even cardioselective drugs may cause serious reduction in ventilatory function (20). Therefore, caution is always required in these circumstances. Another advantage of cardioselective drugs is that selective beta$_2$-agonists, like salbutamol, can be expected to have a bronchodilator effect (21) in their presence. This is dependent on the dose of antagonist; at higher doses, even practolol, 400 mg, and metoprolol, 200 mg, cardioselectivity may be lost and beta$_2$-agonists will become ineffective. As a general rule, then, in this type of patient, even cardioselective beta-adrenoreceptor antagonists should not be used for the management of hypertension or angina pectoris where effective treatment alternatives exist that avoid possible risk.

2. Cardioselective beta-adrenoreceptor blocking drugs would appear theoretically advantageous for the treatment of hypertension, because their use would not produce inhibition of the peripheral beta$_2$-adrenoreceptors in the vasculature which mediate vasodilatation. These receptors are not under neural control, but respond to circulating epinephrine released from the adrenal medulla. At rest, circulating epinephrine levels are low, and all beta-adrenoreceptor antagonists will cause elevated peripheral resistance after acute administration due to increased sympathetic vasoconstrictor (alpha) outflow in response to reduced cardiac output. During chronic therapy, both selective and nonselective drugs will lower diastolic blood pressure at rest or during standing. During stress from strenuous exercise or hypoglycemia, diastolic blood pressure rises during nonselective blockade due to unopposed alpha stimulation from the circulating epinephrine, whereas with cardioselective antagonists, the diastolic blood pressure is either unchanged or falls, because the preserved beta$_2$ vasodilator response balances the alpha effect (22). Despite these differences, all beta-adrenoreceptor blocking drugs seem to lower blood pressure effectively and to about the same degree: It is usually not possible to distinguish between them clinically. The only clinical circumstance under which vascular sparing is known to be of importance is in the insulin-dependent diabetic. In this type of patient, when beta-adrenoreceptor blocking drugs are considered essential for other aspects of medical care, a cardioselective antagonist should be used: Not only will it cause less interference with glycolysis, but it will be less likely to mask the clinical manifestations of hypoglycemia and, in patients with hypertension or cardiac disease, may prevent the potentially serious consequences of a rise in diastolic blood pressure. But again, it must be remembered that at higher doses, these drugs may have lost their cardioselectivity. This may apply to the usual doses required for treatment of hypertension.

Theoretically, at least, cardioselective antagonists should be preferable in patients with Raynaud's phenomenon or ischemic limb disease. Some benefits have been shown but, in the latter group, some of the difficulties associated with beta-adrenoreceptor blockade may be the consequence of reduced cardiac output and limb perfusion, which may not be significantly different between selective and nonselective agents.

METABOLIC EFFECTS

Catecholamines can cause hyperglycemia by stimulating glycolysis in skeletal muscle predominantly via beta-adrenoreceptors and in the liver mainly via alpha-adrenoreceptors. Thus, in normal subjects, the effect can be abolished only by combined alpha- and beta-adrenoreceptor blockade. Resting plasma-glucose and insulin concentrations are not affected by propranolol, and the fall in plasma glucose after insulin administration is also unaffected. However, the rate of rise of blood glucose levels toward normal after insulin-induced hypoglycemia is decreased, and the increase of plasma glycerol is prevented by the administration of propranolol, but either not at all or to a much less extent by the cardioselective drugs atenolol and metoprolol (22, 23). Cardioselective drugs are therefore preferable in insulin-dependent diabetics, who may be liable to hypoglycemia. In addition, as previously stated, these drugs do not attenuate the cardiovascular response to hypoglycemia (see above) to the same extent as do nonselective drugs.

In man, plasma free fatty acid levels rise following adrenergic stimulation, or infusion of epinephrine or isoproterenol at doses similar to those causing an increase in heart rate. There is a concomitant rise in plasma glycerol levels, indicating that the rise in free fatty acids is due to increased lipolysis rather than to reduced peripheral utilization. Administration of propranolol has been shown to reduce plasma free fatty acid levels at rest and after prolonged fasting, as well as during exercise, emotion, or insulin-induced hypoglycemia. Propranolol, but not practolol, blocks the lipolytic activity of isoproterenol. The increase in free fatty acids that occurs during epinephrine infusion is also blocked by propranolol. The lipolytic activity of epinephrine is only blocked by practolol at doses higher than those that affect its cardiovascular manifestations.

The metabolic effects of beta-adrenoreceptor antagonists are less prominent than their hemody-

namic effects, and the incidence of metabolic side effects is low. However, cardioselective drugs offer important potential advantages in insulin-dependent diabetics.

INHIBITION OF RENIN RELEASE

Beta-adrenoreceptor blocking drugs can antagonize sympathetically mediated renin release (24). Propranolol lowers plasma-renin activity in normal and hypertensive subjects and blocks the orthostatic rise in plasma-renin activity on standing. The effect of different beta-adrenoreceptor antagonists on this system is variable. Among the nonselective drugs, propranolol and timolol have most effect, oxprenolol and alprenolol have less effect, and pindolol has least effect. With the cardioselective drugs, atenolol and metoprolol appear to lower renin release, but practolol has little effect. A possible interpretation of these findings is that renin release is mediated by a beta$_1$-receptor and that partial agonist activity (possessed by oxprenolol, alprenolol, pindolol, and practolol) interferes with the beta-adrenoreceptor antagonism.

Currently the relevance of this property to antihypertensive effect is controversial. Laragh (24) has suggested that decrease in renin output by the kidney is a major factor in the antihypertensive effect of beta-adrenoreceptor blocking drugs. (This evidence has been extensively reviewed in session 14.) However, some evidence may be in conflict with this—Renin can be shown to be reduced by propranolol concentrations that do not lower blood pressure, changing hypertensive patients from propranolol to pindolol has been shown to result in a rise in plasma-renin activity while blood pressure control remained adequate (25) and patients with low renin essential hypertension respond to propranolol therapy (26). Thus, the precise relationship of renin and beta-adrenoreceptor blockade in the causation and management of hypertension remains uncertain.

CLINICAL PHARMACOKINETIC PROPERTIES

ABSORPTION

All beta-adrenoreceptor blocking drugs are well absorbed from the gastrointestinal tract except for atenolol and nadolol (Table 4). Only about 50%

Table 4. Clinical pharmacokinetic properties.

Drug	Absorbed amount (% of dose)	Bioavailability (% of dose)	Plasma protein binding (% bound)	*n*-Octanol/ water distribution ratio (pH 7.0)
Acebutolol	~50	—	20–25	1.3
Alprenolol	>90	~10	85	3.1
Atenolol	~50	~50	3	<0.02
Metoprolol	>95	~40	12	0.2
Nadolol	16–25	—	25–30	N/A
Oxprenolol	~80	~40	78	0.7
Pindolol	>90	~85	57	0.2
Practolol	>90	~100	0	<0.02
Propranolol	>90	~30	80–95	4.3
Sotalol	>90	~100	0	<0.02
Timolol	~70	~55	80	0.3

of an oral dose of acebutolol is absorbed, but it appears that this drug may be excreted into the gut. Absorption occurs mainly in the small intestine, and peak plasma drug concentrations are achieved in approximately 2 h, although absorption may be delayed with acebutolol, atenolol, nadolol, and timolol.

BIOAVAILABILITY

Some drugs are metabolized extensively by the liver, and despite complete alimentary absorption, less than the dose administered by mouth may reach the systemic circulation. This is because drug in the portal vein is exposed to hepatic metabolism before it can appear in the systemic circulation. The greater the ability of the liver to extract the drug, the less will be its bioavailability. This is called presystemic or "first pass" elimination. First-pass metabolism is greatest for alprenolol and propranolol, resulting in a bioavailability of 10–30% (Table 4). It also decreases the bioavailability of metoprolol, oxprenolol, and timolol to a certain extent. For practolol and sotalol, the bioavailability is good, since they are completely absorbed and are not metabolized.

Due to genetic and environmental differences, drugs eliminated by hepatic metabolism show large interindividual variations in circulating drug concentrations as well as low bioavailability. These variations may be five- to tenfold after the same single oral dose and 10–20-fold after chronic administration in patient populations with propranolol, alprenolol, pindolol, and metoprolol (27). Thus

beta-adrenoreceptor blocking drugs with substantial first-pass effects must have the dose adjusted for desired effect within the individual patient. Another important consequence of first-pass metabolism is that in patients with portosystemic anastamoses oral drug may be more bioavailable and that in all patients an intravenous dose of the drug may have a much more potent effect than the same dose administered orally, unless the hepatic biotransformation results in the production of active metabolites.

PLASMA PROTEIN BINDING AND SOLUBILITY

The plasma protein binding of beta-adrenoreceptor blocking drugs varies greatly, and one factor that appears to affect the degree of binding is lipid solubility (Table 4). Propranolol and alprenolol have the highest binding; they are also the most lipid soluble. The least lipophilic drugs, atenolol, practolol, and sotalol, show minimal or no protein binding. Variation in plasma binding may explain some the the individual differences in drug responsiveness, since it is free drug that exerts pharmacologic effect. However, with most beta-adrenoreceptor antagonists, a correlation has been shown between beta-adrenoreceptor blockade and plasma total drug concentration (28), so that plasma binding differences between drugs have so far not proved of major clinical significance.

Lipid solubility also influences the volume of distribution of beta-adrenoreceptor blocking drugs and the more lipid-soluble drugs gain easier access to the central nervous system. Some of the side effects of beta-adrenoreceptor antagonists, like vivid dreams, depression, and insomnia, appear to be centrally mediated. There has been a suggestion that these are more common with more lipophilic drugs, like propranolol, than with more water-soluble drugs, like atenolol. However, the exact position is unclear. Lipophilic drugs have not been shown to exert a more powerful antihypertensive effect nor do they appear to demonstrate any specific effect on the psychic manifestations of anxiety: In contrast, atenolol, a hydrophilic drug, has been found to have central effects in man (29).

VOLUME OF DISTRIBUTION, HALF-LIFE, AND DRUG CLEARANCE

Beta-adrenoreceptor antagonists are rapidly distributed in the body. The size of the distribution volume seems to be related to the lipid solubility of the drug, the highest volumes occurring with the most lipophilic drugs (Tables 4 and 5). Apart from atenolol, in all cases the apparent volume of distribution clearly exceeds the physiologic body space, indicating that these drugs accumulate in certain tissues. Animal experiments suggest that tissues in which beta-adrenoreceptor antagonists accumulate include liver, heart, lungs, and kidneys, but also brain for lipophilic compounds.

The method of elimination of beta-adrenoreceptor blocking drugs also appears to relate to their lipid solubilities. Highly lipid-soluble drugs like propranolol and alprenolol are eliminated by hepatic metabolism, whereas more hydrophilic drugs like atenolol, practolol, and sotalol are primarily eliminated by renal excretion. Several of the other drugs, like pindolol and timolol, may undergo both significant biotransformation and renal elimination. Again, the drugs that are most extensively metabolized have the shortest elimination half-lives (about 2–4 h); drugs undergoing renal clearance have the longest half-lives, from 6 h with atenolol to up to 22 h with nadolol (Table 5).

The clearance of a drug is an expression of the efficiency of all elimination processes; it incorporates both the volume of distribution and half-life. In contrast, half-life can only be assessed in light of the volume of distribution. The total body clearances of alprenolol, propranolol, and metoprolol approach the liver blood-flow rate (about 1.5 liter/min), which is consistent with the extensive hepatic metabolism of these compounds. However, atenolol, practolol, and sotalol have been found to have much smaller clearances, which are near the normal creatinine clearance rate (about 0.12 liters/min) and are consistent with elimination by glomerular filtration (Table 5).

Favorable pharmacokinetic characteristics might include a low variability in the plasma concentrations achieved by a given dose and a long elimination half-life to allow infrequent dosing intervals. In addition, in patients with renal or hepatic dysfunction, beta-adrenoreceptor blocking drugs cleared independently from the diseased organ will be preferable. However, in some situations where renal function may be interfered with, e.g., in renal failure or in elderly patients, reduced first-pass effect in the liver may result in greater bioavailability of drugs such as propranolol. This may be partly offset in the elderly by reduced receptor sensitivity.

Table 5. Clinical pharmacokinetic properties.

Drug	Elimination half-life $t_{1/2}$ (h)	V_d (liters/kg)	Total body clearance C (liters/min)
Acebutolol	3–4	2.3–3.0	0.5
Alprenolol	2–3	3.0–3.4	1.0–1.2
Atenolol	6–9	0.7–1.0	0.10
Metoprolol	3–4	5.6	1.1
Nadolol	17–22	2.1	—
Oxprenolol	1–4	1.3	0.2–0.6
Pindolol	2–5	1.2–2.0	0.5
Practolol	10–13	1.6	0.14
Propranolol	2–5	3.3–5.5	0.8–1.2
Sotalol	7–18	1.6–2.4	0.11–0.4
Timolol	2–5	2.0–2.4	0.5

CONCLUSIONS

Many beta-adrenoreceptor blocking drugs are now available, all of which are effective in the management of essential hypertension and angina pectoris. The differential pharmacologic properties of these drugs seem relatively unimportant—Cardioselective drugs are preferable in patients with bronchial asthma or insulin-dependent diabetes, but should be used only when essential, remembering that cardioselectivity may be lost at relatively low dose levels. Partial agonist activity and membrane stabilizing activity do not appear to offer any major advantage, although nonselective drugs with the former property may offer modest benefits in patients with bradycardia or peripheral limb ischemia. In any individual patient with a particular problem even the most potentially beneficial beta-adrenoreceptor antagonist can cause a serious adverse effect. Pharmacokinetically, beta-adrenoreceptor antagonists with low variability of plasma drug concentration at a fixed dose and longer elimination half-lives may be preferred: These are usually drugs with low lipid solubility and predominantly renal clearance.

ous adverse effect. Pharmacokinetically, most beta-adrenoreceptor blocking drugs are well absorbed, but vary in their lipid solubility. The more lipid-soluble drugs tend to be highly protein bound, subject to primarily hepatic clearance with short elimination half-lives and large volumes of distribution: They may show wide interpatient variability in plasma drug concentrations at steady state on a fixed dose. In contrast, the drugs having lower lipid solubility and predominantly renal clearance may have longer half-lives and show less interpatient variation at steady state. This latter group would have advantages in terms of infrequent dosage intervals and more predictable clinical response at fixed doses.

SUMMARY

There are now at least ten different beta-adrenoreceptor blocking drugs available to the prescribing clinician, each of which is promoted by its manufacturer has having advantages over the others. There are a number of possible differences between the drugs. First, although each of these drugs blocks beta-adrenoreceptors competitively, they have variable potency compared with propranolol: This does not appear to be clinically important, however, and each is effective in controlling hypertension and angina pectoris. Membrane stabilizing activity is not present at the plasma drug concentrations required for beta-adrenoreceptor blockade, antiarrhythmic effect, and antianginal efficacy. Drugs having partial agonist activity may not reduce resting heart rate as much as drugs without this property, but the evidence that they reduce cardiac output less at comparable levels of beta-adrenoreceptor blockade is not convincing, nor should they be prescribed in patients with obstructive airway disease, since they prevent the bronchodilator effects of beta$_2$-agonists. Cardioselective beta-adrenoreceptor blocking drugs are preferable in patients suffering from bronchial asthma or insulin-dependent diabetes, but they should only be used if no other effective treatment alternatives exist. Cardioselectivity is, however, a dose-dependent phenomenon and may disappear at relatively modest doses. In any individual patient with a particular problem, e.g., heart failure or asthma, even the most potentially beneficial beta-adrenoreceptor antagonist may cause a seri-

REFERENCES

1. Ahlquist RP (1948) A study of the adrenotropic receptors. Am J Physiol (Lond) 153: 586–600
2. Lands AM, Luduena FP, Buzzo HJ (1967) Differentiation of receptor systems responsive to isoproterenol. Life Sci 6: 2241–2249
3. Barnett DB, Rubb EL, Nohorski SR (1977) Direct evidence for two types of beta-adrenoceptor binding site in lung tissue. Nature 273: 166–168
4. Powell CB, Slater IH (1958) Blocking of inhibitory adrenergic receptors by a dichloro analog of isoproterenol. Pharmacol Exp Ther 122: 480–488
5. Barrett AM (1973) Beta-adrenoceptive antagonists: In: Hamer J (ed) Recent advances in cardiology. Churchill Livingstone, Edinburgh and London, p 289
6. Morales-Aguilera A, Vaughan-Williams EM (1965) The effects on cardiac muscle of β-receptor antagonists in relation to their activity as locak anaesthetics. Br J Pharmacol 24: 332–338
7. Coltart DJ, Meldrum SJ (1970) The effect of propranolol on the human and canine transmembrane action potential. Br J Pharmacol 40: 148P
8. McDevitt DG, Brown HC, Carruthers SG, Shanks RG (1977) Observations on the influence of intrinsic sympathomimetic activity and cardioselectivity on β-adrenoceptor blockade in man. Clin Pharmacol Ther 21: 556–566
9. Choquet Y, Capone RJ, Mason DT, Amsterdam EA, Zelis R (1972) Comparison of the beta-adrenergic blocking properties and negative inotropic effects of oxprenolol and propranolol in patients. Am J Cardiol 29: 257
10. Gibson (1977) Pharmacodynamic properties of β-adrenoceptor blocking drugs in man. In: Avery GS (ed) Drug Treatment: Principles and Practice of Clinical Pharmacology and Therapeutics. Publishing Services Group, Acton, Mass.
11. Franciosa JA, Johnson SM, Tobian LJ (1980) Hae-

modynamic effects of oxprenolol and propranolol in hypertension. Clin Pharmacol Ther 26: 676–681

12. Connolly CK, Batten JC (1970) Comparison of the effect of alprenolol and propranolol on specific airway conductance in asthmatic subjects. Br Med J 2: 515–516

13. Oh VMS, Kaye CM, Warrington SJ, Taylor EA, Wadsworth J (1978) Studies of cardioselectivity and partial agonist activity in β-andrenoceptor blockade comparing effects on heart rate and peak expiratory flow rate. Br J Clin Pharmacol 5: 107–120

14. McDevitt DG (1978) β-adrenoceptor antagonists and respiratory function. Br J Clin Pharmacol 5: 97–99

15. Christenson CC, Boye NP, Erikson H, Hansen G (1978) Influence of pindolol (Visken) on respiratory function. Eur J Pharmacol 13: 9–12

16. Marshall AJ, Roberts CJC, Barritt DW (1976) Raynaud's phenomenon as side-effect of β-blockers in hypertension. Br Med J 1: 1498–1499

17. McNeill RS (1964) Effect of a β-adrenergic blocking agent, propranolol, on asthmatics. Lancet 2: 1101–1102

18. Powles R, Shinebourne E, Hamer J (1969) Selective cardiac sympathetic blockade as an adjunct to bronchodilator therapy. Thorax 24: 616–618

19. Lertora JJL, Mark AL, Johannsen UJ, Wilson WR, Abboud FM (1975) Selective β-adrenoceptor blockade with oral practolol in man. A dose related phenomenon. J Clin Invest 56: 719–24

20. Chang LCT (1971) Use of practolol in asthmatics: A plea for caution. Lancet 2: 321

21. Formgren H (1976) The effect of metoprolol and practolol on lung function and blood pressure in hypertensive asthmatics. Br J Clin Pharmacol 3: 1007–1014

22. Davidson N McD, Corrall RJM, Shaw TRD, French EB (1976) Observations in man of hypoglycaemia during selective and non-selective beta-blockade. Scot Med J 22: 69–72

23. Deacon SP, Barnet D (1976) Comparison of atenolol and propranolol during insulin-induced hypoglycaemia. Br Med J 2: 272–273

24. Laragh JH (1973) Vasoconstriction-volume analysis for understanding and treating hypertension: The use of renin and aldosterone profiles. Am J Med 55: 261–274

25. Stokes GS, Weber MS, Thornell IR (1974) β-blockers and plasma renin activity in hypertension. Br Med J 1: 60–62

26. Hollifield JW, Sherman K, Vander Zwagg R, Shand DG (1976) Proposed mechanism of propranolol's antihypertensive effect in essential hypertension. N Eng J Med 295: 68–73

27. Shand DG (1977) Pharmacokinetic properties of the β-adrenoceptor blocking drugs. In: Avery GS (ed) Cardiovascular drugs, Adis Press, Sydney (β-Adrenoceptor blocking drugs, Vol 2, pp 41–54)

28. McDevitt DG (1977) The assessment of β-adrenoceptor blocking drugs in man. Br J Clin Pharmacol 4: 413–425

29. Salem SAM, McDevitt DG (1980) Central effects of atenolol in man. Clin Pharmacol Ther 27: 283

Session 15B
Potentials for Secondary Cardioprotection in Clinical Trials

Chairman: D. Shand

Postinfarction Intervention Studies with Propranolol and Atenolol: Problems in Design and Interpretation

N. S. Baber and J. A. Lewis

Propranolol, a nonselective beta-adrenergic blocking agent without partial agonist activity, has been tested in eight postinfarction trials, in which mortality or nonfatal reinfarctions have been the major end points (1–8). There is only one published study with atenolol—a cardioselective beta-adrenergic block agent, without partial agonist activity (15).

Differences in the design and execution of these studies makes comparisons between them extremely difficult, but such comparisons are necessary for two reasons:

1. To establish if a decision can be taken at a community level, concerning the routine use of beta-blocking agents in selected patients.
2. To establish whether there are any important differences in the efficacy or safety of betablockers, with different pharmacological profiles.

The most recent trial with propranolol compared the effects of propranolol, 40 mg, three times a day, with placebo in patients who had survived an anterior myocardial infarction 2–14 days (mean 8.5 days) previously (16). The trial was a double-blind randomized prospective study in which patients were followed up at 1, 3, 6, and 9 months. Three hundred-fifty-five patients received propranolol, with a mean duration in trial of 172 days. Three hundred-sixty-five patients received placebo, with a mean trial duration of 169 days. Twenty-three percent were withdrawn from the propranolol group, and 24% from placebo. The total mortality was 7.9% on placebo, and 7.4% on propranolol. There were six cardiac deaths after withdrawal in the propranolol group and seven in the placebo group.

The number of withdrawals for heart failure and the deaths in heart failure were the same in each group. There was a trend for more patients with a history of heart failure in the pretreatment phase to die in the propranolol group than in the placebo group. There was also a trend for patients whose pretreatment systolic pressure above the mean, and for patients with a trial entry diastolic presence above the mean, to have a reduced mortality in the propranolol group. The converse was also true.

Atenolol, in a dose of 50 mg twice a day, has been compared with propranolol and with 40 mg three times daily placebo, in a prospective randomized double-blind trial, in patients with suspected myocardial infarction, within the last 24 h (10). Patients were followed up at three monthly intervals for 1 year. Three hundred-eighty-eight patients were randomized: 132 on propranolol, 127 on atenolol, and 129 on placebo. By 1 year, 58% had been withdrawn from the propranolol group, 61% from the atenolol group, and 54% from the placebo group. Most withdrawals occurred during the first 6 weeks and were mainly for hypotension or bradycardia in the beta-blocker groups. The total and in-trial mortalities are shown in Table 1.

Table 1. Postinfarction trial: Propranolol versus atenolol versus placebo.

	Propranolol	Atenolol	Placebo
No. entered	132	127	129
<6-week mortality			
In-trial	3	2	10 $p < 0.05^a$
Total	10	11	15 N.S.
<1-year mortality			
In-trial	5	4	10 N.S.
Total	17	19	19 N.S.

[a] Fisher's exact test. Comparison of each beta-blocker group with placebo.

These two trials are quite different in design and in mode of patient selection. Essentially, both are "negative," but their results merit closer examination, in view of the more hopeful results obtained with some, but not all the other studies with propranolol, atenolol, practolol, and oxprenolol. Table 2 (a, b) lists these trials.

If it is accepted that beta-blockers do have a

Table 2a. Studies with beta-blocking drugs in patients with myocardial infarction—treatment started <48 h after event.[a]

Author	Drug	Dose (mg/ day)	Total no. of patients	Duration of treat- ment	Mortality		
					Drug	Placebo	p
Snow (1)	Propranolol	30–60	91	28 days	16	35	<0.025
Snow (1)	Propranolol	30–60	107	28 days	13	29	<0.05
Multicentre (4)	Propranolol	80	195	28 days	15	12.6	NS
Balcon et al. (2)	Propranolol	80	114	28 days	23	24	NS
Clausen et al. (3)	Propranolol	40	130	14 days	28	25	NS
Barber et al. (5)	Propranolol	160	99	28 days	19.4	25.5	NS
Sloman and Stannard (6)	Propranolol	60	49	21 days	11.5	17.5	NS
Norris et al. (8)	Propranolol	80	454	21 days	13.7	10.5	NS
Kahler et al. (7)	Propranolol	80	69	21 days	7.9	19.3	NS
Fucella (9)	Oxprenolol	120	220	21 days	13.2	7.9	NS
Briant and Norris (10)	Alprenolol	400	172	3 days	8	7	NS
Reynolds and Whitlock (11)	Alprenolol	400	78	1 year	7.9	7.7	NS
Barber et al. (12)	Practolol	600	298	2 years	27	31	NS
Barber et al. (12) (HR > 100 bpm)	Practolol	600	53	1 year	9	43	<0.05
Mitchell (13)	Propranolol/ Atenolol	120/100	265	42 days	10.2	11.2	NS
Andersen et al. (14)	Alprenolol	5–10 lv 400 oral	480	1 year	25.6	26.4	NS
Andersen et al. (14) (<65 years old)	Alprenolol	5–10 lv 400 oral	480	1 year	9.3	20.4	<0.01
Peltola (unpublished)	Propranolol	60	159	in hospital	20.3	38.1	<0.01

[a] Summary of the major postinfarction studies in which a beta-adrenergic blocking agent has been given within the first 24–48 h of the onset of chest symptoms. Most of the reports listed do not state the mean time or ranges of administration of the beta-blocking agent. The following studies give these data: Barber et al. (12): 50% commenced treatment within 3–4 h (range 7 min to 7 days); Andersen et al. (14): >50% patients commenced treatment under 6 h; Peltola (unpublished): All patients admitted in less than 4 h.

Table 2b. Studies with beta-blocking drugs in patients with myocardial infarction—treatment started > 1 week after event.[a]

	Author	Drug	Dose (mg/day)	Total No. of patients	Duration of treatment (years)	Mortality (%)		
						Drug	Placebo	p
1.	Ahlmark et al. (1974)	Alprenolol	400	162	2	1.5	10.5	<0.05
2.	Wilhelmsson et al. (1974)	Alprenolol	400	230	2	2.6	9.5	<0.05
3a	Multicentre International Study	Practolol	400	3,053	2	3.2	5.1	<0.01
3b	Multicentre International Study (1975) Anterior M.I.	Practolol	400	1,539	2	2.6	5.6	<0.01
4.	Baber et al. (1979)	Propranolol	120	720	0.75	7.9	7.4	NS

[a] Summary of four studies in which a beta-adrenergic blocking agent has been given after recovery from myocardial infarction. The mean starting times, in days (ranges), were as follows: Ahlmark et al. (14); Wilhelmsson et al. (7–21); Multicentre 13 (7–28); Baber et al. 8.4 (2–13). The most convincing reduction in mortality has been demonstrated for patients with anterior infarction, treated with practolol.

role to play in the prophylactic treatment of either early or late myocardial infarction, or both, then the following issues, to account for different trial results, should be considered.

METHODOLOGY

1. Trial size.
2. Harm to specific subgroups outweighing benefit to the group as a whole.
3. Analysis by intention to treat (total mortality), or by death on treatment (in-trial mortality).
4. Differentiation of late from early intervention studies.
5. Patient selection.
6. Mode of death in relation to time after infarction.

PHARMACOLOGICAL

1. Importance of dose in relationship to prevention of sudden death and potentially fatal arrhythmias.
2. Significance of partial agonist activity or cardioselectivity.
3. Changes of metabolism of beta-blockers during myocardial infarction.

Each of these points can be considered separately and a decision can be taken that one is of such importance as to warrant testing in a clinical trial. For example, a high-risk subset could be chosen for study, as was seen in the Practolol Multicentre Trial (17). Patients who had an anterior infarction and a trial entry diastolic blood pressure below the mean (<80 mmHg) had the largest re-

duction in mortality. The converse appeared to be true for the propranolol trial, although the difference between placebo and propranolol groups was not statistically significant.

An alternative approach is to make the assumption that all beta-blockers are likely to be equally effective or ineffective and that it is justifiable to pool all the beta-blocker studies. We have done this for 19 trials (see Table 3 for results). The present status of confidence that can be put in beta-blocking agents in general can also be displayed by plotting the 90% confidence limits for each trial, as was recently illustrated by Freiman et al. (18). This is shown for 18 beta-blocker postinfarction studies in Fig. 1. Three points are worth noting.

1. The results of each trial are scattered around and on either side of the "no difference" line on the x axis.
2. The confidence limits are very wide on most of the trials because of their small size.
3. The upper 90% confidence limit includes the line that represents a 50% reduction in mortality in 14 of the 18 studies and includes the line representing a 25% reduction in 17 of the 18 studies (i.e., it is not possible to rule out the possibilities of this size of reduction, had the individual trials continued).

It is of interest that trial size was the central issue discussed by the authors of both the propranolol and atenolol/propranolol studies described above. Wilcox et al. (15) state that

> In our view practising doctors will conclude that if benefit to patients cannot be shown by a trial such as ours then it cannot be large enough to make a valuable contribution to the management of their patients with suspected myocardial infarction.

Baber et al. (16) note that a reduction of less than 50% (which this trial was designed to show)

Table 3. Pooled results from beta-blocker postinfarction studies.

Type	No. of trials	No. of patients	Mean percentage death rate		Reductions (%)	Significance (%)
			Drug	Placebo		
Overall	19	approx. 7,440	10.5	12.2	14	5
Short-term	13	approx. 2,500	11.7	13.1	10	NS
Long-term	6	approx. 5,000	9.8	11.7	16	5

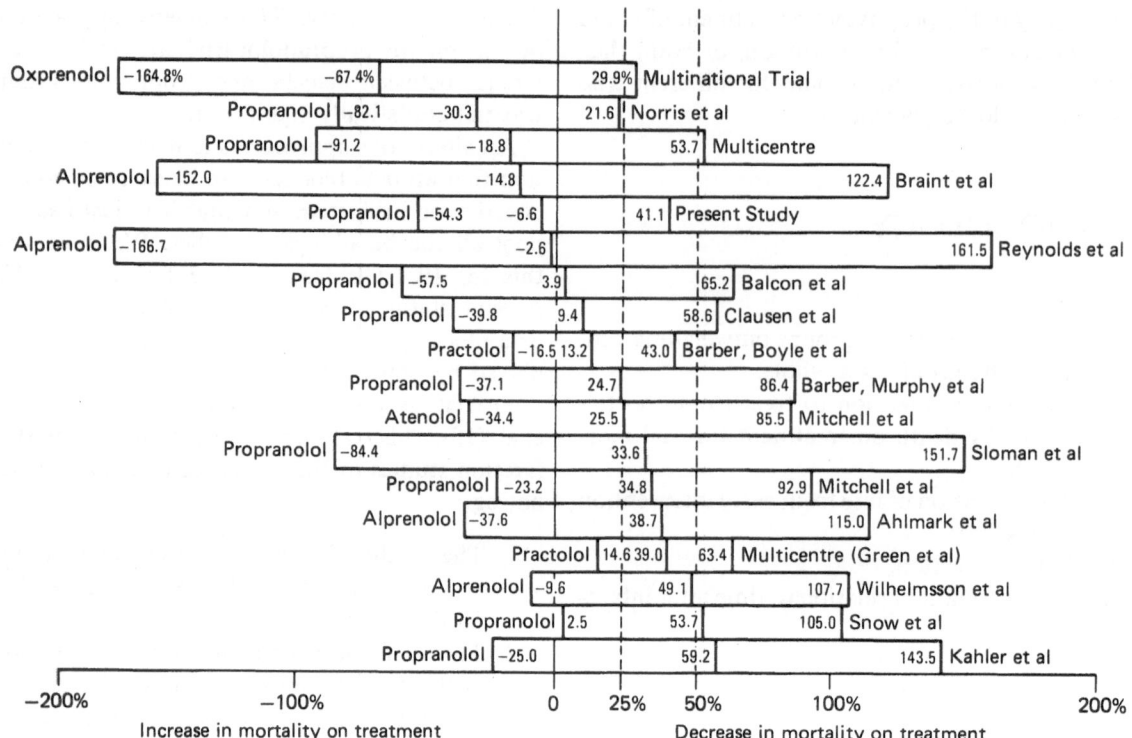

Fig. 1. Eighteen beta-blocker postinfarction studies.

is still possible, within the confidence limits of the study. They also question whether a smaller reduction can lead to a decision on the widespread use of beta-blockers.

In conclusion, our current view is in agreement with that of Braunwald (19), who states that "β-blocking agents are showing promise in the prophylactic treatment of myocardial infarction, but that no definite decisions about them can yet be taken," and with Lovell (20), who concludes that "The implications of the demonstrations of long-term benefit from a beta-blocker are so great that the demonstration must be absolutely conclusive."

SUMMARY

Propranolol has been tested in eight postinfarction trials, in which mortality has been the major end point. There is only one published study with atenolol a new cardioselective beta-blocking agent. In a recent double-blind (DB) late-intervention prophylactic study, 720 patients who had sustained an anterior myocardial infarction during the previous 2–14 day (mean 8.5 days) period were randomized to treatment with propranolol 40 mg tds, or matching placebo. By 9 months, 23% had been withdrawn from the propranolol group and 24% from placebo. The total mortality was 7.9% in placebo and 7.4% in propranolol. The study with atenolol compared this drug, in a dose of 50 mg bd, with propranolol 40 mg tds, and matching placebo, in a DB study in 388 patients started on oral treatment within 24 h of onset of suspected myocardial infarction. Treatment continued for 1 year when the withdrawals were 58% propranolol, 61% atenolol, and 54% placebo. The total annual mortality was 12.9% propranolol, 14.9% atenolol, and 14.7% placebo. As other studies with practolol and alprenolol have shown reductions in mortality, it is important to consider possible reasons why this has not been clearly demonstrated in the two studies described. These reasons include (1) the small size of these trials and consequent wide confidence limits; (2) harm to specific subgroups outweighing benefit to others; (3) importance of route of administration, dose, and blood level in relationship to sudden death; (4) significance of partial agonist activity and cardioselectivity.

REFERENCES

1. Snow PJD (1965) Effect of propranolol in myocardial infarction. Lancet 2: 551
2. Balcon R, Jewitt DE, Davies JPH, Oram S (1966) A controlled trial of propranolol in acute myocardial infarction. Lancet 2: 917
3. Clausen S, Felsby M, Schonan Jorgensen F, Lyager Nielsen B, Roin J, Strange B (1966) Absence of prophylactic effect of propranolol in myocardial infarction. Lancet 2: 920
4. Multicentre International Trial (1966) Propranolol in acute myocardial infarction. Lancet 2: 1435
5. Barber JM, Murphy FM, Merrett JD (1967) Clinical trial of propranolol in acute myocardial infarction. Ulster Med J 35: 127
6. Sloman G, Stannard M (1967) Beta-adrenergic blockade and cardia arrhythmias. Br Med J 4: 508
7. Kahler RL, Brill SJ, Perkins WE (1968) The role of propranolol in the managment of acute myocardial infarction. In: Kattus AA, Ross G, Hall YE (eds) Cardiovascular beta-adrenergic responses. University of California Press, Los Angeles, P 213
8. Norris RM, Caughey, DE, Scott PJ (1968) Trial of propranolol in acute myocardial infarction. Br Med J 2: 398
9. Fucella LM (1968) Report on the double-blind trial with compound Ciba 39, 089-Ba (Trasicor) in myocardial infarction. Quoted by Sowton, E., Beta adrenergic blockade in cardiac infarction. Prog Cardiovasc Dis 10: 561–574
10. Briant RB, Norris RM (1970) Alprenolol in acute myocardial infarction. Double blind trial. New Zeal Med J 71: 135–138
11. Reynolds JL, Whitlock AML (1972) Effects of a beta-adrenergic receptor blocker in myocardial infarction for one year from onset. Br Heart J 34: 252–259
12. Barber JM, Boyle DMCC, Chaturvedi HC, Singh N, Walsh MJ (1975) Practolol in acute myocardial infarction. ACta Med Scand 587: 213–216
13. Mitchell JRA (1978) Tribulations in trials experience gained from Nottingham Study of beta-adrenergic blockage in acute myocardial infarction. Br Heart J 40: (suppl.) 88–94
14. Andersen MP, Frederiksen J, Jürgensen HJ, Pedersen F, Bechsgaard P, Hansen DA, Nielsen B, Pedersen-Bjergaard O, Rasmussen SL (1979) Effect of alprenolol on mortality among patients with definite or suspected acute myocardial infarction. Preliminary results. Lancet 2: 865–867
15. Wilcox RG, Roland JM, Banks DC, Hampton JR, Mitchell JRA (1980) Randomized trial comparing propranolol with atenolol in immediate treatment of suspected myocardial infarction. Br Med J 1: 885
16. Baber NS, Evans DW, Howitt G, Lewis SA, Thomas K, Wilson C (1980) A multi-centre propranolol post-infarction trial in 49 hospitals in the U.K., Italy and Yugoslavia. Br Heart J (in press)
17. Multicentre International Study (1975) Br Med J 3: 735
18. Freiman JA, Chalmers TC, Smith H Jr, Kuebler RR (1978) The importance of beta, the type II error and sample size in the design and interpretation of the randomized control trial. N Engl J Med 299: 690
19. Braunwald E (1980) Treatment of the patient after myocardial infarction. The last decade and the next, Editorial. N Engl J Med 302: 290
20. Lovell RRH (1978) Review of the present status of drug treatment preventing sudden death. Br Heart J 40 (Suppl): 94

Secondary Prevention of Myocardial Infarction with Beta-Adrenoreceptor Blocking Drugs—Alprenolol, Practolol, and Oxprenolol

S. H. Taylor

Beta-adrenoreceptor antagonists possess many properties that are potentially advantageous after acute myocardial infarction (1–4). They reduce left ventricular oxygen consumption (5), enhance the metabolism of ischemic myocardium (6), limit infarct size in animals (7) and in man (8), retard the mobilization of free fatty acids (6), and attenuate ventricular ectopic activity (9). But it has not been easy to translate these theoretical advantages into proof of clinical benefit. Alprenolol, practolol, and oxprenolol are three drugs for which long-term value in survivors of myocardial infarction has been claimed.

SECONDARY PREVENTION STUDIES WITH ALPRENOLOL

Four studies with alprenolol, a nonselective beta-adrenoreceptor blocking drug with partial agonist activity, have so far been reported (see Table 1).

REYNOLDS AND WHITLOCK (10)

This double-blind randomized placebo-controlled study is difficult to interpret for a number of reasons. The small number of patients involved, the fact that patients in this long-term study were survivors of an earlier beta-blocker study and not rerandomized before inclusion, the limited information about the entry characteristics of patients enrolled in each part of the study, the high withdrawal rate (41 patients), and the lack of information of the fate of these withdrawals all combine to obscure any meaningful interpretation even of the negative result.

WILHELMSSON ET AL. (11)

This double-blind randomized placebo-controlled study demonstrated a marginally statistically significant reduction in "sudden death" rate in the alprenolol-treated patients. There was no signifi-

Table 1. Alprenolol in secondary prevention of myocardial infarction—fixed dose: 400 mg/da.

Authors	Trial period (months)	Patients (years of age)	Placebo					Alprenolol				
			No.	With-drawn	RI	M	SD	No.	With-drawn	RI	M	SD
Reynolds and Whitlock (10)	1–12	<70	39	3	10	3	1	38	4	8	3	2
Wilhelmsson et al. (11)	1–24	57–67	116	8	18	14	11	114	8	16	7	3[c]
Ahlmark and Saetre (12)	0.5–24	<66	93[2]	6	15	11	9	69	4	4[c]	5	1[c]
Andersen et al. (13)	0–24	<65 >65	142 100	25 24	— —	29 35	— —	140 98	29 30	— —	13[b] 48	— —

[a] RI, Reinfarction; M, mortality including withdrawals, SD, "sudden death <24 hr. Control (nonplacebo) group.
[b] $p < 0.05$.
[c] $p < 0.01$.

cant difference in total mortality or nonfatal myocardial reinfarction between the two treatment groups.

The small numbers involved, the randomization of the patients some weeks before treatment was commenced, the lack of detailed information of the outcome in the patients withdrawn from the study, and the omission of the results of compliance testing limit the interpretation of this study. However, it does appear to indicate that alprenolol was associated with a reduction in sudden death risk during the 24 months following myocardial infarction.

AHLMARK AND SAETRE (12)

This randomized, but nonblind comparison between alprenolol and a "control" group of patients not receiving the drug is deficient in too many respects for acceptance. Of the 393 patients initially randomized on admission to hospital, only 162 were eventually included in the study. The outcome in the 231 patients not included and in the ten patients withdrawn during the course of the study is not given. The small numbers involved and the large imbalance in the two treatment groups (93 control : 69 alprenolol) underlines the difficulty in interpreting the authors' claims of a "statistically significant" reduction in reinfarction rate, total mortality, and sudden death.

ANDERSEN ET AL. (13)

These investigators reported a double-blind randomized placebo-controlled study of the influence of alprenolol on mortality from the time of admission to a coronary care unit in patients under and over 65 years of age. In the former group, alprenolol was associated with a significant reduction in total mortality if all patients including withdrawals were considered together. However, when considered separately, neither patients who continued in the study nor those who dropped out showed any statistically significant difference in total mortality between active treatment and placebo. The difference in mortality appeared to reside largely with patients who had suffered a first relatively mild (WHO grade 1) infarction. In patients over 65 years of age the study was terminated due to the apparent, but not "statistically significant," increase in total mortality rate in the active treatment group.

This report is limited by its preliminary nature; only 203 patients had completed 1 year of study and 79 other patients had been treated for an average period of only 6 months. No information is given as to the mode of death—sudden or otherwise—or to the incidence of reinfarction.

SECONDARY PREVENTION STUDIES WITH PRACTOLOL

Two studies with practolol, a relative beta 1 selective adrenoreceptor blocking drug with partial agonist activity have been reported (see Table 2).

BARBER ET AL. (14)

The authors of this double-blind randomized placebo-controlled trial claimed to have shown no

Table 2. Practolol in secondary prevention of myocardial infarction—(fixed dose: 600 or 400 mg/da.)

			Placebo					Alprenolol				
	Trial period (months)	Patients (years of age)	No.	With-drawn	Critical end points[a]			No.	With-drawn	Critical end points[a]		
Authors					RI	M	SD			RI	M	SD
Barber et al. (14)	0–24	32–87	147	?	?	46	?	151	?	?	41	?
Multicentre International Study (15)	0.5–24	<70	1520	270	97	124	55	1,533	250	75	96	41[b]

[a] RI, reinfarction; M, mortality including withdrawals; SD, "sudden death" < 24 hr.
[b] $p < 0.01$.

difference in total mortality between active- and placebo-treated groups during the period 0–24 months following acute myocardial infarction.

However, it is impossible to interpret this observation for a number of reasons. Description of patients entered into the study is adequate, and neither the numbers nor outcome in patients withdrawn from treatment is not given. No information is given of the mode of death, and the incidence of reinfarction is omitted as well. A major limitation is also imposed by the small size of this trial, and the information given does not permit separation of acute inhospital and long-term effects of treatment.

MULTICENTRE INTERNATIONAL STUDY (15)

This double-blind randomized placebo-controlled collaborative trial involving 67 hospitals was prematurely terminated due to adverse reactions with practolol. Sudden death, but not total mortality, was statistically significantly reduced, but only in patients with pre-entry anterior infarction. There was no significant change in reinfarction rate between the two treatment groups.

The high withdrawal rate and the increased death rate in these withdrawals, and the reversal in mortality rate at 1 month in patients with inferior infarction (increased before; reduced after) pose problems in interpreting the result of this study.

SECONDARY PREVENTION STUDIES WITH OXPRENOLOL

Oxprenolol is a nonselective beta-adrenoreceptor blocking drug with partial agonist activity. Two double-blind randomized placebo-controlled studies were recently completed by the Coronary Prevention Research Group (Yorkshire, England) (see Table 3). Their objective was to measure the influence of small doses of the drug (80 mg/day) on morbidity and mortality rates following uncomplicated acute myocardial infarction at three stages in the natural history of the disease in patients under age 70 who were treated for 5 years. To achieve an equal number of predicted critical end events in each treatment group, patients were randomized to placebo : oxprenolol in the ratio of 3 : 4.

During the period 2–56 days no statistically significant trend of influence of active treatment on reinfarction, total mortality, or sudden death was observed.

In the long-term study (1–60 months) three groups of patients were included who had suffered an acute myocardial infarction 1–4, 5–12, and 13–60 months previously. Thirty-one percent of patients were withdrawn from the study. There were statistically significant reductions in sudden death and reinfarction rate in patients receiving active treatment, but these reductions were confined to those who commenced treatment in the period 1–4 months after the acute event and were not influenced by the site of the pre-entry infarction.

CONCLUSIONS

The results of the studies reviewed offer unconvincing evidence for the concept that the long-term administration of the beta-blocking drugs may benefit patients following myocardial infarction. No single study has conclusively demonstrated a positive result, and the interpretation of

Table 3. Oxprenolol in secondary prevention of myocardial infarction—coronary prevention research group.

| Trial period | Placebo | | | | | | Oxprenolol (80 mg/day) | | | | | |
| | No. | With-drawn | Critical end events[a] | | | No. | With drawn | Critical end events[a] | | |
			RI	M	SD			RI	M	SD
2–56 days	136	17	8	6	5	177	21	3	9	9
2–60 months	471	141	58	48	25	632	85	67	60	33

[a] RI, Reinfarction; M, Mortality including withdrawals; SD, sudden death.

the seven trials reported with these three drugs is obscured by the deficient design used in the majority. Neither can the results of the separate trials be pooled for analysis. Three trials used designs that exclude them from comparison with other studies, five are limited by insufficient patient numbers, and one was not placebo controlled. The population selection exercised at entry was not stated in any, and the withdrawal rate varied from 6% to 31% in those studies in which it was reported. The fate of the patients withdrawn was rarely given. Stratification for age, sex, severity of pre-entry infarction, and other pre-entry coronary prognostic risk factors were ignored by all.

In five of the seven studies there was an apparent reduction in sudden death, i.e., death within 24 h of the onset of symptoms. However, this beneficial influence was confined to patients under age 65, usually without extensive myocardial damage and treated relatively soon after the initial episode. No benefit was obtained by starting treatment later than 4 months after infarction, and the claims that benefit was confined to patients with anterior infarction or tachycardia were not generally supported. However, total mortality was rarely influenced, if all patients including withdrawals are considered. This apparent change in the mode, but not the risk, of death needs further confirmation. There was no substantial change in reinfarction rate in most of the trials.

The major benefit of the results of the studies to date probably lies in their influence on scientific thinking rather than on their therapeutic enlightenment. It is clinically unimaginative to expect that all patients following myocardial infarction would derive equal benefit from cardiac sympathetic blockade: These studies go some way toward pointing the direction of selection. It is unlikely that all beta-adrenoreceptor blocking drugs will be equally efficacious; it is of interest that all three drugs possess partial agonist activity, but only one was cardioselective. It is therapeutically unreasonable to imagine that fixed doses should be equally efficacious irrespective of body mass and clinicopathological state. No study has yet examined the possible dose–response relationship.

The studies so far reported have been uncritically enthusiastic as to the possible benefits these drugs may confer in the secondary prevention of coronary heart disease. Equally uncritically, the apparent negative results of many of these studies have also been accepted without reasoned evaluation of the statistical conclusions reached. In all but two of these studies, there was a substantial trend toward a reduction in morbidity and mortality, although only rarely did this achieve the usually accepted level of statistical significance. However, to prove lack of benefit of a treatment it is necessary to know the confidence limits of the result; rarely was this given. In small studies a negative result proves nothing. Sufficient therapeutic stimulus therefore remains for further, more adequate, trials in this field, using these drugs. It is probable that the chief impact of future trials will lie in the definition of the patients most likely to achieve benefit, the drugs and doses most effective and least likely to cause adverse side effects during long-term administration, and the optimum length of treatment. It is to be hoped that such pragmatic solutions will be paralleled by advances in our understanding of the mechanisms by which these drugs induce such benefits.

SUMMARY

The evidence relating to the influence of three beta-adrenoreceptor blocking drugs in seven secondary prevention trials has been critically reviewed. Most of the studies had serious design faults or were of inadequate size to validate either their positive or negative claims. Although it remains to be convincingly demonstrated, the evidence suggests that the long-term administration of these drugs may reduce the subsequent risk of sudden death in patients less than 65 years of age with relatively mild first myocardial infarctions.

REFERENCES

1. Forrester J, Chatterjee K, Parmley WW, Swan HJC (1973): Hemodynamic profiles in acute myocardial infarction and their therapeutic implications. Circulation 48 (Suppl IV) IV 59
2. Taylor SH (1973) New perspectives in beta-blockade. In: Burley DM, Fryer JH, Rondel RK, Taylor SH (eds). Ciba Laboratories, Horsham, 107
3. Harris AS, Otero H, Bocage AJ (1971) The induction of arrhythmias by sympathetic activity before and after occlusion of a coronary artery in the canine heart. J. Electrocardiogr 4: 34
4. Khan MI, Hamilton JT, Manning GW (1973) Early arrhythmias following experimental coronary occlusion in conscious dogs and their modification by beta-adrenoreceptor blocking drugs. Am Heart J 86: 347

5. Sonnenblick EH, Ross J, Covell JW, Kaiser GA, Braunwald E (1965) Velocity of construction as a determinant of myocardial oxygen consumption. Am J Physiol 209: 919

6. Opie LH, Thomas M (1976) Propranolol and experimental myocardial infarction: substrate effects. Postgrad Med J 52 (Suppl 4): 124

7. Maroko PR, Kjekshus JK, Sobel BE, et al. (1971) Factors influencing infarct size following experimental coronary artery occlusions. Circulation 43: 67

8. Norris RM, Clarke ED, Sammel NL, Smith WM, Williams B (1978) Protective effect of propranolol in threatened myocardial infarction. Lancet 2: 907

9. Gibson D, Sowton E (1969) The use of beta-adrenergic receptor blocking drugs in dysrhythmias. Prog Cardiovasc Dis 12: 16

10. Reynolds JL, Whitlock RML (1972) Effects of a beta-adrenergic receptor blocker in myocardial infarction treated for one year from onset. Br Heart J 34: 252

11. Wilhelmsson C, Vedin JA, Wilhelmsson L, Tibblin G, Werkö L (1974) Reduction of sudden deaths after myocardial infarction by treatment with alprenolol. Preliminary results. Lancet ii: 1157–1160

12. Ahlmark G, Saetre H (1976) Long-term treatment with beta-blockers after myocardial infarction. Eur J Clin Pharmacol 10:77–83

13. Andersen MP, Bechsgaard P, Frederiksen J, Hansen DA, Jurgensen HJ, Nielson B, Pedersen F, Pedersen-Bjergaard O, Rasmussen SL (1979) Effect of alprenolol on mortality among patients with definite or suspected acute myocardial infarction. Lancet ii: 865–868

14. Barber JM, Boyle DMcC, Chaturvedi NC, Singh N, Walsh MJ (1975) Practolol in acute myocardial infarction. Acta Med Scand (Suppl. 587): 213

15. Green KG, Alderley Park, Chamberlain DA, et al. (1977) Multicentre International Study. Reduction in mortality after myocardial infarction with long-term beta-adrenoceptor blockade.

The Role of Beta-Blockers in Cardioprotection

Curt D. Furberg

Beta-blockers play an important role in the symptomatic treatment of several cardiac conditions. However, their value in the prevention of cardiovascular morbidity and mortality has not been conclusively documented. One major public health question to be answered is: "Do beta-blockers prolong life in subjects who have survived a myocardial infarction?" Several randomized clinical trials (RCTs) have been conducted in order to answer this question. Subsidiary objectives of these studies have been to determine the effect of beta-blockers on cause-specific mortality (or the mode of death) as well as the incidence of recurrent nonfatal myocardial infarction. Although important, one must keep these objectives in perspective—they are of secondary importance to any effect on total mortality.

Adherence to principles in design and analysis that reduce bias increases the credibility of the findings of a trial. All cause mortality is the preferred end point, as it has the advantage of being based on a simple count with no reliance on defini-

tion or interpretation. Accounting for every randomized subject without exception and crediting any end point to the group to which a subject was originally assigned is another principle that is often neglected.

This review is restricted to studies of the effect of chronic beta-blockade on long-term survival following myocardial infarction (Table 1). The results from eight RCTs (1–11) have been reported since 1972. In four RCTs the study drug was alprenolol, in two practolol, in two propranolol, and in one atenolol. Seven trials were placebo controlled and double blind and thus met optimal design standards.

The results as they related to total mortality are shown in Table 2. The presented data account for every randomized subject in his originally assigned group with the exception of two of the studies (A,C), in which the mortality among the subjects withdrawn for analysis was not reported. Treatment was started as soon as possible after hospital admission in trials (F,G,H). In the re-

Table 1. Clinical trials of the long-term value of beta-blockers in survivors of myocardial infarction.

Authors	Year	Study drug	Control group	Randomization	Type of blindness
Reynolds and Whitlock	1972	Alprenolol	plbo[a]	+	DB[c]
Wilhelmsson et al.	1974, 1975	Alprenolol	plbo	+	DB
Ahlmark et al.	1974, 1976	Alprenolol	umt[b]	+	Open
Barber et al.	1975	Practolol	plbo	+	DB
Multicentre International Study	1975, 1977	Practolol	plbo	+	DB
Andersen et al.	1979	Alprenolol	plbo	+	DB
Barber et al.	1980	Propranolol	plbo	+	DB
Wilcox et al.	1980	Propranolol Atenolol	plbo	+	DB

[a] Placebo.
[b] Usual medical therapy.
[c] Double blind.

Table 2. Number of patients randomized, number of deaths from any cause in the beta-blocker, and control groups, respectively, and level of significant difference between the two groups.

Trial	Authors	Random	Total mortality beta-blocker	Total mortality control	Differential
A	Reynolds and Whitlock	87	3	3	N.S.[e]
B	Wilhelmsson et al.	230	5	11	N.S.
C	Ahlmark et al.	393	7	14	N.S.[e]
D	Barber et al.	298	41	46	N.S.
E	Multicentre International Study	3,063	103	128	N.S.
F1	Andersen et al.	282[a]	13	29	$p < 0.01$
F2		198[b]	48	35	N.S.
G	Baber et al.	720	28	27	N.S.
H1	Wilcox et al.	388	17[c]	19	N.S.
H2			19[d]		

[a] ≤65 years of age.
[b] ≥65 years of age.
[c] Propranolol.
[d] Atenolol.
[e] Outcome of subjects withdrawn from the analysis not included.

maining trials, intervention was initiated shortly before or just after hospital discharge for the acute event. The trial by Barber et al. was limited to patients with anterior myocardial infarction (MI).

Seven of the trials showed no statistically significant difference for total mortality between the groups (Table 2). A recent study by Andersen et al. reported a significant difference in one of the two study groups, subject 65 years of age or below at the time of enrollment. The small number of end points is a limitation of at least three of the trials (A–C). In six of the studies (B–F1,H1) there were more deaths in the placebo group than in the beta-blocker group. In the others, there was neither no difference (A,H2) or there were even fewer deaths (F2,G) among the placebo patients.

When cause-specific mortality was analyzed it appeared as if the incidence of sudden death was reduced by beta-blockade (B,C,E). The interpretation of this finding is not totally clear in light of the absence of an effect on overall mortality. There are two possible explanations. First, beta-blockers do indeed reduce the incidence of sudden death in post-MI patients, but the trials were not of sufficient scope to permit this to be reflected in a reduced total mortality. Alternatively, beta-blockers do not reduce the overall risk of dying, but only change the mode of death.

In summary, eight RCTs involving 5,634 post-MI patients have not convincingly shown whether or not beta-blockers are cardioprotective.

SUMMARY

The reports of eight randomized, placebo-controlled clinical trials of the effect of beta-blockers on mortality in post-MI patients are reviewed. Seven of the trials showed no statistically significant difference between the groups. The eighth study reported a difference only in the younger of two age groups. The eighth study reported a difference only in the younger of two age groups. It remains to be convincingly shown whether beta-blockers are cardioprotective.

REFERENCES

1. Reynolds JL, Whitlock RML (1972) Effects of a beta-adrenergic receptor blocker in myocardial infarction treated for one year from onset. Br Heart J 34: 252–259
2. Wilhelmsson C, Vedin JA, Wilhelmsen L, Tibblin G, Werkö L (1974) Reduction of sudden deaths after myocardial infarction by treatment with alprenolol. Preliminary results. Lancet 2: 1157–1160
3. Vedin A, Wilhelmsson C, Werkö L (1975) Chronic alprenolol treatment of patients with acute myocardial infarction after discharge from hospital. Effects on mortality and morbidity. Acta Med Scand (Suppl 575) 1–56
4. Ahlmark G, Saetre H, Korsgren M (1974) Reduction of sudden deaths after myocardial infarction. Lancet 2: 1563

5. Ahlmark G, Saetre H (1976) Long-term treatment with β-blockers after myocardial infarction. Eur J Clin Pharmacol 10: 77–83

6. Barber JM, Boyle D McC, Chaturvedi NC, Singh N, Walsh MJ (1975) Practolol in acute myocardial infarction. Acta Med Scand (Suppl 587) 213–219

7. Multicentre International Study (1975) Improvement in prognosis of myocardial infarction by long-term beta-adrenoreceptor blockade using practolol. Br Med J 3: 735–740

8. Multicentre International Study (1977) Reduction in mortality after myocardial infarction with long-term beta-adrenoreceptor blockade. Supplementary report. Br Med J 2: 419–421

9. Anderson MP, Bechsgaard P, Frederiksen J, Hansen DA, Jürgensen HJ, Nielsen B, Pedersen F, Pedersen-Bjergaard O, Rasmussen SL (1979) Effect of alprenolol on mortality among patients with definitive or suspected acute myocardial infarction. Lancet 2: 865–868

10. Baber NS, Wainwright Evans D, Howitt G, Thomas M, Wilson C (1980) A multi-centre propranolol post-infarction trial in 49 hospitals in the United Kingdom, Italy and Yugoslavia. Br Heart J 44: (1) 96–100.

11. Wilcox RG, Roland JM, Banks DC, Hampson JR, Mitchell JRA (1980) Randomized trial comparing propranolol with atenolol in immediate treatment of suspected myocardial infarction. Br Med J 1: 280: 885–888

DISCUSSION

Dr. Shand (Durham, North Carolina): Therapy is most rational when we use a drug that has an appropriate mechanism of action to reverse a disease process (or one of its manifestations) in a dose that produces the desired effect. In the case of preventing sudden death and reducing overall mortality after myocardial infarction with beta-blocking drugs, none of these conditions has really been fulfilled. The essential problem is that death cannot be used as a clinical end point to monitor effective drug dosage, which is known to vary widely for all other clinical indications. It is interesting to note that none of us would recommend fixed drug dosage in, say, hypertension, yet the perceived need to create uniformity in clinical trials has led to the use of fixed doses in the published trials of secondary prevention. While it is generally felt that most instances of sudden death have their basis in a ventricular arrhythmia, the recent promising data with the antiplatelet drug, sulfinpyrazone, raises the issue of possible mechanism of action, especially as at least one beta-blocker (pro-

pranolol) has been shown to have antiplatelet actions in patients with coronary artery disease. Until the precise mechanism of action of these drugs is established, our approach must necessarily be indirect. At this time it would seem premature to abandon a drug until it is shown to be present in sufficient concentrations to produce a high degree of cardiac beta-blockade and to suppress ventricular arrhythmias. In the case of early negative trials of propranolol, it is now known that the doses used (120 mg/day at most) is likely to have been subtherapeutic in some individuals. One factor that is known to affect dosage requirements is variable plasma levels, and it will be interesting to see the outcome of the current U.S. multicenter trial of propranolol in which dosage is being guided by plasma-level determinations.

One particularly important issue is whether the result obtained with one beta-blocker can be extrapolated to all others. It is a tantalizing coincidence that the most promising drugs—practolol and alprenolol (to which Dr. Taylor's presentation suggests we might add oxprenolol)—have intrinsic sympathomimetic activity, a property that is poorly understood. It seems that we often embark on large-scale, expensive trials before the clinical pharmacology of the drug is fully understood, the current controversy concerning aspirin dosage being a good example. While this is to some extent unavoidable, therapy will never be truly rational until we fully understand the drugs we use, as well as how to use them optimally. With that, I would like to encourage you to begin the discussion.

Dr. Cohn (Minneapolis, Minnesota): Just as an aside to Dr. Shand's opening statement, actually sulfinpyrazone is being purported to be an antiarrhytmic agent, as a mechanism contributing to its claimed efficacy in preventing sudden death. I would like to address a comment and question to the subject of patient selection for the controlled trials of therapy for postmyocardial infarction. Myocardial infarction is a very heterogeneous disease. The acute and long-term mortality varies tremendously depending on the severity of the coronary disease and perhaps most importantly on the severity of the left ventricular dysfunction. The studies reported today have made no distinct attempt that I've seen to categorize patients on the basis of severity of left ventricular dysfunction, and indeed the mortality rates in many of these studies are so low that one would suspect that the patients with poor LV function are being eliminated from the trial. Since that is the very group that has a high subsequent mortality, if one is trying to demonstrate efficacy of any therapy on mortality the study group certainly should include this patient subgroup. So I would like to ask both Dr. Baber and Dr. Taylor whether in their studies patients who had heart failure were screened out before the study was begun, and to ask Dr. Furberg if he is not struck also by the differences in mortality among the different studies and if he wouldn't agree that more would be learned if patients were categorized more carefully before they were entered into the study. Rather than just looking at age and sex, shouldn't we also be looking at the severity of the left ventricular dysfunction?

Dr. Taylor (Leeds, England): In the study I reported earlier, all patients with enlarged cardiothoracic ratios and any other evidence of left ventricular insufficiency were excluded. I think that was understandable when designing a study a decade ago. I should mention that in another study now under way called The European Infarction Study, which uses oxprenolol 320 mg/day versus placebo, all patients are being included even if they have left ventricular dysfunction. The only exclusions are those in which it is impossible to control left ventricular insufficiency by conventional means.

Dr. Baber (Macclesfield, England): I quite agree with you of course. In the late intervention study I first described [Baber MS, Wainwright Evans D, Howitt G, et al. (1980) Br Heart J 44 (1): 96–100], I suspect our selection criteria were very similar to those in Dr. Taylor's study. We did exclude patients having a history of heart failure in their distant medical history, but in the acute phase they could have had heart failure provided it had cleared by the time of entry. If you look at the patients who had a history of heart failure in the acute phase, but who had cleared by the time of randomization, there is a tendency, and only a tendency, for those who were then randomized to propranolol to have a high mortality over the long term so there may be something in this. In the Nottingham study the selection as regards heart failure was pretty rigorous [Wilcox RG, Roland JM, Banks DC, et al. (1980) Br Med J 280 No. 6218 885–888]. They defined heart failure as the need for 80 mg furosemide. I suspect that there was probably a higher risk group of patients going to the study. However, one must remember that

at the time of randomization, the diagnosis was of suspected infarction and a number of patients did not have an infarct. I think this is the quintessence of the problem that you have put your finger on. We want to look at a high risk group, but are we courageous enough to do it?

Dr. Case (New York, New York): I would like to ask any of the panelists if in any of these studies the differential effects of the beta blocker on blood pressure has been determined with respect to the outcome in view of the fact that in both normal subjects and in hypertensive subjects both pressor and depressor responses can occur?

Dr. Baber: Yes, we looked at this in some detail. Again, there are no statistically significant differences, but there are trends which are as follows. If you can look at the blood pressure acutely when our patients came into hospital (i.e., within some hours of onset of chest pain), you will find that those patients in whom systolic pressure was below the mean for the trial who were subsequently randomized onto propranolol tended to do worse than did those who were randomized onto placebo. And if you look at the diastolic pressures at entry to the trial you find again that those patients whose diastolics were lower than the mean of 80 mmHg for the trial, as we would expect 8 days after infarction, those who were then randomized onto propranolol tended to do worse. The converse is also true, i.e., those with blood pressures above the mean did better on propranolol. Now if you recall the practolol Multicenter trial the converse was shown here [Green KG, Chamberlain DA, Fulton RM, et al. (1975) Br Med J 3: 735–740]. Those patients who at entry have a diastolic pressure below the mean tended to do better on practolol, which was a total surprise to the people doing the study. So yes, I think you are right, there may be something in this. Could I just come back to a question you raised, Dr. Shand, which is about ISA. There are three trials that I think are published now with practolol which are negative in terms of reinfarction rate and mortality in Barber's study [Barber JM, Boyle D McC, Chaturvedi HC, et al. (1975) Acta Med Scand 587: 213–216], which has been pointed out, there was one by Thompson from Australia [Thompson PL, Jones AL, Noon D, et al. (1980) Br Ht J (in press)], and there was another one from England [Evemy KL, Pentecost BL (1978) Eur J Card 6: 391–398]. The latter group looked at the short and long-term mortality and ventricular function. In terms of mortality there was no difference in the placebo and the practolol treated patients.

Dr. Logan (Toronto, Canada): Just a comment on Dr. Furberg's using all-cause mortality as an end point. I agree with that, but you have to make sure that all study participants are getting the same form of care. When the modes of healthcare delivery of two study groups are different, as in the Hypertension Detection Follow-up Program Study, for instance, differences in outcome may not necessarily be due to the specific intervention being assessed, but rather may just represent a difference in the type of care being delivered.

Dr. Furberg (Bethesda, Maryland): Mortality from any cause is a preferred endpoint in a clinical trial as it is essentially bias-free. Any attempt to take into account subject compliance to the study regimens when interpreting trial results may be misleading. One must be very cautious if good compliers in one group are to be compared to good compliers in another. We prefer to analyze data with each randomized subject remaining in his originally assigned group. In other words, we compared treatment strategies or, as Dr. Baber puts it, the intention to treat.

Dr. Myers (New South Wales): As Professor Morgan isn't here from Newcastle, I would just like to say that he is involved in the study with other Australian and Scandinavian groups, who are currently looking at the effect of prindolol in this high-risk group of patients with myocardial infarction. It is hoped that this study will provide some of the answers.

Dr. Cohn: I would just like to comment on two additional issues that have come up. One is the question of sudden deaths versus all mortality. As you well know, that has become a real problem with the sulfinpyrazone study in that the sudden death rate was statistically lower in the treated group but not the total death rate. When one begins to analyze sudden deaths one becomes troubled by the definition being used in such studies. Since we don't really know what sudden death is, and depending on the exact definition that one uses it probably is a phenomenon of multiple mechanisms, it is very difficult to use this diagnosis as an end point for a study. The second point, to get back to my earlier comments, is that from the numbers of studies that have been done, the number of patients who have theoretically been put at risk in this kind of study, and the cost of these controlled trials worldwide, it is painfully apparent that a carefully done study that probably would have involved some invasive studies to categorize the patients might have solved this problem a long time ago. We can predict fairly accurately on the basis of wedge pressure at the time of an acute myocardial infarct the mortality over the ensuing year. The patient who has an acute myocardial infarct with a normal wedge pressure has an extremely low chance of dying in the ensuing 12 months, so that you would probably not want to use a therapy in that group. If Dr. Baber is unwilling to give propranolol or a beta-blocker to those who have been in heart failure, then I would submit that the issue is not going to be resolved with a beta-blocker because the study groups will consist of patients who are unlikely to die.

Dr. Logan: As we know, those patients who take their placebo faithfully have a lower incidence of myocardial infarction than do those people who don't. If you alter medication compliance in one group by monitoring plasma drug levels, you may introduce bias into your study.

Dr. Shand: In fact, the study was set up so that that would not happen. Blood samples are being taken in everyone and the dose of placebo is being changed in a way that statistically won't invalidate the trial. The important thing is that we want people to have a chance at adequate therapy—if they comply.

Session 16
Angiotensin-Converting Enzyme Blockade as a Therapeutic Modality

Chairman: J. H. Laragh

Position Paper: Angiotensin-Converting Enzyme Blockade as a Therapeutic Modality

H. R. Brunner, B. Waeber, G. A. Turini, J. P. Wauters,
D. B. Brunner, and H. Gavras

INTRODUCTION

The existence of a renal pressor hormone was first suggested in 1898 by Tigerstedt and Bergman (1), who gave it the name "renin." During the next 80 years, the renin system, as it later became to be known, went through alternating periods of glamour and complete oblivion. As soon as it was discovered, renin was forgotten until 1934, when Dr. Goldblatt reported his classic experiment (2). This experiment opened up a new era for the renin system. Its various components were rapidly characterized (3–9), and it was believed that it played a predominant role in the pathogenesis of hypertensive diseases. The tide changed somewhat during the early 1960s, when methods became available to measure renin activity in the plasma of hypertensive patients. It was then found that renin was only rarely elevated (10, 11) and, so it became somewhat of a curiosity as a pathogenetic factor seeming only to contribute to rare forms of hypertension, such as renovascular hypertension. This was still true in the beginning of the 1970s, when the first inhibitor of angiotensin II, i.e., saralasin, became available (12). Probably because of the intrinsic agonistic effect of saralasin, results obtained with this compound seemed to confirm that renin contributes actively to the maintenance of hypertension only in those rare cases in which it is clearly elevated (13, 14). The more recent development of inhibitors of converting enzyme (15), which converts the inactive angiotensin I to the active pressor hormone angiotensin II, have completely changed the attitude toward renin, since with these compounds, e.g., teprotide, it has been possible to lower blood pressure in a majority of hypertensive patients (16, 17).

Finally, the synthesis of the first orally active inhibitor of converting enzyme (18) has made long-term treatment of hypertension using this specific approach possible, and with this new tool the interest in renin as a factor contributing actively to the maintenance of hypertensive blood pressure levels has risen tremendously.

During the past few years it has been shown that with chronic converting enzyme blockade, either alone or together with sodium depletion, hypertension can be treated effectively (19–23). Furthermore, blockade of the renin system has proved useful in treating congestive heart failure even in nonhypertensive patients (24–28), has been shown to improve regional blood flow in the kidney (29, 30) and the heart (31), and has been reported to have a beneficial effect in experimental hemorrhagic shock (32). Thus, it has now become apparent that the renin-angiotensin system might play a predominant role in regulating regional and total body circulation. This chapter attempts to review some of the results we have obtained using angiotensin-converting enzyme blockade as a therapeutic tool.

CONVERTING ENZYME BLOCKADE IN NORMAL VOLUNTEERS

In 1976 the new converting enzyme inhibitor captopril, or SQ 14225, which is active orally, became available for clinical research. To start out, the pharmacologic properties of this compound were tested in 14 normotensive volunteers (33). A dose–response curve for angiotensin I was drawn up for each subject prior to the first oral ingestion of captopril. After administration of a single dose, the maximum dose of angiotensin I that had been used previously was reinjected several times over the following hours. Increasing doses of captopril (1, 2.5, 5, 10, and 20 mg) were tested in the same way. Figure 1 shows the degree of inhibition of the diastolic pressor response to angiotensin I obtained after injection of these various doses of captopril. Both degree and the duration of converting enzyme inhibition appear to be dose dependent. Thus, 1 mg captopril only permits partial inhibition, whereas higher doses afford an intensified blockade of the renin-angiotensin system. Thus the mechanism of action of this new inhibitor was confirmed in man, since 20 mg captopril sufficed to block the response to angiotensin I completely within 15 min, for more than 2 h and for doses of angiotensin I up to 160, or even 320 ng/kg body weight. Consequently, it should be kept in mind, when treating hypertensive patients, that increasing the dose of captopril, more than 20 mg, probably will not bring about any more blockade of the renin system, but only prolong the duration of the blockade.

Figure 2 illustrates the time course of the blood pressure lowering effect of three different doses of captopril observed in six hypertensive patients on three consecutive days. With 25 mg captopril, mean blood pressure decreased from a control of 130 ± 8 to 125 ± 11 mmHg at 15 min and to 111 ± 7 mmHg at 60 min after administration. Mean blood pressure returned to base-line levels of 127 ± 8 mmHg at 360 min. Blood pressure reduction induced by 100 mg showed a similar pattern, whereas 200 mg clearly had a prolonged antihypertensive effect, since after 6 h blood pressure was still reduced by 9 ± 4%. Thus, as suggested by the initial studies in normal volunteers, the larger doses did not produce a greater blood pressure fall, but rather prolonged its duration.

Blood pressure was reduced in all hypertensive patients whether the blood pressure increase was due to renal or to renovascular hypertension, or was labeled "essential" hypertension. Not surprisingly, patients with high plasma-renin activity had the greatest blood pressure fall from 181/113 ± 7/2 to 134/87 ± 5/3 mmHg, but in those with normal and even low renin levels, blood pressure was also reduced significantly from 177/109 ± 10/4 to 148/95 ± 7/3 mmHg, and from 171/104 ± 12/3 to 152/95 ± 15/4 mmHg, respectively (Fig. 3). In our first 39 hypertensive patients treated with captopril there was a significant correlation between pretreatment plasma-renin activity and the induced immediate fall in diastolic blood pressure ($r = 0.67$, $p < 0.001$). In the two patients with primary hyperaldosteronism and the lowest renins the blood pressure did not decrease following inhibition of angiotensin-converting enzyme. Thus, even if the pretreatment plasma-renin activity does not precisely predict the blood pressure fall that may be induced by captopril administration, there exists a correlation between the capto-

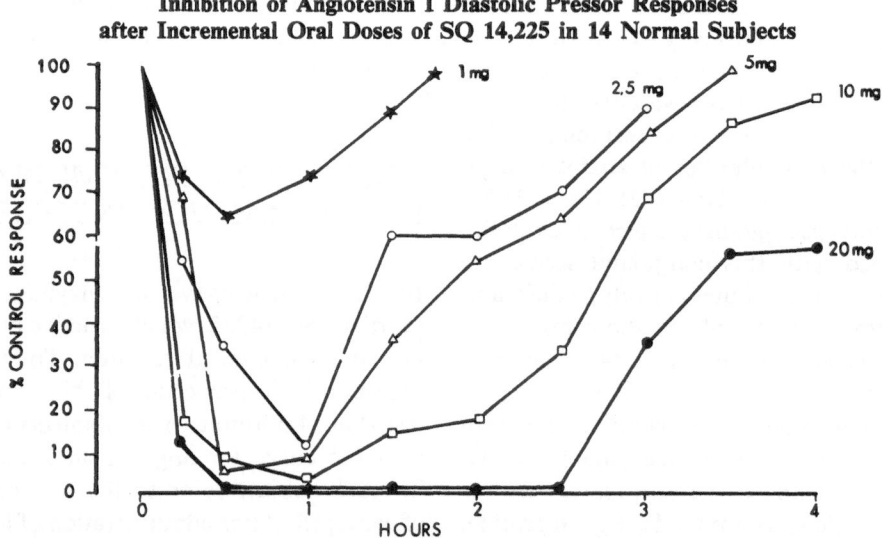

Fig. 1. Inhibition of diastolic pressor responses to angiotensin I in 14 healthy men after incremental doses of captopril. Mean responses of three subjects are shown for each dose of captopril except for 20 mg, where data are derived from two only. [Ferguson et al. (33)]

Antihypertensive Action of 3 Different Single Doses of SQ 14,225

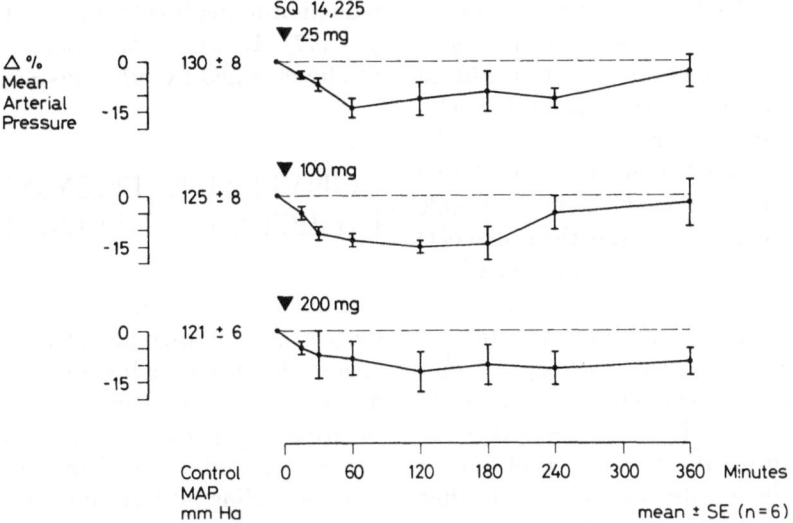

Fig. 2. Magnitude and duration of antihypertensive effect obtained with three different doses of captopril administered on three subsequent days. Note that starting mean arterial pressure (MAP) is different each time. [Brunner et al. (20)]

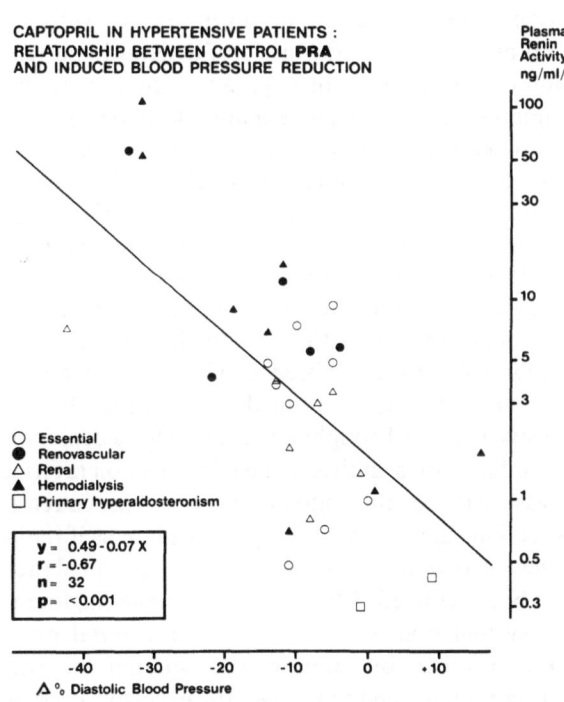

Fig. 3. Correlation between control plasma-renin activity and induced diastolic blood pressure reduction 1 h following the first dose of captopril in 32 patients with different types of hypertension.

pril-induced acute blood pressure reduction and plasma-renin activity. It is, however, less certain whether plasma-renin activity will predict the long-term blood pressure reduction induced by captopril, since in a recent analysis we found that after 4–6 days of therapy the correlation between the induced blood pressure drop and pretreatment plasma-renin activity was less strong. These results taken together suggest that the renin-angiotensin system plays a role even when spontaneous renin secretion is "normal" or low. If the effect of captopril were exclusively due to blockade of angiotensin II production, even low renin levels would be capable of actively participating in raising arterial pressure, e.g., by way of increased sensitivity of the arteriolar receptors to angiotensin II (28). Nevertheless, it is still possible that a mechanism independent of renin is also involved in the antihypertensive action of captopril.

Specificity of its action is one of the main problems of the angiotensin-converting enzyme inhibitor, since this enzyme is one of the physiological pathways responsible for the break down of circulating bradykinin (35). The cardiovascular effects of this latter hormone are complex. In addition to its direct vasodilatory effects, it induces catecholamine secretion by the adrenal medulla (36) and releases prostaglandins from various organs (37–40). In this way, the antihypertensive effect of converting enzyme inhibitors could be mediated both by an accumulation of endogenous bradykinin due to converting enzyme inhibition and by way of increased prostaglandins. In man, plasma bradykinin measurements obtained after teprotide administration are contradictory, both normal (41) and elevated levels (42) having been observed. This may be suggestive of methodological problems. With captopril, it was recently shown that plasma bradykinin levels remained unchanged after chronic converting enzyme inhibition in hypertensive patients (43). Thus it would seem that for the moment measuring this hormone is of limited use in evaluating its possible vasoactive role after converting enzyme inhibition, and all the more so since it is not known whether plasma levels reflect the concentration of this peptide on the vascular receptor. In any event, there seems to be no correlation between the percentage decrease in pressure induced by teprotide in hypertensive patients and the degree to which plasma bradykinin levels increase. However, the fact that plasma kinins do not increase in spite of administration of an angiotensin-converting enzyme inhibitor is not incompatible with the fact that the converting enzyme is identical to kininase II. When purified from human pulmonary tissue, this enzyme actually has a specific affinity for bradykinin 14 times greater than for angiotensin I (44). In other words, total inhibition of the breakdown of bradykinin should necessitate larger doses of a converting enzyme inhibitor than blockade of angiotensin I conversion.

There are several clinical hypotheses against a major role for bradykinin in the pressure drop induced by converting enzyme inhibitors. In normal subjects without sodium depletion and in hypertensive patients with primary hyperaldosteronism, captopril does not modify arterial pressure. Blockade of the renin-angiotensin system by captopril provokes neither tachycardia nor an increase in plasma catecholamines despite a drop in pressure. No tendency toward orthostatic hypotension has been noted in patients chronically treated with this drug. These results are in contrast with the pulse acceleration and large blood pressure fall noted orthostatistically in patients with hyperbradykininism. It is also interesting that teprotide does not reduce arterial pressure in nephrectomized patients (46), although recently one

group of investigators reported a blood pressure reduction in nephrectomized patients with captopril (47). However, this observation contradicts results obtained by other investigators (48).

CONVERTING ENZYME INHIBITION AND DIURETICS

The inverse correlation that exists between the activity of the renin-angiotensin system and sodium balance has been studied extensively both in normal subjects and in patients with various types of arterial hypertension: Plasma-renin levels increase after sodium depletion, but drop following sodium loading (49). An interaction between renin and the sodium factor is also found at the vascular level, since sodium modulates the vasoconstrictor effect of angiotensin II. In other words, arteriolar sensitivity to the action of angiotensin II increases markedly with a sodium overload and is reduced by sodium depletion. The inhibitors of the renin-angiotensin system have made it possible to give a more precise definition of the interdependence between angiotensin II and the sodium factor both in pressure regulation of normotensive subjects (50) and in the pathogenesis of arterial hypertension (51, 52). Thus, the degree to which the renin-angiotensin system participates depends, first of all, on concomitant sodium balance, and the vasopressor component angiotensin II and the sodium factor are revealed by blockade of the renin-angiotensin system. Blockade of the renin system permits the transformation of a given pressure level from a partially or completely renin-dependent situation to a state in which the sodium factor plays the major role. In the absence of renin-angiotensin system blockade, the radical change in the hypertensive patients brought about by sodium depletion often has only a limited beneficial effect on arterial pressure due to the compensatory increase in renin secretion. In fact, everything takes place as if renin levels were abnormally high when sodium balance has been reduced. Blockade of the renin-angiotensin system makes normalization of arterial pressure possible by adding the amount of salt subtraction needed to remove the excessive pressor contribution of the sodium factor.

The lack of normalization of arterial pressure following blockade of the renin-angiotensin system should lead one to suspect sodium retention, which can vary from one patient to the next. Figure 4 shows 12 patients under chronic captopril treatment who needed a diuretic to normalize their arterial pressure. Seven had essential hypertension, while five had hypertension associated with chronic renal failure. During previous treatment consisting of at least beta-blockers and diuretics for all 12 patients, arterial pressure was 178/115 $\pm$ 6/2 mmHg. In hospital, in the absence of any hypertension treatment, arterial pressure was slightly higher at 182/118 $\pm$ 6/4 mmHg. After angiotensin-converting enzyme inhibition for 4–6 days, a pressure drop to 150/96 $\pm$ 6/4 mmHg was obtained ($p < 0.001$). The additional sodium reduction potentiated the hypertensive effect of the renin-angiotensin system inhibition, since arterial pressure was normal at 132/88 $\pm$ 5/3 mmHg after adding a diuretic. Renin secretion was greatly stimulated after converting enzyme inhibition,

probably due to the absence of a negative feedback normally carried out by angiotensin II.

Despite this increase in renin, plasma aldosterone dropped significantly, also reflecting the blockade of angiotensin II production. The sodium subtraction brought about in these patients by diuretics led to a new increase in renin, which should at least have partially neutralized its hypotensive effect. Converting enzyme inhibition rendered this compensatory response of the renin-angiotensin system ineffective and permitted maximum benefit from sodium depletion. In fact, the dose of diuretics used in combination with captopril was less than or equal to that used in association with beta-blockers during the previous conventional treatments when arterial pressure was poorly controlled.

Renin-angiotensin blockade permits precise quantification of the amount of sodium that should be subtracted in order to normalize pressure. After neutralizing the compensatory reaction of the renin-angiotensin system in response to sodium subtraction, the sodium factor becomes the main determinant of arterial pressure, as has been previously observed in nephrectomized patients (53). Figure 5 gives such an example. It depicts results obtained in a 28-year-old patient with severe arterial hypertension and chronic renal failure (serum creatinine levels, 3 mg/d) treated with captopril and diuretics. After converting enzyme inhibition by captopril, there is a close correlation ($r = 0.6$; $p < 0.001$) between diastolic pressure and weight; these two parameters having undergone major changes over eight consecutive months due to modification of his sodium intake and ensuing changes in the dose of diuretics. By contrast, hypertensive patients as well as normal subjects can become hypotensive if an excessive amount of sodium is subtracted while the renin system is blocked. Figure 6 shows the blood pressure behavior after angiotensin-converting enzyme inhibition of a 28-year-old diabetic patient with chronic renal failure (serum creatinine level, 1.7 mg/d). Captopril alone had almost no effect on arterial pressure; it dropped only after adding furosemide 120 mg/ day, and weight had decreased by 4 kg. It even went as low as 90/70 mmHg several days after the patient had been discharged. The patient complained at this time of debilitating weakness and dizziness. These symptoms completely disappeared, however, after stopping diuretics for a short time, which permitted his weight to increase by 0.8 kg. Note that despite the hypotension, the

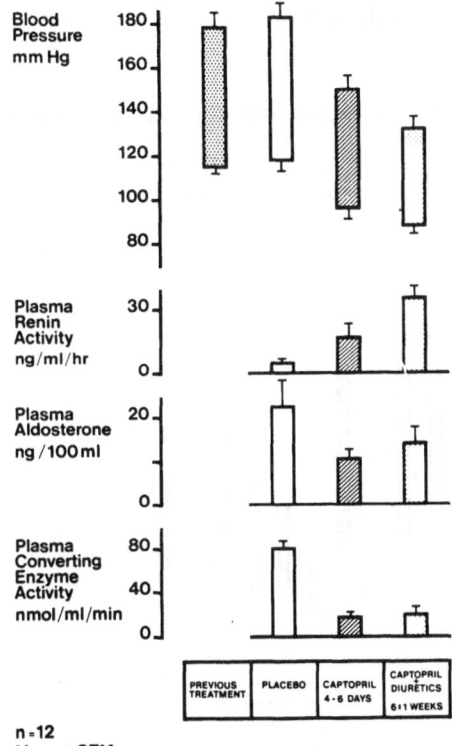

Effect of Captopril and Diuretics on Plasma Renin, Aldosterone and Angiotensin Converting Enzyme Activity

n = 12
Mean $\pm$ SEM

Fig. 4. Effect of captopril alone and in combination with diuretics on blood pressure, plasma-renin activity, plasma aldosterone, and angiotensin-converting enzyme activity. In addition, blood pressure on previous therapy is depicted as the basis for evaluating the efficacy of captopril and diuretics.

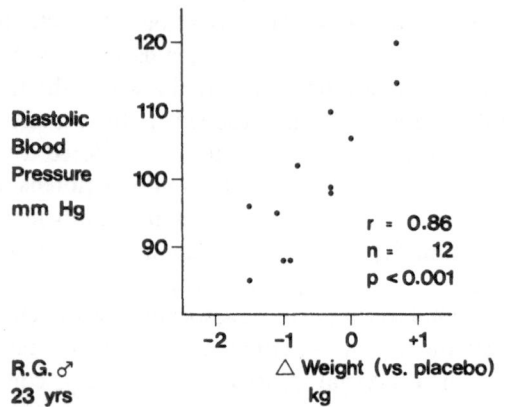

Captopril and Furosemide in a Patient with Chronic Renal Failure: Relationship between Diastolic BP and △ Weight

r = 0.86
n = 12
p < 0.001

R.G. ♂
23 yrs

△ Weight (vs. placebo) kg

Fig. 5. Relationship between furosemide-induced weight changes and diastolic blood pressure in a patient treated with captopril. Weight changes were derived from the weight measured during the placebo period. The observed close correlation between the two parameters suggests that following blockade of the renin system blood pressure becomes sodium dependent.

dose of the converting enzyme inhibitor was never reduced. The fact that these patients show no hypovolemic symptoms when their pressure is normal suggests that the amount of sodium that has to be subtracted to normalize arterial pressure does, in fact, represent a pathologic excess. Thus, the effect of angiotensin-converting enzyme inhibition in a given patient gives more useful information than the determination of peripheral plasma renin activity. Failure to normalize blood pressure by this therapeutic measure alone makes it highly probable that there exists masked sodium retention, which cannot be demonstrated directly by confronting measured renin levels with urinary sodium excretion over 24 h.

COMPARING CAPTOPRIL TO MINOXIDIL

The hypotensive effect of captopril is particularly impressive when compared to that of propranolol and minoxidil, a vasodilator known for its antihy-

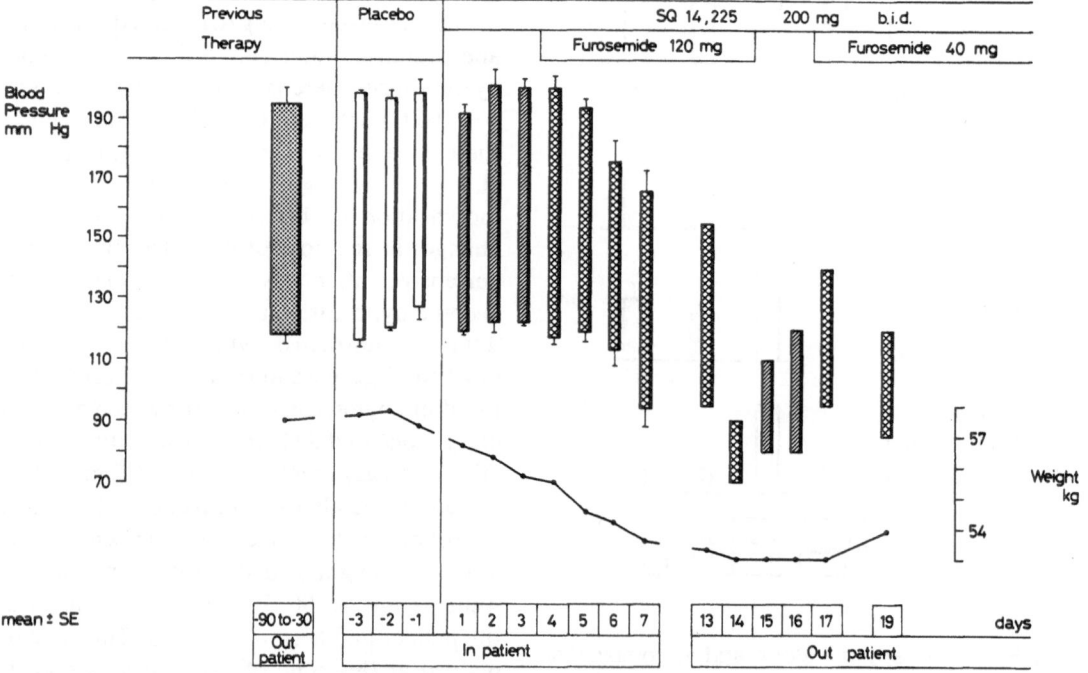

SQ 14,225 Alone and Together with Furosemide in a Hypertensive Patient with Chronic Renal Failure

Fig. 6. Effect of captopril alone and in combination with furosemide on blood pressure and weight in a 28-year-old hypertensive patient with diabetes mellitus and chronic renal failure. With the renin-angiotensin system blocked, blood pressure reduction paralleled the weight loss, reflecting progressive sodium depletion. [Brunner et al. (23)]

pertensive potency (Fig. 7). In a hypertensive patient with chronic renal failure and serum creatinine level of 5.1 mg/d, blood pressure was successfully controlled at 135/86 mmHg by a combination of furosemide and captopril. At the end of the 8th week, captopril had to be discontinued because a skin rash developed. Thereafter, propranolol 320 mg/day was not sufficient to neutralize the compensatory rise in renin induced by the high doses of furosemide; consequently, blood pressure rose again to 200/114 mmHg. Only the subsequent administration of minoxidil, a potent vasodilating drug, was able to reduce blood pressure to 151/95 mmHg, levels similar to those observed during converting enzyme blockade by captopril. However, minoxidil induced a marked sodium retention that led to an increase in weight

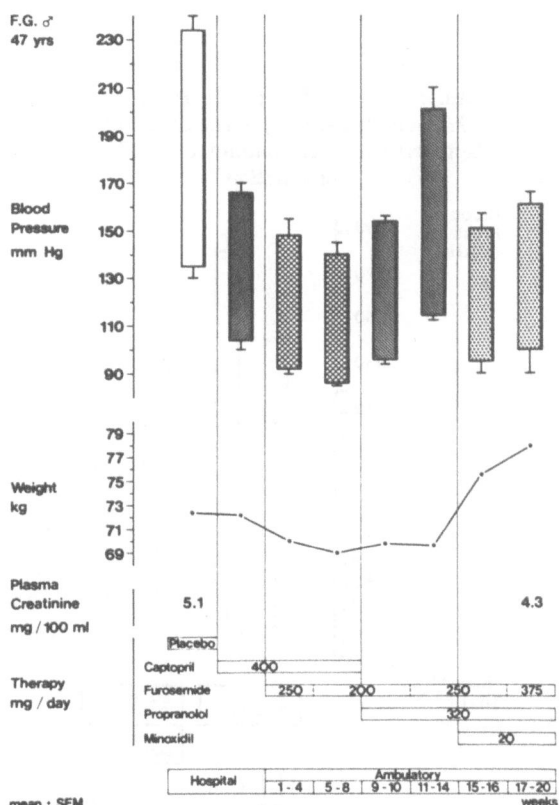

Captopril versus Propranolol and Minoxidil in a Patient with Malignant Hypertension and Chronic Renal Failure

Fig. 7. In this patient with malignant hypertension and chronic renal failure, captopril and furosemide together normalized blood pressure. When captopril had to be replaced by propranolol, blood pressure again rose to hypertensive levels; it could only be brought under control when minoxidil was added.

of more than 4 kg, despite further increases of furosemide. This latter sodium retention was probably the reason why, after 2 months of treatment with minoxidil, blood pressure again began to increase and could not be maintained at normal levels.

CONVERTING ENZYME INHIBITION IN HYPERTENSIVE PATIENTS WITH RENAL FAILURE MAINTAINED ON HEMODIALYSIS

The antihypertensive effect of angiotensin-converting enzyme inhibition by sodium subtraction has also been confirmed in patients undergoing chronic hemodialysis. When arterial hypertension is associated with terminal renal failure, it can usually be corrected by hemodialysis and ultrafiltration of extracellular fluid. Patients who do not respond to this sodium depletion have a tendency toward elevated plasma-renin activity. Binephrectomy has been used as a last resort for controlling arterial pressure in such patients. Eight of our patients undergoing hemodialysis were given chronic captopril treatment because they presented with hypertension that resisted both ultrafiltration and conventional antihypertensive therapy. After 4–6 days of renin-angiotensin system blockade, the blood pressure in these patients before hemodialysis had dropped from 194/113 ± 8/4 to 169/90 ± 10/4 mmHg. However, it was only controlled satisfactorily in the four patients with the highest plasma-renin activity (see Fig. 8). In the remaining patients, sodium subtraction was added to the usual ultrafiltration during dialysis in order to normalize pressure. To do so, 1–2 liters ultrafiltrate were exhanged with an equivalent volume of 5% glucose. This effective sodium subtraction method applied during hemodialysis sessions was generally well tolerated, probably due to the maintainance of an almost constant level of plasma osmolality. The dilution–hyponatremia resulting from this type of manipulation of sodium balance corrects itself gradually up to the next dialysis session, perhaps partly due to extraction of intracellular sodium, which is a fraction of the sodium pool that is difficult to mobilize by other methods. Arterial pressure was normalized in the eight patients to 134/76 ± 7/5 mmHg using captopril alone or associated with this salt subtraction process, without

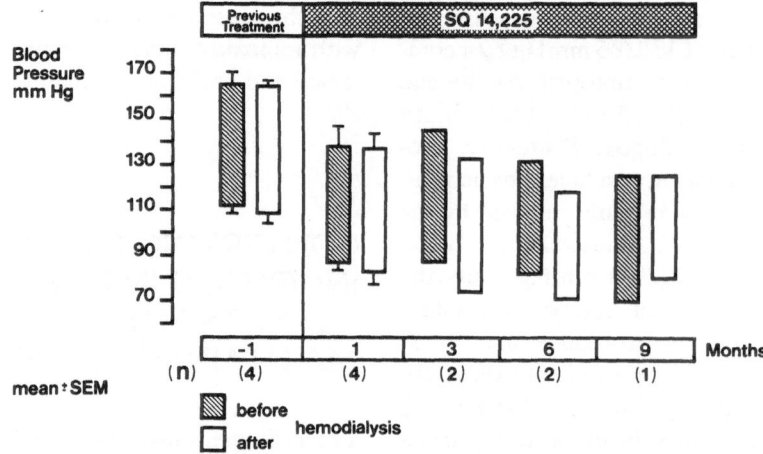

Fig. 8. Results obtained with captopril alone in four patients on maintenance hemodialysis with hypertension resistant to conventional therapy. Predialysis plasma-renin activity was high ranging from 8.9 to 97 ng/ml/h.

ANGIOTENSIN-CONVERTING ENZYME INHIBITION TO TREAT HYPERTENSION CRISIS

Renin-angiotensin system blockade also represents a rational approach to the treatment of hypertensive emergencies. It permits rapid determination of whether or not hypertension is sustained primarily by angiotensin II. Figure 10 shows results obtained after teprotide administration in 18 patients who required emergency treatment for severe hypertension. In 10 patients a reduction in arterial pressure was noted 20 min after intravenous injection of this inhibitor. Based on the observed response of arterial pressure to converting enzyme blockade, a decision was made as to whether or not a salt-free diet and diuretics should be added to the beta-blocking agent. Twenty-four hours later, average arterial pressure in this group of patients had dropped from 152 to 102 mmHg. Since it is now possible to inhibit angiotensin-converting enzyme chronically by oral administration

necessitating any additional and often poorly tolerated weight loss (see Fig. 9).

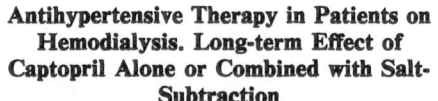

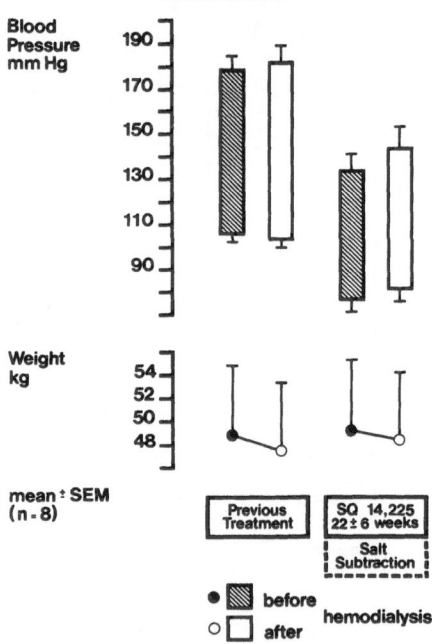

Fig. 9. Effect of captopril alone or combined with salt subtraction on blood pressure and weight of eight patients on chronic hemodialysis resistent to ultrafiltration and conventional therapy.

**Individual Mean B. P. before and 20′ after
I.V. SQ20881, and after 24 h on Chosen
Regimen**

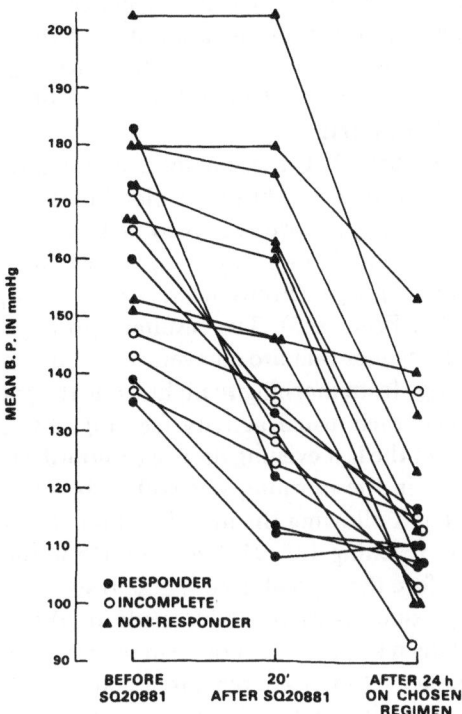

Fig. 10. Decrease in MAP 20 min after i.v. injection of teprotide 1 ng/kg body weight. On the basis of this immediate blood pressure response, individual antihypertensive therapy was chosen. As a result, blood pressure of these 18 patients admitted with a hypertensive crisis was markedly reduced 24 h later. (●) Good response; (○) incomplete response; (▲) no immediate response. [Tifft et al. (54)]

of captopril, the use of this type of antagonist for treatment of hypertensive emergencies has become even more attractive. One can now be sure of complete blockade of the renin-angiotensin system within 15–30 min using captopril, and from this time on constant converting enzyme inhibition can be maintained. If necessary, diuretics are then added until pressure becomes normal. This new approach has proved extremely useful in our experience, since it enabled us to treat most hypertensive emergencies during the few hours following admission and to avoid the use of aggressive antihypertensive drugs, such as nitroprusside and diazoxyde, which should be administered in an intensive care unit.

EFFECT OF RENIN BLOCKADE ON THE HEART

In vitro, angiotensin II has been shown to increase contractility of the isolated papillary muscle (55). In vivo, it has not been possible to demonstrate a positive inotropic effect of angiotensin II, and blockade of the renin system does not seem to reduce cardiac function. Quite the contrary, in normotensive patients with congestive heart failure, administration of saralasin (24), teprotide (25, 26), or captopril (27, 28) markedly improved cardiac function by reducing "preload" and "afterload," thereby raising cardiac index and stroke volume (Fig. 11). Moreover, in the dog, inhibition of angiotensin I conversion has been shown to increase coronary blood flow (31). Thus, blockade of the renin system can decrease the workload

**Captopril in Congestive Heart Failure: Acute Effect
on Hemodynamic Indices**

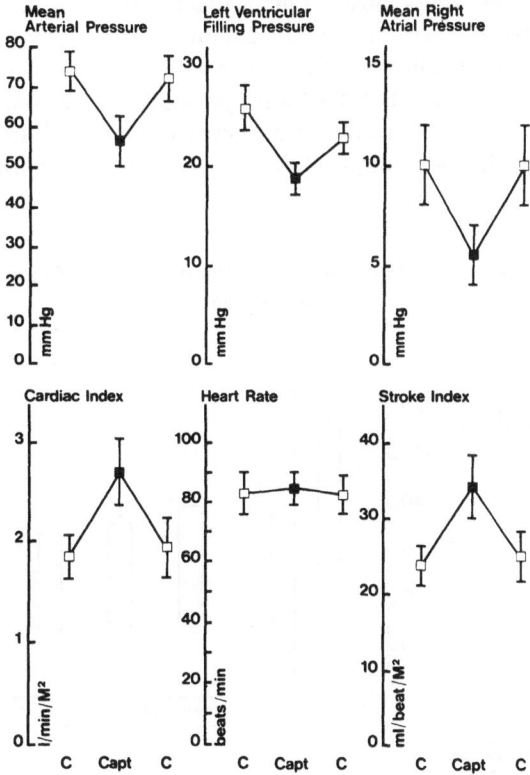

Fig. 11. Hemodynamic correlates of eight normotensive patients with congestive heart failure before (□), during maximum effect of captopril (■), and after return to base line (□).

of the heart, thereby resulting in better pump function and possibly in decreased myocardial oxygen consumption. Simultaneously, coronary blood flow is increased along with enhanced oxygen supply to the myocardium. With these combined effects of angiotensin antagonists, the myocardium can be expected to work under markedly improved conditions.

CLINICAL EXPERIENCE WITH LONG-TERM CONVERTING ENZYME INHIBITION

Chronic converting enzyme inhibition, whether alone or associated with a diuretic, has been used successfully in the long-term treatment of hypertensive patients. It is generally assumed that renin-angiotensin system blockade should be permanently maintained so as to obtain a lasting antihypertensive effect. For this reason, most all investigators have administered captopril in three or four daily doses. Our patients received 100–400 mg/day captopril divided into two daily doses. Figure 12 shows the pressure values measured in 16 patients either during hospitalization or at outpatient checkups over a period of 12 months. During the 4–6 days after initiation of captopril

therapy their arterial pressure had decreased by as much as 176/113 ± 6/4 to 144/90 ± 6/2 mmHg. Thereafter, eight of the patients required a diuretic to maintain the arterial pressure at adequate levels. After 1 year of treatment, overall arterial pressure in all 16 patients was still at 129/88 ± 4/3 mmHg.

To ensure that twice-daily administration of captopril provides continuous blood pressure control, arterial pressure was recorded in 17 of our patients throughout 1 day using a portable, semi-automatic gauge (Protometer, Remler Corporation, San Francisco). The resultant profile shows pressure values that are on average within the normal range from morning to night while the patients go about their usual activity (see Fig. 13). Even 14 h after the last evening dose of captopril, arterial pressure in the morning was still at 140/89 ± 4/4 mmHg. Following the morning dose, it dropped slightly reaching 138/91 ± 4/4 mmHg in the evening before the second dose. These results are surprising, since permanent blockade of the renin-angiotensin system does not seem to occur. In fact, in patients with normal renal function treated with captopril twice daily, plasma converting enzyme activity regained its control value before each dose of captopril (56). Only in patients with chronic renal failure did plasma converting enzyme activity remain partially inhibited 14 h after the last dose of captopril, probably due to renal retention of the drug.

Converting enzyme inhibition seems very well tolerated even over a long period of time. Thus, it has not induced any orthostatic hypotension, and heart rate does not change even in the face of a marked blood pressure decrease. Even if converting enzyme inhibition *per se* does not seem to induce any side effects, several untoward effects have been observed with captopril therapy that probably have to be attributed to the compound. In about 10% of the patients treated with captopril skin rashes developed that most often disappeared when the dose was reduced. In some rare cases, however, treatment had to be discontinued because of persisting skin manifestations. Loss of taste is another unpleasant symptom that is observed frequently. This also was usually present only transiently and disappeared spontaneously, although in some patients it led to interruption of captopril therapy. Proteinuria has also been reported, but thus far it is not clear whether it represents any major clinical problem. Most troublesome are the

Captopril in Hypertensive Patients: Effect of Long-term Therapy

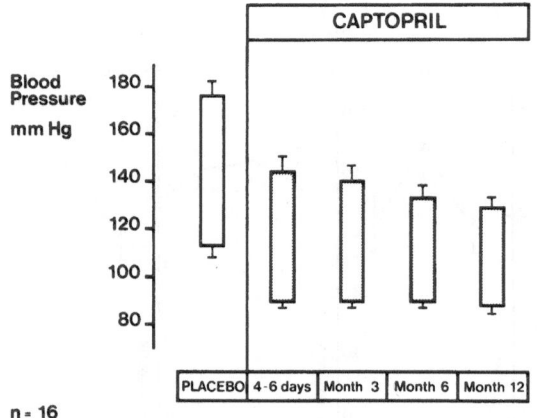

n = 16
Mean ± SEM

Fig. 12. Effect of long-term therapy on hypertensive patients. There was no escape from the antihypertensive action of captopril. Eight of the 16 patients needed additional diuretics.

Captopril Twice Daily in Hypertensive Patients: Blood Pressure Profiles Obtained with a Portable Recorder

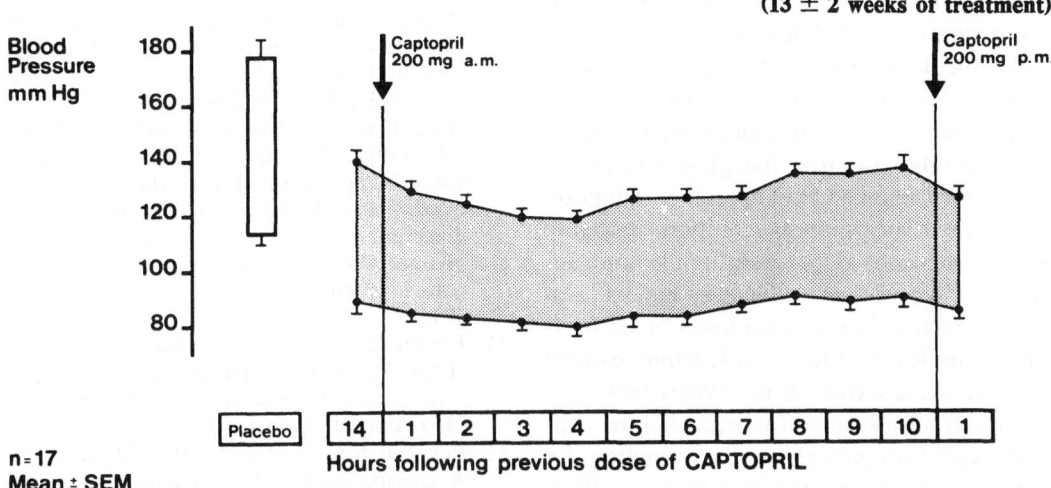

Fig. 13. Blood pressure profiles measured with a portable recorder in 17 ambulatory patients on long-term twice daily administration of captopril. Blood pressure remained controlled throughout the day.

reported cases of leukopenia or even agranolocytosis. In most cases observed thus far, there exists no clear direct causal relationship between captopril and the hematopoietic lesion, but since all cases were observed during the initial phase of captopril therapy, a causal relationship cannot be discarded at the present time. Also troublesome is the observation of several cases of pemphigus that developed during captopril therapy. Therefore, potentially dangerous untoward effects of the compound captopril may present a problem in the near future, but current experience seems to demonstrate that converting enzyme blockade *per se* is extremely well tolerated by all patients, provided they are not excessively salt depleted.

CONCLUSIONS

In conclusion, captopril is the most useful antagonist of the renin-angiotensin system currently available for the treatment of arterial hypertension and congestive heart failure, because it has the advantage of being active when taken orally. Chronic blockade of the renin-angiotensin system seems particularly advantageous, since it permits recognition of those patients who need additional sodium subtraction to normalize their pressure. Following converting enzyme inhibition, diuretics

become particularly effective, probably because compensatory stimulation of the renin-angiotensin system is ineffective and aldosterone levels tend to be reduced while renal blood flow increases. In fact, converting enzyme blockade alone or together with sodium subtraction induced by diuretics or ultrafiltration in hemodialysis patients reduces blood pressure to normal levels in almost all hypertensive patients. Based on the results obtained thus far with angiotensin-converting enzyme inhibitors, it would seem that these agents owe their sustained antihypertensive power primarily to their ability to block endogenous production of angiotensin II. However, whatever the precise mechanism of the blood pressure reduction by converting enzyme inhibitors may be, it appears that blockade of the renin system *per se* causes few if any side effects; hence, this approach to the treatment of hypertensive diseases and congestive heart failure seems extremely promising.

SUMMARY

Captopril, the only orally active inhibitor of the angiotensin-converting enzyme thus far available for clinical use was administered to normal volunteers to assess its efficacy in blocking the pressor response to exogenous angiotensin I. Subsequently, patients with various types of hypertension, including some on chronic hemodialysis, were treated chronically with captopril, 50–200 mg b.i.d. Increasing a single dose beyond 20 mg did not enhance the blocking effect but merely prolonged its duration. The blood pressure reduction observed immediately following administration of the inhibitor was related to base-line plasma-renin activity. Captopril-induced blood pressure reduction did not produce any sodium retention, probably because of reduced aldosterone levels and increased renal blood flow. Whenever blockade of converting enzyme alone did not lower blood pressure to normal levels, additional sodium removal brought it under control. In nonhypertensive patients with refractory congestive heart failure, captopril markedly improved cardiac function by simultaneously decreasing pre- and afterload. With chronic administration, captopril was mostly well tolerated, although during the initial weeks various more or less serious side effects are observed. Specificity of the drug has not yet been established, but many clinical and experimental findings argue in favor of an effect that is predominantly related to blocking the renin system. These data suggest that the renin-angiotensin system actively participates in maintaining blood pressure of hypertensive patients and increases the cardiac load of patients with congestive heart failure. Blockade of the system represents a new, effective approach to the treatment of these disorders.

REFERENCES

1. Tigerstedt R, Bergman PG (1898) Niere und Kreislauf. Schad Arch Physiol 8: 223–271
2. Goldblatt HJ, Lynch RF, Hanzal RF, Sommerville WW (1934) Studies on experimental hypertension. Production of persistent elevation of systolic blood pressure by means of renal ischemia. J Exp Med 59: 347–379
3. Page IH (1939) On the nature of the pressor action of renin. J. Exp Med 70: 520–542
4. Braum-Menendez E, Fasciolo JC, Leloir LF, Munoz JM (1939) La substancia hypertensora de la sangre del rinon isquemiado. Rev Soc Argent Biol 15: 420–430
5. Skeggs LT Jr, Lentz KE, Kahn JR, Shumway NP, Woods KR (1956) Amino acid sequence of hypertension II. J Exp Med 104: 193–197
6. Elliot DF, Pearl WS (1957) The amino acid sequence in a hypertensin. Biochem J 65: 246–254
7. Gross F (1958) Renin und hypertensin, physiologische oder pathologische wirkstoffe? Klin Wochenschr 36: 693–706
8. Laragh JH, Angers M, Kelly WG, Lieberman S (1960) Hypotensive agents and pressor substances. The effect of epinephrine, norepinephrine, angiotensin II and others on the secretory rate of aldosterone in man. JAMA 174: 234–240
9. Biron P, Koiw E, Nowaczynski W, Brouillet J, Genest J (1961) The effects of intravenous infusion of valine-5-angiotensin II and other pressor agents on urinary electrolyte and corticosteroids, including aldosterone. J Clin Invest 40: 338–347
10. Helmer OM (1964) Renin activity in blood from patients with hypertension. Can Med Assoc J 90: 221
11. Brown JJ, Davies DL, Lever AF, Robertson JIS (1964) Variations in plasma renin concentration in several physiological and pathological states. Can Med Assoc J 90: 201–206
12. Pals DT, Masucci FD, Sipos F, Denning JR (1971) A specific competitive antagonist of the vascular action of angiotensin II. Circ Res 29: 664–672
13. Brunner HR, Gavras H, Laragh JH (1973) Angiotensin II blockade in man by Sar[1]-Ala[8]-Angiotensin II for understanding and treatment of high blood pressure. Lancet 2: 1045–1048
14. Streeten DHP, Anderson GH, Freiburg JM, et al. (1975) Use of an angiotensin II antagonist (saralasin) in the recognition of "angiotensinogenic" hypertension. N Engl J Med 292: 657–662
15. Ondetti MA, Williams NJ, Sabo EF, Pluscec J, Weaver ER, Kocy O (1971) Angiotensin-converting enzyme inhibitors from the venom of Bothrops jararaca. Isolation, elucidation of structure and synthesis. Biochemistry 10: 4033
16. Gavras H, Brunner HR, Laragh JH, Sealey JE, Gavras I, Vukovitch RA (1974) An angiotensin converting enzyme inhibitor to identify and treat vasoconstrictor and volume factors in hypertensive patients. N Engl J Med 291: 817–821
17. Case DB, Wallace JM, Keim HJ, Weber MA, Drayer JM, White RP, Sealey JE, Laragh JH (1976) Estimating renin participation in hypertension. Superiority of converting enzyme inhibitor over saralasin. Am J Med 61: 790–796
18. Ondetti MA, Rubin B, Cushman DW (1977) Design of specific inhibitors of angiotensin-converting enzyme: new class of orally active antihypertensive agents. Science 196: 441–444
19. Gavras H, Brunner HR, Turini GA, Kershaw GR, Tifft CP, Cuttelod S, Gavras I, Vukovich RA, McKinstry DN (1978) Antihypertensive effect of the oral angiotensin converting-enzyme inhibitor SQ 14,225 in man. N Engl J Med 298: 991–995
20. Brunner HR, Gavras H, Turini GA, Waeber B, Kershaw GR, Vukovich RA, McKinstry DN (1979) Oral angiotensin-converting enzyme inhibitor in long-term treatment of hypertensive patients. Ann Intern Med 90: 19–23
21. Case DB, Atlas SA, Laragh JH, Sealey JE, Sullivan PA, McKinstry DN (1978) Clinical experience with blockade of the reinin-angiotensin-aldosterone sys-

tem by an oral converting-enzyme inhibitor (SQ 14, 225, captopril) in hypertensive patients. Prog. Cardiovasc Dis 21: 195–206

22. Bravo EL, Tarazi RC (1979) Converting enzyme inhibitor with an orally active compound in hypertensive man. Hypertension 1: 39–46

23. Brunner HR, Waeber B, Wauters JP, Turini GA, McKinstry DN, Gavras H (1978) Inappropriate renin secretion unmasked by captopril (SQ 14,225) in hypertension of chronic renal failure. Lancet 2: 704–707

24. Turini GA, Brunner HR, Ferguson RK, Rivier JL, Gavras H (1978) Congestive heart failure in normotensive man. Haemodynamics, renin and angiotensin II blockade. Br Heart J 40: 1134–1142

25. Curtiss C, Cohn JN, Vrobel T, Franciosa JA (1978) Role of the renin-angiotensin system in the systemic vasoconstriction heart failure. Circulation 58: 763–769

26. Gavras H, Faxon DP, Berkoben H, Brunner HR, Ryan TJ (1978) Angiotensin converting enzyme inhibition in patients with congestive heart failure. Circulation 58: 763–769

27. Davis R, Ribner HS, Keung E, Sonnenblick EH, LeJmtel TH (1979) Treatment of chronic congestive heart failure with captopril an oral inhibitor of angiotensin-converting enzyme. New Engl J Med 301: 117–121

28. Turini GA, Gribic M, Brunner HR, Waeber B, Gavras H (1979) Improvement of chronic congestive heart failure by oral captopril. Lancet 1: 1213–1215

29. Freeman RH, Davis HO, Vitale SJ, Johnson JA (1973) Intrarenal role of angiotensin II. Circ Res 32: 692–698

30. Mimran A, Brunner HR, Turini GA, Waeber B, Brunner DB (1979) Effect of captopril on renal vascular tone in patients with essential hypertension. Clin Sci 57: 421s–423s

31. Gavras H, Liang C, Brunner HR (1978) Redistribution of regional blood flow after inhibition of the angiotensin-converting enzyme. Circ Res 43 (Suppl 1): 59–63

32. Trachte GJ, Lefer AM (1978) Beneficial action of a new angiotensin-converting enzyme inhibitor (SQ 14,225) in hemorrhagic shock in cats. Circ Res 43: 576–582

33. Ferguson RK, Brunner HR, Turini GA, Gavras H, McKinstry DN (1977) A specific orally active inhibitor of angiotensin-converting enzyme in man. Lancet 1: 775–778

34. Brunner HR, Chang P, Wallach R, Sealey JE, Laragh JH (1972) Angiotensin II vascular receptors: their avidity in relationship to sodium balance, the autonomic nervous system and hypertension. J Clin Invest 51: 58

35. Erdös EG (1975) Angiotensin I converting enzyme. Circ Res 36: 247

36. Feldberg W, Levis GP (1964) The action of peptides on adrenal medulla. Release of adrenaline by bradykinin and angiotensin. J Physiol (Lond) 171: 98

37. Ferreira SH, Moncada S, Vane JR (1973) Prosta-

glandins and the mechanism of analgesia produced by aspirin-like drugs. Br J Pharmacol 49: 86

38. McGiff JC, Terragno NA, Malik KU, Lonigro AJ (1972) Release of a prostaglandin E-like substance from canine kidney by bradykinin. Circ Res 31: 36

39. Piper PJ, Vane JR (1969) Release of additional factors in anaphylaxis and its antagonism by anti-inflammatory drugs. Nature 223: 29

40. Terragno DA, Crowshaw K, Terragno NA, McGiff JC (1975) Prostaglandin synthesis by bovine mesenteric arteries and veins. Circ Res 36 (Suppl I): 76

41. Hulthen L, Hökfelt B (1978) The effect of the converting enzyme inhibitor SQ 20,881 on kinins, renin-angiotensin-aldosterone and catecholamines in relation to blood pressure in hypertensive patients. Acta Med Scand 204: 497

42. Williams GH, Hollenberg NK (1977) Accentuated vascular and endocrine response to SQ 20,881 in hypertension. New Engl J 297: 184

43. Johnston CI, Millar JA, McGrath BP, Matthews PG (1979) Long-term effects of captopril (SQ 14,225) on blood pressure and hormone levels in essential hypertension. Lancet 2: 493

44. Nishimura K, Yoshida N, Hiwada K, Ueda E, Kokubu T (1977) Purification of angiotensin I converting enzyme from human lung. Biochim Biophys Acta (Amst) 483: 398

45. Streeten DHP, Kerr KP, Kerr CB, Prior JC, Dalakos TG (1972) Hyperbradykininism: A new orthostatic syndrome. Lancet 2: 1048

46. Case DB, Wallace JM, Laragh JH (1979) Comparison between saralasin and converting enzyme inhibitor in hypertensive disease. Kidney Int 15: 107

47. Man in't Veld AJ, Schicht IM, Derkx FHM, DeBruyn JHB, Schalekamp MADH (1980) Effects of an angiotensin-converting enzyme inhibitor (captopril) on blood pressure in anephric subjects. Br Med J 280: 288–290

48. Leslie BR, Case DB, Sullivan JF, Vaughan ED Jr (1980) Absence of blood pressure lowering effect of captopril in anephric patients. Br Med J 280: 1067–1068

49. Brunner HR, Laragh JH, Baer L, et al. (1972) Essential hypertension: Renin and aldosterone, heart attack and stroke. N Engl J Med 286: 441–449

50. Posternak L, Brunner HR, Gavras H, Brunner DB (1977) Angiotensin II blockade in normal man: Interaction of renin and sodium in maintaining blood pressure. Kidney Int 11: 197

51. Brunner HR, Gavras H, Laragh JH, Keenan R (1974) Hypertension in man. Exposure of the renin and sodium components using angiotensin II blockade. Circ Res 34/35 (Suppl 1): 35

52. Gavras H, Ribeiro A, Brunner HR, Gavras H (1976) Reciprocal relationship between renin dependency and sodium dependency in essential hypertension. New Engl J Med 295: 1278

53. Onesti G, Kim KE, Greco JA, Del Guerico Ed T, Fernandez M, Swartz C (1975) Blood pressure regulation in end-stage renal disease and anephric man. Circ Res 36 (Suppl 1): L45–152

54. Tifft CP, Gavras H, Kershaw GR, Gavras I, Brunner HR, Liang CS, Chonobian AV (1979) Converting enzyme inhibition in hypertensive emergencies. Ann Intern Med 90: 43

55. Koch-Weser J. (1965) Nature of the inotropic action of angiotensin on ventricular myocardium. Circ Res 16: 230–237

56. Waeber B, Brunner HR, Brunner DB, Curtet AL, Turini GA, Gavras H (1980) Discrepancy between antihypertensive effect and angiotensin converting enzyme inhibition by captopril. Hypertension 2: 236–242

Immediate and Delayed Antihypertensive Effects of Angiotensin-Converting Enzyme Inhibition with Captopril

Steven A. Atlas, David B. Case, Patricia A. Sullivan, Jean E. Sealey, and John H. Laragh

INTRODUCTION

Since its introduction as an experimental antihypertensive agent, captopril (Capoten, SQ 14225) has been shown to lower blood pressure effectively in a considerable proportion of patients with essential and renovascular hypertension (1–5). The drug was designed as a specific, potent competitive inhibitor of angiotensin-converting enzyme (6) and, following oral administration to human subjects, it can block almost completely the effects of infused angiotensin I (7). Long-term administration of captopril to hypertensive patients results in a sustained reduction in aldosterone secretion, concomitant potassium retention and, in most cases, natriuresis (8)—effects that can be ascribed to a drug-induced reduction in circulating angiotensin II. Despite these findings, there has been considerable controversy regarding the extent to which its antihypertensive effect is mediated by blockade of the renin-angiotensin system.

This controversy has been fostered in part by the failure of some studies to find a significant relationship between the blood pressure response and pretreatment renin levels (1, 3, 4). But the question of *when* that blood pressure response ought to be assessed has received little attention. It has generally been assumed that the bulk of the antihypertensive effect of lowering angiotensin II ought to occur rapidly, since prompt depressor responses have been observed during short-term infusions of the nonapeptide converting enzyme inhibitor teprotide (SQ 20881) and the angiotensin II antagonist saralasin (9–12). While such an immediate response does occur following oral administration of captopril (2), we have found that this antihypertensive effect is often reversed, although only transiently, during continued administration of the drug.

METHODS

Captopril was administered to 26 untreated hypertensive patients (16 with essential hypertension, six with unilateral, and four with bilateral renal artery stenosis) following 4–5 days on constant sodium (100 mEq) and potassium (60 mEq) intake. Plasma-renin activity (PRA) was measured in the ambulatory position (13, 14) on the last control day. Percentage changes in blood pressure, urinary aldosterone excretion (15), and serum potassium were determined by comparison with the control values (the average of measurements made on the 3 days prior to beginning treatment). Additional details of the methods are given in the legend to Fig. 1 and in ref. 2.

RESULTS AND DISCUSSION

A 10-mg oral dose of captopril was administered in the seated position while blood pressure was monitored at 2-min intervals by Arteriosonde®. Three patients with suppressed PRA and essential hypertension had less than a 5% reduction in mean pressure. Blood pressure fell promptly in the remaining 23 patients, reaching a nadir after 30–90 min (range, 6%–27% fall in mean pressure). For all 26 patients, the magnitude of the blood pressure response to this first dose was inversely related to the pretreatment PRA, which ranged from 0.1 to 28 ng/ml/h ($r = -0.67$, $p < 0.001$).

Following these immediate depressor responses, blood pressure frequently increased transiently toward control levels and remained elevated over the next several days, despite continued administration of the drug at increasing doses. This pattern of response occurred more commonly in those

Time Course of Captopril-induced Changes in
Blood Pressure and Aldosterone Excretion in
Patients with Small (Group I) and Large (Group
II) Immediate Depressor Responses

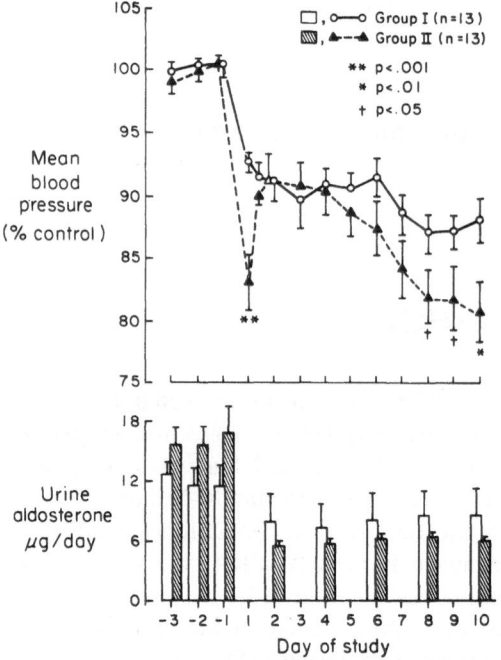

Fig. 1. Time course of captopril-induced changes in blood pressure and aldosterone excretion. Patients were divided into two groups on the basis of their immediate depressor response to the first dose of captopril (Group I, ≤ 10% fall in mean pressure; Group II, > 10% fall in mean pressure). Following the first 10-mg dose, drug dosage was increased at 6-h intervals in order to achieve or maintain a 10% reduction in diastolic pressure or until the maximum dose (600 mg/day) was reached. A stable regimen was achieved by day 4 (Group I, 508 ± 66 mg/day; Group II, 408 ± 56 mg/day). Blood pressure was measured six times/day after 2 min in the standing position, and the mean pressure was calculated as the diastolic pressure plus one-third the pulse pressure; the daily average pressure is expressed as a percentage of the control pressure (average of the 3 days prior to beginning treatment). Vertical bars represent the standard deviation of the mean.

patients who had large immediate depressor responses, being evident in 11 of the 13 patients who had a greater than 10% reduction in mean pressure following the first dose (Fig. 1). This transient resistance to the antihypertensive effect of captopril was clearly not due to a failure to inhibit angiotensin-converting enzyme adequately, since

aldosterone excretion was maximally suppressed by day 2 of treatment and remained so thereafter (Fig. 1).

Because of this phenomenon, the apparent blood pressure response in those patients with large first-dose responses (Group II) was the same during days 2–6 of continuous treatment as in those patients with small (Group I) first-dose responses (Fig. 1). As seen in Table 1, patients with high PRA predominated in Group II (77% versus 15% in Group I). If the blood pressure response were assessed during this period of transient resistance to the drug, one might therefore conclude that blockade of the renin-angiotensin system is not a primary mechanism of the antihypertensive action of captopril (1, 3, 4). Indeed, in the present study there was no correlation between pretreatment PRA and the blood pressure response on days 2 and 4 of treatment (Table 2). However, following day 5 of treatment, blood pressure began to decline further, so that by day 8 there was once again a significant difference between the responses of the two groups (Fig. 1). The maximal antihypertensive effect was generally achieved after 10 days of treatment, although in two patients in Group II it took longer than 1 month. These sustained responses were, like the immediate (first-dose) responses, significantly related to the pretreatment PRA (Table 2).

Of note, patients in Group II, in addition to having higher base-line PRA levels, generally had greater decreases in aldosterone excretion and greater degrees of potassium retention than did patients in Group I (Table 1). The change in each of these parameters was also related to the magnitude of the sustained blood pressure response (Table 2). While it is quite possible that suppression of aldosterone plays some role in the long-term antihypertensive effect of captopril, we have been unable to relate the blood pressure response to the degree of drug-induced natriuresis (2, 8). The degree of aldosterone suppression was also closely correlated with the pretreatment PRA ($r = -0.79$, $p < 0.001$); it is therefore possible that the relationship between the aldosterone and blood pressure responses reflects the fact that each of these variables is dependent on the degree to which angiotensin II has been lowered.

The mechanism responsible for the transient reversal of the antihypertensive action of captopril is unclear. It could perhaps be due to activation of sympathetic reflexes in response to an abrupt

Table 1. Distribution of pretreatment PRA and responses of aldosterone and blood pressure to captopril in patients with small (Group I) and large (Group II) immediate depressor responses.

	No. of patients	
Parameter	Group I	Group II
Pretreatment PRA (ng/ml/h)		
< 2	7	1
2–5	4	2
5–8	1	4
> 8	1	6
Fall in aldosterone excretion after 10 days		
< 30%	5	0
30–50%	6	5
50–70%	1	5
> 70%	1	3
Increase in serum K^+ after 10 days		
< 5%	9	2
5–15%	3	5
15–25%	1	4
> 25%	0	2
Fall in mean pressure after 10 days		
< 10%	4	0
10–15%	6	3
15–20%	3	4
> 20%	0	6
Blood pressure control after 1 year		
Diastolic ≥ 95, captopril + diuretic	3	1
Diastolic < 95, captopril + diuretic	5	1
Diastolic ≥ 95, captopril alone	2	1
Diastolic < 95, captopril alone	3	10

lowering of arterial pressure. Of interest, a similar resistance was probably observed when blood pressure fell transiently in rats given antibodies to angiotensin II (16). Whatever its cause, the resistance to captopril diminishes over a period of days or, at most, weeks. It is important to emphasize that the ensuing magnitude of the sustained antihypertensive effect can be estimated not only from the pretreatment PRA (Table 2), but from the first-dose response as well (17). Therefore, unless the

Table 2. Relationship between the antihypertensive effect of captopril and pretreatment PRA or changes in aldosterone or potassium.

Parameters		% Change in mean pressure after	Correlation coefficient[a]	Significance[a] ($p <$)
X	Versus			
Pretreatment PRA (log)		first dose	−0.67	0.001
		2 days	−0.12	N.S.
		4 days	−0.31	N.S.
		10 days	−0.72	0.001
% change in urine aldosterone		10 days	+0.73	0.001
% change in serum K^+		10 days	−0.59	0.01

[a] Determined by the Spearman test.
N.S., Not significant.

clinical situation dictates otherwise, it is probably best to avoid adding other antihypertensive agents until the maximum effect of captopril has been attained.

In our experience, effective blood pressure control has been maintained in many patients for as long as 3 years. While diuretics often augment its effect, captopril given alone provides effective blood pressure control in most patients who have a good initial response to the drug (Table 1). Although other mechanisms might potentially contribute to the efficacy of converting enzyme inhibitors (18, 19), our observations, coupled with evidence that these agents are ineffective in patients with primary aldosteronism (11) or in anephric subjects (11, 20), suggest that the bulk of captopril's antihypertensive action stems from blockade of the renin-angiotensin system.

SUMMARY

The angiotensin-converting enzyme inhibitor captopril was administered to 26 untreated hypertensive patients. Blood pressure fell promptly following a single oral dose, and the magnitude of these initial depressor responses was inversely related to the pretreatment renin level ($r = -0.67$, $p < 0.001$). Over the next several days, blood pressure frequently increased transiently toward control levels despite increasing doses of the drug and maximal inhibition of angiotensin II formation (as indicated by a sustained reduction in aldosterone excretion). This transient resistance to the antihypertensive action of captopril was especially pronounced in patients who had large initial depressor responses, and during this period there was no correlation between the pretreatment renin and the degree to which blood pressure was lowered. Following day 5, however, blood pressure began to decline again, with a maximal antihypertensive effect generally occurring by day 10 of continuous treatment. The magnitude of this sustained response was similar to that of the first-dose response and was once again inversely related to the baseline renin ($r = -0.72$, $p < 0.001$). The long-term change in blood pressure was also related to the changes in serum potassium ($r = -0.59$, $p < 0.01$) and in aldosterone excretion ($r = +0.73$, $p < 0.001$). These results may explain the failure in some studies to document a relationship between the plasma renin level and the blood pressure response to captopril and suggest that its antihypertensive action is largely explained by blockade of the renin-angiotensin-aldosterone axis.

ACKNOWLEDGMENT

This work was supported in part by grants from the National Institutes of Health (HL 18323-SCR) and the Squibb Institute for Medical Research.

REFERENCES

1. Gavras H, Brunner HR, Turini GA, Kershaw GR, Tifft CP, Cuttelod S, Gavras I, Vukovich RA, McKinstry DN (1978) Antihypertensive effect of the oral angiotensin converting enzyme inhibitor SQ 14225 in man. N Engl J Med 298: 991–995
2. Case DB, Atlas SA, Laragh JH, Sealey JE, Sullivan PA, McKinstry DN (1978) Clinical experience with blockade of the renin-angiotensin-aldosterone system with an oral converting enzyme inhibitor (SQ 14225, captopril) in hypertensive patients. Prog Cardiovasc Dis 21: 195–206
3. Bravo E, Tarazi RC (1979) Converting enzyme inhibition with an orally active compound in hypertensive man. Hypertension 1: 39–46
4. Sullivan JM, Ginsburg BA, Ratts TE, Johnson JG, Barton BR, Kraus DH, McKinstry DN, Muirhead EE (1979) Hemodynamic and antihypertensive effects of captopril, an orally active angiotensin converting enzyme inhibitor. Hypertension 1: 397–401
5. Brunner HR, Gavras H, Waeber B, Kershaw GR, Turini GA, Vukovich RA, McKinstry DN, Gavras I (1979) Oral angiotensin-converting enzyme inhibitor in long-term treatment of hypertensive patients. Ann Intern Med 90: 19–23
6. Ondetti MA, Rubin B, Cushman DW (1977) Design of specific inhibitors of angiotensin converting enzyme. New class of orally active antihypertensive agents. Science 196: 441–444
7. Ferguson RK, Turini GA, Brunner HR, Gavras H (1977) A specific orally active inhibitor of angiotensin-converting enzyme in man. Lancet 1: 775–778
8. Atlas SA, Case DB, Sealey JE, Laragh JH, McKinstry DN (1979) Interruption of the renin-angiotensin system in hypertensive patients by captopril induces sustained reduction in aldosterone secretion, potassium retention and natriuresis. Hypertension 1: 274–280
9. Brunner HR, Gavras H, Laragh JH (1973) Angiotensin II blockade in man by sar[1]-ala[8]-angiotensin II for understanding and treatment of high blood pressure. Lancet 2: 1045–1048

10. Gavras H, Brunner HR, Laragh JH, Sealey JE, Gavras I, Vukovich RA (1974) An angiotensin converting enzyme inhibitor to identify and treat vasoconstrictor and volume factors in hypertensive patients. N Engl J Med 291: 817–821

11. Case DB, Wallace JM, Keim HJ, Weber MA, Drayer JIM, White RP, Sealey JE, Laragh JH (1976) Estimating renin participation in hypertension. Superiority of converting enzyme inhibitor over saralasin. Am J Med 61: 790–796

12. Case DB, Wallace JM, Keim HJ, Weber MA, Sealey JE, Laragh JH (1977) Possible role of renin in hypertension as suggested by renin-sodium profiling and inhibition of converting enzyme. N Engl J Med 296: 641–646

13. Laragh JH, Baer L, Brunner HR, Bühler FR, Sealey JE, Vaughan ED Jr (1972) Renin, angiotensin, aldosterone system in pathogenesis and management of hypertensive vascular disease. Am J Med 52: 633–652

14. Sealey JE, Laragh JH (1977) How to do a plasma renin assay. Cardiovasc Med 2: 1079–1092

15. Sealey JE, Laragh JH (1974) Measurement of urinary aldosterone excretion in man. In: Laragh JH (ed) Hypertension manual. Dun-Donnelley, New York, pp 641–654

16. Brunner HR, Chang P, Wallach R, Sealey JE, Laragh JH (1972) Angiotensin II vascular receptors. Their avidity in relationship to sodium balance, the autonomic nervous system, and hypertension. J Clin Invest 51: 58–67

17. Case DB, Atlas SA, Laragh JH, Sullivan PA, Sealey JE (1980) Use of first-dose response or plasma renin activity to predict the long-term effect of captopril. Identification of triphasic pattern of blood pressure response. J Cardiovasc Pharmacol 2: 339–346

18. Williams GH, Hollenberg NK (1977) Accentuated vascular and endocrine response to SQ 20881 in hypertension. N Engl J Med 297: 184–188

19. Swartz SL, Williams GH, Hollenberg NK, Moore TJ, Dluhy RG (1979) Converting enzyme inhibition in essential hypertension. The hypotensive response does not reflect only reduced angiotensin II formation. Hypertension 1: 106–111

20. Leslie BR, Case DB, Sullivan JF, Vaughan ED Jr (1980) Absence of blood-pressure lowering effect of captopril in anephric patients. Br Med J 1: 1067–1068

Late Resistance to Captopril

Robert C. Tarazi, Emmanuel L. Bravo, and Fetnat M. Fouad

The effectiveness of captopril in the treatment of hypertension has been widely demonstrated by many investigators both in the United States and abroad (1–4). Effective blood pressure control was obtained in both essential and renal hypertensions, both moderate and severe and whether associated with high, normal, or low plasma-renin activity (2, 3). In that respect, comparison of early and late responses to converting enzyme inhibition has demonstrated both similarities and contrasts between the two as regards the correlates of blood pressure control (5, 6). Alterations with time in the pattern of responses to captopril would have important implications for understanding the mechanism(s) of its effectiveness and for its use in daily practice.

There is little doubt that the early blood pressure response to captopril, during the first few hours of its administration, was significantly correlated with the pretreatment level of plasma-renin activity (5). This was shown by different groups using different methods of assessment of renin activity (1, 4, 5). In contrast, maintained blood pressure control after weeks of therapy did not exhibit the same marked dependency on renin status of the patients (6). This contrast is hardly surprising, but it does carry very important practical implications. It is hardly surprising because the mechanisms underlying blood pressure responses need not be the same for acute and long-term treatment. Apart from possible variations in hemodynamic pattern with duration of therapy (7, 8), one must expect a multifactorial interaction of effects and countereffects to the medication used (9). Captopril was no exception to that general rule, but it did show some unexpected aspects in the type of secondary or late resistance to its continued use (6, 10).

BLOOD PRESSURE RESPONSE TO LONG-TERM TREATMENT

The immediate blood pressure response to the first effective dose of captopril was, in our experience, closely related to pretreatment plasma-renin activity (5). The correlation coefficient of that relation was highly significant ($r = 0.737$, $p < 0.001$), and the slope of its regression line not significantly different from that of the correlation obtained in these same patients in response to [Sar^1, Thr^8]AII (5). However, with maintained therapy, many patients lost their blood pressure response to captopril despite progressive increase in dosage to the maximal allowable limit of 450–600 mg/day. Of a total of 32 patients, 24 responded to the initial dose of captopril by a reduction of mean arterial pressure (MAP) by more than 10 mmHg; subsequently, approximately 50% (11 patients) lost this initial response (6, 10). In none of the cases were any of the usual reasons found for secondary resistance to antihypertensive therapy (11). In fact, the secondary to captopril was remarkable, in that it developed in the apparent absence of volume expansion.

VOLUME AND HUMORAL ASPECTS OF LONG-TERM THERAPY

In contrast to most antihypertensive agents, captopril did not lead to significant volume expansion in the vast majority of treated patients, either in our experience (6, 10) or in that of others (12). Of particular importance was the absence of any significant correlation between the blood pressure response to captopril and either change in body weight ($r = -0.091$) or alteration in plasma volume ($r = -0.224$). Our experience in patients was essentially similar in that respect to that in spontaneously hypertensive rats (SHR) (13, 14).

The stability of body weight, ECF, and plasma volume in most patients on captopril (10) might be related to its effects on aldosterone. Bravo and Tarazi (2) have documented a maintained reduction in plasma aldosterone levels to near-normal levels by captopril; this was also observed in long-term therapy of patients in heart failure (15). With longer-term follow-up of patients, a tendency to increased plasma volume was noted only in the group that maintained a good blood pressure response; those in whom initial pressure responses gradually disappeared showed no evidence of volume expansion (6, 10) (Fig. 1). This evolution of arterial pressure and plasma volume levels during captopril therapy was quite different from our experience with other antihypertensive agents, including propranolol. The lack of secondary resistance to beta-blockers has usually been attributed to absence of volume expansion (16, 17). In contrast, secondary resistance to the antihypertensive effect of captopril did develop in the absence of evident volume expansion. In SHR also, gradual loss of blood pressure control necessitating increasing doses of captopril was not associated with either increased body weight (13, 14) or blood volume (14).

This pattern of volume-pressure evolution during therapy is unusual; extracellular fluid and plasma volume expansion have been considered since the very early days of modern antihypertensive therapy to be of primary importance in loss of pressure response to sympatholytics or vasodilators (17–20). Other mechanisms that could theoretically be responsible for loss of pressure control did *not* in fact appear to be operative. Captopril has not been associated with marked cardiac stimulation; there was no evident relationship between blood pressure responses and changes in PRA secondary to converting enzyme inhibition (6, 10). Taken at face value, any rise in PRA would have been of little functional consequence, as suggested by the persistent reduction in plasma aldosterone in treated patients, both responders and nonresponders (2, 6) (Fig. 1).

The variations in blood pressure control with long-term therapy and consequence of late resistance to captopril led to a progressive loss of the correlation between pressure reduction and pretreatment PRA (6, 10). In contrast to the strong correlation between these two indices in the early days of therapy, their relationship became gradually weaker with increased duration of treatment. From an r value of 0.737 ($p < 0.001$) in acute studies, the correlation fell to 0.45 ($p < 0.05$) after a few days and to only 0.03 after 1 month. Hence, the longer-term response to captopril, the response of most significance to clinicians, was *not* in our

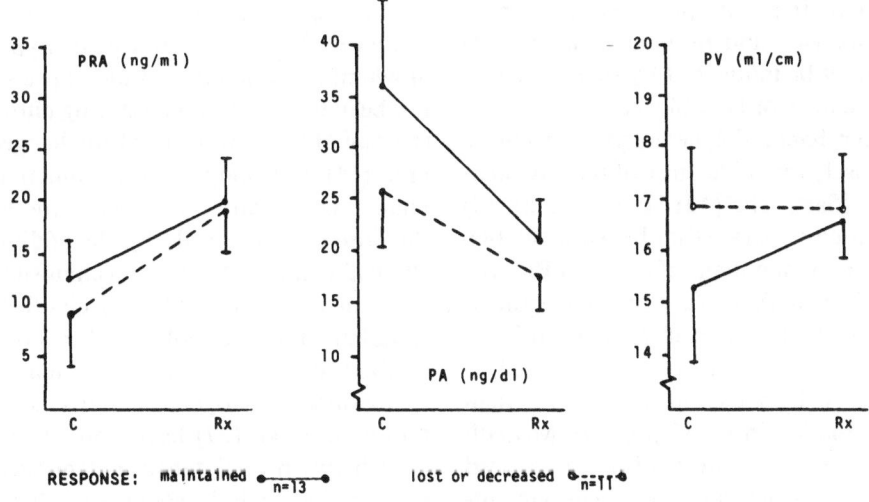

Fig. 1. Changes with long-term treatment (captopril).

experience (2, 6, 10) or in that of others (3, 4, 12) significantly dependent on a high-pretreatment PRA.

HEMODYNAMIC PATTERNS DURING CAPTOPRIL THERAPY

The basic hemodynamic mechanism by which captopril lowers arterial pressure was found in all reported studies to be a lowering of systemic vascular resistance (4, 5, 12, 21). This was observed within $\frac{1}{2}$ to $1\frac{1}{2}$ h oral administration (5) as well as with maintained therapy from 3 to 14 days (12, 21) up to 1 year (22). Similar results were obtained in spontaneously hypertensive rats (2, 14), in rats with acute renovascular hypertension (23), and even in normotensive dogs (24).

The consistency of that hemodynamic response has been contrasted with the variability in changes of peripheral resistance observed with propranolol and other beta-adrenergic blockers (16, 25). These can induce several hemodynamic patterns from decreased output and a rise in resistance to a reduction in total peripheral resistance (TPR) below pretreatment levels depending among other factors on duration of therapy (7, 16). In contrast, the antihypertensive effect of captopril was consistently related to a reduction in TPR. To the extent that hemodynamic changes reflect the factors involved in the action of a drug, these differences between beta-blockers and captopril suggest that the antihypertensive effect of one or both agents cannot be linked *only* to their interference with the renin system. It results probably from more than one mechanism, and its hemodynamic pattern can certainly be influenced by such variables as the cardiac effects of beta-blockade.

On the other hand, the hemodynamic effects of captopril closely resemble those of the angiotensin antagonist [Sar[1], Thr[8]]AII. Fouad et al. (5) demonstrated a close parallelism between the two as regards their predominant effect on TPR, the close relationship of that effect on pretreatment PRA, and the lack of significant changes in heart rate. The same basic features were observed in patients maintained on captopril for more than 1 year. The reduction in blood pressure was still related to the same basic mechanism—a reduced TPR—but a much wider variation in cardiac output was now observed (22). These variations in output among patients were not related, in our opinion, to changes in cardiac performance; heart rate was unchanged and there was no significant difference in clinical status between those with reduced and those with increased cardiac output. The one variable that was related to the level of output was the size of the intravascular volume (22).

Although total blood volume remained unaltered on the average in two different studies of captopril (6, 10, 22), this constancy of the mean covered a variation from an expansion of 9% in a few to a contraction by 24% in some others. Interestingly, those with increased volume also had an unchanged or increased cardiac output, while output was reduced in those who had a reduction in intravascular volume. The result was a modest but significant correlation between total blood volume (TBV) and cardiac output (CO) ($r = 0.44$, $p < 0.05$) (22). The changes in blood volume can be related to a number of variables (26) that need closer study. Of particular importance in this study would be changes in total peripheral resistance, as suggested by our experience with late resistance to captopril (10). Any tendency to expansion of plasma volume was seen in those with maintained pressure control (and hence, presumably, a reduced TPR), whereas plasma volume was unchanged when blood pressure crept up (Fig. 1).

In summary, late resistance to captopril was rather common; it occurred in about 50% of our patients. It was characterized by two seemingly contradictory features: absence of volume expansion, even with marked responsiveness to diuretics or salt depletion. These observations in man are similar to those in spontaneously hypertensive rats in whom a gradual loss of blood pressure response has been uniformly noted during chronic captopril therapy (13, 14) in spite of unchanged blood volume (14) and body weight. Similar to studies in man, this resistance was overcome by increasing the dose or more easily by the addition of hydrochlorothiazide (13). The mechanisms of this late resistance have not yet been clarified. One could speculate about nonvolume effects of sodium (26) or about the interactions between angiotensin and sympathetic neurogenic activity. In that regard, Fiorentini et al. (27) have noted a striking synergism between angiotensin antagonists and alpha-receptor blockade in some patients with resistant hypertension. Continued studies of converting enzyme inhibition will undoubtedly broaden our understanding of the interaction of pressor mechanisms. The long-term effects of captopril thus appear much too complex to be explained on the basis of a single mechanism.

SUMMARY

The initial blood pressure response to captopril is not always maintained on long-term therapy. This was shown both in hypertensive patients and in spontaneously hypertensive rats by the need to increase the dose of the drug or to add diuretic agents in order to maintain adequate blood pressure control, or both. This late resistance was *not* associated with plasma volume expansion or with increase in body weight, differing in that aspect from secondary resistance to most antihypertensive agents. Yet, addition of diuretics often restored blood pressure control, suggesting that nonvolume effects of sodium might be important to that situation. There was no significant difference in plasma aldosterone levels or plasma-renin activity between persistent reponders and those patients who lost their initial blood pressure response to captopril.

ACKNOWLEDGMENT

The studies referred to were supported in part by grants from the National Heart, Lung and Blood Institute (HL-6835) and the Whitaker Foundation.

REFERENCES

1. Case DB, Atlas SA, Laragh JH, Sealey JE, Sullivan PA, McKinstry DN (1978) Clinical experience with blockade of the renin-angiotensin-aldosterone system by an oral converting-enzyme inhibitor (SQ 14225, captopril) in hypertensive patients. Prog Cardiovasc Dis 21: 195–206
2. Bravo EL, Tarazi RC (1979) Converting enzyme inhibition with an orally active compound in hypertensive man. Hypertension 1(1): 39–46
3. Gavras H, Brunner HR, Turini GA, Kershaw SG, Tifft CP, Cuttlelod S, Gavras I, Vukovich RA, McKinstry DN (1978) Antihypertensive effect of the oral angiotensin converting enzyme inhibitor SQ 14,225 in man. N Engl J Med 298: 991–995
4. Fagard R, Amery A, Reybrouck T, Lijnen P, Billet L (1980) Acute and chronic systemic and pulmonary hemodynamic effects of captopril in hypertensive patients. Am J Cardiol (In press)
5. Fouad FM, Ceimo JMK, Tarazi RC, Bravo EL (1980) Contrasts and similarities of acute hemodynamic responses to specific antagonism of angiotensin II ([Sar^1, Thr^8]AII) and to inhibition of converting enzyme (captopril). Circulation 61: 163–169
6. Fouad FM, Tarazi RC, Bravo EL, Saragoca M (1981) Similarities and contrasts between angiotensin II antagonists and the acute and long term effects of captopril. In: Program: Sixth scientific session of the International Society of Hypertension, Goteborg, Sweden, June 11–13, 1979, p 134 (Abst)
7. Tarazi RC (1978) Therapy for multifactorial hypertension. Ann Intern Med 88(5): 705–706
8. Tarazi RC, Fouad FM, Bravo EL (1981) Total peripheral resistance and beta-adrenergic blockade. (This volume)
9. Dustan HP, Tarazi RC, Bravo EL (1975) Hemodynamic adjustments during long-term antihypertensive therapy. In: Milliez P, Safar M (eds) Recent advances in hypertension. Laboratoires Boehringer Ingelheim, France, Vol 2, pp 247–258
10. Tarazi RC, Bravo EL, Fouad FM, Omvik P, Cody RJ Jr (1981) Hemodynamic and volume changes associated with captopril. Hypertension (To be published)
11. Gifford RW Jr, Tarazi RC (1978) Resistant hypertension: Diagnosis and management. Ann Intern Med 88: 661–665
12. Sullivan JM, Ginsburg BA, Ratts TE, Johnson JG, Barton BR, Kraus DH, McKinstry DN, Muirhead EE (1979) Hemodynamic and antihypertensive effects of captopril, an orally active angiotensin converting enzyme inhibitor. Hypertension 1(4): 397–401
13. Sen S, Tarazi RC, Bumpus FM (1980) Effect of converting enzyme inhibitor (SQ 14,225) on myocardial hypertrophy in spontaneously hypertensive rats. Hypertension 2 (2): 169–176
14. Koike H, Ito K, Miyamoto M, Nishino H (1980) Effects of long-term blockade of angiotensin coverting enzyme with captopril (SQ 14,225) on hemodynamics and circulating blood volume in SHR. Hypertension 2(3): 299–303
15. Tarazi RC, Fouad FM, Ceimo JMK, Bravo EL (1979) Renin, aldosterone and cardiac decompensation: studies with an oral converting enzyme inhibitor in heart failure. Am J Cardiol 44: 1013–1018
16. Tarazi RC, Dustan HP, Bravo EL (1979) Hemodynamic effects of propranolol in hypertension. Postgrad Med J 52 (Suppl IV) 52: 92–100
17. Tarazi RC, Dustan HP, Bravo EL (1972) The importance of plasma volume in the treatment of hypertension. In: Schweizer W (ed) Beta-blockers—Present status and future prospects. Hans Huber, Bern Switzerland, pp 102–119

18. Smith AJ (1965) Clinical features of fluid retention complicating treatment with guanethidine. Circulation 31: 485–489

19. Hansen J (1968) Alpha-methyl-dopa (Aldomet) in the treatment of hypertension: effect on blood volume, exchangeable sodium, body weight and blood pressure. Acta Med Scand 183: 323–327

20. Dustan HP, Tarazi RC, Bravo EL (1972) Dependence of arterial pressure on intravascular volume in treated hypertensive patients. N Engl J Med 286: 861–866

21. Cody RJ Jr, Tarazi RC, Bravo EL, Fouad FM (1978) Hemodynamics of orally active converting enzyme inhibitor (SQ 14,225) in hypertensive patients. Clin Sci Mol Med 55: 453–459

22. Bravo EL, Tarazi RC, Fouad FM (1980) Hemodynamic effects of long-term captopril therapy in hypertensive man. In: Proceedings of the Physiological Society of Philadelphia (In press)

23. Ferrone JA, Kardon MB, Walsh GM (1978) Systemic hemodynamic effects of converting enzyme inhibitor (CEI, SQ 14,225) during acute renovascular hypertension. Fed Proc 37: 718 (Abst)

24. Murthy VS, Wldron TL, Goldberg ME (1978) Inhibition of angiotensin converting enzyme by SQ 14,225 in anesthetized dogs: Hemodynamic and renal vascular effects. Proc Soc Exp Biol Med 157: 121–124

25. Tarazi RC (1978) Antihypertensive effect of beta-blockade: Relation of its hemodynamic component to other mechanisms. In: Braunwald E (ed) Beta-adrenergic blockade. A new era in cardiovascular medicine. Excerpta Medica/Elsevier, New York, pp 210–224

26. Tarazi RC (1976) Hemodynamic role of extracellular fluid in hypertension. Circ Res 38 (Suppl II): 72–83

27. Fiorentini R, Fouad FM, Bravo EL, Tarazi RC (1980) Combined adrenoreceptor and angiotensin blockade in resistant hypertension. Clin Pharmacol Ther 27 (2): 253 (Abst)

Converting Enzyme Inhibitors in the Treatment of Heart Failure

Jay N. Cohn, T. Barry Levine, and Joseph A. Franciosa

In congestive heart failure (CHF) systemic vaso-constriction appears to be an important contributor to depressed left ventricular function (1) (Fig. 1). Since plasma-renin activity (PRA) is elevated in many patients with CHF, angiotensin may be a factor in the high systemic vascular resistance (2). The mechanism(s) of stimulation of PRA in CHF is incompletely understood, and in particular it is not known why some individuals have high and some low PRA despite similar hemodynamic derangement. The most reliable correlate of PRA in CHF appears to be the serum sodium concentration (3). Whether low serum sodium is a stimulus for renin release or whether high PRA precipitates hyponatremia is not entirely clear.

Regardless of the mechanism, the high PRA in at least some vasoconstricted patients with CHF made it attractive to assess the possible beneficial effect of inhibiting converting enzyme on the hemodynamics and on the clinical signs and symptoms of CHF. The converting enzyme inhibitors teprotide and captopril therefore were administered acutely in increasing doses in patients with severe chronic CHF to assess the acute varodilator effect and its relationship to plasma-renin activity. Furthermore, a group of patients were placed on chronic captopril therapy to determine in an uncontrolled assessment the possible clinical benefits of this form of therapy.

In response to intravenous infusion of teprotide (0.25–2.0 mg/kg) (4) or a single oral dose of captopril (25–150 mg) (5), a vasodilator effect was characterized by a fall in arterial pressure, systemic vascular resistance, pulmonary wedge pressure, and right atrial pressure in association with increased cardiac output and no change in heart rate. The acute hemodynamic response to these drugs was therefore an improvement in left ventricular performance. The magnitude of the acute

hemodynamic effect was directly related to the control PRA (2) (Fig. 2).

Chronic captopril therapy was initiated in 11 patients not selected on the basis of their acute response to the drug nor to their PRA. During a follow-up period of 3–8 months, clinical improvement was demonstrated by increased exercise tolerance and reduction in heart size (5) Hypotension was prominent in several patients during the early phase of therapy, but this hypotension usually was remarkably well tolerated and tended to disappear with continued therapy. Furthermore, a chronic response to captopril did not appear to be dependent on a high PRA at the time therapy was initiated.

These data suggest that captopril may be an useful additive in the management of moderate

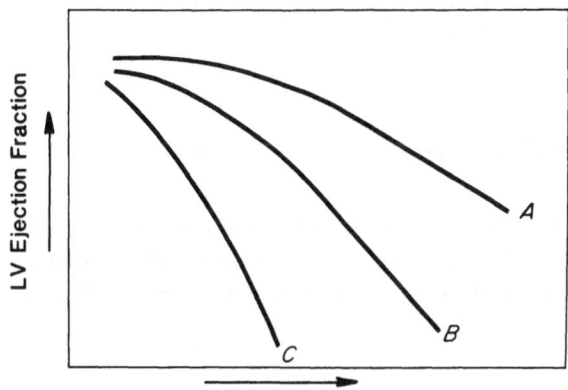

Fig. 1. Relationship between systemic vascular resistance and left ventricular function in the presence of myocardial disease that is mild *(A)*, moderate *(B)*, or severe *(C)*. By reducing systemic vascular resistance, vasodilators can markedly augment ejection fraction.

Plasma Renin Activity and Response to Converting Enzyme Inhibition in Congestive Heart Failure

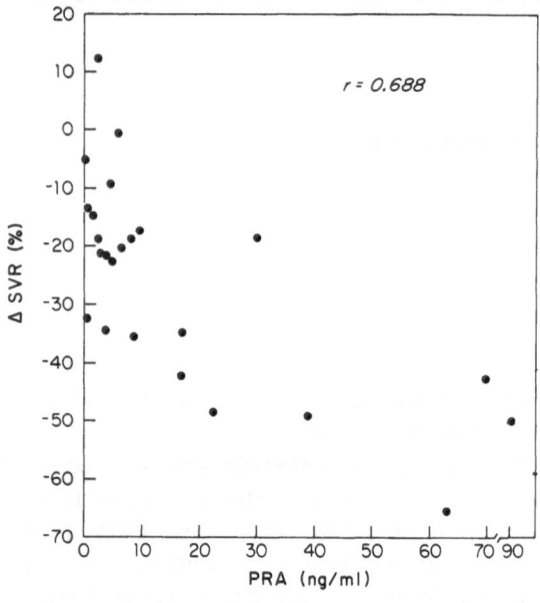

Fig. 2. Relationship between control plasma-renin activity and the fall in systemic vascular resistance induced by acute administration of teprotide or captopril. [Cohn et al. (2)]

to severe CHF. Still unclear is whether its effect can be attributed entirely to angiotensin blockade and whether it should be administered specifically to those patients whose PRA is elevated. Because this class of compounds should inhibit secondary production of aldosterone and should counteract any regional flow abnormalities induced by angiotensin, it may constitute a uniquely effective approach to therapy.

SUMMARY

Vasoconstriction characterized by a high systemic vascular resistance is a hallmark of congestive heart failure, and plasma-renin activity (PRA) is often elevated in this syndrome. Acute infusion of teprotide or oral administration of captopril results in a rise in the depressed cardiac output and a fall in the elevated systemic vascular resistance. The fall in systemic vascular resistance is directly related ($r = 0.61$) to the control PRA. Chronic administration of captopril is associated with improved exercise tolerance, reduced heart size, and symptomatic relief in preliminary uncontrolled studies. These studies suggest that activation of the renin-angiotensin system has a deleterious effect on left ventricular function in heart failure and that inhibition of angiotensin effect by converting enzyme blockade may be a useful approach to therapy in at least some patients.

ACKNOWLEDGMENT

This work was supported in part by grant HL 22977 from the National Heart, Lung and Blood Institute.

REFERENCES

1. Cohn JN (1978) Vasodilator therapy for heart failure: The influence of impedance on left ventricular performance. (Editorial) Circulation 48: 5–8
2. Cohn JN, Mashiro I, Levine TB, Mehta J (1979) Role of vasoconstrictor mechanisms in the control of left ventricular performance of the normal and damaged heart. Am J Cardiol 44: 1019–1022
3. Levine TB, Cohn JN, Vrobel, T, Franciosa JA (1979) High renin in heart failure: A manifestation of hyponatremia. Trans Assoc Am Physicians 92: 203–207
4. Curtiss C, Cohn JN, Vrobel T, Franciosa JA (1978) Role of the renin-angiotensin system in the systemic vasoconstriction of chronic congestive heart failure. Circulation 58: 763–770
5. Levine TB, Franciosa JA, Cohn JN (1980) Acute and long-term response to an oral converting-enzyme inhibitor, captopril, in congestive heart failure. Circulation 62: (1) 35–41

Summary of Worldwide Captopril Experience in Patients with Severe Treatment-Resistant Hypertension

John C. Alexander

This chapter reports on the results of a multicenter trial with captopril in 141 patients selected from among large hypertensive populations in university hospital centers who had not responded to other therapy [supine diastolic blood pressure (SDBP) ≥ 100 mmHg]. Only patients with a history of a SDBP > 120 mmHg were eligible for enrollment in the study. WHO classification was Class III for 54.3% of the patients; 89% were taking three or more antihypertensive drugs and 42% had a serum creatinine greater than 1.5 mg%. The diagnosis was essential hypertension for 67% of the patients, malignant/accelerated for 19%, and renovascular for 10%. Plasma-renin activity (PRA), which was classified by the investigators as low, normal, or high according to the procedure of Laragh (1), was reported for 60 patients; 27.5% of the patients had low values, 40.5% had normal values, and 32.0% had high values.

Treatment was initiated with up to 450 mg/day captopril. If the blood pressure failed to respond, a diuretic was then added. Propranolol could also be added if there was no response to treatment with both captopril and diuretic. Because of the severity of the hypertension in these patients, many investigators proceeded rapidly from treatment with captopril alone to captopril plus diuretic, then to captopril plus a diuretic and propranolol.

After 12 weeks of treatment, 57% of the patients had responded to treatment (mean decrease in SDBP of 23.2%). Of the patients with renovascular hypertension, 91% responded—62% of those with accelerated/malignant hypertension and 50% of those with essential hypertension (Fig. 1). The difference in response between those with renovascular hypertension and essential hypertension was statistically significant ($p < 0.05$). About one-third of patients normalized their blood pressure (SDBP ≤ 90 mmHg) after 12 weeks of treatment. The response rate at week 12 was also correlated with the pretreatment PRA. Of those patients classified as being high renin, 71% responded; 42% of those with normal renin and only 31% of those with low renin responded (Fig. 2). The difference in response between those classified with a high pretreatment PRA and those with a low PRA did not reach statistical significance because of the small number of patients in each group.

Of the patients who responded, 54% were taking captopril plus a diuretic and 37% were taking cap-

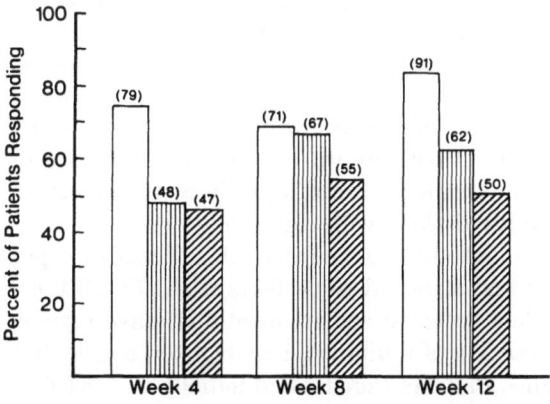

Response Correlated With Diagnosis

Fig. 1. Correlation between the diagnosis and the percentage of patients with treatment-resistant hypertension in whom supine diastolic blood pressure decreased by 10% or more from base line after treatment with captopril. Included were 14 patients with renovascular hypertension, 27 with accelerated or malignant hypertension, and 94 with essential hypertension. There was a significant difference in response between those with renovascular and essential hypertension at weeks 4 and 8 ($p < 0.05$). □, renovascular; ▩, accelerated malignant; ▨, essential.

Response Correlated With PRA

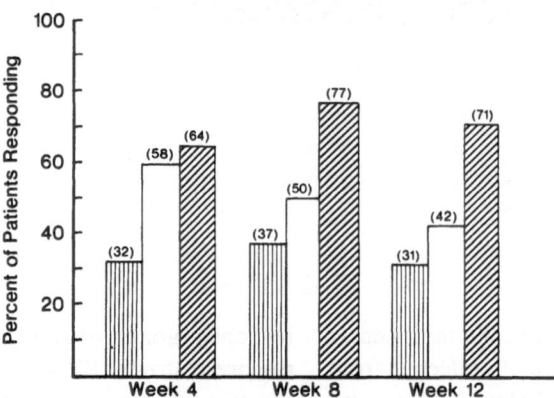

Fig. 2. Correlation between the base-line plasma renin activity (PRA) and the percentage of patients with treatment-resistant hypertension whose supine diastolic blood pressure decreased by 10% or more from base line after treatment with captopril. At week 4, PRA was low for 19 patients, normal for 26, and high for 22. At week 8, PRA was low in 18, normal in 26, and high in 22. By week 12, PRA was low in 16, normal in 12, and high in 14. The only significant difference in response was between those with a high and low PRA at week 8 ($p < 0.05$). ▥, low renin, ☐, normal renin; ▨, high renin.

topril plus a diuretic plus propranolol. Blood pressure was controlled on captopril alone in about 10% of patients. It should be noted that the value of the addition of propranolol to the regimen of patients treated with captopril plus diuretic was not very clear. Only a very few patients seemed to benefit significantly from the addition of propranolol. Some investigators have reported that nearly all patients will respond to aggressive diuretic treatment with large doses of furosemide employed alone with captopril.

This study also compared the efficacy of captopril and standard triple therapy (STT). STT is a widely accepted and frequently effective regimen consisting of a diuretic, beta-blocker, and hydralazine. Patients were treated initially with STT for 1–2 weeks. If their SDBP was greater than or equal to 100 mmHg, they were randomly assigned to continue on STT, or to receive captopril. Data from 96 patients were included in this evaluation: 66 assigned to captopril and 30 to STT. Base-line blood pressure, WHO class, number of previous antihypertensive medications, and the distribution of pretreatment PRA values were similar for both groups. By week 12 of the study, only 10% of the patients responded to STT, as compared to

55% of the patients assigned to captopril ($p < 0.01$). About one-half the responders to captopril required treatment with a diuretic and an additional one-third required concomitant treatment with a diuretic and propranolol.

The data from 24 patients randomly assigned to STT and subsequently crossed over to captopril provide the basis of another important comparison of captopril and STT. While being treated with captopril, 20 of these patients had a decrease in their SDBP, while only 12 showed a decrease in SDBP during treatment with STT.

Captopril, usually in combination with a diuretic or a diuretic and a beta-blocker, was very effective therapy for many patients with severe hypertension who had failed to respond to therapy with the available agents. More than 70% of patients with either high-renin hypertension or renovascular hypertension responded to therapy. Captopril and diuretic appear to be a very effective combination in this patient population. Addition of propranolol was beneficial in only a few patients. The results of this study are consistent with a mechanism of action for captopril that works principally by blockade of the renin-angiotensin system.

SUMMARY

Captopril, alone or in combination with a diuretic or diuretic and a beta-blocker, was used to treat 141 patients with severe, treatment-resistant hypertension. After 12 weeks of treatment, 57% of the patients had responded—91% of those with a diagnosis of renovascular hypertension and only 50% of those with essential hypertension. This difference in response was statistically significant ($p < 0.05$). Patients with a pretreatment PRA classified as high or normal also had a better rate of response than did those with a low PRA. The difference, however, was not statistically significant because of the small number of patients. Most patients required treatment with a diuretic, and about one-third required treatment with a diuretic and beta-blocker. In contrast to the striking therapeutic benefit of combined therapy with captopril and diuretic, addition of a beta-blocker seemed beneficial for only a few patients. The results of this study are consistent with a mechanism of action for captopril that works principally by blockade of the renin-angiotension system.

REFERENCE

1. Laragh JH, Sealey JE, Brunner HR (1972) The control of aldosterone secretion in normal and hypertensive man: Abnormal renin-aldosterone patterns in low renin hypertension. Am J Med 53: 649–66

The Effect of Captopril on Urinary Kinins and Urinary Kallikrein Activity in Essential Hypertension

U.L. Hulthén, J.F. Dymling, M. Bramnert, and B. Hökfelt

Angiotensin-converting enzyme is most likely identical to kininase II (1). This enzyme generates angiotensin II, the most potent vasoconstrictor known (2) By degrading kinins as well, which are potent vasodilators (3), and increasing natriuresis (4), it may be that it increases blood pressure by two separate mechanisms (Fig. 1).

The importance of inhibition of angiotensin conversion for the blood pressure reduction observed in patients with essential hypertension after converting enzyme inhibition with teprotide (5, 6) as well as captopril (7–11) is generally accepted. Studies on the effects of kinins in hypertensive patients have shown increased (12), unchanged (13), as well as decreased (6) blood concentrations after acute administration of teprotide and no change in blood levels during long-term treatment with captopril (11).

The aim of the present study is to investigate the effect of captopril on urinary kinins, which probably reflect intrarenal kinin levels (14, 15) and on urinary kallikrein activity, assumed to reflect intrarenal kinin generation (16), in relationship to its effect on the renin-angiotensin-aldosterone system and blood pressure.

PATIENT GROUPS AND METHODS

PATIENTS

Seven men and two women aged 35–58 were studied. Eight were classified as WHO stages I–II and one as stage III. Endogenous creatinine clearance and urinary catecholamines were normal in all patients. Intravenous pyelography was performed in all patients, and renal angiography in eight of the patients. All were considered to have essential hypertension. No antihypertensive treatment was given for 3 weeks prior to the study.

DESIGN OF THE STUDY

Patients were admitted to a metabolic ward. They were maintained on a diet containing 120 mEq

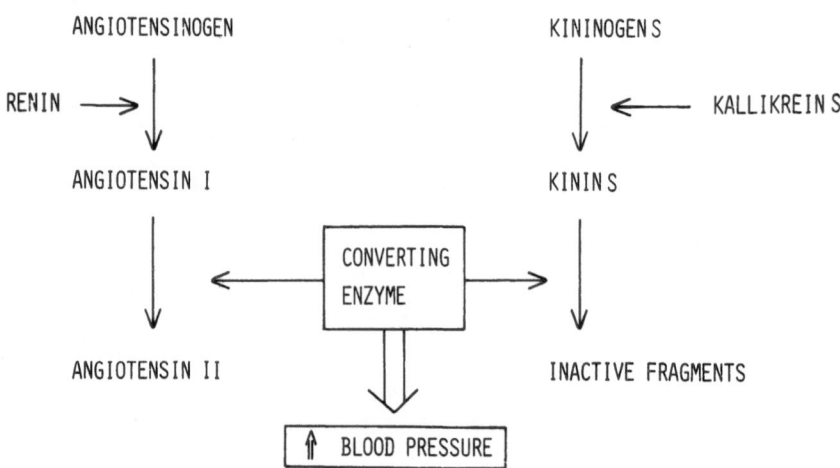

Fig. 1. Mechanism of angiotensin-converting enzyme.

sodium and 95 mEq potassium daily for 11 days. Captopril was administered from day 5 three times daily (7 AM, 3 PM, and 11 PM) in increasing dosages of 75 mg, day 5; 150 mg, day 6; 300 mg, days 7 and 8; and 600 mg, days 9–11. Blood pressure was measured (mean of two recordings) daily at 7 AM, 11 AM, 3 PM, and 7 PM after 10 min in the supine position and 2 min upright. Twenty-four-hour urine samples were collected throughout the study. Immediately after voiding, each portion was divided into two containers, one with 5 ml concentrated galcial acetic acid for preservation of kinins (15), the other without preservatives. Urine was refrigerated during collection. Blood samples were drawn in the supine position through a siliconized cannula at 8.30 AM and after being ambulatory for 1 h at 10 AM on days 4, 8, and 10.

ANALYTIC METHODS

Urinary kinins were extracted with ethanol and measured by radioimmunoassay (RIA) (17). Urinary kallikrein activity was determined as the amount of bradykinin equivalents formed during 15-min incubation with human plasma substrate (15). Plasma-renin activity (PRA) was measured as the amount of angiotensin I generated following 3-h incubation at pH 6.0 (18). Plasma angiotensin II was determined by RIA (19). Urinary aldosterone was assayed according to the method of Ito et al. (20). Serum and urinary sodium, potassium, and creatinine were measured by standard laboratory techniques.

STATISTICAL EVALUATION

Statistical analysis was performed by nonparametric methods. Wilcoxon's two-sample test was used for paired observations and Spearman's rank correlation for calculating correlation coefficients. The values are given as mean ± SEM and the level of significance taken as $p < 0.05$.

RESULTS

During the four control days urinary kinin excretion was directly related to urinary kallikrein activity ($r = 0.44$, $p < 0.02$). On day 4 PRA in the supine as well as in the upright position was posi-

tively correlated to urinary aldosterone ($r = 0.83$, $p < 0.02$ for both). Neither urinary kinins nor urinary kallikrein activity was significantly correlated to either PRA or urinary aldosterone.

During the administration of increasing dosages of captopril, both the supine and upright blood pressures decreased gradually (Fig. 2). The maximal reduction of supine as well as upright mean blood pressure was directly related to basal supine PRA ($r = 0.69$, $p < 0.05$ and $r = 0.79$, $p < 0.02$, respectively) as well as basal upright PRA ($r = 0.76$, $p < 0.05$ and $r = 0.80$, $p < 0.02$, respectively).

PRA in the supine and upright positions increased from 2.6 ± 0.8 and 5.1 ± 1.4 µg/liter/3 h, respectively, to 6.0 ± 2.4 and 13.3 ± 5.0 µg/liter/3 h, respectively; on captopril 300 mg/day and to 7.2 ± 2.5 and 17.6 ± 7.0 µg/liter/3 h, respectively; and on captopril 600 mg/day (Fig. 3). So far plasma angiotensin II has been assayed in seven patients all of whom showed a decrease. Urinary aldosterone decreased during treatment with captopril to levels that were similar on 300 and 600 mg/day (Fig. 4).

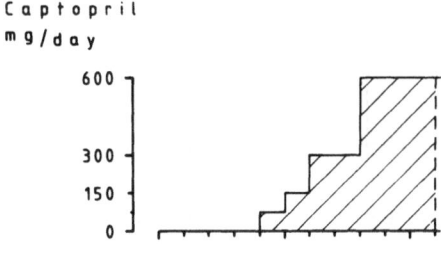
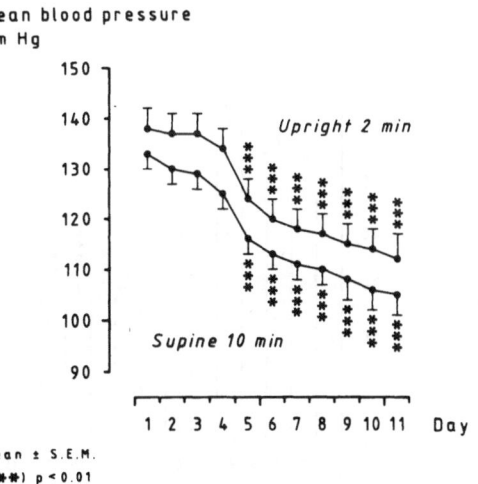

Fig. 2. Effect of captopril on mean blood pressure in supine and upright positions. Mean ± SEM. *** $p < 0.01$.

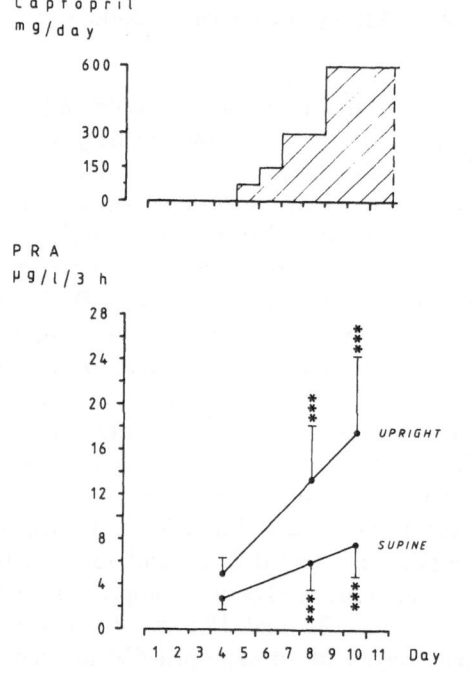

Fig. 3. Effect of captopril on plasma-renin activity in supine and upright positions. Mean ± SEM. *** $p < 0.01$.

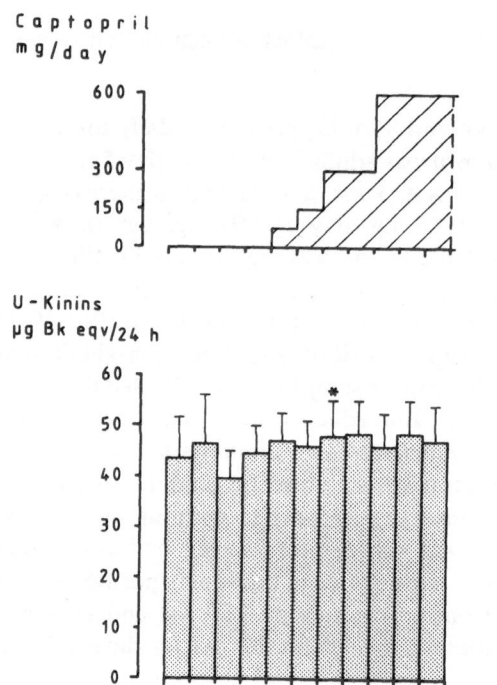

Fig. 5. Effect of captopril on urinary kinins. Mean ± SEM. * $p < 0.05$.

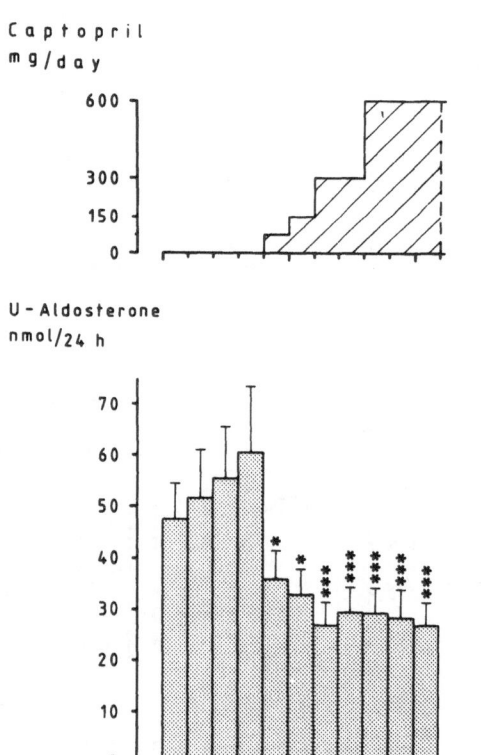

Fig. 4. Effect of captopril on urinary aldosterone. Mean ± SEM $p < 0.05$; *** $p < 0.01$.

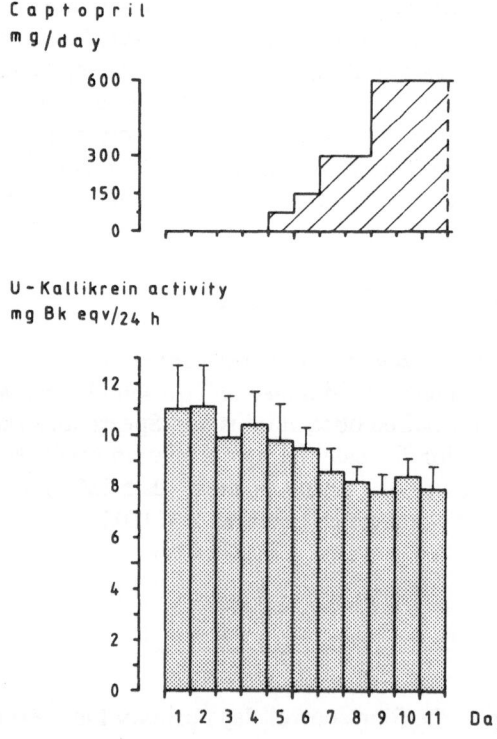

Fig. 6. Effect of captopril on urinary kallikrein activity. Mean ± SEM.

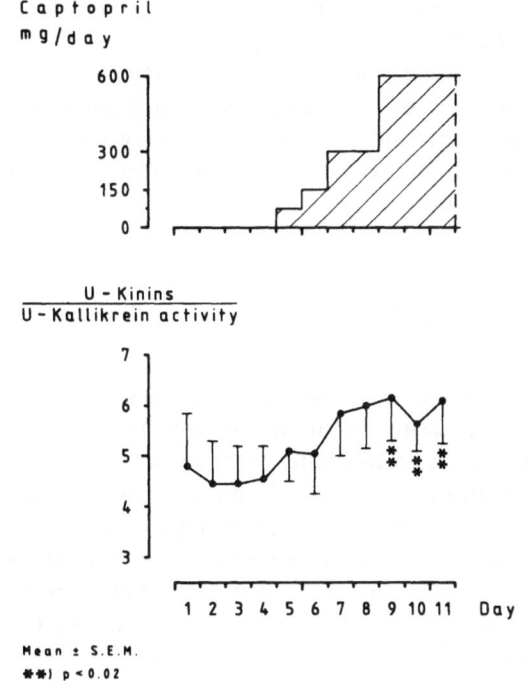

Fig. 7. Effect of captopril on the ratio of urinary kinins to urinary kallikrein activity. Mean ± SEM. ** $p < 0.02$.

Urinary kinin excretion showed no consistent increase during administration of captopril (Fig. 5). By contrast, urinary kallikrein activity decreased numerically, but the reduction was not significant (Fig. 6). The ratio of urinary kinins to urinary kallikrein activity increased significantly from 4.5 ± 0.7 during basal conditions to 6.1 ± 0.9 on captopril 600 mg/day (Fig. 7).

Captopril had no significant effect either on urinary excretion of sodium and potassium or on serum sodium concentration (cumulative sodium balance, 40 ± 44 mEq; cumulative potassium balance, 11 ± 24 mEq) (Figs. 8 and 9). Serum potassium concentration increased from 3.6 ± 0.1 to 4.0 ± 0.1 ($p < 0.05$) (Fig. 9). Endogenous creatinine clearance decreased from 105 ± 6 ml/min/ 1.73 m² body surface area (b.s.) under basal conditions to 94 ± 4 ml/min/1.73 m² b.s. on captopril 600 mg/day (Fig. 10).

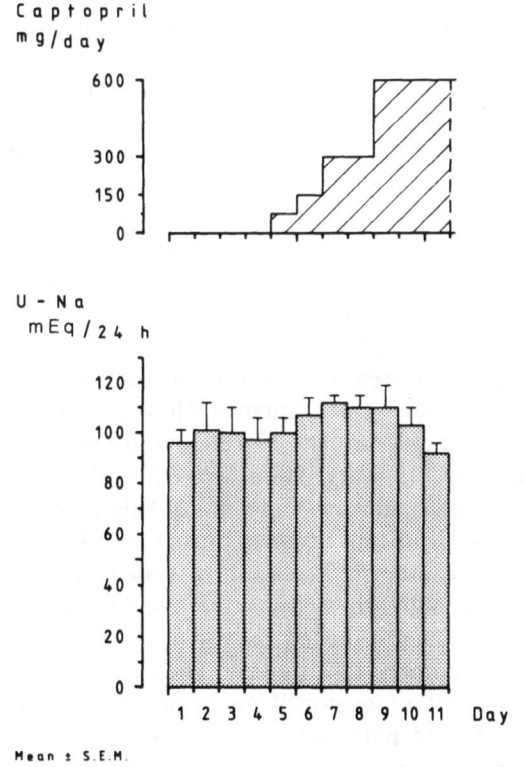

Fig. 8. Effect of captopril on urinary sodium excretion. Mean ± SEM.

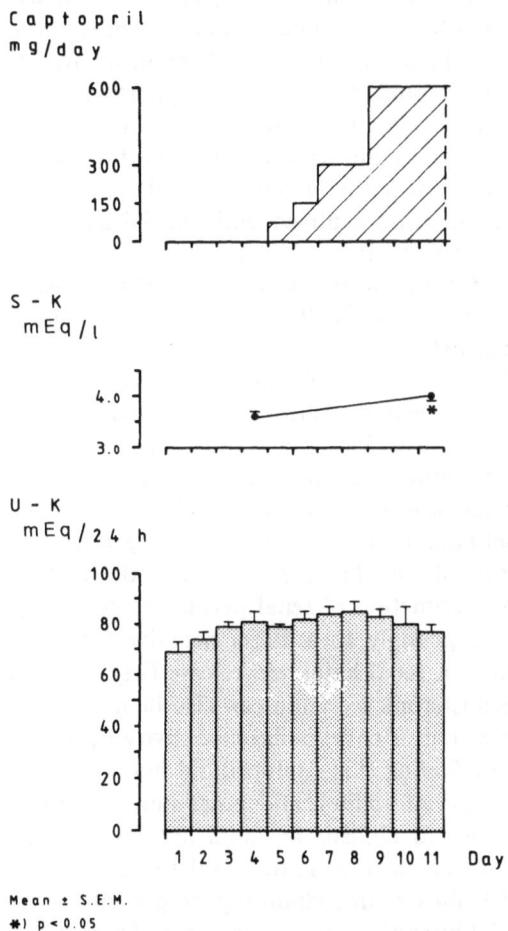

Fig. 9. Effect of captopril on serum potassium concentration and urinary potassium excretion. Mean ± SEM. * $p < 0.05$.

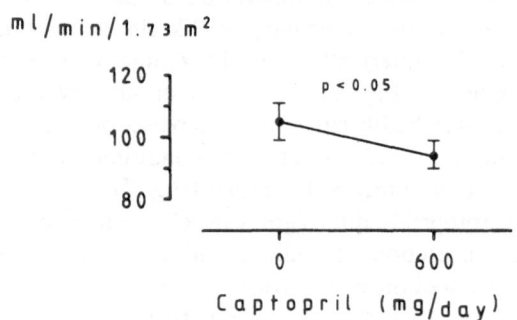

ml/min/1.73 m²

Fig. 10. Effect of captopril on endogenous creatinine clearance.

of potassium from the intracellular to the extracellular compartment took place.

The decrease in endogenous creatinine clearance indicates that the glomerular filtration rate fell during captopril treatment, although an effect of captopril on tubular handling of creatinine cannot be excluded.

DISCUSSION

An earlier study showed a significant positive correlation between urinary kinin concentration and urinary kallikrein activity in fresh urine from normal individuals (15), thereby supporting the concept that both these variables reflect the activity of the renal kallikrein-kinin system. Furthermore, it was shown that kinins are stable for at least 24 h in urine acidified with glacial acetic acid. These data are in accordance with the present finding of a significant positive correlation between kinin levels and kallikrein activity in urine collected before treatment.

The increased ratio of urinary kinins/urinary kallikrein activity during treatment with captopril indicates that kinins accumulated in the kidney on inhibition of kininase II. Kinin levels were not permanently elevated, however, as the release of renal kallikrein seemed to decrease gradually. Secretion of renal kallikrein may have decreased due to the reduction of renal perfusion pressure (21–23) or possibly to a direct negative feedback of kinins on renal kallikrein release (24). Reduction of aldosterone secretion can also be implicated in decreasing urinary kallikrein activity (25).

The finding that captopril did not alter urinary excretion of sodium and potassium in spite of a decrease in aldosterone does not favor a major role for aldosterone in the regulation of natriuresis and kaliuresis in sodium-replete patients with essential hypertension. The increase of serum potassium concentration in spite of unchanged urinary potassium excretion suggests that a redistribution

CONCLUSION

The present study supports the concept that the blood pressure reduction induced by captopril is closely linked to inhibition of angiotensin conversion. Intrarenal kinins do not seem important for this blood pressure reduction to occur, at least not in sodium-replete patients with essential hypertension. The blood pressure reduction following captopril is generally not associated with a natriuresis.

SUMMARY

The effect of captopril on the renal kallikrein-kinin system, as measured by urinary kallikrein activity and urinary kinin excretion, in relationship to its effect on the renin-angiotensin-aldosterone system and blood pressure was studied under metabolic ward conditions in nine sodium-replete patients with essential hypertension (seven men and two women aged 35–58). Before treatment, urinary kinin excretion was directly correlated to urinary kallikrein activity. Increasing dosages of captopril (75–600 mg/day) for 7 days gradually decreased blood pressure, the maximal reduction being positively correlated to basal plasma-renin activity (PRA). During treatment with captopril PRA increased and urinary aldosterone decreased significantly. Urinary kinin excretion showed an inconsistent increase and urinary kallikrein activity an insignificant decrease during the administration of captopril. The ratio of urinary kinins to urinary kallikrein activity increased significantly from 4.5 ± 0.7 during basal conditions to 6.1 ± 0.9 on captopril 600 mg/day. There was no significant effect of captopril on urinary excretion of sodium and potassium, but serum potassium increased significantly. Endogenous creatinine clearance decreased significantly during captopril treatment. These findings suggest that intrarenal accumulation of kinins by kininase II inhibition is not important for the blood pressure reduction during treatment with captopril, probably due to a decrease in the secretion of renal kallikrein. However, the blood pressure reduction appears to be closely linked to inhibition of angiotensin conversion.

REFERENCES

1. Erdös EG (1976) Conversion of angiotensin I to angiotensin II. Am J Med 60: 749–759
2. Khairallah PA, Page IH, Turker KR (1966) Potentiation of vascular myotropic responses by metanephrine and other noncatecholamines. Circ Res XIX: 538–543
3. Fox RH, Goldsmith R, Kidd DJ, Lewis GP (1961) Bradykinin as a vasodilator in man. J Physiol (Lond) 157: 589–602
4. Gill JR Jr, Melmon KL, Gillespie L Jr, Bartter FC (1965) Bradykinin and renal function in normal man: effect of adrenergic blockade. Am J Physiol 209: 844–848
5. Case DB, Wallace JM, Keim HJ, Weber MA, Sealey JE, Laragh JH (1977) Possible role of renin in hypertension as suggested by renin-sodium profiling and inhibition of converting enzyme. New Engl J Med 296: 641–646
6. Hulthén L, Hökfelt B (1978) The effect of the converting enzyme inhibitor SQ 20881 on kinins, renin-angiotensin-aldosterone and catecholamines in relation to blood pressure in hypertensive patients. Acta Med Scand 204: 497–502
7. Atlas SA, Case DB, Sealey JE, Laragh JH, KcKinstry DN (1979) Interruption of the renin-angiotensin system in hypertensive patients by Captopril induces sustained reduction in aldosterone secretion, potassium retention and natriuresis. Hypertension 1: 274–280
8. Brunner HR, Gavras H, Waeber B, Kershaw GR, Turini GA, Vukovich RA, McKinstry DN, Gavras I (1979) Oral angiotensin-converting enzyme inhibitor in long-term treatment of hypertensive patients. Ann Intern Med 90: 19–23
9. Fagard R, Amery A, Lijnen P, Reybrouck T (1979) Haemodynamic effects of Captopril in hypertensive patients: Comparison with saralasin. Clin Sci 57: 131s–134s
10. MacGregor GA, Markandu ND, Roulston JE, Jones JC (1979) Essential hypertension: effect of an oral inhibitor of angiotensin-converting enzyme. Br Med J 2: 1106–1109
11. Johnston CI, McGrath BP, Millar JA, Matthews PG (1979) Long-term effects of Captopril (SQ 14225) on blood pressure and hormone levels in essential hypertension. Lancet 2: 493–496
12. Williams GH, Hollenberg NK (1977) Accentuated vascular and endocrine response to SQ 20881 in hypertension. New Engl J Med 297: 184–188
13. Vinci JM, Horwitz D, Zusman RM, Pisano JJ, Catt KJ, Keiser HR (1979) The effect of converting enzyme inhibition with SQ 20881 on plasma and urinary kinins, prostaglandin E and angiotensin II in hypertensive man. Hypertension 1: 416–426
14. Abe K (1965) Urinary excretion of kinin in man with special reference to its origin. Tohoku J Exp Med 87: 175–184
15. Hulthén UL, Dymling JF, Hökfelt B (1980) Kinins in relation to kallikrein activity, kininogen, electrolytes, aldosterone and catecholamines in urine from normal individuals. Acta Physiol Scand (In press)
16. Carretero OA, Scicli AG (1976) Renal kallikrein: Its location and possible role in renal function. Fed Proc 35: 194–198
17. Hulthén UL, Borge T (1976) Determination of bradykinin in blood by a sensitive radioimmunoassay. Scand J Clin Lab Invest 36: 833–839
18. Haber E, Koerner T, Page LB, Kliman B, Purnode A (1969) Application of a radioimmunoassay for angiotensin I to the physiological measurements of plasma renin activity in normal human subjects. J Clin Endocrinol Metab 29: 1349–1355
19. Kappelgaard AM, Damkjaer Nielsen M, Giese J (1976) Measurement of angiotensin II in human plasma: Technical modification and practical experience. Clin Chim Acta 67: 299–306
20. Ito T, Woo J, Haning R, Horton R (1972) A radioimmunoassay for aldosterone in human peripheral plasma including a comparison of alternate techniques. J Clin Endocrinol Metab 34: 106–112
21. Bevan DR, Macfarlane NAA, Mills IH (1974) The dependence of urinary kallikrein excretion on renal artery pressure. J Physiol (Lond) 241: 34P–35P
22. Hulthén UL, Lecerof H, Hökfelt B (1977) Renal venous output of kinins in patients with hypertension and unilateral renal artery stenosis. Acta Med Scand 202: 189–191
23. Maier M, Binder BR (1973) Dependence of urokallikrein excretion of the perfusion pressure in explanted perfused kidneys. Adv Exp Med Biol 120B: 527–538
24. Karlberg BE, Öhman KP, Nilsson OR, Wettre S (1980) Captopril lowers urinary kallikrein in hypertensive patients. Lancet 1: 150–151
25. Margolius HS, Horwitz D, Pisano JJ, Keiser HR (1974) Urinary kallikrein excretion in hypertensive man, relationships to sodium intake and sodium-retaining steroids. Circ Res 35: 820–825

Session 17
Physiologic Effects and Diagnostic Relevance of Acute Converting Enzyme Blockade

Chairman: D. W. Seldin

Position Paper: Physiologic Effects and Diagnostic Relevance of Acute Converting Enzyme Blockade

David B. Case, Steven A. Atlas, and John H. Laragh

Although the treatment of hypertension has been largely empirical, recent scientific advances have provided improved diagnostic precision in identifying the specific factors or mechanisms involved in sustaining the hypertensive state. Thus, it is now not only possible to measure relevant hormonal levels, but also to antagonize, block, or inhibit their action both acutely for diagnostic purposes and also chronically for long-term control of hypertension. This review will focus on drugs used to block the renin-angiotensin system, in particular the nonapeptide converting enzyme inhibitor teprotide (SQ 20881) and captopril (SQ 14225), an orally active drug that also blocks converting enzyme.

POTENTIAL RELEVANCE OF ACUTE ANGIOTENSIN BLOCKADE

The potential significance of the reinin-angiotensin-aldosterone axis in human hypertension was overlooked for many years, since there were no good or practical methods to assess the activity of the system. The advent of radioimmunoassay for angiotensin I proved more accurate, reproducible, and practical than the bioassay for angiotensin I. However, there remain several distinct problems regarding the use of the measurements of plasma-renin activity by measuring the amount of generated angiotensin I. Even now, there are several methods for incubating plasma samples to generate angiotensin I that differ in pH and selection of inhibitors of angiotensinases which, as a result, do not produce comparable results. Aside from a lack of uniform measurements of plasma-renin activity (PRA), this assay does not actually measure a level of the effector hormone angiotensin II directly. Assays for this hormone are not gener-

ally available and are believed to be unreliable in the range of low values. A measurement of PRA will not, for example, reflect the angiotensin II level if there is any in vivo inhibition of converting enzyme. Other problems with measurements of PRA have been their limited availability and cost. These latter factors have discouraged physicians from recommending the regular use of measurements of PRA or renin-sodium profiles in the routine evaluation of hypertensive patients despite their generally acknowledged diagnostic value.

The option, therefore, of using an acute test dose of a specific angiotensin blocking drug in patients appeared to provide a viable alternative to the measurement of PRA. This was most likely a prominent stimulus to the development of saralasin, an octapeptide analog of angiotensin II designed to act as a competitive inhibitor. It was reasoned that saralasin testing could be used to screen for surgically correctable renovascular hypertension, a condition believed to be partially or completely angiotensin dependent in man. But saralasin testing, or for that matter any acute blocker test of angiotensin II, detects primarily the rapidly reacting action of angiotensin II on arteriolar smooth muscle as a vasoconstrictor as judged by a change in blood pressure.

Acute or single-dose testing, however, does not assess the full coordinated effect of angiotensin II on other target organs. For example, the acute response does not assess the impact of the reduction in aldosterone secretion and the consequent effects on sodium excretion and potassium retention. Moreover, the longer-term effects of angiotensin II on the renal circulation and sodium excretion are not assessed, nor are the effects on the central nervous system and release of antidiuretic hormone. Thus, acute blockade assesses only the rapid-acting components of the renin system and not the slower ones, which may have critical importance in the long-term regulation of arterial pressure. It is conceivable, therefore, that a small depressor response to angiotensin blockade might underestimate the impact of the additional effects of aldosterone, sodium, antidiuretic hormone, and other factors in the maintenance of hypertension.

Another important consideration in analyzing the results of acute angiotensin blockade is that of the immediate physiologic reactions that accompany the effects of pharmacologic blockade. For example, intravenous propranolol lowers renin secretion promptly in addition to reducing cardiac output by about 15%. Nonetheless, even with these two actions which would work toward lowering blood pressure, plasma catecholamines increase and arterial pressure does not change (1). In response to a reduction in cardiac output, sensed by tissues as a threat to perfusion, peripheral resistance rises (active vasoconstriction), with no net change in blood pressure. The induced vasoconstriction in this situation is not likely to be angiotensin mediated, since PRA decreases (1). With angiotensin blockade, there appears to be little change in cardiac output, even with significant depressor responses, to stimulate reflex vasoconstriction and plasma norepinephrine levels measured after 3-day treatment are unchanged from control (2). However, it remains uncertain as to whether there is any acute vasomotor compensation to, but independent of, the vasodilation produced by angiotensin blockade. There is some evidence that over week 1 of long-term treatment with converting enzyme inhibitor that a non-renin-mediated vasoconstrictor effect occurs and then subsides (3, 4).

A final issue related to the interpretation of acute angiotensin blockade studies involves the specificity and the completeness of blockade. This latter issue appears to be a minor problem, since there are for each angiotensin blocking drug a host of studies to indicate dosages that will adequately block the effects of infused angiotensin I or II. The problem of specificity will be discussed with the individual drugs.

Altogether, testing with angiotensin-blocking drugs with a rapid onset of action could conceivably prove more practical clinically than measurements of PRA in determining the extent of participation of the renin system in the hypertension. In some ways, direct physiologic testing with an-

giotensin blockade may prove more accurate than plasma-renin measurements, especially in patients who may be super- or subsensitive to the same amount of angiotensin generated by a given plasma sample. On the other hand, acute testing has its own pitfalls of interpretation.

SARALASIN TESTING: DIFFICULTY IN INTERPRETING

The first angiotensin blocking agent used in human hypertension was saralasin, an octapeptide analog of angiotensin II in which the terminal amino acids were substituted: sarcosine for aspartic acid and alanine for phenylalanine. The initial results demonstrated that the compound did, as predicted, lower blood pressure in high-renin forms of hypertension. The antihypertensive effect, moreover, was potentiated by prior sodium depletion, which served to raise renin levels and to decrease intravascular fluid volume (5, 6). In a second generation of detailed studies with saralasin, the partial agonist potential of the drug was exposed. In low-renin hypertensive patients and also in anephric subjects with no circulating renin, saralasin regularly raised blood pressure (5, 7, 8). In a group of hypertensive patients with similar low levels of PRA, saralasin raised blood pressure in proportion to the positivity of their sodium balance as reflected by increasing 24-h urine sodium excretion rates (7). The rises in blood pressure induced by saralasin can be reduced by sodium depletion with either diuretics or a low-sodium diet (5, 6). Therefore, theoretically it did not seem possible to block the pressor effect of angiotensin interacting with vascular receptors without at the same time introducing a separate pressor effect as a result of interaction of saralasin both with unoccupied receptors and also with those formerly occupied by angiotensin II.

Aside from the problems in interpreting saralasin tests, it did not seem that intravenous infusions of a peptide that had the ability to raise pressure was either practical or safe in screening large numbers of people. However, Dr. David Streeten and his colleagues have studied thousands of hypertensive patients in upstate New York as a service to referring physicians with a minimum of reported difficulties.

CONVERTING ENZYME INHIBITION: BLOCKADE OF ANGIOTENSIN II FORMATION

Although the original studies of Ferriera showed that a peptide mixture from the venom of the viper *Bothrops jararaca* potentiated the action of brady-kinin on smooth muscle (9), Bakhle found that these same peptides inhibited the conversion of angiotensin I to angiotensin II in isolated canine pulmonary tissue (10). Evidence from Ng and Vane (11, 12) supported the idea that the same enzyme both degraded bradykinin and catalyzed angiotensin I conversion. Further studies isolated and purified (13) and later synthesized other pep-tides with this activity (14–17). The nonapeptide SQ 20881 (17) was shown to block the vasopressor effect of angiotensin I (18) and was later found to reduce blood pressure in some hypertensive pa-tients (19). After a larger experience in hyperten-sive patients, it was possible to demonstrate a close direct correlation between the pretreatment level of PRA and the magnitude of the depressor re-sponse (20) (see Fig. 1). Moreover, in untreated

hypertensive patients on the same normal sodium intake, intravenous teprotide (SQ 20881) lowered blood pressure to the greatest extent in the group profiled as high-renin by the renin-sodium index, but did not lower blood pressure significantly in the low-renin subgroup (20) (Fig. 2). In contrast to the experience with saralasin, teprotide did not alter the blood pressure either in anephric patients or in those with primary aldosteronism and low plasma-renin values (7). However, teprotide signif-icantly reduced pressure in more than 90% of pa-tients with normal-renin profiles (7). From these studies, it was possible to predict that inhibition of converting enzyme might be a useful therapeutic approach for common forms of hypertension (20). In addition, the results focused on the potential importance of the renin-angiotensin system in the maintenance of hypertension in the normal and

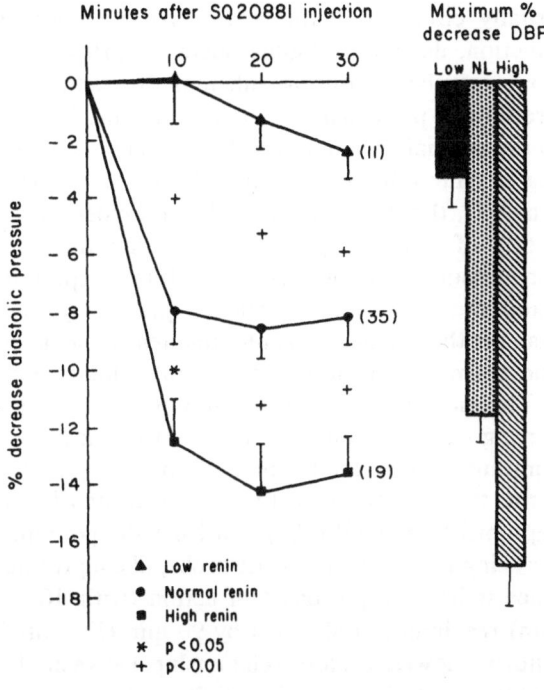

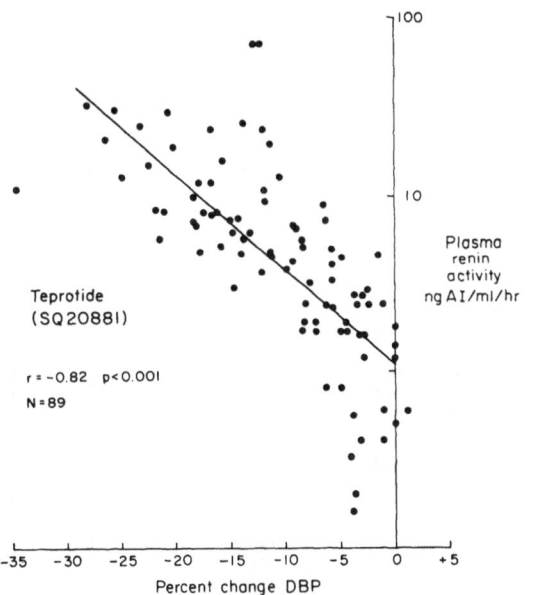

Fig. 1. Effect of intravenous converting enzyme in-hibitor teprotide (SQ 20881) and blood pressure. The percentage change in diastolic blood pressure (DBP) was closely related to the pretreatment level of plasma-renin activity in 89 untreated hypertensive pa-tients.

Fig. 2. Effect of teprotide (SQ 20881) on the blood pressure of hypertensive patients profiled as high-, low, or normal-renin according to renin-sodium profil-ing. *(Left)* The percent decreases in diastolic pres-sure for the 30-min period following injection of the nonapeptide. The numbers of the patients studied in each group are shown in brackets. *(Right)* The maximum induced decrease in pressure. [Case et al. (20), by permission]

high-renin subgroups, but not in untreated low-renin hypertension.

In these latter considerations, the specificity of the drug is called into question, since it blocks the enzyme that also degrades the potent vasodilator bradykinin. Bradykinin is not believed to be a hormone that normally circulates in blood; therefore, plasma levels, however inaccurate their measurement may be, may not be an adequate assessment of whether or not there is excess bradykinin. If bradykinin is generated during converting enzyme blockade, it appears to be in a manner parallel to, and not distinguishable from, the blockade of angiotensin II generation, since the response of blood pressure to the agents is closely related to the base-line renin level. It is curious from a teleologic view that the converting enzyme system located primarily in the pulmonary vascular circuit, immediately proximal to the angiotensin-responsive vasculature, would play a physiologic role in degrading a hormone that does not usually circulate. Perhaps it serves a scavenger function, destroying kinins liberated into the venous circulation during inflammation and thus preventing perturbations in smooth muscle tone in the arterial circulation. If the action of converting enzyme inhibitor is primarily to block angiotensin II, the studies relating the antihypertensive action of captopril provide physiologic meaning for measurements of PRA. Therefore, keeping in mind the limitations mentioned previously, one may use the response to acute angiotensin blockade and plasma-renin measurements interchangeably.

The success of the intravenous nonapeptide converting enzyme inhibitor was very likely a potent stimulus to the development of an orally active form, the first of which to be used in man being captopril (SQ 14225). Captopril has the potential for being used as a diagnostic probe, like teprotide, since it has a rapid onset of action (with 10–15 min) reaching a peak effect by 90 min (3). Initial studies showed a close relationship between the pretreatment plasma-renin activity and the magnitude of the depressor response induced after the first dose of captopril (3, 21). The first dose response of 100 hypertensive patients to captopril in relationship to renin levels is shown in Fig. 3. Even though some of these patients were receiving some form of antihypertensive medication, the relationship was highly significant. Nearly all patients with pretreatment plasma-renin activity of about 3 ng AI/ml/h or greater had substantial

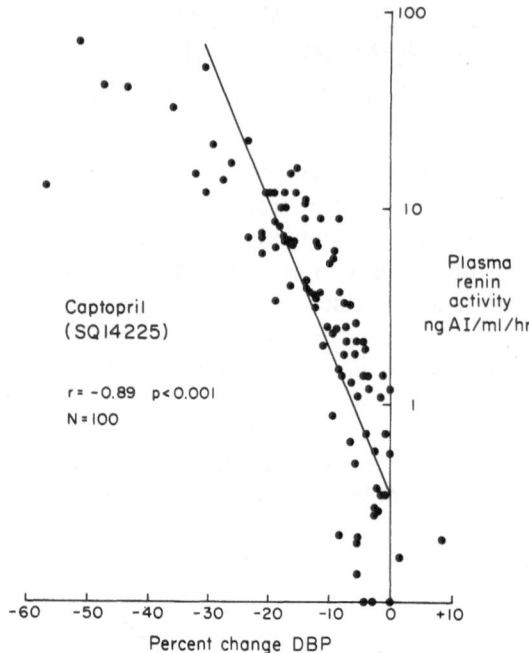

Fig. 3. Effect of oral converting enzyme inhibitor captopril (SQ 14225) in the blood pressures of 100 patients with untreated hypertension. There was a correlation between the induced change in diastolic blood pressure (DBP) and the pretreatment level of plasma-renin activity.

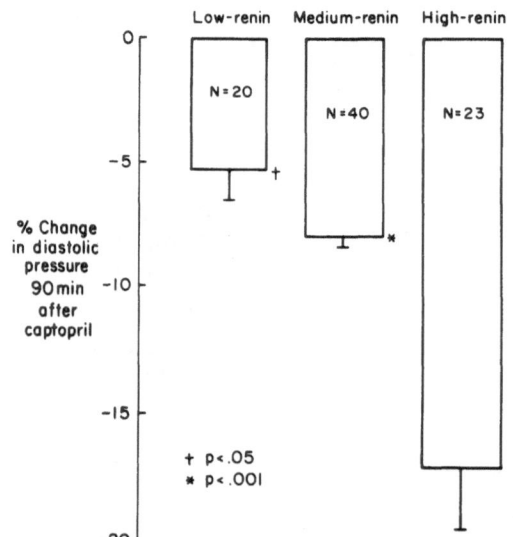

Fig. 4. Acute effect of captopril in renin subgroups studied under the same conditions as patients shown in Fig. 2, i.e., on normal sodium intake, off all medications, and in the seated position. The percentage change in diastolic pressure was greatest in the high-renin group and least in the low-renin group.

decreases in pressure (> 10%), although there was no apparent relationship with renin activity below that level.

In 83 untreated hypertensive patients studied in exactly the same manner as previously described for saralasin and teprotide (5, 7, 20), the responses of patients profiled as low-medium (or normal), and high-renin were significantly different from each other and closely resembled the nonapeptide responses (see Fig. 4). Whereas high-renin patients exhibited a 17.1 ± 1.9 (SEM) % decline in diastolic pressure, those with medium-renin profiles fell only $8.0 \pm 0.8\%$ ($p < 0.001$). The diastolic pressures of low-renin patients decreased $5.3 \pm 1.2\%$, somewhat less than the group of medium-renin patients ($p < 0.05$). Thus the results of captopril testing closely resemble those of teprotide testing in renin-profiled patients.

REACTIVE HYPERRENINEMIA IDENTIFYING RENOVASCULAR HYPERTENSION

Plasma-renin activity rises after angiotensin blockade with saralasin (5, 22, 26), teprotide (20, 27), and captopril (2, 3, 21, 26). Although the rise can be closely correlated with the induced decrease in pressure, thereby representing baroreceptor stimulation of beta-adrenergic renin release, the reduction of angiotensin II or its displacement from receptors may interrupt a direct negative feedback loop of angiotensin II on renin release (28–32). Studies with saralasin (24–26), teprotide (25–27), and captopril (26) have indicated that patients with documented renovascular hypertension exhibit marked reactive hyperreninemia to these drugs, which distinguishes them from patients with essential hypertension, who may exhibit comparable depressor responses. In studies done with patients untreated, on normal sodium intake, and in the seated position, approximately 98% of correctable renovascular hypertension was identified by this renin response, whereas only 12% of high-renin essential and no patients with normal- or medium-renin essential hypertension met the criteria for a positive-reactive renin response (26). The test, however, was usually "false-positive" in patients who were sodium depleted and in some with bilateral renovasular or with accelerated or malignant hypertension (26). Thus, it ap-

pears that ischemic kidneys, which are known to have heavily granulated juxtaglomerular cells, release large amounts of renin with angiotensin blockade. This feature may also help localize ischemic renal tissue during renal vein renin determinations (27). However, if the juxtaglomerular cells are heavily granulated on the basis of malignant hypertension or as a normal physiologic consequence of diuretics or sodium depletion, the discrimination between renovascular and other forms of hypertension may be obscured. Normal sodium intake suppresses renin secretion in normal subjects and in essential hypertension, but does not appear to overcome the ischemic signal for renin generation.

Since it is often impractical to take patients off all antihypertensive therapy, a further series of studies were carried out using captopril in patients already treated with beta-blockers alone (33). It was reasoned that the most potent stimulus for renin release would be mediated by the macula densa in the setting of reduced renal blood flow and glomerular filtration. Patients with essential hypertension, on the other hand, appear to have their renin release more under the control of beta-adrenergic stimulation than do those with renovascular disease, since beta-blockers appear to reduce their renin levels more (34).

Figure 5 illustrates that patients with renovascular hypertension exhibited significant depressor responses to angiotensin blockade with captopril on

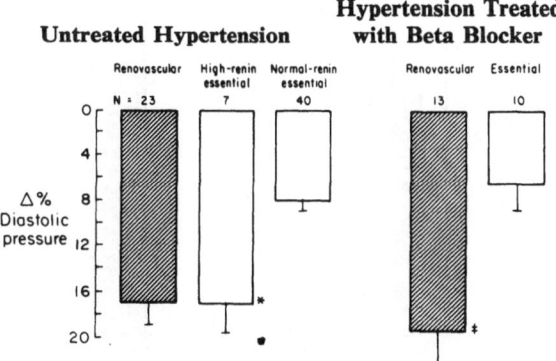

Fig. 5. Captopril tests in untreated hypertensive patients and in others during treatment with beta-blockers. Depressor responses occurred in groups of renovascular hypertension whether or not there was concurrent beta-blocker therapy. These responses were consistently greater in renovascular patients during beta-blocker treatment. $\pm\ p < 005$; $^*p < .001$.

normal sodium intake with or without concurrent beta-blocker therapy. However, in the untreated state, the response of the group of renovascular patients could not be distinguished from that of the group with high-renin essential hypertension. There was a consistently greater depressor response in the group of renovascular than in essential hypertensive patients during beta-blocker therapy. The most unequivocal difference between renovascular and essential hypertension was found in a comparison between the response in PRA measured 90 min after a dose of captopril, particularly during concurrent beta-blocker therapy (Fig. 6). Just as in the untreated state, the mean PRA after captopril for the group of patients with renovascular hypertension treated with beta-blocker was significantly higher than in the group with essential hypertension, with no overlap of values.

Thus it is possible to test for renovascular hypertension with accuracy in patients on normal sodium intake treated with beta-adrenergic blocking drugs by using criteria of depressor responses and reactive hyperreninemia. In fact, it appears that the sensitivity of testing may actually be enhanced by pretreatment with beta-blockers, since renin release resulting from renal ischemia (macula densa and intrarenal baroreceptor mechanisms) does not appear to be suppressed to the extent found in nonischemic kidneys.

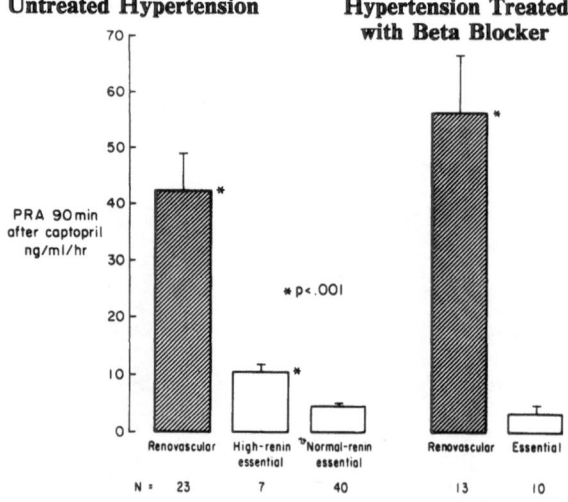

Fig. 6. Levels of plasma-renin activity in renovascular and essential hypertension 90 min after a single dose of captopril. A marked reactive hyperreninemia was found in the group with renovascular hypertension whether or not they were already receiving beta-blocker therapy.

CLINICAL TESTING WITH CONVERTING ENZYME INHIBITORS

On the basis of the studies summarized to this point, the use of PRA measurements or responses to converting enzyme blockade can be used to assess the magnitude of the contribution of angiotensin II in maintaining the hypertension. The finding of angiotensin-dependent hypertension leads to a logical selection of drugs for long-term therapy whose mechanisms of action have been shown to involve inhibition of the renin system. There is ample evidence that these renin-suppressing drugs are effective in high-renin states as well as in a large fraction of patients with normal renin profiles or mild essential hypertension (35–37). In contrast, diuretic agents have been shown to be preferentially effective in low-renin or nonangiotensin-dependent states (38–40).

Testing with converting enzyme inhibitor is a practical method for determining angiotensin-dependent blood pressure and has several advantages when compared to measurements of PRA. The response to the drug is prompt, a feature of cardinal importance in selecting treatment in hypertensive emergencies (41). The prompt response permits selection of initial therapy on a rational basis during the first office visit without having to wait for laboratory results. The test is inexpensive and can be done (with the orally active drugs) in a physician's office. The only risk of the test observed to date is induced hypotension, which can be prevented by testing only on normal sodium intake and without concurrent diuretic treatment.

In addition to guiding initial therapy, the angiotensin-converting enzyme inhibitor test (ACE test) can be used to screen for renovascular hypertension. Thus, in those patients suspected clinically of having underlying renovascular hypertension and also in those with large depressor responses to the first dose, measurement of PRA 90 min after captopril will provide important screening data.

A hypothetical scheme for the integration of the ACE test in the treatment of hypertension is illustrated in Fig. 7. This is one of many possible logical sequences of therapy derived from an orientation that uses drug responses as clues to underlying mechanisms and therefore as guides to the selection of individual medications. The major dif-

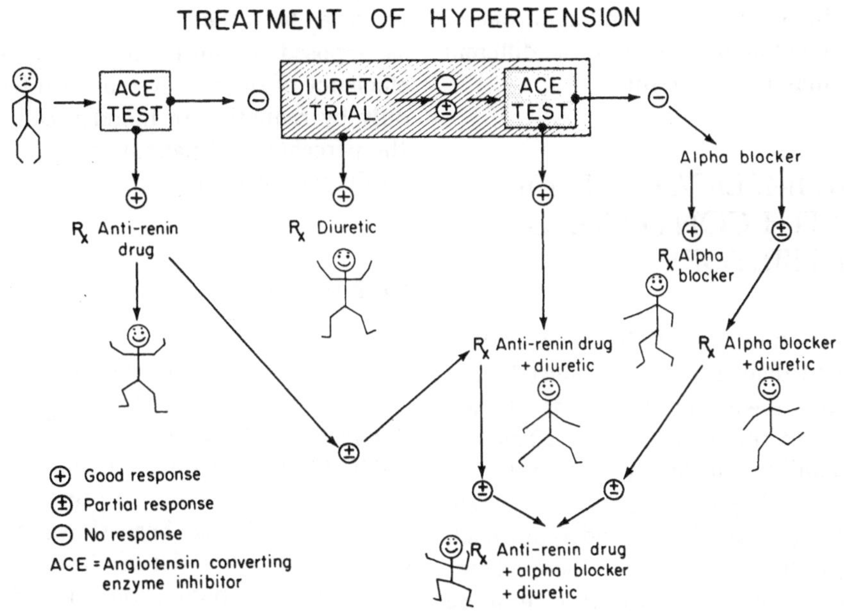

TREATMENT OF HYPERTENSION

⊕ Good response
⊕ Partial response
⊖ No response
ACE = Angiotensin converting
    enzyme inhibitor

Fig. 7. Schema for the treatment of hypertension using the ACE test (single-dose angiotensin-converting inhibitor). See text for details.

ference between this sequence and the stepped-care approach is its individualization of therapy based on observed antihypertensive responses. The initial step in the sequence is an ACE test done under conditions of normal sodium intake and in a representative seated position. A significant depressor response, although possibly not entirely due to blockade of angiotensin II formation, identifies renin-dependent hypertension. The relative magnitude of the response can be judged by the physician in the individual patient with respect to his actual level of pressure achieved as well as his clinical status. A good response signifies the employment of antirenin therapy such as can be achieved by beta-blockers or converting enzyme inhibitors. In this regard, responders to converting enzyme blockade have been shown to respond favorably to beta-blocker therapy (41). In addition, captopril shows evidence that the first dose response predicts the long-term response (4). A good but incomplete response to long-term antirenin therapy can be improved by addition of diuretic or dietary sodium restriction (2, 3, 42).

If there is only a minimal or no response to the initial ACE test, it is unlikely that the hypertension is renin dependent but it may, on the other hand, be sodium or volume dependent. Therefore,

the next diagnostic/therapeutic step is a trial of diuretic therapy for a period of 4–6 weeks. Since about two-thirds of low-renin patients will respond adequately to a diuretic alone (38), there will be only a relatively small percentage of the original number who will then prove poorly responsive to both initial ACE testing and subsequently to an adequate trial of diuretic therapy. That group of nonresponders, according to this schema, would have another ACE test while on diuretic to determine if their unresponsiveness could be due in part to high reactive levels of PRA. If so, the ACE test would reduce blood pressure and suggest the need for combined antirenin and diuretic therapy.

The residual nonresponders to the second ACE test appear to have another mechanism active in sustaining their hypertension—possibly increased alpha-adrenergic tone. Unfortunately, except in pheochromocytoma, there is no clinically useful measurement of this vasoconstrictor mechanism. Hence, this schema shown in Fig. 7 assesses the mechanism by exclusion, i.e., elimination of other mechanisms that can be identified. This group is treated with an alpha-blocker alone (e.g., prazosin, clonidine, or α-methyldopa) with addition of a diuretic if blood pressure control is incomplete or if sodium retention occurs. For the small number of patients incompletely controlled on one or two drugs, the combination of the three different kinds of drugs may be successful.

PRACTICAL IMPLICATIONS OF TESTING WITH CONVERTING ENZYME INHIBITORS

With any innovation of medical diagnosis or therapy, rigorous and deliberate testing must be applied to compare it with the standards already evolved and to determine its relative efficiency, practical applicability, and finally its overall economic impact. The hypothesis presented herein has not, as an integrated scheme, undergone such analysis. The question remains: Are there advantages in a strategy that purports to provide more specific therapy to one based on a commonly effective and time-honored drug (diuretic)?

There are several important matters to be taken into account in this comparison. First, the biochemical and physiological heterogeneity of hypertension has only recently become accepted. Thus, the condition of hypertension in the past was viewed as a relatively uniform condition, appropriately treated with a uniform approach as represented in stepped care. Second, the most recently recommended treatment plan for hypertension did not have the benefit of knowing the significant impact of beta-blockers in the last few years with regard to general effectiveness (36) and possible cardioprotectiveness.

Even though the ACE test is simple and can be used in the daily practice of medicine, its improvement over the present system remains to be determined. In the screening process for secondary hypertension, the ACE test in association with a serum potassium measurement as an index of hyperaldosteronism could form the basis of a very simple, inexpensive screening procedure. The combination of a low serum potassium and no response to a converting enzyme inhibitor is strong evidence for primary aldosteronism. However, low serum potassium plus a depressor response and reactive hyperreninemia are potent indicators of renal hypertension. Even if secondary hypertension is not found, the ACE test guides initial therapy. Moreover, the ACE test by its design seeks out mono-drug therapy before using two or three agents. In contrast, the stepped-care approach selects di-

uretic as base therapy for all and adds on drugs as opposed to substituting them. Ultimately the efficiency of the two systems can be compared not only by reduction of blood pressure, but also by the percentage of patients taking only one or two antihypertensive drugs.

SUMMARY

Acute testing with converting enzyme inhibitor can be used to detect renin-dependent and renin-independent forms of hypertension, which in turn influences the selection of initial long-term therapy. In addition, acute testing with angiotensin blocking agents has been shown to elicit a large, diagnostic reactive rise in plasma-renin activity in renovascular hypertension. These features of converting enzyme inhibition can be incorporated in a hypothetical schema that both tests for secondary forms of hypertension and initiates a sequence of treatment aimed at specific and simple treatment regimens.

REFERENCES

1. Morganti AA, Pickering TG, Lopez-Ovejero JA, Laragh JH (1979) Contrasting effects of acute beta blockade with propranolol on plasma catecholamines and renin is essential hypertension: a possible basis for the delayed antihypertensive response. Am Heart J 98: 490–494

2. Bravo EL, Tarazi RC (1979) Converting enzyme inhibition with an orally active compound in hypertensive man. Hypertension 1: 39–46

3. Case DB, Atlas SA, Laragh JH, Sealey JE, Sullivan PA, McKinstry DN (1978) Clinical experience with blockade of the renin-angiotensin-aldosterone system by an oral converting enzyme inhibitor (SQ 14225, captopril) in hypertensive patients. Prog. Cardiovasc Dis 21: 195–206

4. Case DB, Atlas SA, Laragh JH, Sullivan PA, Sealey JE (1980) Use of first dose response and plasma renin predict the long-term effect of captopril. J Cardiovasc Pharm 2: 339–346

5. Case DB, Wallace JM, Keim HJ, Sealey JE, Laragh JH (1976) Usefulness and limitations of saralasin, a weak competitive agonist of angiotensin II, for evaulating the renin and sodium factors in hypertensive patients. Am J Med 60: 825–836

6. Anderson GH Jr, Dalakos TG, Elias A, Tomycz N, Streeten DHP (1977) Diuretic therapy and response of essential hypertension to saralasin. Ann Int Med 87: 183–187

7. Case DB, Wallace JM, Keim HJ, Weber MA, Drayer JIM, White RP, Sealey JE, Laragh JH (1976) Estimating renin participation in hypertension: Superiority of converting enzyme inhibitor over saralasin. Am J Med 61: 790–796

8. Anderson GH Jr, Streeten DHP, Dalakos TG (1977) Pressor response to 1-sar-8-ala-angiotensin II (saralasin) in hypertensive patients. Circ Res 40: 243–251

9. Ferreira SH (1965) A bradykinin-potentiating factor (BPF) present in the venom of Bothrops jararaca. Br J Pharmacol Chemother 24: 163–169

10. Bakhle YS (1968) Conversion of angiotensin I to angiotensin II by cell-free extracts of dog lung. Nature 220: 919–920

11. Ng KKF, Vane JR (1967) Conversion of angiotensin I to angiotensin II. Nature 215: 762–766

12. Ng KKF, Vane JR (1968) Fate of angiotensin I in the circulation. Nature 218: 144–150

13. Ferreira SH, Greene LJ, Alabaster VA, Josip P, Weaver ER, Kocy O (1970) Activity of various fractions of bradykinin—potentiating factor against angiotensin I-converting enzyme. Nature 225: 379–380

14. Steward JM, Ferreira SH, Greene LJ (1971) Bradykinin-potentiating peptide PCA-Lys-Try-Ala-Pro. Biochem Pharmacol 20: 1557–1567

15. Ondetti MA, Williams NJ, Sabo EF, et al. (1971) Angiotensin-converting inhibitors from the venom of Borthrops jararaca: Isolation, elucidation of structure and synthesis. Biochemistry 10: 4033–4039

16. Cushman DW, Pluscek J, Williams NJ, Weaver ER, Sabo EF, Kocy O, Cheung HS, Ondetti MA (1973) Inhibition of angiotensin-converting enzyme by analogs of peptides from Bothrops jararaca venom. Experientia 29: 1032–1035

17. Cheung HS, Cushman DW (1973) Inhibition of homogenous angiotensin-converting enzyme of rabbit lung by synthetic venom peptides of Bothrops jararaca. Biochim Biophys Acta 293: 451–463

18. Collier, JG, Robinson BV, Vane JR (1973) Reduction of pressor effects of angiotensin I in man by synthetic nonapeptide (BPP$_{9a}$ or SQ 20881) which inhibits converting enzyme. Lancet 1: 72–74

19. Gavras H, Brunner HR, Laragh JH, Gavras I, Vukovich RA (1975) The use of antiotensin-converting enzyme inhibitor in the diagnosis and treatment of hypertension. Clin Sci Mol Med 48: 57S–60S

20. Case DB, Wallace JM, Keim HJ, Weber MA, Sealey JE, Laragh JH (1977) Possible role of renin in hypertension as suggested by renin-sodium profiling and inhibition of converting enzyme. N Engl J Med 296: 641–646

21. McGregor GA, Markander ND, Roulston JE, Jones JC (1979) Essential hypertension: Effect of an oral inhibitor of angiotensin-converting enzyme. Br Med J 2: 1106–1109

22. Baer L, Parra-Carrillo JZ, Radichevich I, Williams GS (1977) Detection of renovascular hypertension with angiotensin II blockade. Ann Intern Med 86: 257–260

23. Wilson HM, Wilson JP, Slaton PE, Foster JH, Liddle GW, Hollifield JW (1977) Saralasin infusion in the recognition of renovascular hypertension. Ann Intern Med 87: 36–42

24. Maxwell MH, Varady P, Zawada ET, Burkhalter JF, Waks U, Marks L (1978) Maximal discrimination of renovascular from essential hypertension by the saralasin test. Clin Sci Mol Med 55: 297S–299S

25. Case DB, Laragh JH (1979) Reactive hyperreninemia following angiotensin blockade with either saralasin or converting enzyme inhibitor: A new approach to screen for renovascular hypertension. Ann Intern Med 91: 153–160

26. Case DB, Atlas SA, Laragh JH (1979) Reactive hyperreninemia to angiotensin blockade identified renovascular hypertension. Clin Sci 57: 313S–316S, 1979.

27. Re R, Noveline R, Escourrou M-T, Athanasoulis C, Burton J, Haber E (1978) Inhibition of angiotensin-converting enzyme for diagnosis of renal-artery stenosis. N Engl J Med 298: 582–586

28. Vander AJ, Geelhoed GW (1965) Inhibition of renin secretion by angiotensin II. Proc Soc Exp Biol Med 120: 399–403

29. DeChamplain J, Genest J, Veyratt R, Boucher R (1966) Factors controlling renin in man. Arch Intern Med 117: 355–363

30. Bunag RD, Page IH, McCubbin JW (1967) Inhibition of renin release by vasopressin and angiotensin. Cardiovasc Res 1: 67–73

31. Shade RE, Davis JO, Johnson JA, Gotshall RW, Spielman WS (1973) Mechanism of action of angiotensin II and antidiuretic hormone on renin secretion. Am J Physiol 224: 926–943

32. Mendelsohn FAO, Johnston CI, Doyle AE Scoggins BA, Denton DA, Coghlan JP (1972) Renin angiotensin II and adrenal corticosteroid relationships during sodium deprivation and angiotensin infusion in normotensive and hypertensive man. Circ Res 31: 728–739

33. Case DB, Sullivan PA, Scahill RM, Heiderich S (1981) The captopril test. (In preparation)

34. Skrabal F, Czaykowska W, Dittrich P, Braunsteiner H (1976) Immediate plasma renin response to propranolol: Differentiation between essential and renal hypertension. Br Med J 2: 144–147

35. Bühler FR, Laragh JH, Baer L, Vaughan ED Jr, Brunner HR (1972) Propranolol inhibition of renin secretion. A specific approach to diagnosis and treatment of renin-dependent hypertensive diseases. N Engl J Med 287: 1209–1214

36. Veterans Administration Cooperative Study Group on Antihypertensive Agents (1977) Propranolol in the treatment of essential hypertension. JAMA 237: 2303–2310

37. Lindner A, Douglas SQ, Adamson JW (1978) Propranolol effects in long-term hemodialysis patients with renin-dependent hypertension. Ann Intern Med 88: 457–462

38. Vaughan ED Jr, Laragh JH, Gavras I, Bühler FR, Gavras H, Brunner HR, Baer L (1973) Volume factor in low and normal renin essential hypertension.

Treatment with either spironolactone or chlorthalidone. Am J Cardiol 32: 523–532

39. Douglas JG, Hollifield JW, Liddle GW (1974) Treatment of low renin essential hypertension. Comparison of spironolactone and a hydrochlorthiazide–triampterene combination. JAMA 227: 518–521

40. Woods JW, Pittman AW, Pullian CC, Werk EE Jr, Waider W, Allen CA (1976) Renin profiling in hypertension and its use in treatment with propranolol and chlorthalidone. N Engl J Med 294: 1137–1143

41. Tifft CP, Gavras H, Kershaw GR, Gavras I, Brunner HR, Liang C-S, Chobanian AV (1979) Converting enzyme inhibition in hypertensive emergencies. Ann Int Med 90: 43–47

42. Johnston CI, McGrath BP, Millar JA, Matthews PG (1979) Long-term effects of captopril (SQ 14,225) on blood pressure and hormone levels in essential hypertension. Lancet 2: 493–496

Does Captopril Decrease Blood Pressure by Mechanisms Other Than Inhibition of Angiotensin II Formation?

Michael J. Antonaccio and Magdi Asaad

The role of the renin-angiotensin-aldosterone system (RAS) in hypertension is still a matter of great controversy. Therefore, it is not surprising that the mechanism of action of captopril, a drug that interferes with the RAS, is also controversial, since it is efficacious in most forms of hypertension regardless of etiology or plasma-renin activity (PRA) (1). Despite the demonstrated specificity of captopril against angiotensin-converting enzyme (ACE) with a consequent decrease in AII levels, several studies suggest a mechanism of action independent of the RAS, and even from ACE inhibition (2–4). As shown in Table 1, there are several lines of evidence that suggest that captopril may have actions other than reducing AII formation. These may be further divided into effects either related or unrelated to ACE inhibition (Table 2).

EFFECTS RELATED TO ACE INHIBITION

KININS

ACE is the same enzyme as kininase II, which degrades kinins. Therefore, it is possible that captopril could act by increasing kinin levels. Direct measurement of kinins after captopril has provided little help, since increases, decreases, and no change have been reported. It is important, however, to note that some investigators report increases in plasma bradykinin levels in normotensive patients whose blood pressure is unchanged after captopril. Conversely, no changes in bradykinin levels have been observed in groups of hypertensive patients in whom blood pressure was significantly reduced by captopril (1). Indirect evidence against the involvement of kinins comes from several other sources:

1. Pretreatment of spontaneously hypertensive rats (SHR) with the kallikrein inhibitor aprotinin did not alter the antihypertensive action of captopril, suggesting that de novo synthesis of kinins is not involved (5).
2. Captopril has no important effect either in the development or in the established state of DOCA-salt hypertension (6–8). Since this is a model of high kallikrein activity, captopril would be predicted to have a profound antihypertensive effect through inhibition of kinin degradation.
3. The hemodynamic consequences of bradykinin administration—direct vasodilation with marked reflex increases in heart rate—are in contrast to the actual changes observed after captopril (5).
4. The reduction in blood pressure after captopril requires several days to return to control levels after discontinuation of drug (1).

Table 1. Does captopril decrease blood pressure by mechanisms other than inhibition of angiotensin II formation?

Reasons for asking:
1. Effectiveness in normal and low reninemic hypertension, such as human essential hypertension, SHR, chronic one- and two-kidney renal hypertension where AII antagonists are ineffective.
2. Dissociation of effects from reductions in AII levels.
3. Dissociation from ACE inhibition.
4. Changes in other factors controlling blood pressure such as kinin levels, salt excretion, and so forth.
5. Effectiveness despite prior AII receptor blockade.
6. Effectiveness in nephrectomized animals and humans.

Table 2. Potential antihypertensive mechanisms of captopril.

Mechanisms related to ACE inhibition	Mechanisms unrelated to ACE inhibition
1. Kinins (plasma, urinary, local)	1. Direct vasodilator
2. Prostaglandins (particularly PGI_2)	2. Receptor antagonist
3. Aldosterone	3. Nonspecific effects (related to -SH?)
4. Central effects	4. Sympathetic blockade (ganglionic, nerves, terminals)
	5. Reflex effects (peripheral and/or central)

Since ACE activity returns to control levels well before blood pressure, and since bradykinin has a very short half-life, significant bradykinin accumulation appears unlikely as a primary antihypertensive mechanism.

PROSTAGLANDIN (PG) RELEASE

Bradykinin releases vasodilating and natriuretic PGs from renal and other tissues, an effect that is enhanced by captopril (9). Therefore, PGs may theoretically play a role in the hemodynamic actions of captopril. However, this now seems unlikely, since pretreatment of SHR with either aspirin or indomethacin does not reduce the antihypertensive, renal vasodilating, and renin-releasing effects of captopril (8, 10). Similar results have also been obtained in dogs (11). In hypertensive patients, PGE_2 levels were not altered by captopril (12).

ALDOSTERONE

Captopril has been consistently shown to decrease aldosterone secretion in hypertensive animals and humans (1). Since this undoubtedly is a consequence related to inhibition of AII formation, it is difficult to determine how much of the antihypertensive action of captopril is directly related to reductions in AII formation in comparison to how much is due to reductions in aldosterone secretion. Certainly the acute antihypertensive effects of captopril in SHR are not due to aldosterone inhibition, since reductions in blood pressure were unaltered after bilateral adrenalectomy, either prior to or following captopril administration (13). In salt-depleted dogs whose blood pressure was markedly reduced by captopril, infusions of aldosterone sufficient to restore predrug plasma levels had no effect on blood pressure, whereas similar infusions with AII completely restored blood pressure to predrug levels (14).

CENTRAL EFFECTS

Although high doses of captopril (>1 mg/kg) directly injected into the cerebral ventricles of SHR or renal hypertensive rats caused modest reductions in blood pressure (15, 16), captopril does not appear to cross the blood brain barrier even after high doses given chronically (17, 18). Thus a significant central effect of captopril appears unlikely.

UNRELATED TO ACE INHIBITION

Several authors have suggested that captopril has an antihypertensive action independent of ACE inhibition. The most compelling evidence derives from studies involving nephrectomized animals or patients. Several investigators have shown that captopril decreases blood pressure in dogs as well as inhibiting the reflexes induced by bilateral carotid artery occlusion (3, 4, 19). These effects were not altered by nephrectomy or prior AII receptor blockade with saralasin. In other studies, captopril did not lower blood pressure in fluid or salt-replete nephrectomized hypertensive patients (20, 21). However, when the patients were fluid or salt depleted, captopril was dramatically antihypertensive in these patients. Therefore, it is undeniable that plasma renin had little to do with the latter efficacy of captopril. But what about the possibility of vascular renin playing a role? Arterial renin concentrations (ARC) in SHR and chronic two-kidney renal hypertensive rats are elevated relative to their normotensive counterparts, despite normal PRA, suggesting a causal role in generating or maintaining the hypertension (8, 22). As shown

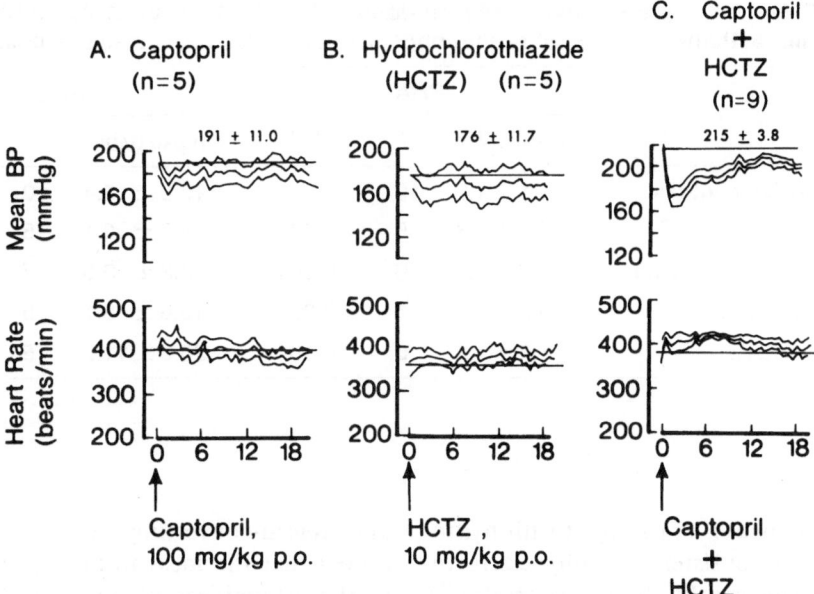

Fig. 1. Effects of captopril on mean blood pressure (mean BP) and heart rate of conscious spontaneously hypertensive rats (SHR). **(a)** Sham bilateral nephrectomy (Nx), salt-replete; **(b)** mean BP after actual bilateral nephrectomy; **(c)** mean BP after actual bilateral nephrectomy in SHR fed a low-salt diet for 2 weeks. (———) MBP before surgery.

in Fig. 1, captopril has only minor antihypertensive effects in nephrectomized versus intact SHR. However, in nephrectomized SHR on a low-salt diet for 2 weeks followed by furosemide, captopril caused significant reductions in mean blood pressure. As shown in Fig. 2, neither captopril nor hydrochlorothiazide alone had any pronounced effect on mean blood pressure of DOCA-salt rats,

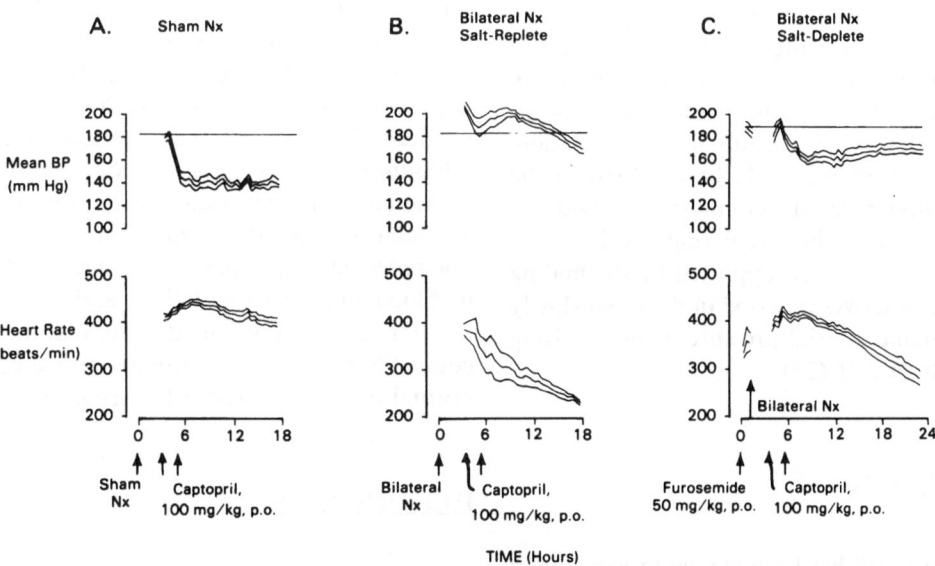

Fig. 2. Mean blood pressure (mean BP) and heart rate of conscious DOCA-salt uninephrectomized hypertensive rats after either **(a)** captopril alone, **(b)** hydrochlorothiazide alone, or **(c)** the combination of hydrochlorothiazide plus captopril. (———) Mean BP before drugs. Abscissa is plotted as time (h).

Table 3. Effect of captopril, hydrochlorothiazide (HCTZ), alone or in combination on plasma-renin activity and arterial renin concentration of DOCA-salt hypertensive rats.

Treatment	PRA			ARC		
	ngAI/ml/hr	N	P	ngAI/g/hr	N	P
Prehypertensive controls	10.1 ± 1.2	12	—	18.0 ± 3.4	10	—
Vehicle	0.5 ± 0.3	5	< 0.001	4.2 ± 2.1	5	< 0.02
Captopril (100 mg/kg p.o.)	0.7 ± 0.3	6	< 0.001	8.3 ± 3.5	5	—
HCTZ (10 mg/kg p.o.)	0.2 ± 0.1	6	< 0.001	15.6 ± 8.1	5	—
Captopril + HCTZ	1.8 ± 1.3	6	< 0.001	26.0 ± 11.8	5	—

whereas the combination of captopril with hydrochlorothiazide was consistently antihypertensive. PRA was not significantly altered by treatment with either captopril or hydrochlorothiazide, alone or in combination (Table 3). In contrast, both captopril and hydrochlorothiazide caused elevations of ARC, the greatest increase occurring with the combination of both drugs. On the basis of these data, it is tempting to suggest that the elevation of ARC by hydrochlorothiazide and the consequent inhibition of local formation of AII by simultaneous captopril administration was responsible for the antihypertensive action of the combination therapy. Similarly, increases in vascular renin activity in nephrectomized salt-depleted SHR or humans might contribute to the hypertension, an effect blocked by captopril. Therefore, we feel that the antihypertensive actions of captopril in normal or low plasma-renin conditions is not inconsistent with its ability to inhibit AII formation. Rather, AII formation might be localized in the vasculature under certain circumstances and not necessarily reflected in circulating levels or by PRA. This suggestion is supported by the finding that AII infusion over a period of days can slowly increase systemic arterial pressure without raising plasma levels of AII (23).

CONCLUSION

Although captopril has been shown to have many effects that do not necessarily correlate with reductions in angiotensin II plasma concentrations, these effects may still be related to inhibition of angiotensin-converting enzyme. Evidence is presented that the local formation of angiotensin II in the arterial vasculature may be important in the regulation of blood pressure, or maintenance of hypertension, or both. It seems likely that captopril may owe some of its antihypertensive actions to inhibition of the renin-angiotensin system in arterial smooth muscle.

SUMMARY

Captopril inhibits angiotensin-converting enzyme (ACE) and consequently decreases angiotensin II formation. However, captopril is an effective antihypertensive agent in most forms of hypertension despite the levels of angiotensin II. Therefore, it is possible that captopril may have actions independent of angiotensin II synthesis or even of ACE inhibition. When the evidence for such possibilities is examined, it seems unlikely that this may occur. Vascular production of angiotensin II, which is not reflected in plasma levels, may be important in blood pressure regulation, and the inhibition of ACE by captopril in the vasculature may account for some of its antihypertensive activity in normal or low reninemic hypertension.

REFERENCES

1. Rubin B, Antonaccio MJ (1980) Captopril. In: Scriabine A (ed) The Pharmacology of Antihypertensive Drugs. Raven Press, New York, pp 21–42
2. Marks ES, Bing RF, Thurston H, Swales JD (1980)

Vasodepressor property of the converting enzyme inhibitor captopril (SQ 14,225): The role of factors other than renin-angiotensin blockade in the rat. Clin Sci 58: 1–6

3. Vollmer RR, Boccagno JA, Harris DN, Murthy VS (1978) Hypotension induced by inhibition of angiotensin-converting enzyme in pentobarbital-anesthetized dogs. Eur J Pharmacol 51: 39–45

4. Jandhyala BS, Nandiwada P, Buckley JP, Kokhandwala MF (1979) Studies on the mechanism of the hypotensive action of SQ 14,225, and angiotensin-converting enzyme inhibitor of anesthetized dogs. Res Commun Chem Pathol Pharmacol 25: 429–446

5. Antonaccio MJ, Rubin B, Horovitz ZP (1980) Effects of captopril in animal models of hypertension. Clin Exp Hyper 2: 613–638

6. Douglas BH, Langford HG, McCaa RE (1979) Response of mineralocorticoid hypertensive animals to an angiotensin I converting enzyme inhibitor. Proc Soc Exp Biol Med 161: 86–87

7. Rubin B, Antonaccio MJ, Horovitz ZP (1980) The antihypertensive effects of captopril in hypertensive animal models. In: Zola P (ed) Angiotensin converting enzyme inhibitors. Horovitz, Urban and Schwarzenberg, Baltimore, Maryland

8. Antonaccio MJ, Assad M, Rubin B, Horovitz ZP (1980) Captopril: Factors involved in its mechanism of action. In: Zola P (ed) Angiotensin converting enzyme inhibitors, Horovitz, Urban and Schwarzenberg, Baltimore, Maryland

9. Murthy VS, Waldron TL, Goldberg ME (1978) The mechanism of bradykinin potentiation after inhibition of angiotensin-converting enzyme by SQ 14,225 in conscious rabbits. Circ Res 43 (Suppl I): 40–45

10. Antonaccio MJ, Harris D, Goldenberg H, High JP, Rubin B (1979) The effects of captopril, propranolol and indomethacin on blood pressure and plasma renin activity in spontaneously hypertensive and normotensive rats. Proc Soc Exp Biol Med 162: 429–433

11. Tobia A, Giardino E (1980) Captopril-induced renal vasodilation in pentobarbital anesthetized dogs. Fed Proc 39: 1189

12. Bravo EL, Tarazi RC (1979) Converting enzyme inhibition with an orally active compound in hypertensive man. Hypertension 1: 39–46

13. Antonaccio MJ, High JP, Rubin B, Schaeffer T (1979) Contribution of the kidneys but not adrenal

glands to the acute antihypertensive effects of captopril in spontaneously hypertensive rats. Clin Sci 57 (Suppl 5): 127S–130S

14. Hall JE, Guyton AC, Smith MJ, Jr, Coleman TC (1979) Chronic blockade of angiotensin II formation during sodium deprivation. Am J Physiol 237: 424–432

15. Stamler JF, Brady MJ, Phillips MI (1980) The central and peripheral effects of captopril (SW 14m225) on the arterial pressure of the spontaneously hypertensive rat. Brain Res 186: 499–503

16. Scholkens BA (1979) Intraventricular injection of the angiotensin converting enzyme inhibitor SQ 14,225 in rats with experimental hypertension. IRCS Med Sci 7: 270

17. Vollmer RR, Boccagno JA (1977) Central cardiovascular effects of SQ 14,225, and angiotensin converting enzyme inhibitor in chloralose anesthetized cats. Eur J Pharmacol 45: 117–125

18. Mann JFE, Rascher W, Dietz R, Schomig A, Gauten D (1979) Effects of an orally active converting-enzyme inhibitor, SQ 14,225, on pressor responses to angiotensin administered into the brain ventricles on spontaneously hypertensive rats. Clin Sci 56: 585–589

19. Harris DN, Heran CL, Goldenberg HJ, High JP, Laffan RJ, Rubin B, Antonaccio MJ, Goldberg ME (1978) Effects of SQ 14,225 an orally active inhibitor of angiotensin-converting enzyme on blood pressure, heart rate and plasma renin activity of conscious normotensive dogs. Eur J Pharmacol 51: 345–349

20. Man in 'T Veld AJ, Wenting GJ, Schalekamp MADH (1979) Does captopril lower blood pressure in anephric patients? Br Med J 2: 1110

21. Man in 'T Veld AJ, Schicht IM, Derkx FHM, de Bruyn JHB, Schalekamp MADH (1980) Effect of an angiotensin converting enzyme inhibitor (captopril) on blood pressure in anephric subjects. Br Med J 1: 288–290

22. Thurston H, Swales JD, Bind RF, Hurst BC, Marks ES (1979) Vascular renin-like activity and blood pressure maintenance in the rat. Hypertension 1: (6) 634–649

23. Bean BL, Brown JL, Casals-Stenzel J, Fraser R, Lever AF, Millar JA, Morton JJ, Petch B, Riegger AJG, Robertson JIS, Tree M (1979) The relation of arterial pressures and plasma angiotensin II concentration. Circ Res 44: 452–458

The Effects of Intravenous Angiotensin II on the Cardiac Baroreceptor Reflex

Eugenie R. Lumbers, Erica K. Potter, D. I. McCloskey, M. J. Ismay, W. B. Lee, and A. D. Stevens

In their original studies in man, Smyth et al. (1) found that when i.v. phenylephrine [an alpha-agonist with no direct cardiac effects (2)] was used to increase arterial pressure, there was a linear relationship between systolic pressure and the pulse interval. However, when they used i.v. angiotensin II to increase arterial pressure, they observed an initial increase in pulse interval as arterial pressure increased, but "later points in the response . . . tended to depart from the regularly linear relation."

Experiments were carried out in conscious sheep and anesthetized mongrel dogs to find out if the reflex cardiac slowing that occurred in response to angiotensin-induced hypertension was different from the reflex cardiac response to phenylephrine-induced hypertension, to find the reasons for this difference, and to see if angiotensin plays a significant role in the regulation of heart rate. Baroreflex sensitivity was measured as the slope of the linear relationship between systolic pressure and pulse interval measured following i.v. injection of phenylephrine (1, 3).

Figure 1(a,c) shows that when i.v. phenylephrine (0.25–2 mg) was used to increase arterial pressure, there was a progressive increase in pulse interval. When i.v. angiotensin (2.5–25 μg) was used to increase arterial pressure, there was no progressive increase in pulse interval (Fig. 2b). Often there was a transient bradycardia, but pulse interval then fell as systolic pressure continued to rise.

After beta-adrenergic blockade with propranolol (15–20 mg i.v., followed by an infusion of 0.36–5 μg/min), the pressor response to i.v. injection of angiotensin was still not associated with a progressive increase in pulse interval, even though the baroreflex sensitivity measured using phenylephrine was increased from 28.8 $\pm$ 4.9 msec/mmHg to 48.2 $\pm$ 6.2 msec/mmHg (SEM)

in nonpregnant sheep and from 12.43 $\pm$ 2.45 msec/mmHg to 20.9 $\pm$ 5.41 msec/mmHg in pregnant sheep (3). After parasympathetic blockade (2–4 mg atropine, followed by an infusion of 0.4 mg/min) and combined parasympathetic and sympathetic blockade, i.v. injections of angiotensin and phenylephrine failed to evoke any reflex bradycardia or tachycardia.

These results suggested that the lack of a baroreceptor-mediated cardiopdepressor reflex when angiotensin was used to raise arterial pressure was due to inhibition by angiotensin II of the reflex vagal excitation that occurs in response to hypertension. This finding was confirmed in experiments in anesthetized dogs in which it was shown that efferent cardiac vagal discharge in single fibers dissected from the right vagus did not increase as systolic pressure increased following injections of angiotensin (Fig. 2, right). When arterial pressure was raised by injection of phenylephrine, there was a progressive increase in vagal discharge (4) (Fig. 2, left).

This action of angiotensin II was exerted beyond the level of the baroreceptors, since the afferent discharge recorded in single baroreceptor fibers dissected from the carotid sinus nerves of three dogs was similar with respect to arterial pressure when arterial pressure was raised by i.v. angiotensin and phenylephrine (4).

In six conscious sheep the pressor effect of 0.22–44 μg/min i.v. angiotensin II was antagonized by a concomitant i.v. infusion of sodium nitroprusside (5) (22–165 μg/min). As the dose of angiotensin II was increased, pulse interval decreased in a dose-dependent manner. This dose-dependent fall in pulse interval was not affected by beta-adrenergic blockade with propranolol. However, it was neither present after treatment with atropine nor after treatment with atropine and propranolol. These results are compatible with

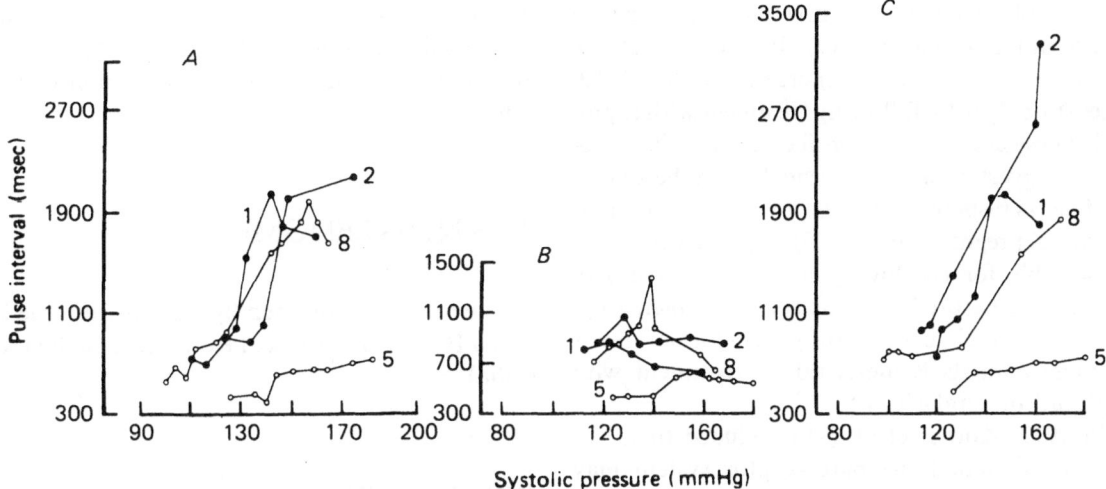

Fig. 1. The relationship between systolic pressure and pulse interval in two nonpregnant ewes (●) and two pregnant ewes (○), when arterial pressure was increased by i.v. injection of phenylephrine **(a,c)** and when arterial pressure was increased by i.v. injection of angiotensin II **(b)**. [Ismay et al. (3), with permission]

the hypothesis that i.v. angiotensin inhibits tonic vagal discharge as well as the increase in vagal discharge evoked by a rise in arterial pressure. They suggest that changes in circulating levels of angiotensin II could modify reflex regulation of heart rate.

This finding was confirmed by showing that the baroreflex sensitivities of five sheep measured using i.v. phenylephrine to raise arterial pressure were depressed during infusions of angiotensin alone

and during infusions of angiotensin in which the pressor action of angiotensin was antagonized by concomitant infusion of sodium nitroprusside (6). Furthermore, the angiotensin antagonist saralasin and the converting enzyme inhibitor captopril modify the cardiac baroreflex. In four pregnant sheep, captopril (10–20 mg, followed by an i.v. infusion of 100 μg/kg/h) produced a fall in systolic pressure of 9.6 $\pm$ 2.8 mmHg that was not associated with a reflex tachycardia. This shift in the

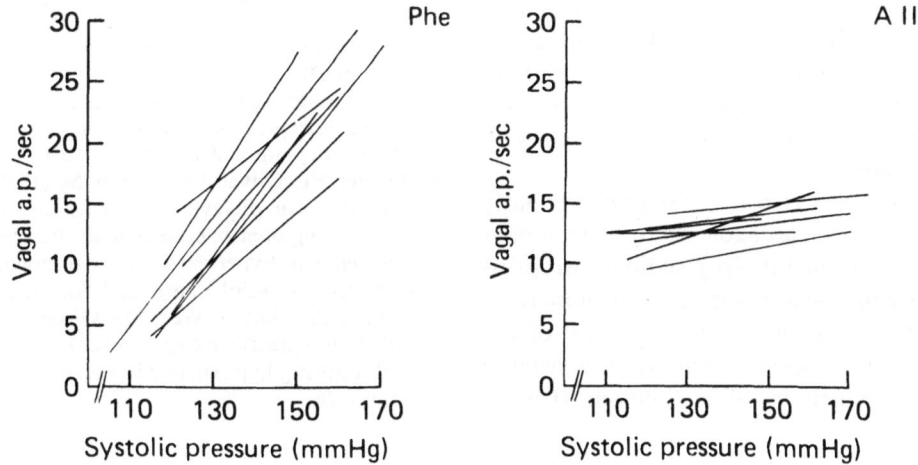

Fig. 2. In the mongrel dog anesthetized with chloralose, the regression lines for cardiac vagal efferent activity (vagal ap/sec) were plotted against systolic pressure for the same periods following i.v. injection of phenylephrine *(left)* and angiotensin *(right)*. There was a progressive increase in vagal discharge when phenylephrine was used to raise arterial pressure. There was no progressive increase in vagal discharge when angiotensin was used to increase arterial pressure. [Lumbers et al. (4), with permission]

location of the baroreflex curve has also been seen in sodium-depleted dogs (7). In pregnant sheep, baroreflex sensitivity was increased by 8.1 ± 5.0 msec/mmHg (SD) following treatment with captopril. These effects of captopril on the cardiac baroreflex suggest that angiotensin II may be one of the factors responsible for the lower baroreflex sensitivity of pregnant animals (3). Angiotensin is also responsible for the low gain (i.e., sensitivity) of the cardiac baroreflex of the sodium-depleted hypertensive rabbit, because the gain of the baroreflex of these animals is increased by treatment with captopril or saralasin (8).

In 1973, Korner et al. (9) concluded that, "In the intact animal the baroreceptor system may thus be considered to change from a fixed-value servocontrol system in which performance depends almost entirely on the output from the arterial baroreceptors during resting conditions to a variable-reference servocontrol system in which other inputs are important determinants of the system's responses to arterial blood pressure stimuli during disturbances." The experiments described demonstrate that one of the other "inputs" referred to in the above statement is the renin-angiotensin system.

SUMMARY

In conscious sheep and anesthetized dogs there was no sustained decrease in heart rate when arterial pressure was increased by i.v. bolus injections of angiotensin II. Intravenous angiotensin II inhibited the increase in efferent cardiac vagal discharge, which is a reflex response to increases in arterial pressure.

When angiotensin II was infused intravenously and its pressor action antagonized by concomitant infusion of a vasodilator drug sodium nitroprusside, angiotensin caused a dose-dependent increase in heart rate and reduced the sensitivity of the cardiac baroreflex response to increases in arterial pressure. These actions of angiotensin II were unaffected by beta-adrenoceptor blockade with propranolol. It was concluded that high levels of angiotensin modify the reflex regulation of heart rate.

ACKNOWLEDGMENT

This work was supported by a grant from the National Health and Medical Research Council (Australia).

REFERENCES

1. Smyth HS, Sleight P, Pickering GW (1969) Reflex regulation of arterial pressure during sleep in man. Circ Res 24: 109–121
2. Varma S, Johnson, SD, Sherman, DD, Youmans WB (1960) Mechanisms of inhibition of heart rate by phenylephrine. Circ Res 8: 1182–1186
3. Ismay MJA, Lumbers ER, Stevens AD (1979) The action of angiotensin II on the baroreceptor response of the conscious ewe and the conscious fetus. J Physiol (Lond) 288: 467–469
4. Lumbers ER, McCloskey DI, Potter ER (1979) Inhibition by angiotensin II of baroreceptor-evoked activity in cardiac vagal efferent nerves in the dog. J Physiol (Lond) 294: 69–80
5. Lee WB, Ismay MJ, Lumbers ER (1980) Mechanisms by which angiotensin II affects the heart rate of the conscious sheep. Cir Res 47(2): 286–292
6. Lee WB, Lumbers ER (1980) Angiotensin and the cardiac baroreflex response to phenylephrine. Clin Exp Pharmacol Physiol (to be published)
7. Clough DP, Conway J, Hatton R, Scott KL (1979) The effect of angiotensin converting enzyme inhibitor on baroreceptor reflexes in conscious dogs during sodium depletion. J Physiol (Lond) 295: 75–76P
8. Korner PI, Oliver JR, Fahim M (1979) Effects of alterations in dietary salt intake and possible role of renin-angiotensin system on the baroreceptor-heart rate reflex in hypertensive and normotensive rabbits. Proc Aust Physiol Pharmacol Soc 10(2): 291
9. Korner PI, Shaw J, West MJ, Oliver JR, Hilder RG (1973) Integrative reflex control of heart rate in the rabbit during hypoxia and hyperventilation. Circ Res 33: 63–76

Captopril in Angiotensin-Salt Hypertension: A Possible Linkage between Angiotensin, Salt, Vascular Disease, and Renomedullary Interstitial Cells

E. E. Muirhead, J. A. Pitcock, B. Brooks, and P. S. Brown

Angiotensin-salt hypertension (ASH) of the rat is induced by removing one kidney, injecting angiotensin subcutaneously each day (0.1 μg/g body wt), and placing the animal on 1% NaCl solution to drink (1, 2). The hypertensive state is derived consistently when the syngeneic rat line, Wistar/GM (3), is used.

In this chapter, we wish to consider a possible relationship between two levels of salt intake to the level of arterial pressure (AP), vascular disease, and the state of the renomedullary interstitial cells (RIC).

TWO LEVELS OF HYPERTENSION VERSUS TWO LEVELS OF SALT INTAKE

In three earlier groups of animals (1–3) (series A), the intake of 1% NaCl solution varied between 30 and 55 ml/day (~4.5–7 mEq Na), most often 30–40 ml/day. The AP was elevated to 150–160 mmHg (control AP 115 ± 2 mmHg). In a recent series of animals (series B, $n = 16$), the 1% NaCl solution intake was 100 ml/day (~15 mEq Na). The AP reached 170–200 mmHg (Fig.1).

The ultimate elevation of the AP was dependent on both factors, angiotensin and salt. Salt without angiotensin plus uninephrectomy elevated the AP slightly (115 ± 2 to 126 ± 2 mmHg), while angiotensin without salt plus uninephrectomy had no effect on the AP. The hypertension was associated with expansion of the extracellular fluid (ECF) volume and elevation of exchangeable Na(2). Other indications of volume expansion included suppressed PRA, decreased aldosterone secretion and reduced JG index.

STATE OF VISCERAL ARTERIAL-ARTERIOLAR VESSELS

Series A displayed hypertrophy and hyperplasia of small visceral arteries (the Folkow-Bevan change) (Fig. 2), but no evidence of acute vascular damage (2) (absence of fibrinoid necrosis, myo-hyalinosis (4), and the onion-skin lesion—renamed musculomucoid intimal hyperplasia (5). The recent group (series B) displayed fibrinoid necrosis and musculomucoid intimal hyperplasia of vessels in the viscera (Figs. 3 and 4). Thus, there was an association between angiotensin, salt intake, AP, and acute vascular disease.

EFFECT OF CAPTOPRIL

The converting enzyme inhibitor, captopril, given by mouth at 3, 30, and 60 mg/kg/day, significantly lowered the AP of animals in series A (6) but failed to lower the AP of animals in series B at doses of 10, 30, and 60–100 mg/kg/day (Figs. 5 and 6).

STATE OF RENOMEDULLARY INTERSTITIAL CELLS (RIC) WITHIN THE REMAINING KIDNEY

STATE OF THE RIC OF ANIMALS IN SERIES A COMPARED WITH THAT OF ANIMALS IN SERIES B (TABLE 1)

The group not responding to captopril (series B) had fewer RIC in the renal papilla (method de-

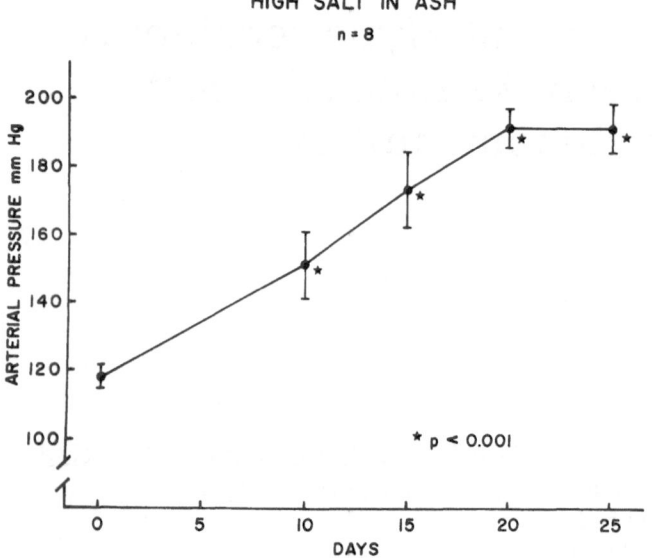

HIGH SALT IN ASH

n = 8

* p < 0.001

Fig. 1. Arterial pressure (AP) elevation of animals in series B (ASH plus high salt intake). The average pressure exceeds 180 mmHg.

scribed in ref. 9) than did the group responding (series A). The number of lipid granules in the RIC was not different between the two groups. There was, however, an outstanding difference in the appearance of the RIC between the two groups. The RIC of series A animals (responders) retained most of the morphologic features of normal RIC, emphasis on the lipid granule–cistern relationship

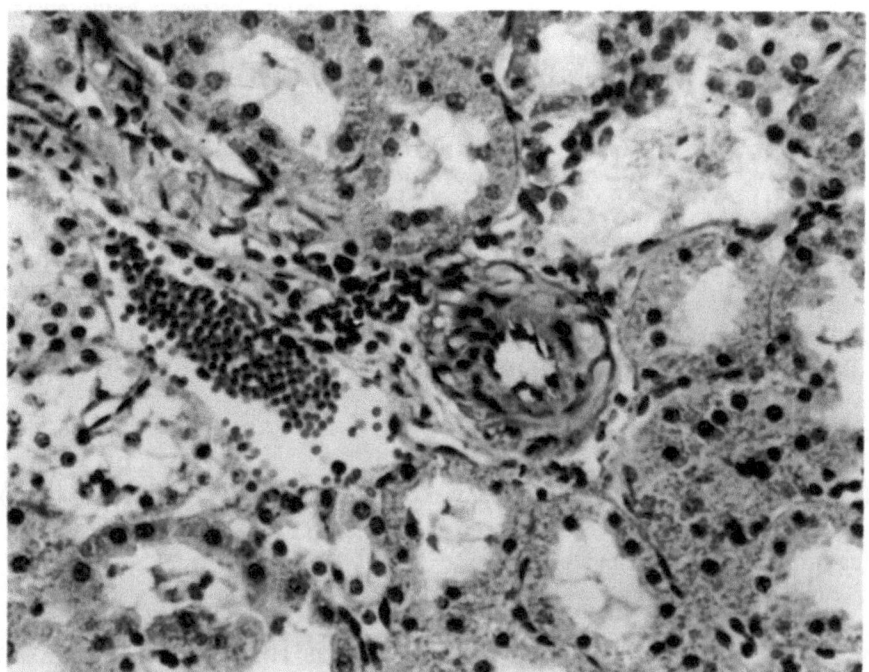

Fig. 2. Small artery in the kidney of an animal in series A [angiotensin = salt hypertension (ASH) plus lower salt intake]. The vessel is thickened due to hypertrophy and hyperplasia of the media (the Folkow-Bevan change). H&E × 175.

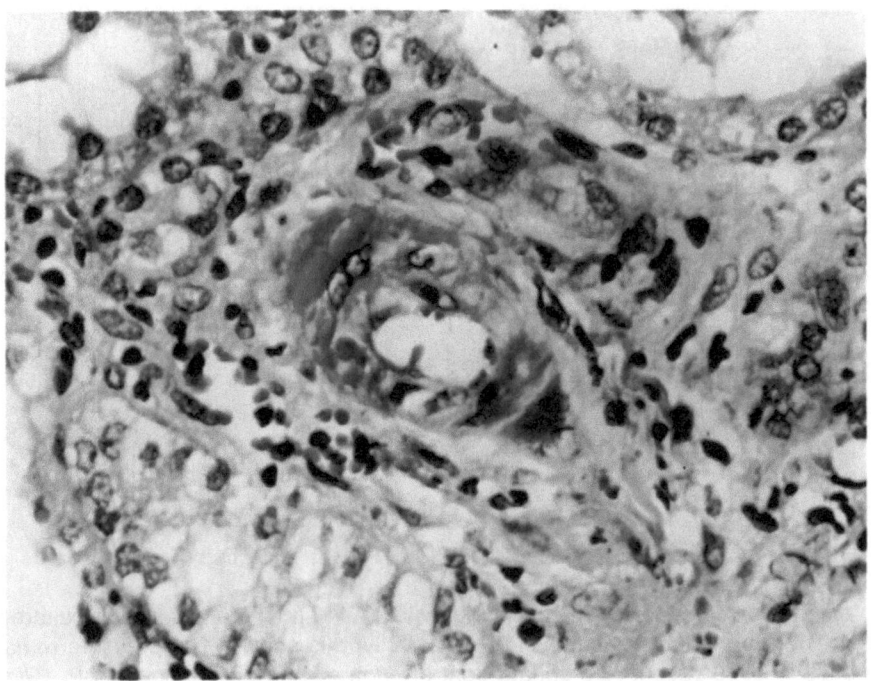

Fig. 3. This small artery in the kidney (series B) displays fibrinoid necrosis. H&E × 175.

(densely osmiophilic and normal looking). The RIC of series B animals (nonresponders) were markedly degenerated (round, having clear cytoplasm, loss of cisterns, pale and moth-eaten granules (Figs. 7 and 8).

EFFECT OF EXTRARENAL RIC

Transplants of fragmented renal medulla and of RIC grown as a monolayer cell culture (into series A animals) lowered the AP of ASH (3, 7)

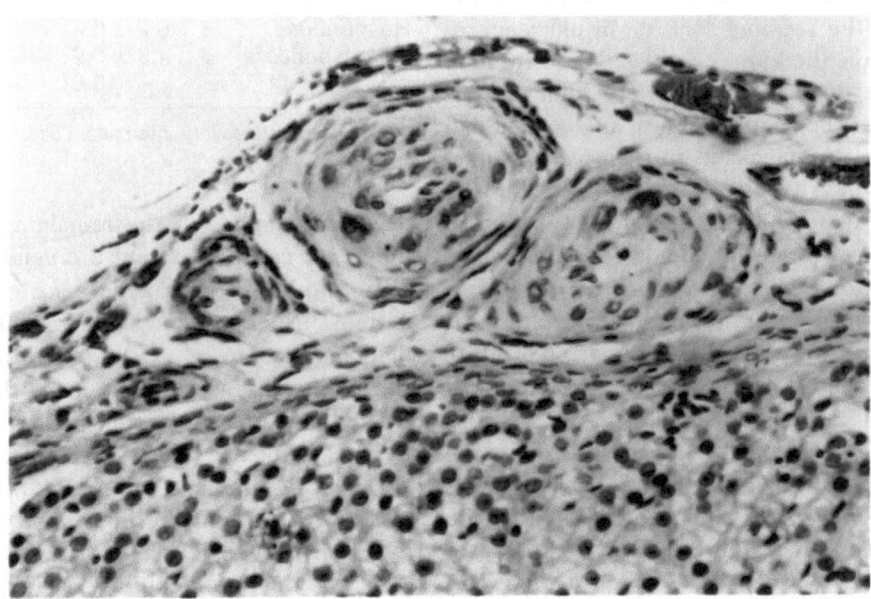

Fig. 4. Three vessels in the adrenal capsule (series B) reveal musculomucoid intimal hyperplasia (onion-skin lesion). H&E × 250.

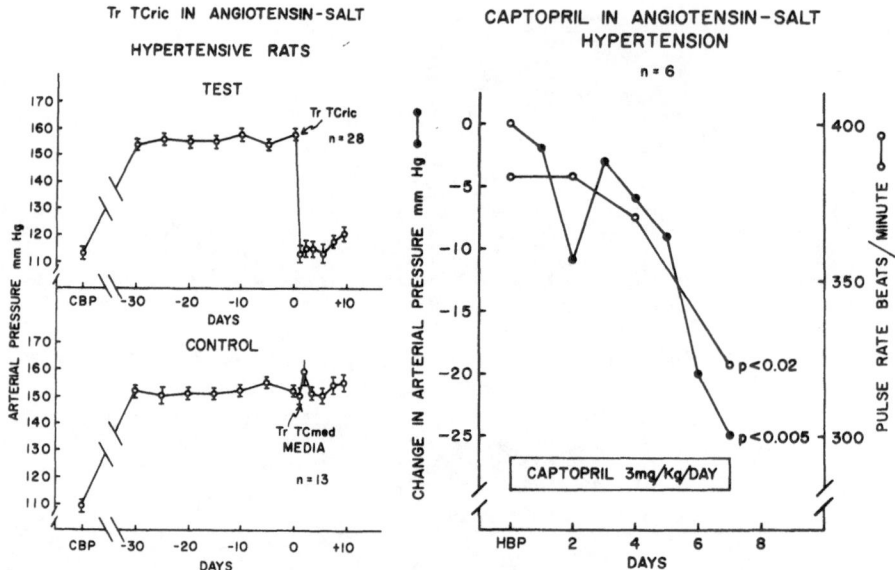

Fig. 5. *(Left, upper)* Lowering of the AP to normal within 24 h after transplants of cultured renomedullary interstitial cells (RIC) in animals having ASH of series A type is shown. The pressure remained depressed for the 8–10 days of observation. Appropriate controls *(lower)* had no change in AP. *(Right)* A significant lowering of the AP by captopril (3 mg/kg/day p.o.) (series A). As the AP was lowered, the pulse rate also was lowered. [Figure *(left)* from Muirhead et al. (1974) The Antihypertensive Action of Renomedullary Interstitial Cells Grown in Tissue Culture. Courtesy of Acta Physiologica Latino Americana. Figure *(right)* from Muirhead et al. (1980) Arch Path Lab Med, p 631. Copyright 1980, American Medical Association.]

(Fig. 5). This effect, on occasion, was rapid (reaching its nadir within 24 h) and in some groups, lasted 2 weeks or longer, i.e., as long as the transplant was viable.

The antihypertensive action of RIC outside the kidney and the seeming lack or insufficiency of activity within the kidney implies a constraining influence on these cells within the kidney. It is proposed that the combination of angiotensin and the elevated salt intake constitute the constraining factors. In other hypertensive settings of the rat, angiotensin alone (8) and salt alone (9) seemed to be injurious to the RIC, making its antihypertensive function defective.

ASH of the rat was low grade when the salt intake was at a lower level (usually 4.5–6.5 mEq/day). Under these conditions (series A), there was an absence of acute vascular disease and a significant response to captopril (6). When the salt intake was high (~15 mEq/day), the hypertensive state was high grade (series B) and associated with acute vascular disease and failure to respond to captopril.

The state of the RIC differed markedly in the two series of animals. The lower salt type had reasonably intact RIC in the papilla of the remaining kidney. The higher salt type had extremely

Table 1. Captopril in angiotensin = salt hypertension.

Group	n	No. RIC/grid[a]	No. granules/cell
Responders	5	6.2 ± 0.4	6.8 ± 0.7
Nonresponders	7	4.9 ± 0.2	6.0 ± 0.8
p		< 0.01	> 0.3

[a] RIC, Renomedullary interstitial cells.

degenerated RIC in the remaining papilla. This difference could represent a crucial point.

In another setting, a decrease of RIC plus an extreme degeneration of the remaining cells was demonstrated to be associated with deficiency of the antihypertensive function of the RIC, as titrated by renopapillary transplantation into hypertensive recipients (9). It is therefore plausible to consider the damage to the RIC in the animals of series B as contributing to the severity of the hypertensive cardiovascular disease due to a deficiency of the renomedullary antihypertensive factor(s).

It is becoming apparent that the RIC within the renal papilla may have their antihypertensive action(s) curtailed under different experimental

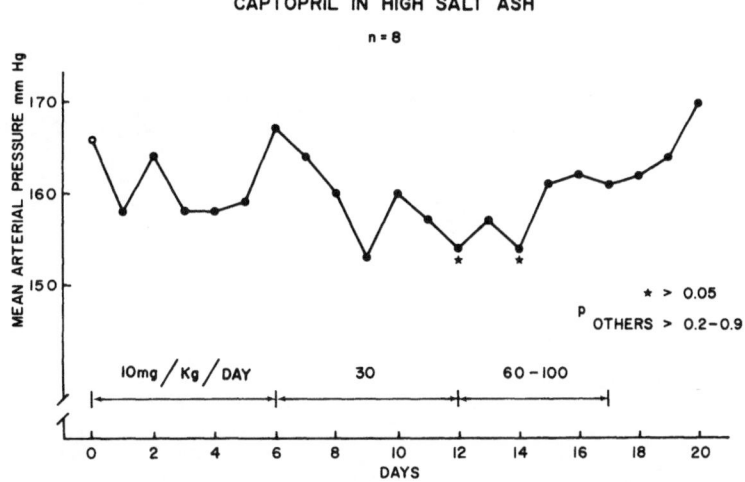

CAPTOPRIL IN HIGH SALT ASH

n = 8

Fig. 6. Failure of captopril to lower the AP of animals of series B at doses of 10, 30, and 60–100 mg/kg/day p.o.

conditions. These include (1) a very high salt intake plus a marked reduction of renal mass (partial nephrectomy-salt hypertension of the rat (9); (2) a high intrarenal angiotensin level (malignant hypertension of the rabbit (10); (3) a very high circulating angiotensin (or renin) level plus reduction of the renal mass (hypertension of the rat due to cultured JG cells (8) and spontaneous hypertension, SHR type, plus unilateral ureteral ligation (11); and (4) a medium angiotensin intake, decreased renal mass plus salt (ASH of the rat). It is suggested that curtailment of the antihyperten-

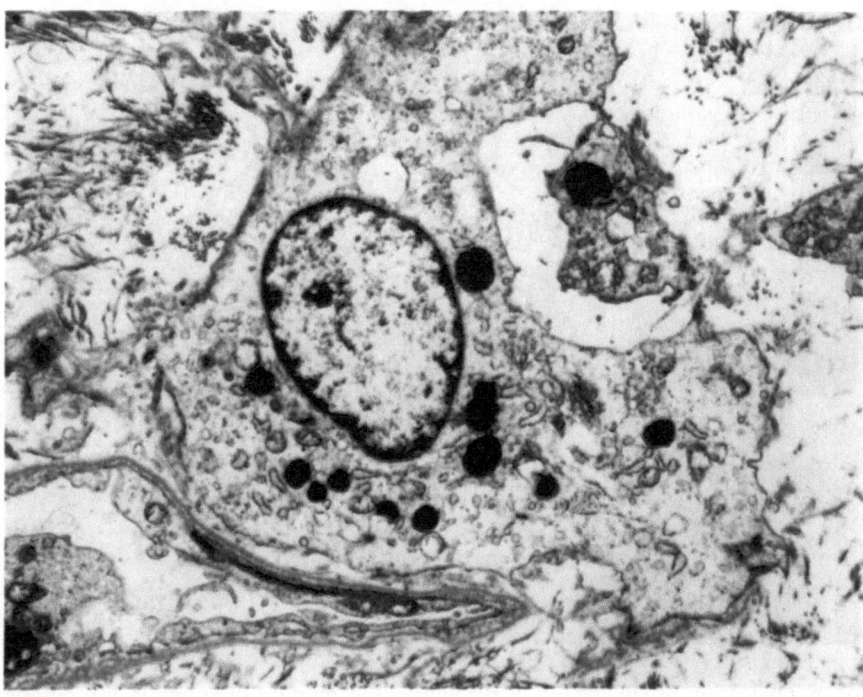

Fig. 7. A RIC from a responder (lower salt group) to captopril (series A). The lipid granules are normal looking, i.e., deeply osmiophilic, and the cisterns and cytoplasmic processors are maintained. EM × 4,000.

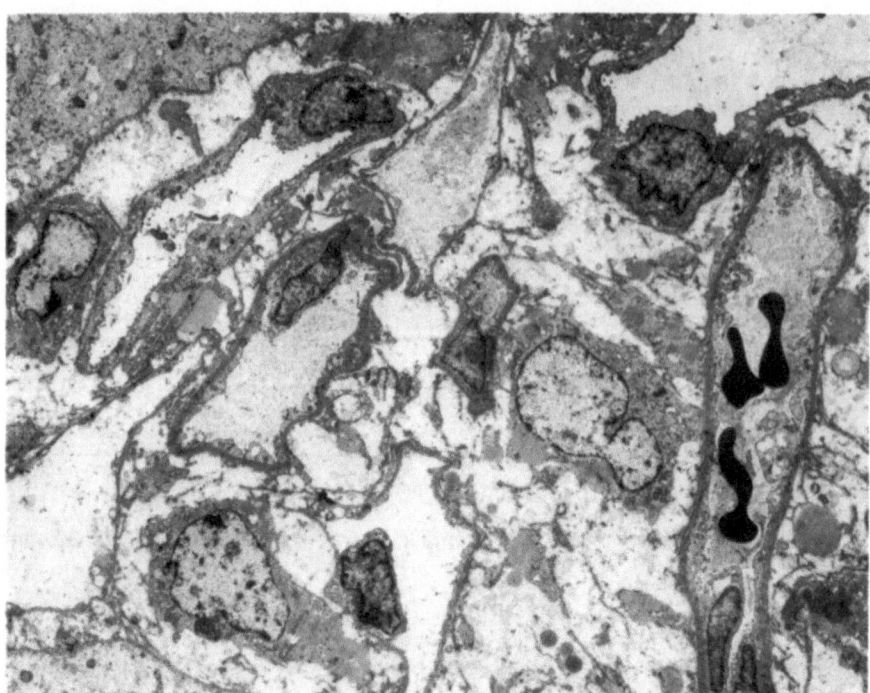

Fig. 8. Lower magnification of RIC from a nonresponder (high salt group) to captopril. The RIC are markedly altered and poorly identifiable. EM × 1,900.

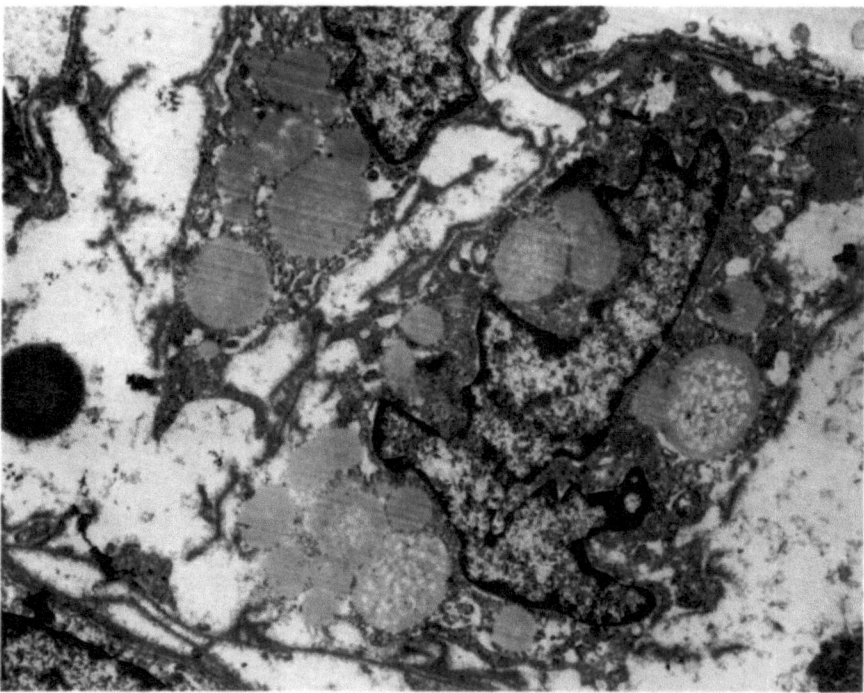

Fig. 9. A higher magnification of RIC of Fig. 8 displaying the marked changes in the cytoplasm, including swollen and pale granules, some having the moth-eaten appearance. The cisterns are not well demonstrated and cytoplasmic processors are absent. In addition, there is an increase in collagenlike material about the cells. EM × 4,000.

Table 2. Renomedullary interstitial cells versus converting enzyme inhibitors in hypertensive states.

RIC[a] decreased and/or damaged: CEI[b] Inactive	RIC Intact, or reasonably so (decreased granules only): CEI Active
Renoprival H[c] PN–SH MH, Goldblatt-type, late SHR plus bilateral nephrectomy[d] ASH, high salt type	SHR, uncomplicated SHR + unilateral hydronephrosis MH, Goldblatt-type, early ASH, lower salt type JGCLH, early

[a] RIC, Renomedullary interstitial cells.
[b] CEI, Converting enzyme inhibitor.
[c] H, Hypertensive state.
[d] Antonaccio et al. (17)

sive function of RIC contributes toward the pathogenesis of the hypertensive states.

Various combinations of three factors seem to be involved in the development of acute hypertensive vascular disease; i.e., fibrinoid necrosis, myohyalinosis, and musculomucoid intimal hyperplasia. These are

1. Elevation of circulating [and possibly arterial] angiotensin (12).
2. Increase in salt intake and salt retention.
3. A deficiency of the antihypertensive function of the RIC.

Moreover, a deficiency of the antihypertensive function of the RIC may be induced by the action of angiotensin and a high salt level within the kidney, i.e., the renal papilla (8–11). Examples of various combinations of these factors associated with acute vascular disease include

1. Extremely high salt intake in the *absence of RIC* and a lower salt intake plus dietary protein and renin, as in the renoprival state of the dog (13–15).
2. Extremely high salt intake plus markedly reduced renal mass, as in partial nephrectomy-salt hypertension (9, 16) (reduced and damaged RIC).
3. Extremely high circulating angiotensin plus a moderate reduction of renal mass (uninephrectomy) and a normal salt intake, as in the hypertension induced by the transplant of juxtaglomerular cells grown in cell culture (evidence for a direct damage induced by angiotensin) (8).

4. Moderate input of angiotensin, a high salt intake, and moderate reduction of renal mass, as in ASH of rat (damaged RIC).

There are indirect, but significant, indications that the converting enzyme inhibitors (CEI) teprotide and captopril exert an antihypertensive action that is, at least partly, mediated by the RIC, perhaps by indirectly stimulating these cells to exert their antihypertensive action. The most plausible explanation for such possibility would consider a decrease in intrarenal angiotensin. The background for this contention is summarized in Table 2. In those hypertensive states in which the RIC are absent or reduced and damaged, the CEI were inactive toward the elevated AP. In hypertensive states in which the RIC were reasonably intact (or normal) in adequate numbers, the CEI lowered the hypertensive AP. Good examples of this association are "lower salt ASH" (CEI active) and "high salt ASH" (CEI inactive).

SUMMARY

Angiotensin-salt hypertension (ASH) of the rat is induced by uninephrectomy, the daily subcutaneous injection of angiotensin (0.1 μg/g body weight), and 1% NaCl to drink. Two levels of hypertension can be derived in ASH, depending on the salt intake. Lower salt intake (~4.5–6.5 mEq Na/day) is associated with (1) a lower level of arterial pressure (150–160 mmHg); (2) the absence of acute vascular disease; and (3) reasonably intact renomedullary interstitial cells (RIC) in the remaining renal papilla. A higher salt intake (~15 mEq Na/day) is associated with (1) a higher grade of hypertension (170–200 mmHg); (2) acute vascular disease (fibrinoid necrosis and the onion-skin lesion); and (3) severe damage to the RIC. Captopril was effective in lowering the blood pressure of the first group (lower salt intake), but failed to alter the blood pressure of the second group (higher salt intake). It is suggested that captopril exerts its antihypertensive action, at least in part, through an effect on the RIC, i.e., stimulating the antihypertensive action of these cells. Other hypertensive models, attended by the absence of or severe damage to the RIC, also fail to respond to captopril and support this interpretation. Various combinations of three factors appear to be involved in the development of acute hypertensive vascular disease, i.e., (1) elevation of circulating angiotensin; (2) increase in salt intake and salt retention; and (3) a deficiency of the antihypertensive function of the RIC.

REFERENCES

1. Muirhead EE, Leach BE, Armstrong F (1973) Angiotensin-salt hypertension. Clin Sci Molec Med 45: 257s–261s
2. Muirhead EE, Leach BE, Armstrong F, Pitcock JA, Brosius WL (1975) Pathophysiology of angiotensin-salt hypertension. J Lab Clin Med 85: 734–745
3. Muirhead EE, Germain GS, Armstrong FB, Brooks B, Leach BE, Byers LW, Pitcock JA, Brown P (1975) Endocrine-type antihypertensive function of renomedullary interstitial cells. Kidney Int 8: S271–282
4. Johnson JG, Muirhead EE Vascular complications of the hypertensive state. In: James C. Hunt (ed) Dialogues in hypertension, hypertension update: Mechanisms, epidemiology, evaluation and management. Health Learning Systems, Bloomfield, N.J., pp 38–51
5. Pitcock JA, Johnson JG, Hatch FE, Acchiardo S, Muirhead EE, Brown P (1976) Malignant hypertension in blacks: Malignant intrarenal arterial disease as observed by light and electron microscopy. Hum Pathol 7: 333–346
6. Muirhead EE, Brooks B, Brosius WL (1980) Antihypertensive action of captopril (SQ 14,225) in angiotensin-salt hypertension. Arch Pathol Lab Med. 104(12): 631–634
7. Muirhead EE, Germain GS, Armstrong FB, Brooks B, Leach BE, Byers LW, Pitcock JA, Brown P (1974) Renomedullary endocrine system: Its antihypertensive action. Trans Assoc Am Phys 87: 288–297
8. Muirhead EE, Rightsel WA, Pitcock JA, Brooks B, Hall MF, Brown P, Brosius WL (1979) Hypertension induced by JG-like cells grown in monolayer tissue culture. Circulation 59–60:II 174 (abst)
9. Pitcock JA, Brown P, Brooks B, Clapp WL, Muirhead EE (1980) Renomedullary deficiency in partial nephrectomy-salt hypertension. Hypertension 2–3: 281–290
10. Muirhead EE, Brooks B, Pitcock JA, Stephenson P (1972) Renomedullary antihypertensive function in accelerated (malignant) hypertension: Observations on renomedullary interstitial cells. J Clin Invest 51: 181–190
11. Muirhead EE, Pitcock JA, Brown P, Brooks B (1980) Models of hypertension due to renal manipulations: Possible linkage between the antihypertensive function of renomedullary interstitial cells and the action of converting enzyme inhibitors. Fed Proc (In press)
12. Swales JD, Thurston H, Queiroz FP, Medina A, Holland J (1971) Dual mechanisms for experimental hypertension. Lancet 2: 1181–1183
13. Muirhead EE, Turner LB, Grollman A (1951) Hypertensive cardiovascular disease: Nature and pathogenesis of arteriolar sclerosis induced by bilateral nephrectomy as revealed by a study of its tinctorial characteristics. Arch Pathol 52: 266–279
14. Muirhead EE, Kosinski M (1962) Renal medulla and renoprival hypertension: Relationship between corticorenal (renin) and medullorenal extracts. Circ Res 11: 674–680
15. Orbison JL, Christian CL, Peters E (1952) Studies on experimental hypertension and cardiovascular disease. Arch Pathol 54: 185–196
16. Koletsky S, Rivera-Velez JM, Pritchard WH (1966) Production of hypertension and vascular disease by angiotensin. Arch Pathol 82: 99–106

Effect of Converting Enzyme Inhibition with Teprotide on Hemodynamics and Cardiovascular Reflexes in Normotensive Subjects

Andreas P. Niarchos and Thomas G. Pickering

INTRODUCTION

Several recent studies, some of which are presented elsewhere in this volume, have provided evidence that the renin-angiotensin-aldosterone system participates in the pathogenesis of elevated arterial pressure in renovascular and essential human hypertension and in some experimental animal models of hypertension. This pathogenetic role of the renin-angiotensin system is now being investigated more precisely because of the availability of the pharmacologic tools that block the renin-angiotensin system in several sites. These agents include saralasin and the similar angiotensin II competitive antagonists, the converting enzyme inhibitors teprotide and captopril, which block the conversion of angiotensin I to angiotensin II, and more recently the antirenin antibodies and the renin-inhibiting peptides that antagonize renin *per se.* It is beyond the scope of this chapter to discuss the specificity of these antagonists, since some may have additional pharmacologic effects; nevertheless, it is generally agreed that the cardiovascular effects of saralasin, converting enzyme inhibitors, and the antirenin agents are mainly attributable to their property to interfere with the renin-angiotensin system.

By contrast, the role of the renin-angiotensin system in regulating normal arterial pressure in normotensive subjects has been least investigated with the exception of the initial studies by Sancho and associates (1), who by administering the converting enzyme inhibitor teprotide to normotensive subjects concluded that the renin-angiotensin system is essential for normal blood pressure maintenance, but only during sodium depletion. Furthermore, cardiovascular reflexes during converting enzyme inhibition have not been studied extensively in normotensive man.

METHODS

The purpose of the present study, in part previously reported elsewhere (2), was to investigate further the role of the renin-angiotensin system in normal blood pressure regulation in eight sodium-repleted and sodium-deprived normotensive subjects. In this study the effects of converting enzyme inhibition were assessed not only on blood pressure and heart rate, but also on cardiac output, peripheral resistance, plasma renin, and plasma catecholamines. The methods and protocol used in this study have been described in detail previously (2). With the subject in the seated position, cardiac output was measured by dye dilution, arterial pressure was recorded via an intraarterial catheter, plasma-renin activity (PRA) was measured by radioimmunoassay (RIA) (3), and catecholamines was measured by the radioenzymatic method of Upjohn Laboratories. All measurements were performed initially on a 150-mEq sodium diet before teprotide and 30 min after i.v. bolus administration of teprotide 1 mg/kg body weight. The hemodynamic and hormonal measurements were repeated 6 days later in six of the eight subjects while on a 10-mEq sodium diet and in whom teprotide was readministered in the same manner. Moreover, in order to study the cardiovascular responses to standing and isometric exercise during converting enzyme inhibition, the hemodynamic measurements were repeated during one-third of the maximum hand grip for 3 min and during standing for 5 min on both normal and low-sodium diets. The paired or unpaired t-test was used for statistical analysis of the results, which are given as mean $\pm$ SEM. A two-tailed p value of less than 0.05 was accepted as significant. Correlation coefficient values were derived by the method of Spearman.

RESULTS

Hemodynamic and Humoral Effects of Teprotide (Seated Position)

The hemodynamic and humoral effects of teprotide 30 min after its administration during the 150-mEq ($n = 8$) and 10-mEq ($n = 6$) sodium intake are summarized in Table 1. The response of mean arterial pressure to teprotide in each individual normal subject is shown in Fig. 1. The decrease in mean arterial pressure by teprotide is due to the decrease in peripheral resistance (Table 1), and this effect is more pronounced with sodium depletion when the renin-angiotensin system is activated, as can be seen in Table 1, which also shows the hemodynamic and humoral responses to sodium depletion in the six normal subjects who were investigated during both diets. During sodium depletion, PRA (and hence angiotensin II) was increased consistently in every subject (by an average of 250%), while plasma epinephrine tended to decrease (by an average of 13%), and plasma norepinephrine was inconsistently and not significantly increased by an average of 31%. The percentage changes induced by teprotide in the hemodynamic variables and PRA during the two diets are shown in Fig. 2. As can be seen, the hemodynamic effects of teprotide were signifi-cantly greater during the 10-mEq sodium intake, but were still present even during the 150-mEq sodium intake.

When data from both studies in all subjects were analyzed together, the maximum decrease in diastolic blood pressure by teprotide correlated significantly with the control plasma renin activity ($r = 0.76$, $p < 0.01$, $n = 14$ measurements); this correlation during the low-sodium intake was $r = 0.81$ ($p < 0.05$, $n = 6$ measurements). The correlation between control PRA and the decrease in total peripheral resistance by teprotide was $r = 0.77$ during the low sodium intake.

Effects of Isometric Exercise

Before teprotide administration and on the 150-mEq sodium intake hand grip increased mean arterial pressure by $26 \pm 3\%$ (from 74 ± 5 to 93 ± 5 mmHg, $p < 0.001$), mainly because of a concurrent increase in cardiac output by $15 \pm 5\%$ (from 4.44 ± 0.30 to 5.13 ± 0.46 liters/min, $p < 0.001$), while the $10 \pm 3\%$ increase in total peripheral resistance was not significant. Cardiac output was increased during hand grip because of an increase in heart rate by $15 \pm 4\%$ (from 66 ± 2 to 76 ± 3 beats/min, $p < 0.001$) not in stroke volume. During the 10-mEq sodium intake, the increase in mean arterial pressure during hand grip was smaller, the average increase being $10 \pm 4\%$ (from

Table 1. Hemodynamic and humoral effects of sodium depletion and teprotide in normotensive subjects.

Effects[a]	150-mEq sodium intale (N = 8)			10-mEq sodium intale (N = 6)		
	Control	30 min post teprotide	p	Control	30 min post teprotide	p
HR (beats/min)	65 ± 3	68 ± 3		69 ± 5	72 ± 6	NS
MAP (mmHg)	75 ± 3	$65 \pm 3(5)$	<0.01	69 ± 2	56 ± 3	<0.005
SV (ml/beat)	73 ± 7	72 ± 8	NS	55 ± 5	62 ± 4	<0.05
CO (liters/min)	4.72 ± 0.36	4.82 ± 0.42	NS	3.91 ± 0.33	4.40 ± 0.3	<0.005
TPR (units)	17 ± 1	14 ± 1	<0.05	18 ± 1	12 ± 1	<0.005
PRA (ng/ml/h)	2.0 ± 0.4	5.23 ± 1.27	<0.01	7.36 ± 1.3	31 ± 4	<0.025
EPI (pg/ml)	74 ± 15	90 ± 24	NS	64 ± 10	91 ± 14	NS
NEPI (pg/ml)	301 ± 35	332 ± 58	NS	367 ± 109	358 ± 83	NS
UNaV (mEq/24 h)	136 ± 6	—	—	13 ± 4	—	
UA (µg/24 h)	10 ± 2	—	—	36 ± 7	—	
UKV (mEq/24 h)	66 ± 6	—	—	67 ± 8	—	
Wt (kg)	74.15 ± 3.44	—	—	72.87 ± 3.51	—	

[a] HR, Heart rate; MAP, mean arterial pressure; SV, stroke volume; CO, cardiac output; TRP, total peripheral resistance; PRA, plasma-renin activity; EPI, plasma epinephrine; NEPI, plasma norepinephrine; UNaV, 24-h urinary sodium excretion; UA, urinary aldosterone; UKV, 24-h urinary potassium excretion; Wt, body weight.

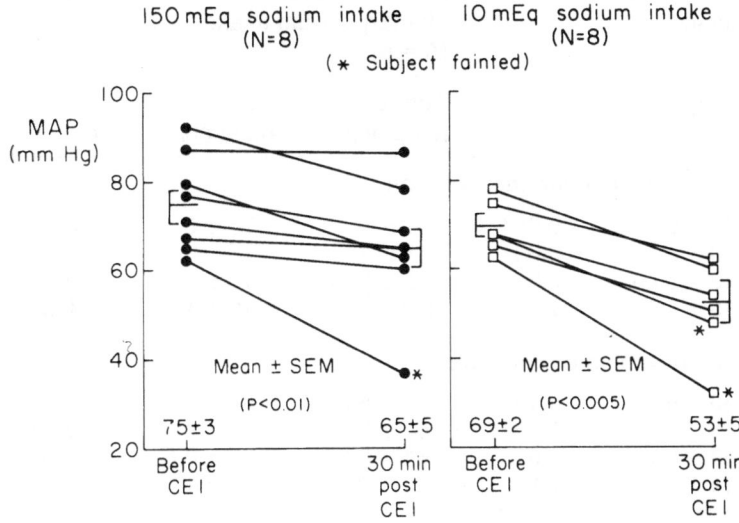

**Effect of the Converting Enzyme
Inhibitor on MAP**

Fig. 1. Mean arterial pressure (MAP) response to the converting enzyme inhibitor (CEI) during the 150- and 10-mEq sodium intake.

68 ± 1 to 75 ± 3 mmHg, $p < 0.05$) because of a concurrent increase in cardiac output by $10 \pm 3\%$ (from 3.75 ± 0.34 to 4.13 ± 0.41 liters/min, $p < 0.05$) without a concomitant change in peripheral resistance. Cardiac output was again increased by the heart rate mechanism after teprotide administration and during the 150-mEq sodium diet when hand grip increased mean arterial pressure

by $28 \pm 3\%$ (from 69 ± 4 to 88 ± 4 mmHg, $p < 0.001$) again via an increase in cardiac output by $38 \pm 16\%$ (from 5.05 ± 0.40 to 6.87 ± 0.72 liters/min, $p < 0.025$) and without any concomitant change in peripheral resistance. On this occasion, the increase in cardiac output was attributable to increases in both heart rate by $17 \pm 4\%$ (from 69 ± 3 to 80 ± 5 beats/min, $p < 0.005$) and in stroke volume by $18 \pm 6\%$ (from 73 ± 4 to 86 ± 5 ml/beat, $p < 0.005$). During the 10-mEq sodium diet and following teprotide hand grip increased again mean arterial pressure by $25 \pm 1\%$ (from 54 ± 3 to 68 ± 4 mmHg, $p < 0.001$), which was mediated by increases in both cardiac output (by 11%) and peripheral resistance (by 19%). Thus teprotide had little consistent effect on the hemodynamic changes during hand grip, which are summarized in Table 2.

The hemodynamic changes induced by hand grip were accompanied by simultaneous changes in plasma catecholamines, which were increased significantly with hand grip but only during converting enzyme inhibition with teprotide at both sodium intakes (Fig. 3).

Hemodynamic Effects of Standing During Converting Enzyme Inhibition with Teprotide

As can be seen from Table 3, the ability to increase heart rate and peripheral resistance, and therefore

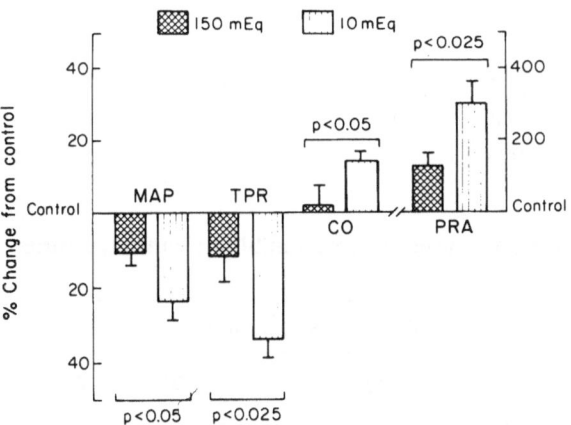

Comparison of the Effect of Converting Enzyme Inhibitor on Hemodynamics and PRA During the 150 and 10 mEq Sodium Intake (N = 6)

Fig. 2. Comparison of the percentage changes produced by teprotide during the 150- and 10-mEq sodium intake. MAP, Mean arterial pressure; TPR, total peripheral resistance; CO, cardiac output; PRA, plasma-renin activity.

Table 2. Hemodynamic effects of isometric exercise before and during converting enzyme inhibition (Mean ± SEM).

Effects[a]	150-mEq sodium intake (N = 8)			10-mEq sodium intake (N = 6)		
	Before hand grip	During hand grip	p	Before hand grip	During hand grip	p
Before converting enzyme inhibition						
HR (beats/min)	66 ± 2	76 ± 3	<0.001	67 ± 5	76 ± 6	<0.02
MAP (mmHg)	74 ± 5	93 ± 5	<0.001	68 ± 1	75 ± 3	<0.05
CO (liters/min)	4.44 ± 0.30	5.13 ± 0.46	<0.001	3.75 ± 0.34	4.13 ± 0.41	<0.05
TRP (units)	17 ± 1	19 ± 1.6	NS	18.6 ± 1.5	19 ± 1.5	NS
During converting enzyme inhibition						
HR (beats/min)	69 ± 3	80 ± 5	<0.005	73 ± 6	80 ± 7	<0.05
MAP (mmHg)	69 ± 4	88 ± 4	<0.001	54 ± 3	68 ± 4	<0.001
CO (liters/min)	5.05 ± 0.46	6.87 ± 0.72	<0.025	4.61 ± 0.26	5.07 ± 0.63	NS
TPR (units)	14 ± 1.6	14 ± 1.8	NS	12 ± 0.5	14 ± 1	NS

[a] HR, Heart rate; MAP, mean arterial pressure; SV, stroke volume; CO, cardiac output; TPR, total peripheral resistance.

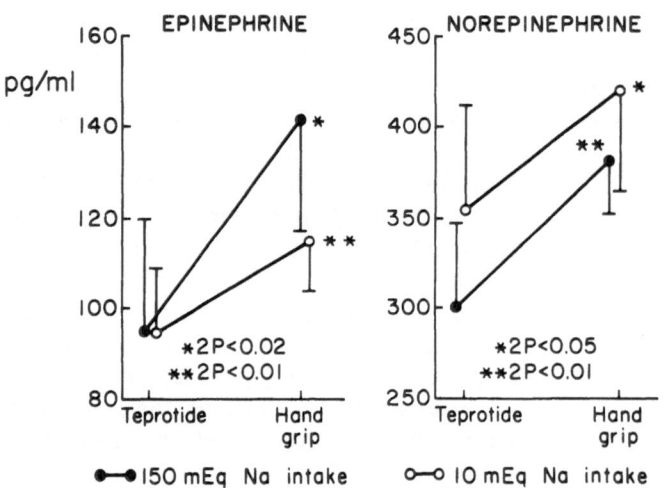

Effect of Isometric Exercise on EPI and NEPI during Teprotide

Fig. 3. Effect of hand grip on plasma catecholamines during converting enzyme inhibition during both the 150- and 10-mEq sodium intake.

Table 3. Hemodynamic effects of standing during converting enzyme inhibition with teprotide (N = 4).

Effects[a]	150-mEq sodium intake			10-mEq sodium intake		
	Sitting	Standing	p	Sitting	Standing	p
HR (beats/min)	67 ± 4	88 ± 6	<0.025	70 ± 6	89 ± 8	NS
MAP (mmHg)	65 ± 1	74 ± 2	<0.01	56 ± 2	61 ± 5	NS
CO (liters/min)	5.31 ± 0.68	4.25 ± 0.28	<0.05	4.37 ± 0.15	3.04 ± 0.18	<0.005
TPR (units)	13 ± 2	18 ± 1	<0.01	12.5 ± 1	20 ± 2	<0.025

[a] HR, Heart rate; MAP, mean arterial pressure; SV, stroke volume; CO, cardiac output; TPR, total peripheral resistance.

to sustain arterial pressure despite the decrease in cardiac output after assuming the upright posture, was preserved; therefore, arterial pressure was maintained during converting enzyme inhibition not only during the normal sodium intake, but when the normal subjects were receiving the low-sodium diet as well. Consequently, no postural hypotension was observed during standing.

DISCUSSION

Hemodynamic Effects of Converting Enzyme Inhibition in Normotensive Subjects

The results of the present study clearly show (Fig. 1) that converting enzyme inhibition with teprotide decreases arterial pressure in normal subjects (in 63% of the subjects investigated) even in the sodium-replete state. Our findings are in agreement with those of MacGregor et al. (11), who have reported elsewhere (4) and in this volume that captopril decreased arterial pressure in normotensive subjects not only during low-sodium intake, but also during normal or even high-sodium intake, although the hypotensive response was the smallest when captopril was given during high-sodium intake.

In the present study the decrease in blood pressure after administration of the inhibitor was due to a decrease in peripheral resistance (peripheral vasodilation) during both the sodium-replete and sodium-depleted states (Table 1). Similar action has been documented in normal dogs (5) and in hypertensive subjects (6). The hemodynamic effects of the inhibitor were enhanced during the sodium-depleted state, when peripheral resistance had increased. The vasoconstriction following sodium and volume depletion is probably mediated mainly via the renin-angiotensin system (5), although other vasoconstrictive hormones, such as catecholamines and arginine vasopressin, may play an important role in sustaining arterial pressure during massive volume depletion or hemorrhage. In the present study, plasma catecholamines were not affected by the 10-mEq sodium intake. On the contrary, plasma renin had increased markedly (by 250%) during sodium depletion, maintaining peripheral resistance and hence arterial pressure despite the concurrent decrease in cardiac output

(Table 2). This hemodynamic pattern was reversed during angiotensin inhibition, but cardiac output was not restored to the level of 150-mEq sodium intake, because volume depletion continued to persist. Because heart rate did not change appreciably during sodium depletion and teprotide administration, the influence of angiotensin II on cardiac output possibly is mediated by its effects on the determinants of stroke volume (venous return, myocardial contractility, coronary blood flow, and afterload).

The increase in stroke volume (and hence cardiac output) caused by the converting enzyme inhibitor during the sodium-depleted state in normal subjects with elevated plasma-renin levels is consistent with our previous findings in hypertensive subjects with elevated PRA (6, 7). The present study was not designed to assess the effects of SQ 20881 on myocardial contractility. However, it is known that although angiotensin II has a positive inotropic effect on the isolated papillary muscle (8, 9), it nevertheless has a negative inotropic effect in the intact heart (10). A myocardial depressant factor has been identified in some shock states and was significantly diminished by the SQ 14225 converting enzyme inhibitor with hemodynamic improvement (11). Moreover, beneficial hemodynamic effects and increased survival during the administration of SQ 20881 converting enzyme inhibitor have been observed on marked hypovolemia caused by extensive hemorrhage (12). Coronary blood flow, not measured in the present study, has been found to increase during angiotensin inhibition with SQ 20881 in the normal sodium-depleted dog (5, 13), and such a mechanism may have contributed to the improvement in cardiac function in the normotensive subjects of the present study.

One of the main determinants of the increase in stroke volume after angiotensin inhibition during the sodium-depleted state in the present study was probably the reduction by the inhibitor in afterload (peripheral resistance) with the consequence of better ventricular emptying. Similar changes in peripheral resistance have been observed in the sodium-depleted normal dog (5). In our study during the sodium-depleted state, the changes in peripheral resistance induced by the inhibitor were related to the control plasma renin activity ($r = 0.77$) as has been observed in hypertensive patients (6, 7). During the sodium-replete state, however, the decrease in afterload caused by the inhibitor, although smaller in magnitude, did not result in an increase in cardiac output, because the concurrent decrease in central venous pressure due to the dilation of the capacitance vessels and consequent decrease in the filling pressure of the heart counteracted the effects of afterload reduction on cardiac output. On the contrary, during the sodium-depleted state, when the filling pressure was maintained during angiotensin inhibition (as can be inferred by the fact that venous pressure increased), stroke volume and cardiac output were increased. Thus, it appears that the increase in cardiac function caused by the converting enzyme inhibitor in the sodium-depleted state has a dual hemodynamic basis: a decrease in afterload and preservation of, or an actual increase in, venous return.

CARDIOVASCULAR REFLEXES DURING CONVERTING ENZYME INHIBITION

In the present study, as well as in previous studies in normal human subjects (1), normal dogs (5), and in hypertensive human subjects (6, 7), the expected compensatory increase in heart rate during the fall in blood pressure after SQ 20881 administration was either minimal or virtually absent. Although the mechanism for this phenomenon needs further investigation, one possible explanation is that inhibition of angiotensin II formation may eliminate the hormone's potentiating (presynaptic) effect on catecholamine release, but this does not appear to be the case in the present study, since plasma catecholamines were not decreased significantly by the inhibitor. Furthermore, it is possible that the gradual decrease in blood pressure somehow modulates baroreceptor responsiveness, or angiotensin inhibition may enhance parasympathetic activity (14).

Although the baroreflex during angiotensin inhibition appears to be not functioning in the supine (7, 15) and seated position (6), our results provide evidence that baroreflex function is normal during converting enzyme inhibition, as can be judged from the tachycardia and vasoconstriction (Table 3) that occur during a short period of standing. Similar findings during short periods of head-up tilt have been reported (15) in hypertensive patients during chronic angiotensin inhibition with the oral converting enzyme inhibitor SQ 14225. However, in other studies in normal subjects (1) and hypertensive patients (16) when prolonged

(30–60 min) head-up tilt was used during angiotensin inhibition combined with volume depletion, marked decreases in blood pressure and fainting occurred. The findings from these later studies are suggestive that a marked reduction in cardiac output caused by the prolonged passive head-up tilt probably contributed to the hypotension induced by angiotensin inhibition.

During isometric exercise with hand grip, the expected normal hemodynamic response (17), i.e., increase in arterial pressure mediated via an increase in cardiac output because of the concurrent increase in heart rate, was preserved during both the 150- and 10-mEq sodium diet and during converting enzyme inhibition with teprotide. However, during the 10-mEq sodium diet and teprotide, the increase in arterial pressure by isometric exercise was partially due to an increase in peripheral resistance in addition to the increase in cardiac output. This vasoconstriction during isometric exercise in the presence of angiotensin II inhibition is probably due to the increased plasma catecholamines (Fig. 3).

CONCLUSIONS

Converting enzyme inhibition with teprotide decreases arterial pressure in normotensive subjects mainly during low-sodium intake and, to a lesser degree, during normal sodium intake. Moreover, cardiovascular responses to standing and isometric exercise remain intact during converting enzyme inhibition. These results taken together suggest that the renin-angiotensin system participates in the maintenance of arterial pressure in normotensive subjects, but it does not appear to play a major role in mediating the cardiovascular responses to standing and isometric exercise.

SUMMARY

The hemodynamic effects of teprotide were investigated in eight normotensive subjects, initially during 150-mEq sodium intake and later on again during 10-mEq sodium intake. Furthermore, the cardiovascular responses during standing and during isometric exercise were investigated in the same subjects before and during converting enzyme inhibition with teprotide. Teprotide decreased mean arterial pressure during both sodium diets by decreasing peripheral resistance. This vasodilatory effect of teprotide was more pronounced during sodium depletion which had resulted in activation of the renin-angiotensin system. Teprotide, however, did not modify the expected normal cardiovascular responses that occur with standing or isometric exercise, or both.

REFERENCES

1. Sancho T, Re R, Burton T, Berger AC, Haber E (1976) The role of the renin-angiotensin-aldosterone system in cardiovascular homeostasis in normal human subjects. Circulation 53: 400–405
2. Niarchos AP, Pickering TG, Case DB, Sullivan P, Laragh JH (1979) Role of the renin-angiotensin system in blood pressure regulation. The cardiovascular effects of converting enzyme inhibition in normotensive subjects. Circ Res 45: 829–837
3. Sealey JE, Laragh JH (1975) Radioimmunoassay of plasma renin activity. Semin Nucl Med 5: 189–202
4. MacGregor GA, Markandu ND, Roulston JE, Jones JC, Morton JJ (1980) The renin-angiotensin-aldosterone system in the maintenance of blood pressure and sodium balance in normotensive subjects. Clin Sci (To be published)
5. Liang CS, Gavras H, Hood WB (1978) Renin angiotensin system inhibition in conscious sodium-depleted dogs. Effects on systemic and coronary hemodynamics. J Clin Invest 62: 874–883
6. Niarchos AP, Pickering TG, Case DB, Wallace JM, Morganti A, Sealey JE, Laragh JH (1978) Preload and afterload reduction during angiotensin II blockade with the converting enzyme inhibitor (Abstract). Am J Cardiol 41: 403
7. Niarchos AP, Roberts AJ, Case DB, Gay WA Jr, Laragh JH (1979) Hemodynamic characteristics of hypertension after coronary artery bypass and effects of the converting enzyme inhibitor. Am J Cardiol 43: 586–592
8. Koch-Weser J (1964) Myocardial actions of angiotensin. Circ Res 14: 337–344
9. Dempsey PJ, McCallum Zt, Kent KM, Cooper T (1971) Direct myocardial effects of angiotensin II. Am J Physiol 220: 477–481
10. Ahmed SS, Levinson GE, Weisse AB, Regan TJ (1975) The effect of angiotensin on myocardial contracticity. J Clin Pharmacol 15: 226–285
11. Trachte GJ, Lefer AM (1978) Beneficial action of a new angiotensin-converting enzyme inhibitor (SQ 14225) in hemorrhagic shock in cats. Circ Res 43: 576–582
12. Morton JJ, Semple PF, Ledinghgan IM, Stuart B, Tehrani MA, Garcia AR, McGarrity G (1977) Effect of angiotensin-converting enzyme inhibitor (SQ 20881) on the plasma concentration of angiotensin I, angiotensin II, and arginine vasopressin in the dog during hemorrhagic shock. Circ Res 41: 301–308
13. Gavras H, Liang CS, Brunner HR (1978) Redistribution of regional blood flow after inhibition of the angiotensin-converting enzyme. Circ Res 43 (suppl I): I59–I63
14. Bravo EL, Tarazi RC (1978) Hemodynamics of an angiotensin II antagonist in normal unanesthetized dogs. Circ Res 43 (Suppl I): 27–31
15. Cody RJ, Tarazi RC, Bravo EL, Fouad FM (1978) Hemodynamics of orally-active converting enzyme inhibitor (SQ 14225) in hypertensive patients. Clin Sci Mol Med 55: 453–459
16. Morganti A, Pickering TG, Lopez-Ovejero JA, Laragh, JH (1980) Endocrine and cardiovascular influences of converting enzyme inhibition with SQ 14225 in hypertensive patients in the supine position and during head-up tilt before and after sodium depletion. J Clin Endocrinol Metab 50: 748–754
17. Nutter DO, Schlant RC, Hurst JW (1972) Isometric exercise and the cardiovascular system. Mod Concepts Cardiovasc Dis XLI: 11–15

DISCUSSION

Dr. Erdos (Dallas, Texas): We have heard a great deal about the effects of captopril in man and animals today, but almost nothing about the properties of the human enzyme it inhibits, although the actions of this compound are attributed to inhibition of converting enzyme or peptidyl dipeptidase (ACE). If we want to learn more about captopril we have to know where the enzyme is located, and which are the properties and the substrates of the human ACE.

Thus, we [T. A. Steward, J. A. Weare, and E. G. Erdos] purified to homogeneity human ACE from lung, where it occurs in vascular endothelium, and from kidney, where tubular epithelium is rich in ACE. We have also detected high concentrations of ACE in the brush border of human intestinal epithelium [Ward et al. (1980) Biochem Pharmacol 29: 1525]. Human kidney has about five times more enzyme per weight than the lung. The homogeneous strongly hydrophobic enzyme cleaves Hip-Gly-Gly, Hip-His-Leu (50 U/min/mg) and Hip-Pre-Arg. The latter two peptides represent the C-terminal end of angiotensin I and bradykinin. Of the biologically active peptide substrates, enkephalins had the highest turnover number, while bradykinin had a higher specificity constant than did angiotensin I or enkephalins.

The isoelectric point of both the lung and kidney enzyme is 5.2, but lung enzyme has other more acidic forms with higher sialic acid content. ACE has an apparent molecular weight of 155,000 and a sedimentation rate of $8.0 \pm 0.1S$. Specific antibodies elicited to human lung or kidney ACE in rabbits reacted with both human enzymes, but not with swine. The intestinal enzyme also has common antigenic determinants with the lung ACE. Gel electrophoresis of peptide fragments of purified human lung and kidney and swine kidney showed that the protein structures of the human enzymes are similar. Human ACE from lung, kidney, and intestine was inhibited by captopril with I_{50} in the order of 10^{-9} M. Thus, when considering the action of captopril in humans, it should be remembered that ACE occurs at sites other than vascular endothelium, in even higher concentrations than in the lung. Furthermore, I believe that measurement of the level of bradykinin in the circulation after captopril administration is as unlikely to yield important information on the local action of this peptide as is measuring acetylcholine or norepinephrine in blood. The effect of bradykinin on carbohydrate metabolism in skeletal muscles or on absorption from the gut are examples of the local actions of peptides that may be potentiated by inhibition of kininase II during captopril therapy.

Dr. Lever (Glasgow, Scotland): I would like to show two figures concerning the second action of captopril. It is a study done by Dr. Tree and Dr. Morton [Tree M, Morton JJ (1979) Clin Sci 58, also Clin Sci (1980)] in our lab on the con-scious dog. Figure 1 shows the protocol. The idea behind the experiment was to infuse angiotensin in stepwise increasing doses so that plasma-angiotensin II concentration increased and blood pressure increased in parallel. The lower line shows the curve we would expect to get in six conscious control dogs. The upper line shows the second curve we might expect to get when the experiment was completed in the same dogs during an infusion of captopril, if captopril lowered blood pressure solely by reducing the plasma concentration of angiotensin II. The reasoning behind this is that if you replace the angiotensin that has been removed by captopril, the dose–response curve should rise along the original curve of the control study. It is a very similar protocol to that used previously in Boston with the earlier converting enzyme inhibitor teprotide. Suppose, instead, that the fall in blood pressure is not wholly explained by the fall in plasma angiotensin II concentration. Then obviously there will be a shift of the curve to the right as shown. The greater the shift, the greater this second mechanism is. Now these are all hypothetical curves. We did the same experiment on the six dogs on two occasions. Figure 2 shows what happens. This is the control study in dogs without captopril. It was repeated on the same dogs on another occasion in a random sequence during captopril infusion. You can see there is a quite considerable displacement of the dose–response curve, which suggests that captopril is lowering blood pressure by more than the one mechanism proposed, namely by reducing plasma-angiotensin II concentration. It does not deny the

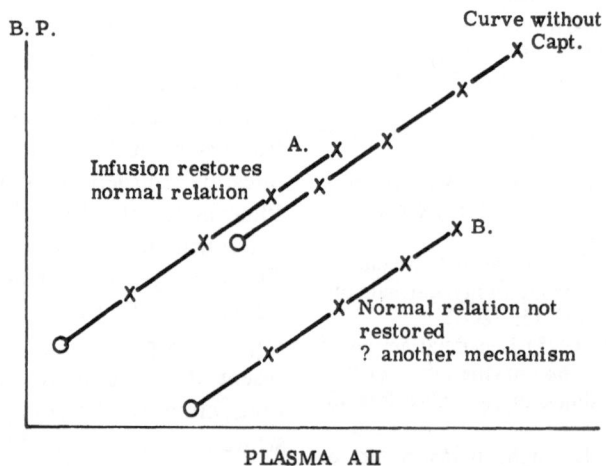

Fig. 1. Angiotensin II dose-response curves—possible effects of captopril.

importance of the reduction of plasma angiotensin II nor does it eliminate a mechanism such as Dr. Antonaccio suggested earlier whereby captopril opposes a vasoconstrictor effect produced from angiotensin II generated locally within the blood vessels. Indeed, I think that this is one very nice explanation for our finding. However, we have repeated the experiment again, but this time given indomethacin. The results so far suggest that a process involving prostaglandin synthesis is responsible for the second hypotensive action of captopril.

Dr. Hollenberg (Boston, Massachusetts): I would like, first, to agree with Dr. Lever. It is very likely that prostaglandins participate in the response to captopril, as indicated by studies performed by Dr. Swartz and Dr. Moore at the Peter Bent Brigham Hospital. Second, in general, the *r* values relating the initial aldosterone level to the change in aldosterone concentration following captopril are about 0.9. I think that's true for all centers and it reflects the fact that the angiotensin is probably responsible for 80% of aldosterone's maintenance. The *r* values relating blood pressure fall to plasma-renin activity run about 0.6 in most centers, suggesting that about one-third of the response to captopril is due to the renin state—perhaps a bit more. Third, I'd really like to comment on the rather dramatic responses of patients with heart failure to converting enzyme. We stud-

ied in collaboration with Dr. Dzau, Dr. Collucci, Dr. Meggs, and Dr. Williams at the Peter Bent Brigham Hospital a series of patients with truly advanced heart failure. All were in a moribund state, resistant to other vasodilator agents. Prior to institution of captopril, it was possible to reduce their edema with furosemide, but only at the price of a rapid increase of the degree of azotemia as well as clinical deterioration of their status. With captopril therapy there were no exceptions. There was a rapid diuresis, clearing of the edema, and normalization of renal function. Their creatinine and PAH clearance, of course, improved very dramatically. This response has been sustained in these patients for up to 16 months now, which supports the concept that the renal vasoconstrictive response in heart failure is angiotensin mediated and suggests very strongly that this agent will be useful in treating these very sick patients.

Dr. Shand (Durham, North Carolina): I enjoyed hearing all the good things about captopril from Dr. Alexander, but I wonder if he might complete the other side of the picture and give us a breakdown on the adverse reactions of the drug.

Dr. Alexander (Princeton, New Jersey): Early on in the clinical program with captopril we observed maculopapular rashes that occurred in about 10% of patients receiving the drug. They seemed to be transient in most patients and were treated either with a reduction in dosage or with

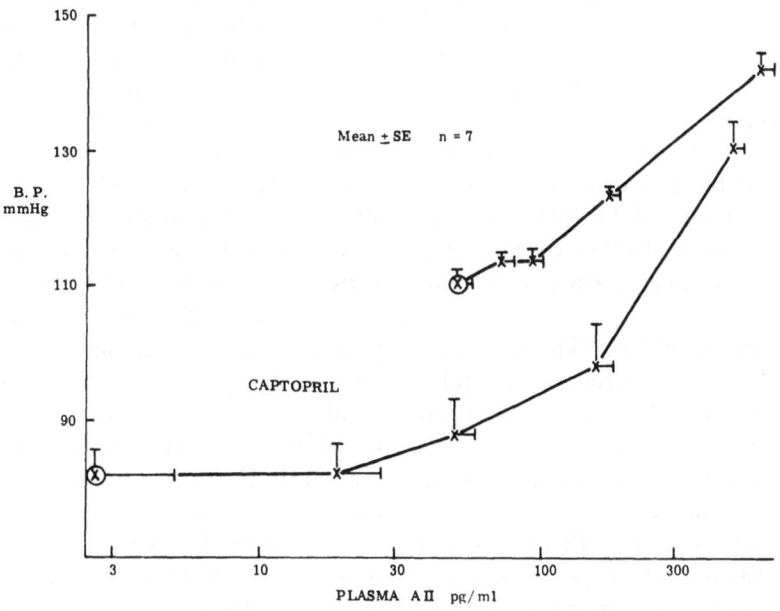

Fig. 2. Angiotensin II infusion with and without captopril.

an antihistaminic. However, some patients had an urticarial component, and a few had angioedema, which required discontinuation of the drug. As we progressed in the clinical program we encountered other problems. A very peculiar thing—a loss or change in taste perception— was observed in about 6% of patients. Once again, this was a transient phenomenon and, in most patients, it disappeared without the patient's having to stop the drug. In a few patients there was a severe loss of taste with weight loss, and the drug had to be discontinued. The rash and taste loss were rapidly reversible upon discontinuation of treatment. More than a year ago, Dr. David Case reported to us two patients in whom proteinuria and membranous glomerulopathy developed. We then started to make a careful study of the protein excretion of all patients. It was extremely difficult to separate the proteinuria possibly related to captopril from proteinuria that was present on pretreatment, or possibly due to the renal disease many patients had. As time has passed, it appears that in around 1% of patients who received the drug proteinuria will develop after 3–9 months of treatment. It is possible that a reduction of the daily dose of captopril could reduce or eliminate this problem. The group at Cornell has permitted some of their patients to continue on the drug and, in general, there has been a diminution or disappearance of protein excretion and no change in creatinine clearance.

Finally, recently we have had reports describing patients in whom agranulocytosis developed. There have been 15 case reports now of patients with agranulocytosis among the 3,000–4,000 patients who have received captopril. It has been difficult to decide in these cases whether captopril caused or aggravated the problem, or whether it was involved at all. Many of the patients were receiving other drugs or had other diseases that had been associated with neutropenia, such as lupus.

Dr. Case (New York, New York): The more serious side effects, such as proteinuria and agranulocytosis, have, in our hands, been reversible when the drug was withdrawn. Proteinuria has completely cleared in 6 patients in whom the drug was continued in the same dosage.

Dr. Niarchos (New York, New York): I would like to ask Dr. Alexander, who says that patients with low renin respond to captopril, what the renin values were?

Dr. Alexander: As I said, in our studies we asked the investigators to use the method of Sealey and Laragh [Am J Med 53: 633–652, 1972] for determination of the renin class. They reported the results to us as normal, high, or low. We do not have information on the precise renin values or the methods employed.

Dr. Menard (Paris, France): I have a brief comment concerning what Dr. Antonnaccio said about the effect of captopril in binephrectomized rats. Arginine-pepstatin is a soluble pepstatin-derivative that blocks renin and other angiotensin I-forming enzymes. Its intravenous injection does not decrease blood pressure in binephrectomized rats on a normal sodium diet, but it does decrease blood pressure in binephrectomized rats on a low-sodium diet. I think this observation fits in with your data and your interpretation. I would like to discuss the effects of captopril on plasma vasopressin and urinary vasopressin, since this hormone could be a participant in the antihypertensive effect of the converting enzyme inhibition. These studies have been performed by Dr. Thibonnier, who has developed a radioimmunoassay of plasma vasopressin in our group. We gave to our patients 1 mg/kg body weight of captopril. On day 1 of the experimental procedure, they ingested a placebo and on day 2 they ingested the active drug. Captopril decreased mean blood pressure, increased plasma-renin activity, and decreased plasma aldosterone. The patients were ten severe hypertensive patients who had been untreated before the experiment. During the first 3 h after this oral administration of captopril there was no change in plasma vasopressin, nor was there an increase that could be due to the decrease in blood pressure or to a fall. When captopril was administered for 7 days, there was a decrease in blood pressure, an increase in PRA, a decrease in plasma aldosterone, and, now, a decrease in urinary vasopressin that was statistically significant after 24-h treatment. These data, I think, suggest that the decrease in urinary vasopressin during the long-term treatment with captopril could participate in the absence of an increase in plasma volume in the presence of the fall in blood pressure. The decrease in aldosterone secretion, but also the decrease in vasopressin production, could avoid sodium and water retention.

Dr. Streeten (Syracuse, New York): I would like to ask Dr. Case two questions. The first is that I think you have in the past interpreted the responses to captopril as indicating that in normal renin essential hypertension renin plays an important role in maintaining the hypertension, since the blood pressure falls in response to captopril. If that is the case, why is it that the plasma-renin activity rises after captopril only in renovascular hypertensive patients and not in the high-renin patients?

Dr. Case: Plasma renin activity rises reactively in patients with essential hypertension too, after captopril as shown previously. However, renin activity rises less in patients with essential hypertension than it does in patients with renovascular hypertension. This may be because the intrarenal receptor for angiotensin II is more sensitive to the negative feedback effect of AII on renin release in renovascular hypertension. I am suggesting that the mechanisms controlling renin release may differ between these conditions.

Dr. Streeten: Apparently, then, you think this is a matter of magnitude of the disorder, and that leads naturally to my second question, which is: Have you any idea of the number of false-negative results you are getting from these renin responses to captopril in your renovascular hypertensives? I think it is well known that you and others have shown that renin does rise in renovascular hypertension after giving these agents, but how many patients of this type are you missing by this procedure, and have you any idea whether you would find them equally well or not as well with saralasin?

Dr. Case: The studies we have done indicate that in people who have had a thorough workup including arteriography, that the false-positive rate is significantly less than 5%. In terms of false-negatives, since we can neither practically nor ethically perform arteriograms on a large group of patients with mild or moderate hypertension who do not have any suggestive features of renovascular disease, it is very hard to determine whether we are missing patients with renovascular hypertension. Aside from the well-established clinical findings, the addition of renal vein renin measurements defines functional renovascular hypertension very well, although it cannot be used as a practical primary screening procedure. I suspect that we may miss those people who have anatomical renal artery stenosis without associated increased renin release from the presumed ischemic kidney. Except for a case report or two, there is no evidence to suggest that the hypertension in this condition improves with surgery.

Dr. MacGregor (London, England): I noticed that no one has talked about the dose of captopril. I think this may be very important in relation to toxic effects. We published some time ago that in a trial of ordinary patients with moderate hypertension 25 mg three times a day was as effective as 100 mg three times a day, and over the last year we have reduced all our patients on captopril to 25 or 12.5 mg three times a day without loss of control of the blood pressure. We no longer see loss of taste, which was a very common side effect in our experience. I wondered whether anyone would like to comment on what their experience has been in terms of dose response to captopril and what dose they would use in light of current knowledge.

Dr. Case: I agree with Dr. MacGregor, although our experience suggests that the mose useful dose range is from 50 to 150 mg per day. Some patients, however, require more.

Dr. Thurston (Leicester, England): If you study dose–response curves to an incremental angiotensin II infusion before and after captopril there is a definite increase in pressor responsiveness. I think the diagram that was shown by Dr. Lever is slightly misleading because he has related measured levels of angiotensin II rather than the infused dose to the absolute blood pressure level. How does the infused dose of angiotensin II relate to the measured levels and the incremental rise in blood pressure?

Dr. Lever: We have now attempted to relate the increment of plasma concentration to the rate of angiotensin infusion, which is what you were asking about. We thought it more relevant to relate the plasma concentration of angiotensin II, the agonist, to its effect. I think it is generally better to do the dose–response curves by relating plasma concentrations of the agonist to their effect, rather than by relating rate of infusions to the effect— much better I would say.

Physician: It has been pointed out that several or quite a large moiety of patients have to be put onto both diuretic and captopril and, as far as I can gather, although this wasn't said, all these patients as described had their captopril first and a diuretic after. Now one of the things that strikes me as a sort of theoretical problem is that if you start a patient with a diuretic you've got two problems, two kinds of diuretics, those of the potassium losing and the potassium sparing. If the patient is on thiazides he might be setting himself up for an acute hypotensive experience on the first dose, as you described in the experiments with sodium-depleted animals. And, on the other hand, it would be quite dangerous in some cases for an inexperienced physician to have been pretreating his patients with potassium-sparing diuretics and then to get another potassium-enhancing influence with captopril. So I wonder if anyone could comment on those particular management problems.

Dr. Case: With respect to starting patients on a diuretic before starting captopril, in our hands, that has been a fairly risky procedure, since the induced degree of volume depletion and hyperreninemia predisposes to hypotensive responses. As a rule, now, we are careful not to pretreat patients with diuretics.

With respect to your second question, we have several patients on captopril with aldactone who have maintained normal levels of serum potassium. There are, however, a few reports of hyperkalemia. This might theoretically be a more relevant problem in patients with reduced renal function. However, it would be unwise to use spironolactone or potassium sparing diuretics in that group, even less wise to use the combination with captopril.

Dr. Seldin (Dallas, Texas): Several people have raised the question of the action of captopril in settings where there is no renin. There is a very exciting paper in *Lancet* by Schalekamp, which appeared in the last several months, in which nephrectomized patients were given captopril in the setting of salt depletion, and uniformly their blood pressures fell. This has been interpreted as evidence possibly for vascular wall renin being inhibited. I wonder if Dr. Antonnacio wants to comment on this matter?

Dr. Antonnacio (Princeton, New Jersey): Yes, I talked to Dr. Schalekamp about that, and we are in agreement. He thinks that it is vascular wall renin, and I think so too.

Dr. Seldin: I gather you have done some studies in rats essentially simulating the whole system that has been shown in man.

Dr. Antonnacio (Princeton, New Jersey): We have done low salt and high salt, but I am afraid I can't tell you the values yet—they are still being measured.

Dr. Seldin: May I make a comment about Dr. Lever's experiments? I would agree with them completely that he has shown that if you infuse angiotensin back, you don't get the same pressor response.

Dr. Muirhead (Memphis, Tennessee): I don't think that was mild sodium depletion in the Schalekamp experiment. I think it was pretty severe.

Dr. Seldin (Dallas, Texas): All right, I'll change the remark about Schalekamp's study to severe sodium depletion.

Dr. Antonnacio: I think Dr. Lever has shown that if he infuses angiotensin II, he has to put back more angiotensin II in the plasma to get the blood pressure back up to the same degree as before captopril. The question is, is that what's important? For instance, what happens to the angiotensin II that is in the kidney after captopril? When you infuse back angiotensin II, do you replace the angiotensin II that has been depleted in the kidney? I doubt it. In addition, the metabolism that occurs is probably quite different under these conditions from that which normally occurs. I think there is an analogy in the noradrenergic system. You can infuse back precursors, but you find that the distribution is quite different, so I think you have to take into consideration distribution, which is probably the most important factor, when you are infusing things back that don't normally get infused.

Dr. Lever: The hypothesis we are testing is that angiotensin II is a blood-borne hormone and that it is exerting a particular effect by a change in the concentration of angiotensin in blood. If we put the peptide back into the blood and change its concentration, I contend that we are testing this hypothesis. I agree with your proposal—I think angiotensin generated in other sites may regulate the peripheral resistance, and it may be that the gap between our two dose–response curves is an indication of the mechanism you propose. But this is a different hypothesis—it is not the mechanism tested by our experiment. Our conclusion is that changes of blood-borne angiotensin II cannot wholly explain the fall of blood pressure after captopril.

Dr. Ganten (Heidelberg, Germany): I would like to make two comments. First, we agree with Dr. Antonaccio that vascular wall renin is elevated in spontaneously hypertensive rats. Inhibition of arterial wall renin therefore is a definite possibility for the antihypertensive action of captopril. Second, I want to call your attention to the possibility that captopril lowers blood pressure by inhibition of the brain renin-angiotensin system. We have previously published data showing that blood pressure can be lowered in spontaneously hypertensive rats by central angiotensin receptor blockade. Dr. Unger from our group has recently presented evidence (Fig. 3) [Horovitz ZP, Goldberg ME (eds) (1980) Angiotensin-converting enzyme inhibitors: Mechanisms of action and clinical implications. Urban and Schwarzenberg, New York] that captopril does have central effects despite the fact that, in cerebrospinal fluid, the conversion of angiotensin I is not inhibited by orally given captopril. The effects of captopril on the brain renin-angiotensin system were indicated by an increase of converting enzyme and of renin in brain tissue following chronic treatment of spontaneously hypertensive rats of the stroke-prone strain (SHRSP) with this inhibitor. In another experiment, captopril was injected into the brain ventricles of SHRSP. A significant decrease of blood pressure was observed (maximum 12.8 ± 1.3 mmHg mean arterial pressure), which started 2–3 min after the captopril injection (5 μg) and lasted for about 20 min (see Fig. 3A).

The central pressor responses to angiotensin I (100 ng) were partially blocked with a maximum of about 70% inhibition after 15 min and returned gradually to control values within 150 min (Fig. 3B). The pressor responses to intravenous angiotensin I were studied in two groups of SHRSP: one group had been injected into the brain ventricles with 5 μg captopril and the other one with the same volume of the vehicle (0.9% NaCl) only. Thus, tachyphylactic effects due to repeated angiotensin I injections at short time intervals could be excluded. The intravenous angiotensin I pressor effects in the group injected centrally with Captopril were at no time significantly different from those injected with control NaCl. The following conclusions can be drawn from these experiments:

1. Blood pressure decreases in response to centrally administered Captopril in SHRSP. This is not the case in normotensive control rats.

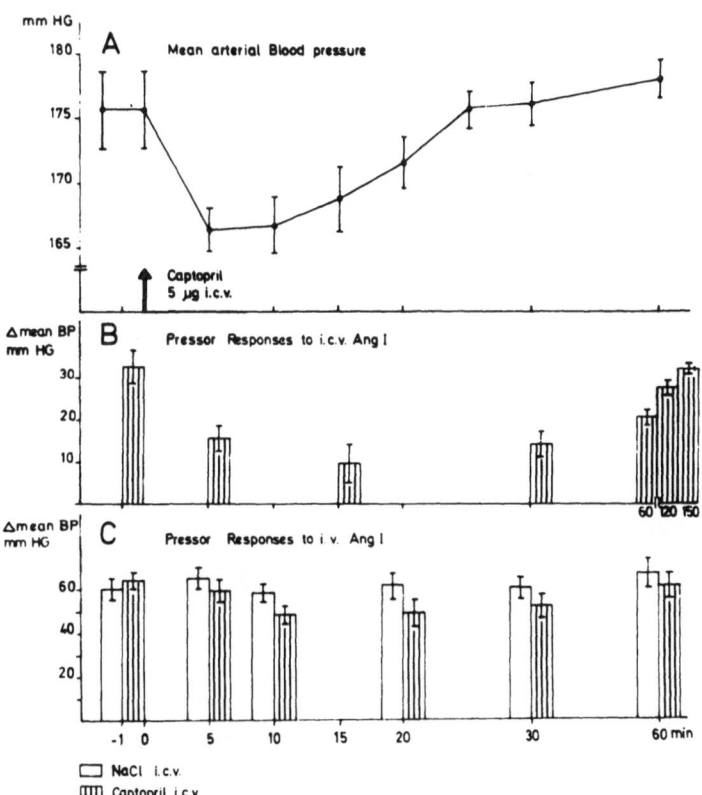

Fig. 3. Changes in mean arterial blood pressure of spontaneously hypertensive rats ($\bar{x}$ ± SEM). Effects of intracerebroventricular (ICV) captopril (5 μg) on systemic blood pressure **(a)** and on the angiotensin-induced pressor responses following central (ICV) **(b)** and peripheral (i.v.) **(c)** angiotensin I (ANG I) administration.

2. Low doses of central captopril (5 µg) cause converting-enzyme inhibition in the CSF and in the brain, but not in the peripheral blood. The fall of blood pressure appears, therefore, to be centrally mediated.

3. In view of the increased renin activity in brain and the suppressed renin in plasma of SHRSP, and in view of the fact that oral captopril does have central effects, these results support a central component in the antihypertensive action of captopril by inhibiting the brain renin-angiotensin system.

Session 18
New Approaches to Renin System Blockade

Chairman: R. L. Soffer

Position Paper: New Approaches to Renin System Blockade

Edgar Haber

Renin has no known direct physiologic effect, but acts only to cleave its substrate angiotensinogen, an alpha II globulin that is synthesized in the liver. The amino acid sequence of the amino terminal 14 residues of renal substrate is known (Fig. 1). Renin cleaves between two leucine residues at positions 10 and 11 to release the decapeptide angiotensin I. Angiotensin I is, in turn, split between residues 8 and 9 by a converting enzyme to yield the active pressor hormone angiotensin II. Aminopeptidases further degrade angiotensin II by removing the amino-terminal aspartic acid. The resultant heptapeptide, sometimes called angiotensin III, is believed by some investigators to be the primary mediator of adrenocortical aldosterone secretion (1). Angiotensin II and III have very short half-lives in the circulation and are further degraded to smaller inactive peptides (2).

RENIN ANTIBODY AS A PHYSIOLOGIC PROBE

The complete purification of hog (3–7) kidney renin has now been accomplished. Because the trained conscious dog has been such a useful model in the examination of the role of the renin system in a variety of deranged physiologic states, we endeavored to purify renin from canine kidney (8) in order to elicit specific antibodies for use as physiologic probes (9). If the antigen were completely homogeneous, the objection raised previously to antibodies as renin inhibitors, i.e., their potential for reaction with other renal components, would be obviated. Furthermore, if antibody Fab fragments were obtained, potential problems with immune complexes or complement activation would be avoided. The kinetics of distribution and excretion of antibody Fab fragments make them ideal tools for both short- and long-term physiologic experiments. Immunogenicity of these antibody derivatives, when administered intravenously, is far less than that of intact antibody preparations (10).

PRODUCTION OF RENIN-SPECIFIC ANTIBODIES

Antidog renin antibodies were raised in goats by initial intramuscular and intradermal injections of the purified enzyme. High-titer antiserum was obtained. At a dilution of 1:20,000, 100 μl antiserum resulted in 50% inhibition of the enzymatic activity of 0.002 Goldblatt units (GU) standardized dog renin.

UTILIZATION OF RENIN-SPECIFIC ANTIBODIES IN PHYSIOLOGIC STUDIES

Dogs were trained to lie quietly on a padded table. One group of animals was anesthetized and subjected to unilateral nephrectomy under sterile conditions. Polyvinyl catheters were implanted chronically into the aorta, renal artery, and inferior vena cava, and the end was exteriorized. An externally inflatable silastic constricting cuff was placed around the renal artery proximal to the renal artery catheter. In some animals, an electromagnetic flow probe was secured around the origin of the renal artery. In a second group of animals, nephrectomy and the placement of the constricting cuff was omitted. Experiments on these trained conscious dogs were started 2 weeks after surgery. Systemic and renal arterial pressures were moni-

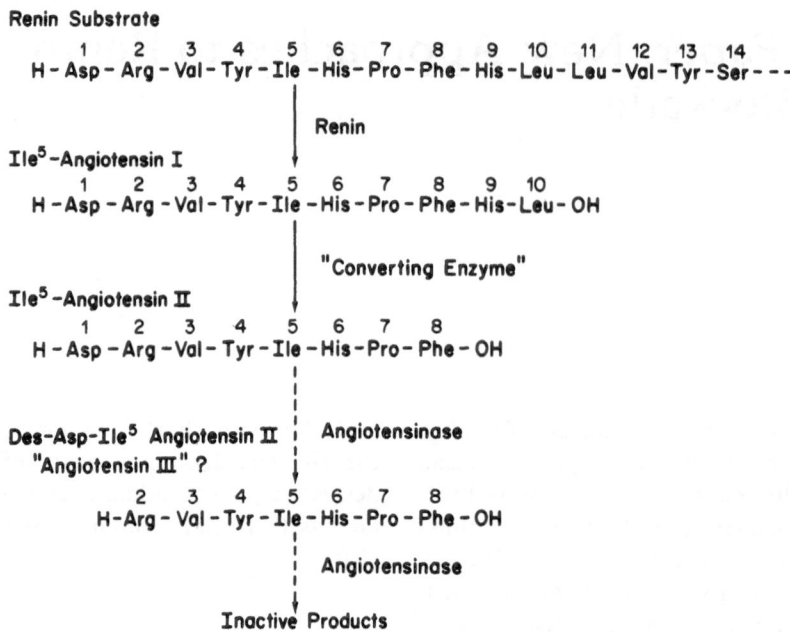

Fig. 1. Biochemistry of the renin-angiotensin system. Ile⁵-angiotensin contains isoleucine in the 5-position and is the form of peptide that occurs in man. The existence of des-Asp¹-angiotensin II as an intermediate in the pathway has not been definitely established. [Oparil S, Haber E (1974) N Engl J Med 291: 389; reprinted by permission]

tored with P23 Statham pressure transducers and recorded on a Grass polygraph; renal blood flow was simultaneously recorded with an electromagnetic flowmeter. Blood samples were collected for determination of plasma renin activity (PRA) by the radioimmunoassay of Haber et al. (11) and expressed as angiotensin I generated (ng ml⁻¹ h⁻¹). Purified renin and antisera were administered as single bolus injections through the inferior vena caval catheter. Renovascular resistance was calculated by dividing mean renal arterial pressure by renal blood flow.

EFFECT OF RENIN-SPECIFIC ANTISERUM ON EXOGENOUSLY ADMINISTERED CANINE RENIN

One GU of purified dog renin given intravenously resulted in a 30-mmHg rise in mean aortic pressure (MAP) and an approximately 50% increase in renovascular resistance. These effects were completely blocked by renin-specific antiserum. The antibodies had no effect on the pressor response to systemic administration of 2 µg angiotensin I or angiotensin II.

The basal PRA of three dogs maintained on an 80-mEq Na, 60-mEq K diet was 0.4 ng ml⁻¹ h⁻¹. Antiserum had no significant effect on MAP in the salt-replete state. Similarly, the nonapeptide angiotensin I converting enzyme inhibitor (<Glu-Trp-Pro-Arg-Pro-Gln-Ile-Pro-Pro-) resulted in only a transient fall in blood pressure of 5 mmHg in these animals.

RENIN-SPECIFIC ANTISERUM IN SODIUM DEPLETION

Four dogs were placed on a 10-mEq Na, 60-mEq K diet and given 80 mg furosemide orally for 5 days. The urinary sodium excretion at steady state was 1 mEq/day, and PRA increased to 3.8 ± 0.4 ng ml⁻¹ h⁻¹. An intravenous bolus of converting enzyme inhibitor (5 mg) decreased MAP by an average of 12 mmHg in these dogs. Administration of preimmune goat serum had no effect on PRA or MAP. Antiserum decreased PRA from 3.8 ± 0.4 to 0.4 ± 0.1 ng ml⁻¹ h⁻¹, paralleled by a prompt fall in MAP from 105 ± 2 to 94 ± 4 mmHg within 30 min. The effectiveness of renin blockade was evidenced by the lack of a pressor response to exogenous renin.

RENIN-SPECIFIC ANTISERUM IN ACUTE RENOVASCULAR HYPERTENSION

Renovascular hypertension was induced in five dogs by inflation of the silastic cuff, which reduced renal artery pressure to 50 mmHg. PRA rose from 3.4 ± 1.8 to 18.3 ± 6.3 ng ml^{-1} h^{-1} within 40 min. Simultaneously, MAP rose from a control level of 102 ± 6 to a plateau of 134 ± 7 mmHg and renal vascular resistance decreased by 11%. Administration of preimmune serum had no significant effect on these parameters. Renin-specific antiserum given 1 h after constriction caused PRA to fall to control levels in 10 min and to 1.3 ± 0.7 ng ml^{-1} h^{-1} in 40 min. The decrease in PRA was accompanied by a similar reduction in MAP to a nadir of 102 ± 6 mmHg and a further decrease of 40% in renal vascular resistance.

The duration of action of the antibody was at least 21 h, as evidenced by continued suppression of PRA and MAP at or below control levels despite maintenance of renal perfusion pressure at 50 mmHg. Beyond this time, PRA and MAP slowly approached their postconstriction, preantiserum levels. This observation regarding duration of action was further supported by the inability of exogenous renin to increase renal vascular resistance for the first 24 h.

STUDIES WITH RENIN-SPECIFIC ANTIBODY FAB FRAGMENT

In spite of a very high degree of selectivity, exhibited by the renin-specific antibody used in these studies, several criticisms may be offered concerning the use of intact antibodies in physiologic studies. First, intact antibodies aggregate with antigens to form multimolecular polymers. These immune complexes together with the complement they bind are known to influence renal function adversely. Second, antigen–antibody aggregates during the course of fixing complement release a variety of mediators that may in themselves be vasoactive

agents. Third, the use of serum introduces a wide variety of substances that may modify vasoreactivity. Fourth, as has been demonstrated above, the effects of antibody are very long lived, hence they do not lend themselves readily to short-term experiments.

To overcome these difficulties, the immune globulin fraction was first purified by DEAE cellulose chromatography in order to isolate IgG. This fraction was then subjected to papain digestion to yield Fab fragments (12). Fab fragments overcome all the disadvantages of antibody. First, they do not form immune complexes of significant size. Second, they do not fix complement when binding antigen. Third, their persistence in the circulation is brief (10).

A recapitulation of experiments in the conscious dog in both sodium-depletion and acute renovascular hypertension utilizing renin-specific Fab indicates qualitatively similar results to those obtained with antiserum. Figure 2 shows a significant hypotensive response in a sodium-depleted dog. The response is more rapid in onset and shorter in duration than that obtained with antiserum.

Figure 3 shows the results of renin-specific antibody Fab fragment infused into an animal subjected to acute renovascular hypertension utilizing the same model described previously. Again, the onset of the hypertensive response is rapid and its duration brief. Thus it appears that renin-specific Fab is a potent blocker of renin activity. It should now be available for further exploration of the various roles that this regulatory enzyme may play in cardiovascular homeostasis.

The general implication of earlier experiments with saralysin and teprotide are confirmed and the results acceptable with considerably more confidence. It is quite clear that renin does not play a major role in maintaining blood pressure in the sodium-replete animal. Sodium deprivation, however, uncovers a very different response. Significant hypotension occurs as soon as the activity of renin is inhibited. Acute renovascular hypertension in the one-kidney canine model also appears to be entirely renin dependent. There is a great deal of work still to be done in exploring other important hypertensive models. Significant questions remain concerning the genesis of chronic renovascular hypertension. What is the difference between the one- and the two-kidney model? Is the form of chronic renovascular hypertension characterized by volume expansion associated with low or normal

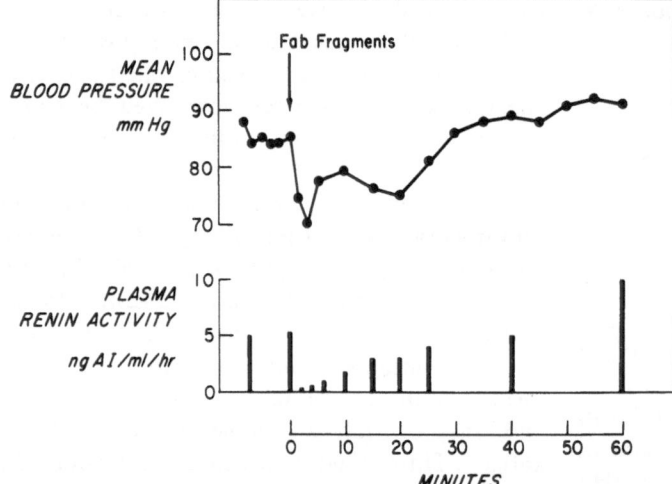

Fig. 2. In an Na⁺-depleted dog, renin-specific antibody Fab causes a transient fall in blood pressure associated with suppression of renin activity in plasma. [Haber E (1980) Clin Sci 59: 7S–19S; reprinted by permission]

plasma renin and aldosterone, renin independent, or are the levels of renin inappropriate for the degree of extracellular volume expansion that exists? What is the role of renin in malignant hypertensive models? How important is renin in the normal maintenance of sodium balance? Is angiotensin really a significant sodium-retaining agent in the normal animal, either through its direct action on the kidney or via the aldosterone pathway? I believe that we now have a tool with which to address these questions directly in the experimental animal with the full confidence that renin alone is inhibited.

RENIN INHIBITORS BASED ON SUBSTRATE ANALOGS

While the antibody Fab fragment appears to be an excellent tool for experimental investigations in animal models, it seems unlikely that the prolonged or repetitive use of antibodies will be possible in humans. Consequently we sought an agent that had both the potential of high selectivity as well as compatibility with human use. As indicated previously, renin is a remarkably fastidious protease with respect to substrate requirements. Could

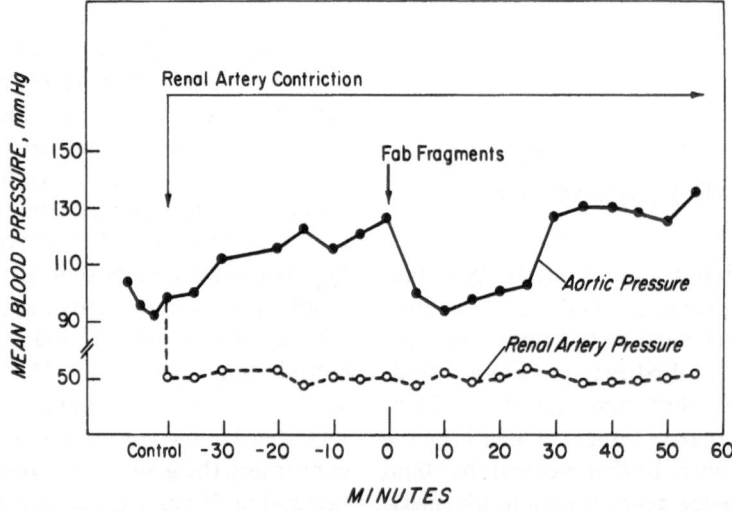

Fig. 3. Renovascular hypertension caused by renal artery constriction (initial aortarenal artery gradient was 50 mmHg) is rapidly reversed by renin-specific antibody Fab. Note the short duration of Fab action. [Haber E (1980) Clin Sci 59: 7S–19S; reprinted by permission]

the unique sequence of amino acids around the cleavage site be used to construct a very specific enzyme inhibitor? Skeggs et al. (13) defined the minimal sequence from natural protein substrate that interacts strongly with renin. The octapeptide sequence extending from histidine-6 through tyrosine-13 (Fig. 1) has kinetic parameters essentially the same as those of the full tetradecapeptide renin substrate (13).

Kokubu et al. (14) synthesized a number of analogs of the tetrapeptide found between residues 10 to 13 (Fig. 1) in the hope of creating an effective inhibitor. While inhibition could be shown, inhibitory constants were only in the millimolar range.

To produce more effective inhibitors, Poulsen et al. (15, 16) synthesized analogs of a larger segment of renin substrate. Peptides were tested as renin inhibitors using a radioimmunoassay (17) to measure decreases in the generation of angiotensin I from either natural protein substrate or the tetradecapeptide. Addition of the octapeptide analogs to the standard assay mixture decreased the rate of formation of angiotensin I. Data from these tests fit the standard Michaelis-Menten equation with a high degree of precision (15). All the synthetic peptides tested were competitive inhibitors.

The native octapeptide sequence is both a competitive inhibitor and a substrate for renin. Edman degradation of the reaction product shows the enzyme quantitatively cleaves the leucyl-leucine bond in the octapeptide (15). The first modifications made in the octapeptide sequence were aimed at producing peptides that would bind, but not be cleaved by renin. Replacement of either leucyl residue (10 and 11 in Fig. 1) with the D-enantiomorph yields inhibitors that are not cleaved by renin. In addition, the [D-Leu6] octapeptide binds renin one order of magnitude (3 μm) more tightly than the parent octapeptide (39 μm).

Since both a high concentration of the inhibitor and tight binding to renin are required to compete with natural substrate, the effectiveness of an inhibitor is best judged by the ratio between solubility and K_i. Addition of a single prolyl residue to [Phe6] octapeptide doubled solubility and decreased K_i so that this ratio increased from 6 to 100 (18). A further improvement in the ratio was obtained by attaching a lysyl residue to the C terminus. Solubility of the Pro-[Phe5, Phe6] octapeptide was increased eightfold with only a doubling of K_i. The solubility/K_i ratio was 420. The pattern of solubility as a function of pH is also changed.

The choice of the lysyl residue was dictated by the desire to increase solubility by adding a charged group without altering the conformation of the inhibitor.

K_i of the various inhibitors can be related to the lipophilicity of amino acid residues at the cleavage site. Replacement of the leucyl residues with phenylalanine yields an analog that binds about 40 times as well as Pro-octapeptide (K_i, 1 versus 39 μm) (19). Pro-[Phe5, Phe6] octapeptide is inactive in vivo. This peptide was cleared from circulation with a half-life considerably less than 1 min. The lysyl analog has a half-life of 3.8 min and is lost from circulation at an exponential rate.

In vivo inhibition of renin by the peptide Pro-His-Pro-Phe-His-Phe-Phe-Val-Tyr-Lys was examined in the monkey *Macaca fascicularis* (20). When infused into normotensive sodium-replete monkeys, no significant change in blood pressure was observed. Purified human renin (7), angiotensin I and II were then injected intravenously at concentrations sufficient to cause pressure rises of 22, 30, and 30 mmHg, respectively. Infusion of the renin inhibitor at a rate of 0.2 mg kg^{-1} min^{-1} blocked the pressor response to human renin ($p < 0.004$), but not that of angiotensin I or II (Fig. 4). These observations indicate that the Pro-[Phe5, Phe6] octapeptidyl-lysine is neither a hypotensive agent in its own right nor does it act as

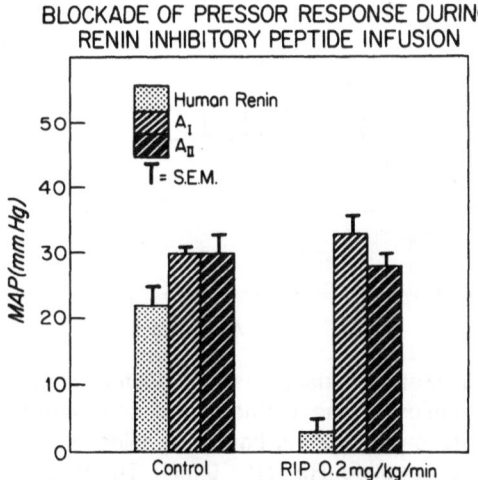

Fig. 4. Pressor response to injections of 2.5 Goldblatt units human renin, 0.3 μg angiotensin 1, or 0.3 μg angiotensin II in the salt-replete *M. fascicularis* in the presence and absence of a constant infusion of Pro-[Phe5, Phe6] octapeptidyl-lysine (0.2 mg kg^{-1} min^{-1}). [Burton et al. (20)]

a converting enzyme inhibitor at the doses used. It appears to block renin specifically.

NA⁺-DEPLETED, NORMOTENSIVE ANIMALS

A total of five studies were performed in sodium-depleted normotensive monkeys. Urinary sodium was 0.62 ± 0.46 (SD) mEq day^{-1}, and PRA was 13.6 ± 5.1 (SD) mg ml^{-1} h^{-1}. Renin inhibitory peptide, given as a 2-mg kg^{-1} intravenous bolus, resulted in a prompt reduction in MAP from 105 $\pm$ 4 to 79 $\pm$ 3 mmHg ($p < 0.004$) (Fig. 5). MAP gradually increased over the ensuing 15 min to a new base line of 100 ± 4 mmHg. The subsequent injection of 1 mg kg^{-1} converting enzyme inhibitor resulted in reduction of MAP to 82 ± 5 mmHg ($p < 0.006$). There is no significant difference be-

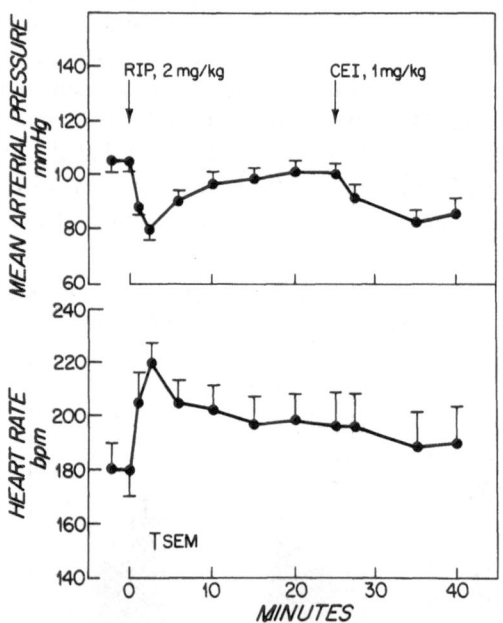

Fig. 5. Mean arterial pressure reduction occurred in five studies of the normotensive sodium-depleted state following a 2-mg kg^{-1} bolus injection of renin inhibitory peptide (RIP) ($p < 0.004$). This was associated with significant cardiac acceleration ($p < 0.003$). The MAP reduction in response to the 1 mg kg^{-1} converting enzyme inhibitor (CEI) ($p < 0.006$) was not significantly different compared with the renin inhibitor peptide response. Abbreviations as described in Methods. [Burton et al. (20)]

tween the hypotensive response to renin inhibitory peptide and that of converting enzyme inhibitor. In this group of monkeys, an important finding was the significant increase of heart rate from 180 $\pm$ 10 to 220 $\pm$ 7 bpm ($p < 0.003$) that occurred during the hypotensive response to renin inhibitory peptide. Following return of MAP to base line, the heart rate remained at an elevated steady-state value of 196 ± 12 bpm ($p < 0.03$ compared with original heart rate of 180 ± 10 bpm). There was no further significant change in heart rate during the hypotensive response to converting enzyme inhibitor.

NA⁺-DEPLETED, HYPERTENSIVE ANIMALS

Renin inhibitory peptide was administered to sodium-depleted, renin-dependent, hypertensive monkeys. In this model, the right kidney was removed and an inflatable cuff was placed around the aorta immediately above the left renal artery. Bolus intravenous injection of peptide produced dose-dependent MAP reductions ranging from 15 mmHg (0.5–1.0 mg kg^{-1}) to 70 mmHg (3.0 mg kg^{-1}). The latter response was associated with a 40-bpm increase in heart rate. To lower MAP gradually, renin inhibitory peptide was given as a graded infusion in 0.2 mg kg^{-1} min^{-1} increments. Six studies were performed (Fig. 6). The base-line MAP was 107 ± 3 mmHg, increasing to 131 ± 3 mmHg ($p < 0.002$) following 1 h of aortic cuff inflation. PRA increased from 12.5 ± 1.7 to 33.2 ± 3.5 mg ml^{-1} h^{-1} ($p < 0.02$). Graded infusion of renin inhibitory peptide was initiated when MAP was stable at this hypertensive level, and prompt reduction of blood pressure occurred. At a dose of 0.4 mg kg^{-1} min^{-1}, the reduction of MAP to 121 ± 2 mmHg was significant ($p < 0.005$). Continued infusion at the rate of 0.6 mg kg^{-1} min^{-1} resulted in reduction of MAP to 107 $\pm$ 4 mmHg ($p < 0.004$ compared to 131 ± 3 mmHg, $p < 0.008$ compared to 121 ± 2 mmHg). When this prehypertensive level of MAP was achieved, the infusion was discontinued. MAP increased to 125 ± 3 mmHg within 5 mins of discontinuation, a hypertensive level not significantly different from 131 ± 3 mmHg. After equilibration at 127 ± 3 mmHg, intravenous administration of

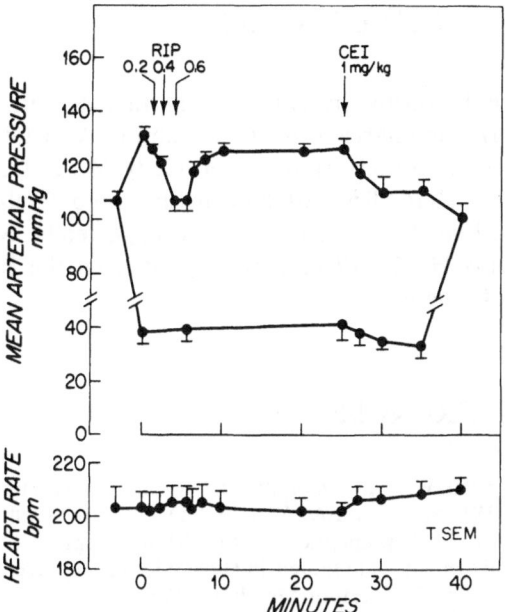

Fig. 6. Following 1 h aortic cuff inflation, mean arterial pressure rose from 107 to 131 mmHg in six studies of renin-dependent hypertension. Renin inhibitory peptide was given as a graded infusion of 0.2-mg $kg^{-1}min^{-1}$ increments. At 0.6 mg $kg^{-1}min^{-1}$, MAP was restored to prehypertensive levels of ($p < 0.004$). After a brief period, infusion was discontinued and MAP increased to 127 mmHg. Converting enzyme inhibitor, 1 mg kg^{-1}, reduced MAP to 111 mmHg ($p < 0.002$). The MAP responses to renin-inhibitory peptide and converting enzyme inhibitor were similar ($p = NS$). Heart rate was consistent throughout. [Burton et al. (20)]

1 mg kg^{-1} converting enzyme inhibitor resulted in reduction of MAP to 111 ± 4 mmHg ($p < 0.002$). The nadir hypotensive response to renin inhibitory peptide and converting enzyme inhibitor were comparable ($P = NS$). Throughout this experiment there was no appreciable change in heart rate.

These experiments closely duplicate the observations previously detailed utilizing renin-specific antibody. The substrate inhibitor peptide acts specifically on renin and does not inhibit the pressor action of either angiotensin I or II. It appears to be well tolerated without any hemodynamic consequences in the normotensive sodium-replete animal. The role of renin in maintaining blood pressure in the sodium-depleted state as well as its importance in acute renovascular hypertension are again clearly demonstrated. The potential of

the peptide lies particularly in its selectivity for human and subhuman primate renin. The substrate analog peptides we have studied have very little inhibitory activity with respect to animal renins (21). Apart from the evident potential for exploring the role of renin in normal human cardiovascular homeostasis and in certain forms of renovascular and renal hypertensive, the opportunity exists for defining the role of this enzyme in the genesis and maintenance of essential hypertension in man. There are highly provocative reports demonstrating a hypotensive effect of the converting enzyme inhibitor captopril in essential hypertension (22). Are these effects related to renin inhibition, to the actions of the converting enzyme inhibitor on kinins, or to yet another system? Utilization of a specific renin inhibitor will serve to clarify this issue.

CONCLUSION

I have attempted to demonstrate the singular value of specific reagents in solving several problems related to the importance of the renin-angiotensin system in physiologic regulation. Renin-specific antibody, particularly antibody Fab fragments, appears to be an extremely potent physiologic tool for demonstrating the role of renin both in normal vascular homeostasis and in the genesis of experimental forms of hypertension. A decapeptide analog of renin substrate is also a specific in vivo inhibitor particularly suited to experiments in subhuman primates and possibly in man. This blocker may permit the dissection of the role of renin in human physiology and in hypertension.

SUMMARY

In order to better define the role of renin both in physiologic control of the circulation as well as in certain pathophysiologic states, it would be desirable to have more specific inhibitors available for both experimental and clinical studies. This chapter describes two specific inhibitors of renin—an antibody to highly purified renal renin and a peptide that is a specific inhibitor of the action of renin on its substrate.

Canine renin was purified to homogeneity [Dzau et al. (8)] and monospecific antibodies raised in goats. Both unpurified antiserum as well as purified antibody Fab fragments were utilized as physiologic probes in the unanesthetized trained dog. The antibody inhibited the pressor action of exogenously administered dog renin, but did not impair the pressor action of either angiotensin I or II. Administration of either antibody or renin-specific Fab had no hemodynamic effect on sodium-replete dogs. However, after sodium depletion, the administration of either antibody or Fab resulted in a significant fall in blood pressure. The depressor response of Fab was more rapid and of shorter duration than that of antibody. Renovascular hypertension was created by inflation of a silastic cuff around the renal artery in an uninephrectomized dog. A 50-ml gradient resulted in a rise of plasma-renin activity and significant hypertension. The administration of either antiserum or renin-specific Fab resulted in a prompt fall in blood pressure to normotensive levels. Again, the onset of hemodynamic changes was more rapid with Fab and of shorter duration than with intact antibody. A renin inhibitor, based on an analog of renin substrate structure, was synthesized. Its sequence was Pro-His-Pro-Phe-His-Phe-Phe-Val-Tyr-Lys. This inhibitor was effective with human and nonhuman primate renin, but was ineffective with renins of other animals tested. In the monkey *Macaca fascicularis* no significant change in blood pressure was obtained upon infusion of the peptide when the animal was sodium replete. However, the pressor effect of purified human renin was inhibited in these animals after infusion of the peptide. The pressor effect of either angiotensin I or angiotensin II was not affected. In sodium-depleted normotensive animals, infusion of the peptide resulted in a significant depressor response. Renovascular hypertension was effected in *M. fascicularis* by uninephrectomy and the constriction of a silastic cuff around the abdominal aorta above the remaining renal artery. Constriction of the cuff resulted in significant systemic hypertension. Infusion of the peptide was promptly followed by a fall in blood pressure to normotensive levels.

Thus, by the use of two different but highly specific inhibitors or renin, the role of the renin-angiotensin system is demonstrated in the maintenance of normal blood pressure during sodium depletion and in the initiation of renovascular hypertension.

ACKNOWLEDGMENT

The following investigators participated in the work summarized in this lecture: A. Clifford Barger, James Burton, Robert Cody, Victor Dzau, Allan Herd, Richard Kopelman, Knud Poulsen, and Eve Slater. This work was supported by NIH grants HL-19517 and by a grant from the Reynolds Industries.

REFERENCES

1. Blair-West JR, Coghlan JP, Denton DA, Funder JW, Scoggins BA, Wright RD (1971) The effects of the heptapeptide (2–8) and hexapeptide (3–8) fragments of angiotensin II on aldosterone secretion. J Clin Endocrinol Metab 32: 575–578
2. Hodge RL, Ng KKF, Vane JR (1967) Disappearance of angiotensin from the circulation of the dog. Nature 215: 138
3. Corvol P, Devaux C, Ito T, Sicard P, Duclox J, Menard J (1977) Large scale purification of hog renin: Physiochemical characterization. Circ Res 41: 616–622
4. Inagami T, Murakami K (1977) Pure renin: Isolation from hog kidney and characterization. J Biol Chem 252: 2978–2983
5. Galen FX, Devaux C, Guyenne T, Menard J, Corvol P (1979) Multiple forms of human renin: Purification and characterization. J Biol Chem 254: 4848–4855
6. Yokosawa H, Inagami T, Haas E (1978) Purification of human renin. Biochim Biophys Res Commun 83: 306–312
7. Slater, EE, Cohn RC, Dzau VJ, Butler VP Jr (1976) Reversal of advanced digoxin intoxication with Fab fragments of digoxin specific antibodies. N Engl J Med 294: 797–800
8. Dazu VJ, Slater EE, Haber E (1979) Complete purification of dog renal renin. Biochemistry 18: 5224–5228
9. Dzau VJ, Kopelman RI, Barger AC, Slater EE, Haber E (1980) Renin specific antibody for study of cardiovascular homeostasis. Science 207: 1091–1093
10. Smith TW, Lloyd BL, Spicer N, Haber E (1979) Immunogenicity and kinetics of distribution and elimination of sheep digoxin-specific IgG and Fab fragments in the rabbit and baboon. Clin Exp Immunol 36: 384–396
11. Haber E, Koerner T, Page LB, Kliman B, Purnode A (1969) Application of a radioimmunoassay for angiotensin I to the physiologic measurements of plasma renin activity in normal human subjects. J Clin Endocrinol Metab 29: 1349–1355
12. Smith TW, Haber E, Yeatman L, Butler VP Jr (1976) Reversal of advanced digoxin intoxication

with Fab fragments of digoxin specific antibodies. N Engl J Med 294: 797–800

13. Skeggs L, Lentz K, Kahn J. Hochstrasser H (1968) Kinetics of the reaction of renin with nine synthetic peptide substrates. J Exp Med 128: 13–34

14. Kokubu T, Hwada K, Ito T, Ueda E, Yamamura Y, Mizoguchi T, Shigezane K (1973) Peptide inhibitors of renin-angiotensinogen reaction system. Biochem Pharmacol 22: 3217–3223

15. Poulsen K, Burton J, Haber E (1973) Competitive inhibitors of renin. Biochemistry 12: 3877–3882

16. Burton J, Poulsen K, Haber E (1975) Competitive inhibitors of renin. Inhibitors effective at physiological pH. Biochemistry 14: 3892–3898

17. Poulsen K, Haber E, Burton J (1976) On the specificity of human renin: studies with peptide inhibitors. Biochim Biophys Acta 452: 533–537

18. Haber E, Burton J (1979) Inhibitors of renin and their utility in physiologic studies. Fed Proc 38: 2768–2773

19. Burton J, Poulsen K, Haber E (1978) Solubility and lipopholicity relationships in the design of renin inhibitors. In: Donaruma LG, Vogol O (eds) Polymer drugs, Academic Press, New York pp 219–238

20. Burton J, Cody RJ Jr, Herd JA, Haber E (1980) Specific inhibition of renin by an angiotensinogen analog: studies in sodium-depletion and renin-dependent hypertension. Proc Natl Acad Sci USA 77(9): 5476–5479

21. Poulsen K, Haber E, Burton J (1976) On the specificity of human renin: Studies with peptide inhibitors. Biochim Biophys Acta 252: 533–537

22. Gavras H, Brunner HR, Turini GA, Kershaw GR, Tifft CP, Cuttelod S, Gavras I, Vukovich RA, McKinstry DN (1978) Antihypertensive effect of the oral angiotensin converting-enzyme inhibitor SQ 14225 in man. New Eng J Med 298: 991–995

Studies on Experimental Hypertension Using Blockers of Renin, Converting Enzyme, and Angiotensin II

F. M. Bumpus

Since the time of Tigerstedt and Bergman it has been known that nephrectomized animals respond to renin with a greater blood pressure rise that is longer lasting than in normal animals. Also, many investigators have observed that the plasma from nephrectomized animals generated angiotensin faster than that from normal animals and have speculated that this is due either to changes in renin substrate or to other unknown factors in the plasma. In our attempts to study this phenomenon, a search for the possibility of an inhibitory substance to renin was initiated. This led to the isolation of a phospholipid substance from the kidney, which proved to be an inhibitor of renin (1). The phospholipid as isolated from the kidney was found to give very little inhibition during the first hour of a 4-h incubation period, and when the lipid was reisolated from the assay mixture after incubation, a new phospholipid was obtained (2). Treatment of the lipid isolated from the kidney with phospholipase A from snake venom, which cleaved saturated fatty acids from the molecule, yielded a lipophospholipid that was shown to have the renin-inhibitory action. This lysophospholipid formed by incubation with phospholipase A or with plasma itself was shown to inhibit renin but to have no effect on the response to angiotensin itself.

This phospholipid when injected into hypertensive rats reduced the blood pressure either in acutely or chronically hypertensive animals. When plasma preinhibitor was administered intramuscularly to acutely hypertensive rats, the blood pressure was reduced in parallel to a reduction in the plasma-renin activity (PRA) (3). A similar phenomenon was noted when the preinhibitor was injected into chronically hypertensive animals—both the blood pressure and the PRA were reduced. It takes time for the reduction in blood pressure, and at the cessation of the injection of the preinhibitor several days are required for a return of the blood pressure to the hypertensive levels. When this preinhibitor was given to normotensive animals, the PRA decreased, while the blood pressure remained unchanged. These results were in agreement with those obtained when hypertensive dogs were made antigenic with renin; however, the renin results remained in question at that time, since impure renin was used to immunize the animals.

Numerous phospholipid renin inhibitors have been synthesized, the most potent of which is a compound designated as URI-73A, an analog of lysophosphidityl ethanolamine as reported by Turcotte et al. (4).

The idea has been developed in utilizing specific angiotensin II antagonists, that in two-kidney hypertensive animals the renin-angiotensin system plays a role in the maintenance of hypertension, but in the one-kidney model it does not. It is generally felt that the one-kidney model is volume dependent rather than renin dependent. We designed experiments to test both a short-term and a long-term one- and two-kidney renal hypertensive models with three types of inhibitors: one blocking renin, one blocking a converting enzyme, and finally the angiotensin II antagonist [Sar^1, Thr^8] A II. Each of these three types of inhibitors was given to the same group of animals at different times and in different order of injection. As expected, all three substances—the synthetic renin inhibitor, URI-73A; the converting enzyme inhibitor, SQ 14225; and the angiotensin II antagonist [Sar^1, Thr^8] AII—all lower blood pressure. The converting enzyme inhibitor produced the greatest drop in pressure, the renin inhibitor almost equally as potent, and the angiotensin II antagonist lowered blood pressure, but not quite to the normotensive levels (4). In the chronic two-kidney model the [Sar¹, Thr⁸] AII had no ability to reduce blood pressure, while the SQ 14225 lowered blood pressure essentially to the normotensive level. While the renin inhibitor lowered blood pressure very significantly in these animals, it did not return all the way to normotensive levels. It must be remembered that the URI-73A does not reduce renin to the undetectable levels in the animals injected. Results are very similar in the one-kidney chronic hypertensive rat of 12 weeks after clipping. Here the [Sar¹, Thr⁸] AII had essentially no effect on the hypertensive animals, while SQ 14225 and the renin inhibitor both lower blood pressure significantly. One might speculate that since the phospholipid renin inhibitor and the converting enzyme antagonist both block the enzyme system from preventing the formation of angiotensin, these experiments would strongly suggest that the renin-angiotensin system is involved. On the other hand, it is difficult to explain why the relatively high levels of [Sar¹, Thr⁸] AII did not lower blood pressure in these animals. If, indeed, the SQ 14225 and the phospholipid are lowering blood pressure by a mechanism other than that related to the renin-angiotensin system, it is difficult to believe that they both would be working through a similar mechanism. It may be that in vivo the angiotensin analog cannot effectively compete with the endogenous natural peptide or that it is not getting to the site of action. Since it is a competitive antagonist, it is possible that its effect can be overcome by increasing amounts of the agonist, while the other two compounds are enzyme inhibitors that prevent the formation of the agonist. There are reports that volume expansion is a contributory factor in the maintenance of low-renin hypertension. This suggests that perhaps changes in volume alone are probably not major factors in the maintenance of chronic hypertension of renal origin. However, since the hypertension is associated with sodium retention, perhaps sodium itself may be playing an important role in the maintenance of hypertension. To determine whether or not large quantities of [Sar¹, Thr⁸] AII would indeed lower blood pressure in chronic hypertensive animals, we infused large quantities of [Sar¹, Thr⁸] AII into chronic two-kidney one-clip hypertensive rats. Following infusion of 125 g/k/min, for several hours the blood pressure dropped and was maintained at a reduced level during the period of infusion, which lasted for 4 days. At the cessation of infusion, the pressure slowly returned toward the hypertensive level, but this required a number of days to reach the original hypertensive level. By contrast, following infusion of [Sar¹, Thr⁸] AII at the same level into one-kidney one-clip chronic hypertensive rats, it was noted that the blood pressure drops for the first 2 days, but while the infusion is still continued the animal seems to escape to the original hypertensive level. Infusion of increased amounts of this antagonist will lower the blood pressure only slightly, and for a short period, at which time the pressure then returns to the original hypertensive state.

These data utilizing a renin inhibitor and converting enzyme inhibitors confirmed the results of the original work with production of antirenin in the hypertensive animal. However, they do not conclusively prove the role of the renin-angiotensin system in these experimental models, particularly because of the inability to reserve the hypertension with the angiotensin II antagonist.

SUMMARY

Antihypertensive comparisons are made using a natural lysophospholipid and its synthetic analogs (renin inhibitor); a converting enzyme inhibitor; SQ 14225; and an angiotensin inhibitor [Sar¹, Thr⁸] angiotensin II. The actions of the renin inhibitor and converting enzyme inhibitor (CEI) were almost parallel with the CEI, produced a slightly greater reduction in blood pressure. In the two-kidney one-clip model with long-term hypertension as well as the one-kidney one-clip rat model, quantities of angiotensin II antagonist, which blocked exogenous angiotensin, did not reduce blood pressure, while extremely high levels (10 μg/k/min) of the antagonist infused into the animals for several days did cause the pressure to drop significantly. The pressure of one-kidney one-clip animal returned to the hypertensive level during infusion, and infusion of greater quantities of inhibitor temporarily reduced pressure. This difference in action is not understood at this time, but it leads to speculation that mechanisms other than angiotensin II may be participating in the chronic model, even though both converting enzyme inhibitors and a renin inhibitor maintain a significant reduction in pressure.

REFERENCES

1. Sen S, Smeby, RR, Bumpus FM (1967) Isolation of a phospholipid renin inhibitor from kidney. Biochemistry 6: 1572
2. Smeby RR, Sen S, Bumpus FM (1968) A naturally occurring renin inhibitor. Circ Res 214: 337
3. Sen S, Smeby RR, Bumpus FM (1969) Plasma renin activity in hypertensive rats after treatment with renin inhibitor. Am J Physiol 216: 499
4. Sen S, Smeby RR, Bumpus FM, Turcotte JG (1979) Role of renin-angiotensin system in chronic renal hypertensive rats. Hypertension 1: 427

Active-Site Specific Inhibitors of Angiotensin-Converting Enzyme

David W. Cushman, Miguel A. Ondetti, and Bernard Rubin

Angiotensin-converting enzyme (kininase II) converts the inactive decapeptide angiotensin I (Asp-Arg-Val-Tyr-Ile-His-Pro-Phe-His-Leu) to the vasopressor and sodium-retaining octapeptide angiotensin II (Asp-Arg-Val-Tyr-Ile-His-Pro-Phe) and inactivates the vasodepressor, sodium-depleting nonapeptide bradykinin (Arg-Pro-Pro-Gly-Phe-Ser-Pro-Phe-Arg) (1, 2). Inhibition of this enzyme is the most effective method now employed for interrupting the pathophysiologic function of the renin-angiotensin-aldosterone system. Converting enzyme inhibitors do not have the agonistic activity encountered with presently available angiotensin II receptor antagonists (3); they bind to their receptor (the enzyme's active site) much more effectively than the peptide (angiotensin I) with which they compete (4), and their target enzyme, unlike renin (5), is not subject to great increases in functional activity in response to reduced blood levels of angiotensin II. The ability of converting enzyme inhibitors to increase blood or tissue levels of bradykinin may be a diagnostic liability, but it is at least potentially a therapeutic asset.

The first inhibitors of angiotensin-converting enzyme with the requisite potency and specificity for use as antihypertensive drugs were naturally occurring peptides from the venom of the Brazilian viper *Bothrops jararaca*. Bradykinin-potentiating peptide 5_a (BPP$_{5a}$, <Glu-Lys-Trp-Ala-Pro) (Fig. 1), the most potent venom peptide inhibitor, is also a substrate for the converting enzyme and is rapidly metabolized in vivo (6, 7). The nonapeptide SQ 28881 (<Glu-Trp-Pro-Arg-Pro-Gln-Ile-Pro-Pro) is not a substrate and has a much longer duration of inhibitory activity in vivo than does the pentapeptide. SQ 20881 (teprotide) specifically inhibits actions of angiotensin I and augments those of bradykinin in vitro and in vivo (4, 6). It is a highly effective antihypertensive drug, but it is active only by parenteral administration (8).

Structure–activity correlations obtained with analogs of the competitive inhibitors BPP$_{5a}$ and SQ 20881 indicated that their carboxyl-terminal tripeptide residues bind to the active site of the enzyme at the same subsites (S_1, S_1', and S_2' in Fig. 1) that are essential for binding and cleavage of peptide substrates, such as angiotensin I and bradykinin. The sequence Trp-Ala-Pro of BPP$_{5a}$ is nearly optimal for binding to this portion of the active site (6). However, both BPP$_{5a}$ and SQ 20881 bind to angiotensin-converting enzyme with much greater affinity than either biologically important peptide substrate, apparently due to additional interactions with adjacent subsites (S_2–S_7) that do not normally participate in substrate binding.

Increasing knowledge of the chemical and enzymatic properties of angiotensin-converting enzyme, including the mechanism of inhibition by snake venom peptides, has recently made it possible to design simple nonpeptide molecules that interact with great affinity and selectivity at the active site of this enzyme (6, 7, 9, 10). Angiotensin-converting enzyme is a carboxypeptidase that splits dipeptides from the carboxyl-terminal ends of its substrates; and the proposed presence of functional zinc ion in this enzyme, as in other carboxypeptidases, was recently confirmed (11). Byers and Wolfenden (12) demonstrated marked competitive inhibition of the well-characterized carboxypeptidase A of bovine pancreas by D-2-benzylsuccinic acid. They postulated that this inhibitor was a biproduct analog, owing its great affinity for the enzyme to multiple active-site–binding interactions characteristic of both products of carboxypeptidase action; the benzyl and 1-carboxyl functions are proposed to bind in the same manner as analogous groups of the amino acid product, and the 4-carboxyl group to bind like the terminal carboxyl group of the other carboxy-

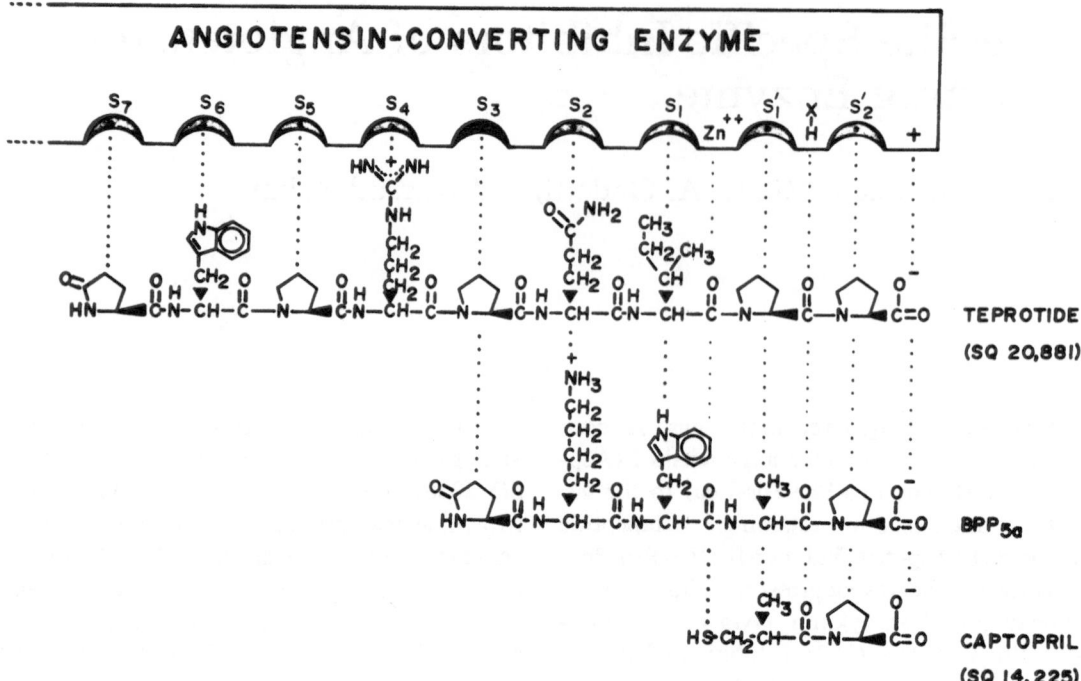

Fig. 1. Postulated interactions of potent competitive inhibitors at the active site of angiotensin-converting enzyme. BPP_{5a} (<Glu-Lys-Trp-Ala-Pro), also a substrate for the enzyme, has a K_i value of 0.06 μM; SQ 20,881 (<Glu-Trp-Pro-Arg-Pro-Gln-Ile-Pro-Pro—) has a K_i value of 0.1 μM; and captopril (D-3-mercapto-2-methylpropanoyl-L-proline) has a K_i value of 0.023 μM. Subsites (circular clefts numbered in both directions from the catalytic center zinc ion) are regions on the enzyme where interactions may occur with side chains of corresponding amino acid residues of peptide substrates or inhibitors.

peptidase product, possibly, as we felt, to the enzyme-bound zinc ion. Applying similar principles, we synthesized succinyl-L-proline as a potential biproduct analog inhibitor of angiotensin-converting enzyme (6, 7, 9, 10). It was only a modest inhibitor of the rabbit lung converting enzyme (I_{50} = 330 μM), but it specifically inhibited the action of angiotensin I on a guinea pig ileum strip and augmented that of bradykinin (9). Addition of a D-2-methyl group, making the resulting inhibitor a biproduct analog of the tightly binding dipeptide Ala-Pro of BPP_{5a}, enhanced inhibitory activity 15- to 20-fold (I_{50} = 22 μM). Replacement of the putative zinc-binding 4-carboxyl function by sulfhydryl led to the extremely potent and specific competitive inhibitor captopril (Fig. 1), which had an I_{50} value of 0.023 μM.

Five important binding interactions are postulated between captopril and the active site of angiotensin-converting enzyme (Fig. 1). Each has been studied extensively by comparing inhibitory activities of analogs with specific structural modifi-

cations (6, 7, 10). Four of the active-site–binding interactions of captopril are essentially the same as those postulated for the terminal dipeptide residue Ala-Pro of BPP_{5a} (Fig. 1), but captopril cannot be cleaved by angiotensin-converting enzyme, and the interaction of its sulfhydryl group with the enzyme-bound zinc ion contributes greatly to its overall enzyme-binding affinity.

Captopril is an extremely potent competitive inhibitor, with a K_i value (enzyme-inhibitor dissociation constant) of 2×10^{-9} M. It has been shown to be markedly specific for inhibition of angiotensin-converting enzyme both in vitro and in vivo, and to be an orally effective antihypertensive drug (4, 6, 13). But only as an inhibitor of angiotensin-converting enzyme is captopril a highly selected compound; as an antihypertensive drug proposed to act by some other mechanism it is a completely random choice, and its antihypertensive action would have to be considered incredibly serendipitous. Thus, although the pathophysiologic consequences of inhibition of angiotensin-converting enzyme may be complex, it is highly probable that all antihypertensive actions of captopril have as a common denominator inhibition of this biologically important enzyme.

SUMMARY

Study of the chemical and enzymatic properties of angiotensin-converting enzyme and of its competitive inhibition by snake venom peptides has elucidated its similarity to the well-characterized zinc metallopeptidase carboxypeptidase A, and permitted development of a hypothetical active-site model. The design and optimization of simple nonpeptide compounds for maximally effective interaction with this proposed active site has culminated in development of a potent and specific orally active inhibitor captopril, an effective antihypertensive drug of novel mechanism.

REFERENCES

1. Skeggs LT, Dorer FE, Kahn JR, Lentz KE, Levine M (1976) The biochemistry of the renin-angiotensin system and its role in hypertension. Am J Med 60: 737–748
2. Erdös EG (1977) The angiotensin I converting enzyme. Fed Proc 36: 1760–1765
3. Case DB, Wallace JM, Keim HJ, Weber MA, Drayer JIM, White RP, Sealey JE, Laragh JH (1976) Estimating renin participation in hypertension: Superiority of converting enzyme inhibitor over saralasin. Am J Med 61: 790–796
4. Cushman DW, Ondetti MA (1980) Inhibitors of angiotensin-converting enzyme for treatment of hypertension. Biochem Pharmacol (To be published)
5. Haber E (1976) The role of renin in normal and pathological cardiovascular homeostasis. Circulation 54: 849–861
6. Cushman DW, Cheung HS, Sabo EF, Rubin B, Ondetti MA (1979) Development of specific inhibitors of angiotensin I converting enzyme (kininase II). Fed Proc 38: 2778–2782
7. Ondetti MA, Cushman DW, Sabo EF, Cheung HS (1979) The design of active-site-directed reversible inhibitors of exopeptidases, In: Kalman TI (ed) Drug action and design: Mechanism-based enzyme inhibitors. Elsevier/North-Holland, New York, pp 271–283
8. Gavras H, Brunner HR, Laragh JH, Sealey JE, Gavras I, Vukovich RA: (1974) An angiotensin-converting enzyme inhibitor to identify and treat vasoconstrictor and volume factors in hypertensive patients. New Engl J Med 291: 817–821
9. Ondetti MA, Rubin B, Cushman DW (1977) Design of specific inhibitors of angiotensin-converting enzyme: New class of orally active antihypertensive agents. Science 196: 441–444
10. Cushman DW, Cheung HS, Sabo EF, Ondetti MA (1977) Design of potent competitive inhibitors of angiotensin-converting enzyme. Carboxyalkanoyl and mercaptoalkanoyl amino acids. Biochemistry 16: 5484–5491
11. Das M, Soffer RL (1975) Pulmonary angiotensin-converting enzyme. Structural and catalytic properties. J Biol Chem 250: 6762–6768
12. Byers LD, Wolfenden R (1972) A potent reversible inhibitor of carboxypeptidase A J Biol Chem 247: 606–608
13. Rubin B, Antonaccio MJ, Horovitz ZP (1978) Captopril (SQ 14,225) (D-3-mercapto-2-methylpropanoyl-L-proline): A novel orally active inhibitor of angiotensin-converting enzyme and antihypertensive agent. Prog Cardiovasc Dis 21: 183–194

Regulation and Properties of Adrenal and Vascular AII Receptors

Greti Aguilera, Alessandro Capponi, and Kevin Catt

The receptor sites for AII in vascular smooth muscle and adrenal gland are the regulatory loci through which the circulating and/or locally formed peptide exerts its characteristic actions on these two major target tissues. The importance of AII in controlling blood pressure regulation, by its acute vasoconstrictor effects and through long-term actions on aldosterone secretion and sodium balance, has been demonstrated in numerous studies and needs no reiteration. The recent use of angiotensin antagonists and converting enzyme inhibitors to block the actions or formation of AII selectively has enabled the extent of angiotensin's role in blood pressure regulation to be accurately defined for the first time (1–3). It is now evident that AII exerts a major modulating effect on arterial pressure control and that it is an important component of the regulatory system that serves to maintain normal blood pressure. This role of AII is particularly evident during sodium depletion, when inhibition of converting enzyme activity causes significant drops of blood pressure in man and experimental animals. The recent recognition that captopril (SQ 14225) lowers blood pressure in many hypertensives without increased plasma renin levels (4, 5), and improves cardiac function in many patients with congestive cardiac failure, has provided further evidence for the role of AII in cardiovascular regulation.

REGULATION OF ADRENAL AII RECEPTORS

The importance of AII in controlling blood pressure indicates the need for more detailed understanding of the mechanisms of action of AII on adrenal and smooth muscle cells. We have recently defined a role for AII in the control of adrenal AII receptors and adrenal sensitivity during changes in sodium balance (6–10). In the rat, the adrenal glomerulosa receptors for AII were shown to be under continuous modulation by changes in sodium intake. Thus, adrenal receptors were increased by low-sodium diet after only 36 h reduced sodium intake, and conversely, were decreased during high-salt diet (6). At each extreme of sodium intake, the change in angiotensin receptors was accompanied by a corresponding shift in adrenal sensitivity to AII, with increased or decreased aldosterone production by glomerulosa cells in vitro during stimulation by the octapeptide. The increases in adrenal receptors and aldosterone responses during sodium restriction were shown by two approaches to be attributable to the trophic effect of AII on the zona glomerulosa cells. First, infusion of AII into normal rats was found to increase adrenal angiotensin receptors and the magnitude of glomerulosa cell responses to angiotensin stimulation (7). Second, blockade of AII formation by infusion of the converting enzyme inhibitor SQ 14225 prevented the increases in adrenal receptors and aldosterone secretion that normally accompany sodium restriction. In animals on normal sodium intake, inhibition of converting enzyme activity also caused a fall in blood AII, adrenal angiotensin receptors, and plasma aldosterone (8–10). These findings have demonstrated that AII has a primary role in controlling aldosterone secretion, both as an acute stimulus and as a long-term regulator of glomerulosa cell function, and indicate that the renin-angiotensin system acts as the major determinant of aldosterone secretion during physiological responses to altered sodium intake.

REGULATION OF SMOOTH MUSCLE AII RECEPTORS

Since the changes in adrenal sensitivity during altered sodium balance are accompanied by reciprocal changes in vascular reactivity, which is decreased in low-sodium states and increased in high-sodium states, it was also of interest to analyze the effects of sodium intake on vascular smooth muscle receptors. In a previous study (6), uterine smooth muscle sites were noted to be reduced after 7 days of sodium restriction, in contrast to the simultaneous enhancement of AII binding in the adrenal glomerulosa zone (Fig. 1). These changes suggested that a parallel form of regulation of AII receptors could occur in vascular smooth muscle, contributing to the divergent effects of changing sodium intake on adrenal and vascular responses to AII. This possibility should obviously be analyzed in vascular smooth muscle or a suitable model, in order to obtain direct information about the relevant receptor sites. However, the characterization of AII receptors in major vessels such as the aorta has been complicated by the relatively small amount of smooth muscle in these tissues (11). We recently observed that the AII receptors of urinary bladder and mesenteric artery exhibit similar binding properties and responses to altered sodium intake, and have employed these tissues for studies on the regulation of vascular AII receptors (12).

Studies on several sources of smooth muscle, including aorta, uterus, bladder, and mesenteric artery, showed relatively low binding to vascular particles, with the highest level in the mesenteric artery. Of the nonvascular tissues apart from the uterus, AII binding was highest in the urinary bladder. The AII sites in bladder and mesenteric artery were similar in terms of ionic dependence, effects of SH-active compounds, and relative binding affinities for AII analogs. In both tissues, des-Asp^1-AII displayed about one-tenth the potency of the octapeptide in displacing ^{125}I-AII from the receptors, indicating a significantly lower affinity for the heptapeptide in smooth muscle. This differs from the adrenal, where the peptides bind with similar affinities. This discrepancy could explain the differential effects the des-Asp^1-heptapeptide on the adrenal, where its activity is similar to that of AII, and on vascular responses, when the heptapeptide is much less active.

In both vascular and vesicular particles, AII receptors were decreased after 4 days of low-sodium intake and were increased by a similar period of high-sodium intake (Fig. 2). These changes in AII binding were due to a true increase and decrease in the number of available AII sites, and not to occupancy by endogenous hormone or to changes in receptor affinity. The specificity of the changes in AII receptors was indicated by

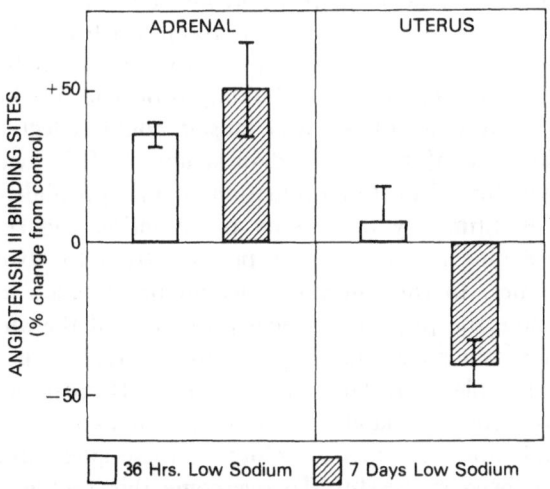

Fig. 1. Reciprocal effects of low sodium intake on adrenal and uterine receptors for AII.

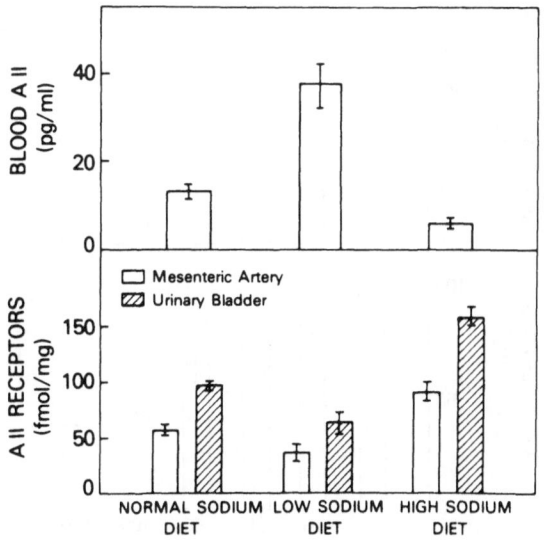

Fig. 2. Effects of low- and high-sodium intake on blood AII concentration and AII receptors in urinary bladder and mesenteric artery.

the absence of alterations in alpha- and beta-adrenergic receptors, measured by binding assays with [³H]dihydroergocryptine and [³H]dihydroalprenolol, respectively. The effects of blood AII concentration on smooth muscle receptors was tested by infusion of AII from osmotic minipumps to elevate the circulating peptide level to that present in sodium restriction. Such rates of AII infusion were accompanied by a decrease in vascular AII sites, with a further fall at higher infusion rates that elevated blood AII beyond the physiological levels seen in sodium deficiency (Fig. 3).

These findings demonstrated that the changes in responsiveness to AII during altered sodium intake are accompanied by parallel changes in vascular receptors for the peptide. These changes in AII sites were the reciprocal of those previously observed in adrenal glomerulosa cells, and provide a mechanism whereby regulation of aldosterone secretion and sodium balance can be achieved with minimal effects on vascular AII receptors. The extent to which regulation of smooth muscle receptors is responsible for the modulation of pressor reactivity remains to be defined, but such changes could obviously exert an important influence in the control of vascular reactivity.

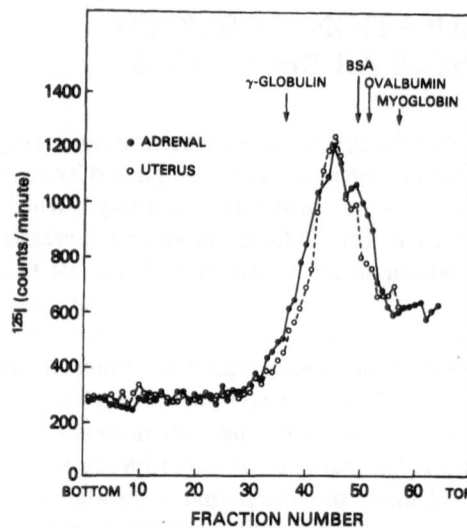

Fig. 4. Density-gradient centrifugation of photoaffinity-coupled AII-receptor complexes extracted from adrenal and uterus with Triton X-100.

PHYSICOCHEMICAL PROPERTIES OF ADRENAL AND SMOOTH-MUSCLE AII RECEPTORS

We have previously shown that adrenal and uterine AII receptors are closely similar in terms of their binding affinities for AII and its analogs (13), with the exception of the des-Asp¹-heptapeptide in rat tissues, as noted above. The latter difference probably reflects more rapid metabolism of des-Asp¹-AII in muscle, and the receptor sites in the two major target tissues appear to be functionally identical. The common binding properties of the AII sites in adrenal and muscle could reflect a similar conformation and/or structure of the two receptors. The full evaluation of this possibility will ultimately depend on the isolation and sequencing of the receptor proteins from the two tissues. In the interim, it would be of value to define the physicochemical properties of the angiotensin receptors extracted from target tissues in soluble form. Unfortunately, the AII receptors are extremely labile during detergent extraction, and most attempts to solubilize these sites have not been successful. To overcome this problem, we sought to couple the labeled peptide covalently to its receptors prior to solubilization and fractionation. This was achieved by photoaffinity labeling,

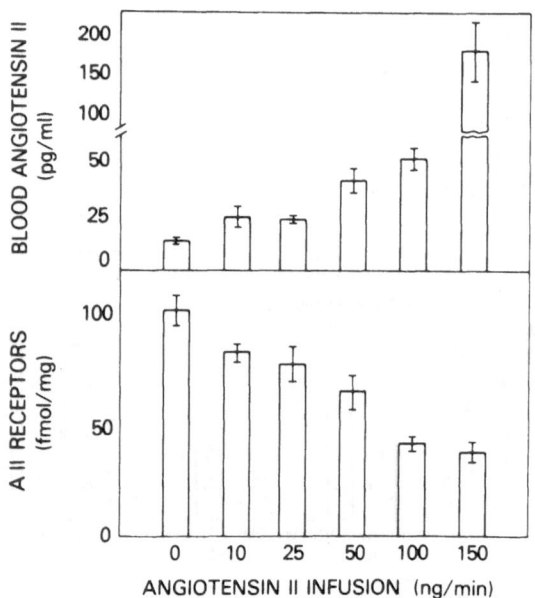

Fig. 3. Elevation of blood AII and down-regulation of vascular AII receptors during infusion of increasing concentrations of AII.

which provided a stable hormone–receptor complex that could be extracted with nonionic detergents and be subjected to physicochemical analysis.

The details of this procedure will be reported elsewhere (14), and involved the preparation of the 2-nitro-5-azidobenzoyl derivative of ^{125}I-labeled AII for receptor-binding studies. The photosensitive AII analog was synthesized as previously described (15), and was shown to retain most of the bioactivity of native AII. After binding and photolysis of the NAB derivative to dog adrenal and uterine receptors, the coupled peptide–receptor complex was extracted with Triton X-100 for analysis by gel filtration and sucrose density gradient centrifugation (Fig. 4). In both tissues, two radioactive species were observed, with molecular weights of 126,000 and 64,500. Analysis of the complexes by SDS-gel electrophoresis revealed a single component of MW 65,000 for adrenal cortex and 68,000 for myometrium, suggesting that the receptors are composed of two subunits of similar size. These observations indicate that the two receptors are similar in physical properties as well as in binding specificity, suggesting that both sites may prove to be of chemical similarity or identity when complete analysis of the binding sites can be performed.

SUMMARY

The angiotensin II (AII) receptors of the adrenal glomerulosa zone and vascular smooth muscle have been shown to undergo simultaneous and reciprocal forms of regulation during changes in sodium intake. Whereas low-sodium intake causes an increase in adrenal sites and a decrease in vascular sites, the opposite changes are induced by high-sodium diet. The effects of low-sodium diet on both adrenal and smooth muscle receptors are reproduced by infusion of AII, indicating that changes in the circulating octapeptide are responsible for regulating AII receptors in the two major target tissues. The reciprocal changes in adrenal and vascular sites contribute to the control of sodium balance by enhancing adrenal sensitivity to AII and decreasing vascular reactivity, so that regulation of aldosterone secretion by AII can occur without changes in blood pressure. In contrast to the divergent regulation of AII receptors in smooth muscle and adrenal during altered sodium intake, the two tissues show almost identical binding properties for AII and analogs. In keeping with their functional similarity, the properties of the sites extracted from adrenal and smooth muscles after photoaffinity labeling with NAB–AII were almost identical, and were consistent with a subunit structure containing a monomer of molecular weight of 65,000. The ability to label and solubilize the AII receptors should permit a more complete analysis of the structure and regulation of the sites present in the two major target tissues concerned in blood pressure regulation.

REFERENCES

1. Johnson JA, Davis JO (1973) Angiotensin II. Important role in the maintenance of arterial blood pressure. Science 179: 906–907
2. Haber E (1976) George C. Griffith Lecture. The role of renin in normal and pathological cardiovascular homeostasis. Circulation 54: 849–861
3. Gavras H, Brunner HR, Vaughan ED, Laragh JH (1973) Angiotensin-sodium interaction in blood pressure maintenance of renal hypertensive and normotensive rats. Science 180: 1369–1372
4. Brunner HR, Gavras H, Waeber B, Kershaw GR, Turini GA, Vukovich RA, McKinstry DN, Gavras I (1979) Oral angiotensin-converting enzyme inhibitor in long-term treatment of hypertensive patients. Ann Intern Med 90: 19–23
5. Niarchos AP, Pickering TG, Case DB, Sullivan P, Laragh JH (1979) Role of the renin-angiotensin system in blood pressure regulation. The Cardiovascular Effects of converting enzyme inhibition in normotensive subjects. Circ Res 45: 829–873
6. Aguilera G, Hauger RL, Catt KJ (1978) Control of aldosterone secretion during sodium restriction: adrenal receptor regulation and increased adrenal sensitivity to angiotensin II. Proc Natl Acad Sci USA 75: 975–979
7. Hauger RL, Aguilera G, Catt KJ (1978) Angiotensin II receptors sites in the adrenal glomerulosa zone. Nature 271: 176–178
8. Aguilera G, Catt KJ (1978) Regulation of aldosterone secretion by the renin-angiotensin system during sodium restriction in rats. Proc Natl Acad Sci USA 75: 4057–4061
9. Catt KJ, Aguilera G, Capponi A, Fujita K, Schirar A, Fakunding J (1979) Angiotensin II receptors and aldosterone secretion. J Endocrinol 81: 37P–48P
10. Aguilera G, Schirar A, Baukal A, Catt KJ (1980) Angiotensin II receptors. Properties and regulation in adrenal glomerulosa cells. Circ Res Suppl I, 46: I–118–127

11. Devynck MA, Meyer P (1976) Angiotensin receptors in vascular tissue. Am J Med 61: 758–767

12. Aguilera G, Catt KJ (1980) Sodium balance and regulation of vascular angiotensin II receptors. Clin Res 28: 549A

13. Capponi AM, Catt KJ (1979) Angiotensin receptors in adrenal cortex and uterus. Binding and activation properties of angiotensin analogues. J Biol Chem 254: 5120–5127

14. Galardy RE, Stafford SS, Schaefer ML, Ho H, LaVorgna KA, Jamieson JD (1978) Biologically active derivatives of angiotensin for labelling cellular receptors. J Med Chem 21: 1279–1283

DISCUSSION

Dr. Laragh (New York, New York): I would like to ask Dr. Catt whether his experiments might provide an explanation for what seems to be happening in at least some forms of hypertension, that is, there seems to be a relatively increased sensitivity of the adrenal to angiotensin, especially in low-renin patients in whom there is an inappropriately high plasma aldosterone level for the angiotensin level. Are these patients with low-renin hypertension reacting to lower AII levels? What would that do to the adrenal glomerulosa receptor response? Would it fit?

Dr. Catt (Bethesda, Maryland): I think it would certainly fit that changes in circulating angiotensin II could in the long run alter the adrenal sensitivity by having a trophic action on the glomerulosa cells. Of course, this is something that was proposed by Ganong a long time ago, and what we have shown has really confirmed the notion that he put forward—that angiotensin II acts as the trophic hormone for the zona glomerulosa. The situation in muscle was rather different because angiotensin is not the trophic hormone for muscle as we all know, and the muscle cells still maintain their function in the absence of angiotensin II. With regard to the hyperplastic effects on the adrenal in man, it is certainly conceivable that that could happen, although one should emphasize that in addition to these receptor changes there are also postreceptor alterations in the responsiveness and we have heard already that the same glands are also more sensitive to ACTH.

Dr. Antonaccio (Princeton, New Jersey): A question for Dr. Bumpus: One of the problems I have always had with renin inhibitors is that they're relatively poor inhibitors from the standpoint of potency. The best ones have an I_{50} of about 0.1 M. That coupled with the fact that they lower blood pressure effectively in DOCA salt rats makes me wonder about their specificity. Have you actually checked this out pharmacologically? Does it have any other mechanism by which it might lower blood pressure?

Dr. Bumpus (Cleveland, Ohio): Yes, we have checked it out, in answer to your question. We have not been able to find anything else. I agree with you that it takes quite a bit of material to inhibit renin, and we never get complete inhibition with it.

Dr. Atlas (New York, New York): I wanted to ask Dr. Haber a question. I believe that you and Victor Dzau have shown that the renin-specific antibody, in lowering blood pressure in dogs, does not produce a reflex tachycardia like converting enzyme inhibitor. I wonder if you have an explanation for why the decapeptide renin inhibitor might do so.

Dr. Haber (Boston, Massachusetts): This question is still under investigation. Your statement is correct—we *have* found a difference between the two in initial experiments, but not in exactly the same model. The experiment has not been done comparing antibody and the peptide inhibitor in the monkey at the same time.

Physician: I've got two questions. Dr. Haber, in your octapeptide analog have you tried inserting diamino acids or other groups to stop the hydrolysis so that you could get greatly enhanced serum half-life? I would like to know about those compounds if you have utilized them. And second to Dr. Cushman, one of the reasons you gave for putting that sulfhydryl group was its affinity for zinc, giving you more localization at that end of the converting enzyme molecule. It's been suggested that maybe some of the side effects and toxicity of the drug are related to this sulfhydryl group. Could you comment on that? Is there any way that you could get away without the sulfhydryl?

Dr. Haber (Boston, Massachusetts): We started out by putting *d*-stereoisomers of acids at the cleavage site. Several compounds with *d*-leucine at positions 5 or 6 in the peptide were reasonably effective inhibitors with inhibitory constants in the 1 μM range, but were ineffective at neutral pH and could only be shown to work in vitro. Experiments in progress now are directed at inserting *d*-stereoisomers of amino acids at both ends of the peptide which will block the actions of either aminopeptidases or carboxypeptidases.

Dr. Cushman (Princeton, New Jersey): In answer to your question about the sulfhydryl, we have been concerned about coming up with alternative zinc-binding groups for a long time. There are a number of such groups that are fairly effective as replacements for sulfhydryl, but I'm not sure that some of them wouldn't be worse than sulfhydryl from a safety point of view. A hydroxamic acid group works fairly well, but I don't think this group would be a very good choice. Certainly compounds that contain phosphorus, such as phosphates or phosphoramides, are fairly effective. Obviously, however, we haven't yet come up with a nonsulfhydryl analog that we are ready to test in the clinic as a replacement for captopril. Apparently one of our competitors will describe such a nonsulfhydryl inhibitor on June 18, at the medicinal chemistry meeting at Troy, New York [see initial published report of this compound in Patchett AA, Harris E, Tristram EW et al. Nature 288: 280–283]. I wouldn't be too surprised, although we have only rumors, if they have come up with an analog of captopril with a nonsulfhydryl ligand for zinc. There is no evidence for any allergic reactions to captopril, although it does form mixed disulfides with plasma sulfhydryl compounds, and perhaps also with those of tissue proteins. Such mixed disulfide formation might even have something to do with the relatively long duration of activity of captopril.

Dr. Catt: I would also like to ask Dr. Cushman about the point he made about the binding of zinc. Somebody mentioned earlier that a side effect of captopril was loss of taste or smell, which I believe is sometimes also related to zinc in some way. Would you expect to see signs of zinc deficiency in people treated with larger doses of captopril for a long time?

Dr. Cushman: I wouldn't, because captopril is not a particularly good zinc-chelating agent. It has only one sulfhydryl group, and should have a second sulfhydryl or another group, such as amino, in order to effectively bind free zinc ion. In this regard, captopril is nothing like penicillamine. Second, I think that alterations in zinc metabolism have been looked for in clinical studies with captopril and haven't been found.

Dr. Soffer (New York, New York): I would like to ask Dr. Haber two questions. One is in regard to the Fab fragments of your antirenin antibodies: How much anticatalytic activity did you recover relative to that in the intact antibody? Second, as I looked at the structure of your renin inhibitor, I thought it likely that it is broken down by converting enzyme, and perhaps as well by kininase I. What do you think?

Dr. Haber: Your first question is exceedingly perceptive. Indeed, there are two mechanisms of renin inhibition. The first is to simply take it out of solution. Thus, a bivalent antibody that can precipitate renin is more effective than a monovalent Fab. The second way is to simply block its catalytic site sterically. Here Fab would be as effective as bivalent antibody. In practice, it loses considerable activity in going from the bivalent to univalent antibody, probably because the only fraction of a heterogeneous antibody pool is directed at the catalytic site. One of the reasons why we are very interested in homogeneous antibodies as produced by cell-fusion methods is that we would like to have a monospecific catalytic site antibody. This general principle has been well demonstrated with other enzymes such as lysozyme in which one can find antibodies that bind to noncatalytic important areas in the molecule and do not inhibit its enzymatic activity. With respect to your second question, Dr. Erdos has had some of our peptide to test.

Dr. Erdos (Dallas, Texas): Dr. Soffer is right, because the renin inhibitor turned out to be a competitive substrate inhibitor of converting enzyme. It inhibited the human enzyme at a concentration in the order of 10^{-6} M in vitro, but the inhibition disappeared fast, presumably owing to the hydrolysis of the peptide by the enzyme as shown by John Weare of our laboratory. Concerning the C-terminal lysine, it could probably be cleaved by human plasma carboxypeptidase N or kininase I. If the L-lysine is replaced with D-lysine, the peptide will be much less susceptible to enzymatic hydrolysis.

Epilogue: After Dinner Science and Friendship

Dr. Charles G. Smith (Revlon Health Care Group): I would like to tell you a little bit about the Revlon Health Care Group and its burgeoning biomedical perspective. We are composed of several major commercial units operating in the health-care field. At Armour, we are involved in immunoglobulin research, in a major program for the collection and fractionation of human plasma, and in peptide synthesis and biological evaluation. Barnes-Hind, a company on the West Coast, is involved in the ophthalmologic–dermatologic fields. Coburn Optical Company produces the equipment for grinding lenses (as well as standard eyeglass lenses) and is studying intraoccular lens implants. Meloy Laboratories is primarily a fundamental research laboratory, located in Virginia. It has a considerable government contract program in immunobiology and viral oncology, a meaningful hybridoma program, and a commercial business in radioimmunoassay (RIA) research and marketing. Meloy is the laboratory that is currently manufacturing interferon, using the resource of human leukocytes from our Armour Division. The National Health Laboratory is a chain of clinical diagnostic laboratories known, I am sure, to some of you. Norcliff-Thayer is our over-the-counter drug company. Technicon, of course, you all know as a fine instrumentation company that recently joined the Revlon Health Care Group. USV Pharmaceutical Corporation is the largest single pharmaceutical member of the family, and it is this group that has launched major programs in hypertension, myocardial function, hypersensitivity diseases, and cyclic nucleotide research.

I will now introduce Mr. John Roelker of the Revlon Health Care Group, who will make some comments on behalf of himself and the Chairman of our Corporation.

Mr. John Roelker: I would like to read a telex from Michel Bergerac, chairman of the Revlon Corporation, who unfortunately is thousands of miles away and wished he were here. It is addressed to John Laragh:

> Dear John:
> I am disappointed that circumstances do not permit me to be here with you this evening to share in the companionship and sense of accomplishment that you and your scientists and colleagues must feel after a day of intellectual stimulation, which must have resulted from the excellence of the contributions. Your efforts and this seminar of distinguished scientists from the United States and abroad cannot help but advance the state of the art and lead to still more progress in the understanding of hypertension and, successfully acting on that understanding, to control and ultimately vanquish this major malady. We are happy to play a part in the development of effective drugs to combat hypertension and are privileged to have had the opportunity to support this important seminar.
> With warm best wishes to you all.

I shall keep my remarks very brief, particularly after the technical excellence of the contributions. The pleasure I have in being here is one I share with the 30,000 people in Revlon, who have worked to permit us to fund research as well as support creative activity in scientific disciplines relating to the health field. And we do this because we believe it is a part of our corporate responsibility. If you will, it is a part of our responsibility in terms of helping the process of what I would like to call, in a way, *disciplined dreaming* in an atmosphere of uninhibited and free exchange—disciplined dreaming, which we hope will lead to a better world for all of us and to more and better therapeutic products. I do not think there is much more to say at this point in time other than the fact that we are delighted to be able to do our share in supporting this kind of activity, an activity that we feel is of great value, more than other things we do as a corporation in terms of advertising or promoting things. We are doing our duty, not only as a corporation, but as good citizens of the health-care world.

Dr. John H. Laragh: This evening has a very simple plan: two speakers, Dr. Andreas Greuntzig and Sir George Pickering. Dr. Greuntzig, possibly, some of you may not know. His achievements have been absolutely singular. What he has done is of great clinical relevance. It complements our discussions on the biochemical and physiologic problems of high blood pressure. Andreas Gruentzig has given the whole frontier of cardiovascular disease a new dimension. He recognized early in his career that the vascular lesions that compromise flow to target organs might be approachable by a mechanical technique if the engineering could be perfected. What he has done in his short career has literally revolutionized the therapy of all cardiovascular disease. Almost single-handedly he has developed a technology that allows him to go into the human subject with a catheter and deal with things like coronary occlusion, renal artery occlusion, and even cerebral vessel blockade as in stroke in a way that has not been heretofore possible. Nonsurgical dilatation of arterial occlusions as a treatment for hypertensions of renal origin, for coronary occlusions, and for peripheral vascular blocks has arrived.

Percutaneous Transluminal Dilatation of Renal Artery Stenosis

A. Gruentzig and U. Kuhlmann

Atherosclerotic and nonatherosclerotic renal artery stenoses are the general causes of renovascular hypertension. Antihypertensive medical therapy can be difficult or can even fail to control blood pressure. In addition, renal failure in generally affected kidneys can be aggravated in the presence of deteriorated bloodflow because of severe arterial stenosis.

In patients with this type of disease, invasive treatment should be considered, such as renovascular surgery. Extended experience with surgery has accumulated over the years. As the results have been reported to be remarkably good, this mode of therapy has been accepted as standard in selected cases. But older patients often fail to respond to surgery (1–3), and mortality ranges between 5 and 9% (1–6). Mortality is even higher in the presence of concomitant impaired renal function or coronary artery disease (2, 3).

As in cases of peripheral and coronary artery disease, angioplasty appears to offer an alternative procedure for treating patients with atherosclerotic stenosis as well as fibromuscular hyperplasia or transplant renal-artery stenosis.

Single observations of inadvertent renal-artery dilatation in 1963 (7) and advertent dilatation with a Teflon catheter in 1971 (6) have been made previously, but only the introduction of the dilatation catheter technique made this method amenable to clinical application. Since its first description (8), the technique has met with increasing interest, and the number of procedures done increases rapidly (9).

Meanwhile a number of promising reports appeared, encouraging the application of the technique (6, 9–20). It might well be that "the technique is the most important advance in the management of ren-o-vascular hypertension since the advent of renin measurements (9)." Nevertheless, the proper role of the method still has to be defined; carefully designed prospective studies are needed to compare this procedure with renal artery surgery (9, 11).

TECHNIQUE

The procedure is basically the same as for peripheral (21, 22) or coronary arteries (23). The passage of the double lumen dilatation catheter, however, can be achieved in two different ways. First, the coaxial guiding catheter system is similar to that used in the coronary arteries. The catheter assembly consists of two catheters. The guiding catheter (F8) is introduced through a French 8 arterial sheath at the groin. Puncture of the ipsilateral femoral artery facilitates selective catheterization of the ipsilateral renal artery.

The guiding catheter is not tapered at the tip and is preshaped as is shown in Fig. 1. For passage through the sheath and introduction into the aorta, the guiding catheter is preloaded with 1.6-mm (0.063 in.) guidewire. The guiding catheter is advanced into the aorta and into the orifice of the renal artery to be dilated. The catheter remains at the orifice, guiding the renal dilatation catheter into the artery. The dilatation catheter has an outer

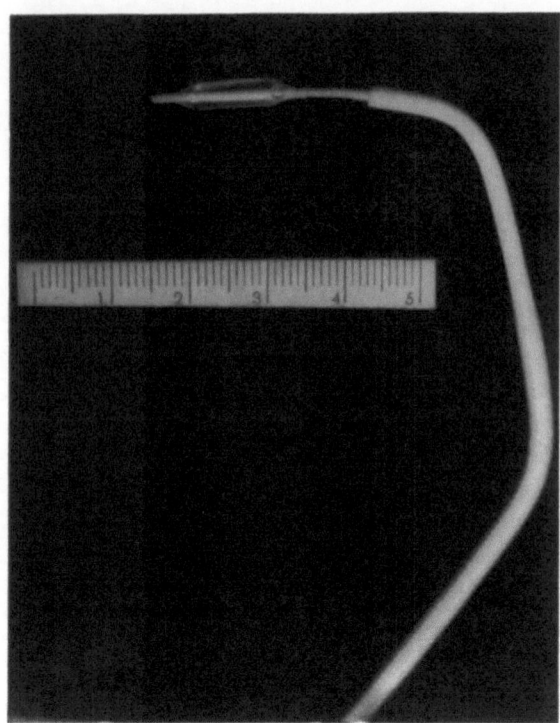

Fig. 1. Guiding catheter.

diameter of French 4.5 and is tapered to about French 3 at the tip. The main lumen of the dilatation catheter is used for contrast material injection and pressure measurements during the procedure. For purposes of comparison, the aortic pressure at the orifice of the renal ostium is recorded through the guiding catheter using a Y connector at the end of the guiding catheter. The balloon is filled with a 50:50 mixture by volume of the contrast agent and sterile normal saline using the second lumen of the dilatation catheter and automatic pressure devices. The balloon segment has a maximal outer diameter of 5 mm, using 5 atm (72.5 psi). If smaller diameters are needed, the 3.7-mm coronary dilatation catheter can be used. It is advisable to use a balloon with a smaller maximal outer diameter than that of the undiseased portion of the renal artery proximal to the point of stenosis. Judgment of the size of the artery from the segment distal to the stenosis is useless because of the common presence of post-stenotic dilatation.

The second method is the catheter–guidewire system, which consists of a double lumen dilatation catheter similar to that used for femoral artery dilatation (21). After placing an angiographic catheter, e.g., Simmons type "sidewinder" (24) into the orifice of the artery, a standard guidewire is first passed through the stenosis followed by the angiographic catheter. During this manipulation, neither pressure recording nor contrast medium injections are available. After passage of the catheter through the area of stenosis, the guidewire is removed, making the catheter available for pressure measurements and contrast medium injections. The guidewire is then gently placed into a side branch of the renal artery. While the guidewire is carefully held in place, the angiographic catheter is removed and exchanged to the dilatation catheter, which then is passed through the stenosis following the route of the guidewire.

Several different types of dilatation catheters are available for the catheter–guidewire technique. But we recommend balloon sizes not larger than 6 mm maximal outer diameter and prefer even smaller sizes. This is to prevent overinflation of the undiseased part of the renal artery with the danger of vessel damage. The coaxial guiding catheter system has the advantage of pressure recording and contrast medium injections while passing, and in addition it must not be advanced into the peripheral renal branches, which could cause irritation of the intima. The disadvantage of the coaxial system is that the guiding catheter limits the balloon size of the dilatation catheter. The maximal balloon size is 5 mm, which can be passed in its deflated and umbrellalike shape fashion through the catheter. In rare cases, a larger balloon might be of use. In these cases, the catheter–guidewire system must be used. The disadvantages of the catheter–guidewire system are the relative blindness while crossing the stenosis and the risk of traumatizing peripheral renal branches as a result of guidewire manipulations. Weighing the advantages and disadvantages of both systems, we prefer the coaxial guiding catheter system, but recommend that both systems be available if one or the other fails.

PROCEDURE

The procedure is carried out in the fasting state and with tranquilizer premedication. After local anesthesia of the groin, insertion of the arterial sheath, and positioning of the guiding catheter, heparin 10,000 U is given to avoid clot formation. In young patients, intrarenal application of nitroglycerin prevents spasm. Selective renal angiogram is obtained in the A-P projection and in angled views if needed. The stenosis is recognized by using the videotape playback. The procedure should not be done without this facility. Once the guiding catheter is positioned at the orifice, the dilatation catheter is very slowly advanced into the artery and manipulated through the stenosis while the renal pressure is monitored through its tip. Simultaneously, the aortic pressure is recorded through the tip of the guiding catheter. Correct pressure measurements are very important because improvement of the distal coronary pressure aids in the decision to terminate the procedure. When the catheter tip traverses the stenosis, the pressure drops. Once the dilatation catheter is properly positioned, the balloon is immediately inflated at pressures of 4 to 5 atm (60 to 75 psi).

The balloon is inflated for approximately 5 to 10 sec by means of the automatic pressure pump. A marked rise in distal pressure after deflation of the balloon indicates the successful dilatation and aids in the decision to terminate the procedure. If the distal pressure fails to respond adequately, the balloon must again be inflated.

ADDITIONAL MANAGEMENT

Additional medical therapy is similar to that recommended for peripheral and coronary artery dilatation (21, 23). Acetylsalicylic acid (300 to 600 mg) should be administered daily beginning prior to the procedure. In case of normalization of blood pressure after dilatation, coumadin is given until the time of restudy, usually 6 to 9 months. Acetylsalicylic acid is discontinued. The value of coumadin treatment for better long-term patency is still under question. We (11) and others (20, 25) prefer coumadin according to the patency in case of peripheral arterial dilatation (21).

In spite of the tendency to alert patients to physical activity the day after peripheral or coronary dilatation, caution is advised in the event of renal dilatation. After successful intervention, the blood pressure normalizes within a few hours; it may result in orthostatic reactions. The mobilization of the patient should therefore be done cautiously. If the blood pressure has not normalized, coumadin therapy is not initiated, but acetylsalicylic acid is continued.

SELECTION OF PATIENTS

Being in the position to pioneer this new procedure, we had to employ rather rigid patient selection similar to those for reconstructive surgery. The basic criterion was the presence of hypertension (>160/95 mm Hg) in spite of adequate medical therapy or intolerable drug side effects. Lateralizing renal vein–renin ratio exceeding 1.5 affected versus unaffected side aided in the decision. However, according to our previous experience with patients undergoing surgery (26), an elevated renin ratio was not a prerequisite for the case selection.

As far as the anatomic criteria are concerned, the stenosis should be severe (>75%), and if there was any uncertainty about the significance of the stenosis, a pressure gradient of (>20 mm Hg across the stenosis) should be present. The pressure measurements have been done with a soft F-3 catheter passed through the diagnostic catheter prior to the procedure.

Morphologically, the technique can be applied to atherosclerotic stenosis as well as to fibromuscular dysplasia—either type, medial, or intimal. The stenosis should not be too proximal including the aortic wall, yet not too far distally including side branches.

For bilateral stenosis, a two-stage procedure is recommended. During the first session, the more severely affected side is treated, whereas the contralateral side is attempted days or weeks afterward. This is not only because the operation time is shortened when one side alone is attempted, but also because less contrast medium is used in cases of impaired renal function; furthermore, endangering the positive results of one side with a complication of the other is to be avoided. The second procedure can be done provided the first procedure goes well and provided that its artery responds favorably to dilatation.

RESULTS

From 1977 to 1980, 33 patients underwent angioplasty in Zurich. In 31 (91%) we have been able to pass the stenosis, inflate the balloon, and effect an improvement in luminal diameter. Twenty-three patients had atherosclerotic stenosis (ASS), as regarded by radiologic criteria (27, 28), and six had stenosis with typical signs of fibromuscular dysplasia (FMD). First, the results of the ASS group: The mean age was 54 years (range 39 to 67 years). All patients had severe hypertension in spite of adequate medical therapy. The blood pressure averaged 203/113 mm Hg. After dilatation, the blood pressure decreased to 141/91 mm Hg and remained at 141/91 mm Hg in the follow-up period. The follow-up period is now an average of 12 months (4 to 24 months).

After dilatation, the pressure gradient across the stenosis measured with the dilatation catheter was reduced, as shown in Fig. 2.

Two patients (9%) had complete recurrence of the stenosis during follow-up, and five showed partial restenosis (22%) at the time of elective control (angiography 6 months later). Four of the partial restenoses have been treated with a second PTA, again with primary success, and the fifth was normotensive with medical therapy, making a second dilatation unnecessary to the present.

Two patients died from cardiovascular disease, and one patient underwent operation for an aortic aneurysm.

The mean age of the FMD group was 38 years (range, 20 to 48 years); average blood pressure was 182/110 mm Hg. Arm blood pressure normalized after dilatation and was 137/87 mm Hg and remained 136/84 mm Hg during follow-up with a mean of 8 months (range, 6 to 9 months). The

pressure changes before and after dilatation and during follow-up are shown in Fig. 3. There was no recurrence.

In two patients dilatation of stenosis of transplanted kidney artery was done with primary success. However, one patient experienced complete recurrence after 4 weeks, requiring surgery, while the other remained improved.

The clinical results are summarized diagrammatically in Fig. 4. Using the criteria of the well-known American Cooperative Study (29), the patients were classified in three classes: (1) cured, (2) improved, and (3) nonimproved, according to blood pressure response and medication after PTA. Cured are patients without medication having normal blood pressure during follow-up; (2) improved are patients with improved diastolic blood pressure after PTA, being less than 110 mm Hg without therapy, or patients with normalization of diastolic blood pressure (>95 mm Hg), but still under antihypertensive drugs; and (3) improved are patients in whom the diastolic pressure remains above 110 mm Hg in spite of therapy.

Of the patients with ASS, most could be improved or even cured. Of the FMD group, four of six patients were cured and the remainder improved. Two typical examples of dilatation of atherosclerotic and nonatherosclerotic stenosis are given in Figs. 5 and 6. Our results are comparable to those in the published literature. The largest series of 153 patients has been compiled in a Euro-

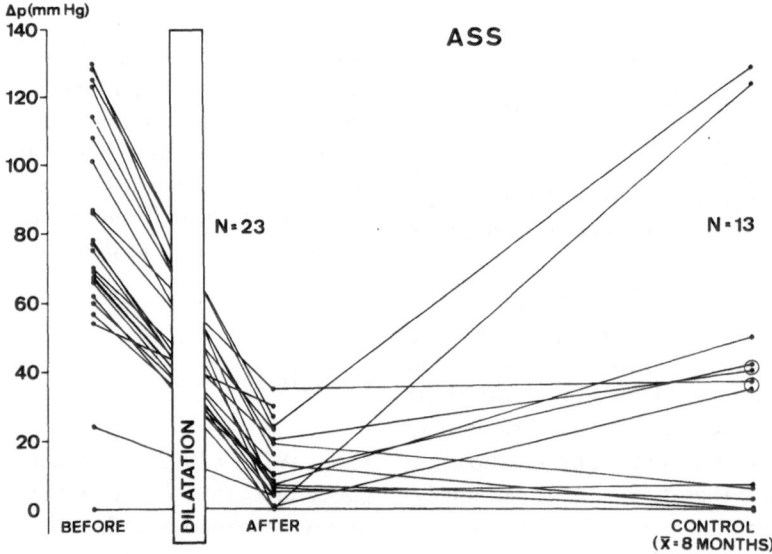

Fig. 2. Pressure gradient across stenosis, measured with dilatation catheter, showing reduction.

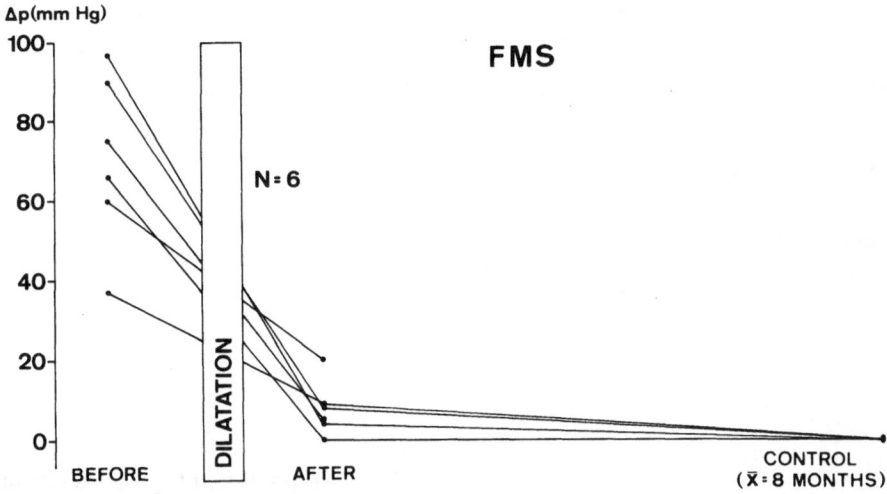

Fig. 3. Pressure gradient across stenosis, showing changes before and after dilatation as well as during follow-up.

pean Cooperative Study (25) reporting a primary success rate of 90%.

However, follow-up data of only a few cases and of a short control period have been available until now (11, 19, 20). Similar definitions for analyzing the follow-up data have been used in these reports, the results of which are rather similar as compared to ours (see Table 1). In comparison with the effect of surgery in case of ASS, the cure and improvement rates were 28%, and 55% respectively, and for FMD 47% and 47%, respectively (26).

Bearing in mind the limited number of cases and limited follow-up of the PTA as well as the

difference in patient population, it is too early to draw definite conclusions. However, we and others (19) believe that in appropriate selected cases, the results of angioplasty are comparable to those obtained through surgery.

Not surprisingly, dilatation is not without complications. In our ASS group, two patients experienced acute deterioration of the already impaired renal function, as a result of contrast medium application. Both patients needed dialysis, and one remained on chronic dialysis. In one patient, orthostatic hypotension caused an episode of transient cerebral ischemia, and in one patient coumadin bleeding occurred during the follow-up period.

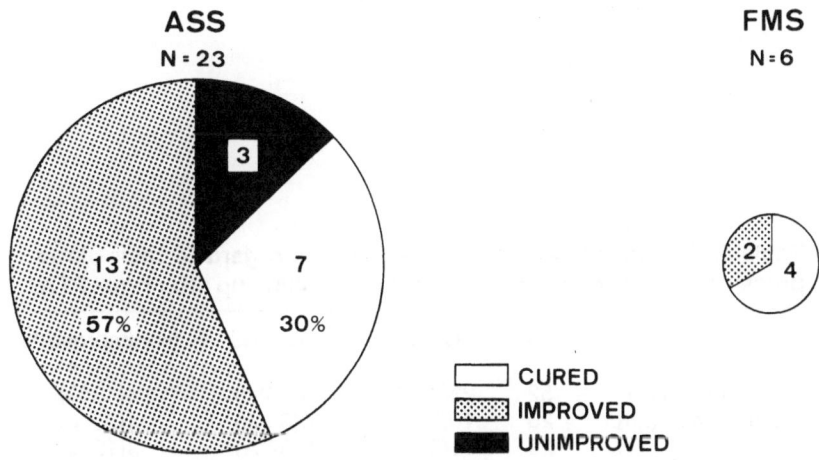

Fig. 4. Follow-up results of renal dilatation.

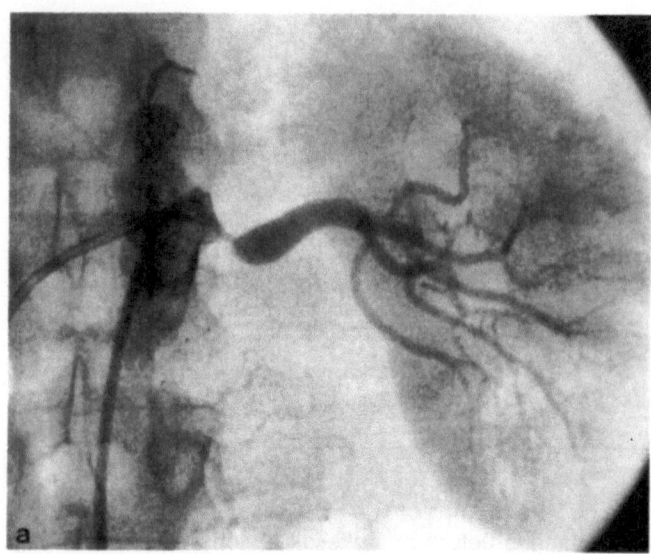

Figs. 5 and 6. Typical examples of dilatation of atherosclerotic and nonatherosclerotic stenosis.

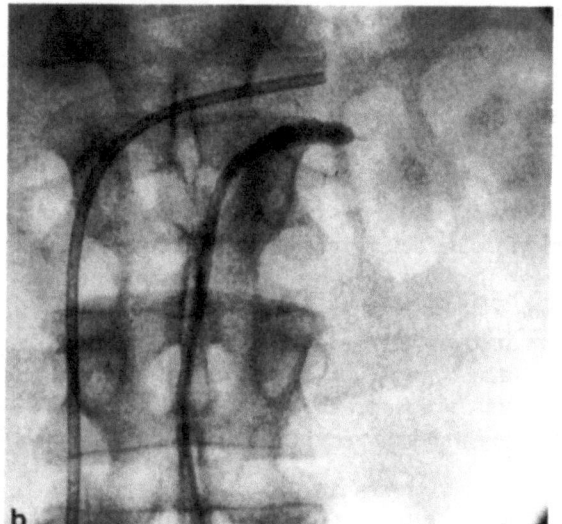

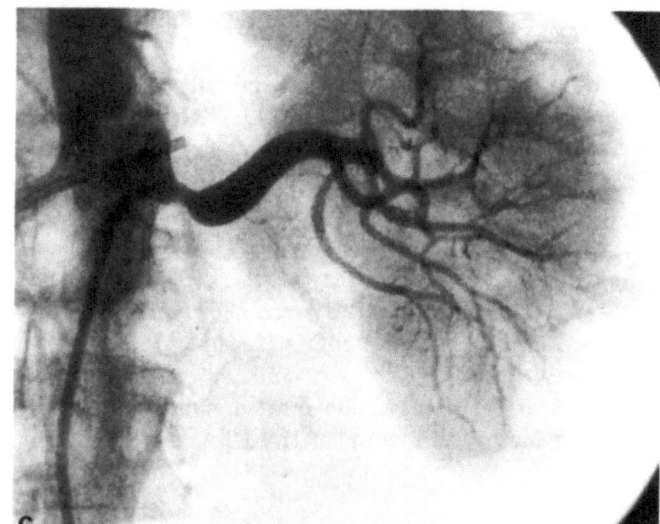

Table 1. Clinical classification of patients in regard to their blood pressure response and medication during follow-up after renal PTA.

	N	Cured	Improved	Nonimproved
Indianapolis (19)	52	23(44%)	25(48%)	4(8%)
Charlottsville (20)	20	10(50%)	6(30%)	4(20%)
Zürich	29	11(38%)	15(52%)	3(10%)
Total	101	44(44%)	46(46%)	11(10%)

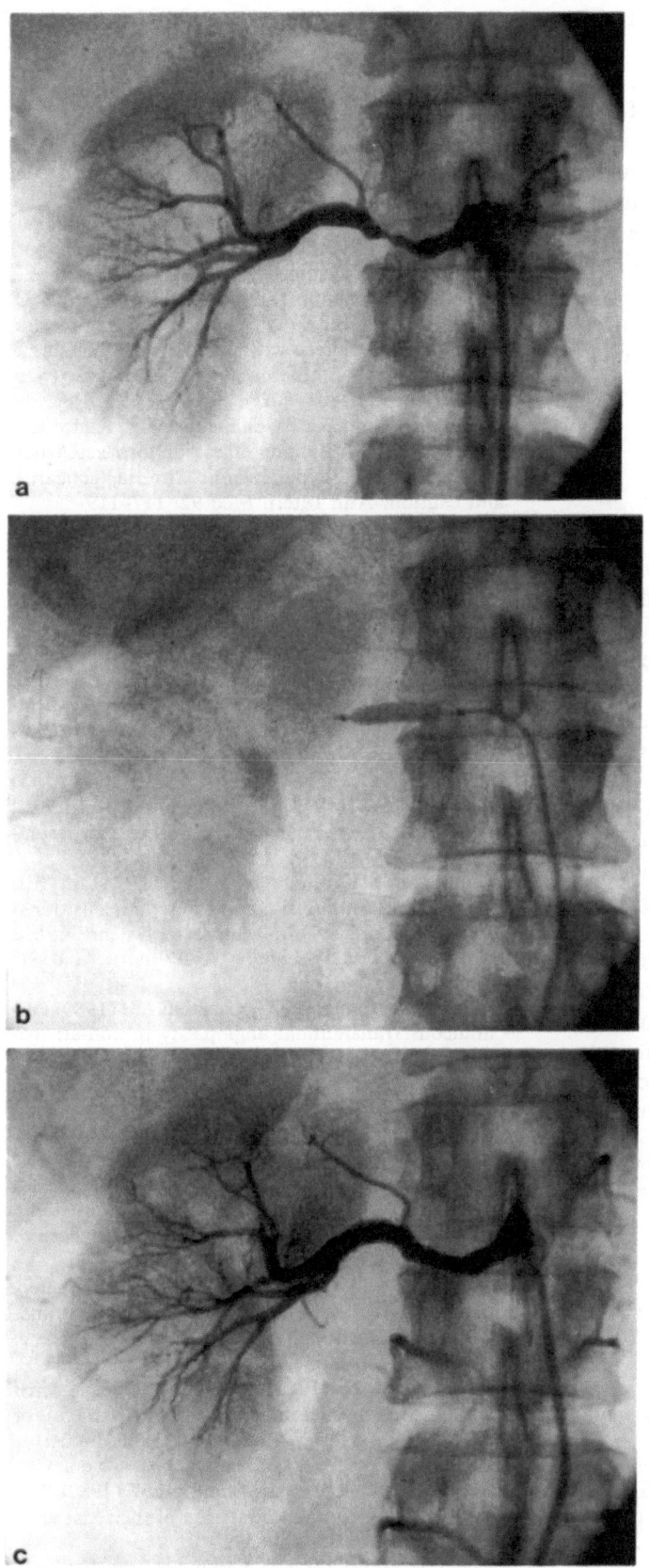

No complications were noted in either the FMD or transplanted group.

Other complications have been reported, e.g., intimal dissection with sudden reclosure (18) renal-artery rupture (25), perforation of the renal artery (19, 20), and hematoma in the unguinal region. Some of these complications might be avoided by means of the coaxial technique and by using smaller balloon sizes. Finally, experience has been accumulated at several centers throughout the world, eliminating the need to approach this procedure in a self-taught fashion. Training can easily be achieved at these centers.

SUMMARY

The results indicate that percutaneous transluminal dilatation of renal artery stenosis is effective in the treatment of renovascular hypertension in properly selected cases. However, as the long-term patency and complication rate, especially in the light of widespread use of the technique, has yet not been established, caution is advised. Therefore, the following rules for patient selection should be applied: (1) The patient remains hypertensive (>160/95 mm Hg) in spite of adequate medical therapy or should have intolerable drug side effects. (2) The patient agrees to have an emergency operation in case of complication. (3) Hemodyamic significance of the stenosis is established before PTA, either by the degree of the stenosis itself, by kidney size, lateralizing renin ratio, 131-iodohippurate clearance study, or trans-stenosis pressure gradient. Under such circumstances, the technique can be applied with reasonable success and patency rates.

REFERENCES

1. Foster JH, Maxwell, MH, Franklin SS, et al. (1975) Renovascular occlusive disease. JAMA 231: 1043–1048
2. Franklin SS, Young JD Jr, Maxwell MH, et al (1975) Operative morbidity and mortality in renovascular disease. JAMA 231: 1148–1153
3. Maxwell MH (1975) Cooperative study of renovascular hypertension. Kidney Int. 8: 5153–5161
4. Shapiro AP, McDonald RH Jr, Scheib E (1976) Renal arterial stenosis and hypertension. Am J Cardiol 37: 1065–1068
5. Stanley JC, Fry WJ (1977) Surgical treatment of renovascular hypertension. Arch Surg 112: 1291–1297
6. Zeitler E (1971) Angiographische Probleme zur Diagnostik und Therapie der renovaskularen Hypertonie. In: Denck H, Flora G, Hilbe G, Piza F, eds. Renovaskulare Hypertonie. Vienna, Verlag der Medizinischen Akademie
7. Colapinto, RF (1980) Inadvertent percutaneous transluminal dilatation of a renal artery with a four-year follow-up. Radiology 135: 605–606
8. Gruentzig A, Kuhlmann U, Vetter W, Lutolf U, Meier B, Siegenthaler W (1978) Treatment of renovascular hypertension with percutaneous transluminal dilatation of atherosclerotic renal-artery stenosis. Lancet 1: 801–802
9. Grim CE, Yune HY, Weinberger MH, Klatte EC, Ryan MP (1980) Balloon dilatation for renal artery stenosis causing hypertension: Criteria, concerns, and caution. Ann Intern Med 92: 117–119
10. Mahler F, Krneta A, Haertel M (1979) Treatment of renovascular hypertension by transluminal renal artery dilatation. Ann Intern Med 90: 56–57
11. Kuhlmann U, Vetter W, Furrer J, Lutolf U, Siegenthaler W, Gruentzig A (1980) Renovascular hypertension: treatment by percutaneous transluminal dilatation. Ann Intern Med 92: 1–6
12. Millan VG, Mast WE, Madias NE (1979) Nonsurgical treatment of severe hypertension due to renal-artery medical fibroplasia. Lancet 1: 993–995
13. Katzen BT, Chang J, Lukowsky GH, Edward G, Abramson EG (1979) Percutaneous transluminal angioplasty for treatment of renovascular hypertension. Radiology 131: 53–58
14. Weinberger MH, Yune HY, Grim CE, Luft FC, Klatte EC, Donohue JP (1979) Percutaneous transluminal angioplasty for renal artery stenosis in a solitary functioning kidney. Ann Intern Med 91: 684–688
15. Martin EC, Diamond NG, Casarella WJ (1980) Percutaneous transluminal angioplasty in non-atherosclerotic disease. Radiology 135: 27–33
16. Diamond NG, Casarella WJ, Hardy MA, Appel GB (1979) Dilatation of critical transplant renal artery stenosis by percutaneous transluminal angioplasty. AJR 133: 1167–1169
17. Sniderman KW, Sos TA, Sprayregen S, et al (1980) Percutaneous transluminal angioplasty in renal transplant arterial stenosis for relief of hypertension. Radiology 135: 23–26
18. Mathias K, Rau W, Kauffmann G (1979) Katheterdilatation einer Arterienstenose nach Nierentransplantation. Dtsch med Wschr 104: 437–8
19. Schwarten ED, Yune, HY, Klatte EC, Grim CE, Weinberger MH (1980) Clinical experience with percutaneous transluminal angioplasty (PTA) of stenotic renal arteries. Radiology 135: 601–604
20. Tegtmeyer CJ, Dyer R, Teates CD, Ayers CR, Carey RM, Wellons A Jr, Stanton LW (1980) Percutaneous transluminal dilatation of the renal arteries. Radiology 135: 589–599
21. Gruentzig A (1977) Die perkutane transluminale

rekanalisation chronischer arterienverschusse mit einer neuen dilatationstechnik. Baden-Baden, G. Witzstrock-Verlag

22. Gruentzig A, Kumpe DA (1979) Technique of percutaneous transluminal angioplasty with the Gruentzig balloon catheter. AJR 132: 547–552

23. Gruentzig A, Senning A, Siegenthaler WE (1979) Non-operative dilatation of coronary-artery stenosis. N Engl J Med 301: 61–68

24. Grable GS, Smith DC (1980) The use of the simmons "sidewinder" catheter in percutaneous transluminal angioplasty of the renal arteries. Radiology 137: 541–543

25. Richter EI, Gruentzig A, Ingrisch H, et al (1980) Percutaneous dilatation of renal stenosis. Ann Radiol (Paris) 23: 275–278

26. Vetter W, Vetter WH, Tenschert W, Kuhlmann U, Studer A, Glanzer K, Pouliadis G, Largiader F, Furrer J, Siegenthaler W (1979) Renovaskuläre Hypertonie. Klin Wochenschr 57: 863–873

27. Abrams HL (1971) Angiography, vol 2, 2nd ed Boston, Little, Brown, pp 860–863

28. Bookstein JJ, Abrams HL, Buenger RE, et al (1972) Radiologic aspects of renovascular hypertension. JAMA 220: 1218–1224

29. Maxwell MH, Bleifer KH, Franklin SS, et al (1972) Cooperative study of renovascular hypertension. Demographic analysis of the study. J. Am Med Assoc 220: 1195

Closing Remarks

Dr. Laragh: This work provides us with a new way of keeping up tissue flow, which is really what life is all about, preserving flow. I thank Dr. Gruentzig and the Revlon Health Care Group again for having allowed us all to get together and hear about this. Finally, Sir George Pickering has agreed to deliver the benediction.

Sir George Pickering: John you have been so kind to invite me. And I would like to thank Chuck Smith and the Revlon Corporation for supporting the scientific sessions. I would like to thank all the contributors, particularly Dr. Gruentzig, for this splendid demonstration of what you can do to arteries that are closed or nearly closed without getting the cutting doctors in to help. I have great respect for the cutting doctors, but if you can keep them out, even better. I suspect that you do not want me to address one of the topics that we have neglected today. And so I shall resist that temptation. Besides, I think the function of an afterdinner speech is not to instruct, it is to entertain.

Now it is past 10 o'clock and I am sure I am speaking for all of you when I say what a wonderful time we have had, and what fun it has been to dwell on our areas of mutual knowledge and have some companionship. It always is fun to meet one's old friends, isn't it? And John, you've made it a wonderful party. Thank you so much.

Index